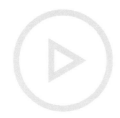

IMPORTANT:

HERE IS YOUR REGISTRATION CODE TO ACCESS
YOUR PREMIUM McGRAW-HILL ONLINE RESOURCES.

For key premium online resources you need THIS CODE to gain access. Once the code is entered, you will be able to use the Web resources for the length of your course.

If your course is using **WebCT** or **Blackboard**, you'll be able to use this code to access the McGraw-Hill content within your instructor's online course.

Access is provided if you have purchased a new book. If the registration code is missing from this book, the registration screen on our Website, and within your WebCT or Blackboard course, will tell you how to obtain your new code.

Registering for McGraw-Hill Online Resources

TO gain access to your McGraw-Hill web resources simply follow the steps below:

1. USE YOUR WEB BROWSER TO GO TO: **http://www.mhhe.com/medicalassisting**
2. CLICK ON **FIRST TIME USER**.
3. ENTER THE REGISTRATION CODE* PRINTED ON THE TEAR-OFF BOOKMARK ON THE RIGHT.
4. AFTER YOU HAVE ENTERED YOUR REGISTRATION CODE, CLICK **REGISTER**.
5. FOLLOW THE INSTRUCTIONS TO SET-UP YOUR PERSONAL UserID AND PASSWORD.
6. WRITE YOUR UserID AND PASSWORD DOWN FOR FUTURE REFERENCE.
   KEEP IT IN A SAFE PLACE.

TO GAIN ACCESS to the McGraw-Hill content in your instructor's **WebCT** or **Blackboard** course simply log in to the course with the UserID and Password provided by your instructor. Enter the registration code exactly as it appears in the box to the right when prompted by the system. You will only need to use the code the first time you click on McGraw-Hill content.

Thank you, and welcome to your McGraw-Hill Online Resources!

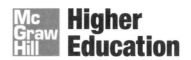

* YOUR REGISTRATION CODE CAN BE USED ONLY ONCE TO ESTABLISH ACCESS. IT IS NOT TRANSFERABLE.

0-07-297145-2 T/A MEDICAL ASSISTING, 2/E

MCGRAW-HILL
ONLINE RESOURCES

REGISTRATION CODE

Z71Y-JXTU-OBRM-QNEI-M6CE

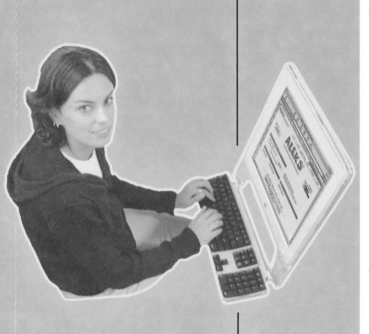

SECOND EDITION

MEDICAL ASSISTING
Administrative and Clinical Competencies

Barbara Ramutkowski, RN, BSN
Pima Medical Institute
Tucson, Arizona

Kathryn A. Booth, RN, MS
Total Care Programming and Wildwood Medical Clinic
Henrico, North Carolina

Donna Jeanne Pugh, RN, BSN
Florida Metropolitan University
Jacksonville, Florida

Sharion K. Thompson, BS, AAB, RMA, CPT
Sanford Brown Institute
Middleburg Heights, Ohio

Leesa G. Whicker, BA, CMA
Central Piedmont Community College
Charlotte, North Carolina

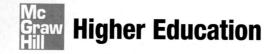

Boston   Burr Ridge, IL   Dubuque, IA   Madison, WI   New York   San Francisco   St. Louis
Bangkok   Bogotá   Caracas   Kuala Lumpur   Lisbon   London   Madrid   Mexico City
Milan   Montreal   New Delhi   Santiago   Seoul   Singapore   Sydney   Taipei   Toronto

The McGraw-Hill Companies

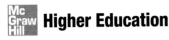 **Higher Education**

MEDICAL ASSISTING: ADMINISTRATIVE AND CLINICAL COMPETENCIES, SECOND EDITION

Published by McGraw-Hill, a business unit of The McGraw-Hill Companies, Inc., 1221 Avenue of the Americas, New York, NY 10020. Copyright © 2005, 1999 by The McGraw-Hill Companies, Inc. All rights reserved. No part of this publication may be reproduced or distributed in any form or by any means, or stored in a database or retrieval system, without the prior written consent of The McGraw-Hill Companies, Inc., including, but not limited to, in any network or other electronic storage or transmission, or broadcast for distance learning.

Some ancillaries, including electronic and print components, may not be available to customers outside the United States.

This book is printed on acid-free paper.

1 2 3 4 5 6 7 8 9 0 QPV/QPV 0 9 8 7 6 5 4

ISBN 0-07-294577-X

Publisher: *David Culverwell*
Senior Sponsoring Editor: *Roxan Kinsey*
Developmental Editor: *Patricia Forrest*
Editorial Coordinator: *Connie Kuhl*
Outside Developmental Services: *Julie Scardiglia*
Senior Project Manager: *Sheila M. Frank*
Senior Production Supervisor: *Laura Fuller*
Media Project Manager: *Sandra M. Schnee*
Media Technology Producer: *Janna Martin*
Designer: *Laurie B. Janssen*
Cover Designer: *Studio Montage*
Lead Photo Research Coordinator: *Carrie K. Burger*
Supplement Producer: *Brenda A. Ernzen*
Compositor: *Interactive Composition Corporation*
Typeface: *10/12 Slimbach*
Printer: *Quebecor World Versailles Inc.*

Cover photo credits: Front (left to right); © Norbert Schafer/CORBIS, © JFPI Studios, Inc./CORBIS, © Photodisc: Medical Perspectives, © Ed Bock/CORBIS, © PhotoDisc: VL59 Medicine Today, © Jose Luis Pelaez, Inc./CORBIS, Total Care Programming, Inc. Back (left to right); © Photodisc: Medicine & Health Care, Total Care Programming, Inc., © Photodisc: VL08 Emergency Room, © Photodisc: Medical Perspectives Photodisc, © Photodisc: V18 Health & Medicines, © Brand X Pictures: Medical Still Life, © Royalty-Free/CORBIS

Library of Congress Cataloging-in-Publication Data

Medical assisting : administrative and clinical competencies / Barbara Ramutkowski . . . [et al.} — 2nd ed.
　　p. cm.
　　Includes index.
　　ISBN 0-07-294577-X
　　1. Medical assistants. 2. Clinical competence. 3. Medical offices—Management. I. Prickett-Ramutkowski, Barbara.

R728.8.M4　　2005
610.73'72069—dc22
　　　　　　　　　　　　　　　　　　　2004040342
　　　　　　　　　　　　　　　　　　　CIP

WARNING NOTICE: The clinical procedures, medicines, dosages, and other matters described in this publication are based upon research of current literature and consultation with knowledgeable persons in the field. The procedures and matters described in this text reflect currently accepted clinical practice. However, this information cannot and should not be relied upon as necessarily applicable to a given individual's case. Accordingly, each person must be separately diagnosed to discern the patient's unique circumstances. Likewise, the manufacturer's package insert for current drug product information should be consulted before administering any drug. Publisher disclaims all liability for any inaccuracies, omissions, misuse, or misunderstanding of the information contained in this publication. Publisher cautions that this publication is not intended as a substitute for the professional judgment of trained medical personnel.

www.mhhe.com

Brief Contents

Contents

Procedures

Preface

Medical Assisting: Administrative and Clinical Competencies, 2nd edition, is a comprehensive textbook for the medical assisting student. It provides the student with information about all aspects of the medical assisting profession, both administrative and clinical, from the general to the specific, it covers the key concepts, skills, and tasks that medical assistants need to know. The book speaks directly to the student, and its chapter introductions, case studies, procedures, and chapter summaries are written to engage the student's attention and build a sense of positive anticipation about joining the profession of medical assisting.

When referring to patients in the third person, we have alternated between passages that describe a male patient and passages that describe a female patient. Thus, the patient will be referred to as "he" half the time and as "she" half the time. The same convention is used to refer to the physician. The medical assistant is consistently addressed as "you."

Patient Education

In this book we focus particularly on patient education and on the role of the medical assistant in encouraging patients to be active participants in their own health care. It is always desirable for patients to be as knowledgeable as possible about their health. Patients who do not understand what is expected of them may become confused, frightened, angry, and uncooperative; educated patients are better able to understand why compliance is important.

Chapter 14 is devoted entirely to patient education. Other chapters cover various aspects of patient interaction—such as Chapter 4, on communicating with the patient, and Chapter 36, on interviewing the patient. Throughout the book, we provide the medical assistant with the information needed to educate patients so that they can participate fully in their health care.

We have also made a consistent effort to discuss patients with special needs. Several chapters in Part 2, Administrative Medical Assisting, and in Part 3, Clinical Medical Assisting, contain special sections of text devoted to the particular concerns of certain patient groups. These groups include the following:

- **Pregnant women.** Pregnancy has profound effects on every aspect of health, all of which must be taken into account when working with pregnant patients.

Where appropriate, we have addressed special concerns for pregnant patients, such as positioning them for an examination, recommending changes in diet, and taking care to avoid harming the fetus with drugs or procedures that would ordinarily pose little or no risk to the patient. Chapter 38, on the general physical examination, includes a separate procedure for meeting the needs of the pregnant patient during an examination.

- **Elderly patients.** Special care is often required with elderly patients. The body undergoes many changes with age, and patients may have difficulty adjusting to their changing physical needs. Several chapters deal with the special needs of elderly patients, such as Chapter 39, which includes an Educating the Patient feature on preventing falls of the elderly.

- **Children.** The special needs of children are complex, because not only their bodies but also their minds and social situations are very different from those of adults. Dealing with children usually means dealing with their parents as well, and medical assistants must hone their communication skills to meet the needs of both patient and parent when working with children. One chapter that focuses on children is Chapter 13, which includes a special text section and a procedure for designing a patient reception area to accommodate children.

- **Patients with disabilities.** Many different diseases and disabilities require extra effort or consideration on the part of the medical assistant. Patients in wheelchairs and patients with diabetes, hemophilia, or visual or hearing impairments all require specific accommodations. For example, Chapter 22 addresses the needs of such patients; it includes a section that discusses the Americans With Disabilities Act and a procedure for making the examination room safe for patients with visual impairments.

- **Patients from other cultures.** Communicating with patients from other cultures, especially when language barriers are involved, poses a special challenge for the medical assistant. In addition, patients from other cultures may have attitudes about medicine or about social interaction that differ sharply from those of the medical assistant's culture. Chapter 4 is one chapter that deals in depth with patients from other cultures. It contains a text section and a Caution: Handle With

Care feature about different cultures' attitudes toward medicine.

Because safety is a primary concern for both the patient and the medical assistant, we have emphasized this aspect of medical assisting work. Every clinical procedure includes appropriate icons, discussed in Chapter 19, for safety precautions required by the Occupational Safety and Health Administration (OSHA) guidelines. These icons for the OSHA guidelines appear in order of use within each procedure. If hand washing is necessary more than once, the hand washing icon appears twice. If biohazardous waste is generated during the procedure, the biohazardous waste container icon will appear, and so on.

Areas of Competence

A key feature of *Medical Assisting* that will enhance its usefulness to both students and instructors is its reference to the areas of competence defined in the 2003 AAMA (American Association of Medical Assistants) Role Delineation Study. The study, which replaces the 1990 DACUM (*Developing A CurriculUM*) analysis, provides a comprehensive list of duties and skills that medical assistants must master at the entry level. The Committee on Accreditation of Allied Health Education Personnel (CAAHEP) requires that all medical assistants be proficient in the 71 entry-level areas of competence when they begin medical assisting work. The opening page of each chapter provides a list of the areas of competence that the chapter covers, and the complete Medical Assistant Role Delineation Chart is provided as an appendix. (A correlation chart also appears in the *Instructor's Resource Binder.*) The chapter-by-chapter listing of areas of competence allows instructors to identify skills that have been covered in the course and helps students find the chapters that cover specific skills and duties.

We have been careful to ensure that the text provides ample coverage of topics used to construct the AMT (Association of Medical Technologists) Registered Medical Assistant (RMA) Exam. A correlation chart appears in the *Instructor's Resource Binder.*

Organization of the Text

Medical Assisting: Administrative and Clinical Competencies, 2nd edition, is divided into three parts. Part 1 provides a basic explanation of the role of the medical assistant in a medical practice. It includes an overview of the profession and covers the different types of medical practices, legal and ethical issues—including important information on HIPAA (Health Information Portability and Accountability Act) regulations—and communication with patients, their families, and coworkers. Part 2 explores the administrative duties of the medical assistant, including basic office work, patient interaction, and the financial responsibilities of a medical practice. Part 3 covers the clinical duties of the medical assistant and includes an overview of the anatomy and physiology of body systems; it also provides information on patient assistance; specialty examinations and medical emergencies; and laboratory and other specialized procedures. Chapter 54, new to this edition, provides the medical assisting student with information about the externship process and how to prepare to find a position as a medical assistant.

The ordering of chapters within each part allows the student and the instructor to build a knowledge base starting with the fundamentals and working toward an understanding of highly specialized tasks. Part 2 introduces the basics of working with office equipment before covering the details of maintaining patient records, scheduling appointments, and processing insurance. Part 3 begins with a grounding in principles of asepsis, a concept that is crucial to all clinical procedures. Subsequent chapters lead the student through the anatomy and physiology of body systems, through general and specialized physical examinations, and eventually into the technical details of laboratory testing, drug administration, electrocardiography, and radiology.

Chapters are also grouped into sections when their subjects relate to a broader topic or area of skills. Each section is set apart, the section opener includes the list of chapters within that section.

Each chapter opens with a page of material that includes the chapter outline and objectives, a list of key terms, and the areas of competence covered in the chapter. The main text of each chapter begins with an overview of chapter content and includes a case study for students to consider as they read the chapter. Chapters are organized into topics that move from the general to the specific. Color photographs, anatomic and technical drawings, tables, charts, and text features help educate the student about various aspects of medical assisting. The text features, set off in boxes within the text, include the following:

- **Case Studies** are provided at the beginning of all chapters. They represent situations similar to those that the medical assistant may encounter in daily practice. Students are encouraged to consider the case study as they read each chapter. Case Study Questions in the end-of-chapter review check students' understanding and application of chapter content.

- **Procedures** give step-by-step instructions on how to perform specific administrative or clinical tasks that a medical assistant will be required to perform. A list of the procedures, which follows the Table of Contents, details the procedures found in each chapter, provides the AAMA competency number associated with each specific procedure, and indicates whether information related to that procedure is included on the student CD.

- **Tips for the Office** boxes provide guidelines on keeping the administration of the medical office running smoothly and efficiently.

- **Educating the Patient** boxes focus on ways to instruct patients about caring for themselves outside the medical office.

- **Diseases and Disorders** boxes give detailed information on specific medical conditions, including how to recognize, prevent, and treat them.
- **Caution: Handle With Care** boxes cover the precautions to be taken in certain situations or when performing certain tasks.
- **Career Opportunities** boxes provide the student with information on various specialized medical professions or duties related to the medical assistant's role within the health-care team.
- **Pathophysiology** boxes, a feature found in each of the chapters on anatomy and physiology, provide students with a list of the most common diseases and disorders of each body system and includes information on the causes, common signs and symptoms, treatment, and where possible, the prevention of each disease.

Each chapter closes with a summary of the chapter material that focuses on the role of the medical assistant. The summary is followed by an end-of-chapter review that consists of the following elements:

- Case Study Questions
- Discussion Questions
- Critical Thinking Questions
- Application Activities
- Internet Activities

A list of further readings, including related books and journal articles, will be provided for each chapter on McGraw-Hill's medical assisting online learning center. The end-of-chapter questions and activities, as well as the additional online resources provide supplementary information about the subjects presented in the chapter and allow students to practice specific skills.

The book also includes a glossary and several appendices for use as reference tools. The glossary lists all the words presented as key terms in each chapter along with a pronunciation guide and the definition of each term. The appendixes include the Medical Assistant Role Delineation Chart, commonly used prefixes and suffixes, Latin and Greek terms, abbreviations and symbols used in medical terminology, and a comprehensive list of professional organizations and agencies.

The Student CD-ROM provides a comprehensive learning program that is correlated to each chapter of the text and reinforces competencies required to become a medical assistant. Short video clips and pictures introduce skills and case studies for application. In addition, numerous interactive exercises and applications are provided for every chapter in the text. The Student CD, included with each student textbook, provides the following menu choices:

- Administrative Practice
- Clinical Practice
- Anatomy and Physiology Review
- Games: Spin the Wheel and Key Term Concentration

- Interactive Review
- Audio Glossary
- Progress Report
- Online Learning Center

The Online Learning Center is a text-specific website that offers an extensive array of learning and teaching tools, including chapter quizzes with immediate feedback, newsfeeds, links to relevant websites, and many more study resources. Log on at www.mhhe.com/medicalassisting

Ancillaries

The *Student Workbook* provides an opportunity for the student to review the material and skills presented in the textbook. On a chapter-by-chapter basis, it provides:

- Vocabulary review exercises, which test knowledge of key terms in the chapter
- Content review exercises, which test the student's knowledge of key concepts in the chapter
- Critical thinking exercises, which test the student's understanding of key concepts in the chapter
- Application exercises, which test mastery of specific skills
- Case studies, which apply the chapter material to real-life situations or problems
- Competency checklists for the procedures in the text

The *Instructor's Resource Binder* provides the instructor with materials to help organize lessons and classroom interactions. It includes:

- A complete lesson plan for each chapter, including an introduction to the lesson, teaching strategies, alternate teaching strategies, case studies, assessment, chapter close, resources, and an answer key to the student textbook
- Procedure competency checklists, reproduced from the *Student Workbook*
- An answer key to the *Student Workbook*
- Charts that show the location in the student textbook, the *Student Workbook,* and the *Instructor's Resource Binder,* of material that correlates with the 2003 AAMA Role Delineation Study Areas of Competence, the SCANS Competencies, the National Health Care Skill Standards, and the AMT Registered Medical Assistant (RMA) Certification Exam Topics
- Power Point Presentations on the IPC CD-ROM

Computer software for the student and instructor is also available. The Student CD-ROM is packaged with each student textbook. The Instructor Resource CD-ROM provides easy-to-use resources for class preparation. The Instructor Resource CD-ROM includes the following:

- ExamView® Pro Test Generator with answer rationales and correlations to AAMA competencies

- PowerPoint® Presentations
- Correlations to AAMA and AMT Standards
- Course syllabi

Together, the Student Edition, the *Student Workbook,* and the *Instructor's Resource Binder* form a complete teaching and learning package. The *Medical Assisting* course will prepare students to enter the medical assisting field with all the knowledge and skills needed to be a useful resource to patients, a valued asset to employers, and a credit to the medical assisting profession.

Acknowledgments

The publisher and authors would like to thank the reviewers and contributors for their assistance in shaping this revision. We appreciate their suggestions, insights, and commitment to providing information that is relevant and valuable to medical assisting students.

In addition, many people and organizations provided invaluable assistance in the process of illustrating the highly technical and detailed topics covered in the text. Their contributions helped ensure the accuracy, timeliness, and authenticity of the illustrations in the book.

We would like to thank the following organizations for providing source materials and technical advice: the American Association of Medical Assistants, Chicago, Illinois; Becton Dickinson Microbiology Systems, Sparks, Maryland; Becton Dickinson VACUTAINER Systems, Franklin Lakes, New Jersey; Bibbero Systems, Petaluma, California; Burdick, Schaumberg, Illinois; the Corel Corporation, Ottawa, Ontario, Canada; Hamilton Media, Hamilton, New Jersey; Nassau Ear, Nose, and Throat, Princeton, New Jersey; Princeton Allergy and Asthma Associates, Princeton, New Jersey; Richmond International, Boca Raton, Florida; Winfield Medical, San Diego, California.

We would like to express our appreciation to the following New Jersey physicians and medical facilities for allowing us to photograph a variety of procedures and procedural settings at their facilities: the Eric B. Chandler Medical Center, New Brunswick; Helene Fuld School of Nursing of New Jersey, Trenton; Mercer Medical Center, Trenton; Mercer County Vocational-Technical Health Occupations Center, Trenton; Plainfield Health Center, Plainfield; Princeton Allergy and Asthma Associates, Princeton; the Princeton Medical Group, Princeton; Robert Wood Johnson University Hospital, New Brunswick; Robert Wood Johnson University Hospital at Hamilton, Hamilton; St. Francis Medical Center, Trenton; St. Peter's Medical Center, New Brunswick; Dr. Edward von der Schmidt, neurosurgeon, Princeton; Wound Care Center/ Curative Network, New Brunswick.

We would also like to thank the following facilities and educational institutions for graciously allowing us to photograph procedures and other technical aspects related to the profession of medical assisting: Total Care Programming, Henrico, North Carolina; Wildwood Medical Clinic, Henrico, North Carolina; Central Piedmont Community College, Charlotte, North Carolina; and Roanoke Rapids Clinic, Roanoke Rapids, Virginia.

Reviewers

Every area of the text was reviewed by practitioners and educators in the field. Their insights helped shape the direction of the book.

Kaye Acton, CMA
    Alamance Community College
    Graham, NC

Jannie R. Adams, PhD, RN, MS-HSA, BSN
    Clayton College and State University,
    School of Technology
    Morrow, GA

Cathy Kelley Arney, CMA, MLT (ASCP), AS
    National College of Business and Technology
    Bluefield, VA

Joseph Balabat, MD
    Drake Schools
    Astoria, NY

Marsha Benedict, CMA-A, MS, CPC
    Baker College of Flint
    Flint, MI

Michelle Buchman
    Springfield College
    Springfield, MO

Patricia Celani, CMA
    ICM School of Business and Medical Careers
    Pittsburgh, PA

Theresa Cyr, RN, BN, MS
    Heald Business College
    Honolulu, HI

Barbara Desch
    San Joaquin Valley College
    Visalia, CA

Herbert J. Feitelberg, BA, DPM
    King's College
    Charlotte, NC

Geri L. Finn
    Remington College, Dallas Campus
    Garland, TX

Kimberly L. Gibson, RN, DOE
    Sanford Brown Institute
    Middleburg Heights, OH

Barbara G. Gillespie, MS
    San Diego & Grossmont Community College Districts
    El Cajon, CA

Cindy Gordon, MBA, CMA
    Baker College
    Muskegon, MI

Mary Harmon
MedTech College
Indianapolis, IN

Glenda H. Hatcher, BSN
Southwest Georgia Technical College
Thomasville, GA

Helen J. Hauser, RN, MSHA, RMA
Phoenix College
Phoenix, AZ

Christine E. Hetrick
Cittone Institute
Mt. Laurel, NJ

Beulah A. Hofmann, RN, MSN, CMA
Ivy Tech State College
Terre Haute, IN

Karen Jackson
Education America
Garland, TX

Latashia Y. D. Jones, LPN
CAPPS College, Montgomery Campus
Montgomery, AL

Donna D. Kyle-Brown, PhD, RMA
CAPPS College, Mobile Campus
Mobile, AL

Sharon McCaughrin
Ross Learning
Southfield, MI

Tanya Mercer, BS, RMA
Kaplan Higher Education Corporation
Roswell, GA

T. Michelle Moore-Roberts
CAPPS College, Montgomery Campus
Montgomery, AL

Linda Oprean
Applied Career Training
Manassas, VA

Julie Orloff, RMA, CMA, CPT, CPC
Ultrasound Diagnostic School
Miami, FL

Delores W. Orum, RMA
CAPPS College
Montgomery, AL

Katrina L. Poston, MA, RHE
Applied Career Training
Arlington, VA

Manuel Ramirez, MD
Texas School of Business
Friendswood, TX

Beatrice Salada, BAS, CMA
Davenport University
Lansing, MI

Melanie G. Sheffield, LPN
Capps Medical Institute
Pensacola, FL

Kristi Sopp, RMA
MTI College
Sacramento, CA

Carmen Stevens
Remington College, Fort Worth Campus
Fort Worth, TX

Deborah Sulkowski, BS, CMA
Pittsburgh Technical Institute
Oakdale, PA

Fred Valdes, MD
City College
Ft. Lauderdale, FL

Janice Vermiglio-Smith, RN, MS, PhD
Central Arizona College
Apache Junction, AZ

Erich M. Weldon, MICP, NREMT-P
Apollo College
Portland, Oregon

Terri D. Wyman, CMRS, CMS
Ultrasound Diagnostic School
Springfield, MA

Contributors

Kaye Acton, CMA
Alamance Community College
Graham, North Carolina

Jannie R. Adams, PhD, RN, MS-HSA, BSN
Clayton College and State University, School
of Technology
Morrow, Georgia

Cathy Kelley Arney, CMA, MLT (ASCP), AS
National College of Business and Technology
Bluefield, Virginia

Russell E. Battiata
National School of Technology
Miami, Florida

Marti A. Burton, RN, BS
Canadian Valley Technology Center
El Reno, Oklahoma

Ann Coleman
Society of Nuclear Medicine
Reston, Virginia

Barbara G. Gillespie, MS
San Diego and Grossmont Community
College Districts
El Cajon, California

Regina Hoffman, PhD
Midlands Technical College
Columbia, South Carolina

Donna D. Kyle-Brown, PhD, RMA
CAPPS College, Mobile Campus
Mobile, Alabama

Cynthia Newby, CPC
    Chestnut Hill Enterprises
Melanie G. Sheffield, LPN
    Capps Medical Institute
    Pensacola, Florida
Cynthia T. Vincent, MMS, PA-C
    Wildwood Medical Clinic
    Henrico, North Carolina
Terri D. Wyman, CMRS, CMS
    Ultrasound Diagnostic School
    Springfield, Massachusetts

MEDICAL ASSISTING

Administrative and Clinical Competencies

One

Introduction to Medical Assisting

"The medical assisting profession is filled with challenges and rewards every day. Everything is important when you are assisting a patient. You should get to know your patient, and his family, if possible, in order to understand the patient's specific needs. This is especially true with an elderly patient. Treat your patient like a family member. Be considerate and concerned, and always maintain a pleasant attitude.

"It is also essential to know your physician well, and how he or she likes to work. Let the physician know all the information the patient has shared with you, to help him or her make a better diagnosis. Keep informed about what the physician has recommended for treatment. The patient will have questions along the way. It's good medicine to be able to give him solid information about his condition and reinforce the doctor's orders when necessary. A skilled physician and an organized, cooperative, receptive medical assistant promote and maintain exceptional patient care."

Sue Haines
Medical Assistant, Princeton, New Jersey

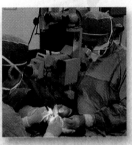

SECTION ONE
Foundations and Principles

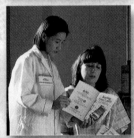

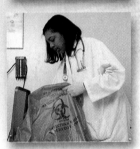

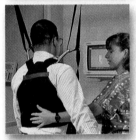

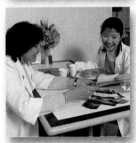

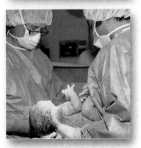

SECTION 1

FOUNDATIONS AND PRINCIPLES

The Profession of Medical Assisting

AREAS OF COMPETENCE

2003 Role Delineation Study

GENERAL

Professionalism

- Display a professional manner and image
- Demonstrate initiative and responsibility
- Prioritize and perform multiple tasks
- Promote the CMA credential
- Enhance skills through continuing education

Communication Skills

- Recognize and respond effectively to verbal, nonverbal, and written communications

Legal Concepts

- Perform within legal and ethical boundaries
- Recognize professional credentialing criteria

KEY TERMS

accreditation

American Association of Medical Assistants (AAMA)

Certified Medical Assistant (CMA)

CLIA (Clinical Laboratory Improvement Amendments)

contaminated

cross-training

externship

HIPAA (Health Insurance Portability and Accountability Act)

managed care organization (MCO)

OSHA (Occupational Safety and Health Act)

portfolio

practitioner

Registered Medical Assistant (RMA)

résumé

CHAPTER OUTLINE

- Growth of the Medical Assisting Profession
- Medical Assistant Credentials
- Membership in a Medical Assisting Association
- Training Programs and Other Learning Opportunities
- Daily Duties of Medical Assistants
- Personal Qualifications of Medical Assistants
- On the Job
- The AAMA Role Delineation Study

OBJECTIVES

After completing Chapter 1, you will be able to:

1.1 Describe the job responsibilities of a medical assistant
1.2 Discuss the professional training of a medical assistant
1.3 Identify the personal characteristics a medical assistant needs
1.4 Define multiskilled health professional
1.5 Explain the importance of continuing education for a medical assistant
1.6 Describe the process and benefits of certification and registration
1.7 List the benefits of becoming a member of a professional association

Introduction

Medical assisting is one of the fastest-growing occupations in allied health care today. Health care is changing at a rapid rate, from advanced technology to implementing cost-effective medicine while maintaining quality patient care. The medical assistant is the perfect complement to this changing industry. Employers are looking for health care professionals who are "generalists." A generalist is someone who is trained in all departments in the facility in which they are employed. Medical assistants who graduate from an accredited institution will gain the skills that enable them to multitask. A multitasking professional is someone who is able to work in the administrative areas, the clinical areas, and the financial areas. Employers are seeking credentialed health care professionals who are dedicated to the profession and the patient.

This chapter will introduce the professional standards that are required in medical assisting.

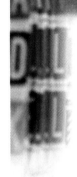

CASE STUDY

Medical assistants are considered generalists in most medical environments. The following scenarios describe how the medical assistant functions as a generalist or multiskilled professional. As you review the scenarios, make note of the many duties the medical assistant performs.

Scenario 1 Kim is 28 years old. She has been working as a medical assistant for 6 years. She is currently working in a family practice office with two doctors, two other medical assistants, and a medical records clerk. Her role is primarily administrative; she is mainly responsible for phone reception and patient check-in and check-out.

A 29-year-old female patient calls complaining of lower back pain. As Kim listens to the patient describe her condition, she determines the severity of the patient's discomfort and schedules a same-day appointment. When the patient arrives at the office, Kim greets her at the front desk, verifies her address and insurance information, and escorts her to an exam room. After the physician completes the exam, the patient is instructed to see Kim on the way out. Kim reviews the patient's prescriptions and schedules a diagnostic test and laboratory work for the patient at another facility. Kim then collects the patient co-pay and gives the patient a receipt. After the patient leaves, Kim prepares the insurance forms for reimbursement and files the patient's chart.

Scenario 2 David is 38 years old. He has been working as a medical assistant for 13 years. He currently works as a clinical medical assistant in an urgent care center that specializes in occupational medicine and basic emergency medicine. He is flexible and works a combination of days, afternoons, and weekends. He normally works with two doctors, two nurses, and four other medical assistants during his shift. The center's patients usually arrive on a walk-in basis.

A 40-year-old man signs in with the receptionist. She helps the patient complete the necessary forms for the medical chart. After the chart is completed, she places the chart at the clinical station. David reviews the medical chart and makes note that the patient, a truck driver, is here for an occupational physical. He obtains the protocol from the trucking company file and verifies the testing requested by the company. He then escorts the patient to an exam room and interviews the patient regarding his medical history. He explains all the testing that will be completed and escorts the patient to the laboratory. David collects a urine drug screen, following precise directions, and collects a blood specimen. David then performs an auditory and visual screening and escorts the patient back to the exam room. The patient is given a gown with instructions on how to put it on. After a few minutes, David obtains an EKG on the patient. The patient is now ready for the physical part of the exam, which is performed by the doctor. David verifies the information again and gives the chart to the doctor. After the doctor is finished with the exam, David returns to the patient, explains how the physical is reported to his employer, and escorts him to the x-ray technician for a chest x-ray. After the patient leaves, David completes the paperwork, submits the laboratory work to an outside reference lab, and submits the x-ray to be read by a radiologist.

As you read this chapter, consider the following questions:

1. How are the two jobs different?
2. How are the two jobs the same?
3. How do these two medical assistants function as multiskilled health-care professionals?

Growth of the Medical Assisting Profession

As a medical assistant you will be an allied health professional trained to work in a variety of health-care settings: medical offices, clinics, and ambulatory care facilities. Your role, with varied and challenging administrative and clinical duties, will be integral to creating a health-care facility that operates smoothly and provides a patient-centered approach to quality health care. Your specific responsibilities will likely depend on the location and size of the facility as well as its medical specialties.

Medical assisting is now one of the fastest-growing occupations. As the health services industry expands, the U.S. Department of Labor predicts that medical assisting will grow at a much faster rate than the average rate for all occupations through the year 2010. The growth in the number of physicians' group practices and other health-care practices that use support personnel will in turn continue to drive up demand for medical assistants.

According to the U.S. Department of Labor Bureau of Statistics, in the year 2000, medical assistants held approximately 329,000 jobs. Of these, 60% were in physicians' offices, and approximately 15% were in hospitals, including outpatient and inpatient facilities. The rest were in nursing homes and the offices of other health **practitioners** (those who practice a profession), such as chiropractors, optometrists, and podiatrists. Some medical assistants worked in other health-care facilities.

Modern health insurance, Medicare, and Medicaid now make medical care available to more people, and the number of physicians is increasing. Thus, more medical assistants will be needed to run these physicians' offices.

The following factors will also increase job opportunities for medical assistants: growth of outpatient clinics and health maintenance organizations (HMOs), and the population increase. Specifically, greater numbers of older people now require a relatively higher level of medical care. Today, the elderly are the fastest-growing segment of the U.S. population. Statistics show that the entire population will grow 22% from 2000 to 2005, but that those aged 65 and older will increase to 78.5%. The older population has unique needs and problems.

History of the Medical Assisting Profession

With the emergence of formal training programs for medical assistants and the continuous changes in health care today, the role of the medical assistant has become dynamic and wide ranging. These changes have raised the expectations for medical assistants. The knowledge base of the modern medical assistant includes:

- administrative and clinical skills
- patient insurance product knowledge (specific to the workers' geographical locations)
- compliance, especially of OSHA and HIPAA guidelines
- exceptional customer service
- practice management
- current patient treatments and education

The medical assisting profession today requires a commitment to self-directed, lifelong learning. Health care is changing rapidly because of new technology, new health-care delivery systems, and new approaches to facilitating cost-efficient, high-quality health care. A medical assistant who can adapt to change and is continually learning will be in high demand.

Creating the American Association of Medical Assistants

The seed of the idea for a national association of medical assistants—to be called the **American Association of Medical Assistants (AAMA)**—was planted at the 1955 annual state convention of the Kansas Medical Assistants Society. The next year, at an American Medical Association (AMA) meeting, the AAMA was officially created. In 1978 the U.S. Department of Health, Education, and Welfare declared medical assisting an allied health profession. In the early 1970s the American Medical Technologists (which has been a national certifying body for laboratory personnel since 1939) began a program to register medical assistants at accredited schools. You will read more about the benefits of joining one of these organizations later in the chapter. Figure 1-1 shows the pins worn by medical assistants who are certified by the AAMA and by those registered by the American Medical Technologists.

The AAMA's Purpose. The AAMA works to raise standards of medical assisting to a more professional level. It is the only professional association devoted exclusively to the medical assisting profession. Its creator and first

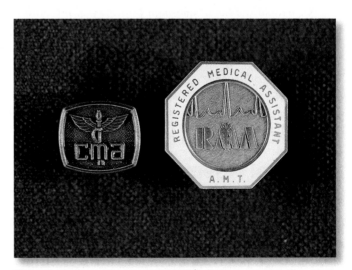

Figure 1-1. The pin on the left is worn by members of the American Association of Medical Assistants. The pin on the right is worn by medical assistants registered by the American Medical Technologists.

president, Maxine Williams, had extensive experience in orchestrating medical assisting projects for the Kansas Medical Assistants Society. She also served as cochair of the planning committee that formed the AAMA.

The AAMA Creed. To maintain the professional standards of the medical assisting profession, the AAMA has developed the following creed, which is reprinted here with the permission of the organization:

> *I believe in the principles and purposes of the profession of medical assisting.*
> *I endeavor to be more effective.*
> *I aspire to render greater service.*
> *I protect the confidence entrusted to me.*
> *I am dedicated to the care and well-being of all people.*
> *I am loyal to my physician-employer.*
> *I am true to the ethics of my profession.*
> *I am strengthened by compassion, courage, and faith.*

AAMA Code of Ethics. The AAMA has also established a code of ethics, which is reprinted here with the permission of the organization:

> The Code of Ethics of AAMA shall set forth principles of ethical and moral conduct as they relate to the medical profession and the particular practice of Medical Assisting.
>
> Members of AAMA dedicated to the conscientious pursuit of their profession, and thus desiring to merit the high regard of the entire medical profession and the respect of the general public which they serve, do pledge themselves to strive always to:

A. render service with full respect for the dignity of humanity

B. respect confidential information obtained through employment unless legally authorized or required by responsible performance of duty to divulge such information

C. uphold the honor and high principles of the profession and accept its disciplines

D. seek to continually improve the knowledge and skills of medical assistants for the benefit of patients and professional colleagues

E. participate in additional service activities aimed toward improving the health and well-being of the community

Medical Assistant Credentials

According to Donald A. Balasa, JD, MBA, AAMA executive director and staff legal counsel, "voluntary credentialing . . . is usually national in its scope and most often sponsored by a nongovernmental, private-sector entity" (Balasa, 1994). Employers today prefer or even insist that their medical assistants have credentialing within their discipline. Understanding why employers are aggressively recruiting credentialed medical assistants is of utmost importance for medical assisting educators as well as all medical assistants. Listed here are some explanations as to why credentialing is becoming so important for a medical assistant's entry into and advancement within the allied health force.

Malpractice

The United States continues to be one of the most litigious nations in the civilized world. Disputes that used to be settled by discussion and mediation are now being referred to attorneys and ending up in courts of law. Lawsuit mania is particularly acute in the world of health care. Employers of allied health professionals have correctly concluded that having credentialed personnel or staff will lessen the likelihood of a successful legal challenge to the quality of work of employees.

Managed Care Organizations

Managed care is a growing trend in today's health-care industry. The cost limitations imposed by **managed care organizations (MCOs)** are causing mergers and buyouts throughout the nation. Small physician practices are being consolidated or merged into larger providers of health care, and the resulting economies of scale can make the delivery of health care more cost-effective. Human resource directors of MCOs place great importance in professional credentials for their employees and therefore are more likely to establish certification or registry as a mandatory professional designation for medical assistants.

State and Federal Regulations

Certain provisions of the **OSHA (Occupational Safety and Health Act)** and the **CLIA (Clinical Laboratory Improvement Amendments)** are making mandatory credentialing for medical assistants a logical step in the hiring process. Presently, OSHA and CLIA do not require that medical assistants be credentialed, but there are various components of these statutes and their regulations that can be met by demonstrating that medical assistants in a clinical setting are certified.

CMA Certification

The **Certified Medical Assistant (CMA)** credential is awarded by the Certifying Board of the AAMA. The AAMA's certification examination evaluates mastery of medical assisting competencies based on the 2003 Role Delineation Study, discussed later in this chapter. The National Board of Medical Examiners (NBME) also provides technical assistance in developing the tests.

CMAs must recertify the CMA credential every 5 years. This mandate requires you to learn about new medical developments through education courses or participation in an examination. Hundreds of continuing education courses are sponsored by local, state, and national AAMA groups. The AAMA also offers self-study courses through its Continuing Education Department. As described in the AAMA's publication *Certified Medical Assistants: Health-Care's Most Versatile Professionals,* the advantages of CMA certification include respect and recognition from peers in the medical assisting profession.

As of June 1998, only applicants of medical assisting programs accredited by the Commission on Accreditation of Allied Health Education Programs (CAAHEP) and the Accrediting Bureau of Health Education Schools (ABHES) are eligible to take the certification examination. The examination is administered nationwide every January and June at more than 100 test sites. The AAMA offers the *Candidate's Guide to the Certification Examination* to help applicants prepare for the examination. This guide explains the test format and test-taking strategies. It also includes a sample examination with answers and information about study references.

RMA Registration

The **Registered Medical Assistant (RMA)** credential is given by the American Medical Technologists (AMT), an organization founded in 1939. RMA credentialing by the AMT ensures that you have taken and passed the AMT certification examination for the Registered Medical Assistant. RMA is a generic term used by the American Registry of Medical Assistants since 1950 and by the AMT since 1984.

The AMT sets forth certain educational and experiential requirements to earn the RMA credential. These include:

- Graduation from an accredited high school or acceptable equivalent.
- Graduation from a medical assistant program or institution accredited by the Accrediting Bureau of Health Education Schools (ABHES), from a medical assistant program accredited by a regional accrediting commission, or from a formal medical services training program of the U.S. Armed Forces. Alternatively, the applicant can have been employed in the profession of medical assisting for a minimum of 5 years, not more than 2 of which may have been as an instructor in a postsecondary medical assistant program.
- Passing the AMT examination for RMA certification.

Major Areas of the RMA/CMA Examinations

The RMA and CMA qualifying examinations are rigorous. Participation in an accredited program, however, will help you learn what you need to know. The examinations cover several distinct areas of knowledge. These include:

- General medical knowledge, including terminology, anatomy, physiology, behavioral science, medical law, and ethics

- Administrative knowledge, including medical records management, collections, insurance processing, and the **Health Insurance Portability and Accountability Act (HIPAA)**
- Clinical knowledge, including examination room techniques, medication preparation and administration, pharmacology, and specimen collection

Membership in a Medical Assisting Association

Professional associations set high standards for quality and performance in a profession. They define the tasks and functions of an occupation. In addition, they provide members with the opportunity to communicate and network with one another. They also present their goals to the profession and to the general public. Becoming a member of a professional association helps you achieve career goals and further the profession of medical assisting.

Professional Support for CMAs

When you become a member of the AAMA, you will have a large support group of active medical assistants. Membership benefits include:

- Professional publications, such as *The CMA*
- A large variety of educational opportunities, such as chapter-sponsored seminars and workshops about the latest administrative, clinical, and management topics (Figure 1-2)

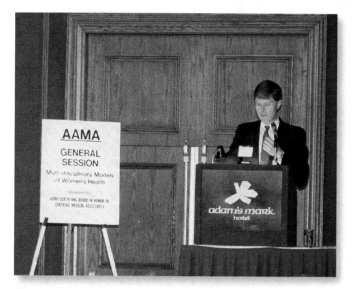

Figure 1-2. Local and state chapters of the AAMA and AMT frequently sponsor seminars and workshops on administrative, clinical, or management topics. In this picture, Donald A. Balasa, executive director and staff legal counsel for the AAMA, addresses a group at the annual AAMA national convention.

- Group insurance
- Legal counsel
- Local, state, and national activities that include professional networking and multiple continuing education opportunities

Professional Support for RMAs

The AMT offers many benefits for RMAs. These include:

- Professional publications
- Membership in the AMT Institute for Education
- Group insurance programs—liability, health, and life
- State chapter activities
- Legal representation in health legislative matters
- Annual meetings and educational seminars
- Student membership

Training Programs and Other Learning Opportunities

Formal programs in medical assisting are offered in a variety of educational settings. They include vocational-technical high schools, postsecondary vocational schools, community and junior colleges, and 4-year colleges and universities. Vocational school programs usually last 1 or 2 years and award a certificate or diploma. Community and junior college programs are usually 2-year associate degree programs.

Accreditation

Accreditation is the process by which programs are officially authorized. Two agencies recognized by the U.S. Department of Education accredit programs in medical assisting: CAAHEP and ABHES.

Accredited programs must cover the following topics: anatomy and physiology; medical terminology; medical law and ethics; psychology; oral and written communications; laboratory, clinical, and administrative procedures; typing; transcription; record keeping; accounting; and insurance processing. High school students may prepare for these courses by studying mathematics, health, biology, typing, office skills, bookkeeping, and computers. You may obtain current information about accreditation standards for medical assisting programs from the AAMA.

Medical assisting programs must also include an externship. An **externship** is practical work experience for a specified time frame in physicians' offices, hospitals, or other health-care facilities.

Additionally, the AAMA lists its minimum standards for accredited programs (called essentials). This list of essentials ensures that all personnel—administrators and faculty—are qualified to perform their jobs.

The AAMA requires that administrative personnel exhibit leadership and management skills. They must also be able to fully perform the functions identified in documented job descriptions. Faculty members must develop and evaluate lesson plans, assess student progress toward the program's objectives, and be knowledgeable regarding course content. They must be qualified through work experience and be able to effectively direct and evaluate student learning and laboratory experiences.

The AAMA also has accreditation requirements for financial and physical resources. Each program's financial resources must meet its obligations to students. Schools must also have adequate physical resources—classrooms, laboratories, clinical and administrative facilities, and equipment and supplies.

The Benefits of Certification/Registration

Certification or registration is not required to practice as a medical assistant. You may practice with a high school diploma or equivalent. Your career options will be greater, however, if you graduate from an accredited school and you become certified or registered.

Graduation from an accredited program helps your career in three ways. First, it shows that you have completed a program that meets nationally accepted standards. Second, it provides recognition of your education by professional peers. Third, it makes you eligible for registration or certification (Heyman, 1993).

A solid medical assisting program provides the following:

- Facilities and equipment that are up to date
- Student to instructor ratio of 20:1
- Job placement services
- A cooperative education program and opportunities for continuing education

Externships

In an externship you will obtain work experience while completing a medical assisting program. You will practice skills learned in the classroom in an actual medical office environment.

Externship Requirements. Externships are mandatory in accredited schools. Each program has its own externship requirements. Familiarize yourself with the program requirements as soon as possible. You may be able to obtain an externship site of your choice either at a practice already affiliated with the school or at a practice you find on your own.

The externship is offered in cooperative medical offices or hospitals for a predetermined period (several weeks to several months). Another experienced medical assistant, nurse manager, or licensed nurse practitioner in the externship office often becomes your mentor. This mentor advises and supervises you during the externship.

Externship Duties.   Your duties will be planned to meet your program's requirements for real-world work experience. Approach the externship with a positive attitude. Accept any guidance, constructive criticism, or praise as a learning experience.

Obtaining a Reference.   Your externship also offers you the opportunity to acquire a good reference. A reference is usually written by your supervisor, who will describe your performance, strengths, and skills. You may use this reference later with prospective employers. Because you may be required to provide a list of references when applying for future jobs, ask your externship mentor to prepare a letter of reference for your **portfolio** (a collection of your résumé, reference letters, and other documents of interest, such as awards for volunteer service in a health-related field). Send a thank-you note to your supervisor for allowing you to do an externship and for writing you a reference. Externships will be discussed in more detail in Chapter 54.

Volunteer Programs

Volunteering is a rewarding experience. Before you even begin a medical assisting program, you can gain experience in a health-care profession through volunteer work. As a volunteer, you will get hands-on training and learn what it is like to assist patients who are ill, disabled, or frightened.

You may volunteer as an aide in a hospital, clinic, nursing home, or doctor's office or as a typist or filing clerk in a medical office or medical record room. Some visiting nurse associations and hospices (homelike medical settings that provide medical care and emotional support to terminally ill patients and their families) also offer volunteer opportunities. These experiences may help you decide if you want to pursue a career as a medical assistant.

The American Red Cross also offers volunteer opportunities for the student medical assistant. The Red Cross needs volunteers for its disaster relief programs locally, statewide, nationally, and abroad.

As part of a disaster relief team at the site of a hurricane, tornado, storm, flood, earthquake, or fire, volunteers learn first-aid and emergency triage skills. Red Cross volunteers gain valuable work experience that may help them obtain a job.

Because volunteers are not paid, it is usually easy to find work opportunities. Just because you are not paid for volunteer work, however, does not mean the experience is not useful for meeting your career goals.

Include information about any volunteer work on your **résumé**—a typewritten document that summarizes your employment and educational history. Be sure to note specific duties, responsibilities, and skills developed during the volunteer experience (Figure 1-3). Résumés are discussed in more detail in Chapter 54.

Multiskill Training

Today many hospitals and health-care practices are embracing the idea of a multiskilled health-care professional (MSHP). An MSHP is a cross-trained team member who is able to handle many different duties.

The AAMA includes the word *multiskill* in its definition of the profession of medical assisting:

> Medical assisting is a multiskilled allied health profession whose practitioners work primarily in ambulatory settings, such as medical offices and clinics. Medical assistants function as members of the healthcare delivery team and perform administrative and clinical procedures. (AAMA, 1991)

An MSHP may be trained to perform certain clinical procedures. She is not, however, trained to make judgments or interpretations concerning a patient's diagnosis or treatment, as a physician would.

Reducing Health-Care Costs.   As a result of health-care reform and downsizing (a reduction in the number of staff members) to control the rising cost of health care, medical practices are eager to reduce personnel costs by hiring multiskilled health professionals. These individuals, who perform the functions of two or more people, are the most cost-efficient employees.

Expanding Your Career Opportunities.   Career opportunities are vast if you are self-motivated and willing to learn new skills. If you continue to learn about new administrative and clinical techniques and procedures, you will be an important part of the health-care team.

As you read this book, look for a boxed feature titled Career Opportunities. This feature highlights additional skills medical assistants can learn and integrate into their jobs to make themselves more marketable as multiskilled health professionals. Following are several examples of positions that are sometimes combined with a medical assistant position:

- Office manager
- Medical laboratory technician
- ECG technician
- Medical transcriptionist
- Medical biller
- Hospital admissions coordinator
- A professional who performs physical exams for applicants to insurance companies
- An administrative assistant at insurance companies (particularly in managed care companies), hospitals, and clinics

If you are multiskilled, you will have an advantage when job hunting. Prospective employers are eager to hire multiskilled medical assistants and may create positions for them.

ALICIA HOLT
114 Herald Avenue
Winston, MO 43840
660-555-1212

POSITION: Full-time medical assistant

EDUCATION:

June 1996–June 1998   Associate Degree in Science, Mayerville Community College
                             Will take the medical assisting certification examination
                             after graduation

September 1991–June 1995   Winston Central High School

WORK EXPERIENCE:

May 1998–June 1998   Medical assistant extern
                             Dr. J. D. Perez, pediatrician,
                             Mayerville Pediatrics, Mayerville, MO

September 1994–present   General office clerk
                             Cunningham Medical Supply Company, Winston, MO

June 1994–September 1994   Waitress
                             Bonelli's Italian Restaurant, Winston, MO

VOLUNTEER EXPERIENCE:

May 1995–present   Recreational aide
                             Watson House for Autistic Children, Mayerville, MO

June 1993–present   Receptionist and information clerk
                             Riverside General Hospital, Atherton, MO

SPECIAL SKILLS:

                             Typing 55 wpm
                             WordPerfect and Excel
                             Medical Transcription
                             CPR (certified)
                             First Aid (certified)

                             References available upon request.

Figure 1-3. This medical assistant's résumé includes information about her volunteer work.

Unit Secretary

To gain medical assistant credentials, you must fulfill the requirements of either the American Association of Medical Assistants (for a Certified Medical Assistant) or the American Medical Technologists (for a Registered Medical Assistant). After obtaining your medical assistant certification or registration, you may wish to acquire additional skills in specialty areas through course work or on-the-job training. Although this course work or training may not lead to an additional certification or degree, it will enable you to expand your role in the medical office and advance your career as the demand for skilled health professionals increases.

Skills and Duties

Unit secretaries work in nursing stations or units in a hospital. They keep the nursing station functioning smoothly and free the nursing staff to focus on patient care. A unit secretary usually reports to a head nurse or a unit manager.

The unit secretary has four main areas of responsibility.

1. *Reception.* The unit secretary greets patients and gives them directions. She welcomes visitors and directs them to the rooms of the patients they wish to visit.

2. *Communication.* The unit secretary answers the phone and responds to pages. She addresses patient requests received over the intercom system, such as a request for a nurse or a doctor to come to the patient's room. The unit secretary also delivers mail and messages to patients. Unit secretaries with a command of medical terminology may be involved in coordinating the scheduling of medical personnel for the unit.

3. *Clerical duties.* The unit secretary updates records in patients' charts, transcribes physicians' orders, adds x-rays and laboratory reports to patients' charts, and processes the necessary paperwork for admissions, discharges, transfers, and deaths. In addition, she provides patient information, such as charts and schedules, to doctors and other hospital staff. The unit secretary also schedules patients' visits to other medical units in the hospital, such as laboratories. She keeps track of supply inventories for the unit, places orders for supplies and equipment as needed, and schedules necessary maintenance and repair services.

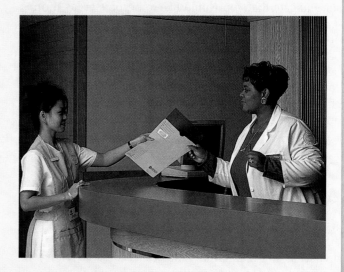

4. *Safety.* In some hospitals the unit secretary may be responsible for checking each room in the unit to make sure that all equipment—such as lamps, televisions, radios, and furniture—is in good working order. Other safety-related duties include keeping work areas free from clutter and making emergency code calls when necessary.

Workplace Settings

Most unit secretaries work at a nursing station or in a unit or ward in a hospital, but some find work in nursing homes. In some locations the work is divided differently than in a hospital. For example, a clinic might employ one person to handle scheduling and telephone reception and another staff member to greet patients and collect check-in information. Thus the clerical duties of the unit secretary might be separate from those of the receptionist.

Education

Unit secretaries need a high school diploma, and they receive their training on the job, although courses are available that provide valuable background. Sometimes a person who volunteers as a unit secretary in a hospital may be promoted to a paid position.

Where to Go for More Information

American Hospital Association
One North Franklin, Suite 2706
Chicago, IL 60606
(312) 422-3000

National Health Council
1730 M Street, NW, Suite 500
Washington, DC 20036
(202) 785-3910

You can gain multiskill training by showing initiative and a willingness to learn every aspect of the medical facility in which you are working. When you begin working within a medical facility, establish goals regarding your career path and discuss them with your immediate supervisor. Indicate that you would like to become **cross-trained** in every aspect of the medical facility. Begin your mastery of the department that you are currently working in and branch out to other departments once you master the skills needed for your current position. This will demonstrate a commitment to your profession as well as a strong work ethic. Cross-training is a valuable marketing tool to include on your résumé.

Daily Duties of Medical Assistants

As a medical assistant you will be the physician's "right arm." Duties include maintaining an efficient office, preparing and maintaining medical records, assisting the physician during examinations, and keeping examining rooms in order. You may also handle the payroll for the office staff (or supervise a payroll service), obtain equipment and supplies, and serve as the link between the physician and representatives of pharmaceutical and medical supply companies. In small practices you will usually handle all duties. In larger practices you may specialize in a particular duty.

Administrative Duties

Your administrative duties may include:

- Greeting patients
- Handling correspondence
- Scheduling appointments
- Answering telephones
- Creating and maintaining patient medical records
- Handling billing, bookkeeping, and insurance processing
- Performing medical transcription
- Arranging for hospital admissions
- Scheduling teleconferences for doctors at different locations to discuss cases
- Supervising personnel
- Developing and conducting public outreach programs to market the physician's professional services
- Negotiating leases of equipment and supply contracts
- Creating a recycling program for the practice (Tips for the Office gives more information on this topic).
- Serving as liaison between the physician and other individuals, such as pharmaceutical sales representatives and lawyers
- Performing as a HIPAA compliance officer

Clinical Duties

Your clinical duties may vary according to state law. They may include:

- Assisting the doctor during examinations
- Asepsis and infection control
- Performing diagnostic tests
- Giving injections, where allowed
- Performing electrocardiograms (ECGs)
- Drawing blood for testing
- Disposing of **contaminated** (soiled, or stained) supplies
- Explaining treatment procedures to patients
- Performing first aid and cardiopulmonary resuscitation (CPR)
- Patient education
- Preparing patients for examinations
- Preparing and administering medications as directed by the physician, and following state laws for invasive procedures
- Facilitating treatment for patients from diverse cultural backgrounds and for patients with hearing or vision impairments, or physical or mental disabilities
- Recording vital signs and medical histories
- Removing sutures or changing dressings on wounds
- Sterilizing medical instruments

Other clinical duties may include instructing patients about medication and special diets, authorizing drug refills as directed, and calling pharmacies to order prescriptions. You may also assist with minor surgery or teach patients about special procedures before laboratory tests, surgery, x-rays, or ECGs.

Laboratory Duties

Your laboratory duties may include:

- Performing tests, such as a urine pregnancy test, on the premises
- Collecting, preparing, and transmitting laboratory specimens
- Teaching patients to collect specific specimens properly
- Arranging laboratory services
- Meeting safety standards and fire protection mandates
- Performing as an OSHA compliance officer

Specialization

You may also choose to specialize in a specific area of health care. For example, podiatric medical assistants make castings of feet, expose and develop x-rays, and assist podiatrists in surgery. Ophthalmic medical assistants help ophthalmologists (doctors who provide eye care) by administering diagnostic tests, measuring and

Recycling in the Medical Office, Hospital, Laboratory, or Clinic

You may easily incorporate recycling procedures into the daily routine of a medical office, hospital, laboratory, or clinic. Medical facilities generate a tremendous amount of recyclable paper material. Recycling may be required by state law. Purchase paper products that can be recycled, or those made of postconsumer recycled materials, and take care in disposing of them (Roseen, 1991).

Some states levy large fines for noncompliance with recycling regulations. It is thus important to have a well-organized office recycling program. There are two essential aspects of recycling: disposal and purchasing. To create a complete recycling program, ensure that materials are disposed of properly and that purchased products have been made from recycled materials.

You may easily call the town's recycling center for guidelines for packaging recycled materials and for a pickup schedule. The recycling center may also provide containers for recyclable materials. You must fulfill all town and state legal recycling requirements.

Most paper products that do not have a glossy coating (like some fax paper) are recyclable. Each recycling center will provide a list of paper materials that can and cannot be recycled.

You must also research disposal techniques for biohazardous materials and follow regulations listed in the office policy manual and OSHA guidelines. These materials cannot be recycled and must be disposed of properly. They must not be mixed with recyclable waste. You will follow the office policy manual and OSHA guidelines for hazardous medical wastes—including blood products, gloves, cotton swabs, body fluids, and sharps (needles or instruments that puncture the skin). These materials must be disposed of following standard guidelines and in a specially designed protective container.

You must keep recycling issues in mind at all times. Always choose products made from recycled materials—including paper (computer paper and letterhead), printer cartridges, pencils, and many other products.

---

recording vision, testing the functioning of eyes and eye muscles, and performing other duties. (Medical specialties and medical assistant specialties are fully discussed in Chapter 2.)

Personal Qualifications of Medical Assistants

There are several personal qualifications that you must have to be an effective and productive medical assistant. You must enjoy working with all types of people, possess good critical thinking skills, and be able to pay attention to detail. Empathy, willingness to learn, flexibility, self-motivation, professionalism, integrity, and sound judgment are other important traits. Additionally, you must have a neat, professional appearance, possess good communication skills, and know how to remain calm in a crisis.

Critical Thinking Skills

You will develop critical thinking skills over time, as you apply knowledge about and experience with human nature, medicine, and office administration to new situations. Critical thinking skills include quickly evaluating circumstances, solving problems, and taking action.

Critical thinking skills are used every day. One example is prioritizing your work—deciding which are the most important tasks of the day and which are less important. On a day where everything seems to be "top priority," you must use your professional judgment, knowledge of office policies, and experience with physicians and coworkers to determine what should get done first, second, third, and so on.

You must use critical thinking skills to assess how to react to emergency situations. If you see a patient suddenly pass out in the physician's waiting room, you must quickly see that the patient receives first aid, notify a physician, and alert the patient's family.

Attention to Detail

The profession of medical assisting requires attention to detail. You must check every detail when administering drugs, processing bills and insurance forms, and completing patient charts.

The need for attention to detail is illustrated in the common request to call a patient's pharmacy to order a prescription. You must accurately relay information from the doctor's prescription to the pharmacist. You must ask the pharmacist to read back the information to ensure that he has heard it correctly. Then you must document, in the chart, what has been ordered and when.

Empathy

Empathy is the ability to "put yourself in someone else's shoes" and to identify with and understand another person's feelings. Patients who are ill, frustrated, or frightened appreciate empathic medical personnel.

Many patients require empathy during a medical crisis. For example, a patient with the flu may describe how coughing has prevented him from getting a full night's sleep. You may display empathy by saying, "I know how the flu can disrupt sleep. I just got over it last week myself. It's important to rest in bed, though, even if you can't always sleep."

Willingness to Learn

You must always display a willingness to learn. You will gain new skills more easily and become better acquainted with the administrative and clinical topics and issues related to the practice in which you work if you are willing to learn. Keep an open mind, listen carefully to the professionals with whom you work, observe procedures carefully, listen actively to others, and do your own homework to learn more about medical topics so you can apply new information to your daily activities. For example, if you work in a pediatric practice, you might take a continuing education class on child development at a local community college, at a YWCA, or in a workshop offered by a professional association such as the AAMA or AMT (Figure 1-4).

Flexibility

You will encounter new people and situations every day. An attitude of flexibility will allow you to adapt and to handle them with professionalism.

An example of the need for flexibility occurs when a physician's schedule changes to include evening and weekend hours. The staff may also be asked to change schedules. You must make it a priority to be flexible and to meet the employer's needs.

Self-Motivation

You must be self-motivated and willing to offer assistance with work that needs to be done, even if it is not your assigned job. For example, if you think of a more efficient way to organize patient check-in, discuss it with your supervisor. She may agree and be willing to give your idea a try. If a coworker is on vacation, offer to pitch in and work extra time to keep the office running smoothly.

Professionalism

You should exhibit courtesy, conscientiousness, and a generally businesslike manner at all times on the job. It is important to act professionally with coworkers, patients,

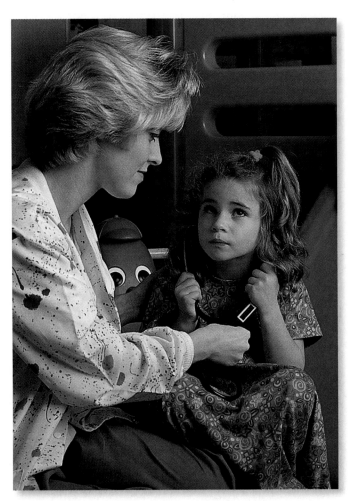

Figure 1-4. A medical assistant who works part-time in a pediatric practice might volunteer one day a week at a preschool to learn more about working with children.

doctors, and others in the work setting. You are an agent of your employer—you represent the doctor or doctors in the practice.

One example of professional behavior includes treating all patients with dignity and kindness. Another is making sure that you have completed and documented all your daily duties before leaving work at the end of each day.

You can start acting like a professional even while you are in the classroom studying to become a medical assistant. Presenting a neat appearance, showing courtesy and respect for peers and instructors, having a good attendance record, and arriving on time to class are all important elements that contribute to professionalism in school and in the workplace.

Neat Appearance

A medical professional always strives to maintain a neat appearance in the workplace. Personal cleanliness is an important part of maintaining a neat appearance. Your appearance is your first impression to your patients, coworkers, and the physicians you work with. Medical facilities and staff are considered "conservative" work environments. Your appearance should reflect a conservative style. Listed here are a few professional guidelines to follow in the medical environment:

- Your uniforms should be clean, pressed crisply, and in good repair. Your uniform should fit your body type and should not be ill-fitting.
- Your shoes should be comfortable, white, clean, and in good condition. Laces should be white and clean. Avoid athletic-looking shoes. Polish your shoes on a daily basis. Only leather shoes that are not open are permitted in a patient treatment area.
- Choose a hairstyle that is flattering and conservative. Hair should be clean and pulled back from your face and off your collar if long. Natural colors for hair are the only acceptable color in a medical environment.
- Your nails should be a short working length, no more than ¼ inch. Nail polish should be pale or clear. A French manicure is acceptable. Acrylic nails should be avoided. Many medical facilities are banning acrylic nails.
- Avoid heavy perfumes and colognes. Many patients and coworkers could be allergic to perfume and cologne.
- Jewelry should be kept to a minimum and in good taste. No more than one ring should be worn. Rings may tear through latex gloves. Ears can be pierced with one hole, and small earrings are appropriate. Any earrings that dangle can be torn off by a patient, such as pediatric patients. Males should not wear earrings in the medical environment.
- Tattoos should never be in a location where they can be seen by a patient.
- Body piercing and tongue piercing is not acceptable in a medical environment. Patients may view this as a visual threat and question your level of competence. Many physicians will rule you out on the first interview if a body piercing (other than ears) is present.
- Bath or shower daily and use an antiperspirant.
- Brush your teeth at least twice daily and schedule regular dental visits to maintain oral health and hygiene.
- Schedule regular checkups with your personal physician.
- Get plenty of rest and eat a well-balanced diet.
- If you are not required to wear a uniform, choose clothing that is conservative and business-appropriate. Avoid fad fashions. Wear low-heeled or flat, polished shoes and a lab coat if working with patients.

Some activities may make it difficult to maintain a neat appearance—replacing the toner in the copy machine, for example, or filling the developing solution in the x-ray machine. Always store a spare uniform or business outfit at your workplace.

Attitude

Your attitude will leave an impression of the type of person you are. In the medical environment, many people depend on you, including coworkers and patients. Your attitude can make or break your career. Professionals always project a positive, caring attitude. They respond to criticism as a learning experience. They take direction from authority without question. They function as a vital member of a medical team. A negative attitude will not be acceptable in a team-oriented medical environment. Many people do not know they have a negative attitude. Ask yourself these questions, and determine if you need to make improvements on your attitude before you begin your new career.

- Do I have repeated conflict with friends or family?
- Have I had a conflict at work that has resulted in voluntary or involuntary termination?
- Do I have conflict with authority figures, such as my instructors?
- Do people make comments about my attitude?

In the workplace environment, professional medical assistants are pleasant, smiling, and conducting themselves in a businesslike and professional manner.

Integrity and Honesty

People with integrity hold themselves to high standards. Everything they do, every task they complete, is performed with a goal of excellence. Individuals with integrity take extreme pride in everything they do. The characteristics of integrity are honesty, dependability, and reliability. Integrity and honesty are key in providing superior customer service to your patients. You must follow through on everything you say you are going to do. For example, if you tell a patient that you are going to return their call regarding a medication, you must call the patient at the time you indicated. Professionals with integrity are honest with the staff and physicians they work with. If you make an error, be honest about it. In order to have integrity, you must be dependable and reliable. Your office staff and physician must be able to trust you and the decisions you make.

Diplomacy

Diplomacy is the ability to communicate with patients, coworkers, managers, and physicians in a manner that is not offensive and that both expresses and inspires cooperation. Communicating with diplomacy is communicating with tact. Medical assistants are often exposed to situations that they may not agree with. A professional has the ability to look at both sides of a situation and to deal with it with courtesy and professionalism.

Proper Judgment

You should demonstrate proper judgment in every task. Before making an important decision, you must carefully evaluate each possible outcome.

An example of a situation that requires proper judgment is assessing when an exception should be made in a doctor's schedule of patients. Suppose the next patient on the schedule is in the waiting room. She is having a routine checkup. An unscheduled patient comes in with chest pains. You use proper judgment and allow the patient with chest pains to see the doctor first.

Communication Skills

Effective communication involves careful listening, observing, speaking, and writing. Communication even involves good manners—being polite, tactful, and respectful. You must use good communication skills during every patient discussion and in every interaction you have with physicians, other staff members, and other professionals with whom your practice does business. (Communication skills are discussed in Chapter 4.)

Remaining Calm in a Crisis

There is always the potential for a crisis or emergency in the health-care field. During a crisis you must remain calm and be prepared to handle any situation.

An example of the need for calm and effective action occurs when a patient appears to suffer a stroke while sitting in the waiting room of a busy medical office. You must quickly direct your peers to alert the doctor and remove the other patients from the room while you begin emergency first-aid measures.

On the Job
Rights of the Medical Assistant

You have the right to be free from any kind of discrimination in the workplace and during the hiring process. These rights are set forth under Title VII of the 1964 Civil Rights Act.

Title VII. The main prohibitions of the civil rights statute are as follows:

> It shall be unlawful employment practice for an employer to fail or refuse to hire or to discharge any individual, or otherwise to discriminate against any individual with respect to his or her compensation, terms, conditions, or privileges of employment, because of such individual's race, color, religion, sex, or national origin, or to limit, segregate, or classify employees or applicants for employment in any way which would deprive or tend to deprive any individual of employment opportunities or

otherwise adversely affect his or her status as an employee, because of such individual's race, color, religion, sex, or national origin. (Lindgren and Taub, 1993)

This law also protects workers from receiving lower pay than the opposite sex for the same work and from denial of a promotion opportunity because of gender.

Sexual Harassment. Title VII also addresses and defines sexual harassment:

> Unwelcome sexual advances, requests for sexual favors, and other verbal or physical conduct of a sexual nature . . . when submission to such conduct is made either explicitly or implicitly a term or condition of an individual's employment, submission to or rejection of such conduct by an individual is used as the basis for employment decisions affecting such individual, or such conduct has the purpose or effect of unreasonably interfering with an individual's work performance or creating an intimidating, hostile, or offensive working environment. (Lindgren and Taub, 1993)

Sexual harassment occurs in a variety of circumstances, and anyone may be sexually harassed. A man or a woman may be the victim or the harasser, and the victim does not have to be of the opposite sex. The victim may be the person being directly harassed or even a coworker who overhears the harassment. The victim has the responsibility to let the harasser know that the conduct is offensive. The victim should also report any instance of sexual harassment to a supervisor or personnel department.

The AAMA Role Delineation Study

In 1996 the AAMA formed a committee whose goal was to revise and update its standards for the accreditation of programs that teach medical assisting. The committee's findings were published in 1997 as the "AAMA Role Delineation Study: Occupational Analysis of the Medical Assisting Profession." The study included a new Role Delineation Chart that outlines the areas of competence you must master as an entry-level medical assistant. The Role Delineation Chart was further updated in 2003.

Areas of Competence

The Medical Assistant Role Delineation Chart, shown in Appendix I, provides the basis for medical assisting education and evaluation. Mastery of the areas of competence listed in this chart is required for all students in accredited medical assisting programs. The chart shows three general areas of competence: administrative, clinical, and general, or trandisciplinary. Each of these three areas is divided into two or more narrower areas, for a total of ten specific areas of competence. Within each area, a bulleted list of statements describes the medical assistant's role.

Uses of the Role Delineation Chart

According to the AAMA, the Role Delineation Chart may be used to:

- Describe the field of medical assisting to other health-care professionals
- Identify entry-level areas of competence for medical assistants
- Help practitioners assess their own current competence in the field
- Aid in the development of continuing education programs
- Prepare appropriate types of materials for home study

Summary

There are many kinds of on-the-job training, training programs, and careers for medical assistants. As you make the decision to become a medical assistant, you must evaluate your skills and the type of position you would like to obtain. An important goal will be to obtain a real-life view of the medical assistant's daily administrative, clinical, and laboratory duties. These skills and duties are outlined under the areas of competence listed in the AAMA Role Delineation Chart.

You must also research how to obtain on-the-job training or choose a training program that will adequately teach you those skills, how to conduct a job search, and whether or not to become a certified or registered medical assistant, and take advantage of the benefits of membership in medical assisting organizations such as the AAMA.

Additionally, you must be aware that the medical assisting profession will continue to change. You will need to stay abreast of changes in technology, procedures, and local, state, and federal regulations governing the way you perform daily duties.

REVIEW

CHAPTER 1

CASE STUDY QUESTIONS

Now that you have completed this chapter, review the case study at the beginning of the chapter and answer the following questions:

1. How are the two jobs different?
2. How are the two jobs the same?
3. How do these two medical assistants function as multiskilled health-care professionals?

Discussion Questions

1. Why are more employers recruiting credentialed medical assistants?
2. Name two of the most important personal qualities required of a medical assistant and explain why each is important for success.
3. What is the purpose of the AAMA Role Delineation Chart?
4. Discuss ways to gain real-world work experience in the field of medical assisting.

Critical Thinking Questions

1. Describe an effective medical assistant, and explain two ways a new medical assistant may learn to be an efficient and effective employee.
2. How will the "aging boom" affect health care and the profession of medical assisting in the future?
3. What is a self-directed, lifelong learner? How can a medical assistant achieve this goal?
4. Why is it important to stay current on changes in technology and health care?

Application Activities

1. With a partner, pick one of the following two situations. Without showing your partner, write a description of how you would display the personal attribute stated at the end of the scenario. After you and your partner have written your descriptions, compare them with each other.

   Patient Situation

   Patient says: "I have such a horrible headache. I've been feeling tired lately too."

   Attribute You Wish to Display

   Empathy

   Patient Situation

   Doctor: "I'm really backed up on paperwork. Could you come in an hour early tomorrow morning to help me organize it? You will be paid for the overtime."

   Attribute You Wish to Display

   Flexibility

2. List several challenging but realistic short-term and long-term goals for a medical assistant.
3. A. Think of all the personal qualifications you possess. List those that will help you as a medical assistant.
   B. List all of the personal qualifications you need to develop or improve in order to work successfully in the career of medical assisting.
   C. Describe the actions you will take to acquire the personal qualifications to become a multiskilled medical assistant.

Types of Medical Practice

AREAS OF COMPETENCE

2003 Role Delineation Study

GENERAL

Professionalism

- Work as a member of the health-care team
- Promote the CMA credential
- Enhance skills through continuing education

Legal Concepts

- Perform within legal and ethical boundaries
- Recognize professional credentialing criteria

CHAPTER OUTLINE

- Medical Specialties
- Working With Other Allied Health Professionals
- Specialty Career Options
- Professional Associations

OBJECTIVES

After completing Chapter 2, you will be able to:

2.1 Describe medical specialties and specialists.
2.2 Explain the purpose of the American Board of Medical Specialties.
2.3 Describe the duties of several types of allied health professionals with whom medical assistants may work.
2.4 Name professional associations that may help advance a medical assistant's career.

KEY TERMS

- acupuncturist
- allergist
- anesthetist
- cardiologist
- chiropractor
- dermatologist
- doctor of osteopathy
- endocrinologist
- family practitioner
- gastroenterologist
- gerontologist
- gynecologist
- internist
- massage therapist
- nephrologist
- neurologist
- oncologist
- orthopedist
- osteopathic manipulative medicine (OMM)
- otorhinolaryngologist
- pathologist
- pediatrician
- physiatrist
- physician assistant (PA)
- plastic surgeon
- primary care physician
- radiologist
- surgeon
- triage
- urologist

Introduction

Medical assistants are an integral part of a health-care delivery team. It is important to recognize the many different physician specialists and allied health professions. Medical assistants are often asked to call and process insurance referrals to different specialties and diagnostic departments. Therefore, a working knowledge of the different specialties and allied health professionals demonstrates professionalism and competence.

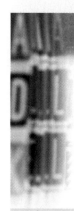

Susan has worked as a medical assistant for 12 years. She is considering furthering her educational background in a different allied health profession. She has a strong interest in nursing and in the laboratory.

As you read this chapter, consider the following questions:

1. What are Susan's career options in nursing? How much further education would she need in order to become a nurse?
2. What are Susan's career options in a laboratory setting? How much further education would she need in order to work in a laboratory?

Medical Specialties

Since the beginning of the twentieth century, some physicians have specialized in particular areas of study. There are now approximately 22 major medical specialties. Within each specialty are several subspecialties. For example, cardiology is a major specialty; pediatric cardiology is a subspecialty. As advances in the diagnosis and treatment of diseases and disorders unfold, the demand for specialized care increases and more medical specialties emerge.

If you graduate from an accredited medical assisting program, you will be well equipped to work with a physician specialist. If you work in the office of a physician specialist, you must continue to learn all the new skills that apply to that specialty. First, however, it is helpful to understand the education and licensing process any medical doctor must undergo to become a board-certified physician.

Physician Education and Licensure

The educational requirements for physicians are rigorous and take several years to complete. To earn the title MD (doctor of medicine), thereby qualifying as a licensed physician, a student must complete a bachelor's degree with a concentration typically in the sciences. Then she must attend a medical school accredited by the Liaison Committee on Medical Education (LCME). Upon completing medical school, she is awarded the degree of MD, but this is not the end of her medical training. She must also pass the U.S. Medical Licensing Examination (USMLE). This examination, commonly known as medical boards, has three parts. Part 1 is usually taken after the second year of medical school, part 2 during the fourth year of medical school, and part 3 during the first or second year of postgraduate medical training.

After medical school an MD begins a residency—a period of practical training in a hospital. The first year of residency is known as an internship. Once it is completed an MD can become certified by the National Board of Medical Examiners (NBME). After completing her internship and passing her medical boards, the MD becomes certified as an NBME Diplomate. If she wishes to specialize in a particular branch of medicine, she must complete an additional 2 to 6 years of residency. She also will apply to the American Board of Medical Specialties (ABMS) to take an examination in her specialty area. After passing the examination, she will be board-certified in her area of specialization. For example, a physician who specializes in pediatrics would receive certification from the American Board of Pediatrics.

The ABMS is an organization of many different medical specialty boards. Its primary purpose is to maintain and improve the quality of medical care and to certify doctors in various specialties. This organization helps the member boards develop professional and educational standards for physician specialists.

Family Practice

Family practitioners (sometimes called general practitioners) are MDs who are generalists and treat all types and ages of patients. They do not specialize in a particular branch of medicine. Many patients seek medical care from a family practitioner and may never have visited a medical specialist. Family practitioners are called **primary care physicians** by insurance companies. The term refers to individual doctors who oversee patients' long-term health care. Some people, however, have internists as their primary care physicians.

A family practitioner sends a patient to a specialist when she has a specific condition or disease that requires advanced care. For example, a family practitioner refers a patient with a lump in her breast to an **oncologist,** a specialist who treats tumors, or to a general surgeon. Either of these doctors may order a mammogram or perform a needle biopsy of the lump to determine if it is malignant.

If you work in a general practice, you will encounter patients with many different conditions and illnesses. As in any medical setting, you must become knowledgeable about preventing the transmission of viruses. This important topic is discussed in several parts of this book.

If you work for a general practitioner, you will often be responsible for arranging patient appointments with specialists. It is important, therefore, for you to know about the duties of each medical specialist. One or more of these specialties may interest you, and you may decide to seek a position as a medical assistant for a physician in that specialty.

Allergy

Allergists diagnose and treat physical reactions to substances, including mold, dust, fur, and pollen from plants or flowers. An individual with allergies is hypersensitive to substances like drugs, chemicals, or elements in nature. An allergic reaction may be minor, such as a rash; serious, such as asthma; or life-threatening, such as swelling of the airways or nasal passages.

Anesthesiology

Anesthetists use medications that cause patients to lose sensation or feeling during surgery. These health-care practitioners administer anesthetics before and during surgery. They also educate patients regarding the anesthetic that will be used and its possible postoperative effects. An anesthesiologist is an MD. A certified registered nurse anesthetist (CRNA) is a registered nurse who has completed an additional program of study recognized by the American Association of Nurse Anesthetists.

Cardiology

Cardiologists diagnose and treat cardiovascular diseases (diseases of the heart and blood vessels). Cardiologists also read electrocardiograms (ECGs) for hospital laboratories. They educate patients about the positive role healthy diet and regular exercise play in preventing and controlling heart disease.

Dermatology

Dermatologists diagnose and treat diseases of the skin, hair, and nails. Their patients have conditions ranging from warts and acne to skin cancer. Dermatologists treat boils, skin injuries, and infections. They remove growths—such as moles, cysts, and birthmarks—and they treat scars and perform hair transplants.

Doctor of Osteopathy

Doctors of osteopathy, who hold the title of DO, practice a "whole-person" approach to health care. DOs feel that patients are more than just a sum of their body parts, and they treat the patient as a whole person instead of concentrating on specific symptoms. Osteopathic physicians understand how all the body's systems are interconnected and how each one affects the other. They focus special attention on the musculoskeletal system, which reflects and influences the condition of all other body systems.

One key concept that DOs believe is that structure influences function. If a problem exists in one part of the body, it may affect the function in both that area and other areas. DOs focus on the body's ability to heal itself, and they actively engage patients in the healing process. By using **osteopathic manipulative medicine (OMM)** techniques, DOs can help restore motion to these areas of the body, thus improving function and often restoring health.

Emergency Medicine

Physicians who specialize in emergency medicine work in hospital emergency rooms. They diagnose and treat patients with conditions resulting from an unexpected medical crisis or accident. Common emergencies include trauma, such as gunshot wounds or serious injuries from car accidents; other injuries, such as severe cuts; and sudden illness, such as alcohol or food poisoning.

Endocrinology

Endocrinologists diagnose and treat disorders of the endocrine system. This system regulates many body functions by circulating hormones that are secreted by glands throughout the body. An example of a disorder treated by an endocrinologist is hyperthyroidism, an abnormality of the thyroid gland. Symptoms include weight loss, shakiness, and weakness.

Gastroenterology

Gastroenterologists diagnose and treat disorders of the gastrointestinal tract. These disorders include problems related to the functioning of the stomach, intestines, and associated organs.

Gerontology

Gerontologists study the aging process. Geriatrics is the branch of medicine that deals with the diagnosis and treatment of problems and diseases of the older adult. A specialist in geriatrics may also be called a geriatrician. As the population of older adults continues to increase, there will be greater need for physicians who specialize in diagnosing and treating diseases of the elderly.

Gynecology

Gynecology is the branch of medicine that is concerned with diseases of the female genital tract. **Gynecologists** perform routine physical care and examination of the female reproductive system. Many gynecologists are also obstetricians.

Internal Medicine

Internists specialize in diagnosing and treating problems related to the internal organs. The internal medicine subspecialties include cardiology, critical care medicine, diagnostic laboratory immunology, endocrinology and metabolism, gastroenterology, geriatrics, hematology, infectious diseases, medical oncology, nephrology, pulmonary disease, and rheumatology. Internists must be certified as specialists in these areas.

Nephrology

Nephrologists study, diagnose, and manage diseases of the kidney. They may work in either a clinic or hospital setting. A medical assistant working with a nephrologist may assist in the operation of a dialysis unit for the treatment of patients with kidney disease. In a rural setting a medical assistant might help a doctor operate a mobile dialysis unit that can be taken to the patient's home or to a medical practice that does not have this technology.

Neurology

Neurology is the branch of medical science that deals with the nervous system. **Neurologists** diagnose and treat disorders and diseases of the nervous system, such as strokes. The nervous system is made up of the brain, spinal cord, and nerves that receive, interpret, and transmit messages throughout the body.

Nuclear Medicine

Nuclear medicine is a fast-growing specialty related to radiology. Both fields use radiation to diagnose and treat disease, but radiology beams radiation through the body from an outside source, whereas nuclear medicine introduces a small amount of a radioactive substance into the body and forms an image by detecting radiation as it leaves the body. The radiation that patients are exposed to is comparable to that of a diagnostic x-ray. Radiology reveals interior anatomy whereas nuclear medicine reveals organ function and structure. Noninvasive, painless nuclear medicine procedures are used to identify heart disease, assess organ function, and diagnose and treat cancer.

Obstetrics

Obstetrics involves the study of pregnancy, labor, delivery, and the period following labor called postpartum (Figure 2-1). This field is often combined with gynecology. A

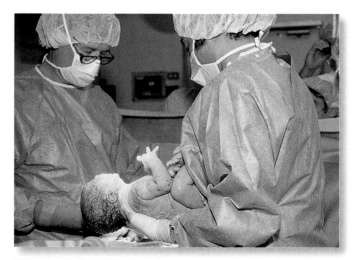

Figure 2-1. Obstetricians who are part of a private practice are usually connected with a specific hospital where they help their patients through labor and delivery.

physician who practices both specialties is referred to as an obstetrician/gynecologist, or OB/GYN.

Oncology

Oncologists, as stated earlier in the chapter, identify tumors, determine if they are benign or malignant, and treat patients with cancer. Treatment may involve chemotherapy, which is the administration of drugs to destroy cancer cells. Treatment may also involve radiation therapy, which kills cancer cells through the use of x-rays. Oncologists treat both adults and children.

Ophthalmology

An ophthalmologist diagnoses and treats diseases and disorders of the eye. This physician specialist examines patients' eyes for poor vision or disease. Other responsibilities include prescribing corrective lenses or medication, performing surgery, and providing follow-up care after surgery. (Ophthalmologists are sometimes confused with optometrists, but the latter are not MDs. Optometrists, however, perform eye exams to determine the general health of the eye and to prescribe corrective eyeglasses or contact lenses.)

Orthopedics

Orthopedics is a branch of surgery that works to maintain function of the musculoskeletal system and its associated structures. An **orthopedist** diagnoses and treats diseases and disorders of the muscles and bones. Some orthopedists concentrate on treating sports-related injuries, either exclusively for professional athletes or for nonprofessionals of all ages. They are called sports medicine specialists.

Otorhinolaryngology

Otorhinolaryngology involves the study of the ear, nose, and throat. An **otorhinolaryngologist** diagnoses and treats diseases of these body structures. This physician specialist is also referred to as an ear, nose, and throat (ENT) specialist.

Pathology

Pathology is the study of disease. It provides the scientific foundation for all medical practice. The **pathologist** studies the changes a disease produces in the cells, fluids, and processes of the entire body (sometimes by performing autopsies, examinations of the bodies of the deceased) to advance the clinical practice of medicine.

There are two basic types of pathologists. Governments and police departments use forensic pathologists to determine facts about unexplained or violent deaths. Anatomic pathologists often work at hospitals in a research capacity, and they may read biopsies (samplings of cells that could be malignant).

Pediatrics

Pediatrics is concerned with the development and care of children and the diseases of childhood. A **pediatrician** diagnoses and treats childhood diseases and teaches parents skills to keep their children healthy.

Physical Medicine

Physical medicine specialists **(physiatrists)** diagnose and treat diseases and disorders with physical therapy. Physical medicine specialists' patients include both adults and children.

Plastic Surgery

A **plastic surgeon** performs the reconstruction, correction, or improvement of body structures. Patients may be accident victims or disfigured due to disease or abnormal development. Plastic surgery involves facial reconstruction, face-lifts, and skin grafting. Plastic surgery is also used to repair problems like cleft lip and cleft palate.

Radiology

Radiology is the branch of medical science that uses x-rays and radioactive substances to diagnose and treat disease. **Radiologists** specialize in taking and reading x-rays.

Surgery

Surgeons use their hands and medical instruments to diagnose and correct deformities and treat external and

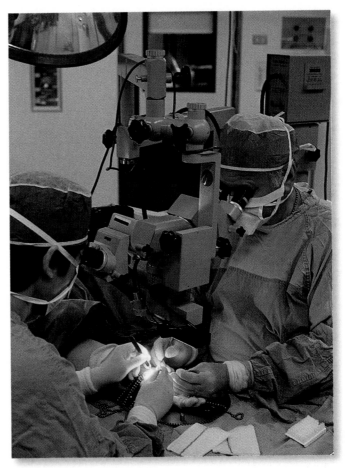

Figure 2-2. Most surgeons specialize in a particular type of surgery, such as heart surgery or hand surgery.

internal injuries or disease (Figure 2-2). They work with many different specialists to surgically treat a broad range of disorders. General surgeons may, for example, perform operations as diverse as breast lumpectomy and repair of a pacemaker. There are also subspecialties of surgery, such as neurosurgery, vascular surgery, and orthopedic surgery.

Urology

A **urologist** diagnoses and treats diseases of the kidney, bladder, and urinary system. A urologist's patients include infants, children, and adults of all ages.

Working With Other Allied Health Professionals

You will always work as a member of a health-care team. That health-care team will include doctors, nurses, specialists, and the patients themselves. You must know the duties of the other allied health professionals in your workplace. Even if you do not work with other allied health professionals in the office, you may contact them through correspondence or by telephone. Understanding the duties of other health-care team members will help make you a more effective medical assistant.

Acupuncturist

Acupuncturists treat people with pain or discomfort by inserting thin, hollow needles under the skin. The points used for insertion are selected to balance the flow of *qi,* or life energy, in the body. The theory of acupuncture relates to Chinese beliefs about how the body works. Qi is composed of two opposite forces called yin and yang. If the flow of qi is unbalanced, insufficient, or interrupted, then emotional, spiritual, mental, and physical problems will result. The acupuncturist works to balance these two forces in perfect harmony. Although there are variations in types of acupuncture—Chinese, Korean, and Japanese—all practitioners will focus on many pulse points along different meridians, the channels through which qi flows.

Chiropractor

Chiropractors treat people who are ill or in pain without using drugs or surgery. They primarily use manual treatments, although they may also employ physical therapy treatments, exercise programs, nutritional advice, and lifestyle modification to help correct the problem causing the pain. The manual treatments, called adjustments, realign the vertebrae in the spine and restore the function of spinal nerves. Chiropractors use diagnostic testing such as x-rays, muscle testing, and posture analysis to determine the location of spinal misalignments, also called *subluxations.* They then develop a treatment plan based on these findings. The treatment plan generally requires several adjustments per week for several weeks or months. Because the treatment does not involve drugs or surgery, the body needs time for healing and correction to occur.

Electroencephalographic Technologist

Electroencephalography (EEG) is the study and recording of the electrical activity of the brain. It is used to diagnose diseases and irregularities of the brain. The EEG technologist (sometimes called a technician) attaches electrodes to the patient's scalp and connects them to a recording instrument. The machine then provides a written record of the electrical activity of the patient's brain. EEG technologists work in hospital EEG laboratories, clinics, and physicians' offices.

Electrocardiograph Technician

The electrocardiograph (ECG) technician is a trained professional who operates an electrocardiograph machine, as pictured in Figure 2-3. An ECG records the electrical

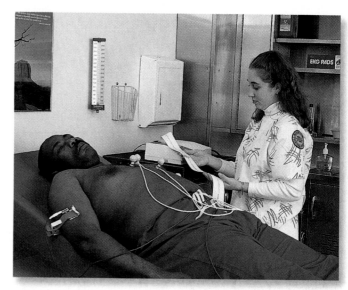

Figure 2-3. The electrocardiograph (ECG) technician is responsible for operating an electrocardiograph machine, which detects heart abnormalities and monitors patients with cardiac problems.

impulses reaching the heart muscles. Physicians and cardiologists use the readings from this machine to detect heart abnormalities and to monitor patients with known cardiac problems. Electrocardiograph technicians work in hospitals.

Massage Therapist

Massage therapists use pressure, kneading, stroking, vibration, and tapping to promote muscle and full-body relaxation as well as to increase circulation and lymph flow. Increasing circulation helps remove blood and waste products from injured tissues and brings fresh blood and nutrients to the areas to speed healing. Massage is one of the oldest methods of promoting healing and is used to treat strains, bruises, muscle soreness or tightness, lower-back pain, and dislocations. It can also relieve muscle spasm, restore motion and function to a body part, and decrease edema.

Medical Records Technologist

There are two types of medical records technologists: the Registered Records Administrator (RRA) and the Accredited Records Technician (ART). These technologists are responsible for organizing, analyzing, and evaluating medical records. Other responsibilities include compiling administrative and health statistics, coding symptoms, and inputting and retrieving computerized health data. These positions involve typing medical reports, preparing statistical reports on patient treatments, and supervising clerical personnel in the medical records department. Accredited records technicians and registered records

Medical Office Administrator

To gain medical assistant credentials, you must fulfill the requirements of either the American Association of Medical Assistants (for a Certified Medical Assistant) or the American Medical Technologists (for a Registered Medical Assistant). After obtaining your medical assistant certification, you may wish to acquire additional skills in specialty areas through course work or on-the-job training. Although this course work or training may not lead to an additional certification or degree, it will enable you to expand your role in the medical office and advance your career as the demand for skilled health professionals increases.

Skills and Duties

A medical office administrator manages the practice of a single physician (solo practice) or of a group practice. His duties are determined, in part, by the size of the practice. If the practice is large, he may have more managerial duties. If it is small, he may act as the receptionist, secretary, and records clerk. (Occasionally, in a solo practice, the practice nurse performs many or all of these functions.) Large group practices with 10 to 15 physicians may have one medical office administrator, while larger group practices with 40 to 50 physicians (such as managed care organizations) may have a highly trained practice administrator who oversees and coordinates the work of several assistant administrators.

The medical office administrator's reception duties begin with greeting and welcoming new patients. He may provide a medical history form for patients and answer any questions they may have. The administrator must have a knowledge of medical terminology in order to answer patients' questions.

This health-care professional coordinates the practice's records and filing. For example, he ensures that x-rays and test results are attached to the appropriate records and that insurance information is up to date. The medical office administrator may also schedule appointments for patients as well as referrals with other specialists. He may also keep track of the medical and nursing staff schedule. Sometimes the administrator is the person who calls patients ahead of time to confirm their appointments.

In a solo or small practice, the medical office administrator may perform general secretarial tasks, such as handling the mail and answering the telephone. He must have strong computer and word processing skills as well as shorthand, typing, and bookkeeping skills. In a large practice the administrator may train and oversee clerical staff and secretaries.

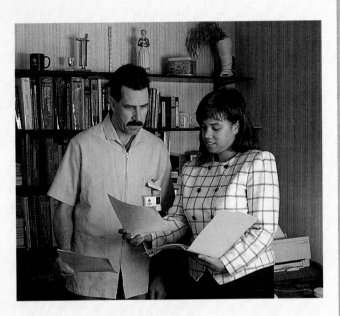

He may also interview and evaluate applicants for clerical jobs.

Workplace Settings

Medical office administrators may work in solo practices, group practices, or medical clinics. Specialized health-care facilities, such as nursing homes, may also employ medical office administrators.

Education

Although medical office administrators may learn the medical terminology they need on the job, they usually acquire their secretarial and clerical background through course work, either in a business/vocational school or in a junior or community college. The educational requirements for a medical office administrator vary with the size of the practice and the extent of the administrator's responsibilities. Upper-level positions require a graduate degree.

Where to Go for More Information

American Academy of Medical Administrators
30555 Southfield Road, Suite 150
Southfield, MI 48076
(313) 540-4310

Medical Group Management Association
104 Inverness Terrace East
Englewood Cliffs, CA 80112
(313) 799-1111

National Association of Medical Staff Services
P.O. Box 23590
Knoxville, TN 37933-1590
(615) 531-3571

administrators work in hospitals, nursing homes, health maintenance organizations, physicians' offices, and government agencies.

Medical Secretary

A medical secretary assists medical, professional, and technical personnel by performing secretarial and clerical support. These functions include taking dictation and typing as well as composing and preparing letters on a word processor. Other functions include maintaining medical and administrative files. A medical secretary may work in a hospital, nursing home, physician's office, or clinic.

Medical Technology

Medical technology is an umbrella term that refers to the development and design of clinical laboratory tests (such as diagnostic tests), procedures, and equipment. Two types of allied health professionals who work in medical technology are the medical technologist and the medical laboratory technician.

Medical Technologist. Medical technologists perform laboratory tests and procedures with clinical laboratory equipment. They examine specimens of human body tissues and fluids, analyze blood factors, and culture bacteria to identify disease-causing organisms. They also supervise and train technicians and laboratory aides. Medical technologists have 4-year degrees and may specialize in areas such as blood banking, microbiology, and chemistry. These technologists are employed in clinics, hospitals, private practices, colleges, pharmaceutical companies, government, research, and industry.

Medical Laboratory Technician. Medical laboratory technicians (MLTs) have 1- to 2-year degrees and are responsible for clinical tests performed under the supervision of a physician or medical technologist. They perform tests in the areas of hematology, serology, blood banking, urinalysis, microbiology, and clinical chemistry. Medical laboratory technicians work in hospital laboratories, commercial laboratories, medical clinics, and physicians' offices.

Medical Transcriptionist

Medical transcriptionists translate a physician's dictation about patient treatments into comprehensive, typed records. Attorneys, insurance companies, and medical specialists need accurate medical records. Medical transcriptionists work in doctors' offices, hospitals, clinics, laboratories, and radiology departments and for medical transcription services and insurance companies. Medical assistants often have medical transcription duties.

Mental Health Technician

A mental health technician, sometimes called a psychiatric aide or counselor, works in a variety of health-care settings with emotionally disturbed and mentally retarded patients. This health professional assists the psychiatric team by observing behavior and providing information to help in the planning of therapy. The mental health technician also participates in supervising group therapy and counseling sessions. This technician may work in a psychiatric clinic, specialized nursing home, psychiatric unit of a hospital, or community health center. Other places of employment include crisis centers and shelters. Training varies widely, from on-the-job training to advanced degrees, depending on job responsibilities and medical setting.

Nuclear Medicine Technologist

A nuclear medicine technologist performs tests to oversee quality control, to prepare and administer radioactive drugs, and to operate radiation detection instruments. This allied health professional is also responsible for correctly positioning the patient, performing imaging procedures, and preparing the information for use by a physician. A nuclear medicine technologist may work in a hospital, public health institution, or physician's office or—with appropriate clinical experience—in a teaching position at a college or university. There are 2- and 4-year training programs. The registration examination is administered by the American Registry of Radiologic Technologists.

Occupational Therapist

An occupational therapist works with patients who have physical injuries or illnesses, psychologic or developmental problems, or problems associated with the aging process. This health professional helps patients attain maximum physical and mental health by using educational, vocational, and rehabilitation therapies and activities. The occupational therapist may work in a hospital, clinic, extended care facility, rehabilitation hospital, or government or community agency. To become an occupational therapist, you need a 4-year degree, followed by a 9- to 12-month internship at an accredited hospital. Then you must pass the national board examination, in order to earn the title of OTR—registered occupational therapist.

Pharmacist

Pharmacists are professionals who have studied the science of drugs and who dispense medication and health supplies to the public. Pharmacists know the chemical and physical qualities of drugs and are knowledgeable about the companies that manufacture drugs.

Pharmacists inform the public about the effects of prescription and nonprescription (over-the-counter) medications. Pharmacists are employed in hospitals, clinics, and nursing homes. They may also work for government agencies, pharmaceutical companies, privately owned pharmacies, or chain store pharmacies. Some pharmacists own their own stores.

There are three levels of pharmacists, each with different training requirements. A pharmacy technician (CPhT) can typically receive on-the-job training. Formal training, although not required by most states, includes certificate programs and 2-year college programs offering associate degrees in science. Voluntary certification is by examination. A registered pharmacist (RPh) requires 5 years of college training with a bachelor's degree in science. Pharmacists must be registered by the state and must pass a state board examination. A doctor of pharmacy (PharmD) requires 6 to 7 years of college training, which may be followed by a residency in a hospital setting.

Phlebotomist

Phlebotomists are allied health professionals trained to draw blood for diagnostic laboratory testing. They work in medical clinics, laboratories, and hospitals. Although medical assistants are also trained to draw blood for standard types of tests, phlebotomists are trained at a more advanced level to be able to draw blood under difficult circumstances or in special situations. For example, if a blood sample is needed for a potassium-level test, it must be drawn in a particular manner that only phlebotomists are trained to do. In most states phlebotomists must be certified by the National Phlebotomy Association or registered by the American Society of Clinical Pathologists.

Physical Therapist

A physical therapist (PT) plans and uses physical therapy programs for medically referred patients. The PT helps these patients to restore function, relieve pain, and prevent disability following disease, injury, or loss of body parts. A physical therapist uses various treatment methods, which include therapy with electricity, heat, cold, ultrasound, massage, and exercise. The physical therapist also helps patients accept their disabilities. A physical therapist may work in a hospital, outpatient clinic, rehabilitation center, home-care agency, nursing home, voluntary health agency, private practice, or sports medicine center. A physical therapist must have a bachelor's degree in physical therapy and must pass a state board examination.

Physician Assistant

A **physician assistant (PA)** is a health-care provider who practices medicine under the supervision of a physician. Physician assistants are licensed by the state in which they practice. PAs are trained in medicine with a curriculum similar in content but shorter in duration than medical school. Most physician assistants are nationally certified and hold the title PA-C. National certification is maintained through cycles of examinations and continuing medical education.

The scope of the physician assistant's practice corresponds to the supervising physician's practice. Duties may include taking patient histories, performing physical examinations, ordering and interpreting laboratory tests, performing procedures, assisting in surgery, diagnosing medical conditions, and developing and carrying out treatment plans. Physician assistants can prescribe medication in most states. PAs work in a wide variety of health-care settings, including hospitals, clinics, private physician offices, schools, prisons, and governmental agencies. They also serve as faculty in physician assistant programs. Medical assistants may work with physician assistants, particularly in outpatient settings.

Radiographer

A radiographer (x-ray technician) is one of the most common positions for individuals whose education is in radiologic technology. The radiographer assists a radiologist in taking x-ray films. These films are used to diagnose broken bones, tumors, ulcers, and disease. A radiographer usually works in the radiology department of a hospital. The x-ray technician may, however, use mobile x-ray equipment in a patient's room or in the operating room. A radiographer may be employed in a hospital, laboratory, clinic, physician's office, government agency, or industry.

Registered Dietitian

Registered dietitians help patients and their families make healthful food choices that provide balanced, adequate nutrition (Figure 2-4). Dietitians are sometimes called nutritionists. Dietitians may assist food-service directors at health-care facilities and prepare and serve food to groups. They may also participate in food research and teach nutrition classes. Dietitians work in community health agencies, hospitals, clinics, private practices, and managed care settings. They may also teach at colleges and universities, and they serve as consultants to organizations and individuals.

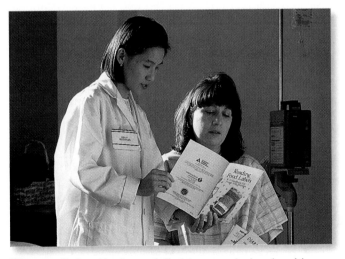

Figure 2-4. Registered dietitians work closely with patients who need to modify their food choices for better health.

Radiologic Technologist

A radiologic technologist is a health-care professional who has studied the theory and practice of the technical aspects of the use of x-rays and radioactive materials in the diagnosis and treatment of disease. A radiologic technologist may specialize in radiography, radiation therapy, or nuclear medicine. Radiologic technologists generally work in hospitals; some work in medical laboratories, medical practices, and clinics.

Respiratory Therapist

A respiratory therapist evaluates, treats, and cares for persons with respiratory problems. The respiratory therapist works under the supervision of a physician and performs therapeutic procedures based on observation of the patient. Using respiratory equipment, the therapist treats patients with asthma, emphysema, pneumonia, and bronchitis. The respiratory therapist plays an active role in newborn, pediatric, and adult intensive care units. The therapist may work in a hospital, nursing home, physician's office, or commercial company that provides emergency oxygen equipment and services to home-care patients.

Nursing Aide/Assistant

Nursing aides assist in the direct care of patients under the supervision of the nursing staff. Typical functions include making beds, bathing patients, taking vital signs, serving meals, and transporting patients to and from treatment areas. Nursing assistants are often employed in psychiatric and acute care hospitals, nursing homes, and home health agencies. On-the-job training can range from 1 week to 3 months.

Practical/Vocational Nurse

Licensed practical nurses (LPNs) and licensed vocational nurses (LVNs) provide nursing care to the sick. Both terms refer to the same type of nurse. Duties involve taking and recording patient temperatures, blood pressure, pulse, and respiration rates. They also include administering some medications under supervision, dressing wounds, and applying compresses. LPNs and LVNs are not allowed, however, to perform certain other duties, such as some intravenous (IV) procedures or the administration of certain medications.

Practical/vocational nurses assist registered nurses and physicians by observing patients and reporting changes in their conditions. LPNs/LVNs work in hospitals, nursing homes, clinics, and physicians' offices and in industrial medicine. To meet the needs of the growing aging population in this country, employment opportunities for LPNs and LVNs in long-term care settings have increased.

LPNs/LVNs must graduate from an accredited school of practical (vocational) nursing (usually a 1-year program).

They are also required to take a state board examination for licensure as LPNs/LVNs.

Associate Degree Nurse

Associate degrees in nursing (ADNs) are offered at many junior colleges and community colleges and at some universities. These programs combine liberal arts education and nursing education. The length of the ADN program is typically 2 years. ADNs are also considered RNs if they pass the state boards.

Diploma Graduate Nurse

Diploma programs are usually 3-year programs designed as cooperative programs between a community college and a participating hospital. The programs combine course work and clinical experience in the hospital.

Baccalaureate Nurse

A baccalaureate degree refers to a 4-year college or university program. Graduates of a 4-year nursing program are awarded a bachelor of science in nursing (BSN) degree. The curriculum includes courses in liberal arts, general education, and nursing courses. Graduates are prepared to function as nurse generalists and in positions that go beyond the role of hospital staff nurses. BSNs are also considered RNs if they pass the state boards.

Registered Nurse

A nurse who graduates from a nursing program and passes the state board examination for licensure is considered an RN, indicating formal, legal recognition by the state. The RN is a professional who is responsible for planning, giving, and supervising the bedside nursing care of patients. An RN may work in an administrative capacity, assist in daily operations, oversee programs in hospital or institutional settings, or plan community health services.

Registered nurses work in a variety of settings. These settings include hospitals, nursing homes, public health agencies, industry, physicians' offices, government agencies, and educational settings. Some RNs continue their education to earn master's or doctoral degrees.

Nurse Practitioner

A nurse practitioner (NP) is an RN who functions in an expanded nursing role. The NP usually works in an ambulatory patient care setting alongside physicians. An NP may work in an independent nurse practitioner practice with no physicians. An independent nurse practitioner takes health histories, performs physical examinations, conducts screening tests, and educates patients and families about disease prevention.

An NP who works in a physician's practice may perform some duties that a physician would, such as administering

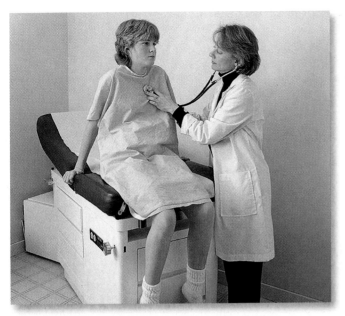

Figure 2-5. Many nurse practitioners work in physicians' offices and are trained to perform routine examinations.

physical examinations and treating common illnesses and injuries (Figure 2-5). For example, in an OB/GYN practice the NP can perform a standard annual gynecologic examination, including taking a Pap smear or a culture to test for yeast infection. The nurse practitioner emphasizes preventive health care.

The NP must be an RN with at least a master's degree in nursing and must complete 4 to 12 months of an apprenticeship or formal training. With specific formal training the student may become a pediatric nurse practitioner, an obstetric nurse practitioner (midwife), or a psychiatric nurse practitioner. The nurse practitioner works with medical assistants.

Specialty Career Options

The various medical specialties can open up many career possibilities for medical assistants. Deciding to specialize may become one of your career goals five or more years from now. Remember that you may need additional training or education for some of these positions. Your hard work will be rewarded, however, as you gain additional job responsibilities.

Choosing an area in which to specialize involves research and careful thought. Local and medical college libraries can supply a great deal of information about the areas in which you may specialize. State employment agencies or schools can help you make career choices.

It is also helpful to check the help-wanted section in local newspapers for information about jobs in specialized areas. Many newspapers separate health-care career opportunities into easy-to-find boxed sections. You may also directly contact companies you would like to work for. Ask about job opportunities, and find out what skills and training the employer requires.

Anesthetist's Assistant

Anesthetist's assistants provide anesthetic care under an anesthetist's direction. Hospitals and high-technology surgical centers frequently employ anesthetist's assistants. These assistants gather patient data and assist in evaluation of patients' physical and mental status. They also record planned surgical procedures, assist with patient monitoring, draw blood samples, perform blood gas analyses, and conduct pulmonary function tests.

Certified Laboratory Assistant

Certified laboratory assistants perform routine procedures in bacteriology, chemistry, hematology, parasitology, serology, and urinalysis. Laboratory assistants work under the supervision of a medical technologist or hospital anatomic pathologist. They work in laboratories at hospitals, clinics, and physicians' offices and in independent laboratories. One-year training programs are offered by hospitals, vocational schools, and community colleges.

Dental Assistant

A dental assistant can practice without formal education or training. In this case, on-the-job training is provided. A dental assistant performs many administrative and laboratory functions that are similar to the duties of a medical assistant. For example, a dental assistant may serve as chair-side assistant, provide instruction in oral hygiene, and prepare and sterilize instruments. To perform expanded clinical and chair-side functions such as those of a hygienist, a dental assistant must have at least 1 year of training in theory and clinical application. This formal education also requires work experience in a dental office.

Dental assistants often work in a private practice. They also work in clinics, dental schools, and local health agencies. Insurance companies hire dental assistants to process dental claims.

Emergency Medical Technician/Paramedic

An emergency medical technician (EMT), sometimes called a paramedic, works under the direction of a physician through a radio communication network. This health professional assesses and manages medical emergencies that occur away from hospitals or other medical settings, such as in private homes, schools, offices, or public areas. An EMT is trained to **triage** patients (to assess the urgency and type of condition presented as well as the immediate medical needs) and to initiate the appropriate treatment for a variety of medical emergencies. While transporting patients to the medical facility, an EMT records, documents, and radios the patient's condition to the physician, describing how the injury occurred. An EMT may work for an ambulance service, fire department, police department, hospital emergency department, private industry, or voluntary care service. Training requirements vary by state but typically require a high school diploma and driver's license, 100 hours of classroom training, and an average of 6 months of practical training on an ambulance squad or in a hospital emergency room.

Occupational Therapist Assistant

Occupational therapist assistants work under the supervision of an occupational therapist. They help individuals with mental or physical disabilities reach their highest level of functioning through the teaching of fine motor skills, trades (occupations), and the arts. Duties include preparing materials for activities, maintaining tools and equipment, and documenting the patient's progress. Occupational therapist assistants must earn a 2-year degree (OTA).

Ophthalmic Assistant

An ophthalmic assistant aids ophthalmologists with the routine functions of the practice. This health professional performs simple vision testing, takes medical histories, administers eyedrops, and changes dressings. There are three levels in this category of allied health professional (from most senior to least senior): ophthalmic technologist, ophthalmic technician, and ophthalmic assistant. Duties are determined by the supervising ophthalmologist. No states currently require certification for these positions.

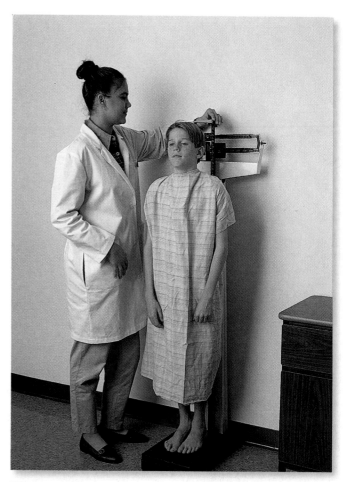

Figure 2-6. If you enjoy working with children, you might consider working as a pediatric medical assistant.

Pathologist's Assistant

Pathologist's assistants work under the supervision of a pathologist. Pathologist's assistants sometimes work with forensic pathologists—professionals who study the human body and diseases for legal purposes, in cooperation with government or police investigations. They may prepare frozen sections of dissected body tissue. Assistants working for anatomic pathologists (professionals who study the human body and diseases in a research capacity) may maintain supplies, instruments, and chemicals for the anatomic pathology laboratory. Pathologist's assistants perform laboratory work about 75% of the workday. Assistants also perform a variety of administrative duties. They work in community hospitals, university medical centers, and private laboratories.

Pediatric Medical Assistant

A pediatric medical assistant assists the pediatrician in administrative and clinical duties (Figure 2-6). These duties include obtaining medical histories and preparing patients for examination. Other duties include performing routine tests, sterilizing supplies and equipment, typing, filing, and clerical work. This health professional also educates patients and their parents or guardians about follow-up care and maintains patients' records. A pediatric medical assistant should be able to communicate well with children. Other helpful skills include patience and organizational skills. Pediatric medical assistants work with pediatricians in private practice, hospitals, and clinics.

Pharmacy Technician

Pharmacy technicians perform specific routine tasks related to record keeping and preparing and dispensing drugs. Duties include preparing medications for administration and making sure patients receive the correct medication. Pharmacy technicians usually work in hospitals or similar facilities under the supervision of a nurse, pharmacist, or other health-care professional. In a commercial pharmacy they work under the pharmacist's supervision. Opportunities are also available with pharmaceutical firms and wholesale pharmaceutical distributors.

Training can be on the job or through certificate programs and 2-year college programs (associate degree).

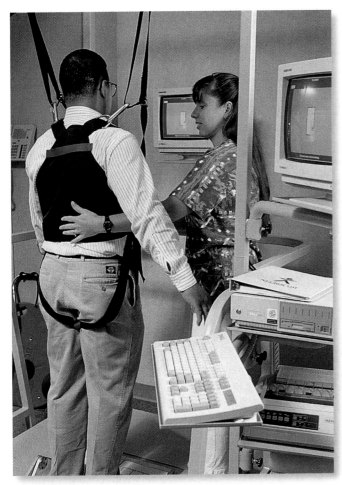

Figure 2-7. Physical therapy assistants provide guidance and support to patients who are recovering from a physical injury or from surgery on a limb or joint.

National certification is voluntary by examination and earns the title CPhT (certified pharmacy technician).

Physical Therapy Assistant

A physical therapy assistant (PTA) works under the direction of a physical therapist to assist with patient treatment. The assistant follows the patient care program created by the physical therapist and physician. This health professional performs tests and treatment procedures, assembles or sets up equipment for therapy sessions, and observes and documents patient behavior and progress (Figure 2-7). A physical therapy assistant may practice in a hospital, nursing home, rehabilitation center, or community or government agency.

Radiation Therapy Technologist

A radiation therapy technologist assists the radiologist. He may, for example, assist with administering radiation treatment to patients who have cancer. He may also be responsible for maintaining radiation treatment equipment. The technologist shares responsibility with the radiologist for the accuracy of treatment records. A radiation therapy technologist may work in a hospital, laboratory, clinic, physician's office, or government agency. Training requires a high school diploma and graduation from a 2- or 4-year program in radiography.

Respiratory Therapy Technician

Respiratory therapy technicians work under the supervision of a physician and a respiratory therapist. Respiratory therapists perform procedures such as artificial ventilation. They also clean, sterilize, and maintain the respiratory equipment and document the patient's therapy in the medical record. Respiratory therapy technicians work in hospitals, nursing homes, physicians' offices, and commercial companies that provide emergency oxygen equipment and therapeutic home care.

Speech/Language Pathologist

A speech/language pathologist treats communication disorders, such as stuttering, and associated disorders, such as hearing impairment. This health professional evaluates, diagnoses, and counsels patients who have these problems. A speech/language pathologist may work in a school, hospital, research setting, or private practice or may teach at a college or university.

Speech/language pathologists usually have a master's degree in speech/language pathology or audiology. Certification and licensing requirements vary by state, usually depending on the work setting (public school, private practice, clinic, and so on).

Surgeon's Assistant

A surgeon's assistant provides patient services under the direction, supervision, and responsibility of a licensed surgeon. This health professional's tasks include obtaining a patient's history and physical data. She then discusses the data with a physician or surgeon to determine what procedures to use to treat the problem. A surgeon's assistant may also assist in performing diagnostic and therapeutic procedures. She must be calm and have good judgment in the high-pressure environment of the operating room. Surgeon's assistants work primarily in hospitals.

Surgeon's assistants are considered a subcategory of physician assistant. Training programs are usually affiliated with 2- and 4-year colleges and with university schools of medicine and allied health. These programs include practical work in the surgery unit of an affiliated hospital.

Professional Associations

Membership in a professional association enables you to become involved in the issues and activities relevant to your field and presents opportunities for continuing education. It is a good idea to become informed about such associations, even those, such as the American Medical Association, that are open to physicians only. The physician you work for may ask you to obtain information about the group's activities and meetings. Table 2-1 summarizes professional associations related to the field of medicine and medical assisting.

American Association of Medical Assistants

The American Association of Medical Assistants (AAMA), as described in Chapter 1, was created to serve the interests

TABLE 2-1 Professional Medical Organizations		
Professional Organization	**Membership Requirements**	**Advantages of Membership**
American Association of Medical Assistants (AAMA)	Interested individuals and those who practice medical assisting may join the AAMA.	Offers flexible continuing education programs; publishes bimonthly *The Professional Medical Assistant;* offers legal counsel, professional recognition, various member discounts
American Association for Medical Transcription (AAMT)	Interested individuals and those who practice medical transcription may join the AAMT.	Educates and develops medical transcriptionists as medical language specialists; offers advice and support for self-employed medical transcriptionists
American College of Physicians (ACP)	Physicians and medical students may join.	Provides education and information resources to the field of internal medicine and its subspecialties
American Hospital Association (AHA)	Institutional health-care providers and other individuals may join.	Provides consultant referral service and access to health-care information resources
American Medical Association (AMA)	Physicians and medical students may join.	Provides large information source; publishes *Journal of the American Medical Association (JAMA);* offers AMA/Net
American Medical Technologists (AMT)	Medical assistants, medical technologists, medical laboratory technicians, dental assistants, and phlebotomy technicians may join.	Offers national certification as Registered Medical Assistant (RMA); offers certification to other health-care professionals, publications, state chapter activities, continuing education programs
American Pharmaceutical Association (APhA)	Pharmaceutical professionals and physicians may join.	Helps members improve skills; active in pharmacy policy development, networking, publishing, research, public education
American Society of Clinical Pathologists (ASCP)	Any professional involved in laboratory medicine or pathology may join.	Resource for improving the quality of pathology and laboratory medicine; offers educational programs and materials; certifies technologists and technicians
American Society of Phlebotomy Technicians (ASPT)	Interested individuals and those who practice phlebotomy may join.	Offers national certification as a phlebotomy technician and continuous education programs

of medical assistants and to further the medical assisting profession. The AAMA offers self-paced continuing education classes; workshops and seminars at the local, state, and national levels; and job networking opportunities. Other benefits include legal counsel, group health insurance, professional recognition, and member discounts.

American Association for Medical Transcription

The American Association for Medical Transcription (AAMT) is the professional organization for the advancement of medical transcription. The AAMT also educates medical transcriptionists as medical language specialists. The AAMT offers advice and support to the many medical transcriptionists who are self-employed.

American College of Physicians

Founded in 1915, the American College of Physicians (ACP) is the largest medical specialty organization in the world. It is the only society of internists dedicated to providing education and information resources to the entire field of internal medicine and its subspecialties.

American Hospital Association

The American Hospital Association (AHA) is the nation's largest network of institutional health-care providers. These providers represent every type of hospital: rural and city hospitals, specialty and acute care facilities, freestanding hospitals, academic medical centers, and health systems and networks. The AHA works to support and promote the interests of hospitals and health-care organizations across the country. Organizations as well as individual professionals may join the AHA. Membership benefits include use of the AHA consultant referral service, accessed, for example, by hospitals that need experts in areas not addressed by in-house personnel. Members also have access to AHA's health-care information resources, including teleconferencing and AHA database services.

American Medical Association

The American Medical Association (AMA) was founded in 1847. Its members include 300,000 physicians from every medical specialty. The AMA promotes science and the art of medicine and works to improve public health. The AMA is the world's largest publisher of scientific and medical information and publishes ten monthly medical specialty journals. The AMA also accredits medical programs in the United States and Canada.

The AMA provides an online service called AMA/Net for physicians and medical assistants, offering up-to-date information about current medical topics. To use the AMA/Net, the medical office must have a computer, telephone, and modem.

American Medical Technologists

American Medical Technologists (AMT) was established in 1939 as a not-for-profit organization. The AMT offers national certification as a Registered Medical Assistant (RMA) to medical assisting practitioners. It also offers certification to medical technologists, medical laboratory technicians, dental assistants, and phlebotomy technicians. Membership benefits include continuing education classes, workshops and seminars, and job networking opportunities.

American Pharmaceutical Association

The American Pharmaceutical Association (APhA), the national professional society of pharmacists, was founded in 1852. The APhA represents the interests of pharmaceutical professionals, and it strives to help individual members improve their skills. The APhA works to advance the field of pharmacy and the safety of patients. The APhA is active in pharmacy policy development, networking, publishing, research, and public education.

Summary

There are many medical settings in which you can serve as a medical assistant. Some settings will be in specialized branches of medicine. It is important to gain an understanding of the major areas of medicine, as well as the various subspecialties, in order to choose and plan for the type of setting in which you would like to work.

Learning about various allied health professionals—such as pharmacists, nurse practitioners, and medical transcriptionists—will help you interact with others on the job. Learning about specialty career options—such as physical therapy assistants, certified laboratory assistants, and ophthalmic assistants—can give you ideas about integrating new skills into your job as a multiskilled health professional.

Joining a professional organization will enable you to stay informed about issues and activities in the medical assisting field and the specialty or subspecialty in which you work. Professional organizations also provide other benefits to members, such as group health insurance; job networking opportunities; state or chapter meetings, seminars, workshops, and guest presentations; and member discounts. Membership in a professional organization helps you be recognized as a professional. Therefore, it is an important addition to your résumé.

REVIEW

CHAPTER 2

CASE STUDY *QUESTIONS*

Now that you have completed this chapter, review the case study at the beginning of the chapter and answer the following questions:

1. What are Susan's career options in nursing? How much further education would she need in order to become a nurse?
2. What are Susan's career options in a laboratory setting? How much further education would she need in order to work in a laboratory?

Discussion Questions

1. Why is geriatrics a growing medical specialty?
2. How might learning about specialty career options help motivate medical assistants in their careers?
3. How do professional organizations help medical assistants perform their job duties?

Critical Thinking Questions

1. How might a medical assistant's experience working with a medical specialist differ from her experience working with a general practitioner, in terms of learning about medicine?
2. If you worked for an obstetrician or OB/GYN, how might you use your spare time to learn more about the specialty and do your job better?
3. Why might a medical assistant be interested in joining a professional association such as the American Hospital Association?

Application Activities

1. Interview a medical assistant, such as a physical therapy assistant, who has chosen a specialty career option. What additional education or training did she need to obtain the position? What are her administrative and clinical duties? What does she like about her job? What does she find most challenging? How did she come to choose the specialty? Report your findings to the class.
2. Create a job-hunting plan for a medical assistant interested in learning about job opportunities in a specialty medical assisting career. Your plan should consist of at least four different ways for the medical assistant to look for jobs.
3. Pick three medical specialties, and identify the skills required for a medical assistant in each specialty.

Legal and Ethical Issues in Medical Practice, Including HIPAA

AREAS OF COMPETENCE

2003 Role Delineation Study

CLINICAL

Fundamental Principles

- Apply principles of aseptic technique and infection control
- Comply with quality assurance practices

Patient Care

- Coordinate patient care information with other health-care providers

GENERAL

Legal Concepts

- Perform within legal and ethical boundaries
- Prepare and maintain medical records
- Document accurately
- Follow employer's established policies dealing with the health-care contract
- Implement and maintain federal and state health-care legislation and regulations
- Comply with established risk management and safety procedures
- Recognize professional credentialing criteria

KEY TERMS

abandonment
agent
arbitration
assault
authorization
battery
bioethics
breach of contract
civil law
contract
crime
criminal law
defamation
disclosure
durable power of attorney
electronic transaction record
ethics
expressed contract
felony
fraud
implied contract
law
law of agency
liable
living will
malpractice claim
misdemeanor
moral values
negligence
Notice of Privacy Practices (NPP)
Privacy Rule
protected health information (PHI)
Security Rule
subpoena
tort
treatment, payments, and operations (TPO)
uniform donor card
use
void

CHAPTER OUTLINE

- Medical Law and Ethics
- OSHA Regulations
- Quality Control and Assurance
- Code of Ethics
- HIPAA
- Confidentiality Issues and Mandatory Disclosure

OBJECTIVES

After completing Chapter 3, you will be able to:

3.1 Define ethics, bioethics, and law.
3.2 Discuss the measures a medical practice must take to avoid malpractice claims.
3.3 Describe OSHA requirements for a medical office.

3.4 Describe procedures for handling an incident of exposure to hazardous materials.

3.5 Compare and contrast quality control and quality assurance procedures.

3.6 Explain how to protect patient confidentiality.

3.7 Discuss the impact that HIPAA regulations have in the medical office.

Introduction

Medical law plays an important role in medical facility procedures and the way we care for patients. We live in a litigious society, where patients, relatives, and others are inclined to sue health-care practitioners, health-care facilities, manufacturers of medical equipment and products, and others when medical outcomes are not acceptable. It is important for a medical professional to understand medical law, ethics, and protected health information as it pertains to HIPAA. There are two main reasons for medical professionals to study law and ethics: The first is to help you function at the highest professional level by providing competent, compassionate health care to patients, and the second is to help you avoid legal problems that can threaten your ability to earn a living.

A knowledge of medical law and ethics can help you gain perspective in the following three areas:

1. *The rights, responsibilities, and concerns of health-care consumers.* Not only do health-care professionals need to be concerned about how law and ethics impact their respective professions, they must also understand how legal and ethical issues affect patients. As medical technology advances and the use of computers increases, patients want to know more about their options and rights as well as more about the responsibilities of health-care practitioners. Patients want to know who and how their information is used and the options they have regarding health-care treatments. Patients have come to expect favorable outcomes from medical treatment, and when these expectations are not met, lawsuits may result.

2. *The legal and ethical issues facing society, patients, and health-care professionals as the world changes.* Every day new technologies emerge with solutions to biological and medical issues. These solutions often involve social issues, and we are faced with decisions, for example, regarding reproductive rights, fetal stem cell research, and confidentiality with sensitive medical records.

3. *The impact of rising costs on the laws and ethics of health-care delivery.* Rising costs, both of health-care insurance and of medical treatment in general, can lead to questions concerning access to health-care services and the allocation of medical treatment. For example, should everyone, regardless of age or lifestyle, have the same access to scarce medical commodities such as transplant organs or highly expensive drugs?

In today's society, medical treatment and decisions surrounding health care have become complex. It is therefore important to be knowledgeable and aware of the issues and the laws that govern patient care.

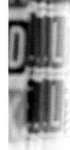

CASE STUDY

A medical assistant is very busy on a Monday morning. She has drawn blood on a patient that she has known for years and has been very comfortable chatting with this patient. The patient is checking out at the front desk in the reception area, and she notices that he forgot his prescription for Dilantin, a medication for seizure control. She rushes up to the front area and, as he is opening the door, says to him, "Mr. Doe, you forgot your prescription for Dilantin."

As you read this chapter, consider the following questions:

1. Does the medical assistant's comment represent a breach of confidentiality?
2. Has any HIPAA rule been violated? If so, which one?

Medical Law and Ethics

In order to understand medical law and ethics, it is helpful to understand the differences between laws and ethics. A **law** is defined as a rule of conduct or action prescribed or formally recognized as binding or enforced by a controlling authority. Governments enact laws to keep society running smoothly and to control behavior that could threaten public safety. **Ethics** is considered a standard of behavior and a concept of right and wrong beyond what the legal consideration is in any given situation. **Moral values** serve as a basis for ethical conduct. Moral values are formed through the influence of the family, culture, and society.

Classifications of Law

There are two types of law that pertain to health-care practitioners: criminal law and civil law.

Criminal Law. A **crime** is an offense against the state committed or omitted in violation of a public law. **Criminal law** involves crimes against the state. When a state or federal criminal law is violated, the government brings criminal charges against the alleged offender, for example, *Ohio v. John Doe*. State criminal laws prohibit such crimes as murder, arson, rape, and burglary. A criminal act may be classified as a felony or misdemeanor. A **felony** is a crime punishable by death or by imprisonment in a state or federal prison for more than one year. Some examples of a felony include abuse (child, elder, or domestic violence), manslaughter, fraud, attempted murder, and practicing medicine without a license.

Misdemeanors are less serious crimes than felonies. They are punishable by fines or by imprisonment in a facility other than a prison for one year or less. Some examples of misdemeanors are thefts under a certain dollar amount, attempted burglary, and disturbing the peace.

Civil Law. **Civil law** involves crimes against the person. Under civil law, a person can sue another person, a business, or the government. Court judgments in civil cases often require the payment of a sum of money to the injured party. Civil law includes a general category of law known as torts. A **tort** is broadly defined as a civil wrong committed against a person or property that causes physical injury or damage to someone's property or that deprives someone of his or her personal liberty and freedom. Torts may be intentional (willful) or unintentional (accidental).

Intentional Torts. When one person intentionally harms another, the law allows the injured party to seek a remedy in a civil suit. The injured party can be financially compensated for any harm done by the person guilty of committing the tort. If the conduct is judged to be malicious, punitive damages may also be awarded. Examples of intentional torts include the following:

- Assault. **Assault** is the open threat of bodily harm to another, or acting in such as way as to put another in the "reasonable apprehension of bodily harm."
- Battery. **Battery** is an action that causes bodily harm to another. It is broadly defined as any bodily contact made without permission. In health-care delivery, battery may be charged for any unauthorized touching of a patient, including such actions as suturing a wound, administering an injection, or performing a physical examination.

- Defamation of character. Damaging a person's reputation by making public statements that are both false and malicious is considered **defamation** of character. Defamation of character can take the form of slander and libel. Slander is speaking damaging words intended to negatively influence others against an individual in a manner that jeopardizes his or her reputation or means of livelihood.
- False imprisonment. False imprisonment is the intentional, unlawful restraint or confinement of one person by another. Preventing a patient from leaving the facility might be seen as false imprisonment.
- Fraud. **Fraud** consists of deceitful practices in depriving or attempting to deprive another of his or her rights. Health-care practitioners might be accused of fraud for promising patients "miracle cures" or for accepting fees from patients while using mystical or spiritual powers to heal.
- Invasion of privacy. Invasion of privacy is the interference with a person's right to be left alone. Entering an exam room without knocking can be considered an invasion of privacy. The improper use of or a breach of confidentiality of medical records may be seen as an invasion of privacy.

Unintentional Torts. The most common torts within the health-care delivery system are those committed unintentionally. Unintentional torts are acts that are not intended to cause harm but are committed unreasonably or with a disregard for the consequences. In legal terms, such acts constitute negligence. **Negligence** is charged when a health-care practitioner fails to exercise ordinary care and the patient is injured. The accused may have performed an act or failed to perform an act that a reasonable person would or would not have performed. Under the principles of negligence, civil liability exists only in cases in which the act is judicially determined to be wrongful. Health-care practitioners, for example, are not necessarily liable for a poor-quality outcome in delivering health care. Practitioners become liable only when their conduct is determined to be malpractice, the negligent delivery of professional services.

Contracts

A **contract** is a voluntary agreement between two parties in which specific promises are made for a consideration. The elements of a contract are important to health-care practitioners because health-care delivery takes place under various types of contracts. To be legally binding, four elements must be present in a contract:

1. Agreement—One party makes an offer and another party accepts it. Certain conditions pertain to the offer:
   - It can relate to the present or the future.
   - It must be communicated.
   - It must be made in good faith and not under duress or as a joke.

- It must be clear enough to be understood by both parties.
- It must define what both parties will do if the offer is accepted.

For example, a physician offers a service to the public by obtaining a license to practice medicine and opening for business. Patients accept the physician's offer by scheduling appointments, submitting to physical examinations, and allowing the physician to prescribe or perform medical treatment. The contract is complete when the physician's fee is paid.

2. Consideration—Something of value is bargained for as part of the agreement. The physician's consideration is providing service; the patient's consideration is payment of the physician's fee.

3. Legal subject matter—Contracts are not valid and enforceable in court unless they are for legal services or purposes. For example, a contract entered into by a patient to pay for services of a physician in private practice would be **void** (not legally enforceable) if the physician was not licensed to practice medicine. **Breach of contract** may be charged if either party fails to comply with the terms of a legally valid contract.

4. Contractual capacity—Parties who enter into the agreement must be capable of fully understanding all its terms and conditions. For example, a mentally incompetent individual or a person under the influence of drugs or alcohol cannot enter into a contract.

Types of Contracts. The two main types of contracts are expressed contracts and implied contracts. An **expressed contract** is clearly stated in written or spoken words. A payment contract is an example of an expressed contract. **Implied contracts** are those in which the acceptance or conduct of the parties, rather than expressed words, creates the contract. A patient who rolls up a sleeve and offers an arm for an injection is creating an implied contract.

Malpractice

Malpractice claims are lawsuits by a patient against a physician for errors in diagnosis or treatment. Negligence cases are those in which a person believes that a medical professional did not perform an essential action or performed an improper one, thus harming the patient.

Following are some examples of malpractice:

- Postoperative complications. For example, a patient starts to show signs of internal bleeding in the recovery room. The incision is reopened, and it is discovered that the surgeon did not complete closure of all the severed capillaries at the operation site.
- *Res ipsa loquitur.* This Latin term, which means "The thing speaks for itself," refers to a case in which the doctor's fault is completely obvious. For example, if a lung cancer patient has to have the right lung removed

and the surgeon instead removes the left lung, the patient will most likely sue the surgeon for malpractice. Another example is a case in which a surgeon accidentally leaves a surgical instrument inside the patient.

Following are examples of negligence:

- Abandonment. A health-care professional who stops care without providing an equally qualified substitute can be charged with **abandonment**. For example, a labor and delivery nurse is helping a woman in labor. The nurse's shift ends, but all the other nurses are busy and her replacement is late for work. Leaving the woman would constitute abandonment.
- Delayed treatment. A patient shows symptoms of some illness or disorder, but the doctor decides, for whatever reason, to delay treatment. If the patient later learns of the doctor's decision to wait, the patient may believe he has a negligence case.

Negligence cases are sometimes classified using the following three legal terms.

1. *Malfeasance* refers to an unlawful act or misconduct.
2. *Misfeasance* refers to a lawful act that is done incorrectly.
3. *Nonfeasance* refers to failure to perform an act that is one's required duty or that is required by law.

The Four Ds of Negligence. The American Medical Association (AMA) lists the following four Ds of negligence:

1. Duty. Patients must show that a physician-patient relationship existed in which the physician owed the patient a duty.
2. Derelict. Patients must show that the physician failed to comply with the standards of the profession. For example, a gynecologist has routinely taken Pap smears of a patient and then, for whatever reason, does not do so. If the patient then shows evidence of cervical cancer, the physician could be said to have been derelict.
3. Direct cause. Patients must show that any damages were a direct cause of a physician's breach of duty. For example, if a patient fell on the sidewalk and damaged her cast, she could not prove that the cast was damaged because it was incorrectly or poorly applied by her physician. It would be clear that the damage to the cast resulted from the fall. If, however, the patient's leg healed incorrectly because of the way the cast had been applied, she might have a case.
4. Damages. Patients must prove that they suffered injury.

To go forward with a malpractice suit, a patient must be prepared to prove all four Ds of negligence.

Malpractice and Civil Law. Malpractice lawsuits are part of civil law. Civil law is concerned with individuals' private rights (as opposed to criminal offenses against public law). Under civil law, a breach of some obligation that causes harm or injury to someone is known as a tort. A tort can be intentional or unintentional. Both negligence and breach of contract are considered torts. Breach of contract is the failure to adhere to a contract's terms. The implied physician-patient contract includes requirements like maintaining patient confidentiality. (Remember that an implied contract is one that is not created by specific, written words, but rather is defined by the conduct of the parties. Usually the parties involved have some special relationship.)

Settling Malpractice Suits.

Malpractice suits often require a trial in a court of law. Sometimes, however, they are settled through arbitration. **Arbitration** is a process in which the opposing sides choose a person or persons outside the court system, often with special knowledge in the field, to hear and decide the dispute. (Your local or state medical society has information about your state's policy on arbitration.) If injury, failure to provide reasonable care, or abandonment of the patient is proved to have occurred, the doctor must pay damages (a financial award) to the injured party.

If the doctor you work with becomes involved in a lawsuit, you should be familiar with subpoenas. A **subpoena** is a written court order addressed to a specific person, requiring that person's presence in court on a specific date at a specific time. If you were directly involved in the patient case that precipitated the lawsuit, you might be subpoenaed. Another important term to know is *subpoena duces tecum,* which is a court order to produce documents. If you are in charge of patient records at the practice, you may be required to locate, assemble, photocopy, and arrange for delivery of patient records for this purpose.

Law of Agency.

According to the **law of agency,** an employee is considered to be acting as a doctor's **agent** (on the doctor's behalf) while performing professional tasks. The Latin term *respondeat superior,* or "Let the master answer," is sometimes used to refer to this relationship. For example, the employee's word is as binding as if it were the doctor's (so you should never, for example, promise a patient a cure). Therefore, the doctor is responsible, or **liable,** for the negligence of employees. A negligent employee, however, may also be sued directly, because individuals are legally responsible for their own actions. Therefore, a patient can sue both the doctor and the involved employee for negligence. The employer, or the employer's insurance company, can also sue the employee.

The American Association of Medical Assistants (AAMA) recommends that you purchase your own malpractice insurance and have a personal attorney. Most likely, in a case of negligence the doctor would be sued (because you as an employee are acting on the doctor's behalf), and you are usually covered by the doctor's malpractice insurance. Even if you are young and think you do not have many assets, you should still obtain your own insurance.

Courtroom Conduct.

Most health-care practitioners will never have to appear in court. If you should be asked to appear, the following suggestions may prove helpful:

- Attend court proceedings as required. Failure to appear in court could result in either charges of contempt of court or the case being forfeited.
- Do not be late for scheduled hearings.
- Bring required documents to court and present them only when requested to do so.
- Before testifying, refresh your memory concerning all the facts observed about the matter in question, such as dates, times, words spoken, and circumstances.
- Speak slowly, clearly, and professionally. Do not use medical terms. Do not lose your temper or attempt to be humorous.
- Answer all questions in a straightforward manner, even if the answers appear to help the opposing side.
- Answer only the question asked, no more and no less.
- Appear well groomed, and dress in clean, conservative clothing.

How Effective Communication Can Help Prevent Lawsuits.

Patients who see the medical office as a friendly place are generally less likely to sue. Physicians, medical assistants, and other medical office staff who have pleasant personalities and are competent in their jobs will have less risk of being sued. Medical assistants can help by:

- Developing good listening skills and nonverbal communication techniques so that patients feel the time spent with them is not rushed
- Setting aside a certain time during the day for returning patients' phone calls
- Checking to be sure that all patients or their authorized representatives sign informed consent forms before they undergo medical or surgical procedures
- Avoiding statements that could be construed as an admission of fault on the part of the physician or other medical staff
- Using tact, good judgment, and professional ability in handling patients
- Refraining from making overly optimistic statements about a patient's recovery or prognosis
- Advising patients when their physicians intend to be gone
- Making every effort to reach an understanding about fees with the patient before treatment so that billing does not become a point of contention

Terminating Care of a Patient

A physician may wish to terminate care of a patient. Terminating care is sometimes called withdrawing from a case. Following are some typical reasons a physician may choose to withdraw from a case:

- The patient refuses to follow the physician's instructions.
- The patient's family members complain incessantly to or about the physician.
- A personality conflict develops between the physician and patient that cannot be reasonably resolved.
- The patient insists on having pain medication refilled beyond what the physician considers medically necessary.
- The patient habitually does not pay or fails to make satisfactory arrangements to pay for medical services. A physician may stop treatment of such a patient and end the physician-patient relationship only if adequate notice is given to the patient.
- The patient fails to keep scheduled appointments. To protect the physician from charges of abandonment, all missed appointments should be noted in the patient's chart.

A physician who terminates care of a patient must do so in a formal, legal manner, following these four steps.

1. Write a letter to the patient, expressing the reason for withdrawing from the case and recommending that the patient seek medical care from another physician as soon as possible. Figure 3-1 shows an example of a letter of termination.
2. Send the letter by certified mail with a return receipt requested.
3. Place a copy of the letter (and the return receipt, when received) in the patient's medical record.
4. Summarize in the patient record the physician's reason for terminating care and the actions taken to inform the patient.

Standard of Care

You are expected to fulfill the standards of the medical assisting profession for applying legal concepts to practice. According to the AAMA, medical assistants should uphold legal concepts in the following ways:

- Maintain confidentiality
- Practice within the scope of training and capabilities
- Prepare and maintain medical records
- Document accurately
- Use appropriate guidelines when releasing information
- Follow employer's established policies dealing with the health-care contract
- Follow legal guidelines and maintain awareness of health-care legislation and regulations
- Maintain and dispose of regulated substances in compliance with government guidelines

---

LETTER OF WITHDRAWAL FROM CASE

Dear Mr._____:

I find it necessary to inform you that I am withdrawing from further professional attendance upon you for the reason that you have persisted in refusing to follow my medical advice and treatment. Since your condition requires medical attention, I suggest that you place yourself under the care of another physician without delay. If you so desire, I shall be available to attend you for a reasonable time after you have received this letter, but in no event for more than five days.

This should give you ample time to select a physician of your choice from the many competent practitioners in this city. With your approval, I will make available to this physician your case history and information regarding the diagnosis and treatment which you have received from me.

Very truly yours,

_____, MD

Figure 3-1. Physicians are required to inform patients in writing if they wish to withdraw from a case.
Source: Medicolegal Forms With Legal Analysis, American Medical Association, © 1991.

- Follow established risk-management and safety procedures
- Recognize professional credentialing criteria
- Help develop and maintain personnel, policy, and procedure manuals

Often laws dictate what medical assistants may or may not do. For instance, in some states it is illegal for medical assistants to draw blood. No states consider it legal for medical assistants to diagnose a condition, prescribe a treatment, or let a patient believe that a medical assistant is a nurse or any other type of caregiver. In addition to what is stated by law, you and the physician must establish the procedures that are appropriate for you to perform.

Administrative Duties and the Law

Many of a medical assistant's administrative duties are related to legal requirements. Paperwork for insurance billing, patient consent forms for surgical procedures, and correspondence (such as a physician's letter of withdrawal from a case) must be handled correctly to meet legal standards. Documentation, such as making appropriate and accurate entries in a patient's medical record, is legally important. You may also maintain the physician's appointment book. This book is considered a legal document. It can prove, for instance, that the physician, if unable to see a patient, arranged for the patient to be seen by another physician in the same practice. In other words, the physician provided a qualified substitute as required by law.

You may also be responsible for handling certain state reporting requirements. Items that must be reported include births; certain diseases such as acquired immunodeficiency syndrome (AIDS) and other sexually transmitted diseases; drug abuse; suspected child abuse or abuse of the elderly; injuries caused by violence, such as knife and gunshot wounds; and deaths. Reports are sent to various state departments, depending on the content of the report. For example, suspected child abuse cases are reported to the state department of social services. Addressing these state requirements is called the physician's public duty.

Phone calls must be handled with an awareness of legal issues. For example, if the physician asks you to contact a patient by phone and you call the patient at work, you should not identify yourself or the physician by name to someone else without the patient's permission. You can say, for example, "Please tell Mrs. Arnot that her doctor's office is calling." If you do not take this precaution, the physician can be sued for invasion of privacy. You must abide by similar guidelines if you are responsible for making follow-up calls to a patient after a surgical procedure.

Documentation

Patient records are often used as evidence in professional medical liability cases, and improper documentation can contribute to or cause a case to be lost. Physicians should keep records that clearly show what treatment was performed and when it was done. It is important that physicians be able to demonstrate that nothing was neglected and that the care given fully met the standards demanded by law. One cliché to remember is "If it is not written down, then it was not done." Pay attention to spelling in charts and keep a medical dictionary handy if you are not sure of a spelling. Today's health-care environment requires complete documentation of actions taken and actions not taken. Medical staff members should pay particular attention to the following situations.

Referrals. Make sure the patient understands whether the referring physician's staff will make the appointment and notify the patient, or whether the patient must call to set up the appointment. Document in the chart that the patient was referred and the time and date of the appointment, and follow up with the specialist to verify that the appointment was scheduled and kept. Note whether reports of the consultation were received in your office, and document any further care of the patient from the referring physician.

Missed Appointments. At the end of the day, a designated person in the medical office should gather all patient charts of those who missed or canceled appointments without rescheduling. Charts should be dated, stamped, and documented "No Call/No Show" or "Canceled/No Reschedule." The treating physician should review these records and note whether follow-up is indicated.

Dismissals. To avoid charges of abandonment, the physician must formally withdraw from a case. Be sure that a letter of withdrawal or dismissal has been filed in the patient's records. All mailing confirmations should be filed in the record, such as the return receipt from certified mail.

All Other Patient Contact. Patient records should include reports of all tests, procedures, and medications prescribed, including prescription refills. Make sure all necessary informed consent papers have been signed and filed in the chart. Make entries into the chart of all telephone conversations with the patient. Correct documentation requires the initials or signature of the person making the notation on the patient's chart as well as the date and time.

Controlled Substances and the Law

You must also follow the correct procedures for the safekeeping and disposal of controlled substances, such as narcotics, in the medical office. It is important to know the right dosages and potential complications of these drugs, as well as prescription refill rules, in order to understand and interpret the directions of the physician in a legally responsible manner. Prescription pads must be kept secure so that they do not fall into the wrong hands.

Quality Control and Assurance

A medical office often has a physicians' office laboratory to perform different types of clinical tests, depending on the physician's specialty and state laws. The Clinical Laboratory Improvement Amendments of 1988 (CLIA '88) lists the regulations for laboratory testing. Physicians must display a certificate from CLIA confirming that their office complies with CLIA regulations. These regulations set standards for the quality of work performed in a laboratory and the accuracy of test results. Congress passed these laws after publicity about deaths caused by errors in the test used to diagnose cancer of the uterus.

According to CLIA '88, there are three categories of laboratory tests: waived tests, moderate-complexity tests, and high-complexity tests. Waived tests, the simplest kind, require the least amount of judgment and pose an insignificant risk to the patient in the event of an error. The laboratory applies for a certificate of waiver from the U.S. Department of Health and Human Services, which grants permission to perform any test on the list of waived tests and to bill it to Medicare or Medicaid. Tests that patients can do at home with kits approved by the department's Food and Drug Administration (FDA), such as the blood glucose test, also fall under this heading.

Most tests are in the moderate-complexity category. Cholesterol testing and checking for the presence or absence of sperm are examples. CLIA lists all waived and moderate-complexity tests and considers all other tests to be of high complexity.

Under CLIA '88, medical assistants are always allowed to perform waived tests. These tests are listed in Figure 3-5. Medical assistants can also perform moderate-complexity tests as long as the physician can ensure that the assistant is appropriately trained and experienced according to federal guidelines. Some state laws may be stricter than the federal laws, so the medical office should check with the state health department to see if there are any local rules about what kinds of tests medical assistants may perform. As you advance in your career, you will most likely be trained to do more and more types of tests, receiving training either by senior staff members or through outside programs.

Elements of the Quality Assurance Program

CLIA '88 also requires every medical office to have a quality assurance (QA) program. This program must include a quality control (QC) program specifically for the laboratory. The goal is to track and improve the quality of all aspects of the medical practice—including patient care, laboratory procedures, record keeping, employee evaluations, finances, legal responsibilities, public image, staff morale, insurance issues, and patient education. Documentation is

Waived Tests

- Dipstick or tablet reagent urinalysis (nonautomated) for the following: bilirubin, glucose, hemoglobin, ketone, leukocytes, nitrite, pH, protein, specific gravity, and urobilinogen
- Fecal occult blood
- Ovulation tests—visual color tests for human luteinizing hormone
- Urine pregnancy tests—visual color comparison determination
- Erythrocyte sedimentation rate—nonautomated
- Hemoglobin—(nonautomated) by copper sulfate
- Blood glucose—by glucose monitoring devices cleared by FDA specifically for home use
- Spun microhematocrit
- Hemoglobin—(automated) by single analyte instruments with self-contained or component features to perform specimen-reagent interaction, providing direct measurement and readout

Figure 3-5. Under CLIA '88, medical assistants are always allowed to perform waived tests.

required by QA regulations, to provide evidence that QA procedures are in place in the office. This documentation becomes extremely important if there is an inspection or a legal dispute.

Any QA program must include the following elements:

- Written policies on the standards of patient care and professional behavior
- A QC program
- Training and continuing education programs
- An instrument maintenance program
- Documentation requirements
- Evaluation methods

Software programs are available to help medical offices develop a QA program and procedures manual.

The Laboratory Program

The laboratory QC program must cover testing concerns such as patient preparation procedures, collection of the specimen (blood, urine, or tissue), labeling, preservation and transportation, test methods, inconsistent results, use and maintenance of equipment, personnel training, complaints and investigations, and corrective actions. The accuracy of the tests, and the instruments and chemicals that are used, must be monitored through QC procedures and documented. (Laboratory QC programs are discussed in more detail in Chapter 45.)

Code of Ethics

Medical ethics is a vital part of medical practice, and following an ethical code is an important part of your job. Ethics deals with general principles of right and wrong, as opposed to requirements of law. A professional is expected to act in ways that reflect society's ideas of right and wrong, even if such behavior is not enforced by law. Often, however, the law is based on ethical considerations.

Bioethics: Social Issues

Bioethics deals with issues that arise related to medical advances. Here are three examples of bioethical issues.

1. A treatment for Parkinson's disease was developed that uses fetal tissue. Some women, upon learning about this treatment, might get pregnant just to have an abortion and sell the fetal tissue. Is this ethical?

2. If a couple cannot have a baby because of a medical condition of the mother, using a surrogate mother is an option some couples choose. The surrogate mother is artificially inseminated with the sperm of the husband and carries the baby to term. The couple then raises the child. Ethically speaking, who is the real mother, the woman who bears the child or the woman who raises the child? If the surrogate mother wants to keep the baby after it is born, does she have a right to do so?

3. When a liver transplant is needed by both a famous patient who has had a history of alcohol abuse and a woman who is a recipient of public assistance, what criteria are considered when determining who receives the organ? Who makes the decision? Ethically, treating physicians should not make the decision of allocating limited medical resources. Decisions regarding the allocation of limited medical resources should consider only the likelihood of benefit, the urgency of need, and the amount of resources required for successful treatment. Nonmedical criteria, such as ability to pay, age, social worth, perceived obstacles to treatment, patient's contribution to illness, or the past use of resources should not be considered.

Practicing appropriate professional ethics has a positive impact on your reputation and the success of your employer's business. Many medical organizations, therefore, have created guidelines for the acceptable and preferred manners and behaviors, or etiquette, of medical assistants and physicians.

The principles of medical ethics have developed over time. The Hippocratic oath, in which medical students pledge to practice medicine ethically, was developed in ancient Greece. It is still used today and is one of the original bases of modern medical ethics. Hippocrates, the fourth-century-B.C. Greek physician commonly called the "father of medicine," is traditionally considered the author of this oath, but its authorship is actually unknown.

Among the promises of the Hippocratic oath are to use the form of treatment believed to be best for the patient, to refrain from harmful actions, and to keep a patient's private information confidential.

The AMA defines ethical behavior for doctors in *Code of Medical Ethics: Current Opinions with Annotations* (Chicago: American Medical Association, 1996). Medical assistants as well as doctors need to be aware of these principles.

> A physician shall be dedicated to providing competent medical service with compassion and respect for human dignity.

This concept means that medical professionals will respect all aspects of the patient as a person, including intellect and emotions. The doctor must decide what treatment would result in the best, most dignified quality of life for the patient, and the doctor must respect a patient's choice to forgo treatment.

> A physician shall deal honestly with patients and colleagues and strive to expose those physicians deficient in character or competence or who engage in fraud or deception.

Medical professionals, including medical assistants, should respect colleagues, but they must also respect and protect the profession and public welfare enough to report colleagues who are breaking the law, acting unethically, or unable to perform competently. Dilemmas may arise where one suspects, but is not able to prove, for instance, that a coworker has a substance abuse problem or another problem that is affecting performance. Ignoring such a situation in medical practice could cost someone's life as well as lead to lawsuits.

In terms of billing, a doctor should bill only for direct services, not for indirect ones, such as referrals. The doctor also should not bill for services that do not really pertain to the practice of medicine, such as dispensing drugs.

It is also unethical for the doctor to influence the patient about where to fill prescriptions or obtain other medical services when the doctor has a personal financial interest in any of the choices.

> A physician shall respect the law and also recognize a responsibility to seek changes in requirements that are contrary to the patient's best interests.

Several legal or employer requirements have come under scrutiny as being contrary to a patient's best interests. Among them are discharging patients from the hospital after a certain time limit for certain procedures, which may be too soon for many patients. Insurance company payment policies have sometimes been criticized as unfair. So have health maintenance organization (HMO) financial policies that may conflict with a doctor's preference in treatment.

CODE OF ETHICS

The Code of Ethics of the AAMA shall set forth principles of ethical and moral conduct as they relate to the medical profession and the particular practice of medical assisting.

Members of the AAMA dedicated to the conscientious pursuit of their profession, and thus desiring to merit the high regard of the entire medical profession and the respect of the general public which they serve, do pledge themselves to strive always to:

A. render service with full respect for the dignity of humanity;

B. respect confidential information obtained through employment unless legally authorized or required by responsible performance of duty to divulge such information;

C. uphold the honor and high principles of the profession and accept its disciplines;

D. seek to continually improve the knowledge and skills of medical assistants for the benefit of patients and professional colleagues;

E. participate in additional service activities aimed toward improving the health and wellbeing of the community;

Figure 3-6. The AAMA's Code of Ethics sets the ethical standard for the profession of medical assisting. (Reprinted with permission of the American Association of Medical Assistants.)

> A physician shall respect the rights of patients, of colleagues, and of other health professionals and shall safeguard patient confidences within the constraints of law.

A document called the Patient's Bill of Rights, established by the American Hospital Association in 1973 and revised in 1992, lists ethical principles protecting the patient. (The text of the Patient's Bill of Rights appears in Chapter 36.) Some states have even passed this code of ethics into law. Among a patient's rights are the right to information about alternative treatments, the right to refuse to participate in research projects, and the right to privacy.

> A physician shall continue to study; apply and advance scientific knowledge; make relevant information available to patients, colleagues, and the public; obtain consultation; and use the talents of other health professionals when indicated.

Keeping up with the latest advancements in medicine is crucial for providing high-quality, ethical care. Most states require doctors to accumulate "continuing education units" to maintain a license to practice. These units are earned by means of educational activities such as courses and scientific meetings. The AAMA requires medical assistants to renew their certification every 5 years, by either accumulating continuing education credits through the AAMA or retaking the certification examination.

> A physician shall, in the provision of appropriate patient care, except in emergencies, be free to choose whom to serve, with whom to associate, and the environment in which to provide medical services.

Ethically, doctors can set their hours, decide what kind of medicine to practice and where, decide whom to accept as a patient, and take time off as long as a qualified substitute performs their duties. Doctors may decline to accept new patients because of a full workload. In an emergency, however, a doctor may be ethically obligated to care for a patient, even if the patient is not of the doctor's choosing. The doctor should not abandon that patient until another physician is available.

> A physician shall recognize a responsibility to participate in activities contributing to an improved community. This ethical obligation holds true for the allied health professions as well.

In addition to knowing the physician's codes of ethics, medical assistants should follow the AAMA's Code of Ethics, which appears in Figure 3-6 and in Chapter 1.

HIPAA

Today, health care is considered a trillion-dollar industry, growing rapidly with technology and employing millions of health-care workers in numerous fields. The U.S. Department of Labor recognizes 400 different job titles in the health-care industry.

On August 21, 1996, the U.S. Congress passed the Health Insurance Portability and Accountability Act (HIPAA). The primary goals of the act are to improve the portability and continuity of health-care coverage in group and individual markets; to combat waste, fraud, and abuse in health-care insurance and health-care delivery; to promote the use of medical savings accounts; to improve access to long-term care services and coverage; and to simplify the administration of health insurance.

The purposes of the act are to:

- Improve the efficiency and effectiveness of health-care delivery by creating a national framework for health privacy protection that builds on efforts by states, health systems, and individual organizations and individuals

- Protect and enhance the rights of patients by providing them access to their health information and controlling the inappropriate use or disclosure of that information
- Improve the quality of health care by restoring trust in the health-care system among consumers, health-care professionals, and the multitude of organizations and individuals committed to the delivery of care

HIPAA is divided into two main sections of law: Title I, which addresses health-care portability, and Title II, which covers the prevention of health-care fraud and abuse, administrative simplification, and medical liability reform.

Title I: Health-Care Portability

The issue of portability deals with protecting health-care coverage for employees who change jobs, allowing them to carry their existing plans with them to new jobs. HIPAA provides the following protections for employees and their families:

- Increases workers' ability to get health-care coverage when starting a new job
- Reduces workers' probability of losing existing health-care coverage.
- Helps workers maintain continuous health-care coverage when changing jobs.
- Helps workers purchase health insurance on their own if they lose coverage under an employer's group plan and have no other health-care coverage available.

The specific protections of this title include the following:

- Limits the use of exclusions for preexisting conditions
- Prohibits group plans from discriminating by denying coverage or charging extra for coverage based on an individual's or a family member's past or present poor health.
- Guarantees certain small employers, as well as certain individuals who lose job-related coverage, the right to purchase health insurance.
- Guarantees, in most cases, that employers or individuals who purchase health insurance can renew the coverage regardless of any health conditions of individuals covered under the insurance policy.

Title II: Prevention of Health-Care Fraud and Abuse, Administrative Simplification, and Medical Liability Reform

HIPAA Privacy Rule. The HIPAA Standards for Privacy of Individually Identifiable Health Information provide the first comprehensive federal protection for the privacy of health information. The **Privacy Rule** is designed to provide strong privacy protections that do not interfere with patient access to health care or the quality of health-care delivery. This act creates, for the first time, national standards to protect individuals' medical records and other personal health information. The privacy rule is intended to:

- Give patients more control over their health information
- Set boundaries on the use and release of health-care records
- Establish appropriate safeguards that health-care providers and others must achieve to protect the privacy of health information
- Hold violators accountable, with civil and criminal penalties that can be imposed if they violate patients' privacy rights
- Strike a balance when public responsibility supports disclosure of some forms of data—for example, to protect public health

Before the HIPAA Privacy Rule, the personal information that moves across hospitals and doctors' offices, insurers or third-party payers, and state lines fell under a patchwork of federal and state laws. This information could be distributed—without either notice or authorization—for reasons that had nothing to do with a patient's medical treatment or health-care reimbursement. For example, unless otherwise forbidden by state or local law, without the Privacy Rule, patient information held by a health plan could, without the patient's permission, be passed on to a lender who could then deny the patient's application for a home mortgage or a credit card or could be given to an employer who could use it in personnel decisions.

Individually identifiable health information includes:

- Name
- Address
- Phone numbers
- Fax number
- Dates (birth, death, admission, discharge, etc.)
- Social Security number
- E-mail address
- Medical record numbers
- Health plan beneficiary numbers
- Account numbers
- Certificate or license numbers
- Vehicle identifiers and serial numbers, including license plate numbers
- Device identifiers and serial numbers
- Web Universal Resource Locators (URLs)
- Internet Protocol (IP) address numbers

The core of the HIPAA Privacy Rule is the protection, use, and disclosure of **protected health information (PHI)**. Protected health information means individually identifiable health information that is transmitted or maintained by electronic or other media, such as computer storage devices. The Privacy Rule protects all PHI held or transmitted by a covered entity, which includes health-care providers, health plans, and health-care clearing-houses. Other covered entities include employers, life insurers, schools or universities, and public health authorities. Protected health information can come in any form or media, such as electronic, paper, or oral, including verbal communications among staff members, patients, and other providers. *Use* and *disclosure* are the two fundamental concepts in the HIPAA Privacy Rule. It is important to understand the differences between these terms.

Use. **Use** refers to performing any of the following actions to individually identifiable health information by employees or other members of an organization's workforce:

- Sharing
- Employing
- Applying
- Utilizing
- Examining
- Analyzing

Information is used when it moves within an organization.

Disclosure. **Disclosure** occurs when the entity holding the information performs any of the following actions so that the information is outside the entity:

- Releasing
- Transferring
- Providing access to
- Divulging in any manner

Information is disclosed when it is transmitted between or among organizations.

Under HIPAA, *use* limits the sharing of information within a covered entity, while *disclosure* restricts the sharing of information outside the entity holding the information.
The Privacy Rule covers the following PHI:

- The past, present, or future physical or mental health or condition of an individual
- Health care that is provided to an individual
- Billing or payments made for health care provided

Information that is not individually identifiable or unable to be tied to the identity of a particular patient is not subject to the Privacy Rule.

Managing and Storing Patient Information. Medical facilities have undergone many changes to the way they manage and store patient information. The Privacy Rule compliance was enforced in April of 2003. Many facilities contracted consultants that specialized in HIPAA and became certified in HIPAA compliance. For the health-care provider, the Privacy Rule requires activities such as:

- Notifying patients of their privacy rights and how their information is used

- Adopting and implementing privacy procedures for its practice, hospital, or plan
- Training employees so that they understand the privacy procedures
- Designating an individual to be responsible for seeing that the privacy procedures are adopted and followed
- Securing patient records containing individually identifiable health information so that they are not readily available to those who do not need them

Under HIPAA, patients have an increased awareness of their health information privacy rights, which includes the following:

- The right to access, copy, and inspect their health-care information
- The right to request an amendment to their health-care information
- The right to obtain an accounting of certain disclosures of their health-care information
- The right to alternate means of receiving communications from providers
- The right to complain about alleged violations of the regulations and the provider's own information policies

Sharing Patient Information. When sharing patient information, HIPAA will allow the provider to use health-care information for **treatment, payment, and operations (TPO).**

- Treatment—Providers are allowed to share information in order to provide care to patients
- Payment—Providers are allowed to share information in order to receive payment for the treatment provided
- Operations—Providers are allowed to share information to conduct normal business activities, such as quality improvement

If the use of patient information does not fall under TPO, then written authorization must be obtained *before* sharing information with anyone.
Patient information may be disclosed without authorization to the following parties or in the following situations:

- Medical researchers
- Emergencies
- Funeral directors/coroners
- Disaster relief services
- Law enforcement
- Correctional institutions
- Abuse and neglect
- Organ and tissue donation centers
- Work-related conditions that may affect employee health
- Judicial/administrative proceedings at the patient's request or as directed by a subpoena or court order

When using or disclosing PHI, a provider must make reasonable efforts to limit the use or disclosure to the minimum amount of PHI necessary to accomplish the intended purpose. Providing only the minimum necessary information means taking reasonable safeguards to protect an individual's health information from incidental disclosure. State laws may impose more stringent requirements regarding the protection of patient information. Health-care providers and staff should only have access to information they need to fulfill their assigned duties. The minimum necessary standard does not apply to disclosures, including oral disclosures, among health-care providers for treatment purposes. For example, a physician is not required to apply the minimum necessary standard when discussing a patient's medical chart information with a specialist at another hospital.

Patient Notification. Since the effective date of the HIPAA Privacy Rule, medical facilities have made major changes in how they inform patients of their HIPAA compliance. You may have noticed, as a patient yourself, the forms and information packets that are now provided by your health-care providers. The first step in informing patients of HIPAA compliance is the communication of patient rights. These rights are communicated through a document called **Notice of Privacy Practices (NPP)**. A notice must:

- Be written in plain, simple language.
- Include a header that reads: "This Notice describes how medical information about you may be used and disclosed and how you can get access to this information. Please review carefully."
- Describe the covered entity's uses and disclosures of PHI.
- Describe an individual's rights under the Privacy Rule.
- Describe the covered entity's duties.
- Describe how to register complaints concerning suspected privacy violations.
- Specify a point of contract.
- Specify an effective date.
- State that the entity reserves to right to change its privacy practices.

The second step in patient notification is to implement a document that explains the policy of the medical facility on obtaining **authorization** for the use and disclosure of patient information for purposes other than TPO. The authorization form must be written in plain language. Some of the core elements of an authorization form include:

- Specific and meaningful descriptions of the authorized information
- Persons authorized to use or disclose protected health information
- Purpose of the requested information
- Statement of the patient's right to revoke the authorization
- Signature and date of the patient

Security Measures. Health-care facilities can undertake a number of measures in order to help reduce a breach of confidentiality, including for information that is either stored or delivered electronically (i.e., stored in computers or computer networks, or delivered via computer networks or the Internet).

HIPAA Security Rule. In February 2003, the final regulations were issued regarding the administrative, physical, and technical safeguards to protect the confidentiality, integrity, and availability of health information covered by HIPAA. The **Security Rule** specifies how patient information is protected on computer networks, the Internet, disks, and other storage media and extranets. The rapidly increasing use of computers in health care today has created new dangers for breaches of confidentiality. The Security Rule mandates that:

- A security officer must be assigned the responsibility for the medical facility's security
- All staff, including management, receives security awareness training
- Medical facilities must implement audit controls to record and examine staff who have logged into information systems that contain PHI
- Organizations limit physical access to medical facilities that contain electronic PHI
- Organizations must conduct risk analyses to determine information security risks and vulnerabilities
- Organizations must establish policies and procedures that allow access to electronic PHI on a need-to-know basis

Computers are not the only concern regarding security of the workplace. The facility layout can propose a possible violation if not designed correctly. All facilities must take measures to reduce the identity of patient information. Some examples of facility design that can help reduce a breach of confidentiality include the security of patient charts, the reception area, the clinical station, and faxes sent and received.

Chart Security. Patient charts can be kept confidential by following these rules:

- Charts that contain a patient's name or other identifiers cannot be in view at the front reception area or nurse's station. Some offices have placed charts in plain jackets to prevent information from being seen.
- Charts must be stored out of the view of a public area, so that they cannot be seen by unauthorized individuals.
- Charts should be placed on the filing shelves without the patient name showing.
- Charts should be locked when not in use. Many facilities have purchased filing equipment that can be locked and unlocked without limiting the availability of patient information.

Notifying Those at Risk for Sexually Transmitted Disease *(continued)*

is transmitted. Alert the patient as to precautions to take so he will not continue to transmit the disease to others. Help the patient understand why it is important for people who may have contracted the disease from him to be told they may have it.

Then, offer to contact the patient's former and current partners. Fully explain each step in the notification process, assuring the patient that his name will not be revealed under any circumstances. Answer any questions and address any concerns about the notification process. If the patient is still reluctant to provide information, give him some time to think about it away from the office, and follow up periodically with a phone call.

Once the patient agrees to reveal names, write down the names and other information, preferably phone numbers. To make sure you have correct information, read it back to the patient, spelling each person's name in turn and reciting the phone number or address. Write down the phonetic pronunciations of any difficult names. Tell the patient when you will make the notifications.

You now are ready to contact these individuals. Professionals who work with STD patients recommend guidelines for contacting current and former partners to alert them about potential exposure to an STD. Note that these guidelines are applicable only to STDs other than AIDS.

Determine how you will contact each individual: in writing, in person, or by phone.

1. If you use U.S. mail, mark the outside of the addressed envelope "Personal." On a note inside, simply ask the person to call you at the medical office. Do not put the topic of the call in writing.

2. If you make the contact in person, ask where you can talk privately. Even if the person appears to be alone, others may still be able to overhear the conversation.

3. If you use the phone, identify yourself and your office, and ask for the specific individual. Do not reveal the nature of your call to anyone but that person. If pressed, tell the person who answers the phone that you are calling regarding a personal matter.

Once on the phone or alone with the person, confirm that you are talking to the correct person. Mention that you wish to talk about a highly personal matter, and ask if it is a good time to continue the discussion. If not, arrange for a more appropriate time.

Inform the individual that she has come in contact with someone who has a sexually transmitted disease. Recommend that the person visit a doctor's office or clinic to be tested for the disease.

Be prepared for a variety of reactions, from surprise to anger. Respond calmly and coolly. Expect to respond to questions and statements such as:

- Who gave you my name?
- Do I have the disease?
- Am I really at risk? I haven't had intercourse recently (or) I've only had intercourse with my spouse.
- I feel fine. I just went to my doctor recently.

Let the person know that you cannot reveal the name of the partner because the information is strictly confidential. Assure the person that you will not reveal her name to anyone either.

Explain that exposure to the disease does not mean a person has contracted it. Encourage the person to get tested to know for sure.

Tell the person that she is still at risk, even if she hasn't had intercourse recently or has had it only with a spouse. Let the person know that someone with whom she came in close contact at some point has contracted the disease.

Even if the person says, "I feel fine," she may still have the disease. Again, stress the importance of getting tested.

Provide your name and phone number for contact about further questions. Recommend local offices and clinics for testing, and provide phone numbers. If the person will come to your office, offer to make the appointment.

Finally, document the results of your call. Log in the original patient's file the date that you completed notification. Include any pertinent details about the notification. Alert the patient when all people on the list have been notified.

The AMA has several standard forms for authorization of disclosure and includes disclosure clauses in many other forms. For example, the consent-to-surgery form includes a clause about consenting to picture taking and observation during the surgery. When using a standard form, cross out anything that does not apply in that particular situation. Medical practices often develop their own customized forms.

Summary

You must carefully follow all state, federal, and individual practice rules and laws while performing your daily duties. You must also follow the AAMA Code of Ethics for medical assistants. It is an important part of your duties to help the doctor avoid malpractice claims—lawsuits by the patient against the physician for errors in diagnosis or treatment.

To perform effectively as a medical assistant, you must maintain an office that follows all OSHA regulations for safety, hazardous equipment, and toxic substances. The office also must meet QC and QA guidelines for all tests, specimens, and treatments. It is your responsibility to follow HIPAA guidelines, to ensure patient privacy and confidentiality of patient records, to fully document patient treatment, and to maintain patient records in an orderly and readily accessible fashion.

REVIEW

CHAPTER 3

CASE STUDY QUESTIONS

Now that you have completed this chapter, review the case study at the beginning of the chapter and answer the following questions:

1. Does the medical assistant's comment represent a breach of confidentiality?
2. Has any HIPAA rule been violated? If so, which one?

Discussion Questions

1. How does the law of agency make it possible for a patient to sue both the medical assistant and the physician for an act of negligence committed by the medical assistant?
2. Under HIPAA, what rights do patients have regarding confidentiality and ownership of their medical records? When does a patient give up the right to confidentiality?
3. Are health-care professionals legally liable for all unsatisfactory outcomes?
4. What are two scenarios that would void a contract between physician and patient?

Critical Thinking Questions

1. What is an example of a bioethical issue? Give two opposing views of the issue.
2. What are two different situations that could turn into a malpractice or abandonment suit if committed by physicians or their medical staff members?
3. Describe implied consent and two ways that a patient can accept treatment by implied consent.

Application Activities

1. Research a controversial topic from the following list:
   Euthanasia
   Surrogacy
   Abortion
   Fetal stem cell research
   Cloning
   Emergency contraceptive (morning-after pill)

Write a three-page report that presents both the pro side and the con side of the issue. Write a closing paragraph that gives your personal opinion and views and how you have been conditioned in that belief, for example, social, cultural, and religious beliefs.

2. Choose teams of four people, and stage debates on the controversial topics listed in question 1. Research your topics thoroughly and present arguments on both sides. Your purpose is to state facts and persuade your audience to your beliefs.

   Rules for the debate:
   - Participants must be courteous and professional
   - Presentations must be factual
   - Opening arguments are four minutes for each side
   - Each side presents, and then for three minutes each side is allowed to counter any fact
   - Closing arguments are five minutes for each side
   - Have the class vote on which side was more persuasive.

3. In a medical law textbook or journal, research a malpractice case. Prepare a 10-minute presentation for the class in which you summarize both sides of the case (patient and caregiver). Include when and where the case took place. Explain how the case was settled and whether the settlement took place in a court of law or through arbitration. Close with your opinion about whether the case was settled fairly.

4. Research a piece of legislation on a health-care issue or practice, either a bill passed in the last 5 years or a bill currently being considered in Washington. What impact has this bill had or might this bill have on the medical assisting profession? Summarize your findings in a one- to two-page report.

CHAPTER 4

Communication With Patients, Families, and Coworkers

AREAS OF COMPETENCE

2003 Role Delineation Study

GENERAL

Professionalism
- Display a professional manner and image
- Demonstrate initiative and responsibility
- Work as a member of the health-care team
- Adapt to change
- Treat all patients with compassion and empathy
- Promote the practice through positive public relations

Communication Skills
- Recognize and respect cultural diversity
- Adapt communications to an individual's ability to understand
- Recognize and respond effectively to verbal, nonverbal, and written communications
- Serve as liaison

Legal Concepts
- Perform within legal and ethical boundaries
- Document accurately

KEY TERMS

active listening
aggressive
assertive
body language
burnout
closed posture
conflict
empathy
feedback
hierarchy
homeostasis
hospice
interpersonal skills
open posture
passive listening
personal space
rapport

CHAPTER OUTLINE

- Communicating With Patients and Families
- The Communication Circle
- Understanding Human Behavior and How It Relates to the Provider-Patient Relationship
- Types of Communication
- Improving Your Communication Skills
- Communicating in Special Circumstances
- Communicating With Coworkers
- Managing Stress
- Preventing Burnout
- The Policy and Procedures Manual

OBJECTIVES

After completing Chapter 4, you will be able to:

4.1 Identify elements of the communication circle.
4.2 Give examples of positive and negative communication.

4.3 List ways to improve listening and interpersonal skills.

4.4 Explain the difference between assertiveness and aggressiveness.

4.5 Give examples of effective communication strategies with patients in special circumstances.

4.6 Discuss ways to establish positive communication with coworkers and superiors.

4.7 Explain how stress relates to communication and identify strategies to reduce stress.

4.8 Describe how the office policy and procedures manual is used as a communication tool in the medical office.

Introduction

The ability to recognize human behaviors and the ability to communicate effectively are vital to a medical assistant and the pursuit for success. This chapter has taken a psychological approach to understanding human behavior and the challenges that influence therapeutic communication in a health-care setting. Patients will often have more interaction with the medical assistant than with any other health-care practitioner in the facility. It is important that patients develop a good rapport and feel confident in the care they are receiving from your office. The medical assistant sets the tone for the communication cycle and must be aware of all the obstacles that can affect human communication. As a medical assistant, you are often exposed to all kinds of patients. You will see patients from different cultures, socioeconomic backgrounds, educational levels, ages, and lifestyles. You must be able to communicate with each patient with professionalism and diplomacy.

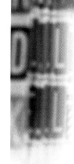

CASE STUDY

Mary is 23 years old and has been a medical assistant for 6 months. She is currently working in a walk-in clinic in a large urban city. She has interviewed three patients this morning. One patient is a homeless transient male who appears to have some type of mental incapacity; the second is a teenage girl who suspects she might be pregnant; and the third is a well-dressed professional male who complains of a sore throat.

As you read this chapter, consider how you would answer the following questions relative to each of the patients:

1. How will Mary adapt her communication style to communicate with each patient?
2. What types of communication roadblocks will she encounter with each one?
3. What types of communication techniques will she use for each patient?

Communicating With Patients and Families

Think about the last time you had a doctor's appointment. How well did the staff and physicians communicate with you? Were you greeted cordially and pleasantly invited to take a seat, or did someone thrust a clipboard at you and say "Fill this out"? If you had a long wait in the waiting room or examination room, did someone come in to explain the delay? Did you become frustrated and angry because nobody told you what was happening?

As a medical assistant, you are a key communicator between the office and patients and families. The way you greet patients, explain procedures, ask and answer questions, and attend to the individual needs of patients forms your communication style. Your interaction with the patient sets the tone for the office visit and can significantly influence how comfortable the patient feels in your practice. Developing strong communication skills in the medical office is just as important as mastering administrative and clinical tasks.

Customer service is the most important part of communication to families and patients. Your mastery of clinical and administrative skills is only a portion of your skills; customer service and communication skills are the other 70%.

A definition of customer service includes the following two points:

1. The patient comes first
2. Patient needs are satisfied

In today's health-care environment, patients are consumers and are more educated than ever before. Patients have more options in choosing a physician or a health-care facility. Patients who feel that they were not given exceptional customer service will choose another physician or facility to meet their needs. Another reason a facility must strive for exceptional customer service is that a medical facility grows rapidly from referral business. A medical facility that acquires a reputation for having an "unfriendly" staff will feel the negative impact from that reputation.

Listed here are some examples of customer service in the physician's office:

- Using proper telephone techniques
- Writing or responding to telephone messages
- Explaining procedures to patients
- Expediting insurance referral requests
- Assisting in billing issues
- Answering questions or finding answers to patient questions
- Ensuring that patients are comfortable in your office
- Creating a warm and reassuring environment

From a business perspective, exceptional customer service is vital to a medical facility's success. Any business that does not provide exceptional customer service will not grow and thrive in today's business economy.

The Communication Circle

As you interact with patients and their families, you will be responsible for giving information and ensuring that the patient understands what you, the doctor, and other members of the staff have communicated. You will also be responsible for receiving information from the patient. For example, patients will describe their symptoms. They may also discuss their feelings or ask questions about a treatment or procedure. The giving and receiving of information forms the communication circle.

Elements of the Communication Circle

The communication circle involves three elements: a message, a source, and a receiver. Messages are usually verbal or written. (As you will see later in the chapter, some messages are nonverbal.) The source sends the message, and the receiver receives it. The communication circle is formed as the source sends a message to the receiver and the receiver responds (Figure 4-1).

Consider this example, in which Simone, a medical assistant who works in a physical therapy office, is speaking with Mrs. Sommer, a patient who is having therapy for a back injury. Watch the communication circle at work.

Simone:	The physical therapist says you're making great progress and that you can start on some simple back exercises at home.

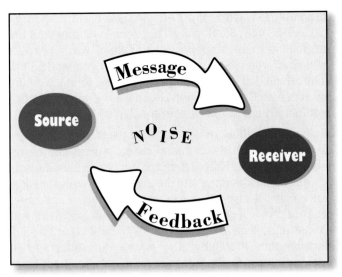

Figure 4-1. The process of communication involves an exchange of messages through verbal and nonverbal means.

	I'd like to go over them with you. Then I'll give you a sheet that illustrates the exercises. How does that sound to you?
Mrs. Sommer:	I'm a little nervous about doing exercises. I still have some pain when I bend over.
Simone:	I understand. It's important, though, to start using those muscles again. Why don't you show me exactly where it hurts. Then we can go over proper body mechanics, such as bending down to pick something up and getting in and out of chairs, the car, and bed. Then we'll just start with one or two of the exercises and save the rest for next time, when you're feeling more ready.
Mrs. Sommer:	Yes, I only feel up to doing a little bit today.

The medical assistant (the source) gives a verbal message (about back exercises) to the patient (the receiver). The patient responds by drawing attention to her pain and uneasiness about certain movements. The patient's response is also a message to the medical assistant, who responds in turn. The giving and receiving of information continues within the communication circle until the exchange is finished.

Feedback. Another word for response is **feedback,** which is verbal or nonverbal evidence that the receiver got and understood the message. When you communicate information to a patient or ask a patient a question, always look for feedback. For example, if you calculate a pregnant patient's due date and tell her she's 12 weeks pregnant, look for a response. If she responds, "Oh, good, that means I'm out of danger of having a miscarriage," you would respond that whereas most miscarriages occur in the first 12 weeks, some risk of miscarriage remains throughout the pregnancy. If she responds, "I thought I was 14 weeks pregnant," you would need to clarify how you worked out your calculation and compare it with hers, to uncover any discrepancy. Good communication in the medical office requires patient feedback at every step.

Noise. Anything that distorts the message in any way or interferes with the communication process can be referred to as noise. Noise refers not only to sounds, such as a siren or jackhammer on the street below the medical office suite. It also refers to room temperature and other types of physical comfort or discomfort, such as pain, and to emotions, such as fear or sadness. If patients are feeling uncomfortable in a chilly or hot room, upset about their illness, or in great pain, they may not pay close attention to what you are saying. Conversely, if you are feeling upset about a personal problem outside work or if you are unwell or preoccupied with all the things you have on your to-do list, you may not communicate well.

As you deal with each patient, try to screen out or eliminate both literal and figurative noise. For example, before you start a conversation with a patient in an examination room, you might ask, "Are you too chilly or too hot? Is the temperature in here comfortable for you?" If there is construction going on outside the building, see if there is a less noisy inner room or office that you might be able to use. If a patient seems nervous or upset, address those feelings before you launch into a factual discussion.

If you are feeling stressed or out of sorts, that feeling constitutes a type of noise. Try to take a "breather" between patients or a break from desk work—walk downstairs, get some fresh air, stretch your legs. Feeling dehydrated or hungry affects your communication efforts too. Limit your caffeine and sugar intake. Drink plenty of water and juice throughout the day. Eat a good lunch and healthful snacks. Leave your personal problems at home.

Humanizing the Communication Process in the Medical Office

As highly structured managed care organizations and technological advances rapidly change the face of health care, many patients feel that health care is becoming impersonal. Every time you communicate with patients, you can counteract this perception by playing a humanistic role in the health-care process. Being humanistic means that you work to help patients feel attended to and respected as individuals, not just as descriptions on a chart. Good communication supports this patient-centered approach.

Make a point of developing and using strong communication skills to show patients that you, the doctors, and other staff members care about them and their feelings. Taking care to treat patients as people helps humanize the communication process in the medical office.

Understanding Human Behavior and How It Relates to the Provider-Patient Relationship

Understanding human behavior is important when you are communicating with patients. Medical assistants are exposed to many different personality types in addition to different illnesses. When you understand why a person is behaving in a certain way, you can adjust your communication style to adapt to that person. Abraham Maslow, a well-known human behaviorist, developed a model of human behavior known as the **hierarchy** (i.e., a classification) of needs. This hierarchy states that human beings are motivated by unsatisfied needs and that certain lower needs have to be satisfied before higher needs, like self-actualization, are met. Maslow felt that people are basically trustworthy, self-protecting, and self-governing and that humans tend toward growth and love. He believed that humans are not violent by nature, but are violent only when their needs are not being met.

Deficiency Needs

According to Maslow, there are general types of needs—physiological, safety, love, and esteem—that must be satisfied before a person can act unselfishly. He called these needs *deficiency needs*.

Physiological Needs. Physiological needs are humans' very basic needs, such as air, water, food, sleep, and sex. When these needs are not satisfied, we may feel sickness, irritation, pain, and discomfort. These feelings motivate us to alleviate them as soon as possible to establish **homeostasis** (that is, a state of balance or equilibrium). Once those feelings are alleviated, we may think about other things.

Safety Needs. People have the need and desire for establishing stability and consistency. These basic needs are security, shelter, and existing in a safe environment.

Love Needs. Humans have a desire to belong to groups: clubs, work groups, religious groups, family, and so on. We need to feel loved and accepted by others. Humans are like pack animals—we place great importance in belonging to society.

Esteem Needs. Humans like to feel that they are important and have worthiness to society. There are two types of self-esteem. The first results from competence or mastery of a task, such as completing an educational program. The second is the attention and recognition that comes from others.

Self-Actualization

The need for self-actualization is "the desire to become more and more what one is, to become everything that one is capable of becoming." To reach this level, a person utilizes many tools to maximize potential, such as education. Successful people have reached this level on the hierarchy ladder.

When working and communicating with patients, remember this hierarchy of human needs and observe what need a patient is deficient in. For example, if an elderly patient has recently lost her husband, she may feel lonely and deficient in the love need. You may see homeless patients who are deficient in their physiological and safety needs. You may have a young girl as a patient who is overweight and has low self-esteem. On the other hand, you may have a high-level executive as a patient who has reached self-actualization. Each of these scenarios would require a communication style adjustment in order for you to effectively communicate with these patients.

Types of Communication

Communication can be positive or negative. It can also be verbal, nonverbal, or written. To help ensure effective communication with patients, familiarize yourself with these different types of communication. (Written communication is discussed in Chapter 7.)

Positive Communication

In the medical office, communication that promotes patients' comfort and well-being is essential. Treating patients brusquely or rudely is unacceptable in the health-care setting. It is your responsibility—not the patient's—to set the stage for positive communication.

When information—even bad news—is communicated with some positive aspect, patients are more likely to listen attentively and respond positively themselves. For example, you might explain to a patient who is about to get an injection, "This will sting, but only for a couple of seconds. When we're through, you're free to go." You would not just say, "This is going to hurt."

Other examples of positive communication are:

- Being friendly, warm, and attentive ("It's good to see you again, Mrs. Armstrong. I know you're on your lunch hour, so let's get started right away.")
- Verbalizing concern for patients ("Are you comfortable?" "I understand it hurts when I do this; I'll be gentle." "This paperwork won't take long at all.")
- Encouraging patients to ask questions ("I hope I've explained the procedure well. Do you have any questions, or are there any parts you would like to go over again?")
- Asking patients to repeat your instructions to make sure they understand
- Looking directly at patients when you speak to them
- Smiling (naturally, not in a forced way)

- Speaking slowly and clearly
- Listening carefully

Negative Communication

Most people do not purposely try to communicate negatively. Some people, however, may not realize that their communication style has a negative impact on others. Look for and ask for feedback to help you curb negative communication habits. Ask yourself, "Do the physicians and my other coworkers seem glad to speak with me? Are they open and responsive to me?" "Do patients seem at ease with me, or are they very quiet, turned off, or distant?" (Note that some patients may respond this way because of the way they feel, not because of the way you are communicating with them.) Here are some examples of negative communication:

- Mumbling
- Speaking brusquely or sharply
- Avoiding eye contact
- Interrupting patients as they are speaking
- Rushing through explanations or instructions
- Treating patients impersonally
- Making patients feel they are taking up too much of your time or asking too many questions
- Forgetting common courtesies, such as saying please and thank you
- Showing boredom

A good way to avoid negative communication is to open your eyes and ears to others in service-oriented workplace settings. The next time you buy something at a store, call a company for information over the phone, or eat out at a restaurant, take note of the way the staff treats you. Do they answer your questions courteously? Do they give you the information you ask for? Do they make you feel welcome? What specifically makes their communication style positive or negative? Remember, you can always improve your communication skills.

Body Language

Verbal communication refers to communication that is spoken. Nonverbal communication is also known as **body language**. Body language includes facial expressions, eye contact, posture, touch, and attention to personal space. In many instances, people's body language conveys their true feelings, even when their words may say otherwise. A patient might say "I'm OK about that," but if she is sitting with her arms folded tightly across her chest and avoids looking at you, she may not mean what she says.

Facial Expression. Your face is the most expressive part of your body. You can often tell whether someone has understood your message simply by his facial expression. For example, when you are explaining a procedure to a patient, look at his expression. Does it seem puzzled? Is his brow wrinkled? Does he look surprised? Facial expressions can give you clues about how to tailor your communication efforts. They also serve as a form of feedback.

Eye Contact. Eye contact is an important part of positive communication. Look directly at patients when speaking to them. Looking away or down communicates that you are not interested in the person or that you are avoiding her for some reason.

There may be cultural differences in the ways patients react to eye contact. In some cultures, for example, it is common to avoid eye contact out of respect for someone who is considered a superior. Thus, children may be taught not to look adults in the eye.

Posture. The way you hold or move your head, arms, hands, and the rest of your body can project strong nonverbal messages. During communication, posture can usually be described as open or closed.

Open Posture. A feeling of receptiveness and friendliness can be conveyed with an **open posture**. In this position, your arms lie comfortably at your sides or in your lap. You face the other person, and you may lean forward in your chair. This demonstrates that you are listening and are interested in what the other person has to say. Open posture is a form of positive communication.

Closed Posture. A **closed posture** conveys the opposite, a feeling of not being totally receptive to what is being said. It can also signal that someone is angry or upset. A person in a closed posture may hold his arms rigidly or fold them across his chest. He may lean back in his chair, away from the other person. He may turn away to avoid eye contact. Slouching is a kind of closed posture that can convey fatigue or lack of caring. Watch for patients with closed postures that may indicate tension or pain. Avoid closed postures yourself—they have a negative effect on your communication efforts.

Touch. Touch is a powerful form of nonverbal communication. A touch on the arm or a hug can be a means of saying hello, sharing condolences, or expressing congratulations. Family background, culture, age, and gender all influence people's perception of touch. Some people may welcome a touch or think nothing of it. Others may view touching as an invasion of their privacy. In general, in the medical setting, a touch on the shoulder, forearm, or back of the hand to express interest or concern is acceptable.

Personal Space. When communicating with others, it is important to be aware of the concept of personal space. **Personal space** is an area that surrounds an individual. By not intruding on patients' personal space, you show respect for their feelings of privacy.

In most social situations, it is common for people to stand 4 to 12 ft away from each other. For personal conversation, you would typically stand between 1½ and 4 ft away from a person. Some patients may feel uncomfortable—and may become anxious—when you stand or sit close to them. Others prefer the reassurance of having people close to

them when they speak. Watch patients carefully. If they lean back when you lean forward or if they fold their arms or turn their head away, you may be invading their personal space. If they lean or step toward you, they may be seeking to close up the personal space.

Improving Your Communication Skills

Sharpening your communication skills should be an ongoing effort and will help you become a more effective communicator. Good communication skills can enhance the quality of your interaction with patients and coworkers alike. Among the skills involved in communication are listening skills, interpersonal skills, therapeutic communication skills, and assertiveness skills.

Listening Skills

Listening involves both hearing and interpreting a message. Listening requires you to pay close attention not only to what is being said but also to nonverbal cues, such as those communicated through body language.

Listening can be passive or active. **Passive listening** is simply hearing what someone has to say without the need for a reply. An example is listening to a news program on the radio; the communication is mainly one-way. **Active listening** involves two-way communication. You are actively involved in the process, offering feedback or asking questions. Active listening takes place, for example, when you interview a patient for her medical history. Active listening is an essential skill in the medical office.

There are several ways to improve your listening skills:

- Prepare to listen. Position yourself at the same level (sitting, standing) as the person who is speaking, and assume an open posture (Figure 4-2).
- Relax and listen attentively. Do not simply pretend to listen to what is being said.
- Maintain eye contact.
- Maintain appropriate personal space.
- Think before you respond.
- Provide feedback. Restate the speaker's message in your own words to show that you understand.
- If you do not understand something that was said, ask the person to repeat it.

Interpersonal Skills

When you interact with people, you use **interpersonal skills.** When you make a patient feel at ease by being warm and friendly, you are demonstrating good interpersonal skills. In addition to warmth and friendliness, valuable interpersonal skills include empathy, respect, genuineness, openness, and consideration and sensitivity.

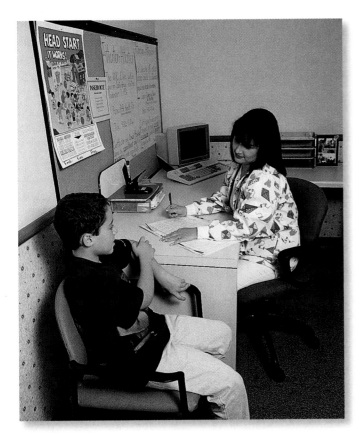

Figure 4-2. Active listening requires two-way communication and positive body language.

Warmth and Friendliness. A friendly but professional approach, a pleasant greeting, and a smile get you off to a good start when communicating with patients. When your approach is sincere, patients will be more relaxed and open.

Empathy. The process of identifying with someone else's feelings is **empathy.** When you are empathetic, you are sensitive to the other person's feelings and problems. For example, if a patient is experiencing a migraine headache and you have never had one, you can still let her know you are trying to imagine, or relate to, her situation. In other words, you can acknowledge the severity of her pain and show support and care. You must, however, always remain objective in your interaction with patients.

Respect. Showing respect can mean using a title of courtesy such as "Mr." or "Mrs." when communicating with patients. It can also mean acknowledging a patient's wishes or choices without passing judgment.

Genuineness. Being genuine in your interactions with patients means that you refrain from "putting on an act" or just going through the motions of your job. Patients like to know that their health-care providers are real people. In a medical setting, being genuine means caring for each patient on an individual basis, giving patients the full attention they deserve, and showing respect for them. Being genuine in your communication with patients encourages them to place trust in you and in what you say.

Openness. Openness means being willing to listen to and consider others' viewpoints and concerns and being receptive to their needs. An open individual is accepting of others and not biased for or against them.

Consideration and Sensitivity. You should always try to show consideration toward patients and act in a thoughtful, kind way. You must be sensitive to their individual concerns, fears, and needs.

Therapeutic Communication Skills

Therapeutic communication is the ability to communicate with a patient in terms that they can understand and, at the same time, feel at ease and comfortable in what you are saying. It is also the ability to communicate with other members of the health team in technical terms that are appropriate in a health-care setting. Therapeutic communication techniques are methodologies that can improve communication with patients.

Therapeutic communication involves the following communication skills:

- Being Silent. Silence allows the patient time to think without pressure.
- Accepting. This skill gives the patient an indication of reception. It shows that you have heard the patient and follow the patient's thought pattern. Some indicators of acceptance include nodding; saying "Yes," "I follow what you said," and other such phrases; and body language.
- Giving Recognition. Show patients that you are aware of them by stating their name in a greeting or by noticing positive changes. With this skill, you are recognizing the patient as a person or individual.
- Offering Self. Make yourself available to the needs of the patient.
- Giving a Broad Opening. Allow the patient to take the initiative in introducing the topic. Ask open-ended questions such as "Is there something you'd like to talk about?" or "Where would you like to begin?"
- Offering General Leads. Give the patient encouragement to continue by making comments such as "Go on" or "And then?"
- Making Observations. Make your perceptions known to the patient. Say things like "You appear tense today" or "Are you uncomfortable when you . . . ?" By calling patients' attention to what is happening to them, you encourage them to notice it for themselves so that they can describe it to you.
- Encouraging Communication. Ask patients to verbalize what they perceive. Make statements such as "Tell me when you feel anxious" or "What is happening?" Patients should feel free to describe their perceptions to you, and you must try to see things as they seem to the patients.
- Mirroring. Restate what the patient has said to demonstrate that you understand.

- Reflecting. Encourage patients to think through and answer their own questions. A reflecting dialogue may go like this:

  Patient: Do you think I should tell the doctor?

  Medical Assistant: Do you think you should?

  By reflecting patients' questions or statements back to them, you are helping patients feel that their opinions about their health are of value.

- Focusing. Focusing encourages the patient to stay on the topic.

- Exploring. Encourage patients to express themselves in more depth. Try to get as much detail as possible about a patent complaint, but avoid probing and prying if the patient does not wish to discuss it.

- Clarifying. Ask patients to explain themselves more clearly if they provide information that is vague or not meaningful.

- Summarizing. This skill involves organizing and summing up the important points of the discussion and gives the patient an awareness of the progress made toward greater understanding.

Ineffective Therapeutic Communication. In the previous section, the focus was on how to communicate effectively in a therapeutic environment. Oftentimes people think they are communicating thoroughly, but they are not. Here are some roadblocks that can interfere with your communication style:

- Reassuring. This type of communication indicates to the patient that there is no need for anxiety or worry. By doing this, you devalue the patient's feelings and give false hope if the outcome is not positive. The communication error here is a lack of understanding and empathy.

- Giving Approval. Giving approval is usually done by overtly approving of a patient's behavior. This may lead the patient to strive for praise rather than progress.

- Disapproving. Being disapproving is done by overtly disapproving of a patient's behavior. This implies that you have the right to pass judgment on the patient's thoughts and actions. Find an alternate attitude when dealing with patients. Adopting a moralistic attitude may take your attention away from the patient's needs and may direct it toward your own feelings.

- Agreeing/Disagreeing. Overtly agreeing or disagreeing with thoughts, perceptions, and ideas of patients is not an effective way to communicate. When you agree with patients, they will have the perception that they are right because you agree with them or because you share the same opinion. Opinions and conclusions should be the patient's, not yours. When disagreeing with patients, you become the opposition to them instead of their caregiver. Never place yourself in an argumentative situation regarding the opinions of a patient.

- Advising. If you tell the patient what you think should be done, you place yourself outside your scope of practice. You cannot advise patients.

- Probing. Probing is discussing a topic that the patient has no desire to discuss.

- Defending. Protecting yourself, the institution, and others from verbal attack are classified as defending. If you become defensive, the patient may feel the need to discontinue communication.

- Requesting an Explanation. This communication pattern involves asking patients to provide reasons for their behavior. Patients may not know why they behave in a certain manner. "Why" questions may have an intimidating effect on some patients.

- Minimizing Feelings. Never judge or make light of a patient's discomfort. It is important for you to perceive what is taking place from the patient's point of view, not your own.

- Making Stereotyped Comments. This type of communication involves using meaningless clichés when communicating with patients. An example of a stereotypical comment is "It's for your own good." These types of comments are given in an automatic, mechanical way as a substitute for a more reasonable and thoughtful explanation.

Defense Mechanisms. When working with patients, it is important to observe their communication behaviors. Patients will often develop *defense mechanisms,* which are unconscious, to protect themselves from anxiety, guilt, and shame.

Here are some common defense mechanisms that a patient may display when communicating with the doctor, medical assistant, or other health-care team members:

- Compensation: Overemphasizing a trait to make up for a perceived or actual failing

- Denial: An unconscious attempt to reject unacceptable feelings, needs, thoughts, wishes, or external reality factors

- Displacement: The unconscious transfer of unacceptable thoughts, feelings, or desires from the self to a more acceptable external substitute

- Dissociation: Disconnecting emotional significance from specific ideas or events

- Identification: Mimicking the behavior of another to cope with feelings of inadequacy

- Introjection: Adopting the unacceptable thoughts or feelings of others

- Projection: Projecting onto another person one's own feelings, as if they had originated in the other person

- Rationalization: Justifying unacceptable behavior, thoughts, and feelings into tolerable behaviors

- Regression: Unconsciously returning to more infantile behaviors or thoughts

- Repression: Putting unpleasant thoughts, feelings, or events out of one's mind

TABLE 4-1	A Comparison of Nonassertive, Assertive, Aggressive, and Nonassertive Aggressive Behavior			
	Nonassertive Behavior	**Assertive Behavior**	**Aggressive Behavior**	**Nonassertive Aggressive Behavior (NAG)**
Characteristics of the behavior	Emotionally dishonest, indirect, self-denying; allows others to choose for self; does not achieve desired goal	Emotionally honest, direct, self-enhancing, expressive; chooses for self; may achieve goal	Emotionally honest, direct, self-enhancing at the expense of another, expressive; chooses for others; may achieve goal at expense of others	Emotionally dishonest, indirect, self-denying; chooses for others; may achieve goal at expense of others
Your feelings	Hurt, anxious, possibly angry later	Confident, self-respecting	Righteous, superior, derogative at the time and possibly guilty later	Defiance, anger, self-denying; sometimes anxious, possibly guilty later
The other person's feelings toward you	Irritated, pity, lack of respect	Generally respected	Angry, resentful	Angry, resentful, irritated, disgusted
The other person's feelings about her/himself	Guilty of superior	Valued, respected	Hurt, embarrassed, defensive	Hurt, guilty or superior, humiliated

Adapted from Alberti, Robert E., and Emmons, Michael, *Your Perfect Right: A Guide to Assertive Behavior,* San Luis Obispo, California: Impact, 1970.

- Substitution: Unconsciously replacing an unreachable or unacceptable goal with another, more acceptable one

Assertiveness Skills

As a professional, you need to be **assertive,** that is, to be firm and to stand by your principles while still showing respect for others. Being assertive means trusting your instincts, feelings, and opinions (not in terms of diagnosing, which only the doctor can do, but in terms of basic communication with patients), and acting on them. For example, when you see that a patient looks uneasy, speak up. You might say, "You look concerned. How can I help you feel more comfortable?"

Being assertive is different from being aggressive. When people are **aggressive,** they try to impose their position on others or try to manipulate them. Aggressive people are bossy and can be quarrelsome. They do not appear to take into consideration others' feelings, needs, thoughts, ideas, and opinions before they act or speak.

To be assertive, you must be open, honest, and direct. Be aware of your body position: an open posture conveys the proper message. When you communicate, speak confidently and use "I" statements such as "I feel . . ." or "I think . . ." (Assertiveness is also discussed later in the chapter in the section on communicating with coworkers.)

Developing your assertiveness skills increases your sense of self-worth and your confidence as a professional. Being assertive will also help you prevent or resolve conflicts more peacefully and increase your leadership ability. People look up to and respect professionals who are assertive in the workplace. See Table 4-1 for a comparison of assertive, nonassertive, and aggressive behaviors.

Communicating in Special Circumstances

If you make an effort to develop good interpersonal skills, most patients will not be difficult to communicate with. You will, however, encounter patients in special circumstances, when they may be anxious or angry. These situations sometimes inhibit communication. Patients from different cultures may pose challenges to communication. Others may have some type of impairment or disability that makes communication difficult. Similarly, young patients, parents with children who are ill or injured, and patients with terminal illnesses may present communication difficulties. Learning about the special needs of these patients and polishing your own communication skills will help you become an effective communicator in any number of situations.

The Anxious Patient

It is common for patients to be anxious in a doctor's office or other health-care setting. This reaction is commonly known as the "white-coat syndrome." There can be many reasons for anxiety. A patient can become anxious because she is ill and does not know what is wrong with her—she may fear the worst. A patient may have recently been diagnosed with an illness that he knows nothing about, which may necessitate a severe lifestyle change. Fear of bad news or fear that some procedure is going to be painful can create anxiety. Anxiety can interfere with the communication process. For example, because of anxiety a patient may not listen well or pay attention to what you are saying.

Some patients—particularly children—may be unable to verbalize their feelings of fear and anxiety. Watch for signs of anxiety. They may include a tense appearance, increased blood pressure and rates of breathing and pulse, sweaty palms, reported problems with sleep or appetite, irritability, and agitation. Procedure 4-1 will help you communicate with patients who are anxious.

The Angry Patient

In a medical setting, anger may occur for many reasons. Anger may be a mask for fear about an illness or the outcome of surgery. Anger may come from a patient's feeling of being treated unfairly or without compassion. Anger may stem from a patient's resentment about being ill or injured. Anger may be a reaction to frustration, rejection, disappointment, feelings of loss of control or self-esteem, or invasion of privacy.

As a medical assistant, you will encounter angry patients and will need to help them express their anger constructively, for the sake of their health. At the same time, you must learn not to take expressions of anger personally; you may just be the unlucky target. A goal with angry patients is to help them refocus emotional energy toward solving the problem. Study the following steps in communicating with an angry patient.

1. Learn to recognize anger and its causes. Anger is easy to recognize in most people, but it can be subtle in others. Patients who speak in a tense tone, are stubborn, or appear to ignore your attempts at communication may be angry.

2. Remain calm and continue to demonstrate genuineness and respect. Communicate that you respect and care about the patient's feelings.

3. Focus on the patient's physical and medical needs.

4. Maintain adequate personal space. Place yourself on the same level as the patient. If the patient is standing, encourage him to sit down. Maintain an open posture to show that you are receptive to listening. Maintain eye contact, but avoid staring at the patient, which can make the person angrier.

5. Avoid the feeling that you need to defend yourself or to give reasons why the patient should not be angry. Instead, listen attentively and with an open mind to what the patient is saying. Most patients' anger will lessen if they know someone is really listening to them and showing an interest in their emotions and needs.

6. Encourage patients to be specific in describing the cause of their anger, their thoughts about it, and their feelings. Be empathic and acknowledge the patient's feelings and perceptions. Follow through with any promises you might make concerning correction of a problem, but avoid totally agreeing or disagreeing with the patient. State what you can and cannot do for the patient.

7. Present your point of view calmly and firmly to help the patient better understand the situation. If patients are receptive to your viewpoint, their perspective may change for the better.

8. Avoid a breakdown in communication. Allow the patient to voice anger. Trying to outtalk the patient or overexplain will only annoy and irritate him. You might also suggest that the patient spend a few moments alone to gather his thoughts or to cool off before continuing any type of communication.

9. If you feel threatened by a patient's anger or if it looks as if the patient's anger may become violent, leave the room and seek assistance from one of the physicians or other members of the office staff. Document any threats in the patient's chart.

Patients of Other Cultures

Our beliefs, attitudes, values, use of language, and views of the world are unique to us, but they are also shaped by our cultural background. In any health-care setting, you will most likely have contact with patients of diverse cultures and ethnic groups. Each culture and ethnic group has its own behaviors, traditions, and values. Rather than viewing these differences as barriers to communication, strive to understand and be tolerant of them.

Remember that these beliefs are neither superior nor inferior to your own. They are simply different. Never allow yourself to make value judgments or to stereotype a patient, a culture, or an ethnic group. Each patient is an individual in her own right.

Different Views and Perceptions. It is common for patients in many cultures to view health-care professionals as superior to themselves intellectually, socially, and economically. Patients from minority ethnic groups may feel that health-care professionals of the majority ethnic group cannot understand them or identify with them. In some cases, unfortunately, they may be right. The professional's attitude of superiority may stem from the feeling that because she knows more about medical issues than the patient does, she is somehow more important than the patient.

PROCEDURE 4.1

Communicating With the Anxious Patient

Objective: To use communication and interpersonal skills to calm an anxious patient

Materials: None

Method

1. Identify signs of anxiety in the patient.
2. Acknowledge the patient's anxiety. (Ignoring a patient's anxiety often makes it worse.)
3. Identify possible sources of anxiety, such as fear of a procedure or test result, along with supportive resources available to the patient, such as family members and friends. Understanding the source of anxiety in a patient and identifying the supportive resources available can help you communicate with the patient more effectively.
4. Do what you can to alleviate the patient's physical discomfort. For example, find a calm, quiet place for the patient to wait, a comfortable chair, a drink of water, or access to the bathroom (Figure 4-3).
5. Allow ample personal space for conversation. Note: You would normally allow a 1½- to 4-ft distance between yourself and the patient. Adjust this space as necessary.
6. Create a climate of warmth, acceptance, and trust.
   a. Recognize and control your own anxiety. Your air of calm can decrease the patient's anxiety.
   b. Provide reassurance by demonstrating genuine care, respect, and empathy.
   c. Act confidently and dependably, maintaining truthfulness and confidentiality at all times.
7. Using the appropriate communication skills, have the patient describe the experience that is causing anxiety, her thoughts about it, and her feelings. Proceeding in this order allows the patient to describe what is causing the anxiety and to clarify her thoughts and feelings about it.
   a. Maintain an open posture.
   b. Maintain eye contact, if culturally appropriate.
   c. Use active listening skills.
   d. Listen without interrupting.
8. Do not belittle the patient's thoughts and feelings. This can cause a breakdown in communication, increase anxiety, and make the patient feel isolated.
9. Be empathic to the patient's concerns.
10. Help the patient recognize and cope with the anxiety.
    a. Provide information to the patient. Patients are often fearful of the unknown. Helping them understand their disease or the procedure they are about to undergo will help decrease their anxiety.
    b. Suggest coping behaviors, such as deep breathing or other relaxation exercises.
11. Notify the doctor of the patient's concerns.

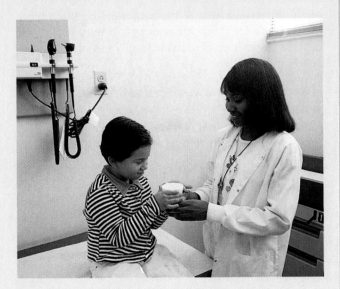

Figure 4-3. You can calm children's anxiety by spending time talking with them, playing a game, reading a story, or just offering a glass of water.

Do your best to treat patients of all cultures and ethnic groups with equal respect. Effective communication cannot take place unless you respect the patient's dignity and maintain the patient's sense of self-worth.

Maintaining an open mind will help you see and understand differences in cultural perceptions to which you must be sensitive. For example, patients may have different views of their role and the role of their families in the

Multicultural Attitudes About Modern Medicine

Patients' cultural backgrounds have a great effect on their attitudes toward health and illness. Patients from different cultural backgrounds often have beliefs about the causes of illness, what symptoms mean, and what to expect from health-care professionals that are different from those of modern medicine. Understanding some of these perceptions, behaviors, and expectations will help you communicate effectively with patients of different cultures.

Beliefs About Causes of Illness

Some cultures have beliefs about the causes of illness that differ sharply from accepted notions in the mainstream culture. As an example, many cultures believe that some illnesses are caused by hot or cold forces in the body. Some believe that winds and drafts cause illness or that illness can be caused by blood that is too thick or too thin. Others believe that having bad feelings toward others can create ill health.

Because of such beliefs, it may be hard to obtain information from patients about possible reasons for their medical problems. It may also be hard for some patients to realize the importance of taking medication to treat certain illnesses. In this case, you may have to be very persuasive and firm when giving the patient instructions for medication usage. It may be helpful or necessary to involve other family members in persuading the patient.

How Symptoms Are Presented and What They Mean

People from different cultures may differ in the way they perceive and report symptoms. Some may express pain very emotionally because their culture may feel that suppressing pain is harmful. In contrast, people from other cultures may not admit that they are in pain, thinking that acknowledging pain is a sign of weakness. People of all cultures may be more likely to report physical symptoms of illness than they are to report psychologic symptoms. Be aware of nonverbal indications of pain or other symptoms.

Treatment Expectations

Patients from other cultures may be totally unaccustomed to some of the practices of modern medicine. Patients of certain ethnic or cultural groups often consult other types of healers before seeing a doctor. They are likely to have different expectations of treatment from each.

Patients from other cultures may be wary of certain treatments because these treatments are so different from what they are accustomed to. This is especially true of some of the medical procedures and interventions considered to be state-of-the-art, such as laser surgery or diabetes management.

When dealing with patients of other cultures, keep in mind their perspectives on health care. Try to avoid generalizations and cultural stereotyping, however, because there can be a variation of attitudes within ethnic groups. Treat each patient as an individual, and you will be providing the best care possible.

---

health-care process. They may view the roles of men and women differently than you do. Patients may also have different views of the cause of their illness and how it should be treated. "Caution: Handle With Care" discusses different cultural views of health care.

The Language Barrier. Patients who cannot speak or understand English may have difficulty expressing their needs or feelings effectively. You may need to speak through an interpreter to gather and convey information or to discuss sensitive issues with a patient. Instead of using medical terms, which can be difficult to translate, try to say the same thing using basic, familiar words and simple phrases.

If the patient comes to the office often, take the time to learn some basic phrases in the patient's native language, such as "How are you feeling today?" and "Is there anything I can get you?" Even if the rest of your conversation must take place in English, your small efforts will be much appreciated.

The Patient With a Visual Impairment

When communicating with a patient who has a visual impairment, be aware of what you say and how you say it. Since people with visual impairments cannot usually rely on nonverbal clues, your tone of voice, inflection, and speech volume take on greater importance.

Following are some suggestions for communicating with a patient who has a visual impairment.

- Use large-print materials whenever possible.
- Make sure there is adequate lighting in all patient areas.
- Use a normal speaking voice.
- Talk directly and honestly. Explain instructions thoroughly.
- Do not talk down to the patient; preserve the patient's dignity.

The Patient With a Hearing Impairment

Hearing loss can range from mild to severe. How you communicate depends on the degree of impairment and on whether the patient has effective use of a hearing aid.

Following are some tips to help you communicate effectively with a hearing-impaired patient.

- Find a quiet area to talk, and try to minimize background noise.
- Position yourself close to and facing the patient. The patient will rely on visual clues such as the movement of your lips and mouth, your facial expression, and your body language (Figure 4-4).
- Speak slowly, so the patient can follow what you are saying.
- Remember that elderly patients lose the ability to hear high-pitched sounds first. Try speaking in lower tones.
- Speak in a clear, firm voice, but do not shout, especially if the patient wears a hearing aid.
- To verify understanding, ask questions that will encourage the patient to repeat what you said.
- Whenever possible, use written materials to reinforce verbal information.

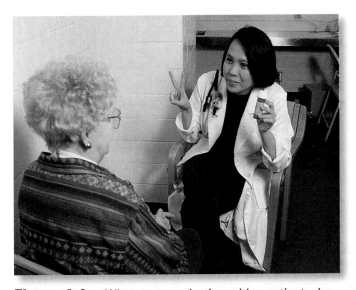

Figure 4-4. When communicating with a patient who has a hearing impairment, position yourself close to the patient and use gestures and effective body language.

The Patient Who Is Mentally or Emotionally Disturbed

There may be times when you will need to communicate with patients who are mentally or emotionally disturbed. When dealing with this type of patient, you need to determine what level of communication the patient can understand. Keep these suggestions in mind to improve communication.

- It is important to remain calm if the patient becomes agitated or confused.
- Avoid raising your voice or appearing impatient.
- If you do not understand, ask the patient to repeat what he said.

The Elderly Patient

Medical assistants now spend at least 50% of their time caring for older patients. Be aware of the vast differences in the capabilities of people of this age group. Do not stereotype all elderly patients as frail or confused. Most are not, and each patient deserves to be treated according to her own individual abilities.

Always treat elderly patients with respect. Regardless of their physical or mental state, elderly patients are adults. Do not talk down to them. Use the title "Mrs." or "Mr." to address older people unless they ask you to call them by their first name.

Denial or Confusion. Some elderly patients deny that they are ill. For example, in a survey of elderly people, the majority of whom had at least one chronic condition, 85% reported that they were in good or excellent health (Bradley and Edinberg, 1990). Patients' perception of how they feel may be quite different from their actual state of health.

The reverse situation can also occur. Elderly patients may overreact to a problem and consider themselves sicker than they really are. They may become dependent, passive, or anxious. Elderly patients may also over- or underestimate their ability to perform certain tasks or to deal with certain limitations.

Elderly patients may be confused if they have some impairment in memory, judgment, or other mental abilities. Signs of confusion can occur with Alzheimer's disease, senility, depression, head injury, or misuse of medications or alcohol. Elderly patients may or may not be aware of their condition. They may have difficulty understanding instructions.

The following tips can help you communicate with elderly patients.

- Act as if you expect the patient to understand.
- Respond calmly to any confusion on the patient's part. Tell the truth. Use facts. Do not go along with misconceptions or make up explanations.
- Use simple questions and terms, but avoid using baby talk or speaking to the patient as if he were a child.

- Explain points slowly and clearly, using concrete terms rather than abstract expressions. Say, for example, "You may feel a pinprick and a sting when I put the needle in" instead of "You may feel some discomfort in your arm."
- Ask the patient to relax and speak slowly.
- If you do not understand the patient, simply say that you cannot understand her well and ask her to repeat what she said. Do not say you understand when in fact you do not. It is important not to belittle the patient. It is equally important to inform yourself about what could be very important information.

The Importance of Touch. Because they often live alone, many elderly patients experience a lack of physical touch. Using touch—offering to hold a patient's hand or placing an arm around his shoulder—communicates that you care about the patient's well-being.

Terminally Ill Patients

Terminally ill patients are often under extreme stress and can be a challenge to treat. It is important that health-care professionals respect the rights of terminal patients and treat them with dignity. It is also important that you communicate with the family and offer support and empathy as their loved one accepts her condition. You should also provide information on **hospice,** which is an area of medicine that works with terminally ill patients and their families. Hospice workers often go to the home of the terminally ill patient or work with patients in facilities. Hospice care is usually staffed with RNs who have specialized training in issues related to death and dying. They work with the family and patient in the beginning, assisting with medications, and they end by making arrangements with the funeral home and coroner.

Elisabeth Kübler-Ross, a world-renowned authority in the areas of death and dying, developed a model of behavior that patients will experience on learning their condition. This is called the Stages of Dying or Stages of Grief. This model is widely used today in work with terminally ill patients.

Kübler-Ross's Stages of Dying include five stages, which usually—but not always—progress in the following order:

1. Denial. Patients are in direct denial or periods of disbelief. This defense is generally temporary.
2. Anger. Patients may suddenly realize what is really happening and respond with anger. They can become difficult patients in this stage and display temper tantrums and fits of rage.
3. Bargaining. Patients attempt to make deals with physicians, clergy, and family members. Patients at this stage may become more cooperative and congenial.
4. Depression. The patient will begin to show signs of depression, such as withdrawal, lethargy, and sobbing.

The patient's body is beginning to deteriorate, and the patient may experience more pain and realize that relationships with family and friends will soon be gone.

5. Acceptance. Patients accept the fact that they are dying. They will begin arrangements for when they expire, making funeral or burial requests. The patient's family needs the most support at this stage.

Even though these stages have been generalized to dying, many experts have applied them to the grieving process as well.

The Young Patient

A doctor's office can be a frightening place for children. They often associate the doctor's office with getting a shot or being sick. Sometimes parents have misled their children about what to expect from a visit to the doctor. When dealing with children, it is better to recognize and accept their fear and anxiety than to dismiss these emotions. When children realize that you take their feelings seriously, they are more apt to be receptive to your requests and suggestions.

Explain any procedure, no matter how basic (such as testing a reflex with a reflex hammer), in very simple terms. Let the child examine the instrument.

Other suggestions include using praise ("You were very brave") and always being truthful. Do not tell children that a procedure will not hurt if it will, or you will lose their trust.

As children get older, you can use more detailed descriptions when explaining procedures. Remember that after the age of 7 or 8, children can tell if they are being talked down to or treated like babies. Encourage them to participate actively in their care, and direct any questions or instructions to them, when appropriate. You should also respect the adolescent's request not to have a parent present during private conversations.

Parents

Parents are naturally concerned about their children and are likely to be worried or anxious when a child is ill. Children often react to a situation based on how they see their parents react. Reassuring parents and keeping them calm can also help children relax.

The Patient With AIDS and the Patient Who Is HIV-Positive

Patients with acquired immunodeficiency syndrome (AIDS) and patients who have the human immunodeficiency virus (HIV), the virus that causes AIDS, have a grave illness to deal with. They also face a society that often stigmatizes them, saying they have only themselves to blame. These patients often feel guilty, angry, and depressed. Many literally hate themselves.

To communicate effectively with these patients, you need accurate information about the disease and the risks involved. Take the initiative to educate yourself about AIDS and HIV. Patients will have many questions. Part of your role as a good communicator will be to answer as many questions as you can. If a patient asks a question you cannot answer, tell the physician, so he can respond quickly.

Above all, remember that HIV is not transmitted through casual or common physical contact, such as brushing by a person in a crowded hall or shaking hands. It is transferred only through bodily fluids. Patients with AIDS and those who are HIV-positive need to know you are not afraid to be near them, to touch them, or to talk to them. Like any patient whose body is being ravaged by a serious illness, these patients need human contact (verbal and physical), and they need to be treated with dignity.

Patients' Families and Friends

Family members or friends sometimes accompany a patient to the office. These individuals can provide important emotional support to the patient. Always ask patients if they want a family member or friend to accompany them to the examination room, however. Do not just assume their preference. Acknowledge family members and friends, and communicate with them as you do with patients. They should be kept informed of the patient's progress, whenever possible, to avoid unnecessary anxiety on their part. You must always protect patient confidentiality, however. Too often, health-care workers think that it is acceptable to discuss patient cases in detail with family members, even without the consent of the patient.

Communicating With Coworkers

The quality of the communication you have with coworkers greatly influences the development of a positive or negative work climate and a team approach to patient care. In turn, the workplace atmosphere ultimately affects your communication with patients.

Positive Communication With Coworkers

In your interactions with coworkers, use the same skills and qualities that you use to communicate with patients. Have respect and empathy; be caring, thoughtful, and genuine; and use active listening skills. These skills will help you develop **rapport,** which is a harmonious, positive relationship, with your coworkers (Figure 4-5).

Following are some rules for communication in the medical office.

- Use proper channels of communication. For example, if you are having problems getting along with a coworker, try first to work it out with her. Do not go

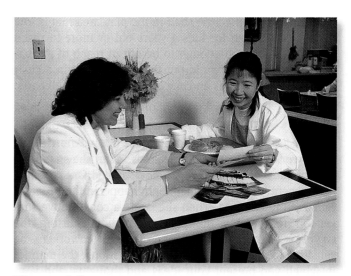

Figure 4-5. Rapport with coworkers is easy to build when you are open, friendly, and thoughtful.

over her head and complain to her supervisor. Your coworker may not have realized the effect of her behavior and may wish to correct it without involving her supervisor. If you go to the supervisor right away, working relationships can become even more strained.
- Have the proper attitude. You can avoid conflict and resolve most problems if you maintain a positive attitude. A friendly approach is much more effective than a hostile approach. Remember that many problems are simply the result of misinformation or lack of communication.
- Plan an appropriate time for communication. If you have something important to discuss, schedule a time to do so. For example, if you want to talk with the office manager about renewing the lease of a piece of office equipment, tell him you would like to discuss that topic and ask him to let you know a time that is convenient.

As an example of good communication with coworkers, consider this exchange between Mai Lee, a medical assistant, and Margot, a coworker in a pediatric practice. Note the way Mai Lee demonstrates assertiveness.

Mai Lee: I know you spent a lot of time choosing the new toys for the reception area. I love the wooden safari animal puzzles.

Margot: Thanks. I think the children really enjoy themselves now.

Mai Lee: I wanted to mention to you, though, that I'm concerned about the toy tea set with miniature cupcakes and sandwiches. Anything that's smaller than a golf ball is a choking hazard to infants and toddlers.

Margot: I don't think the little ones pay much attention to the tea set. It's mostly for older kids.

Mai Lee: Yes, but I'm still afraid that a baby could put one of those pieces in his mouth. What if we

According to some experts on stress, there are five stages that lead to burnout (Miller and Smith). The road to burnout follows this path:

1. The Honeymoon Phase. During the honeymoon phase, your job is wonderful. You have boundless energy and enthusiasm, and all things seem possible. You love the job and the job loves you. You believe it will satisfy all your needs and desires and solve all your problems. You are delighted with your job, your coworkers, and the organization.

2. The Awakening Phase. The honeymoon wanes and the awakening stage starts with the realization that your initial expectations were unrealistic. The job isn't working out the way you thought it would. It doesn't satisfy all your needs, your coworkers and the organization are less than perfect, and rewards and recognition are scarce.

   As disillusionment and disappointment grow, you become confused. Something is wrong, but you can't quite put your finger on it. Typically, you work harder to make your dreams come true. But working harder doesn't change anything and you become increasingly tired, bored, and frustrated. You question your competence and ability, and start losing your self-confidence.

3. Brownout Phase. As brownout begins, your early enthusiasm and energy give way to chronic fatigue and irritability. Your eating and sleeping patterns change, and you indulge in escapist behaviors such as partying, recreational drugs, alcoholism, and binge shopping. You become indecisive and your productivity drops. Your work deteriorates. Coworkers and superiors may comment on it.

   Unless interrupted, brownout slides into later stages. You become increasingly frustrated and angry and project the blame for your difficulties onto others. You are cynical, detached, and openly critical of the organization, superiors, and coworkers. You are beset with depression, anxiety, and physical illness.

4. Full-Scale Burnout Phase. Unless you wake up and interrupt the process or someone intervenes, brownout drifts remorselessly into full-scale burnout. Despair is the dominant feature of this final stage. It may take several months to get to this phase, but in most cases it takes three to four years. You experience an overwhelming sense of failure and a devastating loss of self-esteem and self-confidence. You become depressed and feel lonely and empty.

   Life seems pointless, and there is a paralyzing, "what's the use" pessimism about the future. You talk about "just quitting and getting away." You are exhausted physically and mentally. Physical and mental breakdowns are likely. Suicide, stroke, or heart attack is not unusual as you complete the final stage of what all started with such high hopes, energy, optimism, and enthusiasm.

5. The Phoenix Phenomenon. You can arise from the ashes of burnout (like a phoenix), but it takes time.

First, you need to rest and relax. Don't take work home. If you're like many people, the work won't get done and you'll only feel guilty for being "lazy."

Second, be realistic in your job expectations as well as your aspirations and goals. Whoever you're talking to about your feelings can help you, but be careful. Your readjusted aspirations and goals must be yours and not those of someone else. Trying to be and do what someone else wants you to be or do is a sure-fire recipe for continued frustration and burnout.

Third, create balance in your life. Invest more of yourself in family and other personal relationships, social activities, and hobbies. Spread yourself out so that your job doesn't have such an overpowering influence on your self-esteem and self-confidence.

The Policy and Procedures Manual

The policy and procedures manual is a key written communication tool in the medical office. No discussion of communication in the medical office would be complete without a description of this important document. The manual is used by permanent employees as well as by temporary employees who may be hired when others are ill or on vacation or when there is an unusually heavy workload. The manual covers all office policies and clinical procedures. It is usually developed as a joint effort by the physician (or physicians) and the staff (often the medical assistant).

Policies

Policies are rules or guidelines that dictate the day-to-day workings of an office. Although individual policies vary from office to office, most medical office manuals describe the following policy areas:

- Office purposes, objectives, and goals as set down by the physician(s)
- Rules and regulations
- Job descriptions and duties of staff personnel
- Office hours
- Dress code
- Insurance and other benefits
- Vacation, sick leave, and other time away from the office
- Salary and performance evaluations
- Maintenance of equipment and supplies
- Mailings
- Bookkeeping
- Scheduling of appointments and maintenance of patient records
- OSHA guidelines

The policy section of the manual also typically describes the chain of command for the office, or the person to whom each employee reports. This information is sometimes presented in chart form and called an organizational chart. For example, the receptionist, secretary, medical assistant, and billing person might report to the office manager. The office manager, in turn, might report directly to the physician or physicians. This chain of command varies from office to office, depending on the size and needs of the practice.

Procedures

Detailed instructions for specific procedures are covered in the procedures section of the manual. The areas discussed include clinical procedures and quality assurance programs.

Each clinical procedure should include instructions about the following:

- Purpose of the test, clinical application, and usefulness
- Specimen required and collection method; special patient preparation or restrictions
- Reagents, standards, controls, and media used; special supplies
- Instrumentation, including calibration and schedules
- Step-by-step directions
- Calculations
- Frequency and tolerance of controls; corrective action to be taken if tolerances are exceeded
- Expected values; values requiring special notification; interpretation of values

- Procedure notes (e.g., linearity or detection limits)
- Limitations of method (e.g., interfering substances and/or pitfalls and precautions)
- Method validation
- References
- Effective date and schedule for review
- Distribution

Developing a Manual

Although it is likely that your office will already have a manual, you may be involved in reorganizing, producing, or updating the manual. In any event, it is important to understand how a manual is developed.

Planning. To begin planning a manual, first determine a format, or how you will organize the information. The format depends on the office's needs and organization. Many offices prefer a loose-leaf notebook in which pages can easily be replaced when changes or updates are necessary. Figure 4-8 shows a sample page from a manual.

After determining a format, create an outline, organizing the topics and subtopics. Have it approved by the office manager and physician or physicians. In the procedures section, begin each procedure sheet on a new page. Include the following for each procedure page:

- The style to be used for each procedure, whether quantitative or qualitative

---

MILLSTONE MEDICAL ASSOCIATES

Policy and Procedures Manual

Procedure for Creating a Medical File for a New Patient

GOAL: To create a complete medical record for each new patient containing all necessary personal and medical information

PROCEDURE:
1. Establish that the patient is new to the doctor's office.
2. Ask the patient for all necessary insurance information. If the patient has an insurance card, make a photocopy of it for his file.
3. Ask the patient to fill out the patient information form. Keyboard the information onto a new patient information form, for legibility.
4. Review all information with the patient, to check for accuracy.
5. Label the new patient's folder, according to office procedure. Type either the patient's name (for an alphabetic file) or the correct number (for a numerical file).
6. If filing is done numerically, fill out a cross-reference form on the computer, along with a patient ID card to be stored in a secure location.
7. Add the patient's name to the necessary financial records, including the office ledger, whether on paper or on the computer.
8. After completing the folder label information, place the new patient information form inside the folder, along with any other personal or medical information that pertains to the patient.
9. On the outside of the patient's folder, clip a routing slip.

Figure 4-8. This page from a policy and procedures manual provides the office staff with information about creating a medical file for a new patient.

beepers or pagers, answering machines, and fax machines. How limited would a medical practice become if the recording of the care given to a patient had to done *without* the use of a word processor, computer, or typewriter? What if all patient billing, bank deposits, and payroll management had to be done *without* the use of an adding machine or calculator? Without a shredder, each piece of confidential paper would have to be torn many times before discarding. Possibly the most difficult of all tasks would be the duplication of endless documents by hand because there is no copy machine!

In this chapter you will be learning about the use and maintenance of many important pieces of administrative medical office equipment. Additionally, you just might come away with a new appreciation of the importance they play in the function of the efficient medical practice.

CASE STUDY

Meg is a CMA and is the first to arrive each morning at the busy medical practice where she works. As she unlocks the back door, she is thinking about the entry process. She knows she will set off an alarm as she enters and that she must go immediately to the security alarm box on the nearby wall and type in her security code number to turn off the system.

Meg walks to the front door and unlocks it. As she walks to her desk, she notices the fire extinguisher hanging on the wall. She makes a note to herself to call the maintenance company today to notify them that the expiration date on the extinguisher is this month. They will replace the old one with another extinguisher.

Meg next turns on all the lights. As she walks through the quiet front office, she sees three messages in the fax machine that have come in overnight. She picks them up and scans them quickly before she places them in the center of her desk.

She switches on the copy machines. On the top display is a four-digit number that indicates the number of copies each machine has made this month. Because it is the first of the month, she will call the leasing company today to report that number. Her office is billed based on how many copies are made each month.

Sitting at her desk, Meg turns off the telephone answering machine, which has been in operation throughout the night. There are four messages. As she listens, she makes careful notes before she discards each message and turns off the system. She knows that the phone will start ringing soon.

Meg turns on her computer and reviews all the tasks ahead of her today as a CMA in a busy medical practice. She has received e-mail from another doctor's office asking her to call about a new referral. Another e-mail is requesting medical records.

There is one more thing Meg must check before she settles in to her day's work. She makes her way to the break room and makes a big pot of coffee for all the staff. With a steaming coffee mug in hand, Meg walks back to her desk. Let the day begin!

As you read this chapter, consider the following questions:

1. What factors might go into the choice of an answering machine over the use of an answering service?
2. What backups for system failure might be important for the equipment in a medical office?
3. How could a misdialed phone number on the fax machine impact the life of a patient?
4. Why is routine maintenance of all office equipment important?

Office Communication Equipment

When you think of equipment for a medical office, you probably imagine x-ray machines, blood pressure monitors, and stethoscopes. You will, however, find many other kinds of equipment in a medical practice. Medical offices also use business communication equipment, which includes telephones, facsimile machines, computers, and photocopiers. One of your duties as a medical assistant may be to operate the medical office's communication equipment.

Just as medical equipment has evolved over the years, so has office equipment. The office communication equipment available years ago handled only the most basic tasks. Medical practices may have had a single telephone and a typewriter. If copies of patient records were required,

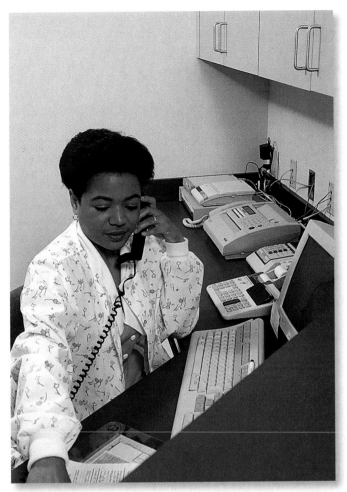

Figure 5-1. Most medical offices today rely on many up-to-date pieces of communication equipment.

medical assistants handwrote a duplicate set or used carbon paper to make additional copies.

Today technology allows almost instantaneous communication of information throughout the world. This instant communication can be critical for the fast-paced medical profession, where information often translates to the need for immediate treatment, sometimes in life-threatening situations. Communicating effectively within a medical office can be as vital as providing the correct treatment to patients—and often ensures that they receive such treatment (Figure 5-1).

Telephone Systems

Although the telephone is a common item in offices, it is one of the most important pieces of communication equipment in a medical practice. Not only is it the instrument patients use to communicate with the office, but it is also the primary means of communication with other doctors, hospitals, laboratories, and other businesses important to the practice.

Multiple Lines. Few practices can function with just one telephone line because if that line is in use, no other calls can come in or go out. Most medical offices have a telephone system that includes two or more telephones and several telephone lines. The six-button telephone is a popular choice in medical practices. This system has four lines for incoming or outgoing calls, an intercom line, and a button for putting a call on hold.

A telephone system can be set up so that incoming calls ring on all the telephones in the office. A more common setup in busy practices is to use a switchboard, a device that receives all calls. The receptionist then routes calls to the appropriate telephone extensions.

Patient Courtesy Phone. Some offices have a patient courtesy phone, which provides an outside local phone line strictly for the use of patients. Long-distance calls should be blocked from this phone. The addition of such a line leaves office lines free for business calls. This phone is located in the reception area. A patient courtesy phone provides a line of communication for patients to call for transportation or to contact work or family as needed. It is helpful to post a sign near the phone to indicate guidelines for its use. Calls are usually limited to two minutes.

Leaving a Message on an Answering Machine or Fax Machine. On occasion, it is also important to send a message to a patient's answering machine or fax machine. It is now required by law, including HIPAA, that you use these pieces of equipment correctly and confidentially. The goal in calling a patient's home is to speak directly to the patient or to leave a message with enough information to get the patient to call back. Be careful to avoid disclosing confidential patient information to anyone but the patient. Your primary concern is to guard the patient's private medical information. *Never* leave any information if you are unsure of the phone number dialed. Additionally, even if you know the number is correct, you cannot ensure that only the intended patient will receive the message. To guard the patient's privacy, *state only the following information:*

- The name of the individual for whom the message is intended
- The date and time of the call
- The name of your office or practice
- Your name as the contact person in the office
- The phone number of your office or practice
- The hours the office is open for a return call
- A request for a return call

Be especially careful of the hasty and indiscriminate use of fax machines. HIPAA law now states that the best format for the use of fax machines involves the use of a locked mailbox at the receiver's end of the transmission. Most in-home users, however, will not have this feature. It is always best to simply fax a request containing only the same information that was recommended for answering machines.

Automated Menu. Instead of using a switchboard, some medical practices route calls by means of an automated menu. Callers listen to the recorded menu and, in response, press a number on their telephone keypad. For example, the menu will say, "Press 2 to speak to Dr. Lowell." The caller presses 2, and the phone rings in Dr. Lowell's office. The Tips for the Office section provides more information on routing calls through an automated menu. If your office uses such a menu, make sure the voice prompts are clear and understandable.

Voice Mail. An automated menu is often used in conjunction with **voice mail,** which is an advanced form of answering machine. If a doctor is out of her office or taking another telephone call, the call is answered by voice mail, and the caller can leave a message. One of the benefits of a voice-mail system is that callers never receive a busy signal.

Answering Machine. Many offices use a telephone answering machine to answer calls after office hours, on weekends and holidays, and when the office is closed for any reason. A typical recorded message announces that the office is closed and states when it will reopen. The message must always indicate how the caller can reach the doctor or the answering service in an emergency.

An answering machine may be programmed simply to play a taped message from the office, or it may also record messages from callers. If callers can leave messages, you should check the answering machine to retrieve them at the start of each day and after the lunch break.

Answering Service. Instead of or in addition to an answering machine, most medical offices use an answering service. Unlike answering machines, answering services provide people to answer the telephone. They take messages and communicate them to the doctor on call. The doctor on call is responsible for handling emergencies that may occur when the office is closed, such as at night or on weekends or holidays.

Upon receiving a call from the answering service, the doctor calls the patient. For example, the doctor may recommend ways for the patient to alleviate her pain and ask her to come into the office the next morning.

Answering services can be used in two ways. The doctor's office may have an answering machine to record calls of a routine nature and give the number of the answering service to call in emergencies. Alternatively, the answering service may have a direct connection to the doctor's office, picking up calls after a certain number of rings day or night or during specific hours.

Although most answering services provide satisfactory, sometimes even outstanding, service, it is good practice to check up on the service every so often by calling it during its coverage hours. This quality check ensures that the service meets office standards and expectations.

Tips for the Office

Routing Calls Through an Automated Menu

An automated menu system answers calls for you and separates requests into categories so that you can deal with them efficiently. You may already be familiar with automated menus, which are widely used by many large businesses. Someone who calls an automated system hears a recorded message identifying the business. The message gives the caller a list of options from which to choose to identify the purpose of the call. The caller selects an option by pressing the corresponding button on her push-button telephone. If she does not have a push-button telephone, her call is automatically routed so that she can talk to a person or leave a voice-mail message.

How does an automated menu system save time and effort in a medical office? You don't have to answer calls as they come in but can instead reserve a block of time in which to listen and respond to messages. This system allows you to complete other work without interruption.

To set up an automated system, you need to plan specific categories from which patients can choose. Categories may include (1) making and changing appointments, (2) asking billing questions, (3) asking medical questions of the doctors or nurses, (4) reporting patient emergencies, and (5) calls from another doctor's office.

When the caller presses the code for a patient emergency, the call rings in the office because it needs to be answered immediately. You or other staff members can respond to calls in the other categories in a timely fashion. Questions for doctors or nurses can be routed immediately to the appropriate voice mail, bypassing you and the office receptionist.

Automated menu systems can be set up by telephone vendors listed in the yellow pages. When choosing an automated telephone system, be careful that callers do not become lost in the process. It is a good idea to set up a system that allows callers to return easily to the main menu. Be sure to build in an option for rotary dial telephones as well. Following up on messages promptly will also help callers feel comfortable with your voice-mail system, so you should check for messages at least once every hour.

Some answering services specialize in medical practices. These medical specialty services will ask the medical practice to give specific directives for the triage of calls. Always ask any service for references before signing a contract for service.

Pagers (Beepers)

Physicians often need to be reached when they are out of the office, so many carry pagers. Pagers or beepers are small electronic devices that give a signal to indicate that someone is trying to reach the physician.

Technology of Paging. Each paging device is assigned a telephone number. When someone calls that number, the pager picks up the signal and beeps, buzzes, or vibrates to indicate that a call has been made. Most pagers have a window that displays the caller's telephone number so that the person who has been paged can return the call promptly. Certain models display a short message. Some pagers store telephone numbers so that the receiver can return several calls without having to write down the numbers.

Paging a Physician. Many telephone messages can wait until the physician returns to the office or calls in for messages. When a message needs to be delivered immediately, however, paging is an efficient response. The paging process is as simple as making a telephone call.

1. A list of pager numbers for each physician in the practice should be kept in a prominent place in the office, such as by the main switchboard. Make sure you know where these numbers are kept. Look up the telephone number for the pager of the physician you need to contact.

2. Dial the telephone number for the pager.

3. You will hear the telephone ringing and the call picked up. Listen for a high-pitched tone, which signals the connection between the telephone and the pager.

4. To operate most pagers, you need to dial the telephone number you wish the physician to call, followed by the pound sign (#), located below the number 9 on a push-button telephone. (Some pager services have an operator and work much like an answering service. Give the operator a message, and the operator will contact the physician.)

5. Listen for a beep or a series of beeps signaling that the page has been transmitted. Then hang up the phone. The physician will call the number at his earliest convenience.

Interactive Pagers (I-Pagers)

Interactive pagers (I-pagers) are designed for two-way communication. The individual carrying the pager is paged in much the same way as the traditional pager. The pager can be set on "Audio" or "Vibrate" to alert the carrier that a message is coming in. However, the interactive pager screen displays a printed message and allows the physician to respond by way of a mini keyboard.

The physician can respond to the printed page by typing a return message (done by typing with the thumbs). The physician can respond back in real time to the office. The office computer and the physician enter into a conversation much like e-mail or an Internet chat room. Many problems can be handled quickly and efficiently in this manner. Additionally, because the I-pager can function silently, the physician can communicate with her office while in a meeting without disturbing others.

Each interactive pager has its own wireless Internet address. The user types in the receiving party's e-mail address and creates a message on a monitor screen. The interactive pager will give the sender the status of his message by indicating on the screen when the message has been sent, received, or read.

I-pagers can communicate with other I-pagers as well. I-pagers also have broadcast capability, meaning the sender can send to more than one receiver at a time. For this reason, practices with multiple physicians may find them very helpful.

Interactive pagers can also send messages to traditional telephones. The message is typed into the pager, and the system "calls" the telephone number. When answered, an electronic-type voice reads the message to the individual who has answered.

Facsimile Machines

Critical documents, such as laboratory reports or patient records, often need to be sent immediately to locations outside the office. Documents can be sent by means of a facsimile machine, or fax machine. A fax machine scans each page, translates it into electronic impulses, and transmits those impulses over the telephone line. When they are received by another fax machine, they are converted into an exact copy of the original document.

A fax machine in a medical office should have its own telephone line. A separate line ensures that transmission of incoming and outgoing faxes will not be interrupted and that the machine will not tie up a needed telephone line when sending or receiving information.

Benefits of Faxing. A fax machine can send an exact copy of a document within minutes. The cost for sending a fax is the same as for making a telephone call to that location. For a short document, this is usually less expensive than an overnight mail service.

Many fax machines have a copier function and can be used as an extra copy machine. This function may only be useful, however, if the machine uses plain paper. The telephone for the fax may also be used as an extra extension for outgoing calls, if needed.

Thermal Paper Versus Plain Paper. Some fax machines print on rolls of specially treated paper called electrothermal, or thermal, paper, which reacts to heat and electricity. Thermal paper tends to fade over time, so documents received on this type of paper may need to be photocopied. Many new models of fax machines use plain paper instead of thermal paper, avoiding the need for making copies. Information is transferred to the plain paper by either a carbon ribbon or a laser beam.

Sending a Fax.   Sending a fax is a simple process. One or more pages of a document can be sent at any given time.

1. Prepare a **cover sheet,** which provides information about the transmission. Cover sheets can vary in appearance but usually include the name, telephone number, and fax number of the sender and the receiver; the number of pages being transmitted; and the date. Often medical practices use preprinted cover sheets, with blanks that can be filled in for each transmission. All cover sheets must carry a statement of disclaimer to guard the privacy of the patient. A **disclaimer** is a statement of denial of legal liability. (A sample cover sheet is shown in Figure 5-2.) A disclaimer should be included on the cover sheet and may read something like the following: "This fax or e-mail contains confidential or proprietary information that may be legally privileged. It is intended only for the named recipient(s). If an addressing or transmission error has misdirected the fax or e-mail, please notify the author by replying to this message. If you are not the named recipient, you are not authorized to use, disclose, distribute, copy, print, or rely on this fax or e-mail and should immediately shred it or delete it from your computer system."

2. Place all pages face down in the fax machine's sending tray or area. Dial the telephone number of the receiving fax machine, using either the telephone attached to the fax machine or the numbers on the fax keyboard.

3. If you use the fax telephone, listen for a high-pitched tone. Then press the "Send" or "Start" button, and hang up the telephone. Your fax is now being sent.

4. If you use the fax keyboard, press the "Send" or "Start" button after dialing the telephone number. This button will start the call.

5. Watch for the fax machine to make a connection. Often a green light appears as the document feeds through the machine.

6. If the fax machine is not able to make a connection, as when the receiving fax line is busy, it may have a feature that automatically redials the number every few minutes for a specified number of attempts.

City Medical Associates
555 London Street Strathspey, PA 19919

Janet Michaels, MD   INTERNAL MEDICINE   Scott J. Michaels, MD

FACSIMILE COVER SHEET

Date: _____

To: _____   From: _____

Fax #: _____   Fax #: _____

# of pages (including this cover sheet): _____

Message: _____

_____

Figure 5-2.   Every document that is sent by fax transmission should include a cover sheet, which provides details about the transmission. A disclaimer should be included on the cover sheet.

7. When a fax has been successfully sent, most fax machines print a confirmation message. When a fax has not been sent, the machine either prints an error message or indicates on the screen that the transmission was unsuccessful.

Receiving a Fax. Faxes can be received 24 hours a day if the fax machine is turned on and has an adequate supply of paper. If the fax machine is not already sending or receiving a fax, the fax telephone rings briefly, signaling the start of a transmission. The transmission begins shortly thereafter, with the machine printing out the document as it is sent. When completed, the machine usually prints a transmission report, with the number of pages, the date and time, and the originating fax number.

Typewriters

Typewriters can be used to create correspondence, interoffice documents, medical forms brought in by patients or sent from insurance companies, and patient bills. Typewritten documents are easier to read than handwritten ones and project a more businesslike appearance.

Models and Features. Although typewriter models differ in features, all use a standard keyboard. Placement of the keys is identical on each typewriter. The arrangement is not alphabetic. Rather, the most frequently used keys are near the middle, where your fingers can most easily reach them, and the least used keys are toward the outside.

A wide variety of typewriter models are available. Most offices use electric or electronic models. Although both are powered by electricity, they differ in their ability to perform certain functions. For example, electronic typewriters can store limited amounts of information for further use, but electric typewriters cannot. Both electric and electronic typewriters provide a wide selection of features, including, but not limited to, automatic carriage return, automatic centering, self-correction, and changeable typefaces or fonts.

Typewriters Versus Word Processors. Typewriters should not be confused with word processors, which perform a similar function but are more sophisticated. Word processors can store entire documents in memory, thereby allowing much greater flexibility in manipulating material than do typewriters. Word processors display documents on a screen or monitor, and these documents can be revised as often as needed before being printed out. Word processors are typically more expensive than typewriters, but they are less expensive than computers and make it easy to generate perfect documents.

Today many medical practices use computers with word processing software. (Chapter 6 discusses the use of computers in a medical office.)

Office Automation Equipment

Using automated equipment enables you to perform a task more easily and quickly than doing it manually. For example, adding numbers on a calculator is a much faster process than doing it on paper. Many of the administrative tasks in a medical practice can be accomplished with automated equipment, giving you more time to perform other procedures.

Photocopiers

A photocopier, also called a copier or copy machine, instantly reproduces office correspondence, forms, bills, patient records, and other documents. Before photocopiers were available, offices used carbon paper to reproduce documents as they were being typed. The number of copies that could be made was limited.

A photocopier takes a picture of the document it is to reproduce and prints it on plain paper using a heat process. Photocopiers use either liquid or dry toner, a form of ink. They can make an unlimited number of copies. Photocopiers do not require treated or otherwise special paper. Various kinds of paper can be used in the machine, including office stationery and colored paper. Many photocopiers accept different sizes of paper, from the standard 8½- by 11-inch paper to 8½- by 14-inch legal paper and even larger.

Photocopiers come in many models, from desktop machines for limited use to industrial models for continual heavy use. The machines vary in features and speed. All styles of machines are available through purchase or lease.

Special Features. Copiers offer a wide range of special features. They may collate (assemble sets of multiple pages in order) and staple pages, enlarge or reduce images, and produce double-sided copies (print on both sides of the page). Some can also adjust contrast and even track the cost of a job via a specific code input into the machine. Although the majority of photocopiers used in medical offices produce black-and-white copies, photocopiers are available that make color copies. Some copiers can make transparencies (text and images printed on clear acetate), which physicians often use for presentations.

One of the more useful features of photocopiers is the help function. Selecting this function displays directions in plain English that explain how to fix a paper jam or deal with other routine copier problems. Some copiers are even programmed to indicate that service is needed.

Making Copies. Although the procedure for making copies differs slightly from machine to machine, most machines can be operated by following these basic steps.

1. Make sure the machine is turned on and warmed up. It will display a signal when it is ready for copying.

2. Prepare your materials, removing paper clips, staples, and self-adhesive flags.

3. Place the document to be copied in the automatic feeder tray as directed, or upside down directly on the glass. The feeder tray can accommodate many pages; you may place only one page at a time on the glass. Automatic feeding is a faster process, and you should use it when you wish to collate or staple packets. Page-by-page copying is advantageous if you need to copy a single sheet or to enlarge or reduce the image. To use any special features, such as making double-sided copies or stapling the copies, you have to press a button on the machine.

4. Set the machine for the desired paper size.

5. Key in the number of copies you want to make, and press the "Start" button. The copies are made automatically.

6. If necessary, press the "Clear" or "Reset" button when your job is finished to prepare the machine for the next user.

7. If the copier becomes jammed, follow the directions on the machine to locate the problem (for example, there may be multiple pieces of paper stuck inside the printer), and dislodge the jammed paper. Most copy machines will show a diagram of the printer and the location of the problem.

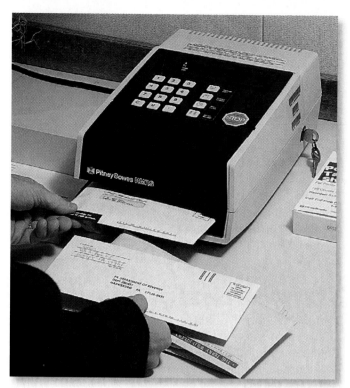

Figure 5-3. The postage meter is a convenient and cost-effective way to apply postage to office correspondence and packages.

Adding Machines and Calculators

For handling tasks such as patient billing, bank deposits, and payroll, medical practices depend on adding machines and calculators. The difference between the two types of machines is minimal. Adding machines typically plug into an outlet and produce a paper tape on which calculations are printed. Calculators are more often battery- or solar-powered, with memory to store figures. Calculators are portable and usually do not produce a paper tape.

Routine Calculations. Both adding machines and calculators are sufficient for routine office calculations. These machines perform basic arithmetic functions, such as addition, subtraction, multiplication, and division. Many of today's models perform such specialized functions as computing percentages and storing data. Some are even computerized.

Checking Your Work. It is easy to hit an incorrect key or to key in a number twice when using an adding machine or a calculator. Therefore, check all mathematical computations. An error on a bill causes problems for both the patient and the office.

If the machine produces a paper tape, check the numbers on the tape against the numbers you are adding. The paper tape is especially useful when adding a long series of numbers. Without a printed record, you must perform the same calculations again to make sure the total is correct.

Postage Meters

Every medical office uses the U.S. Postal Service. Patient bills, routine correspondence, purchase orders, and payments are just some of the items typically sent by mail. (See Chapter 7 for additional information on mailing correspondence.)

Although some medical offices use stamps, most use a postage meter. A postage meter is a machine that applies postage to an envelope or package, eliminating the need for postage stamps (Figure 5-3). There are often two parts to a postage meter: the meter, which belongs to the post office, and the mailing machine, which the practice can own. The meter actually applies the postage, and the mailing machine does the rest, such as sealing the envelope.

Benefits of Using a Postage Meter. There are several advantages to using a postage meter instead of purchasing stamps. It saves frequent trips to the post office. It also saves money for the office by providing the exact amount of postage needed for each item. When you have to use a combination of stamps, you may exceed the required postage. It is unlikely as well as impractical for a practice to keep every denomination of stamps on hand.

Some postage meters can imprint envelopes with the name of your medical practice or with a message at the same time postage is applied. The message appears immediately to the left of the postal mark, at the top of the envelope.

PROCEDURE 5.1

How to Use a Postage Meter

Objective: To correctly apply postage to an envelope or package for mailing, according to U.S. Postal Service guidelines

Materials: Postage meter, addressed envelope or package, postal scale

Method

1. For the postage meter to function, there must be money in your postal account. Contact the company that is managing your account or your local post office for more information.

2. Verify the day's date. U.S. Postal Service guidelines prohibit mailing envelopes and packages that are postmarked with an incorrect date. Check that the postage meter is plugged in and switched on before you proceed.

3. Locate the area where the meter registers the date. Many machines have a lid that can be flipped up, with rows of numbers underneath. Months are represented numerically, with 1 symbolizing January, 2 symbolizing February, and so on. Check that the date is correct. If it is not, change the numbers to the correct date.

4. Make sure that all materials have been included in the envelope or package. Weigh the envelope or package on a postal scale. Standard business envelopes weighing up to 1 oz require the minimum postage (the equivalent of one first-class stamp). Oversize envelopes and packages require additional postage. A postal scale will indicate the amount of postage required.

5. Key in the postage amount on the meter, and press the button that enters the amount. For amounts over $1, you may have to press a "$" button or the "Enter" button twice. This feature verifies large amounts, catching errors in case you mistakenly press too many keys.

6. Check that the amount you typed is the correct amount. Envelopes and packages with too little postage will be returned by the U.S. Postal Service. If you send an envelope or package with too much postage, your practice will not be reimbursed.

7. If you are applying postage to an envelope, hold it flat and right side up (so that you can read the address). Seal the envelope (unless the meter seals it for you). As you face the postage meter, locate the plate or area where the envelope can slide through. This feature is usually near the bottom of the meter. Place the envelope on the left side, and give it a gentle push toward the right. Some models hold the envelope in a stationary position. (If the meter seals the envelope for you, be sure to place it correctly to allow for sealing.) The meter will grab the envelope and pull it through quickly.

8. For packages, you need to create a postage label to affix to the package. Follow the same procedure for a label as for an envelope. Affix the postmarked label on the package in the upper right corner.

9. Check that the printed postmark has the correct date and amount and that it is legible.

Many types of postage meters are available, from basic models for a small office to advanced models for large businesses. The latest machines include automatic date setting, memory to program a large mailing, and display alerts for low postage or the need for ribbon replacement. Some models can apply postage to parcels without the use of labels or tape. Procedure 5-1 shows you how to use a postage meter.

Prepaying for Postage. To use a postage meter, you must prepay the postage. You can take your meter to the post office to add postage, or you can use a postage meter service. A service maintains the postal account for you. Although the money in each account is the property of the U.S. Postal Service, the provider manages the account and adds postage to the meter. Postage can also be added to the meter by telephone or by modem, with data sent directly to the meter over the telephone line. The process takes only a few minutes, and the call is often toll-free. Before postage can be added, however, money must be deposited into an account. Keeping the postage account current ensures that all mail is sent on a timely basis. This task may be one of your responsibilities.

On any meter, you can check the amount of postage used and the amount remaining with the touch of a button. On some models, the meter must have $10 or more for the machine to apply postage to an envelope or package.

Postage Scales

Besides the postage meter, you also need a scale. Postal scales are a good investment because they show both the weight and the amount of postage required. Some postage

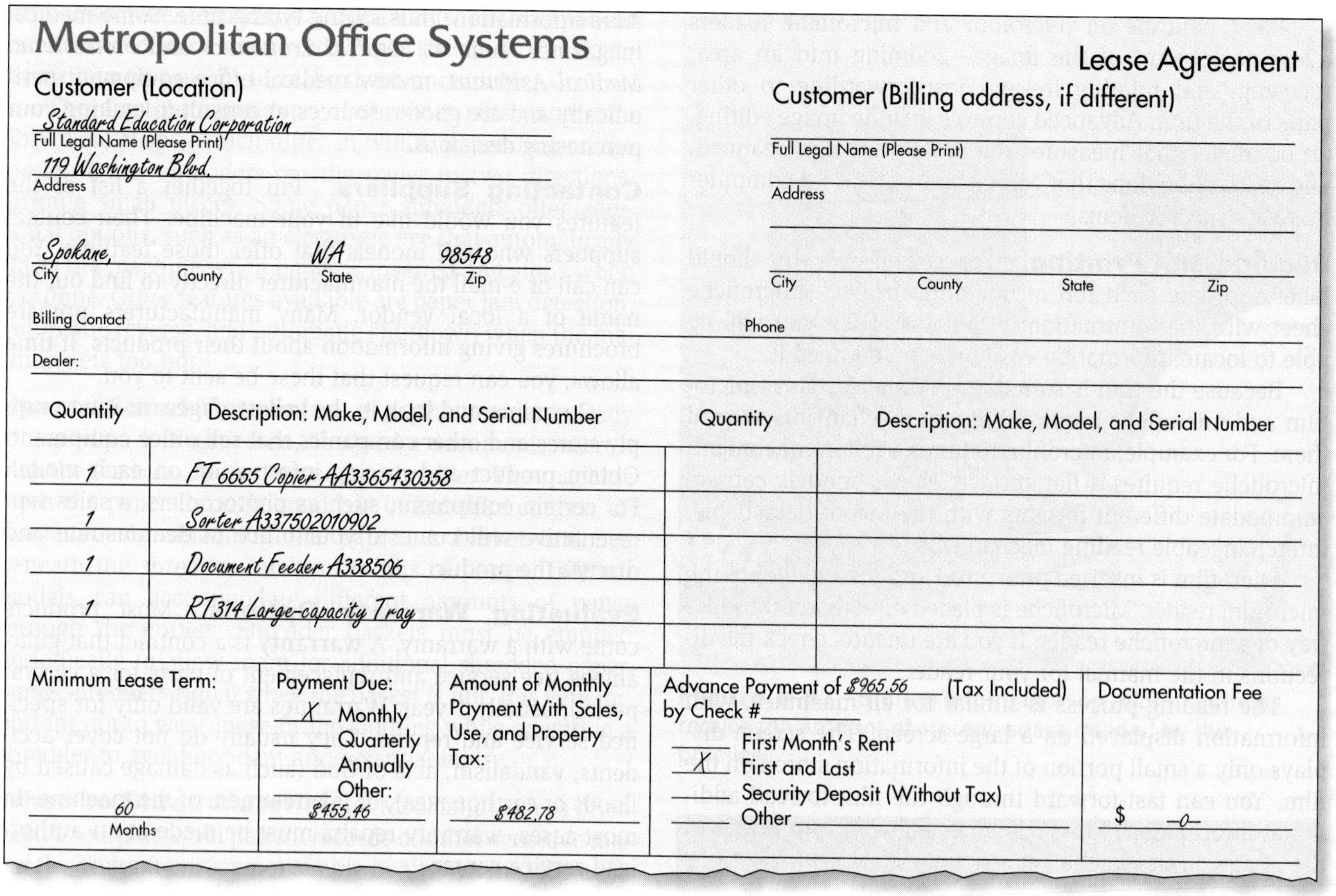

Metropolitan Office Systems

Lease Agreement

Customer (Location)

Standard Education Corporation
Full Legal Name (Please Print)

119 Washington Blvd.
Address

Spokane,   _WA_   _98548_
City   County   State   Zip

Billing Contact

Dealer:

Customer (Billing address, if different)

Full Legal Name (Please Print)

Address

City   County   State   Zip

Phone

Quantity	Description: Make, Model, and Serial Number	Quantity	Description: Make, Model, and Serial Number
1	FT 6655 Copier AA3365430358		
1	Sorter A337502010902		
1	Document Feeder A338506		
1	RT 314 Large-capacity Tray		

Minimum Lease Term:	Payment Due:	Amount of Monthly Payment With Sales, Use, and Property Tax:	Advance Payment of _$965.56_ (Tax Included) by Check #_____	Documentation Fee
60 Months	_X_ Monthly ___ Quarterly ___ Annually ___ Other: $455.46	$482.78	___ First Month's Rent _X_ First and Last ___ Security Deposit (Without Tax) ___ Other _____	$ _–0–_

Figure 5-8. Read lease agreements carefully.

For most large pieces of office equipment, such as photocopiers, there is also an option to **lease** the equipment. Leasing, or renting, usually involves an initial charge and a monthly fee. On average, the initial charge is equal to about two monthly payments.

Lease Agreement. A lease is for a specified time, after which time the equipment is returned to the seller (Figure 5-8). Some leases allow purchase of the equipment at the end of the rental period for an additional payment. The details of the purchase option are covered in the lease agreement.

Advantages of Leasing. When you lease a product, your office does not own it, but you have several advantages. Leasing allows purchasers to keep more of their money. The initial cost of obtaining the machine is a fraction of the full cost of purchasing it. Therefore, the remainder of the money can earn interest in the bank or be used for other expenses. Leasing is advantageous when you do not have enough money to buy the equipment but need the services it provides. In addition, leasing allows businesses to update equipment every few years at the end of each lease period. Updating may not be as affordable if you buy equipment. Often the company that leases the product is also responsible for servicing it. Finally, in most cases, businesses are able to take lease payments as a tax deduction each year.

Leasing is not the best solution for everyone. It is important to weigh the advantages of leasing against the advantages of buying equipment for your medical practice.

Negotiating. Whether you decide to lease or buy equipment, always ask whether the price is firm or if there is room for negotiation. Although most equipment prices are set, terms can sometimes be negotiated on more expensive pieces of equipment. Companies that lease office equipment are often flexible in determining the monthly payment. For example, many companies accept smaller payments to start out, with larger payments near the end, or vice versa.

Some suppliers will match their competitors' prices. Also, if you are purchasing several pieces of equipment at the same time, a supplier may be able to offer some savings on the total cost of the purchase or provide some service, such as delivery, free of charge.

Maintaining Office Equipment

Office equipment must be regularly maintained to provide high-quality service. Daily or weekly maintenance, such as cleaning the glass on the photocopier or replacing toner, can be performed by the office staff. However, more extensive maintenance should be done by the equipment supplier.

Equipment Manuals

The best source of information about maintaining a piece of equipment is the manual that comes with it. This booklet gives basic information about the equipment, including how to set it up, how it works, special features, and problems you may encounter. The information in an equipment manual is extremely valuable. If the manual is lost, call the manufacturer to obtain another one. Equipment manuals should be filed where they can be retrieved easily.

Maintenance and Service Contracts

Equipment suppliers provide standard maintenance contracts when office equipment is purchased. A **maintenance contract** specifies when the equipment will be cleaned, checked for worn parts, and repaired. A standard maintenance contract may include regular checkups as well as emergency repairs.

In addition, some suppliers offer a **service contract,** which covers services that are not included under the standard maintenance agreement. For example, a service contract may cover emergency repairs if they are not covered under standard maintenance. In some cases, service contracts are combined with maintenance contracts in one document.

It is important to keep track of all maintenance performed on your equipment. Many offices keep a maintenance log, where staff members record the date and purpose of each service call. This log is helpful in identifying whether equipment should be replaced because of its need for frequent servicing.

Troubleshooting

You can call a service supplier the minute a piece of equipment stops functioning properly, but you can also take steps to see whether you can determine and correct the problem yourself. This process is called **troubleshooting.** Resolving the problem can save you the cost of a service call that may not be covered by your standard agreement.

The first step in troubleshooting is to eliminate possible simple causes of a problem. For example, if the machine is powered by electricity, make sure that it is plugged into a functioning outlet and that it is turned on. Are all doors and other openings in their correct positions? Are all machine connections firmly in place?

If you cannot discover a simple cause for the problem, it is time to test the machine to determine what it is failing to do. In the case of a malfunctioning photocopier, for example, try making a copy, and note the response. Write down any error messages the machine provides.

Next, consult the equipment manual. Many manuals devote a section to troubleshooting. If you cannot find the solution after reading the manual, call the manufacturer or the place of purchase for additional assistance. Be prepared to explain the steps you have already taken toward resolving the problem.

Backup Systems

Occasionally, more than one piece of equipment can be affected by a problem. For example, if the electricity goes off, all electrical equipment will go out at once. To avoid losing important information and records, it is important to have backup systems in place.

Computers. Computers should be placed on a backup system. The company that services the computer system usually sets this up. Computer backup may occur either automatically off-site over the phone lines or on-site, which may require that a staff member manually plug in a backup tape every night before going home. Computer backup usually occurs at midnight, when the office is not using the system. Computer backup ensures that all information will be retrievable even if the computers suffer a catastrophic failure.

Telephones. The use of cell phones in addition to traditional phones offers a backup to communication in the event that phone service is interrupted. Cell phones are also helpful during emergency weather conditions.

Electricity. A backup generator may supply emergency power for lighting in key hallways and exam rooms. Interior rooms and halls can quickly become very dark and hazardous when the electricity is unexpectedly cut off.

Battery Power. Battery power backup is a key component of security and warning system backups. Audio warning signals sound when it is time to replace the batteries in smoke and security detectors. These systems should be checked every six months.

Fire Extinguishers. Fire extinguishers need to be serviced or replaced once a year to ensure maximum performance. The office may choose to contract with a local company to provide this annual maintenance evaluation.

Equipment Inventory

Each piece of equipment is an asset of a business. It is part of the business's net worth and should be listed on the medical practice's balance sheet. Therefore, taking inventory of office equipment provides relevant information for the practice's money manager. It may also indicate whether old machinery is due for replacement.

There is no set format for taking an office equipment inventory. Figure 5-9 shows one example. Many offices use a master inventory sheet to survey all equipment at a glance. The master sheet usually includes such general information as equipment names and the quantity of each type of equipment.

EQUIPMENT INVENTORY

ITEM	PURCHASE DATE	PURCHASE PRICE
1. TotalOffice oak desk	10/15/02	$295.00
2. TotalOffice rolling desk chair	10/15/02	$119.00
3. TotalOffice 4-drawer file cabinet	1/28/03	$150.00
4. TotalOffice 2-drawer file cabinet	1/28/03	$100.00
5. HYtech Pentium 100 computer	5/29/04	$1150.00
6. HYtech 14-inch monitor	5/29/04	$200.00

Figure 5-9. An equipment inventory sheet includes equipment names and the quantity of each type of equipment.

Many offices also keep more detailed information about each individual piece of equipment in files or on a single sheet of paper. Detailed information may include the following:

- Name of the equipment, including the brand name
- Brief description of the equipment
- Model number and registration number
- Date of purchase
- Place of purchase, including contact information
- Estimated life of the product
- Product warranty
- Maintenance and service contracts

All equipment inventories should be updated periodically.

Summary

In many ways, state-of-the-art office equipment is as important for a medical office as its medical equipment. Although every office does not have the same equipment, common machines include telephones, computers, pagers, fax machines, dictation-transcription equipment, photocopiers, adding machines and calculators, postage meters, check writers, paper shredders, and microfilm or microfiche readers.

As a medical assistant, you may be expected not only to operate this equipment but also to help make purchasing decisions by researching various options. This research includes obtaining information about product features, warranties, and maintenance. Yet another decision is whether to lease or buy the equipment.

Equipment is an asset for a medical office. The office staff needs to maintain a comprehensive inventory of the products leased and purchased. It is important to keep up to date with new technologies that will help the administrative office function smoothly and efficiently.

CHAPTER 5

CASE STUDY QUESTIONS

Now that you have completed this chapter, review the case study at the beginning of the chapter and answer the following questions:

1. What factors might go into the choice of an answering machine over the use of an answering service?
2. What backups for system failure might be important for the equipment in a medical office?
3. How could a misdialed phone number on the fax machine impact the life of a patient?
4. Why is routine maintenance of all office equipment important?

Discussion Questions

1. Why is office equipment important to the medical office? Give at least three examples of pieces of typical office equipment, and describe their use in the medical office.
2. Compare and contrast the advantages and disadvantages of buying and leasing equipment.
3. What are some features of a standard product warranty?
4. Describe a scenario in which an interactive pager might be helpful in a medical office.

Critical Thinking Questions

1. Imagine that you are responsible for the maintenance of the office equipment in a busy medical practice. What weekly, monthly, and yearly checks might you perform? How would you document these checks?

2. You think that your office needs a new photocopier. Explain how you would justify this need to the office manager.
3. You have been asked to create a patient sign to hang on the wall over the courtesy phone. What will your sign say?
4. The fax machine in your office is malfunctioning. Explain the steps you might take to troubleshoot the problem.

Application Activities

1. Your office frequently uses temporary employees to help with copying. The office manager asks you to write directions for the use of the photocopier, to be posted near the machine. Using the computer, create a sign suitable for posting.
2. Your office is moving soon, and you have been asked to assist in the design of a new communication system for the practice. What features would you include in the new system?
3. You have been asked to design a cover sheet for the fax machine for your office. Using the computer, design a form with a disclaimer.
4. Go online and research three different types of photocopiers. Write a report describing each. Be sure to include the equipment name, manufacturer, warranty options, price, advantages to buying or leasing, features, and recommendations for use.

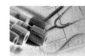

Carpal Tunnel Syndrome

As the number of computers used in the home and workplace has escalated in recent years, the number of cases of carpal tunnel syndrome has also risen dramatically. Carpal tunnel syndrome is a hand disorder that is often associated with computer use. The term for this condition comes from the name for a canal (the carpal tunnel) located in the wrist. Several tendons pass through this tunnel, allowing the hand to open and close.

Carpal tunnel syndrome results from repetitive motion, such as keyboarding, for hours at a time. This motion may cause swelling to develop around the tendons and carpal tunnel. The swelling compresses the nerve. The people most likely to develop carpal tunnel syndrome are workers whose jobs require them to perform repetitive hand and finger motions.

Symptoms

The symptoms associated with carpal tunnel syndrome include the following:

- Tingling or burning in the hands or fingers
- Weakness or numbness in the hands or fingers
- Hands that go to sleep frequently
- Difficulty opening or closing the hands
- Pain that stems from the wrist and travels up the arm

Tips for Prevention

If you use a keyboard for extended periods, you should practice proper techniques to prevent carpal tunnel syndrome.

- While seated, hold your arms relaxed at your sides, and check to make sure that your keyboard is positioned slightly higher than your elbows. As you input, keep your elbows at your sides, and relax your shoulders (see Figure 6-2).
- Use only your fingers to press keys, and do not use more pressure than necessary. Use a wrist rest, and keep your wrists relaxed and straight.

- When you need to strike difficult-to-reach keys, move your whole hand rather than stretching your fingers. When you need to press two keys at the same time, such as "Control" and "F1," use two hands.
- Try to break up long periods of keyboard work with other tasks that do not require computer use.

Tips for Relieving Symptoms

If you have symptoms of carpal tunnel syndrome, try these suggestions for relief.

- Elevate your arms
- Wear a splint on the hand and forearm
- Discuss your symptoms with a physician, who may prescribe medication

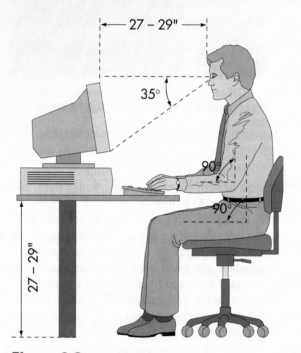

Figure 6-2. Maintaining proper posture and hand positions helps to avoid strain or injury of the back, eyes, neck, or wrist when keyboarding.

simply slide your finger across the touch pad. To click on an item, you push a button similar to that on a mouse or trackball, or you tap your finger on the touch pad.

Modem. This term **modem** is a shortened form of the words *modulator-demodulator*. A modem is used to transfer information from one computer to another over telephone lines. Because modems allow information to be transferred both to and from a computer, they are considered input/output devices. The speed at which a modem transfers data is called the baud rate. Although the current standard modem speed is 28,800 baud, modem speeds are continually being improved. Modems are essential for any medical office that needs to transfer files electronically, as when submitting insurance claim forms.

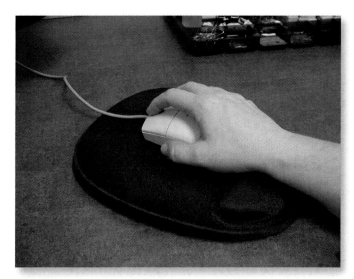

Figure 6-3. Using a mouse, you can point and click to access a variety of functions.

An advanced type of modem is a fax modem. This device allows the computer to send and receive files much as a fax machine does. A fax modem is not quite as versatile as a regular fax machine, however. The information being sent must first be input into the computer. You could not, for example, use a fax modem to send a patient record with handwritten notes on it.

Scanner. A **scanner** is a device used to input printed matter and convert it into a format that can be read by the computer. Scanners are useful in the medical office because patient reports from another doctor, a hospital, or another outside source can be easily entered into the computer. Scanners are also making it possible to move into a paperless medical system. Using a scanner is much faster than keyboarding, or inputting the information with a keyboard. Three types of scanners are available:

1. Handheld scanners are generally the least expensive but are more difficult to use and produce lower-quality results than the other two types.
2. A single-sheet scanner feeds one sheet of paper through at a time and looks similar to a single-sheet printer.
3. A flatbed scanner is the most expensive type of scanner but is the easiest to use and produces the highest-quality input. It works much like a small photocopier: the paper lies flat and still on a glass surface while the machine scans it.

Processing Devices. There are two major processing components inside the system unit, or computer cabinet. The **motherboard** is the main circuit board that controls the other components in the system. The **central processing unit (CPU),** or microprocessor, is the primary computer chip responsible for interpreting and executing programs.

How quickly the computer processes information depends on the type of microprocessor and its speed, which is measured in megahertz (MHz) or gigahertz (GHz). Most microprocessors are known by a number, such as 600 MHz or 3 GHz. A popular microprocessor is the Intel Pentium. Today's microprocessors are commonly measured in gigahertz. One gigahertz equals 1000 megahertz.

Storage Devices. One of the main tasks of a computer is to store information for later retrieval. The computer uses memory to store information either temporarily or permanently. Several types of drives are used for permanent information storage.

Memory. Computers use two types of memory to store data: **random-access memory (RAM)** and read-only memory (ROM). RAM is temporary, or programmable, memory. While you are working on a software program, the computer is accessing RAM. In general, the more RAM that is available, the faster the computer will perform. As software programs become more sophisticated, they require more RAM. Only a few years ago, 32 megabytes (MB) of RAM was the minimum amount needed to run most programs. (Megabytes are a measurement of memory space.) Today, however, many applications require much more RAM.

Read-only memory (ROM) is permanent memory. The computer can read it, but you cannot make changes to it. The purpose of ROM is to provide the basic operating instructions the computer needs to function.

Hard Disk Drive. The hard disk drive is where information is stored permanently for later retrieval. Software programs and important data are usually stored on the hard disk for quick and easy access. The amount of hard disk space needed to store software programs is increasing rapidly. The more software programs you want to store, the larger the hard disk you will need. Older computers have a 500- or 850-MB hard disk. Many newer computers have a hard disk capacity of 20 gigabytes (GB) to 250 gigabytes or more.

Diskette Drive. The diskette drive can read from and write to diskettes (also called disks). Flexible 5¼-inch disks, which were once commonly used, are now outdated. The standard diskette format in current use is 3½-inch disks, which are rigid. These disks are more compact and can store more information than the older, longer disks.

CD-ROM Drive. CD-ROMs look just like audio compact discs, but they contain software programs. The term **CD-ROM** stands for "compact disc—read-only memory." The main advantage of a CD-ROM over a diskette is its ability to store huge amounts of data.

CD-ROM drives have become standard equipment on most personal computers. Although many software packages are available on both CD-ROM and diskettes, some large programs are available only on CD-ROM. These programs include multimedia applications such as medical encyclopedias. **Multimedia** refers to software that uses more than one medium—such as graphics, sound, and text—to convey information.

Tape Drive. This storage device is used to back up (make a copy of) the files on the hard disk. The information is copied onto magnetic tapes that resemble audiotapes. If the hard drive malfunctions, you will have a copy of the information on these tapes. It is possible to back up the information onto diskettes. Most hard disks, however, contain so much information that a large number of diskettes would be required to back up all the data. With most tape drives, the entire contents of the hard disk can be stored on one or two tapes. Store these tapes at night in a fireproof container.

Output Devices. Output devices are used to display information after it has been processed. A monitor and a printer are two output devices needed in the medical office.

Monitor. A computer monitor looks like a television screen. It displays the information that is currently active, such as a word processing document, an Internet link, or e-mail. Monitors are available in color; all of the software programs that are used today, including multimedia applications, require a color monitor to run.

Color monitors vary in the number of colors they can display and in the resolution of the images. *Resolution* refers to the crispness of the images and is measured in dot pitch. The lower the dot pitch, the higher the resolution. For example, a monitor with a 0.26 dot pitch displays sharper images than a monitor with a 0.39 dot pitch. Using a high-resolution monitor can help you avoid eye strain.

Printer. A printer is required to produce a **hard copy,** which is a readable paper copy or printout of information (see Figure 6-4). You will need a printer to print out correspondence, patient reports, bills, insurance claims, and other documents. Printer resolution is noted in terms of dots per inch (dpi). The higher the dpi, the better the print quality. Printer output varies, depending on the type of printer and the model. The three most commonly used printers are dot matrix, ink-jet, and laser.

1. **Dot matrix printers** create characters by placing a series of tiny dots next to one another. The dot matrix printer is the only type that is an impact printer, which means that it makes an impression on the paper as it prints. Although it is the least expensive of the three types, the dot matrix printer is slower and noisier and produces a lower-quality output than the other types. Because it is an impact printer, however, it is the only type that is capable of producing multiple copies with carbon paper or other multicopy forms.

2. **Ink-jet printers** also form characters using a series of dots, but they are nonimpact printers in which the dots are created by tiny drops of ink. Many ink-jet printers are capable of printing in both black and color. Because of their high-quality output and affordable prices, ink-jet printers are popular for home and small-office use.

3. **Laser printers** are high-resolution printers that use a technology similar to that of photocopiers. Of the three printer types, laser printers are the fastest and produce the highest-quality output. Laser printers are more expensive than dot matrix or ink-jet printers. Prices have dropped significantly over the years, however, so laser printers may be affordable even for small medical offices.

Because each type of printer has advantages and disadvantages, some medical offices may purchase more than one type. For example, a medical office may have a dot matrix printer for creating internal memos and multipage insurance forms and a laser printer for creating documents whose quality resembles that of typeset documents.

A current trend in printers is the "all-in-one" model, which functions not only as an ink-jet printer but also as a fax machine, scanner, and photocopier. This type of machine may be convenient for a small medical office that requires each of these functions but does not have space for four separate devices. In addition, purchasing an all-in-one unit is usually more economical than purchasing the machines separately.

Software

Computer software is generally divided into two categories: operating system and application software. The operating system controls the computer's operation. Application software allows you to perform specific tasks, such as scheduling appointments.

Operating System. When you turn on a computer, the operating system starts working, providing instructions that the computer needs to function. Because most medical practices use IBM-compatible personal computers, the

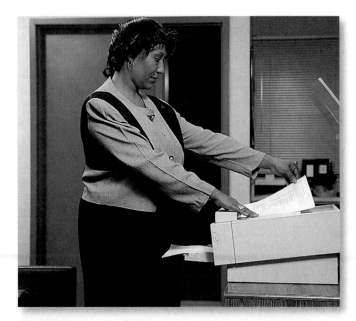

Figure 6-4. You may need to print out hard copies of documents to send to patients, vendors, insurance companies, or other doctors' offices.

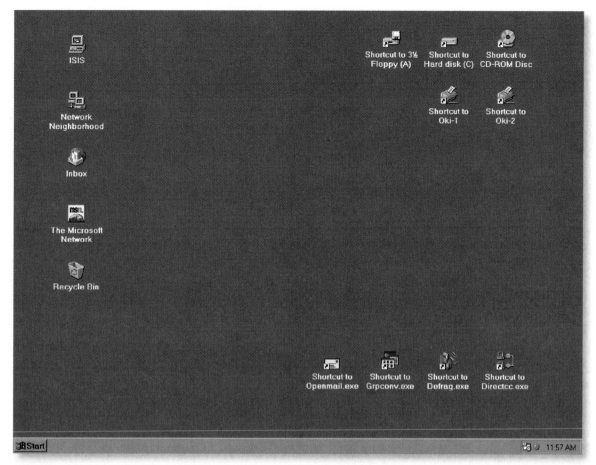

Figure 6-5. The Windows 2000 operating system employs a graphical user interface. Icons identify programs or other menu choices.

operating systems discussed here are DOS (disk operating system) and Microsoft Windows and Windows 2000. IBM-compatible computers are most suitable for businesses that use computers primarily to manipulate words. Apple computers are used by businesses, such as advertising agencies or design firms, that are extensively involved in graphics, visual images, or desktop publishing.

DOS. DOS is the original operating system created for IBM and IBM-compatible computers. It uses a command line interface—you must learn and use commands to perform certain tasks. For example, to copy a file from a hard drive to a diskette drive, you must type a command that instructs the computer to copy the file.

Windows. This operating system employs a graphical user interface (GUI) instead of a command line interface. With a GUI, menu choices are identified by **icons,** or graphic symbols. For example, the "Print" command is usually identified by a button with a tiny illustration of a printer on it. To print a document, you move the pointing device until the arrow is on the printer icon and then click the button.

An important advantage of the Windows operating system over DOS is that it is easier to learn because you do not have to remember commands. Another benefit of Windows is that it is a **multitasking** system—users can run two or more software programs simultaneously. You

could, for example, enter patient information into a **database,** a collection of records created and stored on the computer, while a word processing program is running in the background. DOS is not a multitasking system; you can run only one application at a time.

Windows 2000. This operating system, introduced in 2000, is similar to Windows but has many additional features (see Figure 6-5). In most businesses, Windows 2000 is quickly becoming the standard operating system for IBM and IBM-compatible computers. Most new computers are shipped with Windows 2000 preinstalled, and many software programs are being written to run exclusively under this operating system.

Applications. Most of the software sold in stores is application software. It is used for a specific purpose, or application. Word processing, database, and accounting software are just a few examples of the wide variety of applications available.

Using Computer Software

Computer software has been developed for nearly every office function imaginable. Using software, you can complete tasks with greater speed, accuracy, and ease than with a manual system. Learning how to use the software correctly, however, is the key to getting the most out of your computer system.

Word Processing

In the medical office, as in any office, word processing is a common computer application. It has replaced the typewriter for writing correspondence and reports, transcribing physicians' notes, and performing many other functions. Correcting errors is easy on a word processor, and you can save documents for later retrieval and modification. Procedure 6-1 shows you how to use a word processing program to create a form letter. A form letter can be merged with a patient mailing list to create letters that are personalized with patients' names.

Database Management

A database is a collection of records created and stored on a computer. In a medical office, databases are used to store patient records such as billing information, medical chart data, and insurance company facts. These records can be sorted and retrieved in many ways and for a variety of

purposes. You may be asked to find, add to, or modify information in a database. For example, you might use a database to determine all the patients covered by a particular insurance company.

Accounting and Billing

Accounting and billing software is extremely useful in an office environment. It enables you to perform many tasks, including keeping track of patients' accounts, creating billing statements, preparing financial reports, and maintaining tax records. (You will learn more about accounting and billing functions in Chapters 17 and 18.)

Appointment Scheduling

Instead of writing in an appointment book, you can use software to schedule appointments. Some scheduling packages allow you to enter patient preferences, such as day of the week and time, and then to list available appointments based on that information. If the office system is on a network, scheduling software is particularly valuable, because more than one user can access the appointment schedule at a time.

PROCEDURE 6.1

Creating a Form Letter

Objective: To use a word processing program to create a form letter

Materials: Computer equipped with a word processing program, printer, form letter to be input, 8½-by-11-inch paper.

Method

1. Turn on the computer. Select the word processing program.

2. Use the keyboard to begin entering text into a new document.

3. To edit text, press the arrow keys to move the cursor to the position at which you want to insert or delete characters, and enter the text. Use the "Insert" mode to add characters or the "Typeover" mode to type over and replace existing text.

4. To delete text, position the cursor to the left of the characters to be deleted and press the "Delete" key. Alternatively, place the cursor to the right of the characters to be deleted and press the "Backspace" key (the left-pointing

arrow usually found at the top right corner of the keyboard).

5. If you need to move an entire block of text, you must begin by highlighting it. In most Windows-based programs, you first click the mouse at the beginning of the text to be highlighted. Then you hold down the left mouse button, drag the mouse to the end of the block of text, and release your finger from the mouse. The text should now be highlighted. Choose the button or command for cutting text. Then move the cursor to the place where you want to insert the text, and select the button or command for retrieving or pasting text.

6. As you input the letter, it is important to save your work every 15 minutes or so. Some programs do this automatically. If yours does not, use the "Save" command or button to save the file. Be sure to save the file again when you have completed the letter.

7. Print the letter using the "Print" command or button.

Electronic Transactions

Using a computer equipped with a modem and communications software, you can perform several types of electronic transactions. This technology enables you to send and receive information instantaneously rather than waiting the days or weeks required for regular mail. Common electronic transactions include sending insurance claims and communicating with other computer users.

Sending Insurance Claims. Insurance claims can be submitted directly from the medical office to an insurance company. This procedure enables claims to be processed quickly and efficiently. (Processing insurance claims is discussed in Chapter 15.)

Communicating. The ability to communicate and share information with other computer users and systems is important in many medical offices. This communication may take place through electronic mail, online services, and the Internet. The Tips for the Office section gives ideas for saving time and money while you are online.

Electronic Mail. Commonly known as e-mail, **electronic mail** is a method of sending and receiving messages through a network. Through e-mail, you can communicate with computer users in your own office, across town, or on the other side of the world.

Online Services. These services, known as *servers,* provide a means for health-care professionals to communicate with one another. Most online services contain forums that

---

Tips for the Office

Saving Time and Money Online

If the medical office where you work is computerized, the system most likely has a modem for sending e-mail and transferring files electronically. The modem may also be used to access various online services and the Internet, a global network of computers. If this access is not currently available in the medical office, it probably will be in the near future. You may even be asked to help choose an online service or Internet provider for the office.

These services, known as *Internet Service Providers (ISPs)* allow access to a network of servers that provides a means for health-care professionals to communicate with one another. Unless the people using these services are careful, however, this access can be very costly. In general, the more time you spend online, the more expensive the service becomes. For this reason, knowing how to use these communications systems wisely is a valuable asset.

Choosing an Online Service

Compare several services for the following features:

- Free trial membership. Many services offer a free 1-month membership to try out the service. The trial periods enable office staff members to test several services to determine which one best suits their needs.
- Local access telephone number. Make sure the service provides an access number within the local dialing area of the office. If it does not, the office will be charged long-distance telephone rates each time someone goes online. These fees are separate from the online service's rates and can add up quickly.
- Volume discount plan. If the office will be using the online service often, find a provider that

offers a discount for frequent usage. Rather than charging a per-hour rate over the first 5 hours of use, for example, these services charge a flat rate for 20 or 30 hours of use per month. Some offer unlimited use for a flat rate.

- Extra fees. Although access to most of the information found in online services is included in the membership fee, some providers charge extra for premium or extended services. If you want to read or print out the full text of an article in a medical journal, for example, some providers charge an additional fee. Make sure you consider these extra fees when comparing costs of online services.
- Availability of health-care information. Some online services provide discussion groups (commonly known as chat rooms) and resources that would be useful to the medical office. Other services may not offer as much relevant information. By comparing several services, you can determine which service best meets the needs of the practice.

Sending and Receiving E-Mail

When using e-mail, follow these guidelines to manage your online time efficiently.

- Compose messages off-line. Most services allow you to write e-mail messages before you actually go online. When you have finished writing the message, you simply log onto the service and click a button to send the e-mail. This technique will save a great deal of online time, especially if you must frequently send lengthy messages.

continued ⟶

- Read messages off-line. When you receive an e-mail message, you do not have to read it immediately. You will spend less time online if you save the message on the hard disk to read or print out later.
- Use computerized address books. As part of the e-mail system, most services provide an online address book in which you can store frequently used e-mail addresses. Instead of wasting time searching for an e-mail address in a standard card file, you simply click on the person's name in the address book, and the mail is automatically sent to that person. You can also use the address book to send the same e-mail message to several people at once.

Doing Research

Although a great deal of valuable information can be found through online services and the Internet, searching for this information can be time-consuming. Here are some tips to make the most of your online time.

- Use the favorite places feature. Keep a list of favorite places, or sites that you visit frequently. Instead of trying to remember a long Internet address or searching for the location of information you found last week, you simply add these sites to your list of favorite places and click on the name to visit them.
- Refine your searches. Searching for *arthritis,* for example, might produce hundreds of references that you would have to read through to determine their relevance. Narrowing your search to *juvenile rheumatoid arthritis,* on the other hand, would produce fewer references but would provide more exact matches.
- Download files. *Download* means to transfer a file to the hard disk. Instead of reading through information while you are online, you can usually save online time by downloading the files and retrieving them later (after you have logged off the online service).

offer information and discussion groups focusing on a wide range of medical topics. Health-care workers can learn about the latest medical research and technology or exchange ideas with others in their field. In addition, some online services provide access to medical databases such as MEDLINE, created by the National Library of Medicine. Users can search MEDLINE for records and abstracts from thousands of medical journals from around the world.

Internet. The **Internet** is a global network of computers. Through the Internet, you can communicate with millions of computer users around the world. In addition, many large medical facilities, universities, and other organizations—such as the National Institutes of Health and the Centers for Disease Control and Prevention—provide medical resources, databases, and other information on the Internet. Users can visit such Internet sites as the Virtual Hospital, sponsored by the University of Iowa, and the Cyberspace Hospital, sponsored by the National University of Singapore. At these sites you may find multimedia textbooks, presentations, and links to other related sites on the Internet. Table 6-1 describes these and other popular medical resources available on the Internet.

Research

The advent of CD-ROM technology has revolutionized the world of research. Not only can an immense amount of information be contained on one compact disc, but the CD-ROM usually provides additional information in the form of videos and sound (see Figure 6-6). A CD-ROM encyclopedia, for example, might also provide spoken pronunciations of medical terms. This type of software may help patients—especially children—understand the human body as well as various medical conditions.

Software Training

Software programs may seem quite complex. Most people need a period of training before they feel comfortable using the application. Several methods of training—some from outside sources and some provided by the software manufacturer—are available.

Classes. Many computer vendors offer training classes for the software packages they sell. In addition, community colleges and high schools sometimes offer adult education classes for a variety of applications, including word processing and communications. These classes may be at the beginner, intermediate, or advanced level.

Tutorials. Many software packages come with a **tutorial,** which is a small program designed to give users an overall picture of the product and its functions. The tutorial usually provides a step-by-step walk-through and exercises in which you can try out your newly acquired knowledge.

TABLE 6-1 Medical Resources on the Internet

Organization	Web Address	Description
American Medical Association	http://www.ama-assn.org	News announcements and press releases; articles from *JAMA* and other AMA journals; links to other medicine-related Internet sites
Cyberspace Hospital	http://ch.nus.sg	Various departments and services, organized like a real hospital; medical bulletins; capability for users to search for information on medical topics
HealthWeb	http://hsinfo.ghsl.nwu.edu/healthweb/index.html	Starting point for searching the Internet because it contains links to a wide variety of medical resources
National Institutes of Health	http://www.nih.gov	Medical news and current events; press releases; biomedical information about health issues; scientific resources; links to Internet sites of related government agencies
National Library of Medicine	http://www.nlm.nih.gov	Internet site for world's largest biomedical library; research and development activities; connections to online medical information services
New England Journal of Medicine	http://www.nejm.org	Articles and abstracts; archives of past issues
U.S. Department of Health and Human Services	http://www.os.dhhs.gov	Programs and activities of this agency; links to divisions of agency, including Centers for Disease Control and Prevention, Food and Drug Administration, and National Institutes of Health
Virtual Hospital	http://vh.radiology.uiowa.edu	Information on a variety of health issues, medical resources, tutorials, and multimedia textbooks

Documentation. Nearly all software manufacturers provide some type of documentation with their programs. Documentation is usually in the form of written instruction manuals or online help that is accessed from within the program.

Manuals. Some manuals provide detailed information on software operation and may include an index and sections on troubleshooting and commonly asked questions. Other manuals may simply give installation instructions and brief information on program basics. This type of manual may refer users to the software's online help.

On-Line Help. In most software applications, users access the online help screen by clicking on a "Help" button or by pressing a certain function key, such as "F1." The online help usually provides a "Contents" section (shown in Figure 6-7), in which you can browse for topics. An index, in which you can search for key words, is also provided.

Technical Support. A software company's technical support service is designed to assist you with problems that go beyond the scope of the user's guide or manual. A call to technical support is important when you encounter a problem that cannot be solved by simple problem-solving techniques. By calling a toll-free number, you can access a knowledgeable team who will listen to the description of the problem and suggest solutions over the phone.

Before calling technical support:

- Check the system for errors to the best of your ability. Check your manual for answers. Ask your supervisor for assistance.

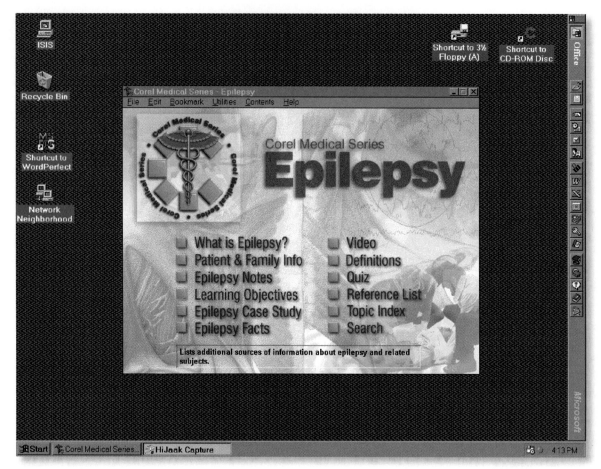

Figure 6-6. A CD-ROM provides features, such as video and sound, that are not possible in a standard printed book.

- Have the software registration number available.
- Be prepared to follow the instructions of the technical support personnel.
- Plan to call from a location that gives ready access to the computer with the problem.

Technical support is also helpful when you are upgrading software. Some software companies automatically notify their customers of available upgrades. The technical support service is always a good source of information regarding the latest products and their applications.

Selecting Computer Equipment

Perhaps you are working in a medical office that is not yet computerized. If the decision is made to convert to a computerized system, you may be asked to help select equipment. Even if your office already uses computers, the system will probably need to be upgraded at some point to provide more functions. In either situation, you may be asked for your input in selecting software, adding a network, or choosing a vendor.

The first step for helping in the selection process is to learn as much as you can about hardware and software. You can get information by taking an introductory computer class at an adult school or community college; by reading computer magazines or books; or by talking to friends, relatives, or coworkers who use computers.

Converting to a Computerized Office

When an office converts from a manual system to computers, staff members should determine how the new computer system will be used. The objective is to obtain a system that not only meets current office needs but that can also be expanded and upgraded to meet future needs. To get the longest use from a computer system, a good general guideline is to buy the most advanced system possible within the allowed budget.

Upgrading the Office System

Computer hardware is changing and improving at such a rapid pace that a new system seems to become outdated

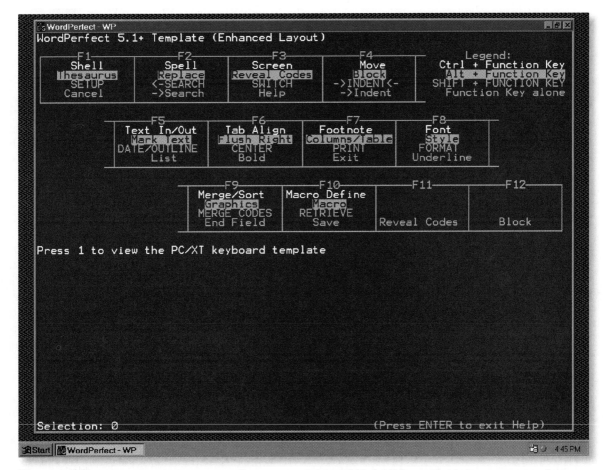

Figure 6-7. An online help system allows you to access helpful information when you are using a software program.

almost as soon as it is purchased. In addition, more-advanced software is introduced every day, and this software requires more-advanced hardware to run. Consequently, an office system purchased only a year or two ago may need to be upgraded. Sometimes an upgrade simply requires replacement or addition of certain components. For instance, a laser printer can take the place of a dot matrix printer, or a CD-ROM drive can be added. In other cases, such a solution is not possible or cost-effective, so an entirely new system must be purchased.

Selecting Software

After a decision is made regarding the type of software needed, such as an accounting program, a specific product must be chosen. To make an informed decision, you can read software reviews in computer magazines or trade publications. You might also check with other medical offices to get opinions on software packages. A crucial step in selecting software is to make sure the office computer system meets the minimum system requirements listed on the software box. For example, a medical encyclopedia may require a 486 SX processor, Windows 98, 16 MB of RAM, 30 MB of available hard disk space, and a CD-ROM drive.

Adding a Network

There are several advantages to adding a network to the computer system in a medical office. A computer network enables users to share software programs and files and allows more than one person to work on the same patient's information at one time. While you are working on a patient's insurance claim, for example, another assistant might be inputting billing information. Some medical offices are virtually paperless. They use a highly sophisticated network with a notebook or desktop computer in every examination room (Figure 6-8). Doctors input information into patients' computerized charts. If a doctor is in her office and a patient is waiting, a staff member at the front desk sends an e-mail message to the doctor's desktop computer, and a beep sounds as an alert. Networks also allow large medical facilities to communicate with employees via e-mail. For instance, an internal memo about changes in office policies may be sent by e-mail to all employees.

Choosing a Vendor

When purchasing computer equipment, you should look for a reputable vendor who not only offers a reasonable price but also provides training, service, and technical

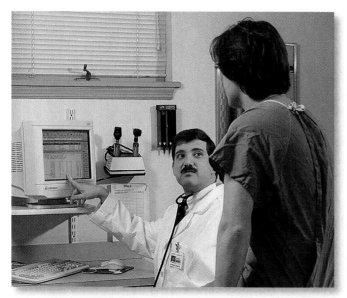

Figure 6-8. Some medical offices use highly sophisticated computer networks.

support. A first step might be to check with personnel in other medical offices that use a computer system. Find out which dealer they use and if they are satisfied with the system, salespeople, and support. You can also ask dealers for names of references—medical offices that have purchased systems from them. It is a good idea to get cost estimates from at least three vendors, and it is preferable to buy all hardware components from the same vendor.

Security in the Computerized Office

Although security measures are important in any office, they are especially important in a computerized medical office. Great care must be taken to safeguard confidential files, make backup copies on a regular basis, and prevent system contamination.

Safeguarding Confidential Files

Much of the information collected in a medical office is confidential. Just as with paper records, confidential information stored on the computer should be accessible only to authorized personnel. Two common ways to provide security in a computerized office are to employ passwords and to install an activity-monitoring system.

Passwords. In many hospitals and physicians' offices, each employee who is allowed access to computerized patient files is given a password. The employee must enter the password into the computer when using the files. Access codes or passwords only allow the user into approved areas according to the individual's job description. If you are given a password, do not divulge it to anyone else

unless your office manager asks you to do so. If an employee leaves or is fired, that person's password should be immediately erased from the system.

Activity-Monitoring Systems. In conjunction with passwords, some health-care facilities use a computer system that monitors user activity. Whenever someone accesses computer records, the system automatically keeps track of the user's name and the files that have been viewed or modified. In this way, problems or security breaches can be traced back to specific employees.

Making and Storing Backup Files

For securing important computer files, it is essential to routinely make diskette or tape backups of them (see Figure 6-9). How often backups are made varies among medical offices; your supervisor will tell you the policy for your office. Just as important as making the backups is storing them properly. Backup files should not be stored near the original files. Ideally, they should be kept outside the medical office—perhaps at the physician's home—so that they will be secure in case of fire, burglary, or other catastrophe at the office.

Preventing System Contamination

Another important security issue in the computerized medical office is computer viruses. Computer viruses are

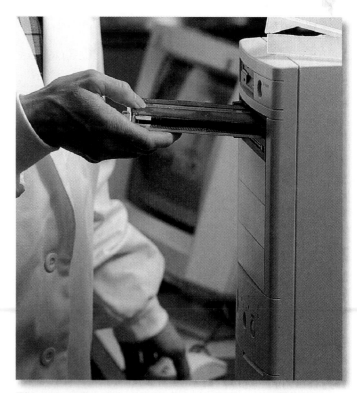

Figure 6-9. It is important to back up computer files and store them properly.

programs written specifically to contaminate the hard disk by damaging or destroying data.

One way that viruses can be passed from computer to computer is through shared diskettes that have been infected. Another way is through infected files retrieved from online services, the Internet, and electronic bulletin boards. Several software programs are available to detect and correct computer viruses. Most are fairly inexpensive but provide an invaluable service.

Computer System Care and Maintenance

Like a car, a computer needs routine care and maintenance to stay in sound condition. The computer user's manual outlines the steps required. Also, a good general rule is not to eat or drink near the computer. Crumbs and spilled liquids can damage the system components and storage devices.

System Unit

The system unit should be placed in a well-ventilated location, with nothing blocking the fan in the back of the cabinet. To keep the system's delicate circuitry from being damaged by an electrical power surge, you should use a power strip with a surge protector. You plug the computer into the power strip, and then plug the power strip into the electrical outlet.

Monitor

The computer monitor needs to be protected from screen burn-in, which may happen if the same image stays on the computer screen for an extended time. To prevent burn-in, you can use a **screen saver,** which automatically changes the monitor display at short intervals or constantly shows moving images. All Windows operating systems come equipped with screen savers. A wide variety of screen savers are also available as separate software packages.

To protect their screens, many newer monitors "power down" after a certain period of inactivity. If no one uses the computer for 30 minutes, for example, the monitor screen goes blank. To resume using the computer after the screen saver has been activated or the monitor has powered down, you simply touch any key or move the mouse.

Printer

Maintenance of a printer generally consists of replacing the ribbon, ink cartridge, or toner cartridge. You can tell when the ribbon or cartridge needs to be changed because the ink on your printouts becomes very light.

Replacement is usually a simple process, described in the printer manual.

Information Storage Devices

Diskettes, CD-ROMs, and magnetic tapes are highly sensitive devices. Even a small scratch may cause permanent damage or make it impossible to retrieve data. To avoid problems, handle and store disks and tapes properly.

Diskettes. Diskettes should be kept away from magnetic fields, such as a paper clip holder that has a magnet in it. They should also be kept out of direct sunlight and away from extreme temperatures. Although 3½-inch disks are sturdy they should be handled with care. They should be labeled appropriately and stored in a durable storage case.

CD-ROMs. Figure 6-10 shows the proper way to handle a CD-ROM. When you pick it up, touch only the edges or the edge and the hole in the center. CD-ROMs should be stored in the clear plastic case in which they are packaged, sometimes called a jewel case. If a CD-ROM becomes dusty or smudged with fingerprints, you can clean it by rubbing it gently with a soft cloth. Always rub from the center to the outside. *Never* rub in a circular motion.

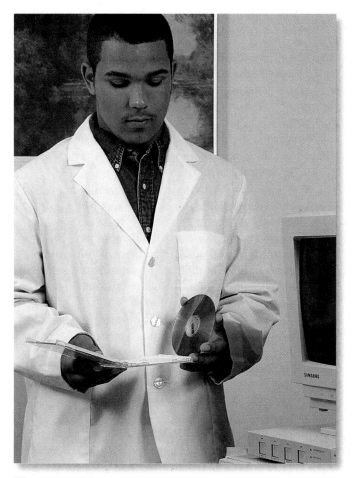

Figure 6-10. When handling a CD-ROM, be careful not to touch the flat surface of the disc.

Dental Office Administrator

To gain medical assistant credentials, you must fulfill the requirements of either the American Association of Medical Assistants (for a Certified Medical Assistant) or the American Medical Technologists (for a Registered Medical Assistant). After obtaining your medical assistant certification or registration, you may wish to acquire additional skills in specialty areas through course work or on-the-job training. Although this course work or training may not lead to an additional certification or degree, it will enable you to expand your role in the medical office and advance your career as the demand for skilled health professionals increases.

Skills and Duties

A dental office administrator carries out clerical and administrative duties for a dentist or a dental group. His duties may vary with the size of the practice. In a large practice he may oversee the clerical staff. In a small practice he may have more varied tasks, including staffing the reception desk, maintaining records, and performing other support services.

The duties of a dental office administrator mostly fall into the following six categories:

1. Communication. In many offices, this task is the administrator's main responsibility. He answers the telephones and manages the correspondence for the practice, which may include billing.

2. Reception. The office administrator greets and welcomes patients. He must have a knowledge of dental terminology in order to assist patients with dental paperwork.

3. Scheduling. The dental office administrator coordinates patient appointments and may schedule referrals with other specialists, such as orthodontists. He may also maintain the schedules of the dental hygienists and other office staff. Sometimes the administrator is responsible for calling patients to confirm appointments ahead of time.

4. Records and filing. The administrator may manage the patient records and other files. He attaches dental x-rays to the appropriate records and maintains up-to-date insurance information to ensure accurate billing.

5. Support duties. The dental office administrator has a range of other duties that vary from practice to practice. Typically, he is responsible for managing office supplies. He often needs to type or take shorthand. He also uses computer and word processing skills. Specialized skills, such as bookkeeping, may also be helpful.

6. Supervision. In a large dental practice, the administrator trains and oversees clerical staff and secretaries.

Workplace Settings

Dental office administrators may work in a private practice, a group practice, or a dental clinic.

Education

Dental office administrators often learn the dental and medical terminology they need on the job. They may acquire secretarial training by taking courses, either in a business/vocational school or in a junior or community college. A high school diploma is usually required. Further education may be necessary in a practice where the administrator must supervise other staff members.

Where to Go for More Information

American Academy of Dental Practice
   Administrators
1063 Whippoorwill Lane
Palatine, IL 60067
(312) 934-4404

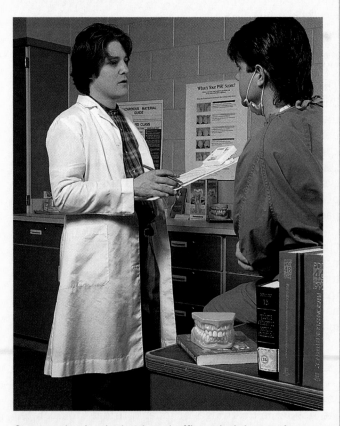

Communication is the dental office administrator's most important task.

Magnetic Tapes. These tapes should be treated much as you would treat audiotapes. They should be stored in a relatively cool, dry place, away from magnetic fields.

Computers of the Future

Computers are evolving at such a rapid pace that it is virtually impossible to predict the changes that will take place even in the next few years. Some important new technologies, however, have already been introduced in the medical office and will be improved in the near future. Telemedicine, CD-R technology, and speech recognition technology are only three examples of new computer technologies. Undoubtedly, more will be explored and developed every year.

Telemedicine

Telemedicine refers to the use of telecommunications to transmit video images of patient information. These images are already used to provide medical support to physicians caring for patients in rural areas. Some experts feel that telemedicine has great potential and that advancements in computer technology will make telemedicine more popular in the future.

CD-R Technology

While CD-ROMs can only be *read* by the computer, CD-R (compact disc–recordable) media can be read *and* written to. CD-R technology allows you to use compact discs like diskettes—to store data and information. Recordable CDs, however, can store much more information than diskettes can. Although CD-R technology is currently available, it is not yet widely used because it is still fairly expensive.

Speech Recognition Technology

This technology enables the computer to comprehend and interpret spoken words. The user simply speaks into a microphone instead of inputting information with a keyboard or a scanner. Because every human voice is different, however, and the English language is vast and complex, this technology is difficult to perfect. As speech recognition technology becomes more advanced, more accurate, and less expensive, it will most likely gain widespread acceptance. It has a great deal of potential, including the ability to virtually eliminate the need for medical assistants to transcribe physicians' notes.

Summary

Most medical offices have already converted from a paper-based system of record keeping to a computer-based one. You should familiarize yourself with the types of computers available and the hardware and software components that make up a computer system. A variety of software programs are used in the medical office, including word processing, database management, accounting and billing, appointment scheduling, and electronic transactions, such as submitting insurance claims. Other computer technology you need to know about includes modems, scanners, and CD-ROM software.

Whether you are converting to a computerized office or simply upgrading an existing system, learn the guidelines for selecting computer hardware and software. In a computerized office it is also important to know how to secure computerized files and to care for and maintain computer equipment.

REVIEW

CHAPTER 6

CASE STUDY QUESTIONS

Now that you have completed this chapter, review the case study at the beginning of the chapter and answer the following questions:

1. Are you more like Chris or Alicia? What background do you bring to the study of computers that makes you feel the way you do?
2. Why is it important for an office to continue to use the manual system at the same time that it converts to a computerized system?
3. Who should be trained in the use of a new computer system in a medical practice? Why?
4. Which group do you think would be the most difficult to train in an average medical practice?
   a. Those who think like Chris?
   b. Those who think like Alicia?
   c. The physicians?

   What would be the best way to approach the group you just identified?

Discussion Questions

1. Compare and contrast the three kinds of printers. What are the advantages of each?
2. What do you think is in the future in the development of computers? Describe your vision of the typical medical office and its use of computers 25 years from now.
3. A new computer system has just been installed at your office. How would you encourage and assist a fellow employee in learning the new system?

Critical Thinking Questions

1. A technical problem is detected on the computer at your desk. What would you do? Explain in detail.
2. A fellow employee asks to use your password to the computer because she has forgotten hers. How do you respond and why?
3. Summarize the proper care and maintenance of computer diskettes and CDs. How does proper care reduce problems?

Application Activities

1. Go online and research the purchase of a new software package for a medical encyclopedia. Which would you recommend for purchase by your office and why?
2. Look through computer magazines or trade journals for descriptions or reviews of the latest software upgrades for your computer system. Describe what new benefits the upgrades offer and how each feature would benefit a medical practice.
3. Research one of the technological advances mentioned in this chapter—telemedicine, CD-R technology, or speech recognition technology—to learn more about it. Find out how the technology benefits the medical office. Write and present a full report on your topic.

CHAPTER 7

Managing Correspondence and Mail

AREAS OF COMPETENCE

2003 Role Delineation Study

ADMINISTRATIVE

Administrative Procedures

- Perform basic administrative medical assisting functions

GENERAL

Communication Skills

- Recognize and respond effectively to verbal, nonverbal, and written communications
- Utilize electronic technology to receive, organize, prioritize, and transmit information

KEY TERMS

annotate

clarity

concise

courtesy title

dateline

editing

enclosure

full-block letter style

identification line

key

letterhead

modified-block letter style

proofreading

salutation

simplified letter style

template

CHAPTER OUTLINE

- Correspondence and Professionalism
- Choosing Correspondence Supplies
- Written Correspondence
- Effective Writing
- Editing and Proofreading
- Preparing Outgoing Mail
- Mailing Equipment and Supplies
- U.S. Postal Service Delivery
- Other Delivery Services
- Processing Incoming Mail

OBJECTIVES

After completing Chapter 7, you will be able to:

7.1 List the supplies necessary for creating and mailing professional-looking correspondence.

7.2 Identify the types of correspondence used in medical office communications.

7.3 Describe the parts of a letter and the different letter and punctuation styles.

7.4 Compose a business letter.

7.5 Explain the tasks involved in editing and proofreading.

7.6 Describe the process of handling incoming and outgoing mail.

7.7 Compare and contrast the services provided by the U.S. Postal Service and other delivery services.

Introduction

Communication skills are important in every profession. Written materials are tangible demonstrations of an office staff's ability to communicate and conduct business.

Others often evaluate the entire medical practice by the work of one employee. When a letter, form, or document is carelessly prepared and sent into the community, the physician may be judged as "careless." However, when a letter or general business correspondence is constructed in a neat, concise, and well-organized fashion, the physician is often judged to be organized and competent. The skill demonstrated in the creation of a simple business letter reflects on the medical skills of the physician and the practice. Professional image is conveyed in written correspondence.

Because written documents also serve as legal records, all documents must be prepared with great care and attention to detail. The administrative role of the medical assistant includes the creation of documents that are consistently accurate and clear.

In this chapter you will learn how to write effectively. You will develop skills in composing a business letter. You will learn different styles and formats of writing and will learn how to professionally manage all forms of correspondence commonly used in an ambulatory care setting.

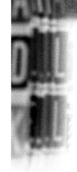

CASE STUDY

Paula and Tom are medical assistants whose duties include making sure the daily correspondence is created and on the physician's desk before they go home at the end of the day. Today, they are working together to complete these tasks.

Paula will key into the computer letters of referral to other physicians. She is using a template saved within the computer to easily and quickly turn out many different letters. She is simply keying in different fields of information with the specifics for each patient referral. She then prints out a draft copy for proofreading and review by the physician or office manager. Once reviewed, corrected, and approved, she will print out the final letters onto the more expensive letterhead of the office. She will also copy the address from the letters and complete a mailing envelope for each letter.

Tom is assisting as he takes each completed letter and attaches all materials noted as enclosures to each letter. He then folds each letter and its enclosures carefully and inserts them into the properly addressed envelope. Next, he determines the weight of each envelope and the best choice for mailing it. He sorts the mailing into separate piles for different mail handling. The routine mailing is run through the stamp machine. The appropriate forms for the specialty mailing are created and attached. Tom makes sure copies of all mailings are carefully placed in the patient's chart. Both Paula and Tom know the importance of careful and accurate handling of all patient correspondence.

As you read this chapter, consider the following questions:

1. Why is it important to accurately and carefully prepare correspondence for an ambulatory setting? What could the poor management of documents and correspondence mean to a medical practice?
2. What are the differences between the language used in an informal or casual letter and that used in a formal or professional business letter?
3. What are some appropriate shortcuts that can assist in the daily management of correspondence and mailing?
4. What are some factors to consider in choosing the best mode of delivery for letters and parcels?

Correspondence and Professionalism

As in any business, correspondence from health-care professionals to patients and colleagues must be handled carefully, with appropriate attention to content and presentation. By learning how to create, send, and receive correspondence and other types of mail, you can ensure positive, effective communication between your office and others. Well-written, neatly prepared correspondence is one of the most important means of communicating a professional image for the medical office (Figure 7-1).

Choosing Correspondence Supplies

The first step in preparing professional-looking correspondence is choosing the right supplies. Many offices already have most of these supplies on hand. However, you may

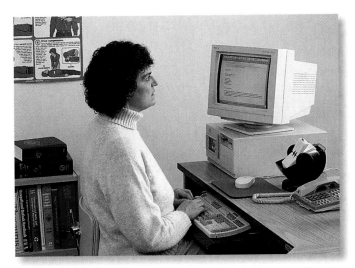

Figure 7-1. The correspondence that goes out of and comes into a medical office is vital to a well-run practice.

be responsible for choosing and ordering such supplies. You may need to make decisions about letterhead paper, envelopes, labels, invoices, and statements.

Letterhead Paper

Letterhead refers to formal business stationery on which the doctor's (or office's) name and address are printed at the top. In most cases, the office phone number is listed, along with the names of all the associates in the practice. Letterhead is used for correspondence with patients, colleagues, and vendors.

The fiber content of paper is the amount of wood pulp in the paper. Letterhead paper can be cotton fiber bond (sometimes called rag bond) or sulfite bond. Cotton fiber bond contains cotton pulp along with chemically treated wood pulp. It is usually more expensive than other types of paper. Cotton bond contains a watermark, which is an impression or pattern that can be seen when the paper is held up to the light. A watermark indicates that the paper is of high quality. The most popular cotton bond used for letterhead is 25% cotton because it is economical, but all higher grades can be used.

Sulfite bond is made from chemically treated wood pulp. It is smoother than cotton bond and less expensive. Sulfite bond comes in five grades, numbered one through five. Grade one is a cost-effective bond for letterhead. This grade of sulfite bond also has a watermark. You often cannot tell the difference between this grade of sulfite bond and cotton bond.

The finish of a paper refers to the paper's look and feel. Papers with a smooth finish are the most popular type for letterheads. They are less expensive and work well with most printers. Another type of finish used in high-quality letterhead is linen laid. This type has a rougher feel because it is embossed with a design, much like linen fabric.

Envelopes

Envelopes are used for correspondence, invoices, and statements. Typically, business letterhead, matching envelopes, and sometimes invoice and statement letterhead are printed together.

Familiarize yourself with the several types of envelopes used in the medical office.

- The most common envelope size used for correspondence is the No. 10 envelope (also called business size). It measures 4⅛ by 9½ inches.
- Envelopes used for invoices and statements can range from No. 6 (3⅝ by 6½ inches) to No. 10. These envelopes commonly have a transparent window that allows the address on the invoice or statement to show through, saving time and reducing the potential for errors involved in retyping the address.
- Smaller payment-return envelopes—preaddressed to the doctor's office—are often included along with a bill, for the patient's convenience.
- Tan kraft envelopes, also called clasp envelopes, are available in many sizes and are used to send large or bulky documents.
- Padded envelopes are used to send documents or materials, such as slides, that may be damaged in the normal course of mail handling.
- The stock and quality of the envelope should always match the stationery. An office typically has two grades of envelopes with a return address. One is a less expensive stock and quality of paper with a block format return address printed in black. The second is a more expensive stock and quality of paper with a block format return address printed in black or a dark color.

Labels

Address labels, printed from a computerized mailing list, can greatly speed the process of addressing envelopes for bulk mailings. For example, you may have to send a notice of a change in office hours or a quarterly office newsletter to a large number of patients in a practice.

You may choose to set up a system for frequently used labels. Many practices write referrals and other business letters to the same addresses again and again. For fast and easy access, it is helpful to print out labels a full page at a time of the same address. Pages of labels can then be stored in alphabetized folders near the transcription desk.

Invoices and Statements

There are several different types of invoices and statements in use today. They include:

- Preprinted invoices (used to send an original bill)
- Preprinted statements (used to send a reminder when an account is 30 or more days past due)

- Computer-generated invoices and statements
- Superbills (discussed in Chapter 17)
- Data mailers

Written Correspondence

A letter is a form of communication—much like holding a conversation in person. The recipient will form an impression of the physician or the office based on the letter. Therefore, letters must be clear and well written and must politely convey the appropriate information.

Commonly used paragraphs and even entire letter formats, or **templates,** are used repeatedly in some practices. It is handy to save these bodies of text in the computer for quick and easy repeated access. With very few keystrokes, the material can be selected and displayed quickly. Then minor changes specific to the letter or document can be added.

It is also helpful to use the cut, paste, and copy features in word processing software to quickly piece together a correspondence that uses sentences or paragraphs from other documents. Large and small bodies of text can easily be moved from document to document, saving time for the medical assistant.

Types of Correspondence in the Medical Office

As a medical assistant, you will be responsible for preparing routine letters at the physician's request. You may transcribe some letters from the physician's dictation and compose others from notes.

The purpose of most letters is to explain, clarify, or give instructions or other information. Correspondence includes letters of referral; letters about scheduling, canceling, or rescheduling appointments; patient reports for insurance companies; instructions for examinations or laboratory tests; answers to insurance or billing questions; and cover letters or form letters to order supplies, equipment, or magazine subscriptions.

Parts of a Business Letter

Figure 7-2 illustrates the parts of a typical business letter. Details about format may vary from office to office.

Dateline. The **dateline** consists of the month, day, and year. It should begin about three lines below the preprinted letterhead text on approximately line 15. The month should

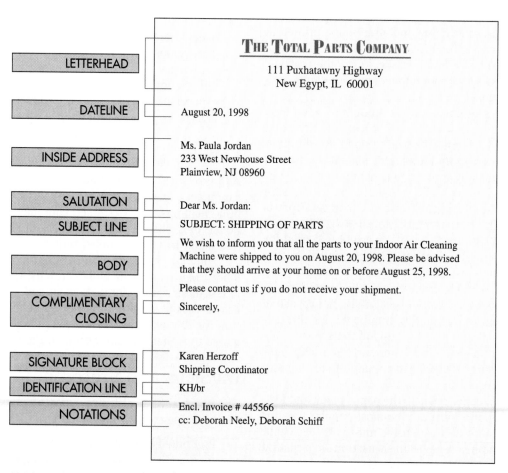

Figure 7-2. Knowing the parts of a typical business letter enables medical assistants to create written communications that reflect well on the office.

always be spelled out, and there should be a comma after the day.

Inside Address. The inside address contains all the necessary information for correct delivery of the letter. In general, you should:

- **Key,** or type, the inside address on the left margin. It should be two, three, or four lines in length.
- Include a **courtesy title** (Dr., Mr., Mrs., and so on) and the intended receiver's full name. Note: If Dr. is used, it is not followed by MD after the name. For example, either of these forms is acceptable: Dr. John Smith; John Smith, MD. This form is not acceptable: Dr. John Smith, MD.
- Include the intended receiver's title on the same line with the name, separated by a comma, or on the line below it.
- Include the company name, if applicable.
- Use numerals for the street address, except the single numbers one through nine, which should be spelled out—for example, Two Markham Place.
- Spell out numerical names of streets if they are numbers less than ten.
- Spell out the words *Street, Drive,* and so on.
- Include the full city name; do not abbreviate.
- Use the two-letter state abbreviation recommended by the U.S. Postal Service (USPS) (Table 7-1).

TABLE 7-1	USPS State Abbreviations		
State	**Abbreviation**	**State**	**Abbreviation**
Alabama	AL	Montana	MT
Alaska	AK	Nebraska	NE
Arizona	AZ	Nevada	NV
Arkansas	AR	New Hampshire	NH
California	CA	New Jersey	NJ
Colorado	CO	New Mexico	NM
Connecticut	CT	New York	NY
Delaware	DE	North Carolina	NC
District of Columbia	DC	North Dakota	ND
Florida	FL	Ohio	OH
Georgia	GA	Oklahoma	OK
Hawaii	HI	Oregon	OR
Idaho	ID	Pennsylvania	PA
Illinois	IL	Puerto Rico	PR
Indiana	IN	Rhode Island	RI
Iowa	IA	South Carolina	SC
Kansas	KS	South Dakota	SD
Kentucky	KY	Tennessee	TN
Louisiana	LA	Texas	TX
Maine	ME	Utah	UT
Maryland	MD	Vermont	VT
Massachusetts	MA	Virginia	VA
Michigan	MI	Washington	WA
Minnesota	MN	West Virginia	WV
Mississippi	MS	Wisconsin	WI
Missouri	MO	Wyoming	WY

- Leave one space between the state and the zip code; include the zip + 4 code, if known.

Attention Line. An attention line is used when a letter is addressed to a company but sent to the attention of a particular individual. If you do not know the name of the individual, call the company directly to inquire the name of the appropriate contact person. A colon between the word *Attention* and the person's name is optional.

Salutation. When addressing a person by name, use a **salutation,** a written greeting such as "Dear," followed by Mr., Mrs., or Ms., and the person's last name. The salutation should be keyed at the left margin on the second line below the inside address. A colon should follow. When you do not know the name, it is becoming common practice to use the business title or department in the salutation, as in "Dear Laboratory Director" or "Dear Claims Department." This also avoids confusion if you do not know the gender of a person with a name such as Pat or Chris.

Subject Line. A subject line is sometimes used to bring the subject of the letter to the reader's attention. The subject line is not required. However, if it is used, it should be keyed on the second line below the salutation. The subject line may be flush with the left margin, indented five spaces, or centered to the page.

Body. The body of the letter begins two lines below the salutation or subject line. The text is single-spaced with double-spacing between paragraphs.

If the body contains a list, set the list apart from the rest of the text. Leave an extra line of space above and below the list. For each item in the list, indent five to ten spaces from each margin. Single-space within items, but leave an extra line between items. A bulleted list has a small, solid, round circle before each item.

Complimentary Closing. The closing is placed two lines below the last line of the body. "Sincerely" is a common closing. "Very truly yours" and "Best regards" are also acceptable closings in business correspondence.

Signature Block. The signature block contains the writer's name on the first line and the writer's business title on the second line. The block is aligned with the complimentary closing and typed four lines below it, to allow space for the signature.

Identification Line. The letter writer's initials followed by a colon or slash and the typist's initials are sometimes included in the letter. These initials are called the **identification line.** This line is typed flush left, two lines below the signature block.

Notations. Notations include information such as the number of **enclosures** that are included with the letter and the names of other people who will be receiving copies of the letter (sometimes referred to as cc's, or carbon copies).

If there are enclosures, a notation should appear flush left, one or two lines below the identification line (or one or two lines below the signature block, if no identification line is present). You may abbreviate the word *Enclosure* by typing "Enc," "Encl," or "Encs" (with or without punctuation, depending on the style of the letter you are writing). The copy notation, "cc," appears after the enclosure notation and includes one or more names or initials.

Punctuation Styles

Two different styles of punctuation are used in correspondence: open punctuation and mixed punctuation. A writer should use one punctuation style consistently throughout a letter.

Open Punctuation. This style uses no punctuation after the following items when they appear in a letter:

- The word *Attention* in the attention line
- The salutation
- The complimentary closing
- The signature block
- The enclosure and copy notations

Mixed Punctuation. This style includes the following punctuation marks used in specific instances:

- A colon after *Attention* in the attention line
- A colon after the salutation
- A comma after the complimentary closing
- A colon or period after the enclosure notation
- A colon after the copy notation

Letter Format

Follow these general formatting guidelines for all letters.

- With paper 8½ inches wide, it is common to use 1-inch margins on the left and right.
- Roughly center the letter on the page according to the length of the letter. (Most word processing programs can do this centering automatically.) For shorter letters, you can use wider margins and start the address farther down the page. For longer letters, use standard margins but start higher up on the page.
- Single-space the body of the letter. Double-space between paragraphs or parts of the letter.
- Use short sentences (no more than 20 words on average).
- Have at least two sentences in each paragraph.
- Divide long paragraphs—more than 10 lines of type—into shorter ones.

For multipage letters, use letterhead for the first page and blank paper for the subsequent pages. (When you order letterhead, be sure to order blank paper of the same type as the letterhead for subsequent sheets.) Using a

1-inch margin at the top, include a heading with the addressee, date, and page number on all pages following the first one. Resume typing or printing the text about three lines below the heading.

Letter Styles

Different letter styles are used for different purposes. Your office is likely to have a preferred style in place. The four most common letter styles are full-block, modified-block, modified-block with indented paragraphs, and simplified.

Full-Block Style. The **full-block letter style,** also called block style, is typed with all lines flush left. Figure 7-3 shows an example of the block letter style. This style may include a subject line two lines below the salutation. Block-style letters are quick and easy to write because there are no indented paragraphs to slow the typist. Block style is one of the most common formats used in the medical office.

Modified-Block Style. The **modified-block letter style** is similar to full block but differs in that the dateline, complimentary closing, signature block, and notations are aligned and begin at the center of the page or slightly to the right. This type of letter has a traditional, balanced appearance.

Modified-Block Style With Indented Paragraphs. This style is identical to the modified-block style except that the paragraphs are indented.

Simplified Style. The **simplified letter style** is a modification of the full-block style and is the most modern letter style. Figure 7-4 shows an example of the simplified letter style. The salutation is omitted, eliminating the need for a courtesy title. A subject line in all-capital letters is placed between the address and the body of the letter. The subject line summarizes the main point of the letter, but does not actually use the word *subject*. All text is typed flush left. The complimentary closing is omitted, and the sender's name and title are typed in capital letters in a single line at the end of the letter. Note that this letter style always uses open punctuation, so it is both easy to read and quick to type. In most situations in a medical office, however, the simplified letter style may be too informal.

Effective Writing

To create effective, professional correspondence that reflects well on the practice, be sure that you use an appropriate style, clear and concise language, and the active voice. Following are some general tips to help you write effective letters.

- Before you write, know the type of person to whom you are writing. Is the letter to a physician, a patient, a vendor, or fellow staff members? Decide if the tone should be formal or more relaxed.

- Know the purpose of the letter before you begin, and make sure your letter accurately conveys that purpose.
- Be **concise.** Use short sentences. Be brief. Be specific. Do not use unnecessary words. Use the simplest way to say what you mean.
- Show **clarity** in your writing; state your message so that it can be understood easily.
- Use the active voice whenever possible. Voice shows whether the subject of a sentence is acting or is being acted upon. Here is an example of the active voice:

  "Dr. Huang is seeing 18 patients today."

  Here is an example of the same sentence, written in the passive voice:

  "Eighteen patients will be seen by Dr. Huang today."

  Note that the active voice is more direct and livelier to read.
- Use the passive voice, however, to soften the impact of negative news:

  "Your account will be turned over to a collection agency if we do not receive payment promptly."

  It would sound harsher to say:

  "We will turn over your account to a collection agency if we do not receive payment promptly."
- Always be polite and courteous.
- Always check spelling and the accuracy of dates and monetary figures.

Editing and Proofreading

Editing and proofreading take place after you create the first draft of a letter. Editing involves checking a document for factual accuracy, logical flow, conciseness, clarity, and tone. Proofreading involves checking a document for grammatical, spelling, and format errors. When possible, ask another person to proofread your work as well. *Never* skip over the very important steps of editing and proofreading!

Tools for Editing and Proofreading

Reference books can help you prepare letters that appear professional. Keep the following tools available.

Dictionary. An up-to-date dictionary gives you more than definitions of words. A dictionary tells you how to spell, divide, and pronounce a word and what part of speech it is, such as a noun or adjective.

Medical Dictionary. It is nearly impossible for even the most experienced health-care professional to be familiar with every medical term. A medical dictionary will serve as a handy reference for terms with which you are unfamiliar or about which you would like more information.

Becoming familiar with some of the prefixes and suffixes commonly used in medical terms can help you

ABC PUBLISHERS, INC.

July 10, 1998

Ms. Lara Erickson
2594 Hughes Boulevard
Hamilton City, NJ 08999

Dear Ms. Erickson:

SUBJECT: SHIPMENT DELAY

Thank you for contacting us regarding your order for *Smith and Doe's New Medical Dictionary*. Due to an unexpectedly heavy demand for the book, we are experiencing delays in processing and shipping orders.

We expect to ship your book in four weeks, around August 15. Because of this delay, we offer you the option of canceling your order with a full refund. If you would like to cancel at this point, please fill out and return the enclosed postcard. If we do not hear from you, your order will be shipped when ready.

We are sorry for any inconvenience this delay may cause you. Please be assured that ABC Publishers values its customers and always endeavors to fulfill orders in a timely fashion.

Sincerely yours,

Andrew Williams

Andrew Williams
Customer Service Manager

AW/cjc
Enclosure

---

117 New Avenue New York, NY 10000

Figure 7-3.   The full-block letter style is quicker and easier to type than other styles.

ABC PUBLISHERS, INC.

July 10, 1998

Ms. Lara Erickson
2594 Hughes Boulevard
Hamilton City, NJ 08999

SHIPMENT DELAY

Thank you for contacting us regarding your order for *Smith and Doe's New Medical Dictionary*. Due to an unexpectedly heavy demand for the book, we are experiencing delays in processing and shipping orders.

We expect to ship your book in four weeks, around August 15. Because of this delay, we offer you the option of canceling your order with a full refund. If you would like to cancel at this point, please fill out and return the enclosed postcard. If we do not hear from you, your order will be shipped when ready.

We are sorry for any inconvenience this delay may cause you. Please be assured that ABC Publishers values its customers and always endeavors to fulfill orders in a timely fashion.

Andrew Williams

ANDREW WILLIAMS, CUSTOMER SERVICE MANAGER

AW/cjc
Enclosure

117 New Avenue New York, NY 10000

Figure 7-4.   The simplified letter style is considered by some executives to be the most readable style for correspondence.

understand the meanings of many words. Appendix B lists some common medical prefixes and suffixes.

Physicians' Desk Reference (PDR). The *PDR* may be thought of as a dictionary of medications. Published yearly, it provides up-to-date information on both prescription and nonprescription drugs. You can consult the *PDR* for the correct spelling of a particular drug or for other information about its usage, side effects, contraindications, and so on.

English Grammar and Usage Manuals. These manuals answer questions concerning grammar and word usage. They usually contain sections on punctuation, capitalization, and other details of written communication.

Word Processing Spelling Checkers. Most word processing programs used in medical offices have built-in spelling checkers. There are also programs designed specifically to check spelling in medical documents. These spelling checkers include most common medical terms that would not be found in a regular software program.

Spelling checkers pick up many spelling errors and often give you suggestions for correct spellings. If you indicate the choice you meant to input, the program automatically replaces the misspelled word. These programs may not detect all spelling errors, however. They should not be relied on as the only means of checking a document. For example, spelling checkers cannot tell you that you used the wrong word if you type the word *form* instead of *from,* because *form* is also a correctly spelled word.

You may be able to add words that are not currently recognized by the spelling checker in your computer. Use this feature to add medical terms. A word of caution is important here! Before you add the word to the computer's dictionary, be sure to look up the exact spelling in a medical dictionary. The computer will recognize only the spelling you add. If you place the *wrong* spelling in the computer, your spelling checker will not correct it.

When you type e-mails, take special care to use correct grammar and punctuation. Spelling checkers are available in most e-mail programs and should be used at the completion of the e-mail. The e-mail spelling checker does not automatically point out mistakes as you type.

Some software packages offer grammar-checking and style-checking features. These programs can identify certain problems, but the person using them still needs to know basic rules of grammar and style to correct errors.

Editing

The **editing** process ensures that a document is accurate, clear, and complete; free of grammatical errors; organized logically; and written in an appropriate style. It is a good idea to leave some time between the writing and editing stages so that you can look at the document in a fresh light. As you edit, you must examine language usage, content, and style.

Language Usage. Learn basic grammar rules. When in doubt, refer to a grammar handbook or reference manual. Make sure all sentences are complete. Ask yourself, Is this the best way to convey what I want to say? Do my word choices reflect the overall tone of the document? For example, in a business letter, you would avoid choosing phrases that are too colloquial or cute, such as "Thanks a million" or "Take it easy."

Content. A letter should contain all the necessary information the writer intends to convey. If you are editing someone else's letter and something appears to be missing, check with the writer. She may have omitted information by mistake.

The content of a letter should follow a logical thought pattern. Create a clean, concise letter by:

- Stating the purpose of the letter in the first sentence
- Discussing one topic at a time
- Changing paragraphs when you change topics
- Listing events in chronological order
- Sticking to the subject
- Selecting your words carefully
- Reading over what you have written before printing

Style. Use a writing style that is appropriate to the reader. A letter written to a patient is likely to require a different style than one written to a physician.

Proofreading

Proofreading means checking a document for errors. After you edit a document, put it aside for a short time before proofreading it. Ideally, have a coworker proofread your work. There are three types of errors that can occur when preparing a document: formatting, data, and mechanical.

Formatting Errors. These errors involve the positioning of the various parts of a letter. They may include errors in indenting, line length, or line spacing. To avoid these errors, take the following two steps:

1. Scan the letter to make sure that the indentions are consistent, that the spacing is correct, and that the text is centered from left to right and top to bottom.
2. Make sure you have followed the office style.

Data Errors. Data errors involve mistyping monetary figures, such as a balance on a patient statement. Verify the accuracy of all figures by checking them twice or by having one or two coworkers check them.

Mechanical Errors. Mechanical errors are errors in spelling, punctuation, spacing between words, and division of words. Mechanical errors also include reversing words or characters, typing them twice, or omitting them altogether. Here are some tips to help you avoid mechanical errors.

- Learn basic spelling, punctuation, and word division rules. When in doubt, be sure to check a manual on English usage. Table 7-2 presents some basic rules concerning the mechanics of writing. Figure 7-5 lists

Commonly Misspelled Medical Terms and Other Words

Medical Terms

abscess	dissect	leukocyte	prescription
aerobic	eosinophil	malaise	prophylaxis
anergic	epididymis	menstruation	prostate
anesthetic	epistaxis	metastasis	prosthesis
aneurysm	erythema	muscle	pruritus
anteflexion	eustachian	neuron	psoriasis
arrhythmia	fissure	nosocomial	psychiatrist
asepsis	flexure	occlusion	pyrexia
asthma	fomites	ophthalmology	respiration
auricle	glaucoma	oscilloscope	rheumatism
benign	glomerular	osseous	roentgenology
bilirubin	gonorrhea	palliative	scirrhous
bronchial	hemocytometer	parasite	serous
calcaneus	hemorrhage	parenteral	specimen
capillary	hemorrhoids	parietal	sphincter
cervical	homeostasis	paroxysm	sphygmomanometer
chancre	humerus	pericardium	squamous
choroid	ileum	perineum	staphylococcus
chromosome	ilium	peristalsis	surgeon
cirrhosis	infarction	peritoneum	vaccine
clavicle	inoculate	pharynx	vein
curettage	intussusception	pituitary	venous
cyanosis	ischemia	plantar	wheal
defibrillator	ischium	pleurisy	
desiccation	larynx	pneumonia	
diluent	leukemia	polyp	

Other Words

absence	assistance	controversy	eligible
accept	associate	corroborate	embarrass
accessible	auxiliary	counsel	emphasis
accommodate	balloon	courtesy	entrepreneur
accumulate	bankruptcy	defendant	envelope
achieve	believe	definite	environment
acquire	benefited	dependent	exceed
adequate	brochure	description	except
advantageous	bulletin	desirable	exercise
affect	business	development	exhibit
aggravate	category	dilemma	exhilaration
all right	changeable	disappear	existence
a lot	characteristic	disappoint	fantasy
already	cigarette	disapprove	fascinate
altogether	circumstance	disastrous	February
analysis	clientele	discreet	fluorescent
analyze	committee	discrete	forty
apparatus	comparative	discrimination	grammar
apparent	complement	dissatisfied	grievance
appearance	compliment	dissipate	guarantee
appropriate	concede	earnest	handkerchief
approximate	conscientious	ecstasy	height
argument	conscious	effect	humorous

(continued)

Figure 7-5. Familiarize yourself with these commonly misspelled words, and check their spelling carefully whenever you use them.

- With a regular business-size envelope, fold the letter in thirds. Fold the bottom third up first, then the top third down, and insert the letter.
- With a window envelope, use an accordion fold. Fold the bottom third up. Then, fold the top third back so that the address appears in the window, and insert the enclosure.

Before folding the letter, double-check that it has been signed, that all enclosures are included, and that the address on the letter matches the one on the envelope. Any enclosures that are not attached to the letter should be placed inside the folds so that they will be removed from the envelope along with the letter.

Mailing Equipment and Supplies

The proper equipment and supplies will help you handle the mail efficiently and cost-effectively. In addition to letterhead, blank stationery for multipage letters, and envelopes, you will need some standard supplies. The USPS provides forms, labels, and packaging for items that need special attention, such as airmail, Priority Mail, Express Mail, certified mail, or registered mail. Private delivery companies, such as United Parcel Service (UPS), also provide shipping supplies to their customers.

Airmail Supplies

In the past, any piece of mail that was transported by air was designated as airmail. Today nearly all first-class mail outside a local area is routinely sent by air. However, airmail services are still available for some packages and for most mail going to foreign countries.

If you are sending an item by airmail, attach special airmail stickers, available from the post office, on all sides. (The word *AIRMAIL* can also be neatly written on all sides.) Special airmail envelopes for letters can be purchased from the USPS.

Envelopes for Overnight Delivery Services

For correspondence or packages that must be delivered by the next day, a number of overnight delivery services are available through the USPS and private companies. Most companies require the use of their own envelopes and mailing materials. Make sure you keep adequate supplies on hand.

Postal Rates, Scales, and Meters

Postal rates and regulations change periodically, and every medical office should have a copy of the latest guidelines. These guidelines are available from the USPS. Postal scales and meters are described in Chapter 5.

U.S. Postal Service Delivery

The USPS offers a variety of domestic and international delivery services for letters and packages. Following are some of the services you will be most likely to use in a medical office setting.

Regular Mail Service

Regular mail delivery includes several classes of mail as well as other designations such as Priority Mail and Express Mail. The class or designation determines how quickly a piece of mail is delivered.

First-Class Mail. Most correspondence generated in a medical office—letters, postcards, and invoices—is sent by first-class mail. Items must weigh 11 ounces or less to be considered first-class. (An item over 11 ounces that requires quick delivery must be sent by Priority Mail, which is discussed later in the chapter.) The cost of mailing a first-class item is based on its weight. The standard rate is for items 1 ounce or less that are not larger than $6\frac{1}{8}$ inches high and $11\frac{1}{2}$ inches wide. Additional postage is required for items that are heavier or larger. Postage for postcards is less than the letter rate. First-class mail is forwarded at no additional cost.

Second-Class Mail. Second-class mail is not used by most medical offices. This class of mail is designed for the delivery of newspapers and periodicals only.

Third-Class Mail. Third-class mail is also known as bulk mail. It is not often used in medical offices. Bulk mail is used for the mailing of books, catalogs, and other printed material that weighs less than 16 ounces. This class of mailing is available only to authorized mailers.

Fourth-Class Mail. Fourth-class mail is also called parcel post. It is used for items that weigh at least 1 pound but not more than 70 pounds and that do not require speedy delivery. Rates are based on weight and distance. There is a special fourth-class rate for mailing books, manuscripts, and some types of medical information.

Priority Mail. Priority class is useful for heavier items that require quicker delivery than is available for fourth-class mail. Any first-class item that weighs between 11 ounces and 70 pounds requires Priority Mail service. Although the rate for Priority Mail varies with the weight of the item and the distance it must travel, the USPS offers a flat rate for all material that can fit into its special Priority Mail envelope. The USPS guarantees delivery of Priority Mail items in 2 to 3 days.

Express Mail. Express Mail is the quickest USPS service. Different types are available, including next-day and second-day delivery. Express Mail deliveries are made 365 days a year. Rates vary, depending on the weight and the specific service. A special flat-rate envelope is also available. Items sent by Express Mail are automatically insured against loss or damage. You can drop off packages at the post office or arrange for pickup service.

Special Postal Services

The USPS offers a variety of special mail delivery services in addition to the regular classes of mail. These services may require an additional fee above and beyond the cost of postage.

Special Delivery. Use special delivery if you want an item delivered as soon as it reaches the recipient's post office. Delivery of the item is typically made before the regularly scheduled mail delivery. Special delivery service is available within certain distance limits and during certain hours.

Certified Mail. Certified mail offers a guarantee that the item has been received. The item is marked as certified mail and requires the postal carrier to obtain a signature on delivery (Figure 7-7). The signature card is then returned to the sender. The card should be added to the patient's file. This documentation is evidence that the document was not only mailed but also received. The receiver's name is clearly printed along with the signature. The certified mail signature card becomes a legal document, which may be important in court.

Return Receipt Requested. You may request a return receipt to obtain proof that an item was delivered. The receipt indicates who received the item and when. You can obtain a return receipt for various types of mail.

Registered Mail. Use registered mail to send items that are valuable, irreplaceable, or otherwise important. Registered mail provides the sender with evidence of mailing and delivery. It also provides the security that an item is being tracked as it is transported through the postal system. Because of this tracking process, delivery may be slightly delayed.

To register a piece of mail, take it to the post office, and indicate the full value of the item. Both first-class mail and Priority Mail can be registered.

International Mail

The USPS offers both surface (via ship) and airmail service to most foreign countries. Information on rates and fees is available from the post office.

There are various types of international mail, which are similar to the domestic classes. The USPS also provides international Express Mail and Priority Mail services, along with special mail delivery services such as registered mail, certified mail, and special delivery.

Tracing Mail

If a piece of registered or certified mail does not reach its destination by the expected time, you can ask the post office to trace it (Figure 7-8). You will need to present your original receipt for the item.

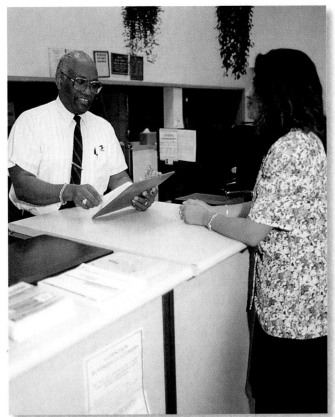

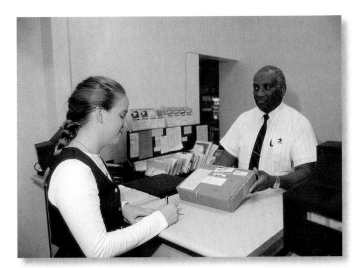

Figure 7-7. If no one is in the office when the mail is delivered, the medical assistant may need to go to the post office to sign for a certified letter or package.

Figure 7-8. Tracing an item is a service that post offices perform when important items are delayed or do not reach their destinations.

Other Delivery Services

In addition to the USPS, other companies provide mail and package delivery services. The costs and types of services vary.

United Parcel Service

United Parcel Service (UPS) delivers packages and provides overnight letter and express services. You can either drop off packages at a UPS location or have them picked up at your office. Fees vary with the services provided, such as ground or air. Packages are automatically insured against theft or damage.

Express Delivery Services

Companies such as Federal Express and Airborne Express provide several types of quick delivery services for letters

PROCEDURE 7.2

Sorting and Opening Mail

Objective: To follow a standard procedure for sorting, opening, and processing incoming office mail

Materials: Letter opener, date and time stamp (manual or automatic), stapler, paper clips, adhesive notes

Method

1. Check the address on each letter or package to be sure that it has been delivered to the correct location.

2. Sort the mail into piles according to priority and type of mail. Your system may include the following:
   - Top priority. This pile will contain any items that were sent by overnight mail delivery in addition to items sent by registered mail, certified mail, or special delivery. (Faxes and e-mail messages are also top priority.)
   - Second priority. This pile will include personal or confidential mail.
   - Third priority. This pile will contain all first-class mail, airmail, and Priority Mail items. These items should be divided into payments received, insurance forms, reports, and other correspondence.
   - Fourth priority. This pile will consist of packages.
   - Fifth priority. This pile will contain magazines and newspapers.
   - Sixth priority. This last pile will include advertisements and catalogs.

3. Set aside all letters labeled "Personal" or "Confidential." Unless you have permission to open these letters, only the addressee should open them.

4. Arrange all the envelopes with the flaps facing up and away from you.

5. Tap the lower edge of the envelope to shift the contents to the bottom. This step helps to prevent cutting any of the contents when you open the envelope.

6. Open all the envelopes. (It is more efficient to open all the envelopes first and then to remove the contents.)

7. Remove and unfold the contents, making sure that nothing remains in the envelope.

8. Review each document, and check the sender's name and address.
   - If the letter has no return address, save the envelope, or cut the address off the envelope, and tape it to the letter.
   - Check to see if the address matches the one on the envelope. If there is a difference, staple the envelope to the letter, and make a note to verify the correct address with the sender.

9. Compare the enclosure notation on the letter with the actual enclosures to make sure that all items are included. Make a note to contact the sender if anything is missing.

10. Clip together each letter and its enclosures.

11. Check the date of the letter. If there is a significant delay between the date of the letter and the postmark, keep the envelope. (It may be necessary to refer to the postmark in legal matters or cases of collection.)

12. If all contents appear to be in order, you can discard the envelope.

13. Review all bills and statements.
    - Make sure the amount enclosed is the same as the amount listed on the statement.
    - Make a note of any discrepancies.

14. Stamp each piece of correspondence with the date (and sometimes the time) to record its receipt. If possible, stamp each item in the same location—such as the upper right corner. (It may be necessary to refer to the date in legal matters or in cases of collection.)

How to Spot Urgent Incoming Mail

How can you tell if a piece of incoming mail is urgent? First-class mail marked "Urgent" tells you that it requires immediate attention. Here are some other signals to look for.

Overnight Mail

Any package that has been sent by an overnight carrier or by USPS Express Mail should be considered urgent and should be opened immediately.

Certified Mail

Certified mail requires your signature on delivery. The sender used certified mail to be sure that the item would be sent to the proper person.

Registered Mail

Items sent by registered mail typically are valuable, irreplaceable, or otherwise important. Registered mail provides the sender with evidence of mailing and delivery.

Special Delivery

An item sent by special delivery is likely to be delivered sometime before the normal mail delivery—possibly even on a Sunday or holiday. The sender requested special delivery to ensure that the item would be delivered promptly after it was received at the addressee's post office.

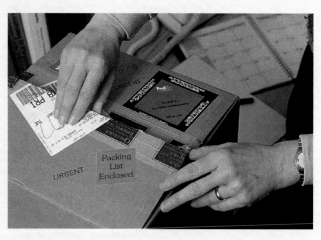

Figure 7-9. Urgent materials receive top priority upon arrival at an office.

---

and packages. Rates vary according to weight, time of delivery, and in some cases, whether you have the package picked up at your office or drop it off at one of the company's local branches.

Messengers or Couriers

When items must be delivered within the local area on the same day, local messenger services are an option. Many messenger companies are listed in the yellow pages of the telephone book.

Processing Incoming Mail

Mail is an important connection between the office and other professionals and patients. Often an office has an established procedure for handling the mail. It is best to set aside a specific time of the day to process all the incoming mail at once rather than trying to do a little bit at a time.

Although it sounds simple, processing mail involves more than merely opening envelopes. In general, it involves the following steps: sorting, opening, recording, annotating, and distributing.

Sorting and Opening

The first step in processing mail is to sort it. Mail is typically sorted according to its priority. Sort mail in an uncluttered area to avoid mixing it with other paperwork. Follow a regular sorting procedure each time so that you do not miss any steps. Procedure 7-2 outlines suggested steps for sorting and opening the mail. The Tips for the Office section discusses how to recognize urgent incoming mail.

Recording

It is a good idea to keep a log of each day's mail. This daily record lists the mail received and indicates follow-up correspondence and the date it is completed. This method helps in tracing items and keeping track of correspondence.

Annotating

Because you will be reading much of the incoming mail, you may also be encouraged to annotate it. To **annotate** means to underline or highlight key points of the letter or to write reminders, comments, or suggested actions in the margins or on self-adhesive notes. Annotating may involve

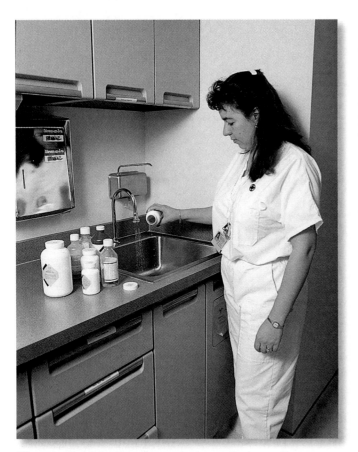

Figure 7-10. Certain nontoxic medical supplies must be carefully disposed of according to medical office policy.

Handling Drug and Product Samples

Many physicians receive a number of drug and product samples in the mail. Handling procedures vary from office to office. Samples of nonprescription products, such as hand creams or cough drops, may be displayed in the patient treatment area for patients to take.

The physician may ask that you put samples of any new prescription drugs in the consultation room for him to evaluate. Store other drug samples in a locked cabinet reserved solely for such samples. Sort and label the samples by category, such as antibiotics, sedatives, painkillers, and so on. Never give samples to patients unless specified by the physician. If the physician directs you to give samples to a patient, make sure to write this information in the patient's chart and date the entry.

When a box of samples is half empty, it is common practice to destroy half of the remaining samples by pouring liquids down the drain and putting pills in a garbage disposal. Samples should not be put in the trash. (The remaining samples that have not been destroyed may be used at the physician's direction.) Once a month, any samples that are past their expiration date should be destroyed (Figure 7-10).

Summary

As a medical assistant, you are responsible for many of the tasks involved in writing correspondence and processing outgoing and incoming mail in the medical office. Proper and efficient management of correspondence and mail is essential to promoting a positive, professional office image.

Choosing the proper letterhead and envelopes helps to ensure professional-looking correspondence. Knowing the parts of a letter and the various letter styles and formats used in the business environment today helps you create effective correspondence. Knowing how to edit and proofread and how to use writing reference books helps ensure that your letters are understandable and well written.

Familiarity with the types of mail services available enables you to choose the proper services to meet the office's mailing needs. Following proper procedures and recommended USPS guidelines ensures that office mail will be received in the most timely manner.

Handling incoming mail is also an important responsibility. Following an established procedure allows you to process and route the mail efficiently.

pulling a patient's chart or any previous related correspondence from a file and attaching it to the letter.

Distributing

The next step is to sort letters into separate batches for distribution. These batches might include correspondence that requires the physician's attention, payments to be directed to the person in charge of billing, and correspondence that requires your attention. Each batch should be presented to the appropriate person in a file folder or arranged with the highest-priority items on top. You may be given specific instructions on how to distribute magazines, newspapers, and advertising circulars.

CASE STUDY QUESTIONS

Now that you have completed this chapter, review the case study at the beginning of the chapter and answer the following questions:

1. Why is it important to accurately and carefully prepare correspondence for an ambulatory setting? What could the poor management of documents and correspondence mean to a medical practice?
2. What are the differences between the language used in an informal or casual letter and that used in a formal or professional business letter?
3. What are some appropriate shortcuts that can assist in the daily management of correspondence and mailing?
4. What are some factors to consider in choosing the best mode of delivery for letters and parcels?

Discussion Questions

1. Why is it important to closely follow the basic rules of writing when creating a business letter?
2. Name and describe the five steps involved in processing incoming mail.
3. Explain the differences between certified mail, first-class mail, and registered mail.

Critical Thinking Questions

1. What is your weakest area in writing? How might you improve? Create and complete a project that helps you improve your weakest area.
2. The physician tells you to make sure that all patient letters that address withdrawing the services of the practice are "well documented." What does the physician mean? What would you do?
3. Imagine that your coworker is out sick. You must make sure all the work is handled. Which is more important—typing referral letters or sorting the mail? Why? How might you proceed if you are responsible for both but don't have the time to complete both?
4. Make flash cards from Table 7-1 and Table 7-3, and quiz one of your classmates. Which states or terms do you find difficult?

Application Activities

1. You are employed in Dr. Angelo Carillo's office. A young patient of yours, Rodney Sills, has broken his wrist, and Dr. Carillo says that Rodney will be unable to participate in gym class for 10 weeks. Create a letter notifying his gym instructor of the situation.
2. Prepare a No. 10 business envelope using the USPS guidelines for addressing envelopes. Include the following information.

Return address:
Dr. Angelo Carillo, 123 Winding Way, Suite 2, Rockland, NJ 09876

Mailing address:
ABC Insurance, 987 Hill Street, Marrakesh, CA 01234

Attention:
Susan Jones, Claims Department

Special Instructions:
Certified Mail

3. Using proper letter formatting technique and the basic rules of writing reviewed in this chapter, correct the following letter:

September 18th, 1997

Mountainside Hospital
Samuel Adams, Educational Coordinator
1 Mountainside Lane
San Francisco, California, 94112

Dear mr. Adams:
I am writing in response to your letter of the 10th. I am very interested in presenting a talk at your Health Fare in February. I am aviulable to speak on either the 20th or the 21st.

If there is any flexibility in scheduling, I would prefer to present my talk in the afternoon. Also, please let me know how long I should prepare to speak. I am including a copy of an article I recently wrote on the same subject for the local paper.

I am looking forward to hearing from you.
Sincerly,
Enclosure
Dr. Angelo Carillo
AC/SCB

Typical Supplies in a Medical Office

Administrative Supplies

Appointment books, daybooks

Back-to-school/back-to-work slips

Clipboards

Computer supplies

Copy and facsimile (fax) machine paper

File folders, coding tabs

History and physical examination sheets/cards

Insurance forms: disability, HMO and other third party payers, life insurance examinations, Veterans Administration, workers' compensation

Insurance manuals

Local welfare department forms

Patient education materials

Pens, pencils, erasers

Rubber bands, paper clips

Social Security forms

Stamps

Stationery: appointment cards, bookkeeping supplies (ledgers, statements, billing forms), letterhead, second sheets, envelopes, business cards, prescription pads, notebooks, notepads, telephone memo pads

Clinical Supplies

Alcohol swabs

Applicators

Bandaging materials: adhesive tape, gauze pads, gauze sponges, elastic bandages, adhesive bandages, roller bandages (gauze and elastic)

Cloth or paper gowns

Cotton, cotton swabs

Culture tubes

50% dextrose solution

Disposable sheaths for thermometers

Disposable tips for otoscopes

Gloves: sterile, examination

Hemoccult test kits

Iodine or Betadine pads

Lancets

Lubricating jelly

Microscopic slides and fixative

Needles, syringes

Nitroglycerin tablets

Safety pins

Silver nitrate sticks

Suture removal kits

Sutures

Thermometer covers

Tongue depressors

Topical skin freeze

Urinalysis test sticks

Urine containers

Injectable medications: diazepam (Valium), diphenhydramine hydrochloride (Benadryl), epinephrine (Adrenalin), furosemide (Lasix), isoproterenol (Isuprel), lidocaine (Xylocaine: 1%, 2%, and plain), meperidine hydrochloride (Demerol), morphine, phenobarbital, sodium bicarbonate, sterile saline, sterile water

Other medicines, chemicals, solutions, ointments, lotions, and disinfectants, as needed

General Supplies

Liquid hypoallergenic soap

Paper cups

Paper towels

Tampons

Tissues: facial, toilet

Figure 8-2. Familiarize yourself with the typical supplies in a medical office.

systematically. Keep a list of these items, and update it as needed. This supply list is usually kept in the office procedures manual. Appropriate sections of the list may be posted on the cabinets where those items are stored.

To help keep track of supplies, categorize them according to the urgency of need. Although all supplies in your office are necessary, some supplies are more important than others. Figure 8-2 can help you determine vital, incidental, and periodic supplies for your office.

Vital Supplies. These items are absolutely necessary to ensure the smooth running of the practice. They include paper examination table covers and prescription pads. Without these items, the physician would be unable to work in a clean examination environment or to readily prescribe medication for patients during office visits. Another type of vital supply is an item that requires a special order, such as a printed form. Special orders take time to obtain, so they must be ordered well before supplies run low.

Incidental Supplies. These supplies are needed in the office but do not threaten the efficiency of the office if the supply runs low. Incidental supplies include staples and rubber bands, which can be purchased quickly and easily at a local stationery store.

Periodic Supplies. These supplies require ordering only occasionally. For example, you will order appointment books only once or twice a year, probably in small numbers. The urgency of ordering some periodic items can depend on the size of the office. A multiphysician office, for example, would require more appointment books than a single-physician office. Another example of a periodic item might be holiday cards to send to the physician's colleagues and patients.

Storing Office Supplies

Storing office supplies requires good organizational skills and attention to detail. Many people in an office use these supplies, so the items should be stored neatly and in an orderly way. In addition, it is important to store supplies safely to prevent loss or theft, damage, or deterioration.

Location. In a small medical office, supplies are generally kept near the areas of the office where they are used. Administrative supplies are usually stored behind or adjacent to the reception area, with clinical supplies stored near the examination rooms. If the practice has a laboratory, pertinent supplies are stored in or near the laboratory. Offices that have separate supply rooms offer more storage space.

Small medical offices may not have ample space for storage. It may be tempting to store boxes on the floor behind the air conditioning unit, stacked up close to the ceiling, or in potentially hazardous locations, such as near a source of heat. It is essential that supplies be stored according to the guidelines described by JCAHO (Joint Commission for Accreditation of Health Organizations).

Items may not be stored on the floor; instead, they must be raised off the floor, as on a crate or shelf, to avoid contamination by water. Items stored close to the ceiling are considered a fire hazard. JCAHO standards require that supplies stored on the top shelf of a closet or storage area be at least 18 inches below the ceiling.

Avoid storing any boxes or supplies near a water heater, air conditioning unit, heater, or stove. Many expendable items and their packaging are combustible and can quickly become a fire hazard. Air conditioning units may drip water on the floor. If boxes of expensive forms are stored nearby, they can quickly become ruined as water seeps unnoticed into the packaging.

Storage Cabinets. Each storage cabinet should be labeled with a list of its contents. Keep all stock of one item together. Store small items together according to type.

Finding supplies is easier if you keep small items at eye level. Put large, bulky goods, such as reams of stationery, on lower shelves. Label boxes and containers clearly so that all employees can readily find what they need and so that the inventory process is easier.

As you initially arrange items on storage shelves, label the shelves. Reserve enough space to completely stock each item. Do not put anything but the appropriate item in each designated space. This easy system allows for a quick review when you reorder supplies.

To reduce the risk of errors on reorders, keep each item's original label attached to it. Cover the label with clear tape, if necessary. If you must replace a worn label, do it immediately when needed, making sure the new label has the same detailed information as the old one. Bottles with pouring spouts should be labeled on the side opposite the spout to prevent the liquid from dripping onto the label. Use a laundry marking pen to label linens with the name of your office. Linen services usually premark linens with the name of the company or the practice.

Many items have a shelf life after which they are no longer usable. By not overordering and by rotating supplies—using older ones first—your office will be able to use items during their shelf life. This is true not only for perishable items such as medications, but also for linens and paper, which can deteriorate. Keep in mind when stocking medications or chemicals that a more recent shipment may have an earlier expiration date than a previous shipment. Always check expiration dates when storing supplies. Be careful to arrange them so that items with earlier expiration dates are in front of those with later dates.

Administrative Supplies. In addition to such expendable items as pens, pencils, and paper clips, paper products are important to a medical office. In general, paper products should be stored flat in their original boxes or wrappings to prevent pages from bending or curling. However, information booklets may be stored upright to save space. Envelopes and other paper goods with gummed surfaces must be kept dry to prevent them from sticking together.

Clinical Supplies. The rules of good housekeeping and asepsis (see Chapter 19) apply to storage areas for clinical supplies. These areas must be kept clean and protected from damage and exposure to the elements.

All dressings and most bandaging materials must be kept sterile. For example, gauze that may be used to bandage an open wound must be sterile. Elastic rolled bandages, which do not touch open wounds, must be clean but not necessarily sterile.

Chemicals, drugs, and solutions should be kept in a cool, dark place because light causes some substances to deteriorate. Store all liquids in their original containers. Line cabinets with plastic-coated shelf paper, and wipe it frequently with a damp cloth.

Store poisons and narcotics separately from other products. Narcotics must be stored securely out of sight in a locked cabinet. Never store strong acids near alkaline solutions or flammable items near sources of heat. Solutions that will be stored for a considerable length of time should have a small amount of space at the top of the bottle to allow for heat expansion.

Some liquids should be stored in the refrigerator. Check each item for specific storage instructions. If storage space is limited, consider eliminating some items—especially bulky ones that are rarely used or items that patients can purchase at surgical supply stores.

Clinical refrigerators may be needed to store certain clinical supplies that require refrigeration. Never store food items and clinical items in the same refrigerator. A clinical refrigerator must be kept at a constant temperature to properly maintain the chemical integrity of lab supplies. Monitoring and recording the date and temperature of the clinical refrigerator should be completed once a week or per office protocol.

Taking Inventory of Medical Office Supplies

The list of supplies your office uses regularly and the quantities you have in storage constitute the office **inventory.** Keeping track of the office's inventory is a job that requires careful planning, attention to detail, and basic math skills. Accurate inventory activity ensures that the office never runs out of much-needed supplies.

Understanding Your Responsibilities

It is important to have an understanding with the doctor or doctors in the practice about the extent of your responsibilities for maintaining supplies. Some doctors are more involved with the details of running an office than others. Your responsibilities may grow as you become more experienced. The doctor, however, usually takes care of certain duties, such as meeting with drug company representatives or authorizing large purchases.

Generally you will be responsible for overseeing the flow of supplies bought and used, calculating the budget for supplies, selecting supplies and vendors, following correct purchasing and payment procedures, and storing the goods properly.

The Inventory Filing System. To oversee the flow of inventory efficiently, you will need a filing system (see Procedure 8-1). This system consists of several elements:

- The list of supplies (discussed earlier in the chapter)
- An itemized inventory
- An inventory card or record page for each item
- A list of the names and addresses of current vendors

- A file of current catalogs from vendors (including some vendors not currently used, for comparison shopping)
- A want list of brands or items that the office does not currently use but may want to try in the future
- Files for **invoices,** or bills from vendors, and completed order forms
- Reorder reminder cards to indicate when an in-stock item should be reordered
- Color-coded, removable self-adhesive flags to indicate "Need to Order" or "On Order"
- An inventory and ordering schedule
- Order forms for each vendor (may be multiple-copy forms, fax forms, electronic forms, or e-mail forms)

The Inventory Card or Record Page. The inventory card or record page for each item or category of items may be a 4-by-6-inch index card or a page in a loose-leaf binder (Figure 8-3). These separate cards or pages make it easy to group together the items that need to be ordered at any given time. Records kept on the card or page help you monitor how quickly items are used and how much should be ordered each time.

Some information may change. As you become more proficient at monitoring inventory or as the practice grows or diminishes in size, you may find that quantities, vendors, or reorder quantities need to be adjusted. With the help of the doctor, you will be able to determine the ideal quantity of each item to have on hand, depending on the size of the practice, the available storage space, and the ordering schedule.

It is important to check the storage areas regularly, preferably at specific times, and to count the items on hand. When the supply of an item begins to run low, you (or another staff member) should flag the inventory card or record page to indicate the need to reorder it at the next regular ordering time.

Color-coded, removable self-adhesive flags on the inventory card or record page are an efficient way to track inventory. A red flag, for example, might indicate that a supply needs to be ordered. A yellow flag might be substituted when the item has been ordered.

Reorder Reminder Cards. Reorder reminder cards (Figure 8-4) are usually brightly colored cards inserted directly into stock on the supply shelf to indicate when it is time to reorder an item. For example, if you have determined that four boxes of staples is a sufficient quantity to keep on hand and your office supply orders are filled in 2 business days, you might place the reorder reminder card between the third and fourth boxes of staples. The reorder quantity on the inventory card or record page for staples would indicate "four boxes."

The reorder reminder cards also remind other staff members to tell you when an item is in short supply. In some offices, the medical assistant labels the reminder card with the name and bar code number of the supply

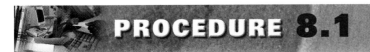

PROCEDURE 8.1

Step-by-Step Overview of Inventory Procedures

Objective: To set up an effective inventory program for a medical office

Materials: Pen, paper, file folders, vendor catalogs, index cards or loose-leaf binder and blank pages, reorder reminder cards, vendor order forms

Method

1. Define with your physician/employer the extent of your responsibility in managing supplies. Know whether the physician's approval or supervision is required for certain procedures, whether any systems have already been established, and if the physician has any preference for a particular vendor or trade-name item. If your medical practice is large, determine which medical assistant is responsible for each aspect of supply management.

2. Know what administrative and clinical supplies should be stocked in your office. Create a formal supply list of vital, incidental, and periodic items, and keep a copy in the office's procedures manual.

3. Start a file containing a list of current vendors with copies of their catalogs.

4. Create a want list of brands or products the office does not currently use but might like to try. Inform other staff members of the list so that they can make entries.

5. Make a file for supply invoices and completed order forms. (Keep these documents on file for at least 3 years.)

6. Devise an inventory system of index cards or loose-leaf pages for each item. List the following data for each item on its card:
   - Date and quantity of each order
   - Name and contact information for the vendor and sales representative
   - Date each shipment was received
   - Total cost and unit cost, or price per piece for the item
   - Payment method used
   - Results of periodic counts of the item
   - Quantity expected to cover the office for a given period of time
   - Reorder quantity (the quantity remaining on the shelf that indicates when reorder should be made)

7. Have a system for flagging items that need to be ordered and those that are already on order. For example, mark their cards or pages with a self-adhesive tab or note. Make or buy reorder reminder cards to put into the stock of each item at the reorder quantity level.

8. Establish with the physician a regular schedule for taking inventory. Every 1 to 2 weeks is usually sufficient. As a backup system for remembering to check stock and reorder, estimate the times for these activities. Mark them on your calendar, or create a tickler file on your computer.

9. Order at the same times each week or month, after inventory is taken. However, if there is an unexpected shortage of an item, and more than a week or so remains before the regular ordering time, place the order immediately.

10. Fill in the vendor's order form (or type a letter of request). Order by telephone, fax, or e-mail, if possible, to expedite the order. Be sure to follow procedures that have been approved by the physician or office manager. When placing an order, have all the necessary information at hand, including the correct name of the item and the order and account numbers. Record the order information in the inventory file for that item. Be sure to obtain from the vendor an estimated arrival time for the order, and mark that date and order number on your calendar.

11. When you receive the shipment, record the date and the amount received on the item's inventory card or record page. Check the shipment against the original order and the packing slip inside the package to ensure that the right items, sizes, styles, packaging, and amounts have arrived. If there is any error, immediately call the vendor, with the catalog page and the inventory card or record page at hand.

12. Check the invoice carefully against the original order and the packing slip, making sure that the bill has not already been paid. Sign or stamp the invoice to show that the order was received.

13. Write a check to the vendor to be signed by the physician. Be sure to show the physician the original order, packing slip, and invoice. Record the check number, date, and amount of payment on the invoice, and initial it or have the physician do so. Write the invoice number on the front of the check.

14. Mail the check and the vendor's copy of the invoice to the vendor within 30 days, and file the office copy of the invoice with the original order and packing slip.

| (ITEM NAME) | *Exam Table Paper 21"* | | | | | | | | | | | | | |

ORDER QUANTITY _12_ **REORDER POINT** _4_

ORDER	QTY	REC'D	UNIT COST	PRICE	PREPAID	ON ACCT.	ORDER	QTY	REC'D	UNIT COST	PRICE	PREPAID	ON ACCT.
1/4	12	1/8	$12.25	$147.00	Check 1214	X							
2/5	12	2/9	$12.25	$147.00	Check 2110	X							

INVENTORY COUNT

	JAN.	FEB.	MAR.	APR.	MAY	JUNE	JULY	AUG.	SEPT.	OCT.	NOV.	DEC.
DATE ____	7	10										
DATE ____												

ORDER SOURCE

Smith Physician's Supply Co.

493 Carlton Avenue

South Union, NJ 07422

908-899-6123 Contact: Martin Kohn

UNIT PRICE

12 - $147.00

36 - $441.00

Figure 8-3. The inventory card or record page is the primary inventory-tracking tool in managing medical office supplies.

item, such as "staples 002345." This method allows any staff member to pull the card when the last box of staples before the reminder card is taken from the supply shelf. The staff member can then place the card in a "To Be Ordered" envelope. Some offices can reorder simply by scanning the bar code. Staff members in some offices request supplies by writing them in an order book or on an order list.

Inventory Reminder Kits. Some mail-order supply vendors sell inventory kits, complete with cards and tabs or flags. Computerized inventory systems are also available. Shelves still need to be checked and counts logged on to the computer, however. Therefore, smaller offices generally do not benefit as much as larger ones from a computerized inventory system.

Scheduling Inventory and Ordering

Establish a regular schedule for counting the supplies in the office. Taking inventory every 1 or 2 weeks is usually sufficient. Estimating when you will probably need to reorder a particular item—and putting that date on your calendar or in your appointment book—is also helpful. You and the physician can determine how often storage areas should be checked.

Established Ordering Times. You should have established ordering times, such as the same day each week or month, after inventory is taken. For example, you might take inventory the first Tuesday of every month and order supplies the first Thursday of every month.

A regular schedule for taking inventory and ordering helps all staff members remember when they must give their requests to you. Although you may need to adjust the ordering time occasionally, try to adhere to the schedule to avoid the expense and inconvenience of rush orders.

When to Order Ahead of Schedule. When you take inventory, and the spare supply of an item has not reached but is close to the placement of the reorder reminder card, you must decide whether you should reorder then or wait until the next regular ordering time. You will probably find it is more efficient to go ahead and order rather than wait. Ordering early assures you that the supply will not be depleted before the next regular ordering time.

Ordering ahead of schedule can be especially important if there is a large demand for a particular product and manufacturers' production levels have not caught up with that demand. This situation can occur if there has been an outbreak of a particular flu or virus, or if the Food and Drug Administration has determined that a certain product is harmful, resulting in higher demand for an alternative product.

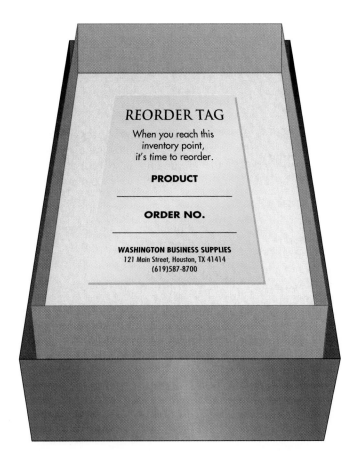

Figure 8-4. Reorder reminder cards are usually brightly colored cards inserted directly into the spare stock of an item on the supply shelf to indicate when it is time to reorder the item.

Unanticipated Shortage of a Supply Item. If the supply of an item reaches the reorder reminder card, and there is still a long time before the next regular ordering time, place the order immediately so that you do not risk running out of the item.

To help you oversee inventory effectively, finish one container before opening a new one. Keep all stock of the same item in one place. The need to count inventory of an item in more than one location or container increases the likelihood of errors. If an item is kept in more than one location, as in the case of multiple examination rooms, inventory is best maintained per room.

As a medical assistant, you want to be sure that there are always sufficient quantities of supplies to keep the office running efficiently. It is unwise to stock spare supplies in too great a quantity, however, because the administrative budget is not likely to support such expenditures. In addition, spare quantities of supplies can be a storage problem.

Ordering Supplies

Ordering supplies requires a procedure to deal with vendors and to order and check supplies. You can avoid common purchasing mistakes by understanding the most efficient way to order supplies for your office.

Locating and Evaluating Supply Vendors

A vendor will most likely already be in place when you join a practice. You should, however, be aware of competitors' prices, services, and other incentives intended to attract your office as a customer. Sometimes the incentives—such as bonus supplies with certain purchases—can represent sizable savings. Remember also that your time has a dollar value to the practice, and services that save you time are worth comparing when evaluating vendors.

Obtaining recommendations from other medical offices is a good way to locate office-supply dealers who sell items at reasonable prices and are also reputable. **Reputable** vendors fulfill orders accurately with quality items, deliver products in good condition, and charge fair prices. Keep in mind when evaluating vendors that the physician may have preferences for certain trade names or vendors.

Gathering Competitive Prices. The costs of maintaining a medical practice are continually rising. Saving money on supplies through careful purchasing strategies is one way to help your physician/employer reduce spending. The medical assistant is often largely responsible for comparison pricing, ordering, and establishing and maintaining relationships with vendors. Your awareness of the most up-to-date information about vendors and supplies is valuable to your physician/employer. Discuss prices with the physician, who in turn may want to discuss them with an accountant.

Setting Up a Supply Budget. The average medical practice spends 4% to 6% of its annual gross income on administrative, clinical, and general supplies. If an office is spending more than 6%, it may be time to reevaluate the office's spending practices. Remember, though, that any budget is only a guide. A budget is meant to serve your office, not the reverse. You and your physician/employer may need to adjust the supply budget based on prices and discounts available from vendors.

Comparing Vendors. To collect competitive data from vendors, contact them by telephone or in writing to request catalogs and other forms of product information. If you are not in charge of routing mail, make sure that supply-related mail, such as product catalogs and sale notices, is routed to you. Catalogs usually include basic information, such as the dealer's name, address, and telephone number, order numbers for items, and vendor policy (Figure 8-5). When investigating a vendor, obtain the following information:

- Prices—costs for supplies, delivery, and any other services; special discounts; minimum quantities applicable; bonus supplies with purchases

BY PHONE

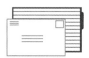

Call our toll-free number:
(800) BIBBERO
(800-242-2376)
Monday thru Friday,
6:00 A.M. – 5:00 P.M. (PST)

BY MAIL

Complete order form and mail to:
Bibbero Systems, Inc.
1300 N. McDowell Blvd.
Petaluma, CA 94954-1180

BY FAX

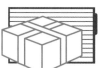

Complete order form and transmit via
FAX to : 800-242-9330
Our FAX line is open 24 hours daily.

SHIPPING POLICY

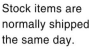

Stock items are normally shipped the same day.

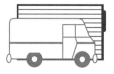

FREE DELIVERY

Free delivery on pre-paid orders totaling $300.00 or more.

Fill out the enclosed order form located in the center of this catalog, and return in the enclosed postage-paid envelope to:

Bibbero Systems, Inc.
1300 N. McDowell Blvd.
Petaluma, CA 94954-1180

If you are in a hurry, call us toll free at: 800-242-2376 or FAX us at 800-242-9330. Our Customer Service Department will be happy to assist you.

For items requiring custom imprinting, please enclose with your order the following information, either typed or printed: Name, Specialty, Address, City/State & Zip Code, Telephone Number and State License Number.

Send us your specifications for any type of special form - Patient Registration, History Forms, Dividers, Charts, etc. – and we will furnish quotes at no charge. We can print single page or multiple part forms.

Please Note: All custom printed orders are subject to an overrun or underrun variance of 10%.

Stock orders received by 11:00 A.M. are normally shipped the same day. Out-of-stock items are automatically back ordered. Custom printed orders normally leave our plant within 10-15 working days after proof approval.

Combined stock and custom printed orders are shipped together, if requested. All orders are shipped via the best method available to your location. Common carriers are used for large volume orders. Overnight air and 2nd day delivery services are available on request.

All orders prepaid by check, Visa, MasterCard or American Express totaling $300.00 or more will be shipped freight free within the continental U.S. This offer excludes furniture, cabinets, and special order items. We regret that the high cost of shipping outside the 48 contiguous states prohibits us from extending this service; we will use the most economical shipping method available to your location.

TERMS

Full payment is due upon receipt of merchandise. Accounts are considered overdue after thirty (30) days and will be subject to a 1% monthly service charge. A service charge of $10.00 will be applied to all returned checks. For information regarding special financial arrangements, please contact our Credit Department at 800-242-2376.

GUARANTEE!

Your Satisfaction Guaranteed!

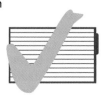

We guarantee our stock products. Return any of our stock products within 60 days of purchase for full credit, exchange or refund of your purchase price. After 60 days, your return will be subject to prior approval and a 15% restocking charge. All returns must have an authorization number. Call our Customer Service Department at 800-242-2376 for your authorization number and enclose it with your return. Opened and/or partially used packages cannot be returned. Personalized items, made to order, special orders and unlocked or opened software cannot be returned.

We accept Visa, MasterCard, & American Express for all your purchases.

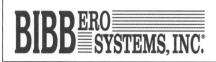

Figure 8-5.   Examine supply catalogs carefully to find out vendors' company policies.

- Quality—product descriptions, illustrations, trade names, recommendations for use, durability, guarantees
- Service—availability of products, delivery time and procedures, sales representative availability, damaged-goods policy
- Payment policies

Competitive Pricing and Quality

Part of your responsibility in managing office supplies is to stay informed about the pricing and quality of competitors to your vendors. Savings can add up quickly, and ongoing comparison pricing can save the practice hundreds of dollars a year.

Unit Pricing. Because many medical items come in a variety of package sizes, you need to be aware of how much the office is actually paying per item. To calculate an item's **unit price,** divide the total price of the package by the quantity, or number of items. For example, if a package of 12 pens costs $12, the unit price, or price per pen, is $1 ($12 divided by 12 pens). If another vendor provides the same type of pen in a package of 18 for $17.10, the unit price is 95 cents ($17.10 divided by 18 pens). The second set of pens is the better buy.

Unit prices are generally lower at larger quantities. Therefore, it makes sense to place one large order for a nonperishable item to cover the office until the next ordering time. Generally, however, you should not order more than a year's supply of any one item, particularly if the item is custom-printed. Addresses, insurance codes, or additions to medical staff can change. When placing quantity discount orders, always consider the following factors: whether the supply can be used within a reasonable time, the possibility of spoilage or deterioration, the amount of storage space in the office, and whether the doctor will continue to use the item. Avoid overspending by not ordering more of an item than is reasonable or necessary.

Rush Orders. Unexpected rush orders usually cost the office more money than regularly scheduled orders. (In some cases, a vendor may not charge extra to a steady customer, but these cases would be exceptions.) To avoid rush orders, be aware of approximately how long the vendor takes to deliver an order. You can obtain this information from the vendor policy and by keeping accurate records of your own experience with deliveries.

Mail-Order Companies. Using large, established mail-order companies often saves money for the medical office, but there may be less control over orders and a greater potential for hidden costs. The neighborhood pharmacy may also offer discounts, but ordering from wholesalers or directly from the manufacturer is usually more economical. The Tips for the Office section provides helpful information about cost-efficient ordering by telephone or fax or through an online service.

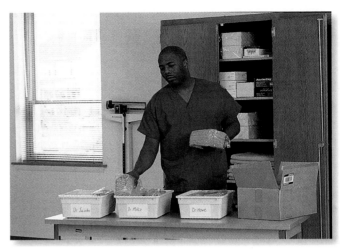

Figure 8-6. Ordering jointly with other offices can cut expenses for everyone.

Purchasing Groups. **Purchasing groups** are groups of physicians that order supplies together to obtain a quantity discount. For example, several medical offices associated with a nearby hospital may order through the hospital. In return for this convenience, the physicians pay dues and guarantee the vendors a certain amount of business. Some programs require members to spend a certain percentage of their supply budget through the group. Groups may also require that members not disclose the group's prices to other physicians. The larger medical practices that participate in these groups save an average of 20% on supplies. The savings are not usually significant for small offices.

Group Buying Pools. If a medical office wants to use local vendors instead of, or in addition to, a purchasing group or if it is too small to benefit from a purchasing group, it can still pool resources with other area offices to qualify for quantity discounts. Even if the offices are ordering different items, discounts are based on the total order, and savings can range from 10% to 20%. Under this arrangement the offices must usually take responsibility for distributing the items among themselves. A buying pool is convenient for medical practices that are in the same building or office complex (Figure 8-6).

Benefits of Using Local Vendors

There are many potential vendors, including local dealers, mail-order companies, and nearby pharmacies. Try to establish good credit and business relationships with reputable local vendors. These companies often charge a little more than mail-order companies. Still, spending most of the office's supply budget through one favored local dealer often results in discounts, special service in the event of an emergency, and information about upcoming sales and specials. Local dealers may also offer more personal assistance, perhaps even a salesperson's help with taking inventory, to compete with larger vendors whose business is

Tips for the Office

Ordering by Telephone or Fax or Online

You may occasionally purchase office supplies at a local retail outlet, but most often you will order them without leaving your office. Three common ways to do so are by telephone, by facsimile (or fax) machine, and through an online service. Here are tips to help make sure every order—no matter which option you choose—is successfully placed.

Ordering by Telephone

1. Clear communication is a must when ordering by telephone. Speak slowly, and enunciate your words carefully to make sure you are understood. It is also a good idea to spell each word of the practice's name and the address to ensure proper delivery. Use expressions like "S as in Sam, P as in people" to clarify your spelling.

2. Ask the representative taking your order to repeat the order. Check that every item is included with the appropriate price, quantity, style, and color.

3. Confirm the expected delivery date so that you will know if something is late. Also confirm how payment will be made, to prevent unexpected delays.

4. Record the name and telephone number of the person who takes the order in case there is a problem with the order. Get an order number (sometimes called a confirmation number) in case you have to call back with a question or a change in your order.

5. If possible, avoid placing telephone orders on Mondays and Fridays, when call volume is typically high.

Ordering by Fax

1. When ordering by fax, use the form provided by the vendor if one is available. This form uses the format to which the supply company is accustomed and will speed the processing of your order.

2. Type your order, or write it neatly and legibly, to prevent miscommunication. Fill out the form completely. Make sure you indicate quantities, descriptions, and prices (including shipping) for each item you order.

3. Proofread your order before you send it. Checking the accuracy of the order now will save time later.

4. Follow up by telephone to make sure your order was received and understood and to confirm the delivery date and payment requirements.

Ordering Online

1. Ordering online requires a computer and a modem connection to the Internet or to an online service. Before ordering online, make sure you are fully familiar with the equipment and the process, or have your supervisor or the supply company's sales representative oversee your initial orders.

2. Type your name and address accurately.

3. If pictures of supplies are not available online, consult the company's printed catalog or CD-ROM catalog. If you do not have access to a catalog, read the online text descriptions carefully, checking trade names and specifications, to select the appropriate merchandise. If you have questions, consult the supply company by telephone.

4. When you have completed the selections, the online service will display your order so that you can confirm it. Check that all the information is accurate, including your name, address, and telephone number.

5. If you have an account with the company, you may type in your account number to place the order. Otherwise, you may wish to arrange to make payment on delivery. If you prefer to pay by credit card, first make sure that the company is reputable and that it uses a security system that prevents your number from being read by anyone unauthorized to do so.

If, despite your best efforts, your order is processed incorrectly, take appropriate action immediately. Although ordering by telephone or fax or online is convenient, it still requires additional time to package items that must be returned.

By law, orders that you place must be fulfilled within a reasonable time. The Federal Trade Commission (FTC) monitors purchases by telephone, fax, and online services to protect consumers. The FTC requires supply companies to provide merchandise within 30 days or to give you the option of canceling the order and receiving a full refund.

based primarily on catalog sales. The extra service may be worth the higher cost.

Buying from local vendors can also provide a public relations benefit for physicians; it means keeping business in the community. However, specialty items may need to be ordered from other vendors. For example, letterhead should be ordered from a reliable printer, whether that printer is located in the community or out of state.

Payment Schedules

Another factor that affects the cost of supplies is the payment schedule. Many vendors do not charge for handling if an order is prepaid. Others offer a discount for enclosing a check with an order. Some delay billing for 30 to 90 days, allowing the physician to keep the money in the bank, collecting interest for a longer period.

The vendor's invoice usually describes payment terms. Two examples of payment terms are:

1. If the invoice says "Net 30," you have 30 days in which to pay the total amount.
2. "1% 10 Days Net 30" means that you will get a savings of 1% of the total price by paying within 10 days.

Copies of all bills and order forms for supplies should be kept on file for at least 7 years in case the practice is audited by the Internal Revenue Service (IRS).

Storage Space as a Cost Factor

When you plan purchases, you need to consider the available storage space. Ideally, there should be enough space in the office to allow occasional large purchases for quantity discounts. If there is not, a vendor might allow you to take partial shipments on a large order. The vendor might also allow you to pay for the partial shipments with partial payments, but you will probably have to request this plan.

Ordering Procedures

Ordering procedures for supplies vary from office to office but always involve these tasks: completing paperwork, checking orders received, correcting errors in shipments, and making payment.

Order Forms. Before ordering merchandise, you should inquire about a vendor's ordering options, discuss them with the physician, and determine which method is best for the office. Many vendors now accept telephone, fax, and e-mail as well as traditional written order forms. Many vendors will also send a sales representative to your office to help you decide which items to purchase and to show you how to complete an order form accurately. Sometimes the sales representative can give you better deals than those described in the catalog. Whatever form you use, be sure to keep a copy of each order you submit.

Before you place an order, gather all the necessary information, such as correct names of items, item numbers, and order and account numbers. This information helps ensure the accuracy of the order. Immediately after placing the order, note all order information on the inventory card or record page for that item.

Purchase Requisitions. You will need to follow any special ordering procedures established in your medical office. The specific procedures and the medical assistant's level of authority vary from one office to another. Sometimes placing an order requires a **requisition** (a formal request from a staff member or doctor), which is given to the medical assistant who does the actual ordering. The doctor's approval may be necessary for large purchases—for example, for orders that total more than $300. Recurring orders may not require the doctor's approval, but you may need to get approval before ordering a new brand or quantities of a particular item over a certain amount.

In a group practice where doctors order different items and several staffers are in charge of ordering, procedures for ordering can be complicated. One common way to simplify matters is to use **purchase orders,** forms that authorize a purchase for the practice. Figure 8-7 shows a sample purchase order. Purchase orders are usually preprinted with consecutive numbers. The medical assistant submits approved purchase orders to the vendor for fulfillment. This method is most often used for expensive items, such as office equipment, but some large practices also use purchase orders for supplies.

Checking Orders Received. When the shipment of supplies arrives, record on the inventory card or record page the date received as well as the quantity of each item. Check the shipment against the order form to make sure the correct items—in the correct sizes, styles, packaging, and quantity—have been delivered.

Then check the contents against the packing slip (a description of the package contents) enclosed in the package. This checking takes time, but catching even one error is worth the time taken. If several people on a staff have ordering responsibility, they can share the task.

Material Safety Data Sheets. Every chemical item ordered in a medical practice must have a **Material Safety Data Sheet (MSDS)** on file in the office. This sheet is provided by the manufacturer of the product and describes the chemical breakdown of the product as well as safety cautions and procedures to follow in using it. Items that require MSDS include, but are not limited to, all soaps, cleansers, waxes, reagents, clinical testing products, inks, toners, and any product that can be splashed or rubbed on the skin or eyes. JCAHO, OSHA (Occupational Safety Hazards Association), and other surveying organizations will require MSDS on all products used in the medical practice. The purpose of the sheet is to provide important

PURCHASE ORDER

Submitted by: _____

Order Number: _____

Date Ordered: _____

Date Required: _____

SHIP TO: Dr. Carlotta Montoni
201 Oak Walk, Suite 32
Gilead, PA 19034

PHONE: 215-610-4120

	ITEM	DESCRIPTION/MODEL	COLOR	SIZE	QUANTITY	PRICE EACH	TOTAL
1.							
2.							
3.							
4.							
5.							
6.							
7.							
8.							
						TOTAL	

Approved: _____ Date: _____

Figure 8-7. A purchase order, when approved by the physician or office manager, is an authorization from the practice for a purchase.

safety information about the item that may be critical in the event of unintended exposure or potentially dangerous reactions.

For fast and easy access, organize these sheets in a notebook in alphabetical order. As new items are ordered and delivered, add the MSDS into the master notebook. As a medical assistant, you must always check the MSDS notebook when stocking the supply shelves to ensure that all items stocked are included in the notebook. If MSDS information is not included with the item, either immediately request the information from the vendor or go online to print information directly from the product manufacturer.

Correcting Errors. All errors in a shipment should be reported immediately to the vendor so that the records can be corrected and missing supplies can be delivered. When you call to report errors, be sure you have all the paperwork in front of you. You will need the invoice number, order date, name of the person who placed the order, name of the person who took the order, and a list of questions or a description of the complaint. If a catalog was used in ordering, have it open to the appropriate page. Always record the name and title of the person you speak with when reporting the error.

Invoices. Typically the vendor sends an invoice to the medical office, either accompanying the merchandise or separately. This invoice also should be checked carefully against the original order and the packing slip. Be sure to check the arithmetic as well. Then sign or stamp the invoice to confirm that the order was received. If an item you order is temporarily out of stock, the vendor usually sends an invoice stamped "Back Ordered." Later, when the item is back in stock, the vendor will ship it to your office.

Make sure the invoice has not already been paid. It is a good habit to record the check number, date, and amount of payment on the invoice. You may initial it or have the doctor initial it.

Disbursements. An invoice is paid with a **disbursement** (payment of funds) to a vendor. Disbursements may be made in cash or by check or money order. Usually you will write a check to the vendor and have the physician sign it. Be sure to show the physician the original order, packing slip, and invoice. On the front of the check, record the invoice number. Finally, mail the check to the vendor with the vendor's copy of the invoice. File the office copy of the invoice, along with the original order and the packing slip, according to your inventory filing system (Figure 8-8).

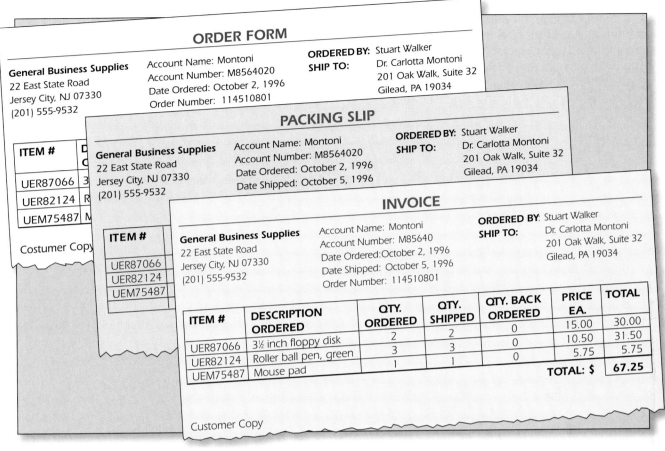

ORDER FORM

General Business Supplies
22 East State Road
Jersey City, NJ 07330
(201) 555-9532

Account Name: Montoni
Account Number: M8564020
Date Ordered: October 2, 1996
Order Number: 114510801

ORDERED BY: Stuart Walker
SHIP TO: Dr. Carlotta Montoni
201 Oak Walk, Suite 32
Gilead, PA 19034

ITEM #	D C
UER87066	3
UER82124	R
UEM75487	M

Costumer Copy

PACKING SLIP

General Business Supplies
22 East State Road
Jersey City, NJ 07330
(201) 555-9532

Account Name: Montoni
Account Number: M8564020
Date Ordered: October 2, 1996
Date Shipped: October 5, 1996

ORDERED BY: Stuart Walker
SHIP TO: Dr. Carlotta Montoni
201 Oak Walk, Suite 32
Gilead, PA 19034

ITEM #
UER87066
UER82124
UEM75487

INVOICE

General Business Supplies
22 East State Road
Jersey City, NJ 07330
(201) 555-9532

Account Name: Montoni
Account Number: M85640
Date Ordered:October 2, 1996
Date Shipped: October 5, 1996
Order Number: 114510801

ORDERED BY: Stuart Walker
SHIP TO: Dr. Carlotta Montoni
201 Oak Walk, Suite 32
Gilead, PA 19034

ITEM #	DESCRIPTION ORDERED	QTY. ORDERED	QTY. SHIPPED	QTY. BACK ORDERED	PRICE EA.	TOTAL
UER87066	3½ inch floppy disk	2	2	0	15.00	30.00
UER82124	Roller ball pen, green	3	3	0	10.50	31.50
UEM75487	Mouse pad	1	1	0	5.75	5.75
					TOTAL: $	67.25

Customer Copy

Figure 8-8. Check the information on the vendor invoice against the original order and the packing slip to make sure there are no errors.

If you make a cash disbursement, obtain a receipt to keep on file. If you are the one responsible for maintaining the practice's financial records and presenting them to the accountant, you may also be responsible for recording the payment information in the office's accounting books.

Avoiding Common Purchasing Mistakes

Even the most watchful professional can make purchasing mistakes. The best you can do is to educate yourself about common mistakes and try to avoid them. For example, be aware of the possibility of dishonest telephone solicitations. A caller may claim to be a sales representative for the manufacturer of the office photocopier, offering bargains on paper or toner. The caller may require advance payment to be sent to a post office box. The bargains may never arrive.

The best way to deal with these solicitations is to tell the caller that your office does not purchase supplies by telephone. If a telephone offer appears to be legitimate and to offer substantial savings, ask for the name and telephone number of the firm so that you can return the call at a more convenient time. Then you can verify the number with the telephone company and check the firm's name with the Better Business Bureau.

Another disreputable tactic some vendors use is bait and switch: the price of one item is lowered to attract the customer, but that item is always "sold out" and the customer is encouraged to buy a more expensive one. A vendor may also mislead you by raising the price of an item you have been ordering without informing you. Always confirm the current price, check invoices as they come in, and record everything in the item's file. Having your inventory card or record page open while ordering will prompt you to notice and question price changes. If there is an honest error, a reputable firm will readily and courteously correct it.

Problems can also be avoided by carefully supervising a new vendor's sales representative until a comfortable, professional rapport has been established. Discuss your inventory system with representatives, and ask them questions about their procedures.

Summary

A typical medical practice uses both administrative and clinical office supplies. Supplies can be categorized as vital, incidental, and periodic.

Keeping track of supplies involves creating supply lists and taking inventory. You must know the storage requirements for various kinds of supplies. An inventory filing system can help you organize office supply tasks. Maintaining adequate supplies and well-organized storage space contributes to the smooth running of the office.

You will also locate, evaluate, and establish and maintain working relationships with vendors. It is important to be adept at comparison pricing and to stay abreast of competitors' product quality, pricing policies, and services.

Just as cost-effectiveness is stressed in medical care, it is important to look for ways to control costs when ordering supplies. Checking orders carefully and avoiding dishonest telephone solicitations are two examples of ways to control costs.

Introducti

The medical assista
maintaining patient
evaluation and tre
records are critical
accurate and compl
easily be compromi

Patient records
describe these facet

- Personal inform
- Physical and m

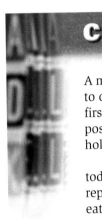

CA

A ma
to op
first s
possi
holds

A
today
repor
eat ir
the p

an at
chart

- S
- (
-
- I

he e
recor

As y

1.
2.
3.
4.
5.

CASE STUDY QUESTIONS

Now that you have completed this chapter, review the case study at the beginning of the chapter and answer the following questions:

1. What is an *expendable* item? What items would you list on the expendable administrative supply list? The clinical supply list? The general supply list?
2. What factors would you consider about each office as you determine the appropriate supplies?
3. How would you recommend that the supplies be stored with inventory management in mind?

Discussion Questions

1. As a new employee, what questions would you want to ask about the process of ordering supplies within the office?
2. What supplies do you think are the most important in a medical practice and why?

Critical Thinking Questions

1. During a routine inventory inspection, you notice that the supply of prescription pads is extremely low for typical office use. Could there be a problem within the office other than just the need to order more pads from the printer? What would you do?

2. You share the responsibility of ordering supplies with another medical assistant in the office. You are checking supplies and ordering regularly, but the other employee is allowing items to become completely depleted. What would you do?
3. The Sunday paper runs an ad indicating that a local supply vendor is going out of business soon. How do you shop for a new vendor? How could you make the most out of the closeout specials advertised?

Application Activities

1. Using vendor catalogs, make a list of ten typical office supply items for a medical practice. Create a fictional office supply list and ordering schedule (including quantities and prices) for the practice.
2. Select a supply company catalog, and become familiar with it. Imagine that you are a sales representative for that company, and make a presentation to your class as if it were a typical medical practice. Your goal is to have the medical office choose your company as its vendor. Be prepared to answer questions about how your company handles various customer concerns.
3. Make a diagram of an office supply cabinet, indicating how you would label and store items for maximum efficiency. Try to use several of the inventory elements discussed in the chapter.

CHA

Mai

KEY TE

documentati
informed co
noncomplia
objective
patient reco
POMR
sign
SOAP
subjective
symptom
transcription
transfer

Community Health Center • 6508 South Street • Kokomo, IN 46902
(317) 555-1234 • Fax: (317) 555-1245

Patient Registration
Patient Information

Name: _____ Today's Date: _____

Address: _____

City: _____ State: _____ Zip Code: _____

Telephone (Home): _____ (Work): _____ (Cell): _____

Birthdate: _____ Age: _____ Sex: M F No. of Children _____ Marital Status: M S W D

Social Security Number: _____ Employer: _____ Occupation: _____

Primary Physician: _____

Referred by: _____

Person to Contact in Emergency: _____

Emergency Telephone: _____

Special Needs: _____

Responsible Party

Party Responsible for Payment: _____ Self _____ Spouse _____ Parent _____ Other

Name (If Other Than Self): _____

Address: _____

City: _____ State: _____ Zip Code: _____

Primary Insurance

Primary Medical Insurance: _____

Insured party: _____ Self _____ Spouse _____ Parent _____ Other

ID#/Social Security No.: _____ Group/Plan No.: _____

Name (If Other Than Self): _____

Address: _____

City: _____ State: _____ Zip Code: _____

Secondary Insurance

Secondary Medical Insurance: _____

Insured party: _____ Self _____ Spouse _____ Parent _____ Other

ID#/Social Security No.: _____ Group/Plan No.: _____

Name (If Other Than Self): _____

Address: _____

City: _____ State: _____ Zip Code: _____

Figure 9-2. The patient registration form is often the first document used in initiating a patient record.

The Medical Center at Springfield
Medical History

Name _____ Age _____ Sex _____ S M W D
Address _____ Phone _____ Date _____

Occupation _____ Ref. by _____
Chief Complaint _____

Present Illness _____
_____
_____
_____
_____
_____

History —Military _____
   —Social _____
   —Family _____
   —Marital _____
   —Menstrual _____ Menarche _____ Para. _____ LMP _____
   —Illness Measles Pert. Var. Pneu. Pleur. Typh. Mal. Rh. Fev. Sc. Fev. Diphth. Other
   —Surgery _____
   —Allergies _____
   —Current Medications _____

Physical Examination

Temp. _____ Pulse _____ Resp. _____ BP _____ Ht. _____ Wt. _____
General Appearance _____ Skin _____ Mucous Membrane _____
Eyes: _____ Vision _____ Pupil _____ Fundus _____
Ears: _____
Nose: _____
Throat: _____ Pharynx _____ Tonsils _____
Chest: _____ Breasts _____
Heart: _____
Lungs: _____
Abdomen: _____
Genitalia: _____
Rectum: _____
Pelvic: _____
Extremities: _____ Pulses: _____
Lymph Nodes: _____ Neck _____ Axilla _____ Inguinal _____ Abdominal _____
Neurological: _____
Diagnosis: _____
_____
_____

Treatment: _____
_____
_____

Laboratory Findings: _____
Date _____ Blood _____
_____
_____
_____

Date _____ Urine _____
_____
_____
_____
_____

Figure 9-3. In some doctors' offices, the medical history form and the physical examination form are combined.

THE OAK HILLS MEDICAL CENTER
Oak Hills, MA

CONSENT TO OPERATION, ADMINISTRATION OF ANESTHETICS,
AND RENDERING OF OTHER MEDICAL SERVICE

Patient: _____ Age: _____

Date: _____ Time: _____

1. I AUTHORIZE AND DIRECT _____ , with the associates
and assistants of his/her choice, to perform upon myself the following operation
_____
_____
_____

   If any unforeseen conditions arise in the course of the operation or in the postoperative period, calling in their judgment for other operations or procedures, I further request and authorize them to do whatever is deemed advisable for my health and well-being.

2. The positive and negative aspects of autologous blood transfusions (receiving my own blood donated prior to surgery), designated blood transfusions (donated in advance by family/friends for my use), or homologous blood transfusions (from general donor population) have been explained to me. I understand autologous and designated transfusions can be accommodated only for nonemergency surgery.

6. I certify that I understand the above consent to operation and that the explanations referred to have been made.

_____   _____
Witness (of signature only)   Signature

Figure 9-4. Patients are asked to sign informed consent forms to confirm that they understand the treatment offered.

medications administered in the hospital; and the disposition, or outcome, of the case. Elements of the form may include the following:

- Date of admission
- Brief history
- Date of discharge
- Admitting diagnosis
- Operations and procedures or hospital course (course of action taken in the hospital)
- Complications
- Instructions to the patient for follow-up care after discharge from the hospital
- Physician's signature

Correspondence With or About the Patient.
All written correspondence from the patient or from other doctors, laboratories, or independent health-care agencies should be kept in the patient's chart. Each piece of correspondence should be marked or stamped with the date the doctor's office received the document.

Information Received by Fax

Some information—such as laboratory results, physician comments, or correspondence—may be received by fax transmission. Always request that the original be mailed if possible. If the original is not available, make a photocopy of the fax. Fax copies made on thermal paper, as opposed to those made from a plain-paper fax, fade over time and may become unreadable.

Dating and Initialing

You must be careful not only to date everything you put into the patient chart but also to initial the entry. This system makes it easy to tell which items the assistant enters into the chart and which items others enter. In many practices the physician initials reports before they are filed to prove that he saw them.

Initiating and Maintaining Patient Records

Besides the receptionist, you will often be the first health-care professional that new patients talk with when they visit a doctor's office. During your first contact with a patient, you will initiate a patient record. Recording information in the medical record is called **documentation.** Complete, thorough documentation ensures that the doctor will have detailed notes about each contact with the patient and about the treatment plan, patient responses and progress, and treatment outcomes.

Initial Interview

You usually perform the following tasks on your own, depending on the doctor's practice and your experience and background. Familiarize yourself with each task.

Completing Medical History Forms. You will help new patients fill out medical history forms or questionnaires. You may retrieve current patients' records from the files to update them. Type the patient's name and other identifying information on the first page and on all subsequent pages of the form.

You may interview patients to fill in some of the remaining blanks about medical history. Some doctors prefer to ask patients questions themselves. Others believe that people sometimes talk more freely with an assistant than they do with the doctor.

Documenting Patient Statements. You will record any signs, symptoms, or other information the patient wishes to share. Document this information in the patient's words, not your interpretation of the words. Record these data in specific detail. For example, if the patient drinks alcohol, you should record the number of drinks per week, the type of liquor consumed, and whether the drinking has affected the patient's behavior and health.

Conduct the interview in a private room or in a semiprivate office away from the reception area, as shown in Figure 9-5. Patients usually do not like to discuss their medical or personal problems in front of others. Your opinion of the patient, such as "the patient seems mentally unstable," is your own and should not be discussed or documented. The Tips for the Office section will help you take information from elderly patients.

Documenting Test Results. Put a copy in the chart of any test results, x-ray reports, or other diagnostic results that the patient has brought with him. You may also record this information on a separate test summary sheet in the chart.

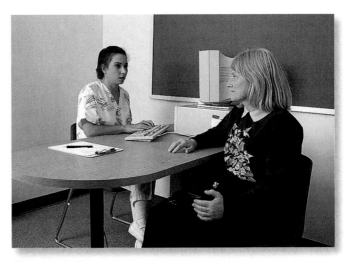

Figure 9-5. Conduct interviews with patients in a private or semiprivate room to make them feel more comfortable.

Examination Preparation and Vital Signs. In many instances, you will prepare patients for examination. You will record vital signs, medication the patient is currently taking, and any responses to treatment. Before you leave a patient, ask, "Is there anything else you would like the doctor to know?" The patient may be more comfortable sharing further information with you than with the doctor.

Follow-Up

After you record the initial interview and background information, the doctor decides what entries will be made regarding examinations, diagnosis, treatment options and plans, and comments or observations about each case. You then maintain the patient record by performing the following duties.

- Transcribe notes the doctor dictates about the patient's progress, follow-up visits, procedures, current status, and other necessary information.
- Post laboratory test results or results of examinations in the record or on the summary sheet.
- Record telephone calls from the patient and calls that the doctor or other office staff members make to the patient (Figure 9-6). Telephone calls can be an important part of good follow-up care. Calls must be dated, and the content of the conversations must be documented. You must initial the entry. Even if the doctor did not reach the patient, the call should be recorded and dated. State whether the doctor got an answer, left a message on an answering machine or with a person, and so on. Legally, if an item is not in the record, it did not happen.
- Record medical instructions or discharge instructions the doctor gives. At the doctor's request, you may counsel or educate the patient regarding treatment regimen or home-care procedures the patient must

Talking With the Older Patient

If you work in a practice that specializes in geriatrics or in any practice with older patients, certain communication skills will help you in your job. You may find yourself in various situations in which knowing how to talk with the older patient will be a necessary skill. Taking a medical history or helping a patient describe her symptoms are two such situations. The following tips will help you and the patient communicate with each other more effectively.

1. Make sure you select a private setting for the patient interview.

2. Many older patients are hard of hearing, but *not deaf.* Speak slightly more slowly than you normally would. Speak clearly and loudly (but do not shout—shouting will insult and anger an older patient who does hear well). Enunciate well, and use a lower tone of voice (elderly people lose the ability to hear high-frequency sounds first). If the patient asks you to repeat a question, rephrase it instead of repeating it verbatim.

3. Look at the patient directly so that she knows you care about what she has to say and so that you can make sure she understands what you tell or ask her.

4. You can show respect for the patient's age by addressing the patient with Mr., Mrs., Ms., or Miss, unless the patient asks to be called by his or her first name.

5. Be patient. Some older patients live alone or in relative isolation and may be out of practice with the two-way communication skills that make a conversation or interview go smoothly. The simple act of being interviewed, even for what may seem to you a straightforward medical history, may unsettle the older patient. For example, he may need to stop and think of a word here and there. Do not supply the word.

Wait and let the patient think of it on his own. Also, do not rush through your questions. Rushing will only make the patient feel anxious and incompetent if she feels she cannot keep up with you.

6. Practice active listening skills. Pay attention to the patient's verbal and nonverbal cues. Do not interrupt the patient. After the patient finishes giving each answer, repeat it, to give him a chance to correct you if you misheard or misunderstood.

7. If you are interviewing the patient to obtain a medical history, explain before you begin the type of questions you will ask and how the information will be used.

8. If you need to use medical terminology, try also to express the same information in lay terms. For example, you might ask, "Do you use a diuretic or pill to help you eliminate fluids?"

9. Be cheerful and friendly but not sugary-sweet. Do not talk down to older patients; they are not stupid.

10. Avoid sounding surprised or excited by any answer to a question or to any information the patient gives.

11. Under no circumstances use endearments such as dear, honey, or sweetie.

12. Look for ways to make a connection so that the patient feels relaxed and comfortable. In the course of taking a patient's history, you might find out that he enjoys swimming. Maybe you do, too—and you can describe a beautiful lake you once went swimming in.

13. Show an interest in the patient as a person. Ask about something she is interested in. For example, a patient might be wearing a piece of handmade jewelry. Ask where it came from. She might have a wonderful story to tell.

follow. This information must be entered into the record, dated, and initialed. Some offices make carbon copies or photocopies of patient instructions.

The Six Cs of Charting

To maintain accurate patient records, always keep these six Cs in mind when filling out and maintaining charts: Client's (patient's) words, Clarity, Completeness, Conciseness, Chronological order, and Confidentiality.

1. *Client's words.* Be careful to record the patient's exact words rather than your interpretation of them. For instance, if a client says, "My right knee feels like it's thick or full of fluid," write that down. Do not rephrase the sentence to say, "Client says he's got fluid on the knee." Often the patient's exact words, no matter how odd they may sound, provide important clues for the physician in making a diagnosis.

2. *Clarity.* Use precise descriptions and accepted medical terminology when describing a patient's condition.

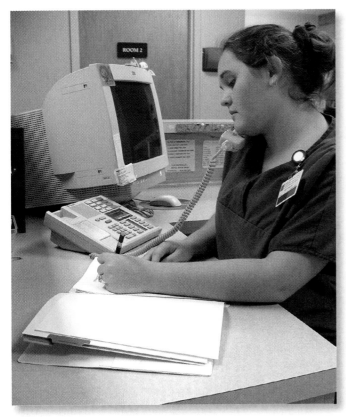

Figure 9-6. All telephone conversations to and from the patient must be logged in the patient record.

For instance, "Patient got out of bed and walked 20 feet without shortness of breath" is much clearer than "Patient got out of bed and felt fine."

3. *Completeness.* Fill out completely all the forms used in the patient record. Provide complete information that is readily understandable to others whenever you make any notation in the patient chart.

4. *Conciseness.* While striving for clarity, also be concise, or brief and to the point. Abbreviations and specific medical terminology can often save time and space when recording information. For instance, you can write "Patient got OOB and walked 20 ft w/o SOB." OOB and SOB are standard abbreviations for "out of bed" and "shortness of breath," respectively. Every member of the office staff should use the same abbreviations to avoid misunderstandings. Table 9-1 lists some common medical abbreviations.

5. *Chronological order.* All entries in patient records must be dated to show the order in which they are made. This factor is critical, not only for documenting patient care but also in case there is a legal question about the type and date of medical services.

6. *Confidentiality.* All the information in patient records and forms is confidential, to protect the patient's privacy. Only the patient, attending physicians, and the medical assistant (who needs the record to tend to the patient and/or to make entries into the record) are allowed to see the charts without the patient's written consent. Never discuss a patient's records, forward them to another office, fax them, or show them to anyone but the physician unless you have the patient's written permission to do so.

Types of Medical Records

You should be familiar with the different approaches to documenting patient information. The most common methods are conventional/source-oriented and problem-oriented medical records.

Conventional, or Source-Oriented, Records

In the conventional, or source-oriented, approach, patient information is arranged according to who supplied the data—the patient, doctor, specialist, or someone else. The medical form may have a space for patient remarks, followed by a section for the doctor's comments.

These records describe all problems and treatments on the same form in simple chronological order. For example, a patient's broken wrist would be recorded on the same form as her stomach ulcer. Although easy to initiate and maintain, this system presents some difficulty in tracking the progress of a specific ailment, such as the patient's ulcer. The doctor has to search the entire record to find information on that one problem.

Problem-Oriented Medical Records

One way to overcome the disadvantages of the conventional approach is to use the problem-oriented medical record **(POMR)** system of keeping charts. This approach, developed by Lawrence L. Weed, MD, makes it easier for the physician to keep track of a patient's progress. The information in a POMR includes the database; problem list; educational, diagnostic, and treatment plan; and progress notes.

Database. The database includes a record of the patient's history; information from the initial interview with the patient (for example, "Patient unemployed—second time in past 12 months"); all findings and results from physical examinations (such as "Pulse 105 bpm, BP 210/80"), and any tests, x-rays, and other procedures.

Problem List. Each problem a patient has is listed separately, given its own number, and dated. You then identify a problem by its number throughout the record. You can also list work-related, social, or family problems that may be affecting the patient's health. For instance, the problem list for the example patient who is unemployed might include, "Severe stomach pain, worse at night and after eating."

You can alert the doctor to the fact that the patient has lost two jobs within 1 year. Such radical life changes can

TABLE 9-1 Common Medical Abbreviations

Abbreviation	Meaning	Abbreviation	Meaning
AIDS	acquired immunodeficiency syndrome	inj.	injection
a.m.a.	against medical advice	IV	intravenous
b.i.d./BID	twice a day	MI	myocardial infarction
BP	blood pressure	MM	mucous membrane
bpm	beats per minute	NPO	nothing by mouth
CBC	complete blood count	NYD	not yet diagnosed
C.C.	chief complaint	OOB	out of bed
CNS	central nervous system	OPD	outpatient department
CPE	complete physical examination	OR	operating room
CV	cardiovascular	PH	past history
D & C	dilation and curettage	PT	physical therapy
Dx	diagnosis	Pt	patient
ECG/EKG	electrocardiogram	q.i.d./QID	four times a day
ER	emergency room	ROS/SR	review of systems/systems review
FH	family history	s.c./subq.	subcutaneously
Fl/fl	fluid	SOB	shortness of breath
GBS	gallbladder series	S/R	suture removal
GI	gastrointestinal	stat	immediately
GU	genitourinary	t.i.d./TID	three times a day
GYN	gynecology	TPR	temperature, pulse, respirations
HEENT	head, ears, eyes, nose, throat	UCHD	usual childhood diseases
HIV	human immunodeficiency virus	VS	vital signs
I & D	incision and drainage	WNL	within normal limits
ICU	intensive care unit		

often provoke strong physical reactions. In this patient's case the elevated blood pressure may be related to the job losses, and stress may be causing the stomach pain.

When you document problems, be careful to distinguish between patient signs and symptoms. **Signs** are objective, or external, factors—such as blood pressure, rashes, or swelling—that can be seen or felt by the doctor or measured by an instrument. **Symptoms** are subjective, or internal, conditions felt by the patient, such as pain, headache, or nausea. Together, signs and symptoms help clarify a patient's problem.

Educational, Diagnostic, and Treatment Plan. Each problem should have a detailed educational, diagnostic, and treatment summary in the record. The summary contains diagnostic workups, treatment plans, and instructions for the patient. Here is an example.

Problem 2, Stomach Pain, 2/2/XX [date]

- *Upper GI exam negative, CBC normal.*
- *Prescribed over-the-counter antacid, 2 tablets by mouth t.i.d. after each meal.*
- *Set up appointment for patient with Dr. R. Neil at stress-management clinic (Broughten Professional Center) for Monday, February 4, at 4:30 p.m.*
- *Patient's anxiety is high. Recheck in 1 week.*

Progress Notes. Progress notes are entered for each problem listed in the initial record. The documentation always includes—in chronological order—the patient's condition, complaints, problems, treatment, and responses to care. Here is an example.

Problem 2, Stomach Pain, 2/9/XX. Patient enrolled in stress-reduction class. Reports stomach pain has diminished—"I can eat without pain; only a little discomfort at night." Vital signs improved: pulse 85 bpm, BP 115/70, respiration 20. Reduced antacid to one tablet by mouth two times daily after meals. Anxiety much reduced. Recheck anxiety level in 2 weeks.

SOAP Documentation

Many medical records, such as the POMR, emphasize the **SOAP** approach to documentation, which provides an orderly series of steps for dealing with any medical case. SOAP documentation lists the patient's symptoms, the diagnosis, and the suggested treatment. Information is documented in the record in the following order.

1. S: **Subjective** data come from the patient; they describe his or her signs and symptoms and supply any other opinions or comments.
2. O: **Objective** data come from the physician and from examinations and test results.
3. A: *Assessment* is the diagnosis or impression of a patient's problem.
4. P: *Plan* of action includes treatment options, chosen treatment, medications, tests, consultations, patient education, and follow-up.

Whether you keep conventional or POMR charts, you can include all these steps for each problem. Figure 9-7 shows an example of SOAP notes. If you abbreviate any term when entering data into the records, use only approved medical abbreviations. For example, use "5 g" instead of "5 grams." Several resources, including those published by JCAHO and the American Medical Association, list approved medical abbreviations for measurements, instructions for taking medication, and other topics. Keep these references readily available in the office.

Appearance, Timeliness, and Accuracy of Records

You must ensure that the medical records are complete. They must also be written neatly and legibly, contain up-to-date information, and present an accurate, professional record of a patient's case.

Neatness and Legibility

A medical record is useless if the doctor or others have difficulty reading it. You should make sure that every word and number in the record is clear and legible. Follow these tips to keep charts neat and easy to read.

- Use a good-quality pen that will not smudge or smear. Blue ink is required by HIPAA. Use highlighting pens to call attention to specific items such as allergies. Be aware, however, that unless the office has a color copier, most colored ink will photocopy black or gray. Highlighting-pen marks may not be visible on a photocopy.
- If you type notes, be sure the typewriter ribbon is dark enough to make clear letters, as shown in Figure 9-8.
- Make sure all handwriting is legible. Take time to write names, numbers, and abbreviations clearly.
- Never use correction fluid in medical records.

Timeliness

Medical records should be kept up to date and should be readily available when a doctor or another health-care professional needs to see them. Follow these guidelines to ensure that a doctor can find the most recent information on a patient when it is needed.

- Record all findings from examinations and tests as soon as they are available.
- If you forget to enter a finding into the record when it is received, record both the original date of receipt and the date the finding was entered into the record.
- To document telephone calls, record the date and time of the call, who initiated it, the information discussed, and any conclusions or results. You can either enter the telephone call directly into the record or make a note referring the doctor to a separate telephone log kept in the record.
- Establish a procedure for retrieving a file quickly in case of emergency. Should the patient be in a serious accident, for example, the emergency doctor will need the patient's medical history immediately.

Accuracy

The physician must be able to trust the accuracy of the information in the medical records. You must make it a priority always to check the accuracy of all data you will enter in a chart. To ensure accurate data, follow these guidelines.

- Never guess at or assume knowledge of names, procedures, medications, findings, or any other information about which there is some question. Always check all the information carefully. Make the extra effort to ask questions of the physician or senior staff member and to verify information.
- Double-check the accuracy of findings and instructions recorded in the chart. Have all numbers been copied accurately? Are instructions for taking medication clear and complete?
- Make sure the latest information has been entered into the chart so that the physician has an accurate picture of the patient's current condition.

OUTLINE FORMAT PROGRESS NOTES

| Patient Name | Hansen | Christopher | M. | Date of Birth | 3 / 1 / 65 | Chart # | H234 |
| | LAST | FIRST | MIDDLE | | | | |

Prob. No. or Letter	DATE	**S** Subjective	**O** Objective	**A** Assess	**P** Plans	Page _1_
	6/16/04	Patient complaining of pain in lower right quadrant. Has been running fever of between 100.5°F and 101.3°F since Sunday morning. Has queasy feeling in stomach and has been unable to eat since yesterday morning.				
			BP 125/75. Temperature 101.2°F. Abdominal exam revealed rebound tenderness and distension in lower right quadrant.			
				Appendicitis		
					1. Admit to hospital 2. Surgically remove appendix.	
						Paul martin

Start each Progress Note (Subjective, Objective, Assessment, and Plans) at the appropriate shaded column to create an outline form. Write through the intervening columns to the right margin of the page.

© 1976 BIBBERO SYSTEMS, INC., PETALUMA, CA   PROGRESS NOTES   TO REORDER CALL TOLL FREE: (800)BIBBERO (800 242-2376)
FORM # 26-7215-01

Figure 9-7.   The SOAP approach to documentation is one way to organize information in a patient record.

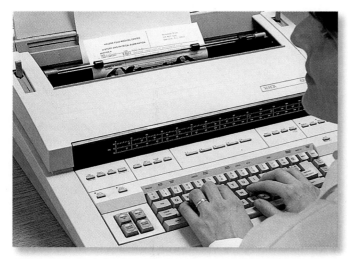

Figure 9-8. Typewritten notes and forms are clear and legible.

Procedure 9-1 explains how to correct a medical chart.

Professional Attitude and Tone

Part of creating timely, accurate records is maintaining a professional tone in your writing when recording information. Record information from the patient in his own words. Also record the doctor's observations and comments as well as any laboratory or test results. Do not record your personal, subjective comments, judgments, opinions, or speculations about a patient's words, problems, or test results. You may call attention to a particular problem or observation, for example, by attaching a note to the chart. Do not, however, make such comments part of the patient's record.

Computer Records

In some offices the computer is used for more than just storing financial, billing, and insurance information. Some hospitals, clinics, and even individual physicians use computer software to create and store patient records.

Advantages of Computerizing Records. In a setting in which several terminals in a network are connected to a main computer, computerizing medical records presents several advantages. A physician can call up the record on her own or another computer monitor whenever the record is needed, review or update the file, and save it to the central computer again (see Figure 9-9).

Computerized records can also be used in teleconferences, where people in different locations can look at the same record on their individual computer screens at the same time. Records can also be sent by modem to the physician's home computer so that the physician will have a patient's records on hand for calls after hours. Computer access to patient records is also helpful for health-care providers with satellite offices in different cities or different parts of a city.

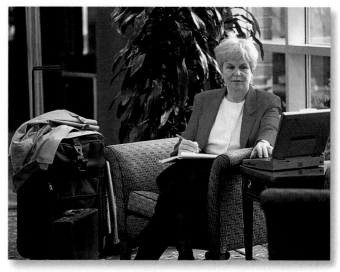

Figure 9-9. Computerized medical records, laptop computers, and the Internet provide physicians with easy access no matter where they are.

Computers are useful for tickler files (files that need periodic attention). For example, they can alert staff members about patients who are due for yearly checkups and patients who require follow-up care. Some hospitals have begun to use electronically scanned images of patients' thumbprints to keep track of records. This system saves time and helps maintain the security of patient records.

Security Concerns. Many health-care professionals have concerns about protecting the confidentiality of patient records in computer files. See Chapter 6 for more information on computer confidentiality.

Medical Transcription

Your knowledge of abbreviations, medical terminology, and medical coding will be invaluable when transcribing a doctor's notes or dictation (either recorded or direct). **Transcription** means transforming spoken notes into accurate written form. These written notes are then entered into the patient record. As is the case with information in medical charts, all dictated materials are confidential and should be regarded as potential legal documents. They are part of the patient's continuing case history. They often include findings, treatment stages, prognoses, and final outcomes. Always date and initial all transcription pages.

Strive to make transcribed material accurate and complete. Good grammar, spelling, and an accurate use of medical abbreviations and terminology are important in maintaining patient records. Use the medical dictionary and the medical computer spelling check to verify the spelling or meaning of words. Ask the physician only if you cannot find something in a reference source. Above-average typing or word processing accuracy and speed are also important.

Medical Transcriptionist

To gain medical assistant credentials, you must fulfill the requirements of either the American Association of Medical Assistants (for a Certified Medical Assistant) or the American Medical Technologists (for a Registered Medical Assistant). After obtaining your medical assistant certification or registration, you may wish to acquire additional skills in specialty areas through course work or on-the-job training. Although this course work or training may not lead to an additional certification or degree, it will enable you to expand your role in the medical office and advance your career as the demand for skilled health professionals increases.

Skills and Duties

A medical transcriptionist creates written health records for patients based on the physician's dictation or notes. The records may be typewritten or input on a computer. Some transcriptionists work for a single physician; others work for a small or large group.

To create a patient record, the transcriptionist listens to an audiocassette containing information dictated by the physician. Typical information on the tape includes the physician's diagnosis and treatment of the patient. Using dictation equipment, the transcriptionist can slow down or stop and start the cassette tape as she types.

The medical transcriptionist must have excellent typing skills and a good command of medical terminology to make sure that medical terms are used accurately and spelled correctly. She will often need to edit the physician's notes to make sure that the language follows Standard English grammar and usage. Sometimes she must also reorganize the physician's comments to create an understandable and easy-to-follow medical record. After she finishes transcribing the record, the medical transcriptionist checks it for correct spelling and punctuation. This last step is called proofreading.

Workplace Settings

Medical transcriptionists may work in the medical records department of a hospital or in a nursing home, clinic, laboratory, physician's practice, insurance company, or emergency or immediate health-care center. Some transcriptionists work for medical transcribing firms; others are self-employed and work out of their homes.

Education

Medical transcriptionists usually complete a training program at a 4-year college or university, junior or community college, vocational institute, or adult education center. They receive instruction in medical terminology, physiology, pharmaceuticals, laboratory procedures, and medical treatments. Some transcriptionists concentrate on a particular specialty area, such as pathology, and acquire specialized training in that area. Medical transcriptionists can become certified if they meet the qualifying standards of the American Association for Medical Transcription.

Where to Go for More Information

American Association for Medical Transcription
P.O. Box 576187
Modesto, CA 95355

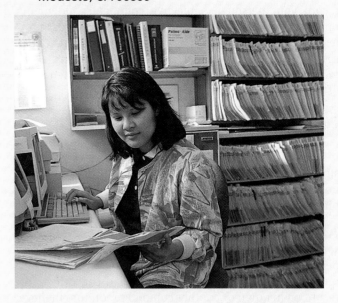

Transcribing Recorded Dictation

Often the doctor or another health-care provider dictates into a recording device or voice-mail dictation center. (This equipment is described in Chapter 5.) The following tips can help ensure fast, accurate transcription.

- Make sure that your workstation is free from clutter and that your desk and chair are at comfortable heights for proper support of your back, arms, and legs. Keep at hand all materials you may need for the transcription process—patient records, correspondence, and references for abbreviations and terminology.

- Adjust the transcribing equipment's speed, tone, and volume to obtain the best-quality sound at a rate of speed that matches your abilities.

- Listen once all the way through the dictation tape, noting instructions, corrections, or special cues. This step helps you plan how to put the material in the correct order. It also ensures accuracy.
- Write down the exact elapsed time on the transcribing equipment's digital counter where difficult phrases, garbled statements, or other problems occur on the tape. Then you can quickly find the problems again and seek the correct information from the doctor.
- While transcribing, listen carefully to the rise and fall of the doctor's voice, which can provide clues about where to place punctuation and where to end sentences.
- If a statement is particularly long or highly technical, simply transcribe it word for word. It may make sense in written form. Never try to guess at the meaning of a word or phrase.
- Finally, reread the finished transcription to make sure that all punctuation, capitalization, spelling of names and terms, and paragraph indentions have been done correctly. You should be able to arrange ideas in their logical order and ensure proper sentence structure. Note any items that are still unclear, and ask the doctor to check them as soon as possible. Never enter questionable material into patient records. Any incorrectly transcribed information can become a legal liability for the doctor should the records be used in a lawsuit.
- All transcribed doctor's notes for the patient's chart should be initialed by the doctor.

Transcribing Direct Dictation

At times the physician may wish to dictate material directly to you. He may want to get observations, comments, or treatment options into the record immediately rather than waiting until a more convenient time to dictate the material into a recorder. Follow these guidelines.

- Use a writing pad with a stiff backing or place the pad on a clipboard to make it easier to write quickly. Use a good ballpoint pen that will not smear or drag on the paper.
- Use incomplete sentences and phrases to keep up with the physician's pace. For example, say "Patient home Friday, recheck 2 wks" instead of "The patient is going home on Friday. We should see him again in 2 weeks."
- Use abbreviations for common phrases (*w/o* for "without," *s/b* for "should be," and so on); for medical terms (*q.d.* for "every day," *mg* for "milligrams," and so on); and for medications or chemicals.
- If a term, phrase, prescription, or name is unclear, ask for clarification right away (say "Excuse me, could you repeat that phrase, please?").
- If the physician speaks with a pronounced accent, ask her to speak more slowly than normal.

- Read the dictation back to the physician to verify all terms, names, figures, and other information for accuracy.
- Enter the notes into the patient record, and date and initial the notes.

Transcription Aids

Keep a library of medical, secretarial, and transcription reference books and medical terminology texts near the transcription workstation. Abbreviations can save time, but you should use only those that are accepted as standard. Reference books will help you find the correct word quickly and easily and help you apply proper grammar, style, and usage to the copy.

Correcting and Updating Patient Records

In legal terms, medical records are regarded as having been created in "due course." All information in the record should be entered at the time of a patient's visit and not days, weeks, or months later. Information corrected or added some time after a patient's visit can be regarded as "convenient" and may damage a doctor's position in a lawsuit.

Using Care With Corrections

If changes to the medical record are not done correctly, the record can become a legal problem for the physician. A physician may be able to more easily explain poor or incomplete documentation than to explain a chart that appears to have been altered after something was originally documented. You must be extremely careful to follow the appropriate procedures for correcting patient records.

Mistakes in medical records are not uncommon. The best defense is to correct the mistake immediately or as soon as possible after the original entry was made. Procedure 9-1 shows you how to correct the patient record.

Updating Patient Records

All additions to a patient's record—test results, observations, diagnoses, procedures—should be done in a way that no one could interpret as deception on the physician's part. In a note accompanying the material, the physician should explain why the information is being added to the record. In some cases the material may simply be a physician's recollections or observations on a patient visit that occurred in the past. Each item added to a record must be dated and initialed. Sometimes a third party may be asked to witness the addition.

Most hospitals and clinics have detailed guidelines for late entries to a patient's chart. You must follow these guidelines carefully to avoid potential legal problems (see Procedure 9-2).

HANDLING INCOMING TELEPHONE CALLS

	Route to doctor immediately	Take message for doctor	Route to nurse or assistant
Emergencies: bleeding, drug/allergic reaction, difficulty breathing, injury, pain, poisoning, shock, unconsciousness, incoherence or hysteria	X		
Calls from other physicians	if possible		
Patient progress report		X	
Patient request for laboratory report		X (if abnormal)	Melissa (if normal)
Patient questions re medication		X	
Patient questions re billing or insurance			Jerry
Patient complaints			Melissa
Appointments			Melissa
Prescription renewals or refills		X	
Office business			Jerry
Personal business		X	
Salespeople			Jerry

Figure 11-1. A routing list identifies which office staff member is responsible for each type of incoming call.

title, however, the name of the individual who has that particular responsibility should be specified.

Types of Incoming Calls

In dealing with incoming telephone calls, you will encounter a variety of questions and requests from numerous people. Many incoming calls are from patients. You will also receive calls from other people, including attorneys, other physicians, pharmaceutical sales representatives, and other salespeople.

Calls From Patients

Patients call the medical office for a variety of reasons, including rescheduling appointments and requesting prescription renewals. If you will be discussing clinical matters over the telephone, it is a good idea to pull the patient's chart. The information in the chart may enable you to address any problems quickly. Having the chart handy also allows you to document the conversation immediately.

Always keep in mind that the physician is legally responsible for your actions, including relaying information to patients over the telephone. The office policy manual typically specifies what you may and may not discuss with patients. If you are uncertain about giving particular

information to a patient, it is best to have the physician return the patient's call.

Appointment Scheduling. Follow office procedures for making or changing appointment times over the telephone. (Scheduling appointments is discussed in Chapter 12.)

Billing Inquiries. If a patient calls about a billing problem, you will need to pull the patient's chart and billing information. With this information, you can compare the charges with the actual services performed.

If a patient claims to have been overcharged, check to see if the correct fee was charged. If you find that an error was made, apologize, and tell the patient the office will send a corrected statement. Ask the patient to wait for the new statement before sending payment. If in fact the proper fee was charged, it may be helpful to speak to the physician before responding to the patient. The physician may be able to tell you if there were special circumstances regarding the visit or charge in question. Allowing the patient to pay the bill in installments is usually an acceptable option.

If a patient is dissatisfied, document all comments, and relay the information to the physician. If a bill has not been paid, ask if there are special circumstances affecting the patient's ability to pay. Always give this information to the physician or office manager.

Requests for Laboratory or Radiology Reports.
If a patient calls the office requesting the results of tests, pull the patient's chart to see if the report has been received. If it has not, suggest that the patient call back in a day or two. Some offices will call the laboratory or radiology office for the results.

In some offices you may be authorized to give laboratory results by telephone if they are normal, or negative, so the patient does not have to wait for results to be mailed. Make a note on the patient's chart if you provide any information about test results. If a test result is abnormal, the physician will need to speak with the patient. In such a case tell the patient that the office has received the results and that the physician will call as soon as possible. Then place the patient's chart and the telephone message on the physician's desk.

Questions About Medications. One of the most common types of calls from patients involves questions about medication. A patient may ask about using a current prescription or may want to renew an existing prescription.

Prescription Renewals. Calls for prescription renewals occur frequently and may come from the patient's pharmacy or from the patient. A pharmacist usually calls to check before dispensing refills if more than a year has passed since the original prescription was written. If the physician has indicated on the patient's chart that renewals are approved, you may authorize the pharmacy to renew a prescription. In any other case, only the physician may authorize renewals. If the physician authorizes a renewal, you may be asked to telephone it in to the patient's pharmacy.

Old Prescriptions. Patients may call to ask if they can use a medication that was prescribed for a previous condition. In these instances, recommend that the patient come in for an appointment. Explain why the medication should not be used: it may be old and no longer effective, the current problem may not be the same as the previous one, the medication may not be helpful, and using the medication may mask the current condition's symptoms and make a diagnosis difficult.

If the patient does not want to make an appointment, relay the information to the physician. The physician will probably want to speak with the patient.

Reports on Symptoms. Sometimes patients call the office about symptoms they wish to discuss with the physician. Here are tips for handling such calls.

- Listen attentively to the patient.
- If the patient is in real distress, try to schedule an appointment that day or as soon as possible.
- Write down all the patient's symptoms completely, accurately, and immediately. In many instances the physician may be able to suggest simple emergency relief measures that you can relay to the patient. These measures may make the patient comfortable until the time of the appointment.

Progress Reports. Physicians often ask patients to call the office to let them know how a prescribed treatment is working. In these instances route the call to the physician, and log the call in the patient's medical record immediately. You may also be responsible for making routine follow-up calls to patients to verify that they are following treatment instructions.

Requests for Advice. Although a patient may ask you for your medical opinion, do not give medical advice of any kind. Explain that you are not trained to make a diagnosis or licensed to prescribe medication. Stress that the patient must see the physician. If the patient cannot come into the office, assure her that the physician will return the call or that you will call back after discussing the problem with the physician. Occasionally a patient wants to speak only with the physician, not other staff members. You must honor this request.

In some cases the physician may feel that a patient's symptoms warrant immediate attention and will insist on seeing the patient before prescribing any treatment. If the patient refuses to come to the office, note the reason on the chart, and suggest a visit to the emergency room or to a nearby physician. For legal reasons, it is important to document such conversations completely in the patient's chart, including the refusal of treatment.

Complaints. Even when an office provides the highest-quality care, complaints still occur. When a patient calls with a complaint, such as a billing error, it is important to listen carefully, without interrupting. Take careful notes of all the details, and read them back to the caller to ensure that you have written them down correctly. Let the caller know the person to whose attention you will bring the complaint and, if possible, when to expect a response.

Always apologize to the caller for any inconvenience the problem may have caused, even if the problem occurred through no fault of the office. Make sure the proper person receives the information about the complaint.

Sometimes a patient who calls with a complaint is angry. Responding to this type of call can be difficult and uncomfortable. Your first priority is to stay calm and try to pacify the caller. Follow these guidelines when dealing with an angry caller.

- Listen carefully, and acknowledge the patient's anger. By understanding the problem, you will be better able to work toward a solution.
- Remain calm, and speak gently and kindly. Do not act superior or talk down to the patient. Do not interrupt the patient. Do not return the anger or blame.
- Let the patient know that you will do your best to correct the problem. This message will convey that you care.
- Take careful notes, and be sure to document the call.
- Do not become defensive.
- Never make promises you cannot keep.

- Follow up promptly on the problem.
- Inform the physician immediately if an angry patient threatens legal action against the office.

Emergencies.   Emergency calls must be immediately routed to the physician. Emergency situations include serious or life-threatening medical conditions, such as severe bleeding, a reaction to a drug, injuries, poisoning, suicide attempts, loss of consciousness, or severe burns. Figure 11-2 lists symptoms and conditions that require immediate help.

Symptoms and Conditions That Require Immediate Medical Help

- Unconsciousness
- Lack of breathing or trouble breathing
- Severe bleeding
- Pressure or pain in the abdomen that will not go away
- Severe vomiting or bloody stools
- Poisoning
- Injuries to the head, neck, or back
- Choking
- Drowning
- Electrical shock
- Snakebites
- Vehicle collisions
- Allergic reactions to foods or insect stings
- Chemicals or foreign objects in the eye
- Fires, severe burns, or injuries from explosions
- Human bites or any deep animal bites
- Heart attack. Symptoms include chest pain or pressure; pain radiating from the chest to the arm, shoulder, neck, jaw, back, or stomach; nausea or vomiting; weakness; shortness of breath; pale or gray skin color.
- Stroke. Symptoms include seizures, severe headache, slurred speech.
- Broken bones. Symptoms include being unable to move or put weight on the injured body part. The injured part is very painful or looks misshapen.
- Shock. Symptoms include paleness; feeling faint and sweaty; weak, rapid pulse; cold, moist skin; confusion or drowsiness.
- Heatstroke (sunstroke). Symptoms include confusion or loss of consciousness; flushed skin that is hot and may be moist or dry; strong, rapid pulse.
- Hypothermia (a drop in body temperature during prolonged exposure to cold). Symptoms include becoming increasingly clumsy, unreasonable, irritable, confused, and sleepy; slurred speech; slipping into a coma with slow, weak breathing and heartbeat.

Figure 11-2.   Emergency calls require swift but careful handling.

If someone calls the office on behalf of a patient who is experiencing any of these symptoms or conditions, you may instruct the caller to dial 911 to request an ambulance. Procedure 11-1 describes the steps for handling emergency calls. The physician should be called to the telephone immediately to offer assistance.

Other Calls

Besides calls from patients, a medical office receives many other types of calls. For example, family members and friends of patients may call the physician at the office. The physician will let you know how to handle these calls. Remember that a patient's information is confidential. HIPAA requires medical providers to obtain authorization from the patient before any information can be disclosed. This is usually in the form of a written authorization, signed by the patient, that indicates what type of information may be given out and to whom. The following are guidelines for managing calls from attorneys, other physicians, and salespeople.

Attorneys.   Refer to the procedures listed in your practice's office policy manual regarding how to handle calls from attorneys. Follow the office guidelines closely, and ask the physician how to proceed if you receive a call that does not fall within the guidelines. Remember, never release any patient information to an outside caller unless the physician has asked you to do so.

Other Physicians.   Patients at your practice may be referred to surgeons, specialists, and other physicians for consultations. Consequently, you may receive calls from those physicians' offices. Route those calls to the physician if the caller requests that you do so. Always remember to ask if the call is about a medical emergency. Also keep in mind that you may not give out any patient information—even to another physician—unless you have a written, signed release from the patient.

Salespeople.   As a medical assistant, you will probably be the contact for salespeople, unless the office policy manual states that another staff member should handle this duty. On the telephone, ask the salesperson to send you information about any new products or equipment. Pharmaceutical sales representatives may want to meet with the physician. Forward such messages to the physician with a request to let you know when to schedule the appointment. Many physicians see pharmaceutical sales representatives on certain days at certain times. Sometimes they limit the number of representatives they will see in one day. Make sure you know your office policy.

Using Proper Telephone Etiquette

Handle all telephone calls politely and professionally. Use proper telephone **etiquette,** or good manners, so you feel confident in your role of providing quality care and

PROCEDURE 11.1

Handling Emergency Calls

Objective: To determine whether a telephone call involves a medical emergency and to learn the steps to take if it is an emergency call

Materials: Office guidelines for handling emergency calls; list of symptoms and conditions requiring immediate medical attention; telephone numbers of area emergency rooms, poison control centers, and ambulance transport services; telephone message forms or telephone message log

Method

1. When someone calls the office regarding a potential emergency, remain calm. This attitude will help calm the caller and enable you to gather necessary information in the most efficient manner.

2. Obtain the following information, taking accurate notes:
   a. The caller's name
   b. The caller's relation to the patient (if it is not the patient who is calling)
   c. The patient's name
   d. The patient's age
   e. A complete description of the patient's symptoms
   f. If the call is about an accident, a description of how the accident or injury occurred and any other pertinent information
   g. A description of how the patient is reacting to the situation
   h. Treatment that has been administered
   i. The caller's telephone number and the address from which the call is being made

   It may be necessary for you to put the call on hold or to hang up so that you can call for medical assistance. Before you do so, however, be sure to read the information back to the caller to ensure that you have written it down correctly.

3. Read back the details of the medical problem to verify them.

4. If necessary, refer to the list of symptoms and conditions that require immediate medical attention to determine if the situation is indeed a medical emergency.

If the Situation Is a Medical Emergency

1. Put the call through to the doctor immediately, or handle the situation according to the established office procedures.

2. If the doctor is not in the office, follow established office procedures. They may involve one or more of the following:
   a. Transferring the call to the nurse practitioner or other medical personnel, as appropriate
   b. Instructing the caller to dial 911 to request an ambulance for the patient
   c. Instructing the patient to go to the nearest emergency room
   d. Instructing the caller to telephone the nearest poison control center for advice and supplying the caller with its telephone number
   e. Paging the doctor

If the Situation Is Not a Medical Emergency

1. Handle the call according to established office procedures.

2. If you are in doubt about whether the situation is a medical emergency, treat it like an emergency. It is better to be overly cautious than to let an emergency go untreated. The doctor should be the one to decide how to handle these situations. You must always alert the doctor immediately about an emergency call, even if the patient declines to speak with the doctor.

---

assistance. Adhering to the guidelines that follow will help ensure that your telephone conversations are pleasant and constructive.

Your Telephone Voice

When you speak on the telephone, your voice represents the medical office. It must effectively present your message. Because you cannot rely on body language or facial expressions to help you communicate over the telephone, it is important to make the most of your telephone voice. Use the following tips to make your voice pleasant and effective.

- Speak directly into the receiver. Otherwise, your voice will be difficult to understand.
- Smile. The smile in your voice will convey your friendliness and willingness to help.

- Visualize the caller, and speak directly to that person.
- Convey a friendly and respectful interest in the caller. You should sound helpful and alert.
- Use language that is nontechnical and easy to understand. Never use slang.
- Speak at a natural pace, not too quickly or too slowly.
- Use a normal conversational tone.
- Try to vary your pitch while you are talking. **Pitch** is the high or low level of your speech. Varying the pitch of your voice allows you to emphasize words and makes your voice more pleasant to listen to.
- Make the caller feel important.

Pronunciation. Proper **pronunciation** (saying words correctly) is one of the most important telephone skills. Sometimes last names are difficult to pronounce. Ask patients, "How do you pronounce your name?" to make them feel welcome and important. When clarifying the spelling of a word or name, it is common practice to state the letter and then a word that begins with the letter. Examples include D as in dog, V as in Victor, M as in Mary, N as in Nancy, and B as in balloon.

Enunciation. **Enunciation** (clear and distinct speaking) is the opposite of mumbling. Good enunciation helps the person you are speaking to understand you, which is especially important when you are trying to convey medical information.

Speaking clearly over the telephone is very important because the speaker cannot be seen. Correct interpretation of the message is determined by hearing the words precisely. Activities such as chewing gum, eating, or propping the phone between the ear and shoulder hinder proper enunciation.

Tone. Because you are not face-to-face with the caller, the most important measurements of good telephone communication are voice quality and tone. Always speak with a positive and respectful tone.

Making a Good Impression

In a sense your telephone duties include public relations skills. How you handle telephone calls will have an impact on the public image of the medical practice.

Exhibiting Courtesy. Using common courtesy is a characteristic of professional office personnel. Courtesy is expressed by projecting an attitude of helpfulness. Always use the person's name during the conversation, and apologize for any errors or delays. When ending the conversation, be sure to thank the caller before hanging up.

Giving Undivided Attention. Do not try to answer the telephone while continuing to carry out another task. This practice may lead to errors in message taking and may give the caller the impression that you are uncaring or uninterested. Give the caller the same undivided attention you would if the person were in the office. Listen carefully to get the correct information.

Putting a Call on Hold. Although you should try not to put a caller on hold, there will be times when it is unavoidable. You may receive a call on another line, or a situation in the office may prevent you from devoting your full attention to the caller. Sometimes you may have to check a file or ask someone else in the office a question on behalf of the caller. Before putting a call on hold, however, always let the caller state the reason for the call. This step is essential so that you do not inadvertently put an emergency call on hold.

The medical office may have a standard procedure for placing a call on hold. Typically you will ask the caller the purpose of the call, state why you need to place the call on hold, explain how long you expect the wait to be, and ask the caller if this wait is acceptable. If you think the wait will be long, offer to call back rather than asking the caller to hold. Being kept on hold too long or too often makes people think the staff is inattentive to their needs.

If you know you can return to the line shortly, you can put the caller on hold, then attend to the problem. If you need to answer a second call, get the second caller's name and telephone number, and put that call on hold until you have completed the first call. You can then return to the second call.

Handling Difficult Situations. At times it will be impossible to give your undivided attention to a caller because of a pressing issue or emergency in the office. If the call itself is not an emergency one, it is best to ask if you can call back. Explain that you are currently handling an urgent matter, and offer to return the call in a few minutes. Most people will appreciate your honesty. Return the call in a reasonable amount of time, and be sure to apologize for the inconvenience.

Remembering Patients' Names. When patients are recognized by name, they are more likely to have positive feelings about the practice. Using a caller's name during a conversation makes the caller feel important. If you do not recognize a patient's name, it is better to ask "Has it been some time since you've seen the doctor?" rather than to ask if the patient has been to the practice before.

Checking for Understanding. When communicating by telephone, you do not have visual signals to convey the caller's feelings and level of understanding of the information you are discussing. Consequently, you must ask certain questions in the right way. If a call is long or complicated, summarize what was said to be sure that both you and the caller understand the information. Ask if the caller has any questions about what you have discussed.

Communicating Feelings. Whenever information is conveyed over the telephone, feelings are also communicated. When dealing with a caller who is nervous, upset, or angry, try to show empathy (an understanding of the other person's feelings). Communicating with empathy helps the caller feel more positive about the conversation and the medical office.

Ending the Conversation. It is not useful to let a conversation run on if you can effectively complete the call sooner. Before hanging up, however, take a few seconds to complete the call so that the caller feels properly cared for and satisfied. You can complete the call by summarizing the important points of the conversation and thanking the caller. Then let the caller hang up first. When you put the receiver down, never slam it—even if the caller has already hung up. Remember that all your actions reflect the professional image of the medical practice. Patients in the waiting room may see you when you are talking on the telephone.

Taking Messages

Always have paper and a pen or pencil near the telephone so that you are prepared to write down messages (Figure 11-3). Proper documentation protects the physician if the caller takes legal action. A record of telephone calls should also be included in a patient's file as part of a complete medical history.

Documenting Calls

Documenting telephone calls is essential in a medical office. You can use telephone message pads or a telephone log book (Figure 11-4). Again, remember that many calls (for example, those concerning clinical problems or referrals)

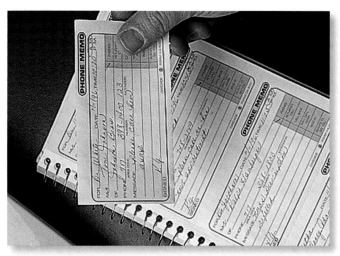

Figure 11-4. When using a telephone message pad or telephone log, be sure to fill out the form completely and accurately.

and the actions or decisions they lead to need to be documented in patients' charts. Every entry into a patient's chart is considered a legal document; therefore the information must be accurate and legible. Accurate documentation helps guard against lawsuits.

Telephone Message Pads. You can use telephone message pads, which often come in brightly colored paper, to record the following information:

- Date and time of the call
- Name of the person for whom you took the message
- Caller's name
- Caller's telephone number (including area code and extension, if any)
- A description or an action to be taken, including comments such as "Urgent," "Please call back," "Wants to see you," "Will call back," or "Returned your call"
- The complete message, such as "Dr. Stephenson wants to reschedule the committee meeting."
- Name or initials of the person taking the call

The Telephone Log. Some medical offices use spiral-bound, perforated message books with carbonless forms to record messages. The top copy, or original, of each message is given to the appropriate person, and a copy is kept in the book for future reference.

Tips for Taking Messages. The following suggestions will help you provide accurate documentation for incoming messages:

- Always have a pen or pencil and paper on hand.
- Jot down notes as the information is given.
- Verify information, especially the spelling of patient or caller names and the correct spelling of medications.
- Verify the correct callback number.

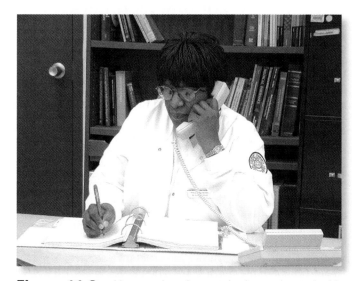

Figure 11-3. Use one hand or a telephone rest to hold the telephone so that the hand you write with is free to take messages.

PROCEDURE 11.2

Retrieving Messages From an Answering Service

Objective: To follow standard procedures for retrieving messages from an answering service

Materials: Telephone message pad or telephone log

Method

1. Set a regular schedule for calling the answering service to retrieve messages. Having a regular schedule ensures that you do not miss any messages.

2. Call at the regularly scheduled time(s) to see if there are any messages.

3. Identify yourself, and state that you are calling to obtain messages for the practice.

4. For each message, write down all pertinent information on the telephone message pad or telephone log. Be sure to include the patient's name and telephone number, time of call, message or description of the problem, and action taken, if any.

5. Repeat the information, confirming that you have the correct spelling of all names.

6. When you have retrieved all messages, route them according to the office policy.

- When taking a phone message for the physician, never make a commitment on behalf of the physician by saying, "I'll have the physician call you." An appropriate response would be, "I will give your message to the physician."

Ensuring Correct Information

When you are taking a message, be sure to get the proper spelling of the caller's name. Repeat the spelling to the caller to make sure it is correct. If it is necessary to pull the patient's chart, ask for the patient's date of birth, in case there are two patient's with the same name. When you have taken down all the necessary information, repeat the key points to the caller for verification.

Maintaining Patient Confidentiality

Do not repeat information over the telephone when the information is confidential. This point is especially important if patients or others in the office may overhear the conversation. You must also maintain patient confidentiality when handling written telephone messages. If a confidential message must be brought to the doctor's attention, do not leave it on the doctor's desk where it can be seen by someone else. Instead, put the message in a file folder marked "Confidential," and place the folder on the desk. Follow the same procedure when handling confidential faxes.

Telephone Answering Systems

An office telephone system can range from a single telephone line to a complex multiline system. Most medical offices use one or more of the following pieces of equipment and services to provide efficient management of telephone calls: an automated voice mail system, an answering machine, and an answering service. These systems are described in Chapter 5. One of your telephone responsibilities may be to retrieve messages from the practice's answering service. Procedure 11-2 describes how to do so.

Placing Outgoing Calls

You will often be required to place outgoing calls on behalf of the medical office. You may need to return calls, obtain information, provide patient education, or arrange patient consultations with other physicians.

Locating Telephone Numbers

Before you can place an outgoing call, of course, you must have the correct telephone number. If you are calling a patient, the telephone number should be in the patient's chart. To find other telephone numbers, you may need to consult a telephone directory or call for directory assistance.

The medical office should have at least one telephone directory, or telephone book, for the local calling area and perhaps additional directories for surrounding areas. Use these books to locate telephone numbers for outside calls. The office may also have a card file with commonly used telephone numbers, as shown in Figure 11-5, or these numbers may be listed in the office policy manual.

If you need to find a long-distance telephone number, many offices use the directory assistance service. You can reach this service by dialing 1-[area code]-555-1212. Use directory assistance only when you have exhausted other options, however, because most long-distance carriers charge a fee each time you use the service.

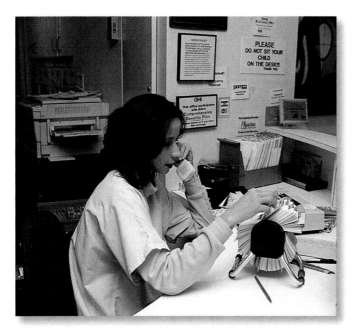

Figure 11-5. Keeping a card file on the desk allows you to easily find frequently used telephone numbers.

Applying Your Telephone Skills

You can apply the telephone skills you use for answering incoming calls when placing outgoing calls. Here are additional tips for handling outgoing calls.

- Plan before you call. Have all the information you need in front of you before you dial the telephone number. Plan what you will say, and decide what questions to ask so that you will not have to call back for additional information.
- Double-check the telephone number. Before placing a call, always confirm the number. If in doubt, look it up in the telephone directory. If you do dial a wrong number, be sure to apologize for the mistake.
- Allow enough time, at least a minute or about eight rings, for someone to answer the telephone. When calling patients who are elderly or physically disabled, allow additional time.
- Identify yourself. After reaching the person to whom you placed the call, give your name, and state that you are calling on behalf of the doctor.
- Ask if you have called at a convenient time and whether the person has time to talk with you. If it is not a good time, ask when you should call back.
- Be ready to speak as soon as the person you called answers the telephone. Do not waste the person's time while you collect your thoughts.
- If you are calling to give information, ask if the person has a pencil and piece of paper available. Do not begin with dates, times, or instructions until the person is ready to write down the information.

Arranging Conference Calls

It may be necessary for you to schedule conference calls with patients, hospitals, or other doctors to discuss tests or surgical results. When dealing with several people, suggest several time slots in case someone is not available at a particular time. Also keep in mind the various time zones in the country. Make sure that all the conference-call participants are given the proper time in their time zone to expect the call.

Telephone Triage

Some physicians delegate to other staff members some of the clinical decision making that is done over the telephone. In these instances, **telephone triage** is used as a process of deciding what necessary action to take. The word *triage* refers to the screening and sorting of emergency incidents. Performing triage correctly is an important skill. You should learn as much as possible about triage techniques.

Learning the Triage Process

Proper training of office staff is vital in providing safe, sound, and cost-effective medical care over the telephone. An increasing number of medical practices are preparing guidelines for the telephone staff to follow when patients call the office with specific medical problems or questions.

Guidelines are often written for common questions, such as how to deal with sniffles and fevers during cold and flu season or how to make a child with chickenpox more comfortable. Members of the telephone staff must realize, however, that their responsibility is to determine whether a caller needs additional medical care. They cannot diagnose or treat the patient's problem.

Office guidelines outline the specific information the telephone staff must obtain from the patient. In general, this information is the same type as that obtained during an office visit. It should include the patient's age, symptoms, when the problem began, and the patient's level of anxiety about the problem.

Categorizing Patient Problems and Providing Patient Education

After the patient information is obtained, the guidelines help the staff categorize the problem according to severity. The telephone staff then decides if the problem can be handled safely with advice over the telephone, whether the patient needs to come into the office, or whether the problem requires immediate attention at an emergency room.

If a problem is deemed appropriate for telephone management, the guidelines may include recommendations for nonprescription treatment that may relieve symptoms and anxiety. This information falls under the category of patient education. Advise the caller that recommendations are based on the symptoms and are not a diagnosis. Remember that only the doctor is authorized to make a diagnosis and prescribe medication. Ask the caller to repeat any instructions you give, and tell the patient to call back within a specified time if symptoms worsen. Be sure to document the conversation in the patient's chart.

Taking Action

Clinical triage involves determining the extent of medical emergencies and deciding on the appropriate action. If a caller is having chest pains, you would be performing a type of triage by instructing him to go to the emergency room as soon as possible. Telephone triage is also used in handling common minor medical problems and questions. Whatever the nature of the problem, the situation must be dealt with appropriately to protect the health and safety of the patient.

Telecommunications

An automated system is used in many hospitals and larger ambulatory care settings. When a call is answered, a recorded voice identifies departments or services the caller can reach by pressing a specified number on the telephone keypad. This telephone system and menu provides a convenient way for patients or callers to reach the direct service or department needed.

Facsimile (Fax) Machines

Facsimile machines, often referred to as fax machines, are commonly used in physicians' offices. A fax is sent over telephone lines from one fax modem to another. Fax machines may be used to send referrals, reports, insurance approvals, or medication refill approvals. Per HIPAA guidelines, a patient's confidentiality must be protected by placing the fax machine in a secure location that only authorized personnel can access. Federal and state laws also must be followed in maintaining or faxing medical records. The physician's office should develop guidelines to follow when faxing information about patients.

Summary

The telephone is an important communication tool in the medical office. Your telephone manner will reflect the professionalism of the office. Medical offices commonly receive several types of calls, and there are varying ways to handle these calls.

Special attention should be given to documenting incoming telephone calls and ensuring accuracy. HIPAA guidelines must be followed to maintain patient confidentiality. This applies to telephone conversations and computer monitors as well as medical records. Telephone etiquette involves practicing proper pronunciation and enunciation, using common courtesy and a respectful tone of voice, giving undivided attention to callers, and accommodating patients' requests and needs. Placing outgoing calls requires the same careful attention as taking incoming calls. Telephone triage is the art of determining the level of urgency of each call and how it should be handled or routed.

CHAPTER 11

CASE STUDY QUESTIONS

Now that you have completed this chapter, review the case study at the beginning of the chapter and answer the following questions:

1. What would your first response to the patient be?
2. Explain how you would handle this situation.
3. What type of incoming call was this?
4. What type of condition did this patient's symptoms indicate?
5. What are some other symptoms of this condition?

Discussion Questions

1. What is the purpose of screening calls that come into the medical office?
2. Why is proper telephone etiquette so important in the medical office?
3. Name five of the most common types of calls received in the medical office that can be handled by the medical assistant. Name two that must be handled by the physician.
4. Describe what a routing list is and what it is used for.
5. Name five symptoms or conditions that require immediate medical help.
6. What is the best way to clarify the pronunciation or spelling of a patient's name?
7. What act does *HIPAA* stand for, and what is the purpose of the act?

Critical Thinking Questions

1. Outline the skills needed by a medical assistant who is responsible for answering incoming calls to a medical office.
2. Describe how you would handle a situation in which an angry patient calls to complain that he was overcharged for a recent office visit.

3. Imagine that you need to call a patient to tell her that she has to return to the office to have some blood redrawn because an insufficient amount of blood was drawn the first time. What would you say to the patient? What would you do if she refused to have the blood redrawn?
4. A 21-year-old female patient had lab tests performed. The patient's mother calls and requests to know her daughter's lab results. What should you do?
5. List the five Cs of communication and define what each means.

Application Activities

1. With a partner, role-play a scenario in which a patient calls the medical office to report symptoms. The patient then claims not to have time to come to the office for an appointment but instead asks for medical advice from the medical assistant. How should the medical assistant respond? When you have finished role-playing, discuss other ways the medical assistant could have dealt with the problem.
2. When speaking with patients on the telephone, how might you demonstrate the following qualities? Give several examples for each quality.
   a. concern
   b. attentiveness
   c. friendliness
   d. respect
   e. empathy
3. Create a one-page training sheet or chart for new personnel illustrating how to handle emergency calls coming into the medical office.
4. Define telephone triage. Give examples of three different patient calls and how you would triage each call.

CHAPTER 12

Scheduling Appointments and Maintaining the Physician's Schedule

KEY TERMS

- advance scheduling
- agenda
- cluster scheduling
- double-booking system
- itinerary
- locum tenens
- matrix
- minutes
- modified-wave scheduling
- no-show
- open-hours scheduling
- overbooking
- time-specified scheduling
- underbooking
- walk-in
- wave scheduling

AREAS OF COMPETENCE

2003 Role Delineation Study

ADMINISTRATIVE

Administrative Procedures
- Schedule, coordinate, and monitor appointments
- Schedule inpatient/outpatient admissions and procedures

GENERAL

Professionalism
- Prioritize and perform multiple tasks

CHAPTER OUTLINE

- The Appointment Book
- Appointment Scheduling Systems
- Arranging Appointments
- Special Scheduling Situations
- Scheduling Outside Appointments
- Maintaining the Physician's Schedule

OBJECTIVES

After completing Chapter 12, you will be able to:

12.1 Explain the importance of the appointment book in maintaining the schedule in the medical office.

12.2 Identify common scheduling abbreviations.

12.3 Identify and describe different types of appointment scheduling systems.

12.4 Discuss ways to arrange appointments for patients.

12.5 Explain how to handle special scheduling situations.

12.6 Explain how to properly document no-shows and late patients.

12.7 Describe how to schedule appointments that are outside the medical office.

12.8 Discuss ways to keep an accurate and efficient physician schedule.

Introduction

As a medical assistant, you need to know all aspects of how to create and utilize an appointment book. In this chapter you will learn to identify the different types of scheduling systems, how each is used, and which type of practice each system would work best in. You will also learn how to handle many types of scheduling situations within the office, including patient appointments,

emergencies, pharmaceutical representatives, and the scheduling of outside appointments with other medical facilities. Legal aspects of the appointment book are discussed, and proper documentation is stressed. Additional topics include appointment cards, reminder mailings, reminder calls, and recall notices for patients.

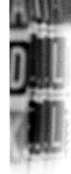

CASE STUDY

A 71-year-old female patient has a routine follow-up appointment with the physician regarding her medications. Her appointment is at 9:00 A.M. and lasts about 15 minutes. As the patient is checking out at the reception desk, she trips and falls, hitting her head on the corner of the reception desk. There is a bleeding wound on her forehead, and she complains of a headache. The physician and another medical assistant obtain a stretcher and move the patient to an exam room to access her injuries. It is expected that this emergency will take at least 45 minutes to handle. You are managing the schedule for the day. The physician has a full schedule for this morning and has already worked in a couple of additional appointment times for patients who need to be seen this morning for acute problems.

The next scheduled appointment is for a 24-year-old male who needs an employment physical for a new job he is to start next week. He must have the physical performed prior to his first day. His appointment is scheduled for 9:15 A.M. and is expected to last 30 minutes. At 9:45 A.M., two patients are scheduled for the same 15-minute appointment. One has a sore throat, and the other is scheduled for a wound check. The afternoon schedule has two appointment openings: the first at 2:00 P.M., which is for 15 minutes, and the second at 4:15 P.M., also for 15 minutes.

As you read this chapter, consider the following questions:

1. How would you adjust the schedule to allow for the emergency without falling behind schedule?
2. If it is necessary to reschedule patients, who should be rescheduled and when?
3. Would you explain anything to the patients in the waiting room about the emergency? If so, what would you say?

The Appointment Book

Time is a treasured commodity for both patients and physicians. Scheduling appointments in an organized fashion shows respect for everyone's time and creates an efficient patient flow. A well-managed appointment book is the key to establishing this efficiency.

Although most patients understand that they will probably have to wait in the reception area before they are seen by the physician, few patients are willing to wait more than 20 minutes. Offices that routinely have long waiting times can end up with dissatisfied patients and other problems. Some patients, in an attempt to avoid a long wait, may deliberately arrive after their scheduled appointment times. Accommodating these latecomers can throw the office schedule off track. Other patients may become resentful and decide to seek medical care with a competing practice.

Even in a well-run office, however, unexpected events can disrupt the schedule. Some patients arrive early, some arrive late, and others do not arrive at all. Some

appointments take longer than expected, for example, if the physician needs to spend extra time with a patient. In addition, emergency appointments sometimes need to be squeezed into the schedule. For these reasons, making an office schedule flow smoothly can be a challenge.

Preparing the Appointment Book

Before you can begin scheduling appointments, you need to prepare the appointment book. The first step is to establish the **matrix,** or basic format, of the appointment book. In order to create the matrix, you need to block off times on the schedule during which the doctor is not available to see patients. Time would be blocked off the schedule, for example, when the doctor was away for the following reasons.

- Hospital rounds
- Surgery
- Lunch

- Vacation days
- Holidays
- Scheduled meetings (for example, pharmaceutical, medical supply company, or in-service meetings)

The day's schedule is then built around this matrix. See Figure 12-1 for an example of a matrix.

Obtaining Patient Information

When the matrix has been established, you can begin scheduling appointments. You must obtain and enter certain patient information for each appointment. At some practices personnel enter the information into both traditional paper appointment books and computerized systems. Then, if the computer fails to work for some reason, the office has the book for reference. Some doctors who have been in practice for many years are used to the appointment book method and do not want to give it up for a computer system. Other offices are completely computerized. Using either the book or computer method, obtain the necessary patient information:

- Patient's full name. Obtain the correct spelling of the patient's name.
- Home and work telephone numbers. Repeat phone numbers to ensure accuracy.
- Purpose of the visit. Use a brief description and utilize approved abbreviations when possible. Do not create your own abbreviations.
- Estimated length of the visit.

Commonly Used Abbreviations

If you are the person who maintains the appointment book, you will find that certain procedures and conditions occur frequently. To save space and time when entering information, use these abbreviations:

BP	blood pressure check
can	cancellation
c/o	complains of
cons	consultation
CP	chest pain
CPE	complete physical examination
ECG	electrocardiogram
FU	follow-up appointment
GI	gastrointestinal
I & D	incision and drainage
inj	injection
lab	laboratory studies
N & V	nausea and vomiting
NP	new patient
NS	no-show patient
P & P	Pap smear (Papanicolaou smear) and pelvic examination
Pap	Pap smear
PMS	premenstrual syndrome
pt	patient
PT	physical therapy
re	recheck
ref	referral
RS	reschedule
Rx	prescription
sig	sigmoidoscopy
SOB	shortness of breath
S/R	suture removal
STD	sexually transmitted disease
surg	surgery
US	ultrasound

Determining Standard Procedure Times

If you are to schedule appointments efficiently, you must have an estimate of how long visits will take. Working with the physician or physicians in your practice, create a list of standard procedure times. Also indicate on the list how much time to allow for tests that are commonly performed in the practice. This list, kept beside the appointment book, helps you identify which openings are appropriate for the procedure or test involved. The lengths and types of tests and procedures will depend on the practice. Following are typical lengths of common procedures:

Complete physical examination	30–60 minutes
New patient visit	30 minutes or more
Follow-up office visit	5–10 minutes
Emergency office visit	15–20 minutes
Prenatal examination	15 minutes
Pap smear and pelvic examination	15–30 minutes
Minor in-office surgery, such as a mole removal	30 minutes
Suture removal	10–20 minutes

A Legal Record

The appointment book is considered a legal record. Some experts advise holding on to old appointment books for at least 3 years. Because the appointment book could be used as evidence in legal proceedings, entries must be clear and easy to read. Management consultants suggest that because the appointment book is a legal medical document, the schedule should be written in blue ink and never with a pencil. Never erase a name or use correction fluid to blot the name out. Instead, draw a single line through the name and beside it write "can" for canceled or "NS" for a no-show patient. Also write the date, time, and reason (if known) why the appointment was missed or canceled, then initial the entry. This information should also be documented in the patient's chart.

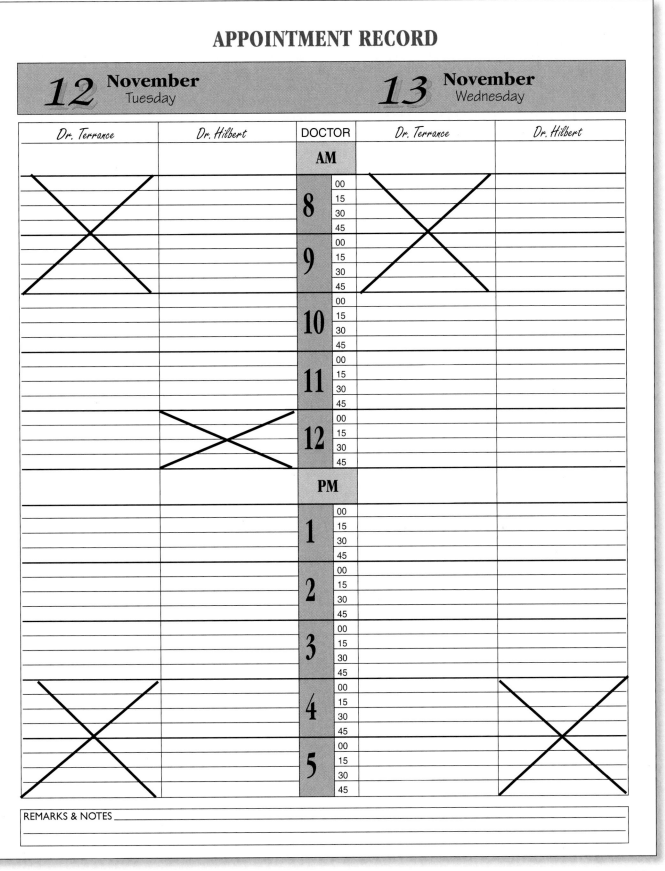

APPOINTMENT RECORD

Dr. Terrance	Dr. Hilbert	DOCTOR		Dr. Terrance	Dr. Hilbert

Figure 12-1. It is important to establish a matrix in the appointment book so that appointments are not scheduled for times when the doctor will be out of the office.

Some offices permit the use of pencil to allow for changes or corrections if necessary. If pencil is used, at the end of each day you or another designated staff member should write directly over the penciled entries in ink to create a permanent document.

Appointment Scheduling Systems

There are several possible appointment scheduling systems. The method chosen usually depends on the type of practice and the physician's preferences. No matter which method your office uses, it should be regularly reviewed to see whether it is meeting its goals: a smooth flow of patients and minimal waiting time.

Open-Hours Scheduling

In the **open-hours scheduling** system, patients arrive at their own convenience with the understanding that they will be seen on a first-come, first-served basis, unless there is an extreme emergency. Depending on how many other patients are ahead of them, they may have a considerable wait. The open-hours system eliminates the problems caused by broken appointments (because there are no appointments), but it increases the possibility of inefficient downtime for the doctor. In addition, with this system the medical assistant cannot pull patients' charts before they arrive.

Most private practices have replaced the open-hours system with scheduled appointments. Open-hours systems are sometimes still used by rural practices and by practices specializing in urgent care, such as emergency centers. An open-hours system still requires the use of an appointment book, to record patients as they come into the office. You must also still establish a matrix so that you will know when a doctor is out of the office.

Time-Specified Scheduling

Time-specified scheduling (also called stream scheduling) assumes a steady stream of patients all day long at regular, specified intervals. Most minor medical problems, such as sore throats, earaches, or blood pressure follow-ups, usually require only 10- to 15-minute appointment slots. More time may be required for appointments such as physical examinations, which usually require 60 minutes, or new patient visits, which usually require 30 minutes (Figure 12-2). When a visit requires more time, you simply assign the patient additional back-to-back slots.

Wave Scheduling

Wave scheduling works effectively in larger medical facilities that have enough departments and personnel to provide services to several patients at the same time. This method of scheduling is based on the reality that some patients will arrive late and that others will require more or less time than expected with the physician. Wave scheduling has the flexibility to allow for appointments that require more time than anticipated or for patients who miss appointments. The goal of wave scheduling is to begin and end each hour with the overall office schedule on track. You determine the number of patients to be seen each hour by dividing the hour by the length of the average visit. If the average is 15 minutes, for example, you schedule four patients for each hour. An example of wave scheduling would be:

10:00 A.M.	Patient A	555-5683	Sore throat
10:15 A.M.	Patient B	555-7322	Low back pain
10:30 A.M.	Patient C	555-4673	FU B/P
10:45 A.M.	Patient D	555-2854	B12 inj

You ask all four to arrive at the beginning of the hour and have the physician see them in the order of their actual arrival. The main problem with wave scheduling is that patients may realize they have appointments at the same time as other patients. The result may be confusion and possibly annoyance or anger.

Modified-Wave Scheduling

The wave system can be modified in several ways. With **modified-wave scheduling,** as shown in Figure 12-3, patients might be scheduled in 15-minute increments. Another option is to schedule four patients to arrive at planned intervals during the first half hour, leaving the second half hour unscheduled. Appointments that are anticipated to require more time should be scheduled at the beginning of the hour. Appointments that are expected to be less time-consuming should be scheduled in 10- to 20-minute time slots. This method allows time for catching up before the next hour begins.

Double Booking

With a **double-booking system,** two or more patients are scheduled for the same appointment slot. Unlike the wave or modified-wave system, however, the double-booking system assumes that both patients will actually be seen by the doctor within the scheduled period. If the types of visits are usually short (5 minutes, for example), it is reasonable to book two patients for one 15-minute opening. If both patients require the entire 15 minutes, however, the office falls behind schedule. Double-booking scheduling works most effectively in practices in which more than one patient can be attended to at a time.

Double booking can be helpful if a patient calls with a problem and needs to be seen that day but no appointments are available. You could double-book this patient with an already scheduled patient. In such cases you should explain that the caller might have to wait a bit before being seen by the doctor.

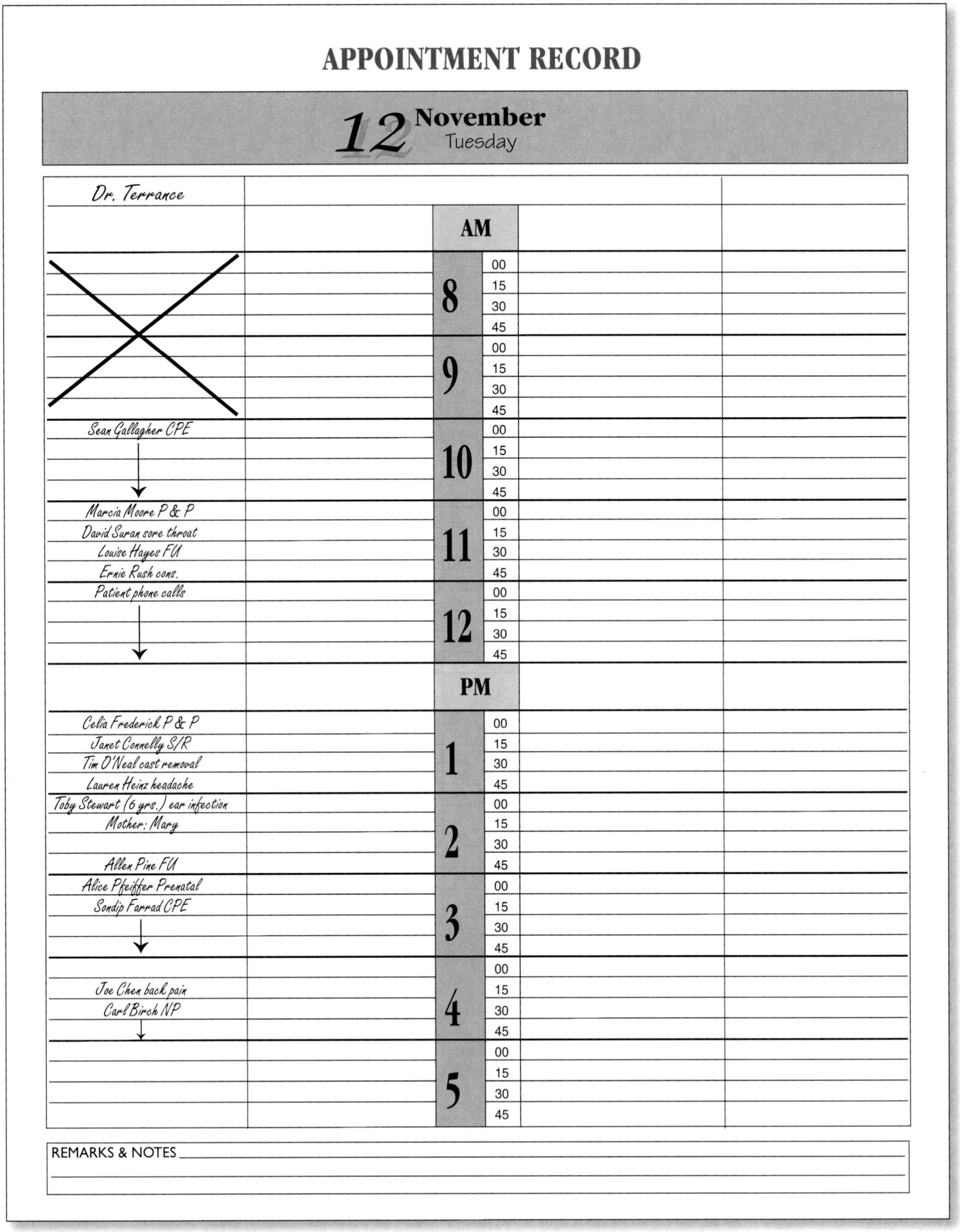

APPOINTMENT RECORD

12 November
Tuesday

Dr. Terrance

		AM		
		8	00	
			15	
			30	
			45	
		9	00	
			15	
			30	
			45	
Sean Gallagher CPE		**10**	00	
			15	
↓			30	
			45	
Marcia Moore P & P		**11**	00	
David Suran sore throat			15	
Louise Hayes FU			30	
Ernie Rush cons.			45	
Patient phone calls		**12**	00	
			15	
			30	
↓			45	
		PM		
Celia Frederick P & P		**1**	00	
Janet Connelly S/R			15	
Tim O'Neal cast removal			30	
Lauren Heinz headache			45	
Toby Stewart (6 yrs.) ear infection		**2**	00	
Mother: Mary			15	
			30	
Allen Pine FU			45	
Alice Pfeiffer Prenatal		**3**	00	
Sondip Farrad CPE			15	
			30	
↓			45	
		4	00	
Joe Chen back pain			15	
Carl Birch NP			30	
↓			45	
		5	00	
			15	
			30	
			45	

REMARKS & NOTES _____

Figure 12-2. Time-specified appointment scheduling is commonly used in the medical office.

is that the scheduling information can be accessed from all terminals located within the practice. Computerized systems can also help staff members identify patients who often are late, forget their appointments altogether, or cancel. In addition, the computer can identify patients who may require additional time with the physician because of special needs.

Arranging Appointments

Whether you are arranging appointments in person or by telephone, be polite and courteous. In scheduling an appointment, try to offer the patient a choice between two different dates, with either a morning or afternoon time slot. Once the patient decides on the date and time, always confirm the appointment by repeating it to the person before printing it in the schedule. If you are scheduling the appointment in person, write the appointment date and time on an appointment card to give to the patient. Whenever possible, try to accommodate the patient's needs while still maintaining a smoothly flowing schedule.

New Patients

A patient who has not been established at a medical practice is considered a new patient. Appointments for new patients are most often arranged over the telephone. Be sure to obtain all the necessary information, including the correct spelling and pronunciation of the person's name, home address, daytime telephone number, and date of birth. When arranging the appointment, keep in mind that some physicians prefer to schedule new patients at certain times of the day, such as first thing in the morning. When scheduling an appointment for a new patient, make sure to allow enough time for filling out forms. Have the new patient arrive 15 to 30 minutes early to do this.

Return Appointments

It is always good practice to ask patients returning to the reception area if they need to schedule another appointment. Getting them to make the appointment then will save you from having to do so by telephone later on. When patients call to arrange appointments, use the telephone techniques outlined in Chapter 11.

Appointment Reminders

Some patients may have trouble remembering their next appointment, especially if they arrange it far in advance. To help patients keep track of their appointments, you can use several types of appointment reminders.

Appointment Cards. In many offices the medical assistant fills out and hands the patient an appointment reminder card, like the one shown in Figure 12-5. To reduce the chance of error, enter the appointment in the appointment book first, then fill out the card. Otherwise, when the

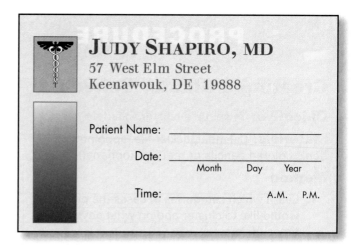

Figure 12-5. Before patients leave the office, be sure to give them an appointment card if they are scheduled to return to the office.

patient takes the appointment card, you have to rely on your memory when entering the appointment in the book.

Reminder Mailings. When making a follow-up appointment in person, you can ask the patient to address to himself a postcard on which you have written the next appointment's date and time. This postcard serves as a backup in case the patient loses the original appointment reminder card. Place the postcard in the tickler file under the day when it should be sent (usually a week before the appointment). Reminder mailings can also be sent to patients who make appointments over the telephone. In this case, of course, you must address the postcard for the tickler file yourself. Reminder mailings are useful when appointments are made many months in advance or are for geriatric patients.

Reminder Calls. Depending on office policy and available time, you might also call patients 1 or 2 days before their appointments to confirm the scheduled time. This technique can be especially helpful for patients with a history of late arrivals or for **no-shows** (patients who do not call to cancel and do not come to the appointment). Writing patients' phone numbers next to their names in the appointment book makes it convenient for you to make reminder appointment calls.

Recall Notices. Many offices book appointments no more than a few weeks in advance. If your office has such a policy, you need a way to make sure patients do not forget to call for appointments that are 6 months—or even a year—away from their last appointments.

Suppose, for example, that the physician tells a patient she should have an annual breast examination. How can you help her remember to call to schedule one at the appropriate time? One way is to use a system of recall notices. In a tickler file enter the patient's name under the month when she should call the office. When the time arrives, send a form letter reminding her that she will soon be due for a breast examination and asking her to call for an appointment.

Special Scheduling Situations

Although a great deal of scheduling is routine, creativity and flexibility are necessary for scheduling some special cases. These special situations often involve patients, but they may also involve physicians.

Patient Scheduling Situations

On some days all patients will keep their appointments and arrive on time. On many other days, however, patients may walk in without appointments, arrive late for scheduled appointments, or miss appointments entirely. Being prepared for these possibilities allows you to handle them better and to keep the office schedule running as smoothly as possible.

Emergencies. Your training as a medical assistant will help you recognize the signs of an emergency. In some instances you will refer the caller to the nearest hospital emergency room or instruct the caller to call Emergency Medical Services for an ambulance. In other instances you will ask the caller to come to the office right away. It is vital that doctors see emergency patients before patients who are already in the waiting area or on the schedule. It is best to explain to waiting patients that there has been an emergency (without giving details). This announcement helps them understand and accept the delay and also gives them an opportunity to reschedule their appointments. The Tips for the Office section provides guidelines for scheduling emergency appointments. Procedure 11-1 in Chapter 11 details how to handle emergency calls.

Referrals. Sometimes other doctors refer patients to the practice for second opinions or special consultations. Patients seeking second opinions before deciding on surgery should be fit into the schedule as soon as possible. Other referred patients should also be seen quickly, as a matter of professional courtesy to the referring doctor as well as good business practice.

If a physician in your office refers a patient to another doctor, your first step should be to check your office's policy and procedure manual. Many office manuals contain a

Tips for the Office

Scheduling Emergency Appointments

As a multiskilled medical assistant, you will be well prepared to tell the difference between acute conditions that are emergencies and those that are not. Guidelines on types of emergencies to be seen in the office and types to be referred elsewhere will vary. If you have any doubt, interrupt the physician to ask for instructions.

Even with buffer times built into the daily schedule, emergencies are still disruptive to most practices. Your ability to stay calm, respond quickly, and remain flexible will be of great comfort to the emergency patient and to others in the waiting area. Read the following story to see how an emergency situation can be handled skillfully.

The Situation

It is 4:15 P.M. in a busy family practice. The telephone rings. The caller is the father of a 10-year-old boy. Maria, the medical assistant, can hear the panic in his voice. His son Kyle has injured his knee while playing football with friends. Kyle cannot straighten the knee, and it is quite swollen.

Maria consults the physician, who suspects torn cartilage. The physician tells Maria to have the father wrap ice in a towel, apply it to Kyle's knee, and bring him in immediately. Maria relays this advice to the father and asks him how soon he can get to the office.

"It will take about 25 minutes," he replies.

The office schedule includes a buffer time opening at 4:30, but based on the father's estimate, Kyle cannot possibly arrive until 4:40. Maria notes that Mrs. Griffin, a good-natured retiree, is scheduled to come in for her weekly blood pressure check at 4:45 P.M. Hers is the last scheduled appointment of the day.

The Solution

Mrs. Griffin lives about 5 minutes from the office. Maria calls her home and explains that there has been an emergency. She offers Mrs. Griffin three choices: she can come in at 4:30 and be seen then; she can arrive at the usual time and expect to wait; or she can be rescheduled for tomorrow.

"No problem," Mrs. Griffin says cheerfully. "I'll come right over."

Mrs. Griffin arrives at 4:35. At 4:40, Kyle hobbles in, supported by his father. Maria greets them and offers Kyle a chair on which to prop his foot.

Mrs. Griffin's blood pressure check is complete at 4:45. Kyle waits only 5 minutes before he is seen.

Thanks to Maria's quick thinking, the office stays on schedule—essentially by switching one appointment for another.

listing of referral physicians and facilities, including the names of facilities or specialty physicians, their addresses, and their phone numbers. If possible, give the patient two referral names to choose from, along with the referral phone numbers and addresses. When choosing the referral names of either physicians or facilities, be sure that the facility accepts the patient's insurance.

Fasting Patients. Some procedures and tests require patients to fast (refrain from eating or drinking anything beginning the night before). Scheduling these patients as early in the day as possible shows consideration for their needs. When scheduling appointments that require the patient to fast, be sure to inform the patient of the need to fast and when fasting should start.

Patients With Diabetes. Like fasting patients, patients with diabetes can use extra consideration when you schedule their appointments. In general, patients who take insulin must eat meals and snacks at regular times. This routine keeps their blood sugar from dropping too low—a condition that can result in confused thinking or even loss of consciousness. Therefore, you might want to avoid scheduling patients with diabetes for slots in late morning, close to lunchtime. If the schedule is running late by the time these patients arrive, they will be waiting in your reception area at a time when they really need to eat.

If the physician sees several patients with diabetes, you might also ask him about keeping appropriate snacks on hand to offer these patients in emergencies. Most patients with diabetes, however, carry their own emergency snacks with them to treat low blood sugar.

Repeat Visits. Some patients need regular appointments, such as for prenatal checkups or physical therapy. If possible, schedule these appointments for the same day and time each week. Establishing a routine helps patients remember their appointments and simplifies the office schedule.

Late Arrivals. If the practice has patients who are routinely late and gentle reminders to be on time have not helped, you might try booking them toward the end of the day. Even if a patient arrives late for a late-afternoon appointment, the doctor has already seen most of the day's patients and the late patient will not disrupt the schedule. Document late arrivals or missed appointments in the patient's chart. With documentation, patients who are habitually late can be called to discuss the reasons for their lateness. The goal of the discussion should be to find a solution so that patients can make their appointments on time and the schedule will run smoothly.

Walk-Ins. From time to time, a patient (or a person who has not visited the practice before) may arrive without an appointment and still expect to see the doctor. These people are called **walk-ins.** Office policies on how to handle walk-ins vary. If the person is experiencing an emergency, handle the situation as you would handle any emergency. Otherwise, you might politely explain that the

doctor is fully booked for the day and offer to schedule an appointment in the usual manner. If, by chance, the doctor is available and willing to see the walk-in, you should still ask the person to call to schedule appointments in the future. If your physician's office has a policy of no walk-ins, post a sign in the lobby or waiting area stating that patients are seen by appointment only.

Cancellations. When patients call to cancel appointments, thank them for calling, and try to reschedule the appointment while they are on the telephone. If patients say they will call later to reschedule, note this information in the appointment book.

You should also write "canceled" in the appointment book and draw a single line through the patient's name. To avoid confusion, cancel the first appointment *before* entering the patient's rescheduled appointment. Remember that the appointment book is a legal record. If you forget to cross out the name at the time of the first appointment, it may later seem that the doctor saw the patient twice. It is also important to note the cancellation in the patient's medical record. This notation can protect the practice from possible legal action. For example, a patient whose incision became infected could not blame the doctor if the patient canceled an appointment for a dressing change.

You may be able to fill slots created by cancellations by calling patients who have appointments scheduled for later in the day or week. Some patients may be willing to come in earlier than planned. When you make appointments, you can ask patients if they would be interested in coming in earlier if openings occur. Placing the names of interested patients in a tickler file can save time later.

Missed Appointments. It is important for legal reasons to document a no-show in the appointment book and patient record. Always inform the physician of any missed appointments in case the patient's condition requires a follow-up. The physician may want you to call the patient with a polite reminder that the patient has missed an appointment and needs to reschedule. There may have been a misunderstanding about the time, or the patient may simply have forgotten the appointment. Some offices, especially ones that use computerized scheduling systems, send out form letters when patients miss appointments. If failure to keep the appointment could endanger the patient's health, mention this possibility to the patient, or ask the physician to tell the patient over the telephone.

Physician Scheduling Situations

Not all scheduling problems result from patients. Sometimes physicians disrupt the office schedule. They may be called away on an emergency, may be delayed at the hospital, or may simply arrive late. In any event, the appointment schedule may get off track.

Physicians are only human and may occasionally be late for appointments. Some physicians are frequently late, however, either when arriving in the morning or when returning from lunch or from regular meetings. If this situation occurs in your office, you might approach it in several ways.

At a staff meeting you could mention that the morning or afternoon schedule often seems to get off to a late start. Then you might ask if anyone has suggestions for improving this situation. The physician may recognize that she is the cause of the problem and decide to resolve it.

If the physician does not take responsibility for the problem, however, you may need to adjust the office schedule to handle the situation. Suppose, for example, that the first patient appointment slot is at 8:30 A.M., but the physician usually does not arrive until 8:35 A.M. You could simply avoid scheduling patients between 8:30 and 8:45 A.M. If a physician is often 15 minutes late returning from lunch or from meetings, you might leave open the first appointment slot after the normal arrival time. In effect, you build buffer time into the schedule.

Scheduling Outside Appointments

You may be responsible for arranging patient appointments outside the medical office. These appointments may include:

- Consultations with other physicians
- Laboratory work
- X-rays
- Other diagnostic tests
- Hospital stays
- Surgeries

Before scheduling these appointments, ask the doctor for an order that identifies the exact procedures to be performed and specifies when the results will be needed. Always verify the patient's type of insurance before choosing which facility or physician the referral will be sent to. Insurance companies that are HMOs (health maintenance organizations) often will arrange the referral themselves. The medical assistant or secretary sending the referral completes the necessary forms and faxes them to the insurance company. The insurance company will authorize the referral and notify the office when approved. Sometimes referrals, if not urgent, can take 30 days or longer to approve.

Once authorization has been obtained, then talk with the patient to find convenient appointment times. This habit is not only courteous but also gives patients a sense of control over situations they may find a bit frightening. Some doctors' offices may have you call the outside laboratory or hospital with all information concerning the patient and then give the patient the number to call to set up the appointment. This approach is often easier for patients. They then have the telephone number in case they need to reschedule.

If you are calling to make the appointment for the patient, tell the medical assistant, scheduling secretary, or admissions clerk what consultation, test, or procedure is required. Then find out what your office or the patient must do to prepare for the appointment. For example, the admitting doctor may need to complete a preadmission evaluation for a patient who is to be hospitalized.

When arrangements have been made, inform the patient, and note on the chart that you have done so. You may also provide the patient with a completed referral slip or, in the case of laboratory work, a laboratory request slip. Procedure 12-2 explains how to schedule and confirm

PROCEDURE 12.2

Scheduling and Confirming Surgery at a Hospital

Objective: To follow the proper procedure for scheduling and confirming surgery

Materials: Calendar, telephone, notepad, pen

Method

1. Elective surgery is usually performed on certain days when the doctor is scheduled to be in the operating room and a room and an anesthetist are available. The patient may be given only one or two choices of days and times. (For emergency surgery the first step is to reserve the operating room.)

2. Call the operating room secretary. Give the procedure required, the name of the surgeon, the time involved, and the preferred date and hour.

3. Provide the patient's name (including maiden name, if appropriate), address, telephone number, age, gender, Social Security number, and insurance information.

4. Call the admissions office. Arrange for the patient to be admitted on the day of surgery or the day before (depending on the surgery to be performed). Ask for a copy of the admissions form for the patient record.

5. Some hospitals want patients to complete preadmission forms. In such cases request a blank form for the patient.

6. Confirm the surgery and the patient's arrival time 1 business day before surgery.

Common Items on a Physician's Schedule

Payments, Dues, and Fees

- Association dues
- Health insurance premium
- Payment for laundry service
- Liability insurance premium
- Life insurance premium
- Office rent
- Property insurance premium
- Paychecks for staff
- Payment for janitorial services
- Payment for leased equipment
- Taxes
  - *–Quarterly federal tax payments*
  - *–Quarterly state tax payments*
  - *–Annual federal and state tax filing deadline*

Time Commitments

- Committee meetings
- Conventions

Renewals and Accreditations

- Facility accreditation
  - *–State requirements*
  - *–Certificate of necessity*
  - *–Laboratory registration*
  - *–Federal requirements*
  - *–Ambulatory surgical centers*
  - *–Physician office laboratory*
- Medical license renewal
- Narcotics licenses renewal
- Drug Enforcement Agency registrations
- CME accreditations

Figure 12-8. Make time to meet with the physician regularly to review scheduling commitments.

Summary

Properly scheduling appointments in the medical office ensures a steady, efficient flow of patients. Setting up a matrix in the appointment book is the first step in scheduling appointments.

There are various appointment scheduling systems, including open-hours scheduling, wave scheduling, and cluster scheduling. Arranging appointments involves scheduling new and return patients and includes appointment reminder techniques. Special scheduling situations may occur, such as emergencies, referrals, and missed appointments. These situations may involve either patients or physicians. You may also be responsible for scheduling outside appointments for patients, as for testing or surgery.

Maintaining the physician's schedule includes such responsibilities as making travel arrangements and planning meetings. Meeting regularly with the physician helps ensure the smooth running of the office.

CASE STUDY QUESTIONS

Now that you have completed this chapter, review the case study at the beginning of the chapter and answer the following questions:

1. How would you adjust the schedule to allow for the emergency without falling behind schedule?
2. If it is necessary to reschedule patients, who should be rescheduled and when?
3. Would you explain anything to the patients in the waiting room about the emergency? If so, what would you say?

Discussion Questions

1. Describe situations that could cause the office to run behind schedule.
2. List the different types of appointment scheduling systems and briefly describe each.
3. Why is it important to note missed appointments and cancellations in the patient record and in the appointment book?
4. What is a matrix and why is it necessary?
5. List how long each of the following appointments should be scheduled for:
   a. earache
   b. CPE
   c. wound check
   d. Pap
   e. suture removal
   f. establish NP w/Rx prn
6. List the information that should be documented in the appointment book when scheduling.
7. Discuss how you would feel in a situation in which you had an extended wait in a physician's office. What could the medical assistant or office personnel do to ease your frustration?

Critical Thinking Questions

1. A patient has called to cancel her appointment for the third time. How should you handle this situation?
2. The physician is running about an hour and a half behind schedule and the schedule is completely filled. Describe how you would handle this problem.

3. Describe how you would handle a situation in which a patient calls for an appointment but is reluctant to disclose the purpose of the visit. What can you say to help the patient realize that it is advantageous to describe the nature of the visit?
4. Right after lunch, a patient walks into the office and requests to see the physician. The patient does not have an appointment and is complaining of pain in her stomach that will not go away. She has vomited a few times and looks very pale. How should you handle this situation?
5. Describe the best scheduling system for the following types of physician offices:
   a. A large practice with four physicians and with x-ray and lab facilities that are available anytime
   b. A small practice with two physicians and with lab facilities that are available only between 8:00 A.M. and 10:00 A.M.

Application Activities

1. A patient arrives at 10:00 A.M. for an appointment. When you check the schedule, the patient is not listed for an appointment for today. The patient produces an appointment card that clearly states that he has an appointment on this date at 10:00 A.M. You check tomorrow's schedule and realize that the patient is scheduled for the next day at 10:00 A.M. The medical office staff member who filled out the appointment card had made a mistake. The schedule for today is completely full and is already running behind. The patient is leaving the country for two months tomorrow morning and must see the physician today. What should you do?
2. A patient is a no-show for an appointment today. List where this should be documented. Discuss why it is important to document a no-show appointment.
3. Dr. Thompson, the only physician in your office, is out of town at a medical meeting. She is due back tomorrow morning. At 4:00 P.M., Dr. Thompson calls to say that a blizzard has closed the airport, and she will be forced to stay away for another day. You look at tomorrow's schedule. She has a full patient load. What should you do?

Do not refer to the patient reception area as the "waiting room." The term has a negative connotation and implies that the patient and family members should expect a long wait. A more positive descriptive term to use is the "reception area."

Medical Office Contact Information.

As a convenience to patients, the business cards of all the physicians practicing at the location should be available. These cards are best placed at the reception window or desk, where patients can access them easily.

Lighting.

Most medical offices use fairly bright lighting in the reception area, allowing patients to see their surroundings easily. Subdued lighting, like that sometimes used in restaurants, could be hazardous because it could cause patients to trip over or bump into hard-to-see objects. In addition, bright lighting is essential for reading, which is a common activity in the patient reception area. Bright lighting also conveys an impression of cleanliness.

Lighting should not be so bright that it becomes bothersome, however. Extremely bright light can be harsh on the eyes and create an annoying glare. A specialist, such as an electrician or lighting showroom salesperson, can help determine the appropriate level of lighting for the patient reception area.

Room Temperature.

Patients will be uncomfortable if the reception area is too hot or too cold. In an uncomfortable setting, waiting time can seem much longer than it really is. Therefore, maintaining an average, comfortable temperature is important.

The thermostat should be kept at a temperature that feels comfortable to you and to the office staff. You might periodically survey patients to see if they are comfortable and adjust the setting accordingly. Many elderly people feel cold because of lowered metabolisms. You may want to increase the temperature setting for a geriatric practice or if the office sees a large number of elderly patients.

Music.

Many medical offices pipe music through speakers to the reception area as well as elsewhere in the office. The music provides a soothing background sound. Because the music is meant to calm patients, it should be chosen accordingly. Classical music, light jazz, and soft rock are appropriate choices, whereas heavy metal and rap music are not. Some offices use prepared tapes or compact discs. Others tune in to a local radio station.

The music should reflect the interests of the patients. If the office serves an older population, you might choose oldies or classical music. Try soft rock for an obstetrics/gynecology practice or children's folk music for a pediatric practice.

Decor

The patient reception area gets its distinctive look from the way it is decorated. With the appropriate elements, the decor can create whatever impression is desired—warm and friendly, modern and elegant, and so on. Some suggestions follow. It is wise to consult a professional decorator, if possible.

Colors and Fabrics.

Colors and fabrics are the primary elements that make up a room's decor. Colors can be used throughout the room—on walls, furniture, carpeting, and other items. Fabrics are used primarily on furniture and draperies.

When using several colors, it is important to decorate in color families to avoid a jarring, unprofessional look. A **color family** is a group of colors that work well together. Colors fall within two basic areas, cool and warm. Using all cool colors—like white, blue, and mauve—creates a more harmonious impression in the reception area than mixing cool colors with warm ones like red, orange, and hot pink. When choosing the color family, consider the mood you want to create. Bright colors produce a lively atmosphere, whereas softer, muted colors create a relaxing one.

Fabrics, too, add to the atmosphere in the room. Heavy fabrics like velvet or brocade are more formal, whereas lightweight or sheer fabrics create a soft, delicate appearance. Patterns on fabrics or wallpaper can immediately change the mood of the room. No matter what the design, fabrics should be easy to clean and maintain.

Many medical offices are carpeted, and carpets come in a variety of colors and patterns. Carpeting is attractive, and it helps reduce noise. Carpet also provides a comfortable cushion when people walk through the office.

Carpeting should be easy to clean and durable enough to handle a large volume of patient traffic. Wall-to-wall carpeting is preferable to scatter rugs, which can cause injuries if someone slips on or trips over them and falls.

Professional services can be contracted to deliver a clean, fresh entry carpet on a regular basis. These rubber-backed carpets lie directly on any floor surface and are commonly used at entranceways and hallways or areas of heavy traffic to catch soil from being "walked" into the rest of the office. Unlike scatter rugs, these heavyweight professional carpets lay flat and are not a hazard for tripping or falling. The service brings a fresh carpet and removes the soiled carpeting as scheduled.

Specialty Items.

Some offices include specialty items, or accessories, as part of the decor (Figure 13-2). Examples of such items include coatracks, aquariums, plants, paintings, sculptures, mobiles, and children's toys. Some items are meant to add a finishing touch, completing the desired atmosphere. Others may help to interest waiting patients by providing an activity, such as watching the fish in an aquarium.

Choosing Accessories. Although specialty items enhance the office decor, keep the number of accessories to a minimum. Too many pieces can give the room a cluttered look. Try to select specialty items that will be pleasing or helpful to patients. A clock is one example. Another useful item is a coatrack, which helps prevent clutter by providing a place for coats, umbrellas, and briefcases. Avoid accessories such as scented candles or potpourri that may be offensive to some people or cause allergic reactions.

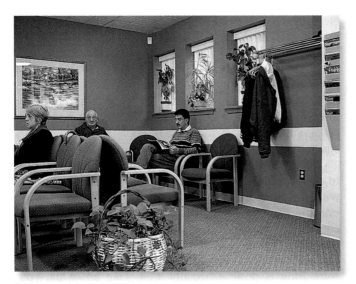

Figure 13-2. Specialty items—such as plants, paintings, and coatracks—enhance the patient reception area.

Keeping Safety in Mind. When selecting specialty items for the medical office, be sure to consider the issue of safety. Follow these guidelines to avoid potential hazards in the patient reception area.

- Do not include any item smaller than a golf ball. Small items present a choking hazard for young children.
- Avoid objects that can be easily pulled apart and then swallowed.
- Avoid easily breakable items, such as glass vases, that might cause cuts or other injuries to patients.
- Choose furniture with rounded, not sharp, corners. Coffee tables or other low tables with sharp corners can be a hazard especially to the elderly and to small children.
- Secure heavy wall hangings, shelves, and coatracks to the wall so that there is no risk of their falling.
- It is preferable to display artificial plants rather than living ones. Living plants may irritate patients who have allergies or present a poisoning hazard if parts of the plants are eaten by toddlers.
- If possible, build large, heavy items (such as fish tanks) into the wall to avoid climbing children and the danger of the items falling.
- Make sure all items in the reception area get a careful daily dusting before patients arrive. Artificial flowers and plants will need to be washed upside-down in soap and water occasionally to remove any potential allergens such as dust.

Furniture

Buying furniture for a patient reception room requires thoughtful planning. Although the office in which you work will no doubt be furnished already, it is a good idea to learn the steps and decisions involved in choosing

furniture. You may be included in future purchasing decisions if the office expands or moves to a new location or if the doctor wants to redecorate.

Furniture styles vary to suit the office decor. Most important, seating furniture should be firm, comfortable, and easy to get in and out of. In addition, washable and fireproof fabric on the furniture minimizes care and maximizes safety.

The reception area should have enough furniture so that all patients and family members or friends who accompany them can sit, no matter how busy the office schedule. Forcing people to stand while they wait for an appointment makes the wait seem much longer. The American Medical Association (AMA) suggests that seating be sufficient to accommodate the number of patients, family members, and friends who may be in the office during a 2-hour time period. When calculating this number, be generous in allowing for family members. In some types of practices, such as pediatrics, all patients are accompanied by at least one parent or guardian and sometimes siblings as well.

Arranging Furniture. The furniture arrangement can make the office seem comfortable or uncomfortable. If furniture is too close together, patients do not have sufficient space to move around easily or to stretch their legs. They may feel cramped. To ensure that patients have adequate room, a good rule of thumb is to allow 12 square feet of space per person. By this measurement, a 120-square-foot room (10 feet by 12 feet) can accommodate ten people comfortably.

The furniture arrangement should allow maximum floor space. Patients should be able to stretch out their legs when seated and to walk around the waiting room if they wish (Figure 13-3). Placing chairs against the wall usually produces the greatest amount of floor area. Additional seating in the middle of the room can be placed back-to-back to conserve space. Seats should be grouped so that families or friends can sit together. Remember to reserve room for

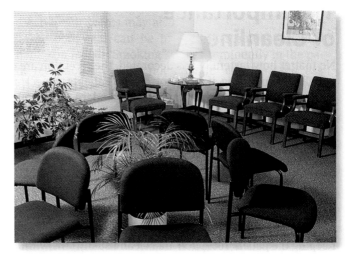

Figure 13-3. The furniture in a patient reception area can be arranged in a variety of ways.

body fluids such as blood and urine. It also includes any potentially hazardous waste generated in the treatment of patients, such as needles, scalpels, cultures of human cells, and dressings.

Although infectious waste is not commonly generated in the patient reception area, it can be—as when a patient vomits or bleeds on the rug or on furniture. If that situation should occur, you must clean up the waste promptly.

Infectious waste must be handled in accordance with federal law. Your office may choose to purchase commercially prepared hazardous waste kits for use in cleaning up spills. After cleaning infectious waste from the patient reception area, deposit it in a biohazard container. Disinfect the site to eliminate possible contamination of other patients.

OSHA Regulations

Federal safety precautions for the workplace are mandated by the Occupational Safety and Health Administration (OSHA), a government agency. OSHA has developed general guidelines for most businesses as well as special rules for health-care practices. To determine whether the requirements are being met, OSHA periodically inspects medical offices. If the rules are not followed, medical offices may be required to pay penalties in addition to correcting the problem. All employees in a medical office must be thoroughly trained in following OSHA guidelines.

Among the OSHA requirements is regular cleaning of walls, floors, and other surfaces. OSHA requires the use of disinfectants to combat bacteria as part of a routine cleaning schedule. In addition, OSHA mandates that broken glass, which may be contaminated, be picked up using a dustpan and brush or tongs. It should not be picked up by hand, even if one wears gloves.

The Physical Components

No one arrangement of a reception area is necessarily better than another. As long as the arrangement provides clear pathways and comfortable places to sit, the reception area will be functional.

Office Access

The path patients must take to get from the parking area or street to the office and then back out again is called the office **access.** Some offices have easy access and some do not (Figure 13-4).

Parking Arrangements. Although some patients walk to the medical office or take public transportation, the majority of patients probably travel by car. Patients who drive to the office need a place to park.

The office can offer either on-street parking or a parking lot. On-street parking requires patients to fend for themselves. They may have to put money into parking meters, and parking spaces may be difficult to find. Both the money

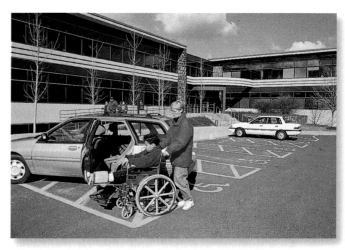

Figure 13-4. Patients should have easy, clear access from the parking lot to the medical office door.

required and the potential problems in finding parking spots limit the ease with which patients can gain access to the office.

A free parking lot improves office access. Parking lots should be well lit for safety. To determine the number of parking spaces the office needs, calculate the average length of time a patient spends in the office from arrival to departure and the number of appointments scheduled during that time period. Allow one parking spot per appointment if most patients drive to the office and fewer if many use public transportation. In your count be sure to include parking spaces for office staff. Periodically reevaluate the office's parking needs because they may change over time. All offices must also provide handicapped parking space for patients.

Entrances. The entrance to the office should be clearly marked so that patients can find the office easily. The name of the practice and of the doctor or doctors should be on the door or beside the door. Just outside the doorway should be a doormat to help control the amount of dirt tracked into the office. If the office door opens directly to the outside, people inside will feel a sudden change in temperature each time the door is opened in hot or cold weather. A foyer or double door arrangement helps minimize the effects of the weather and helps keep the office at a consistent, comfortable temperature.

Doorways must be wide enough to accommodate patients using wheelchairs and walkers. Hallways should be extra wide to allow patients in wheelchairs to turn around or to allow two wheelchairs to pass one another. The Americans With Disabilities Act, discussed later in this chapter, requires that doorways have a minimum width of 32 inches and that hallways have a minimum width of 5 feet. Well-lit hallways, without obstructions, are required.

Safety and Security

Safety and security are important concerns in any public building, and they are especially important in a doctor's office. To ensure safety of the patients and staff, such as protection from hazardous wiring or poorly lit hallways, there are guidelines for businesses, some of which pertain to the patient reception area. In addition, the medical office must be secure from burglary.

Building Exits. Make sure you and the office staff are familiar with all building exits. It may be necessary to leave the office quickly, as during a fire, flood, or other emergency. You and other staff members must be prepared to assist and direct patients toward the exits in such a situation.

Ideally, the office should have at least two doorways that lead directly to the outside or to a hallway that leads to stairs. This arrangement affords patients and staff members the speediest, most direct route outside in case of an emergency. All exits must be clearly labeled with illuminated red "Exit" signs. These signs normally have a backup power system, such as a battery, so that they will remain lit even during a power outage.

Having two or more exits also allows staff members to enter and leave the office during nonemergency situations without disrupting people in the patient reception area. Deliveries can be made at the second entrance, further minimizing interruptions.

Smoke Detectors. By law, a medical office is required to install smoke detectors that sound an alarm when triggered by heat or smoke. The office staff should be trained in the proper procedure if the smoke alarm sounds—including how to evacuate patients from the building efficiently. Smoke detectors must be checked regularly to ensure that they are operating properly.

Security Systems. No matter where the medical office is located, a security alarm system is a wise investment, even if the office building is patrolled by security personnel. A security alarm system offers valuable protection for the confidential patient information housed in a medical office. After the alarm system is installed, all office staff members should thoroughly familiarize themselves with it. They should be able to arm and disarm it easily and know what to do if it is accidentally activated. Each member of the staff should have her or his own individually assigned security access number. This number is required to authorize locking or unlocking the system. Like a credit card, bank, or other security PIN (personal identification number), it should never be shared.

Keeping Patients Occupied and Informed

Many patients who come into a medical office are ill, anxious, and concerned about their health. While they wait in the reception area, they need a way to stay occupied so that the time seems to pass quickly. In addition, patients may want to be informed about a particular medical condition or about general health issues. To meet these patient needs, most medical offices provide reading materials in the patient reception area. They may also offer television or educational videotapes.

Reading Materials

The most common activity in a patient reception area is probably reading. Although some patients bring their own books or magazines, most patients expect to find reading materials at the medical office (Figure 13-5). Magazines and books are probably the most popular types of reading materials, but a variety of others may also be available.

Magazines and Books. Choosing the right mix of reading material to interest all patients is a challenge. You may know doctors' offices that have a wonderful selection of magazines and books and others that have a poor selection. Your judgment of the selection, however, is based on how those publications match your interests. The Tips for the Office section gives guidelines on selecting magazines for the medical office. In addition to reading materials for adults, most offices also have children's books and magazines for younger patients and family members.

You or someone on the office staff should be sure to screen publications for medical content. You can then alert the doctors to articles that might stimulate patients' questions.

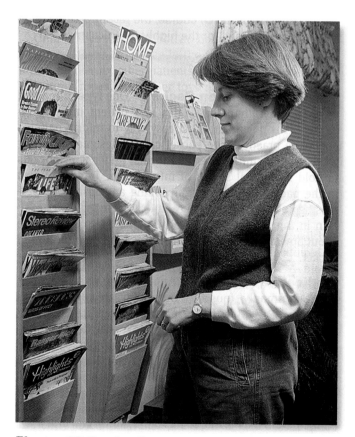

Figure 13-5. Reading materials can be organized on tables or in a wall rack.

needs. The patient reception area should be as comfortable as possible for patients with arthritis, failing eyesight, and other common ailments of the elderly. Make sure there are a few straight-backed chairs, which are easier to get into and out of than soft sofas. Arms on chairs provide support when sitting and standing for patients who are unsteady. In addition, straight-backed chairs offer greater back support than low chairs or couches with sinking cushions. These chairs should be located near the front door and near the examination rooms.

Place reading materials within easy reach of the chairs so that elderly patients do not have to get up from their chairs for them. Have large-print books and magazines available, if possible, for patients with poor eyesight. You might also offer magnifying glasses for patients who like to use them. In addition, make sure that the print on all office signs is large and easy to read. The patient reception area and restrooms should be well lit to help everyone, including elderly patients, see more clearly.

Special Situations

Patients in a medical practice are usually a diverse group of people. Their interests, needs, and medical conditions can have an impact on the design of the reception area.

Patients From Diverse Cultural Backgrounds.
The United States has long been called a melting pot because of its mixture of people and cultures. Each culture lends its own special qualities, and together the cultures combine to create a unique blend of people called Americans.

You may work in a neighborhood that has a distinct culture or one in which many cultures are represented. To help patients feel comfortable, make the reception area reflect aspects of their cultural backgrounds whenever possible. This effort will help patients feel more welcome.

Suppose, for example, that the medical office where you work serves many Hispanic patients. Posting signs in Spanish and English acknowledges the fact that both languages are spoken in that neighborhood. Providing reading materials, such as newspapers and magazines, in a second language—for both adults and children—is another way to show respect and interest. Decorating the

office for Spanish holidays in addition to American ones demonstrates that you care about what is important to patients. Displaying artwork created by local artists and artisans is another idea.

Patients Who Are Highly Contagious.
Patients may have to come into the physician's office when they are highly contagious. This fact is a concern for all patients, but it is especially critical for patients who are immunocompromised. Immunocompromised patients have an immune system—which protects against disease—that is not functioning at a normal level. Because these patients do not have the normal ability to fight off disease, they are at greater risk than the average person for becoming sick. Patients undergoing chemotherapy and patients with AIDS, for example, have compromised immune systems.

To protect patients who are immunocompromised, as well as other patients and staff members, you may need to separate a highly contagious patient from them. Instead of having contagious patients wait in the reception area, for example, you might bring them directly into an examination room to wait. By screening patients for highly contagious conditions and taking precautions, you can minimize the chances of exposing other people unnecessarily.

Summary

The patient reception area is where patients are received before they are seen by the physician. The area's appearance creates an immediate and lasting impression on patients. Patients may notice elements such as temperature, lighting, decor, and cleanliness, all of which influence their perception of the practice.

Offices with well-planned, pleasant reception areas provide a comfortable experience for waiting patients. Important elements include easy access from the outside, safety measures that meet federal requirements, and appropriate furnishings, reading material, and other entertainment to make the wait as enjoyable as possible. Special accommodations for patients who are young, elderly, differently abled, and from diverse cultural backgrounds help create a welcoming environment.

In

He
Th
age
Pe
the
In
inf
dec

CASE STUDY QUESTIONS

Now that you have completed this chapter, review the case study at the beginning of the chapter and answer the following questions:

1. What basic elements are *required* in every patient reception area? What other nonessential elements are nice to include as well?
2. Why is it important to think of the front patient area as the "patient reception area" and not the "waiting room"?
3. What special accommodations in the reception area are important to patients with disabilities?

Discussion Questions

1. What is the Americans With Disabilities Act, and what impact does it have on the patient reception area and patient bathrooms?
2. What is the Older Americans Act, and what impact does it have on the patient reception area and patient bathrooms?
3. What psychological affect does a cheerful, inviting reception room have on the patient?

Critical Thinking Questions

1. What special difficulties might patients in wheelchairs have in a small, overcrowded reception area?
2. Who is responsible if a patient or family member or friend is hurt in the reception area or bathroom? What could be the possible consequences?
3. What would be the best design for a pediatric reception area and bathroom? Describe it.

Application Activities

1. Design a reception area bulletin board for a family practitioner's office. List at least six items to include, and draw a rough sketch for placing these items on a rectangular bulletin board.
2. Develop a daily checklist for closing down a patient reception area at the end of the day. Be sure to include any housekeeping chores.
3. Visit a patient reception area at a clinic or a doctor's or dentist's office. Notice the decor, furniture arrangement, specialty items, and reading materials. Note what you like and dislike about the area. Then write down suggestions for improvement. Compare your results with those of your classmates.

Th

Pati
fice
mec
prog
ease
hea
tien
tien
und
cate
prac

Whenever possible, these guidelines should be recommended to patients of all ages. Good health should be a top priority in life. Although it is best to incorporate healthful behavior before illness develops, remind patients that it is never too late to work toward improving their health.

Protection From Injury

Many accidents happen because people fail to see potential risks and do not develop plans of action. Following safety measures at home, at work, at play, and while traveling can help prevent injury. A discussion of ways to avoid accidents and injury should be part of the educational process. Tips for preventing injury at home and at work are listed in Figure 14-3.

Facts from the latest National Safety Council data (2003) provide information on in-home deaths of people of all ages. These facts indicate that the home is not as safe as people think. According to this data, people are most likely to die in the home in the following ways:

- Falls (33%)
- Poisoning by solids (29%)
- Fires and burns (10%)
- Suffocation by ingestion (5%)
- Drowning (3%)
- Mechanical suffocation (2%)
- Poisoning by gases or vapors (1%)
- All other (15%)

Another essential aspect of educating patients about injury prevention is teaching them about the proper use of medications. A prescription includes specific instructions for taking the medication. Emphasize to the patient that these instructions must be followed exactly. In addition, the patient must not change the dosage or mix medications of any kind without first checking with the physician. Patients who do not adhere to these rules run the risk of potentially dangerous side effects. Tell patients to report to the physician any unusual reactions experienced when taking medications.

When providing a patient with a new prescription, always ask the patient if he has told the doctor about all the medications he is already taking, including herbs and over-the-counter (OTC) medications. If the patient tells you that he has not, immediately inform the physician before the

Tips for Preventing Injury

At Home

- Install smoke detectors, carbon monoxide detectors, and fire extinguishers.
- Keep all medicines, chemicals, and household cleaning solutions out of reach of children. Purchase products in childproof containers. Lock or attach childproof latches to all cabinets, medicine chests, and drawers that contain poisonous items.
- Keep chemicals in their original containers, and store them out of children's reach.
- Install adequate lighting in rooms and hallways. Install railings on stairs.
- Use nonskid backing on rugs to help prevent falls, or remove rugs altogether.
- In the bathroom use nonskid mats or strips that stick to the tub floor.
- Stay with young children when they are in the bathroom.
- Don't rely on bathseats or rings as a safety device for babies and children.
- Set the water temperature on the water heater at 120 degrees F.
- Practice good kitchen safety: Store knives and kitchen tools properly. Unplug small appliances when not in use. Wipe up spills immediately.
- Shorten long electrical cords and speaker wires, or secure them with electrical tape. Avoid plugging too many electrical appliances into the same outlet.

- Never use appliances in the bathtub or near a sink filled with water.
- Exercise caution when using electrical appliances. Use outlet covers when outlets are not in use.
- To reach high places, use proper equipment, such as stepladders, not chairs.
- Use child gates.

At Work

- Use appropriate safety equipment and protective gear, as required.
- Lift heavy objects properly: Bend at the knees, not at the waist. As you straighten your legs, bring the object close to your body quickly. That way, strong leg muscles do the lifting, not weaker back muscles. Never attempt to move furniture on your own. Request that a member of the office building maintenance staff be engaged to do so.
- Use surge protectors on computer equipment to prevent overloading outlets.
- Make sure hallways, entrance areas, work areas, offices, and parking lots are well lit.
- If your job involves desk work, practice proper posture when sitting. Do not sit for long periods of time. Get up and stretch, or walk down the hall and back.

Figure 14-3. You can help patients stay healthy by instructing them about ways to avoid injury.

patient leaves the office. Medications taken together can change the desired drug response. The physician needs to know about *all* drugs as well as herbal preparations and OTC medications that the patient is taking.

Preventive Measures

Preventive health care is an area in which patient education plays a vital role. Patients need to know that they can decrease their chances of getting certain illnesses and diseases by taking preventive measures and avoiding certain behaviors. Preventive techniques can be described on three levels: health-promoting behaviors, screening, and rehabilitation.

Health-Promoting Behaviors. The first level of disease and illness prevention involves adopting the health-promoting behaviors described in the section titled Healthful Habits. This primary level of prevention also includes educating patients about the symptoms and warning signs of disease. One example is informing patients about the warning signs of cancer. The first letters of these warning signs spell the word *caution*. They are as follows:

- **C**hange in bowel or bladder habits
- **A** sore that does not heal
- **U**nusual bleeding or discharge
- **T**hickening or lump in a breast or elsewhere
- **I**ndigestion or difficulty in swallowing
- **O**bvious change in a wart or mole
- **N**agging cough or hoarseness

Screening. The second level of disease prevention is screening. **Screening** involves the diagnostic testing of a patient who is typically free of symptoms. Screening allows early diagnosis and treatment of certain diseases. Examples of screening tests include mammography and Pap smears for women and prostate examinations for men.

Annual screening is important to health maintenance. Although the requirements may differ according to the age and condition of the patient, most annual screenings usually include:

- Routine blood work
- Urinalysis
- Chest x-ray
- EKG (electrocardiogram)
- Physical examination (PE)

Rehabilitation. The third level of disease prevention involves the rehabilitation and management of an existing illness. At this level the disease process remains stable, but the body will probably not heal any further. The objective is to maintain functionality and avoid further disability. Examples of this level of prevention include stroke rehabilitation programs, cardiac rehabilitation, and pain management for a condition such as arthritis.

The Patient Information Packet

When patients come to the medical practice, they need to learn not only about health and medical issues but also about the medical office itself. The patient information packet explains the medical practice and its policies. Unlike most other patient education materials, the patient information packet deals mainly with administrative matters rather than with medical issues.

The patient information packet may be as simple as a one-page brochure or pamphlet. It may be a multi-page brochure, however, or a folder with multiple-page inserts.

Benefits of the Information Packet

The patient information packet is a simple, effective, and inexpensive way to improve the relationship between the office and the patients. It provides important information about the practice and the office staff. This information helps patients feel more comfortable with the qualifications of the health-care professionals involved in their care. The packet may help clarify the roles that each office staff member has in patient care.

The information packet also informs patients of office policies and procedures. Patients will learn the doctor's office hours, how to schedule appointments, the office's payment policies, and other administrative details. This information helps limit misunderstandings about these procedures.

The patient information packet also benefits the office staff. It is both an excellent marketing tool and an aid to running the office more smoothly. Providing patients with a prepared information packet saves staff time by answering a number of potential patient inquiries. The information packet is also a good way to acquaint new office staff members with office policies.

Contents of the Information Packet

Regardless of what material the information packet contains, it must be written in clear language so that patients are able to read and understand it. All materials should be written at a sixth-grade level for reading ease of all patients. Information should not be presented in a technical medical style. Because you may be responsible for preparing portions of the policy packet, you should be familiar with the contents of a typical packet.

Introduction to the Office. A brief introduction serves to welcome the patient to the office. It may be helpful to summarize the office's philosophy of patient care. The office's **philosophy** means the system of values and principles the office has adopted in its everyday practices.

Physician's Qualifications. The packet commonly contains information about the physician's professional qualifications and training. It includes details about

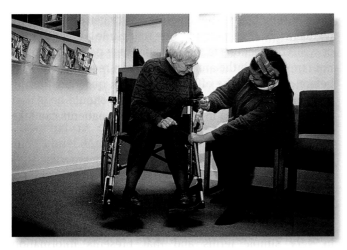

Figure 14-5. When instructing elderly patients, remember that each patient is an individual with unique needs.

instructions are an essential aspect of patient care. Patients can refer to the instructions as necessary or can ask a relative to do so.

- Adjust procedures as needed. When demonstrating a procedure to elderly patients, keep in mind any physical limitations they may have, and adjust the procedure accordingly. Make sure patients understand the instructions by asking them to perform the procedure for you.

Patients With Mental Impairments

Patients with impaired mental functions include those with **dementia,** Alzheimer's disease, mental retardation, drug addictions, and emotional problems. These patients can be challenging to deal with because communication may be difficult. Tact and empathy are important. A key to dealing with these patients is to speak at their level of understanding. Again, you must try to meet patients' needs without talking down to them.

Patients With Hearing Impairments

Patients with hearing impairments may have conditions ranging from mild impairment to total hearing loss. It is a common mistake to treat these patients as though they have mental impairments. Although you may have difficulty communicating with these patients, remember that their inability to hear has nothing to do with their level of intelligence. The Educating the Patient section provides techniques for educating patients who have hearing impairments.

Patients With Visual Impairments

As with hearing impairment, the level of visual impairment can vary significantly from patient to patient. Determining the severity of a patient's condition allows you to tailor your instruction to the patient's needs.

Educating the Patient

Instructing Patients With Hearing Impairments

Educating patients who have hearing impairments need not be difficult if you pay a little extra attention in the following areas.

- Try to eliminate all background noise. Talk in a quiet room, if possible.
- Make sure the room is well lit.
- Face the patient, and make sure the patient can see your mouth. Having the patient watch your mouth movements can help him understand what you are saying.
- Speak loudly and clearly, but do not shout.
- Use visual aids as necessary.
- Tell patients to let you know right away if they cannot hear you or do not catch something you have said. Even patients who do not have hearing impairments often appear to understand what a medical professional is saying rather than admit they are confused. It is a good idea to ask patients to repeat information to you to check their understanding. Also, periodically ask if they

would like you to go over any particular part of the explanation or instructions again.

An additional point to keep in mind when dealing with patients who have hearing impairments is that loss of hearing can cause them to withdraw and feel isolated. Being empathic and patient greatly enhances the educational process.

Elderly Patients With Hearing Loss

Most people experience a gradual loss of hearing as they get older. In addition to the preceding suggestions, try to talk in a lower pitch whenever possible. As people get older, they often have more trouble understanding higher tones.

Patients Who Wear Hearing Aids

When talking to a patient who wears a hearing aid, it is best to speak at a normal level. Many hearing aids make a normal voice louder but filter out loud noises. If you raise your voice, the hearing aid may filter it out. Consequently, the patient may hear only broken speech.

For those with mildly impaired vision, the approach may be as simple as providing instructional materials printed in large type. In addition, you can demonstrate procedures in a well-lit area and close to the patients. For more severe visual impairment, adjust the level of instruction appropriately. For example, to demonstrate how to use a particular knob on a wheelchair, you might actually place the patient's hand on the knob and discuss its function.

When speaking to someone who has a visual impairment, remember to use a normal tone of voice. A patient with a visual impairment does not necessarily also have a hearing impairment. Although you should never talk down to patients, you need to verify that they understand all verbal instructions. Have the patient repeat all instructions to you.

Giving procedural instructions may be a challenge, depending on the patient's ability to perform certain tasks. Suggest that patients ask a family member or friend to help them with procedures they have trouble doing on their own.

Multicultural Issues

Patients who come from diverse cultures often have different beliefs about the causes and treatment of illness. These differences may affect their treatment expectations and their willingness to follow instructions or agree to have certain procedures performed on them. There may also be communication problems if the patient does not understand English well. Communicating with patients in these situations is discussed in Chapter 4.

Patient Education Prior to Surgery

One instance in which patient education is vital to a successful outcome is the instruction given before a patient undergoes a surgical procedure. Although exact instructions vary according to the procedure, their purpose is to prepare the patient for the procedure and to aid the patient during the recovery period. Instructions may include verbal, written, and demonstrative techniques.

The Role of the Medical Assistant

Patients generally receive information about the need for surgery and its nature from the physician. Educating and preparing patients for surgery will probably be your responsibility, however. You may provide support and explanations to patients. You must verify that they understand any information they may have been given by other members of the health-care team. Preoperative instruction may include discussion of postoperative care issues, such as temporary dietary restrictions.

You may also be responsible for determining whether patients have all the information they need before surgery, from both an educational and a legal standpoint. All patients who are undergoing a surgical procedure must first sign an informed consent form. As stated in Chapter 9, this legal document provides specific information about the surgical procedure, including its purpose, the possible risks, and the expected outcome. The informed consent form, along with documentation of all preoperative instruction, must be put in the patient's chart.

Benefits of Preoperative Education

Preoperative education has many benefits. It increases patients' overall satisfaction with their care. It helps reduce patient anxiety and fear, use of pain medication, complications following surgery, and recovery time. Letting the patient know what to expect during the surgery and afterward allows the patient to participate in all aspects of the surgical procedure.

Types of Preoperative Teaching

Three types of teaching should occur during the preoperative period: factual, sensory, and participatory. The combination of these teaching methods gives the patient an overall understanding of the surgical procedure.

Factual. Factual teaching informs the patient of details about the procedure. You should tell the patient what will happen during the surgery, when it will happen, and why the procedure is necessary. Factual information also includes restrictions on diet or activity that may be necessary both before and after surgery. Procedure 14-2 describes how to inform patients of guidelines for surgery.

Sensory. Give patients a description of the physical sensations they may have during the procedure. All five senses may be involved: feeling, seeing, hearing, tasting, and smelling.

Participatory. Participatory teaching includes demonstrations of techniques that may be necessary or helpful during the postoperative period. Aspects of postoperative care include cleaning the wound, changing the dressing, and applying ice packs.

During this phase of teaching, you need to first describe the technique to the patient and then demonstrate it. The patient should repeat the demonstration for you. This practice is called **return demonstration.** If any aspects of the technique are unclear to the patient, you should demonstrate the technique again. The patient should be capable of performing the procedure properly. This process of teaching a new skill by having the patient observe and imitate is called **modeling.**

Using Anatomical Models

An anatomical model is a useful tool in preoperative education. As shown in Figure 14-6, looking at a lifelike model—and being able to see the actual body structures—helps patients better understand their condition. A model also allows patients to see how the surgical procedure will help correct their problem.

explain in their own words what they have learned. In addition, have them engage in return demonstrations.

Additional Educational Resources

Besides the resources available in the medical office, a vast number of outside resources are available for patient education. You can use these resources to obtain information for your own use in patient education, or you can mention them to patients who are looking for additional information. Following are several sources of patient education materials:

- Libraries and patient resource rooms. Most public libraries have an assortment of books, magazines, and electronic databases pertaining to health and medical topics. Many hospitals provide patient resource rooms, which include a variety of educational materials—such as books, brochures, and videotapes—for public use.

- Computer resources. A great deal of up-to-date medical information can be accessed through online services and CD-ROMs. The Internet is another widely used source of medical information.

- Community resources. Many local social service agencies provide specialized health information related to such topics as nursing home care, visiting nurses' care, counseling, and rehabilitation. Most of these agencies are listed in the telephone book. Area hospitals, the library, and the local chamber of commerce are other good sources for these services.

- Associations. Thousands of health organizations and associations can be contacted for information about preventive health care and virtually every known disease or disorder. The names, addresses, and telephone numbers of these organizations are provided in several directories, which are available at most libraries. Figure 14-7 provides a sample list of patient resource organizations.

Career Opportunities

Occupational Therapy Assistant

To gain medical assistant credentials, you must fulfill the requirements of either the American Association of Medical Assistants (for a Certified Medical Assistant) or the American Medical Technologists (for a Registered Medical Assistant). After obtaining your medical assistant certification or registration, you may wish to acquire additional skills in specialty areas through course work or on-the-job training. Although this course work or training may not lead to an additional certification or degree, it will enable you to expand your role in the medical office and advance your career as the demand for skilled health professionals increases.

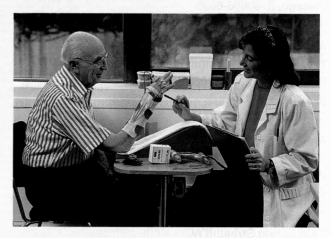

Skills and Duties

An occupational therapy assistant helps patients learn, or relearn, basic and special skills they need to function in their daily lives. Patient interaction is the focus of the occupational therapy assistant's job. An occupational therapy assistant works under the supervision of an occupational therapist.

Occupational therapists teach many different types of skills to many different types of patients. These skills include the following:

- Basic life skills, such as dressing and feeding oneself or moving about at home. For example,

patients with partial paralysis or nerve damage resulting from a stroke may need this type of help.

- Vocational skills, such as typing. These skills will help patients with disabilities get jobs to support themselves.

- Designing and supervising arts and crafts activities. These activities serve as recreation and help patients develop fine motor skills in a nonthreatening, pleasant atmosphere.

- Helping accident victims who have an injured limb or a prosthetic device learn new ways to

continued ⟶

Occupational Therapy Assistant *(continued)*

perform simple tasks. A patient with a prosthetic hand, for example, may need help learning to open jar lids.

- Working with patients who have behavioral or emotional disturbances. Occupational therapy may help these patients express their feelings in constructive ways, by building an interest in music, drama, or art.

The occupational therapy assistant also performs a number of clerical and administrative tasks. He checks inventories, orders supplies, and helps maintain the equipment in his workplace. He may also be responsible for paperwork, including writing reports on therapy sessions with patients.

Workplace Settings

Occupational therapy assistants often work in hospitals. They may also find work in clinics or long-term care facilities, such as retirement communities with assisted-care services, nursing homes, or rehabilitation centers. Some occupational therapists are employed in educational settings, including occupational workshops and schools for children with special needs.

Education

Community colleges and vocational schools offer 2-year programs for an associate degree in occupational therapy assisting. By completing a program approved by the American Occupational Therapy Association and passing a qualifying test, you can become a Certified Occupational Therapy Assistant (COTA).

Where to Go for More Information

The American Occupational Therapy Association
4720 Montgomery Lane
P.O. Box 31220
Bethesda, MD 20824-1220
(301) 948-9626

American Society of Hand Therapists
401 North Michigan Avenue
Chicago, IL 60611
(312) 321-6866

Summary

Patient education plays a key role in many aspects of patient care. Knowledgeable patients are able to take an active approach to their own medical care. They are also likely to be aware of the benefits of activities that promote and protect their health.

There are many reasons for patient education in the medical office. Patients need to understand their medical conditions and to be prepared for necessary procedures. Many opportunities exist to educate patients about the benefits of good health. In addition, patients need to be informed of the policies of the medical office.

Many educational resources are available to both medical assistants and patients. The key for medical assistants is to take advantage of all opportunities to educate patients and to match this teaching to the needs of individual patients.

REVIEW

CASE STUDY *QUESTIONS*

Now that you have completed this chapter, review the case study at the beginning of the chapter and answer the following questions:

1. What might be important to consider when creating an educational plan for a patient? How might the plan vary according to the individual?
2. What factors could block effective patient education?
3. What specific behaviors do you associate with talking down to a patient?
4. Why are good listening skills an important part of teaching?

Discussion Questions

1. Why is it important to educate patients about how to take care of themselves?
2. Patients spend less time in the hospital than ever before. How does this change the role of private medical offices and the role of medical assistants in those practices?
3. What are some good ways to get patients to read printed materials?

Critical Thinking Questions

1. A patient and her grown daughter meet with the physician in your medical office. She receives some bad news and is crying. The daughter is trying to comfort her. It is your job now to explain what will happen next in her care, including procedures and appointment schedules for some important tests in the hospital. How will you proceed?

2. You are measuring the vital signs of an overweight woman. She becomes visibly upset when you ask her to step on the scale. The office has many brochures with tips on promoting good health and exercise. How might you bring up the subject of proper diet and exercise?

Application Activities

1. Develop an educational plan for the overweight patient mentioned in the critical thinking questions. Have another student assume the role of the patient, and practice implementing your plan. Ask the other student to evaluate your teaching method.
2. Write the section of a patient information brochure that describes the general roles of the medical office staff. Exchange your writing sample with that of another student, and critique each other's work.
3. With a partner, role-play a medical assistant giving procedural instructions to a patient with a hearing impairment. Then switch roles, and offer suggestions for improving each other's teaching techniques.

SECTION 3

FINANCIAL RESPONSIBILITIES

CHAPTER 15

Processing Health-Care Claims

KEY TERMS

allowed charge
assignment of benefits
balance billing
benefits
birthday rule
capitation
Centers for Medicare and
    Medicaid Services
    (CMS)
CHAMPVA
clearinghouse
coinsurance
coordination of benefits
co-payment
deductible
disability insurance
electronic data
    interchange (EDI)
exclusion
fee-for-service
fee schedule
formulary
health maintenance
    organization (HMO)
liability insurance
lifetime maximum benefit
managed care
    organization (MCO)
Medicaid
Medicare
Medicare + Choice Plan
Medigap
Original Medicare Plan
participating physicians
preferred provider
    organization (PPO)
premium
referral
remittance advice (RA)
resource-based relative
    value scale (RBRVS)
third-party payer
TRICARE
X12 837 Health Care
    Claim

AREAS OF COMPETENCE

2003 Role Delineation Study
ADMINISTRATIVE
Administrative Procedures
- Understand and apply third-party guidelines
- Obtain reimbursement through accurate claims submissions
- Monitor third-party reimbursement
- Understand and adhere to managed care policies and procedures

CLINICAL
Patient Care
- Coordinate patient care information with other health-care providers

GENERAL
Communication Skills
- Utilize electronic technology to receive, organize, prioritize, and transmit information

Legal Concepts
- Follow employer's established policies dealing with the health-care contract
- Implement and maintain federal and state health-care legislation and regulations

CHAPTER OUTLINE

- Basic Insurance Terminology
- Types of Health Plans
- The Claims Process: An Overview
- Fee Schedules and Charges
- Preparing and Transmitting Health-Care Claims

OBJECTIVES

After completing Chapter 15, you will be able to:

15.1 List the basic steps of the health insurance claim process.

15.2 Describe your role in insurance claims processing.

15.3 Explain how payers set fees.

15.4 Define Medicare and Medicaid.

15.5 Discuss TRICARE and CHAMPVA health-care benefits programs.

15.6 Distinguish between HMOs and PPOs.

Introduction

Health-care claims are a critical part of the reimbursement process. Accurate claims sent to payers mean that physicians receive the maximum appropriate payment for the services they provide. Patients are also concerned with their health-care plans, asking "How much will my insurance pay?" "How much will I owe?" "Why are these doctor's fees different from my previous doctor's fees?"

You will handle questions such as these every day. Not only must you correctly prepare health-care claims, but you will also review patients' insurance coverage, explain the physician's fees, estimate what charges payers will cover, and prepare claims for patients. This chapter prepares you for these tasks by explaining the types of health-care insurance patients have, how payers set the charges they pay for providers' services, and how to transmit complete and accurate claims. This chapter also gives you the information you need about patients' financial responsibilities for services so that you can figure out how much patients should pay and how much will be billed to their health-care plans.

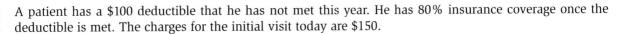

CASE STUDY

A patient has a $100 deductible that he has not met this year. He has 80% insurance coverage once the deductible is met. The charges for the initial visit today are $150.

As you read this chapter, consider the following questions:

1. How much should this patient pay?
2. How much will he owe for his next visit this year, which is expected to have a charge of $200?
3. Assuming that the patient in the case study has a managed care policy, what type of policy does he probably have?
4. What term would you use to describe the part of the payment that is based on 20% of the charges?
5. If you did not know whether the deductible had been met, what procedure would you follow?

Basic Insurance Terminology

The first step in understanding insurance is to learn some basic terminology. Medical insurance, which is also known as health insurance, is a written contract in the form of a policy between a policyholder and a health plan (insurance carrier). The policyholder may also be called the insured, the member, or the subscriber.

Under the insurance policy, the policyholder pays a **premium.** In exchange, the health plan provides **benefits**—payments for medical services—for a specified time period. The policy may cover dependents of the policyholder, such as a spouse or children. The contract may specify a **lifetime maximum benefit,** which is a total sum that the health plan will pay out over the patient's life.

There are actually three participants under insurance contracts. The patient (policyholder) is the *first party,* and the physician who provides medical services is the *second party.* A patient-physician contract is created when a physician agrees to treat a patient who seeks medical services. Through this unwritten contract, the patient is legally responsible for paying for services. The patient may have a policy with a health plan, the *third party,* which agrees to carry the risk of paying for those services and therefore is called a **third-party payer.**

Depending on the type of health plan, the policyholder may pay a **deductible**—a fixed dollar amount that must be paid or "met" once a year before the third-party payer begins to cover medical expenses. The patient may also have to pay **coinsurance,** a fixed percentage of coverage charges after the deductible is met. The coinsurance rate presents the health plan's percentage of the charge followed by the insured's percentage, such as 80-20. The patient often must pay a **co-payment,** a small fee that is collected at the time of the visit. The health plan then pays the covered amount of the charges.

Some expenses, such as routine eye examinations or dental care, may not be covered under the insured's contract. Uncovered expenses are **exclusions.** Many plans offer a prescription drug benefit. Such benefits usually require the use of drugs that are listed on the plan's **formulary,** a list of approved brands.

Two special types of insurance are liability insurance and disability insurance. **Liability insurance** covers injuries that are caused by the insured or that occurred on the insured's property. If an individual (or company) has home, business, automobile, or health liability insurance, the injured person can claim benefits under the insured's policy. To obtain details about coverage, contact the liability insurance company.

Disability insurance is a type of insurance that may be provided by an employer for its employees or purchased privately by self-employed individuals. Disability insurance is activated when the insured is injured or disabled. When the insured cannot work, the insurance company pays the insured a prearranged monthly amount that covers the insured's normal expenses. Generally, disability is far more expensive than life, home, or automobile insurance.

Types of Health Plans

All insurance companies have their own rules about benefits and procedures. Many companies also have their own manuals, printed or online, which you must keep handy in the office for reference. Representatives of the insurance companies are available to work with you, however, to answer questions and help ensure that claims are correctly filed. Their business depends on it. Never hesitate to contact an insurance company. Many have toll-free numbers and Web sites for just this purpose.

There are many sources of health plans in the United States. The majority of individuals with insurance are covered by group policies, usually through their employers. Some people have individual plans. Many are covered under a government plan. Still others—over 40 million Americans—have no health-care insurance.

Fee-for-Service and Managed Care Plans

There are two major types of health plans: fee-for-service plans and managed care plans. **Fee-for-service** plans, the oldest and most expensive type, repay policyholders for costs of health care due to illnesses and accidents. The policy lists the medical services that are covered. The amount charged for services is controlled by the physician who provides them. The benefit may be for all or part of the charges.

Managed care plans, in contrast, control both the financing and the delivery of health care to policyholders.

They enroll policyholders, and they also enroll physicians and other providers, controlling the delivery of health care. The **managed care organizations (MCOs)** that set up managed care health plans reach agreements with physicians and other health-care providers that control fees. Most people who are insured through their employers are covered by some form of a managed care plan.

Physicians who enroll in managed care plans are called **participating physicians.** They have contracts with the MCOs that stipulate their fees, the credentials they must have, and their responsibilities and that also explain the MCO's duties. For example, the MCO must usually publish the participating physicians' names in booklets and on a Web site so that policyholders can choose a provider from the list.

Managed care plans pay their participating physicians in one of two ways—either by contracted fees or a fixed prepayment called **capitation.** In a capitated managed care plan, providers are paid a fixed amount per month to provide necessary, contracted services to patients who are plan members. The rate the provider is paid is based on several factors, including the number of plan members in the insured pool and their ages. The capitated rate per enrollee is paid to the provider even if the provider does not provide any medical services to the patient during the time period covered by the payment. Similarly, the provider receives the same capitated rate if a patient is treated more than once during the time period. In other plans, negotiated per-service fees are paid. These fees are less than the regular rate for a service that the provider normally charges.

As shown in Figure 15-1, more than half of all health plans are **preferred provider organizations (PPOs).** A PPO is a managed care plan that establishes a network of providers to perform services for plan members. In exchange for the PPO sending them patients, the physicians agree to charge discounted fees. Plan members may usually choose to receive care from other doctors or providers outside the network, but they pay a higher charge for these visits.

Another common type of managed care system is a **health maintenance organization (HMO).** Physicians with HMO contracts are often paid a capitated rate, or they may be employees of the organization who are paid salaries. Patients who enroll in an HMO pay premiums and usually also pay a co-payment, oftentimes $10, at the time of the office visit. No other fees are required for any covered service that a member needs. In HMOs, patients must usually choose from a specific group of health-care providers for care. If they seek services from a provider who is not in the health plan, the HMO does not pay for the care. Patients also pay for excluded services.

Medicare

Several federal programs provide health care. The largest is **Medicare,** which provides health insurance for citizens aged 65 and older. Certain patients under the age of 65 may

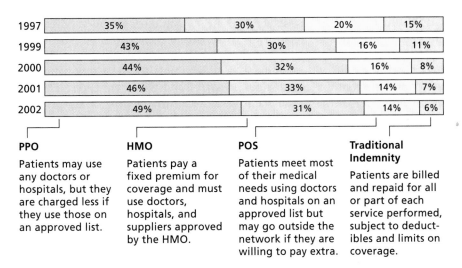

Figure 15-1. Types of health plans.

Source: Mercer's National Survey of Employer Sponsored Health Plans, 2003.
Copyright 2003, The Managed Care Information Center.

also be entitled to Medicare. Such patients include those who are blind or widowed or who have serious long-term disabilities, such as chronic joint pain or kidney failure. The Medicare program is managed by the **Centers for Medicare and Medicaid Services (CMS).**

Part A. Medicare has two parts. Part A is hospital insurance, which is billed by hospitals (or other health-care facilities). It pays most of the benefits for the following individuals:

- A patient who has been hospitalized (as an inpatient) up to 90 days for each benefit period. A benefit period begins the day a patient goes into the hospital and ends when that patient has not been hospitalized for 60 days.

- A patient who has been an inpatient in a skilled nursing facility (SNF) for no more than 100 days in each benefit period. A benefit period is usually 1 calendar year.

- A patient who is receiving medical care at home.

- A patient who has been diagnosed as terminally ill and needs hospice care. Medicare defines *terminally ill* as having a prognosis (prediction of the probable course of a disease in an individual and the chances of recovery) of 6 months or less to live. A hospice is a medical organization that provides pain relief to terminally ill patients and otherwise supports these patients and their families.

- A patient who requires psychiatric treatment. Currently Medicare covers only 190 days of psychiatric hospitalization in a patient's lifetime.

- A patient who requires respite care. Medicare provides for a respite, or short break, for the person who cares for a terminally ill patient at home. The terminally ill patient is moved to a care facility for the respite.

Anyone who receives Social Security benefits is automatically enrolled in Part A and does not have to pay a premium. Individuals aged 65 or older who are not eligible for Social Security benefits may enroll in Part A, but they must pay premiums for the coverage.

Part B. Part B helps pay for a wide range of procedures and supplies. For example, it covers physician services, outpatient hospital services, diagnostic tests, clinical laboratory services, and outpatient physical and speech therapy as long as these services are considered medically necessary. Individuals entitled to Part A benefits automatically qualify for Part B benefits. In addition, U.S. citizens and permanent residents over the age of 65 are also eligible. Part B is a voluntary program; eligible persons may or may not take part in it. However, those desiring Part B must enroll, because coverage is not automatic. Unlike Part A, Part B coverage is not premium-free. In 2003, Part B coverage cost $58.70 per month, and the premium usually increases annually.

Each Medicare enrollee receives a health insurance card. This card lists the beneficiary's name, sex, effective dates for Part A and Part B coverage, and Medicare number. The Medicare number is assigned by CMS and usually consists of the Social Security number followed by a numeric or alphanumeric suffix.

Types of Medicare Plans. Medicare beneficiaries can choose from among a number of insurance plans, including traditional fee-for-service and Medicare + Choice, which consists of a group of different plans.

Fee-for-Service: The Original Medicare Plan. The Medicare fee-for-service plan, referred to by Medicare as the **Original Medicare Plan,** allows the beneficiary to choose any licensed physician certified by Medicare. Each time the beneficiary receives services, a fee is billable. Part of this fee is generally paid by Medicare and part is due from the beneficiary. An annual deductible of $100 is the patient's responsibility. Medicare then pays 80% of approved charges and the patient is responsible for the remaining 20%.

To pay these bills, individuals enrolled in Medicare Part B Original Medicare Plan often buy additional insurance called a **Medigap** plan. These plans frequently reimburse the patient's Part B deductible and additional procedures that Medicare does not cover. If Medicare does not pay a claim, Medigap is not required to pay the claim either. Although private insurance carriers offer Medigap plans, coverage and standards are regulated by federal and state law. In exchange for Medigap coverage, the policyholder pays a monthly premium. A number of different options are available. These choices are labeled A through J. Monthly premiums vary widely across the different plan levels as well as within a single plan level, depending on the insurance company selected. While coverage varies from policy to policy, a set of core benefits is common to all Medigap plans, including the Part B coinsurance amount (usually 20% of approved charges) after the deductible ($100).

Medicare + Choice Plans.   Medicare also offers a group of plans called the **Medicare + Choice Plans.** Beneficiaries can choose to enroll in one of three major types of plans instead of the Original Medicare Plan:

1. Medicare Managed Care Plans
2. Medicare Preferred Provider Organization Plans (PPOs)
3. Medicare Private Fee-for-Service Plans

Medicare Managed Care Plans charge a monthly premium and a small co-payment for each office visit, but not a deductible. Like private payer managed care plans, Medicare managed care plans often require patients to use a specific network of physicians, hospitals, and facilities. Some plans offer the option of receiving services from providers outside the network for a higher fee. However, they offer coverage for services not reimbursed in the Original Medicare Plan, such as physical examinations and inoculations. Participants are generally required to select a primary care provider (PCP) from within the network. The PCP provides treatment and manages the patient's medical care through referrals.

In the *Medicare Preferred Provider Organization Plan (PPO)*, patients pay less to use doctors within a network, but they may choose to go outside the network for additional costs, such as a higher co-payment or higher coinsurance. Patients do not need a PCP, and referrals are not required.

Under a *Medicare Private Fee-for-Service Plan*, patients receive services from the provider they choose, as long as Medicare has approved the provider or facility. The plan is operated by a private insurance company that contracts with Medicare to provide services to beneficiaries. The plan sets its own rates for services, and physicians are allowed to bill patients the amount of the charge not covered by the plan. A co-payment may or may not be required.

Medicaid

Medicaid, also run by CMS, is a health-benefit program designed for low-income, blind, or disabled patients; needy families; foster children; and children born with birth defects. Medicaid is a health cost assistance program, not an insurance program. The federal government provides funds to all 50 states to administer Medicaid, and states add their own funds. Every state has a program to assist with medical expenses for citizens who meet its qualifications. Such programs may have different names and slightly different rules, but they provide basically the same assistance. This assistance includes:

- Physician services
- Emergency services
- Laboratory services and x-rays
- SNF care
- Early diagnostic screening and treatment for minors (those aged 21 and younger)
- Vaccines for children

Accepting Assignment.   A physician who agrees to treat Medicaid patients also agrees to accept the established Medicaid payment for covered services. This agreement is called accepting assignment. If the physician's fee is higher than the Medicaid payment, the patient cannot be billed for the difference. The physician can bill the patient for services that Medicaid does not cover, however.

Medi/Medi.   Older or disabled patients who have Medicare and who cannot pay the difference between the bill and the Medicare payment may qualify for Medicare and Medicaid. This type of coverage is known as Medi/Medi. In such cases, Medicare is the primary payer, and Medicaid is the secondary payer.

State Guidelines.   Medicaid benefits can vary greatly from state to state. It is important to understand the Medicaid guidelines in your state so that your office's Medicaid reimbursement is prompt and trouble-free. Here are some suggestions:

- Always ask for a Medicaid card from all patients who state that they are entitled to Medicaid. Do not submit a claim to Medicaid if the patient cannot prove Medicaid membership. Doing so may constitute fraud. You may contact Medicaid to verify eligibility.
- Check the patient's Medicaid card, which is issued monthly and shows the patient's eligibility for services or procedures (Figure 15-2). Eligibility is based on how much income the patient reported for the previous month.
- Ensure that the physician signs all claims. Then send them to the state's Medicaid-approved contractor (which pays on behalf of the state) or to the state department that administers Medicaid (for example, the state department of social services or public health). Check the regulations with the state Medicaid office if you are unsure where to send the claim.
- Unless the patient has a medical emergency, Medicaid often requires authorization before services are

INDIANA MEDICAID
AND OTHER MEDICAL ASSISTANCE PROGRAMS

100341842799   001

Danny L Owens
07/19/62

Figure 15-2. A Medicaid card gives the patient's name and identification (or Social Security) number.

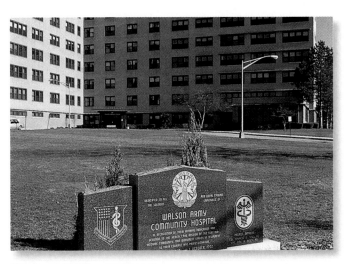

Figure 15-3. TRICARE covers health-care services for family members of military personnel and military retirees at facilities such as the military base hospital pictured here.

performed. Authorization must be obtained from the state Medicaid office in advance.

- Check the time limit on claim submissions. It can be as short as 2 months or as long as 1 year. Verify deadlines with your local Medicaid office.
- Meet the deadlines. If a Medicaid claim is submitted after the time limit, the claim may be rejected.
- Treat Medicaid patients with the same professionalism and courtesy that you extend to other patients. Simply because a patient qualifies for Medicaid assistance does not mean that the patient is in any way inferior to those with private insurance.

TRICARE and CHAMPVA

The U.S. government provides health-care benefits to families of current military personnel, retired military personnel, and veterans through the TRICARE and CHAMPVA programs. Unless you work in a military-related facility, you will probably see TRICARE and CHAMPVA patients only for emergency services or for nonemergency care that a military base cannot provide.

TRICARE.   Run by the Defense Department, **TRICARE** is not a health insurance plan. Rather, it is a health-care benefit for families of uniformed personnel and retirees from the uniformed services, including the Army, Navy, Marines, Air Force, Coast Guard, Public Health Service, and National Oceanic and Atmospheric Administration (Figure 15-3). TRICARE offers families three choices of health-care benefits:

1. TRICARE Prime, a health maintenance organization
2. TRICARE Extra, a managed care network of health-care providers that families can use on a case-by-case basis without a required enrollment
3. TRICARE Standard, a fee-for-service plan

Another program, TRICARE for Life, is aimed at Medicare-eligible military retirees and Medicare-eligible family members. TRICARE for Life offers the opportunity to receive health care at a military treatment facility to individuals aged 65 and older who are eligible for both Medicare and TRICARE.

In the past, individuals became ineligible for TRICARE once they reached age 65, and they were required to enroll in Medicare to obtain any health-care coverage. Beneficiaries could still seek treatment at military treatment facilities, but only if space was available. Under TRICARE for Life, enrollees in TRICARE who are aged 65 and older can continue to obtain medical services at military hospitals and clinics as they did before they turned 65. TRICARE for Life acts as a secondary payer to Medicare; Medicare pays first, and the remaining out-of-pocket expenses are paid by TRICARE.

CHAMPVA.   **CHAMPVA** (Civilian Health and Medical Program of the Veterans Administration) covers the expenses of the families (dependent spouses and children) of veterans with total, permanent, service-connected disabilities. It also covers surviving spouses and dependent children of veterans who died in the line of duty or as a result of service-connected disabilities.

TRICARE and CHAMPVA Eligibility.   You must verify TRICARE eligibility. All TRICARE patients should have a valid identification card. To receive TRICARE benefits, eligible individuals must be enrolled in the Defense Enrollment Eligibility Reporting System (DEERS), a computer database.

Eligibility for CHAMPVA is determined by the nearest Veterans Affairs medical center. Contact this center if any questions arise. Patients can choose the doctor they wish after CHAMPVA eligibility is confirmed.

Under TRICARE and CHAMPVA, participating doctors have the option of deciding whether to accept patients on a case-by-case basis. Make sure you know the policy of the doctor or doctors in your office on this issue.

Blue Cross and Blue Shield

Many people think that Blue Cross and Blue Shield (BCBS) is one large corporation. Rather, it is a nationwide federation of nonprofit and for-profit service organizations that provide prepaid health-care services to BCBS subscribers. Each local organization operates under its own state laws, and specific plans for BCBS can vary greatly.

Workers' Compensation

Workers' compensation insurance covers accidents or diseases incurred in the workplace. Federal law requires employers to purchase and maintain a certain minimum amount of workers' compensation insurance for their employees. Workers' compensation laws vary from state to state. In most states, workers' compensation includes these benefits:

- Basic medical treatment.
- A weekly amount paid to the patient for a temporary disability. This amount compensates workers for loss of job income until they can return to work.
- A weekly or monthly sum paid to the patient for a permanent disability.
- Death benefits.
- Rehabilitation costs to restore an employee's ability to work again.

Not all medical practices accept workers' compensation cases. Make sure you know your office's policy. Records management of workers' compensation varies by state. Typically, you will be responsible for the following administrative tasks when a workers' compensation patient contacts the practice for the first time.

- Call the patient's employer and verify that the accident occurred on the employer's premises.
- Obtain the employer's approval to provide treatment.
- Ask the employer for the name of its workers' compensation insurance company. (Employers are required by law to carry such insurance. It is a good policy to notify your state labor department about any employer you encounter that does not have workers' compensation insurance, although you are not required to do so.) You may wish to remind the employer to report any workplace accidents or injuries that result in a workers' compensation claim to

the state labor department within 24 hours of the incident.
- Contact the insurance company and verify that the employer does indeed have a policy with the company and that the policy is in good standing.
- Obtain a claim number for the case from the insurance company. This claim number is used on all bills and paperwork.

At the time the patient starts treatment, create a patient record. If the patient is already one of the practice's regular patients, create a separate record for the workers' compensation case.

The Claims Process: An Overview

From the time the patient enters a doctor's office until the time the insurer pays the practice for that office visit and associated services, several steps are carried out. In brief, the doctor's office performs the following services:

- Obtains patient information
- Delivers services to the patient and determines the diagnosis and fee
- Records payment from the patient and prepares health-care claims
- Reviews the insurer's processing of the claim, remittance advice, and payment

Most medical assistants use a medical billing program to support administrative tasks such as:

- Gathering and recording patient information
- Verifying patients' insurance coverage
- Recording procedures and services performed
- Filing insurance claims and billing patients
- Reviewing and recording payments

Billing programs streamline the important process of creating and following up on health-care claims sent to payers and bills sent to patients. For example, a large medical practice with a group of providers and thousands of patients may receive a phone call from a patient who wants to know the amount owed on an account. With a billing program, the medical assistant can key the first few letters of the patient's last name and the patient's account data will appear on the screen. The outstanding balance can then be communicated to the patient.

Billing programs are also used to exchange health information about the practice's patients with health plans. Using electronic data interchange (EDI), similar to the technology behind ATMs, information is sent quickly and securely.

Abbreviations Related to Diagnosis

AHF	Acute heart failure
Ca	Cancer
CC	Chief complaint
CHF	Congestive heart failure
CO	Complains of
COPD	Chronic obstructive pulmonary disease
CVA	Cerebrovascular accident
DJD	Degenerative joint disease
DVT	Deep vein thrombosis
Dx	Diagnosis
ESRD	End-stage renal disease
ESRF	End-stage renal failure
FAS	Fetal alcohol syndrome
FBD	Fibrocystic breast disease
FM	Fibromyalgia
FUO	Fever of unknown origin
Fx	Fracture
GI	Gastrointestinal
HA	Headache
HPV	Human papillomavirus
Hx	History
JRA	Juvenile rheumatoid arthritis
RO	Rule out
SOM	Serous otitis media

Abbreviations Related to Procedures

AKA	Above-knee amputation
BKA	Below-knee amputation
Bx	Biopsy
CABG	Coronary artery bypass graft
CT	Computed tomography
CXR	Chest x-ray
D & C	Dilation and curettage
ERCP	Endoscopic retrograde cannulation of pancreatic (duct)
I & D	Incision and drainage
IF	Internal fixation
IVP	Intravenous pyelogram
MRI	Magnetic resonance imaging
PE	Physical examination
PET	Positron emission tomography
PFT	Pulmonary function test
PTCA	Percutaneous transluminal coronary angioplasty
T & A	Tonsilectomy and adenoidectomy
TKA	Total knee arthroplasty
Tx	Treatment

Figure 15-4. Common abbreviations used in claim forms processing.

Obtaining Patient Information

You will need certain information to be able to complete insurance claims for the patients of the medical practice where you work. This information is usually completed on a patient registration form, as shown in Chapter 9.

Basic Facts. When the patient first arrives, obtain or verify the following personal information:

- Name of patient
- Current home address
- Current home telephone number
- Date of birth (month, day, and the four digits of the year)
- Social Security number
- Next of kin or person to contact in case of an emergency

Obtain the following insurance information:

- Current employer (may be more than one)
- Employer address and telephone number
- Insurance carrier and effective date of coverage
- Insurance group plan number
- Insurance identification number (frequently the patient's Social Security number)
- Name of subscriber or insured

Depending on state law, obtain the following release signatures:

- Patient's signature on a form authorizing release of information to the insurance carrier
- Patient's signature on a form for assignment of benefits

Eligibility for Services. After you obtain personal and insurance information and release signatures from the patient, scan or copy the patient's insurance card, front and back, to include in the patient's record. Also verify the effective date of insurance coverage because services performed before this date may be excluded from claims. To reduce possible payment problems, remind the patient before a service is performed if it might not be covered.

Coordination of Benefits. **Coordination of benefits** clauses are legal clauses in insurance policies that prevent duplication of payment. These clauses restrict payment by insurance companies to no more than 100% of the cost of covered benefits. In many families, husband and wife are both wage earners. They and their children are frequently eligible for health insurance benefits through both employers' plans. In such cases the two insurance companies coordinate their payments to pay up to 100% of a procedure's cost. A payment of 100% includes the policyholder's deductible and co-payment. The *primary*, or main, plan is the policy that pays benefits first. Then the *secondary*, or supplemental, plan pays the deductible and co-payment. To determine which plan is the primary, the **birthday rule** is followed. It states that the insurance policy of the policy-holder whose birthday comes first in the calendar year is the primary payer for all dependents.

For example, suppose a husband and wife are both employed and have work-sponsored insurance plans that cover their spouses and their three children. The husband's birthday is July 14 and the wife's birthday is June 11. Because of the birthday rule, the wife's insurance plan is the primary payer, and the husband's is the secondary payer. If a husband and wife were born on the same day, the policy that has been in effect the longest is the primary payer.

The birthday rule is applied in most states in which dependents are covered by two or more medical plans. Different states may have different rules, however. You should check with your state's insurance commission whenever you are in doubt. Table 15-1 describes widely used guidelines.

Delivering Services to the Patient

To ensure accuracy in claims processing, any services delivered to the patient in the office by the physician or other members of the health-care team must be entered into the patient record. **Referrals** to outside physicians or specialists must be entered into the record.

Physician's Services. The physician who examines the patient notes the patient's symptoms in the medical record. The physician also notes a diagnosis and treatment plan (including prescribed medications) and specifies if and when the patient should return for a follow-up visit.

TABLE 15-1 Determining Primary Coverage

- If the patient has only one policy, it is primary.

- If the patient has coverage under two plans, the plan that has been in effect for the patient for the longest period of time is primary. However, if an active employee has a plan with the present employer and is still covered by a former employer's plan as a retiree or a laid-off employee, the current employer's plan is primary.

- If the patient is also covered as a dependent under another insurance policy, the patient's plan is primary.

- If an employed patient has coverage under the employer's plan and additional coverage under a government-sponsored plan, the employer's plan is primary. An example of this is a patient enrolled in a PPO through employment who is also on Medicare.

- If a retired patient is covered by the plan of the spouse's employer and the spouse is still employed, the spouse's plan is primary, even if the retired person has Medicare.

- If the patient is a dependent child covered by both parents' plans and the parents are not separated or divorced (or have joint custody of the child), the primary plan is determined by which parent has the first birth date in the calendar year (the birthday rule).

- If two or more plans cover the dependent children of separated or divorced parents who do not have joint custody of their children, the children's primary plan is determined in this order:

  1. The plan of the custodial parent
  2. The plan of the spouse of the custodial parent (if the parent has remarried)
  3. The plan of the parent without custody

Patient's Name	Insurance Company	Claim Filed		Payment Received		Difference (owed by patient)
		Date	Amount	Date	Amount	

Figure 15-5. After submitting a claim to an insurer, track each claim in an insurance claim register, such as the one pictured here.

After completing the visit with the patient, the physician writes the diagnosis, treatment, and sometimes the fee on a charge slip and instructs the patient to give you the charge slip before leaving.

Medical Coding. The next step is to translate the medical terminology on the charge slip into precise descriptions of medical services and procedural and diagnostic codes on the health-care claim. This step, which is critical to the provider and to reimbursement, is the topic of Chapter 16.

Referrals to Other Services. You may be asked to secure authorization from the insurance company for additional procedures. If so, contact the insurance company to explain the procedures and obtain approval and an authorization number. Enter this referral number in the billing program.

Frequently you will be asked to arrange an appointment for the referred services, particularly if the physician believes they are urgently needed. For example, a physician may send a patient for a specialist's evaluation or x-ray on the same day the patient visits your office.

Preparing the Health-Care Claim

Everyone who receives services from a doctor in the practice where you work is responsible for paying the practice for those services. When the patient brings you the charge slip from the doctor, you may perform one or more of the following procedures, depending on the policy of your practice:

- Prepare and transmit a health-care claim on behalf of the patient directly to the insurance company.
- Accept payment from the patient for the full amount. The patient will submit a claim to the insurance carrier for reimbursement.
- Accept an insurance co-payment.

Filing the Insurance Claim. If you are going to transmit the claim directly to the payer, you will prepare an insurance claim, usually electronically. After the physician reviews the claim, you will transmit the claim to the insurance carrier for payment. The billing program will create a log of transmitted claims, or a register such as the one shown in Figure 15-5 may be maintained.

Time Limits. Claims must be filed in a timely manner. Time limits for filing claims vary from company to company. For example, some insurers will not pay a claim unless it is filed within 6 months of the date of service. The limits for commercial payers such as Blue Cross and Blue Shield vary from state to state.

Medicare states that for services rendered from January 1 to September 30, claims must be filed by December 31 of the following year; for services rendered from October 1 through December 31, claims must be filed no later than December 31 of the second year following the service.

Medicaid states that claims must be filed no later than 1 year from the date of service. The time frame for refiling rejected claims varies by state. In Indiana, for example, if you filed a claim for a service performed on January 2, 2006, and the claim was rejected on May 31, 2006, you would have until May 31, 2007, to refile the claim.

Although Medicare and Medicaid allow quite a long time for claims to be filed, it is poor business practice to wait so long. In the typical medical practice, claims are transmitted within a few business days after the date of service. Many large practices file claims every day or twice a week.

Insurer's Processing and Payment

Your transmitted claim for payment will undergo a number of reviews by the insurer. Currently, much of the review process occurs electronically.

Review for Medical Necessity. The insurance carrier reviews each claim to determine whether the diagnosis and accompanying treatment are compatible and whether the treatment is medically necessary, as explained in Chapter 16.

Review for Allowable Benefits. The claims department also compares the fees the doctor charges with the benefits provided by the patient's health insurance policy. This review determines the amount of deductible or coinsurance the patient owes. This amount—that is, what the patient owes—is called subscriber liability.

Payment and Remittance Advice. After reviewing the claim, the insurer pays a benefit, either to the subscriber (patient) or to the practice, depending on what recipient the claim requested. With the payment, the insurer sends **remittance advice (RA),** also called an explanation of benefits. A patient who receives the payment gets the original RA, and the practice receives a copy (and vice versa). For each service submitted to an insurer, the RA form gives the following information:

- Name of the insured and identification number
- Name of the beneficiary
- Claim number
- Date, place, and type of service (coded)
- Amount billed by the practice
- Amount allowed (according to the subscriber's policy)
- Amount of subscriber liability (co-payment or deductible)
- Amount paid and included in the current payment
- A notation of any services not covered and an explanation of why they were not covered (for example, many insurance plans do not cover a woman's annual gynecologic examination and only a certain dollar amount of well-baby visits for infants)

Reviewing the Insurer's RA and Payment

Verify all information on the RA, line by line, using your records for each patient represented on the RA. In a large practice, you will frequently receive payment and an RA for several patients at one time. An example of a Medicare RA, which is called a Medicare Remittance Notice, is shown in Figure 15-6.

If all numbers on the RA agree with your records, you can make the appropriate entries in the insurance follow-up log for claims paid. In a small practice, the insurance follow-up log is used to track filed claims, using such information as patient name, date the claim was filed, services the claim reflects, notations about the results of the claim, and any balance due from the patient. Larger practices tend to track claims on computer in a file called, for example, "Unpaid Claims." If all the numbers do not agree, you will need to trace the claim with the insurance company.

When a claim is rejected, the RA states the reason. You will need to review the claim, examining all procedural and diagnosis codes for accuracy and comparing the claim with the patient's insurance information. You will probably need to contact the insurance company by telephone to resolve the claim problem.

Fee Schedules and Charges

Physicians establish a list of their usual fees for the procedures and services they frequently perform. The usual fees are those that they charge to most of their patients most of the time under typical conditions. These fees are listed on the office's **fee schedule.**

Medicare Payment System: RBRVS

Third-party payers also set the fees they are willing to pay providers, and often these fees are less than the physician's fee schedule. Most payers base their fees on the amounts that Medicare allows because the Medicare method of fee setting takes into account important factors other than only the usual fees.

The payment system used by Medicare is called the **resource-based relative value scale (RBRVS).** The RBRVS establishes the relative value units for services, replacing providers' consensus on fees (the "usual" or historical charges) with amounts based on resources (what each service really costs to provide).

There are three parts to an RBRVS fee:

1. The nationally uniform relative value. The relative value of a procedure is based on three cost elements: the physician's work, the practice cost (overhead), and the cost of malpractice insurance. For example, the relative value for a simple office visit, such as to administer a flu shot, is much lower than the relative value for a complicated encounter such as planning the treatment of uncontrolled diabetes in a patient.

2. A geographic adjustment factor. A geographic adjustment factor is used to adjust each relative value to reflect a geographical area's relative costs, such as office rents.

3. A nationally uniform conversion factor. A uniform conversion factor is a dollar amount used to multiply the relative values to produce a payment amount. It is used by Medicare to make adjustments according to changes in the cost-of-living index.

When RBRVS fees are used, providers receive considerably lower payments than when usual fees are used. Each part of the RBRVS—the relative values, the geographic adjustment, and the conversion factor—is updated each year by CMS. The year's Medicare fee schedule (MFS) is published by CMS in the *Federal Register*.

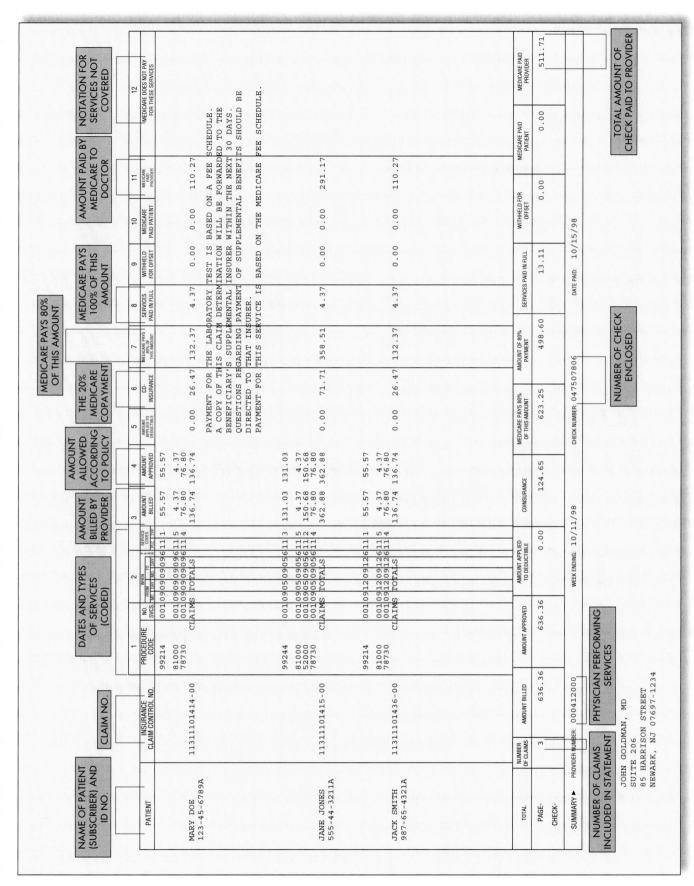

Figure 15-6. The insurer sends the remittance advice form to the medical practice.

Payment Methods

Most third-party payers use one of three methods for reimbursing physicians:

1. Allowed charges
2. Contracted fee schedule
3. Capitation

Allowed Charges. Many payers set an **allowed charge** for each procedure or service. This amount is the most the payer will pay any provider for that work. The term *allowed charge* has many equivalent terms, including *maximum allowable fee*, *maximum charge, allowed amount, allowed fee*, or *allowable charge*.

The physician's usual charge is often greater than a plan's allowed charge. If the physician participates in the plan, only the allowed charge can be billed to the payer. The plan's rules govern whether the provider is permitted to bill a patient for the part of a usual charge that the payer does not cover. Billing a patient for the difference between a higher usual fee and a lower allowed charge is called **balance billing.** Under most contracts, participating providers may not bill the patient for the difference. Instead, the provider must write off the difference, meaning that the amount of the difference is subtracted from the patient's bill and never collected.

For example, Medicare-participating providers may not receive an amount greater than the Medicare-allowed charge that is based on the Medicare fee schedule. The Original Medicare Plan is responsible for paying 80% of this allowed charge (after patients have met their annual deductible). Patients are responsible for the other 20%.

Here is an example of a Medicare billing. A Medicare-participating provider reports a usual charge of $200 for a service, and the Medicare-allowed charge is $84. The provider must write off the difference between the two charges. The patient is responsible for 20% of the allowed charge, not of the provider's usual charge:

Provider's usual fee:	$200.00
Medicare-allowed charge:	$84.00
Medicare pays 80%	$67.20
Patient pays 20%	$16.80

The total that the provider can collect is $84. The provider must write off the difference between the usual fee and the allowed charge, or $116.00 in this example.

Contracted Fee Schedule. Some payers, particularly PPOs, establish fixed fee schedules with their participating physicians. The terms of the plan determine what percentage of the charges, if any, the patient owes and what percentage the payer covers. Participating providers can typically bill patients their usual charges for procedures and services that are not covered by the plan.

Capitation. The fixed prepayment for each plan member in capitation contracts is determined by the managed care plan that initiates contracts with providers. The plan's contract with the provider lists the services and procedures that are covered by the cap rate. For example, a typical contract with a primary care provider might include the following services:

- Preventive care, including well-child care, adult physical exams, gynecological exams, eye exams, and hearing exams
- Counseling and telephone calls
- Office visits
- Medical care, including medical care services such as therapeutic injections and immunizations, allergy immunotherapy, electrocardiograms, and pulmonary function tests
- The local treatment of first-degree burns, the application of dressings, suture removal, the excision of small skin lesions, the removal of foreign bodies or cerumen from the external ear

These services are covered in the per-member charge for each plan member who selects the PCP. Noncovered services can be billed to patients using the physician's usual rate. Plans often require the provider to notify the patient in advance that a service is not covered and to state the fee for which the patient will be responsible.

Calculating Patient Charges

The patients of medical practices have a variety of health plans, so they have different financial responsibilities. In addition to premiums, patients may be obligated to pay deductibles, co-payments, coinsurance, excluded and over-limit services, and balance billing.

All payers require patients to pay for excluded (noncovered) services. Physicians generally can charge their usual fees for these services. Likewise, in managed care plans that set limits on the annual usage (or other period) of covered services, patients are responsible for usage beyond the allowed number. For example, if one preventive physical examination is permitted annually, additional preventive examinations are paid for by the patient.

Communications With Patients About Charges

When patients have office visits with a physician who participates in the plan under which they have coverage, such as a Medicare-participating (PAR) provider, they generally sign an **assignment of benefits** statement. When this occurs, the provider agrees to prepare health-care claims for patients, to receive payments directly from the payers, and to accept a payer's allowed charge. Patients are billed for charges that payers deny or do not pay. When patients have encounters with nonparticipating (nonPAR) providers, the procedure is usually different. To avoid the difficulty of collecting payments at a later date from a patient, practices may require that the patient either (1) assigns benefits or (2) pays in full at the time of services.

Many times patients want to know what their bills will be. For example, suppose a patient receives a bill for $100 from your practice. She calls to say that she has paid her deductible for the year, so her insurance company should have paid 80% of the bill. You call the patient's insurance company and learn that she still has to pay $100 to meet her deductible. If she pays the $100 bill in full, her deductible will then be met. You would have to explain these facts to the patient.

To estimate patients' bills, you should check with the payer to find out:

- The patient's deductible amount and whether it has been paid in full, the covered benefits, and coinsurance or other patient financial obligations
- The payer's allowed charges for the services that the provider anticipates providing

If the patient's request comes after the appointment, the encounter form can be used to tell the payer what procedures are going to be reported on the patient's claim to determine the likely payer reimbursement.

Patients should always be reminded of their financial obligations under their plans, including claim denials, according to practice procedures. The practice's financial policy regarding payment for services is usually either displayed on the wall of the reception area or included in a new patient information packet. The policy should explain what is required of the patient and when payment is due. For example, the policy may state the following:

- For unassigned claims: Payment for the physician's services is expected at the end of your appointment, unless you have made other arrangements with our practice manager.
- For assigned claims: After your insurance claim is processed by your insurance company, you will be billed for any amount you owe. You are responsible for any part of the charges that are denied or not paid by the carrier. All patient accounts are due within 30 days of the date of the invoice you receive.
- For managed care members: Co-payments must be paid before patients leave the office.

It is also a good practice to notify patients in advance of the probable cost of procedures that are not going to be covered by their plan. For example, many private plans as well as Medicare do not pay for most preventive services, such as annual physical examinations. Many patients, however, consider preventive services a good idea and are willing to pay for them. Patients should be asked to agree in writing to pay for any noncovered services. A letter of agreement should also specify why the service will not be covered and the cost of the procedure. In the case of Medicare, a form called the Advance Beneficiary Notice (Figure 15-7) is given to the patient to sign. It explains the charges that the patient is likely to have to pay.

Preparing and Transmitting Health-Care Claims

Health-care claims are a critical communication between medical offices and payers on behalf of patients. Processing claims is a major task in most offices, and the numbers can be huge. For example, a 40-physician group practice with 55,000 patients served annually typically processes 1000 claims daily!

HIPAA Claims and Paper Claims

Two types of claims are in use: (1) the predominant HIPAA electronic claim transaction and (2) the older CMS-1500 paper form. The electronic claim transaction is the HIPAA Health-Care Claim or Equivalent Encounter Information; it is commonly referred to as the "HIPAA claim." Its official name is **X12 837 Health Care Claim.** The paper format is the "universal claim" known as the CMS-1500 claim form (or the HCFA-1500).

As of October 2003, Medicare mandates the X12 837 transaction for all Medicare claims except those from very small practices. Third-party payers may continue to accept paper transactions. But practices that elect to use paper claims must have two versions of their medical billing software: one to capture the necessary data elements for HIPAA-compliant electronic Medicare claims and an older version to generate CMS-1500 claims. Also, under HIPAA regulations, only medical offices that do not handle any other HIPAA-related transactions can still use paper claims. It is anticipated that eventually, for cost reasons, all payers will require electronic submissions and add this provision to their contracts with providers.

Preparing HIPAA Claims. The information entered on claims is called data elements. Many elements, such as the patient's personal and insurance information, are entered in the billing program before patient's appointments, based on forms patients fill out and on communications with payers. After patients' office visits, their claims are completed when the medical assistant enters the billing transactions—the services, charges, and payments—as detailed on the superbill (encounter form). The medical assistant then instructs the software to prepare claims for editing and transmission.

Follow these tips when entering data in medical billing programs:

- Enter data in all capital letters
- Do not use prefixes for people's names, such as Mr., Ms., or Dr.
- Unless required by a particular insurance carrier, do not use special characters such as hyphens, commas, or apostrophes
- Use only valid data in all fields; avoid words such as "same"

| Patient's Name: | Medicare # (HICN): |

ADVANCE BENEFICIARY NOTICE (ABN)

NOTE: You need to make a choice about receiving these health care items or services.

We expect that Medicare will not pay for the item(s) or service(s) that are described below. Medicare does not pay for all of your health care costs. Medicare only pays for covered items and services when Medicare rules are met. The fact that Medicare may not pay for a particular item or service does not mean that you should not receive it. There may be a good reason your doctor recommended it. Right now, in your case, **Medicare probably will not pay for –**

Items or Services:

Because:

The purpose of this form is to help you make an informed choice about whether or not you want to receive these items or services, knowing that you might have to pay for them yourself. Before you make a decision about your options, you should **read this entire notice carefully**.

- Ask us to explain, if you don't understand why Medicare probably won't pay.
- Ask us how much these items or services will cost you (**Estimated Cost: $_____**), in case you have to pay for them yourself or through other insurance.

PLEASE CHOOSE **ONE** OPTION. CHECK **ONE** BOX. **SIGN & DATE** YOUR CHOICE.

☐ **Option 1. YES.   I want to receive these items or services.**
I understand that Medicare will not decide whether to pay unless I receive these items or services. Please submit my claim to Medicare. I understand that you may bill me for items or services and that I may have to pay the bill while Medicare is making its decision. If Medicare does pay, you will refund to me any payments I made to you that are due to me. If Medicare denies payment, I agree to be personally and fully responsible for payment. That is, I will pay personally, either out of pocket or through any other insurance that I have. I understand I can appeal Medicare's decision.

☐ **Option 2. NO.   I have decided not to receive these items or services.**
I will not receive these items or services. I understand that you will not be able to submit a claim to Medicare and that I will not be able to appeal your opinion that Medicare won't pay.

_____   _____
Date   **Signature of patient or person acting on patient's behalf**

NOTE: Your health information will be kept confidential. Any information that we collect about you on this form will be kept confidential in our offices. If a claim is submitted to Medicare, your health information on this form may be shared with Medicare. Your health information which Medicare sees will be kept confidential by Medicare.

OMB Approval No. 0938-0566   Form No. CMS-R-131-G   (June 2002)

Figure 15-7. Advance Beneficiary Notice.
Source: Centers for Medicare and Medicaid Services.

The X12 837 transaction requires many data elements, and all must be correct. Most billing programs or claim transmission programs automatically reformat data such as dates into the correct formats. These data elements are reported in five major sections:

1. Provider
2. Subscriber (the insured or policyholder)
3. Patient (who may be the subscriber or another person) and payer
4. Claim details
5. Services

Not all data elements are required. Some are considered situational and are required only when a certain condition applies. When it does apply, then that data element also becomes required. For example, if a claim involves pregnancy, the date of the last menstrual period is required. If the claim does not involve pregnancy, that date should not be reported.

Before the HIPAA mandate for standard transactions, some payers required additional records, such as their own information sheet, when providers billed them. Some payers also used their own coding systems. The HIPAA Electronic Health Care Transactions and Code Sets (TCS) mandate means that health plans are required to accept the standard claim submitted electronically.

Other standard transactions also support the claim process, such as advising the office of claim status, payment, and other key information. These transactions standards apply to the treatment, payment, and operations information that is exchanged between medical offices and health plans. Each electronic transaction has both a title and a number. Each number begins with X12, which is the number of the EDI format, followed by a unique number that stands for the transaction. Here are some examples of titles and numbers that medical assistants may encounter while processing X12 837 health-care claims:

Number	Title
X12 276/277	Claim status inquiry and response
X12 270/271	Eligibility inquiry and response
X12 278	Referral authorization inquiry and response
X12 835	Payment and remittance advice
X12 820	Health plan premium payments
X12 834	Enrollment in and withdrawal from a health plan

Preparing Paper Claims. The process for preparing paper claims is similar to the X12 837 claim. Usually, the medical billing program is updated with information about the patient's office visit. Then the program is instructed to print the data on a CMS-1500 paper form, shown in Figure 15-8. This claim may be mailed or faxed to a third-party payer.

Because of the HIPAA mandate, the paper claim is not widely in use; however, the information it contains is essentially very similar to the X12 837. For this reason, you should study Procedure 15-1, Completing the CMS-1500 Claim Form. This exercise will give you a good understanding of the data elements needed on all claims.

The CMS-1500 contains 33 form locators, which are numbered items. Form locators 1–13 refer to the patient and the patient's insurance coverage. Form locators 14–33 contain information about the provider and the transaction information, including the patient's diagnoses, procedures, and charges.

Transmission of Electronic Claims

Practices handle the transmission of electronic claims—which may be called electronic media claims, or EMC—in a variety of ways. Some practices transmit claims themselves; others hire outside vendors to handle this task for them.

Claims are prepared for transmission after all required data elements have been posted to the medical billing software program. The data elements that are transmitted are not seen physically, as they would be on a paper form. Instead, these elements are in a computer file.

Three major methods are used to transmit claims electronically: direct transmission to the payer, clearinghouse use, and direct data entry.

Transmitting Claims Directly. In the direct transmission approach, medical offices and payers exchange transactions directly. To do this, providers and payers need the necessary information systems, including a translator and communications technology, to conduct **electronic data interchange (EDI)**.

Using a Clearinghouse. Many offices whose medical billing software vendors do not have translation software must use a **clearinghouse** in order to send and receive data in the correct EDI format. Clearinghouses can take in nonstandard formats and translate them into the standard format. To ensure that the standard format is compliant, the clearinghouse must receive all the required data elements from the physician. Clearinghouses are prohibited from creating or modifying data content.

Medical offices may use a clearinghouse to transmit all their claims, or they may use a combination of direct transmission and a clearinghouse. For example, they may send claims directly to Medicare, Medicaid, and a few other major commercial payers, and use a clearinghouse to send claims to other payers.

Using Direct Data Entry. Online direct data entry (DDE) is offered by some payers. It uses an Internet-based service into which employees key the standard data elements. Although the data elements must meet the HIPAA standards requirements regarding content, they do not have to be formatted for EDI. Instead, they are loaded directly in the health plans' computer.

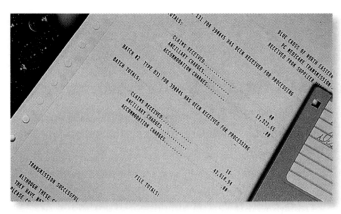

Figure 15-9. Print out the claims report to check for any errors that might make the payer reject a claim.

- Missing payer name and/or payer identifier, required for both primary and secondary payers.

Many offices use a specialized software program called a "claim scrubber" to check claims before they are released and to allow errors to be fixed. Clearinghouses also apply software checks to claims they receive and transmit back reports of errors or missing information to the sender.

Claims Security

Electronic data about patients are stored on a computer system. Most medical offices use computer networks in which personal computers are connected to a local area network (LAN), so users can exchange and share information and hardware. The LAN is linked to remote networks such as the Internet by a router that determines the best route for data to travel across the network. Packets of data traveling between the LAN and the Internet—such as electronic claims—must usually pass through a firewall, a security device that examines information (for example, e-mails) that enter and leave a network, determining whether to forward them to their destination.

The HIPAA rules set standards for protecting individually identifiable health information when it is maintained or transmitted electronically. Medical offices must protect the confidentiality, integrity, and availability of this information. A number of security measures are used:

- Access control, passwords, and log files to keep intruders out
- Backups (saved copies of files) to replace items after damage to the computer
- Security policies to handle violations that do occur

Medical assistants participate in the protection of patients' health information. One way is to select a good password for your computer. Here are tips:

- Always use a combination of letters and numbers that are not real words and also not an obvious number string such as 123456 or a birth date.
- Do not use a user ID (log-on or sign-on) as a password. Even if it has both numbers and letters, it is not secret.
- Select a mixture of both upper case and lower case letters if the system can distinguish between them, and if possible, include special characters such as @, $, or &.
- Use a minimum of six or seven alphanumeric characters. The optimal minimum number varies by system, but most security experts recommend a length of at least six or seven characters.
- Change passwords periodically, but not too often. Forcing frequent changes can actually make security worse because users are more likely to keep passwords written down.

Summary

Part of your responsibilities as a medical assistant will be to make sure that health-care claims are processed accurately. When accurate claims are sent to payers, physicians receive the maximum appropriate payment for the services they provide.

As a medical assistant, you will handle patients' questions about their health-care plans and claims. You will review patients' insurance coverage, explain the physician's fees, estimate what charges payers will cover, estimate how much patients should pay, and prepare complete and accurate health-care claims for patients.

REVIEW

CASE STUDY QUESTIONS

Now that you have completed this chapter, review the case study at the beginning of the chapter and answer the following questions:

1. How much should this patient pay?
2. How much will he owe for his next visit this year, which is expected to have a charge of $200?
3. Assuming that the patient in the case study has a managed care policy, what type of policy does he probably have?
4. What term would you use to describe the part of the payment that is based on 20% of the charges?
5. If you did not know whether the deductible had been met, what procedure would you follow?

Discussion Questions

1. How do HMOs and PPOs compare?
2. What are the differences between Medicare Part A and Part B?
3. Why do insurers coordinate benefits?
4. What is the difference between TRICARE and CHAMPVA?

Critical Thinking Questions

1. How is the increasing cost of medical procedures affecting the insurance industry?
2. How does managed care help control the cost of health insurance?
3. What are the advantages of electronic claims?

Application Activities

1. Apply the birthday rule in this situation:

   Both parents of the patient have health-care coverage through their employers. The father's birthday is October 6 and the mother's is November 23. Which plan is primary for the child?

2. A patient's insurance policy states:

   Annual deductible: $300
   Coinsurance: 70-30

   This year, the patient has made payments totaling $533 to all providers. Today, the patient has an office visit (fee: $80). The patient presents a credit card for payment of today's bill. What is the amount that the patient should pay?

3. A patient is a member of an HMO with a capitation plan and a $10 copay. The usual charges for the day's services would be $480. What does the patient pay?

4. A patient is a member of a PPO health plan that has a 20% discount from the provider and a 15% co-payment. If the day's usual charges are $210, what are the amounts that the plan and the patient each pay?

Internet Activities

1. Visit the BCBS Internet site. Use e-mail to post a question about insurance processing. Check back in a couple of days and report to the class.
2. Visit the CMS Web site and research the current plans available to Medicare beneficiaries.

Processing Health-Care Claims   **277**

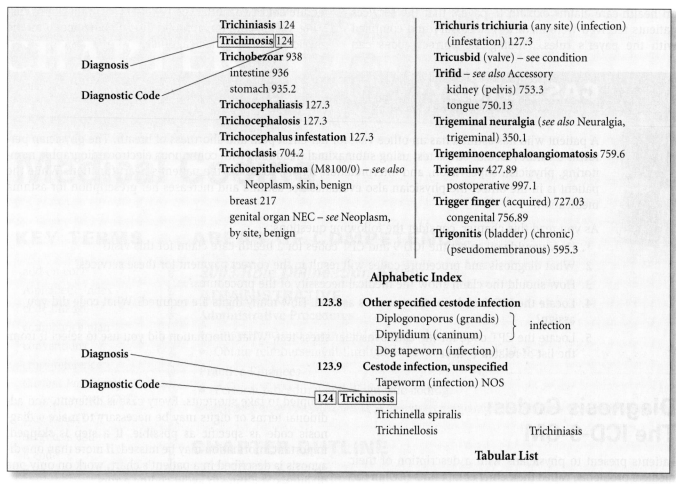

Figure 16-1. ICD alphabetic index and tabular list.

Source: International Classification of Diseases, Ninth Revision, Clinical Modification, 2004, Volumes 1 and 2.

Although the official order of the volumes puts the Tabular List before the Alphabetic Index, the correct use is to examine the Alphabetic Index when you are researching a term and then to verify your selection in the Tabular List. For this reason, commercial printers usually reverse the order, printing the Alphabetic Index at the front and the Tabular List behind it.

The Alphabetic Index

The Alphabetic Index contains all the medical terms in the Tabular List. For some conditions, it also has common terms that are not found in the Tabular List. The index is organized by the condition, not by the body part in which it occurs. For example, you would find the term *wrist fracture* by looking under *fracture* (the condition) and then, below it, *wrist* (the location), rather than by looking under *wrist* to find *fracture.*

The assignment of the correct code begins with looking up the medical term that describes the patient's condition in the Alphabetic Index. The following example illustrates the index's format. Each main term is printed in boldface type and is followed by its code number. For example, if the diagnostic statement is "the patient presents

with blindness," the main term *blindness* is located in the Alphabetic Index.

Blindness (acquired) (congenital) (Both eyes) 369.00
  blast 921.3
    with nerve injury—see Injury, nerve, optic
  Brightis—see Uremia
  color (congenital) 368.59
    acquired 368.55
    blue 368.53
    green 368.52
    red 368.51
    total 368.54
  concussion 950.9
  cortical 377.75

Any other terms that are needed to select correct codes are printed after the main term. These terms may show the cause or source of the disease, or describe a particular type or body site for the main term. In this shortened example, the main term *blindness* is followed by five additional terms, each indicating a different type—such as color blindness—for this medical condition.

Other helpful terms may also be shown. In the example, any of the terms *acquired, congenital,* and *both eyes* may be in the diagnostic statement, such as "the patient presents with blindness acquired in childhood."

Some entries use **cross-references.** If the cross-reference *see* appears after a main term, you *must* look up the term that follows the word *see* in the index. The *see* reference means that the main term where you first looked is not correct; another category must be used. In the previous example, to code *Brightis,* the term *Uremia* must be located.

The Tabular List

The diseases and injuries in the Tabular List are organized into chapters according to the source or body system. There are also two kinds of supplementary codes. The organization of the Tabular List and the ranges of codes each chapter covers are shown in Table 16-1.

Code Structure. ICD-9-CM diagnosis codes are made up of three, four, or five digits, and a description. The system uses three-digit categories for diseases, injuries, and symptoms. Many of these categories are divided into four-digit codes. Some codes are further subdivided into five-digit codes. For example:

415 Acute pulmonary heart disease *[three digits]*

415.1 Pulmonary embolism and infarction *[four digits; more specific]*

415.11 Iatrogenic pulmonary embolism and infarction *[five digits; most specific]*

When listed in the ICD-9, four- and five-digit diagnosis codes should be reported on claims because they represent the most specific diagnosis documented in the patient medical record. If available, the use of fourth and fifth digits is not optional; payers require them. For example, Centers for Medicare and Medicaid Services (CMS) rules state that a Medicare claim will be rejected when the most specific code available is not used.

TABLE 16-1 Tabular List Organization

Classification of Diseases and Injuries	
Chapter	**Categories**
1 Infectious and Parasitic Diseases	001–139
2 Neoplasms	140–239
3 Endocrine, Nutritional, and Metabolic Diseases, and Immunity Disorders	240–279
4 Diseases of the Blood and Blood-Forming Organs	280–289
5 Mental Disorders	290–319
6 Diseases of the Central Nervous System and Sense Organs	320–389
7 Diseases of the Circulatory System	390–459
8 Diseases of the Respiratory System	460–519
9 Diseases of the Digestive System	520–579
10 Diseases of the Genitourinary System	580–629
11 Complications of Pregnancy, Childbirth, and the Puerperium	630–679
12 Diseases of the Skin and Subcutaneous Tissue	680–709
13 Diseases of the Musculoskeletal System and Connective Tissue	710–739
14 Congenital Anomalies	740–759
15 Certain Conditions Originating in the Perinatal Period	760–779
16 Symptoms, Signs, and Ill-Defined Conditions	780–799
17 Injury and Poisoning	800–999
Supplementary Classifications	
V Codes—Supplementary Classification of Factors Influencing Health Status and Contact with Health Services	V01–V83
E Codes—Supplementary Classification of External Causes of Injury and Poisoning	E800–E999

V Codes and E Codes. Two additional types of codes follow the chapters of the Tabular List:

1. **V codes** identify encounters for reasons other than illness or injury, such as annual checkups, immunizations, and normal childbirth. A V code can be used either as a primary code for an encounter or as an additional code.

2. **E codes** identify the external causes of injuries and poisoning. E (for external) codes are used for injuries resulting from various environmental events, such as transportation accidents, accidental poisoning by drugs or other substances, falls, and fires. An E code is never used alone as a diagnosis code. It always supplements a code that identifies the injury or condition itself. E codes are often used in collecting public health information.

Both V and E codes are alphanumeric; they contain letters followed by numbers. For example, the code for a complete physical examination of an adult is V70.0. The code for a fall from a ladder is E881.0.

ICD-9-CM Conventions

A list of abbreviations, punctuation, symbols, type faces, and instructional notes appears at the beginning of the ICD-9. These items, called **conventions,** provide guidelines for using the code set. Here are some important conventions:

NOS—This abbreviation means "not otherwise specified," or "unspecified." It is used when a condition cannot be described more specifically. In general, codes with *NOS* should be avoided. The physician

PROCEDURE 16.1

Locating an ICD-9-CM Code

Objective: To analyze diagnoses and locate the correct ICD code.

Materials: Patient record, ICD-9-CM

Method

1. Locate the statement of the diagnosis in the patient's medical record.
   First, find the diagnosis. This information may be located on the superbill (encounter form) or elsewhere in the patient's chart.

   Example: A patient's medical record reads:
   CC: Chest and epigastric pain; feels like a burning inside. Occasional reflux. Abdomen soft, flat without tenderness. No bowel masses or organomegaly.
   Dx: Peptic ulcer.

   The diagnosis is peptic ulcer.

   Then, if needed, decide which is the main term or condition of the diagnosis.

   Example: In the above diagnosis, the main term or condition is *ulcer.* The word *peptic* describes the type of ulcer.

2. Find the diagnosis in the ICD's Alphabetic Index. Look for the condition first. Then find descriptive words that make the condition more specific. Read all cross-references to check all the possibilities for a term and its synonyms.

   Example: The diagnosis is sebaceous cyst. Look under *cyst,* the condition, rather than *sebaceous,* the descriptive word. Many entries

   in the Alphabetic Index are cross-referenced. For example, *sebaceous* is followed by instructions in parentheses that say "(*see also* Cyst, sebaceous)." Observe all cross-reference instructions.

3. Locate the code from the Alphabetic Index in the ICD's Tabular List.
   Remember, the number to check is a code number, not a page number. The Tabular List gives codes in numerical order. Look for the number in bold-faced type.

4. Read all information to find the code that corresponds to the patient's specific disease or condition.
   Study the list of codes and descriptions. Be sure to pick the most specific code available. Check for the symbol that shows that a five-digit code is required.

5. Record the diagnosis code on the insurance claim and proofread the numbers.
   Enter the correct diagnosis code on the health-care claim, checking that
   - The numbers are entered correctly. If two numbers are transposed, the payer will receive the wrong diagnosis. Proofread the numbers on the computer screen or on the printed claim form.
   - The codes are complete. If the phone rang in the middle of coding a diagnosis, the last number of the code may have been omitted.
   - The highest (most specific) code is used.

should be asked to help select a more specific code, if possible.

NEC—This abbreviation means "not elsewhere classified." It is used when the ICD-9 does not provide a code specific enough for the patient's condition.

[ ] Brackets—Used around synonyms, alternative wordings, or explanations.

( ) Parentheses—Used around descriptions that do not affect the code, that is, nonessential or supplementary terms.

: Colon—Used in the Tabular List after an incomplete term that needs one of the terms that follow to make it assignable to a given category.

} Brace—Encloses a series of terms, each of which is modified by the statement that appears to the right of the brace.

Includes—This note indicates that the entries following it refine the content of a preceding entry. For example, after the three-digit diagnosis code for acute sinusitis, the word *includes* is followed by the types of conditions that the code covers.

Excludes—These notes, which are boxed and italicized, indicate that an entry is not classified as part of the preceding code. The note may also give the correct location of the excluded condition.

Use additional code—This note indicates that an additional code should be used, if available.

Code first underlying disease—This instruction appears when the category is not to be used as the primary diagnosis. These codes may not be used as the first code; they must always be preceded by another code for the primary diagnosis.

A New Revision: The ICD-10-CM

The tenth edition of the ICD was published by the World Health Organization in the mid-1990s. In the United States, the new *Clinical Modification* (ICD-10-CM) is being reviewed by health-care professionals. It is expected to be adopted as the HIPAA-required diagnosis code set before 2010. Major changes include the following:

- The ICD-10 contains more than 2000 categories of diseases, many more than the ICD-9. This creates more codes to permit more specific reporting of diseases and newly recognized conditions, such as SARS.

- Codes are alphanumeric, containing a letter followed by up to five numbers. The sixth digit is added to capture clinical details. For example, all codes that relate to pregnancy, labor, and childbirth include a digit that indicates the patient's trimester.

- Codes are added to show which side of the body is affected when a disease or condition can be involved with the right side, the left side, or bilaterally.

It is generally acknowledged that experienced ICD-9 coders will require only brief training to work effectively and efficiently with ICD-10.

Procedure Codes: The CPT

After an office visit, each procedure and service performed for a patient is reported on health-care claims using a **procedure code.** These codes represent medical procedures, such as surgery and diagnostic tests, and medical services, such as an examination to evaluate a patient's condition. Medical assistants often verify procedure codes and use them to report physicians' services.

The most commonly used system of procedure codes is found in the *Current Procedural Terminology,* a book published by the American Medical Association (AMA) that is commonly known as **CPT.** CPT is the HIPAA-required code set for physicians' procedures.

An updated edition of the CPT is published every year to reflect changes in medical practice. Newly developed procedures are added, and old ones that have become obsolete are deleted. These changes are also available in a computer file because some medical offices use a computer-based version of the CPT.

Medical offices should have the current year's CPT available for reference and keep forms up to date. Previous years' books should also be kept in case there is a question about health-care claims that were previously submitted.

Using the CPT

CPT codes are five-digit numbers, organized into six sections:

Section	Range of Codes
Evaluation and Management	99201–99499
Anesthesiology	00100–01999
Surgery	10021–69990
Radiology	70010–79999
Pathology and Laboratory	80048–89356
Medicine	90281–99602

Except for the first section, the CPT reference book is arranged in numerical order. Codes for evaluation and management are listed first, out of numerical order, because they are used most often.

Each section opens with important guidelines that apply to its procedures. This material should be checked carefully before a procedure code is chosen. The sections of the CPT are divided into categories. These in turn are further divided into headings according to the type of test, service, or body system. Code number ranges included on a particular page are found in the upper right corner. This helps to locate a code quickly after using the index. An example is shown in Figure 16-2.

Locate correct procedure codes by first looking up the term in the CPT's index. Bold-faced main terms may be followed by descriptions and groups of indented terms. The correct code is selected by reviewing each description and indented term under the main term.

Although it may seem tempting to record the procedure code directly from the index, resist the shortcut. Explanations and notes in the guidelines and main sections

Surgery

General

(10000-10020 have been deleted. To report see 10060, 10061)

10021 Fine needle aspiration; without imaging guidance
➲ CPT Assistant Aug 02:10; CPT Changes: An Insider's View 2002

10022 with imaging guidance
➲ CPT Changes: An Insider's View 2002

(For radiological supervision and interpretation, see 76003, 76360, 76393, 76942)

(For percutaneous needle biopsy other than fine needle aspiration, see 20206 for muscle, 32400 for pleura, 32405 for lung or mediastinum, 42400 for salivary gland, 47000, 47001 for liver, 48102 for pancreas, 49180 for abdominal or retroperitoneal mass, 60100 for thyroid, 62269 for spinal cord)

(For evaluation of fine needle aspirate, see 88172, 88173)

Integumentary System

Skin, Subcutaneous and Accessory Structures

Incision and Drainage

(For excision, see 11400, et seq)

10040 Acne surgery (eg, marsupialization, opening or removal of multiple milia, comedones, cysts, pustules)

10060 Incision and drainage of abscess (eg, carbuncle, suppurative hidradenitis, cutaneous or subcutaneous abscess, cyst, furuncle, or paronychia); simple or single

10061 complicated or multiple

10080 Incision and drainage of pilonidal cyst; simple

10081 complicated

(For excision of pilonidal cyst, see 11770-11772)

10120 Incision and removal of foreign body, subcutaneous tissues; simple

10121 complicated

(To report wound exploration due to penetrating trauma without laparotomy or thoracotomy, see 20100-20103, as appropriate)

(To report debridement associated with open fracture(s) and/or dislocation(s), use 11010-11012, as appropriate)

10140 Incision and drainage of hematoma, seroma or fluid collection
➲ CPT Changes: An Insider's View 2002

(If imaging guidance is performed, see 76360, 76393, 76942)

10160 Puncture aspiration of abscess, hematoma, bulla, or cyst
➲ CPT Changes: An Insider's View 2002

(If imaging guidance is performed, see 76360, 76393, 76942)

10180 Incision and drainage, complex, postoperative wound infection

(For secondary closure of surgical wound, see 12020, 12021, 13160)

Excision—Debridement

(For dermabrasions, see 15780-15783)

(For nail debridement, see 11720-11721)

(For burn(s), see 16000-16035)

11000 Debridement of extensive eczematous or infected skin; up to 10% of body surface

+ 11001 each additional 10% of the body surface (List separately in addition to code for primary procedure)

(Use 11001 in conjunction with code 11000)

11010 Debridement including removal of foreign material associated with open fracture(s) and/or dislocation(s); skin and subcutaneous tissues
➲ CPT Assistant Mar 97:1, Apr 97:10, Aug 97:6

11011 skin, subcutaneous tissue, muscle fascia, and muscle
➲ CPT Assistant Mar 97:1, Apr 97:10, Aug 97:6

11012 skin, subcutaneous tissue, muscle fascia, muscle, and bone
➲ CPT Assistant Mar 97:1, Apr 97:10, Aug 97:6

11040 Debridement; skin, partial thickness
➲ CPT Assistant Fall 93:21, May 96:6, Feb 97:7, Aug 97:6

11041 skin, full thickness
➲ CPT Assistant Fall 93:21, May 96:6, Feb 97:7, Aug 97:6

11042 skin, and subcutaneous tissue
➲ CPT Assistant Winter 92:10, May 96:6, Feb 97:7, Aug 97:6

11043 skin, subcutaneous tissue, and muscle
➲ CPT Assistant May 96:6, Feb 97:7, Apr 97:11, Aug 97:6

11044 skin, subcutaneous tissue, muscle, and bone
➲ CPT Assistant Fall 93:21, Mar 96:10, May 96:6, Feb 97:7, Apr 97:11, Aug 97:6

(Do not report 11040-11044 in addition to 97601, 97602)

Figure 16-2. Examples of CPT codes, surgical section.

Source: American Medical Association, *Current Procedural Terminology,* copyright 2003.

more accurately lead to finding main numbers and modifiers that reflect the services performed. That is the only way to ensure reimbursement at the highest allowed level.

Add-On Codes. A plus sign (+) is used for **add-on codes,** indicating procedures that are usually carried out in addition to another procedure. For example, code 90471 covers one immunization administration, and code 90472 covers administering an additional shot. Add-on codes are never reported alone. They are used together with the primary code.

Modifiers. One or more two-digit **modifiers** may be assigned to the five-digit main number. Modifiers are written with a hyphen after the five-digit number and before the two-digit number. The use of a modifier shows that some special circumstance applies to the service or procedure the physician performed. For example, in the surgery section, the modifier *-62* indicates that two surgeons worked together, each performing part of a surgical procedure during an operation. Each physician will be paid part of the amount normally reimbursed for that procedure code. Appendix A of the CPT explains the proper use of each modifier. Some section guidelines also discuss the use of modifiers with the section's codes.

Category II Codes, Category III Codes, and Unlisted Procedure Codes. Category II codes are used to track health-care performance measures, such as programs and counseling to avoid tobacco use. Category III codes are temporary CPT codes for emerging technology, services, and procedures. When no code is available to completely describe a procedure, a code for an unlisted procedure is selected. Unlisted procedure codes are used for new services or procedures that have not yet been assigned codes in CPT. When these codes are used, which is rare, a written explanation of the procedure or service is needed.

Evaluation and Management Services

To diagnose conditions and plan treatments, physicians use a wide range of time, effort, and skill for different patients and circumstances. Evaluation and management codes **(E/M codes)** are often considered the most important of all CPT codes, because they can be used by all physicians in any medical specialty.

The E/M section guidelines explain how to code different levels of these services. Three key factors documented in the patient's medical record help determine the level of service:

1. The extent of the patient history taken
2. The extent of the examination conducted
3. The complexity of the medical decision making

Payers also want to know whether the physician treated a **new patient** or an **established patient.** Physicians often spend more time during new patients' visits than during visits from established patients, so the E/M codes for the two types of patients are separate. For reporting purposes, the CPT considers a patient "new" if that person has not received professional services from the physician within the past three years. An established patient is one who has seen the physician within the past three years. (Note that the current visit need not be for a problem treated previously.) Emergency patients are not classified as either new or established patients.

The CPT has a range of five codes each for new-patient or established-patient encounters. The lowest-level code is often called a Level I code; the highest-level code is a Level V code. For example, code 99213 is the Level III code for an established patient's office visit.

The location of the service is also important because different E/M codes apply to services performed in a physician's office, a hospital inpatient room, a hospital emergency room, a nursing facility, an extended-care facility, or a patient's home.

Surgical Procedures

Figure 16-2 illustrates a series of codes from the integumentary part of the surgical section. Codes listed in the surgery section represent all the procedures that are normally a part of that operation, including local anesthesia, the surgery itself, and routine follow-up care. This combination of services is called a surgical package. Payers assign a fee to each of these codes that pays for all the services provided under them.

The period of time that is covered for follow-up care is called the **global period.** For example, the global period for repairing a tendon might be set at 15 days. A global period for major surgery such as an appendectomy might be set at 100 days. After the global period ends, additional services can be reported separately for payment.

To make the coding process more efficient, medical offices often list frequently used CPT codes on superbills. After seeing the patient, the physician checks off the appropriate procedures or services. An example of a dermatology practice's superbill is shown in Figure 16-3. This sample superbill lists the E/M codes for new and established patient office visits as well as common procedures for the office.

Laboratory Procedures

Organ or disease-oriented **panels** listed in the pathology and laboratory section of the CPT include tests frequently ordered together. An electrolyte panel, for example, includes tests for carbon dioxide, chloride, potassium, and sodium. Each element of the panel has its own procedure code. However, when the tests are performed together, the code for the panel must be used rather than the separate procedure codes.

appropriate reimbursement for reported services by submitting correct health-care claims. These claims, as well as the process used to create them, must comply with the rules imposed by federal and state law and with payer requirements.

Code Linkage

On correct claims, each reported service is connected to a diagnosis that supports the procedure as necessary to investigate or treat the patient's condition. Insurance company representatives analyze this connection between the diagnostic and the procedural information, called **code linkage,** to evaluate the medical necessity of the reported charges. Correct claims also comply with many other regulations from government agencies.

The possible consequences of inaccurate coding and incorrect billing include:

- Denied claims
- Delays in processing claims and receiving payments
- Reduced payments
- Fines and other sanctions
- Loss of hospital privileges
- Exclusion from payers' programs
- Prison sentences
- Loss of the physician's license to practice medicine

To avoid errors, the codes on health-care claims are checked against the medical documentation. A code review checks these key points:

- Are the codes appropriate to the patient's profile (age, gender, condition; new or established), and is each coded service billable?
- Is there a clear and correct link between each diagnosis and procedure?
- Have the payer's rules about the diagnosis and the procedure been followed?
- Does the documentation in the patient's medical record support the reported services?
- Do the reported services comply with all regulations?

Insurance Fraud

Almost everyone involved in the delivery of health care is a trustworthy person devoted to patients' welfare. However, some people are not. For example, according to the Department of Health and Human Services (HHS), in one year alone, the federal government recovered more than $1.3 billion in judgments, settlements, and other fees in health-care fraud cases. Fraud is an act of deception used to take advantage of another person or entity. For example, it is fraudulent for people to misrepresent their credentials or to forge another person's signature on a check.

Claims fraud occurs when physicians or others falsely represent their services or charges to payers. For example,

a provider may bill for services that were not performed, overcharge for services, or fail to provide complete services under a contract. A patient may exaggerate an injury to get a settlement from an insurance company or ask a medical assistant to change a date on a chart so that a service is covered by a health plan.

A number of coding and billing practices are fraudulent. Investigators reviewing physicians' billings look for patterns like these:

- Reporting services that were not performed.
  Example: A lab bills Medicare for a general health panel (CPT 80050), but fails to perform one of the tests in the panel.
- Reporting services at a higher level than was carried out.
  Example: After a visit for a flu shot, the provider bills the encounter as an evaluation and management service plus a vaccination.
- Performing and billing for procedures that are not related to the patient's condition and therefore not medically necessary.
  Example: After reading an article about Lyme disease, a patient is worried about having worked in her garden over the summer and requests a Lyme disease diagnostic test. Although no symptoms or signs have been reported, the physician orders and bills for the Lyme disease test.
- Billing separately for services that are bundled in a single procedure code.
  Example: When a physician orders a comprehensive metabolic panel (CPT 80053), the provider bills for the panel as well as for a quantitative glucose test, which is in the panel.
- Reporting the same service twice.

Note that HIPAA calls for penalties for giving remuneration to anyone eligible for benefits under federal health-care programs. The forgiveness or waiver of co-payments may violate the policies of some payers; others may permit forgiveness or waiver if they are aware of the reasons for the forgiveness or waiver, such as the patient's inability to pay. Routine forgiveness or waiver of co-payments may constitute fraud under state and federal law. The physician practice should ensure that its policies on co-payments are consistent with applicable law and with the requirements of their agreements with payers.

Compliance Plans

To avoid the risk of fraud, medical offices have a **compliance plan** to uncover compliance problems and correct them. A compliance plan is a process for finding, correcting, and preventing illegal medical office practices. Its goals are to:

- Prevent fraud and abuse through a formal process to identify, investigate, fix, and prevent repeat violations

is l
Th
de
pri
un
me
fra

In

Inj
tox
giv
or
wit
uat
do

Medical Coder, Physician Practice

Medical coding specialists work in a number of health-care settings, including medical practices, hospitals, government agencies, and insurance companies. Coders who work in physician practices review patients' medical records and assign diagnosis and procedure codes. They are knowledgeable about the coding rules and procedures for physicians' work, which are different than those for coding hospital services. The position of medical coding specialist is growing in importance in physician practices. Accurate coding is a critical part of ensuring that claims follow the legal and ethical requirements of Medicare and other third-party payers as well as HIPAA regulations.

Medical office employees may gain required health-care work experience and then attain coding positions through coding education from seminars or college classes. Certification as a professional coder offers an excellent route to success as a medical coder in the medical practice setting. Some employers require certification for employment; others state that certification must be earned after a certain amount of time in the position, such as six months. Coding classes followed by examinations are used to obtain certification. Three physician-office coding certifications are available. All require a high school diploma or equivalent.

- The American Health Information Management Association offers the Certified Coding Associate (CCA) credential and the Certified Coding Specialist—Physician-based (CCS-P) credential. The CCA is an entry-level title; completion of either a training program or six months' job experience is recommended. The CCS-P requires at least three years of coding experience.

- The American Academy of Professional Coders offers the Certified Professional Coder (CPC) credential, also requiring coursework and on-the-job experience.

Medical assistants who hold these credentials and have coding experience may advance to coding management and coding compliance auditor positions. Becoming expert in a specialty such as surgical coding also offers advancement opportunities.

relating to reimbursement for health-care services provided

- Ensure compliance with applicable federal, state, and local laws, including employment laws and environmental laws as well as antifraud laws
- Help defend physicians if they are investigated or prosecuted for fraud by showing the desire to behave compliantly and thus reduce any fines or criminal prosecution

When a compliance plan is in place, it demonstrates to payers such as Medicare that honest, ongoing attempts have been made to find and fix weak areas of compliance with regulations. The development of this written plan is led by a compliance officer and committee with the intention to (1) audit and monitor compliance with government regulations, especially in the area of coding and billing, (2) develop written policies and procedures that are consistent, (3) provide for ongoing staff training and communication, and (4) respond to and correct errors.

Although coding and billing compliance are the plan's major focus, it covers all areas of government regulation of medical practices, such as equal employment opportunity (EEO) regulations (for example, hiring and promotion policies) and OSHA regulations (for example, fire safety and handling of hazardous materials such as blood-borne pathogens).

Summary

The ICD-9-CM is used for diagnostic coding in the United States. ICD-9 codes are required for reporting patients' conditions on health-care claims. Codes are made up of three, four, or five numbers and a description. New codes are issued annually, and current codes should be used because they can affect billing and reimbursement.

The ICD-9 has two volumes that are used in medical practices: the Tabular List (Volume 1) and the Alphabetic Index (Volume 2). To find a code, use the Alphabetic Index first. Its main terms may be followed by related terms. The codes themselves are organized into 17 chapters and are listed in numerical order in the Tabular List. Code categories consist of three-digit groupings of a single disease or a related condition. Further clinical detail is shown by four- or five-digit codes. The conventions used in the ICD-9 must be observed to correctly select codes.

V codes identify encounters for reasons other than illness or injury and are used for healthy patients receiving routine services, for therapeutic encounters, for a problem that is not currently affecting the patient's condition, and for preoperative evaluations. E codes, which are never used as primary codes, classify the injuries resulting from various environmental events.

CPT provides a standardized list of five-digit procedure codes for medical, surgical, and diagnostic services. Add-on codes and modifiers may also be selected.

CPT is divided into six sections: (1) evaluation and management, (2) anesthesiology, (3) surgery, (4) radiology, (5) pathology and laboratory, and (6) medicine. The three main factors that influence the level of service for coding purposes are the type and extent of (1) history, (2) examination, and (3) medical decision making. Surgical packages and laboratory panels should be coded as single procedures rather than broken into component parts.

The Health Care Common Procedure Coding System (HCPCS), used to code Medicare services, has codes from CPT as well as Level II national codes.

Diagnoses and procedures must be correctly linked when services are reported for reimbursement because payers analyze this connection to determine the medical necessity of the charges. Correct claims also comply with all applicable regulations and requirements. Codes should be appropriate and documented as well as compliant with each payer's rules.

A medical practice compliance plan addresses compliance concerns of government and private payers. Furthermore, having a formal process in place is a sign that the practice has made a good-faith effort to achieve compliance in coding.

CASE STUDY QUESTIONS

Now that you have completed this chapter, review the case study at the beginning of the chapter and answer the following questions:

1. How would you select the ICD-9 and CPT codes for a health-care claim for this visit?
2. What diagnosis and procedure codes will result in the correct payment for these services?
3. How should the claim show the medical necessity of the procedures?
4. Locate the ICD-9 code for the patient's asthma. How many digits are required? What code did you assign?
5. Locate the CPT code for the cardiovascular stress test. What information did you use to select it from the list of related codes?

Discussion Questions

1. What are the differences among the three code sets discussed in the chapter?
2. Are *see* cross-references in the Alphabetic Index of the ICD-9 followed by codes? Why?
3. Would you expect to locate codes for the following services or procedures in CPT? What range or series of codes would you investigate?
   a. Routine obstetric care including antepartum care, cesarean delivery, and postpartum care
   b. Echocardiography (cardiac)
   c. Radiologic examination, nasal bones, complete
   d. Home visit for evaluation and management of an established patient
   e. Drug test for amphetamines
   f. Anesthesia for cardiac catheterization
4. Why are both the ICD-9 and CPT codes updated each year?

Critical Thinking Questions

1. What is the proper order in which to select a diagnosis code?
2. Why is it necessary to report the most specific diagnosis codes available?
3. What could result if a medical assistant enters an incorrect diagnosis code on a claim?

4. How can improving physicians' documentation of diagnoses and procedures help ensure compliance?
5. A patient asked a medical assistant to help her out of a tough financial spot. Her medical insurance authorized her to receive four radiation treatments for her condition, one every 35 days. Because she was out of town, she did not schedule her appointment for the last treatment until today, which is one week beyond the approved period. The health plan will not reimburse her for this procedure. The patient asks the MA to change the date on the record to last Wednesday so that it will be covered, explaining that no one will be hurt by this change, and anyway, she pays the insurance company plenty.

   What type of action is the patient asking the MA to do? How should the request be handled?

Application Activities

1. A. A female patient is taking a medication that is known to affect the lining of the endometrium. She received an endometrial biopsy and pelvic ultrasound to monitor changes. What type of ICD-9 code is used to describe the medical need for these services?

   B. A patient fell off a ladder while on the job, spraining his left ankle and fracturing the right femur. In addition to the main code, what type of ICD-9 code is used to report his diagnosis?
2. Study Table 1 in the guidelines for the evaluation and management section of CPT. What code range is used for emergency department services? Now turn to Appendix A. Is it correct to use modifier -21 with E/M codes? Modifier -51?
3. Underline the main term in each of the following diagnoses and then determine the correct ICD-9 codes.
   a. cerebral atherosclerosis
   b. spasmodic asthma with status asthmaticus
   c. congenital night blindness
   d. recurrent inguinal hernia with obstruction
   e. incomplete bundle branch heart block
4. Find the following codes in the index of CPT. Underline the key term you used to find the code.
   a. Intracapsular lens extraction
   b. Coombs test
   c. X-ray of duodenum
   d. Unlisted procedure, maxillofacial prosthetics
   e. DTAP immunization

REVIEW

CHAPTER 16

 Internet Activities

1. Both the American Health Information Management Association (AHIMA) and the American Academy of Professional Coders (AAPC) are national associations that certify medical coders and provide information on coding issues. Visit their Web sites and investigate the ways these associations keep their members up-to-date about changes in procedural coding. Also review the activities of these organizations in your local area.

2. Access the Web site of the National Center for Health Statistics and locate information on the current year's ICD-9-CM new codes. Also research and report on the status of ICD-10-CM.

3. Visit the American Medical Association's Web site and search on the terms *Category II* and *Category III*. Review the latest codes in these categories.

Patient Billing and Collections

AREAS OF COMPETENCE

2003 Role Delineation Study

ADMINISTRATIVE

Practice Finances
- Apply bookkeeping principles
- Manage accounts receivable

CHAPTER OUTLINE

- Basic Accounting
- Standard Payment Procedures
- Standard Billing Procedures
- Standard Collection Procedures
- Credit Arrangements
- Common Collection Problems

KEY TERMS

accounts payable
accounts receivable
age analysis
class action lawsuit
credit
credit bureau
cycle billing
damages
disclosure statement
legal custody
open-book account
punitive damages
single-entry account
statement
statute of limitations
superbill
written-contract account

OBJECTIVES

After completing Chapter 17, you will be able to:

17.1 Discuss the importance of accounts receivable to a medical practice.
17.2 Explain how to accept and account for payment from patients.
17.3 Prepare an invoice.
17.4 Manage a billing cycle efficiently.
17.5 Describe standard collection techniques.
17.6 Explain how to perform a credit check.
17.7 Identify credit arrangements.
17.8 Recognize common collection problems.

Introduction

Medical assisting is a multifaceted career. As such, a person in that career may be required to take on many duties in the medical office that are administrative in nature. The medical office has customers who have various payment arrangements, such as third-party payers (usually insurance carriers) and payment plans, and who may also have large outstanding balances. A proper understanding and administration of billing—for both third-party payers and patients—as well as payment collection methods is therefore required.

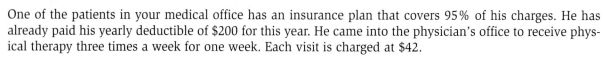

CASE STUDY

One of the patients in your medical office has an insurance plan that covers 95% of his charges. He has already paid his yearly deductible of $200 for this year. He came into the physician's office to receive physical therapy three times a week for one week. Each visit is charged at $42.

As you read this chapter, consider the following questions:
1. What is the total owed for this patient's visits?
2. How much of the total is not covered by insurance and should be billed to the patient?

Basic Accounting

In any business, basic accounting involves managing accounts receivable and accounts payable. **Accounts receivable** is the term for income, or money, owed to the business. **Accounts payable** is the term for money owed by the business. In a medical practice, accounts receivable represents the money patients owe in return for medical services. Accounts payable describes the money the medical practice must pay out to run the practice.

Billing and collections are vitally important tasks because they convert the practice's accounts receivable into readily available income, or cash flow, from which the accounts payable can be paid. Unless billing and collections are carried out effectively, a practice might have plenty of money due in accounts receivable without having enough cash flow for accounts payable.

There are methods of improving billing and collection procedures to increase income for the practice. You will need to know about standard payment, billing, and collection procedures as well as about credit arrangements and common problems in collecting payment.

Standard Payment Procedures

Most physicians prefer to collect payment from patients at each office visit. Immediate payment not only brings income into the practice faster, but it saves the cost of preparing and mailing bills and collecting on past-due accounts. For these reasons, many physicians' offices post a small sign at the reception desk that states, for example, "Payment is requested when services are rendered unless other arrangements are made in advance."

As a medical assistant, you are responsible for collecting these payments. If the patient cannot pay at the time of the visit, it is your responsibility to bill for the physician's services. A bill, the paperwork sent to patients to inform them of payment or balance due, is referred to as an invoice.

Determining Appropriate Fees

A fee schedule is a price list for the medical practice. Figure 17-1 shows an example. The fee schedule lists the services the doctor offers and the corresponding charges for those services. Fees are not randomly assigned. They reflect the cost of services, the doctor's experience, charges of other doctors in the area, and other factors. Sometimes the fee allowed by insurance policies is a determining factor. The practice may use a particular system to determine how much to charge for each service. Following are descriptions of these systems.

Usual and Customary Fees. A usual fee is the fee a doctor charges for a service or procedure. A customary fee is either the average fee charged for a service or procedure by all comparable doctors in the same region or the ninetieth percentile of all fees charged by comparable doctors in the same region for the same procedure. There is a growing tendency, however, to determine fees by national rather than regional trends.

Relative Value Unit. Section 121 of the Social Security Act Amendments of 1994 required CMS to develop a methodology for a resource-based system. This system was created to determine practice expense relative value units (RVUs) for all Medicare physician fee schedule services. Effective January 1, 1999, Phase 1 of resource-based practice expense was put into effect.

For each medical service, an RVU is assigned that reflects the following factors:

- The doctor's skill and time required
- The professional liability expenses related to that service, such as malpractice insurance
- The overhead costs associated with that service

The RVUs are converted to dollar amounts. These dollar amounts form the basis of the RVU fee schedule. This schedule creates uniform payments that are adjusted for geographic differences.

This methodology has reduced the growth rate of spending for doctors' professional services, related services and supplies, and other Medicare Part B services.

Processing Charge Slips

Fees must be determined in order to create a charge slip, the original record of the doctor's services and the charges for those services. Figure 17-2 shows an example of a

John Q. Davis, MD
Adult and Pediatric Urology-Infertility

SERVICE RENDERED	CPT	FEE
Initial OV	99204	$100.00
Follow-up Visit	99214	$65.00
Fertility Consultation	99243	$140.00
Office Consultation	99244	$140.00
Hospital Admission	99223	$150.00
Hospital Consultation	99254	$150.00
ER Visit	99284	$75.00–$150.00
Hospital Visit	99232	$55.00
Urinalysis w/ Micro	81000	$14.00
Culture	87086	$45.00
Stone Analysis	32360	$60.00
Venipuncture	36415	$10.00

SERVICE RENDERED	CPT	FEE
Condyloma Treatment	54050	$40.00
Cystoscopy	52000	$300.00
Catheterization	93975	$45.00
Vasectomy	55250	$775.00
Ultrasonic Guide Needle Biopsy	76942	$395.00
Prostate Biopsy	55700	$325.00
Biopsy Gun	A9270	$45.00
Uroflowmeter	51741	$80.00
Renal Ultrasound	76775	$295.00
Scrotal Ultrasound	76870	$295.00
Acidic Acid	99070	$20.00
Foley Catheter Starter Set	A4329	$35.00

Figure 17-1. The fee schedule shows the charges for services provided by the practice.

DATE	DESCRIPTION–CODE	CHARGE	PAYMENT	CURRENT BALANCE

(918) 555-9680   Tax ID No. 11-0004004

Patricia Belden, MD
111 Roosevelt Boulevard
Lawrence, OK 77527

99205 Office Visit, New Patient	36425 Venipuncture	59025 NST
99215 Office Visit, Established Patient	57454 Colposcopy with Biopsy	54150 Circumcision
99213 Office Visit, Established, Brief	57511 Cryosurgery	58300 IUD Insertion
88155 Pap	58100 Endometrial Biopsy	57170 Diaphragm Fitting
84703 Urine Pregnancy Test	56600 Vulva Biopsy	

NAME_____ DX _____ No. 0005807

Figure 17-2. A charge slip shows the services performed for a patient and the charges for those services.

charge slip. Charge slips are also called fee slips or transaction slips. They are usually numbered consecutively. They may be preprinted with common services and charges for the practice. Charge slips are used in several ways.

Some doctors keep a pad of charge slips on their desk. After seeing a patient, they fill in the services and charges on the charge slip. They give the charge slip to the patient and ask the patient to give it to you on the way out of the office.

In other offices, you may write the patient's name on the charge slip and give the slip to the doctor along with the patient's medical record. The doctor then fills in the services performed and asks you to fill in the charges according to the fee schedule. If questions arise about the fee for a particular service, you can refer to the fee schedule and tell the patient how much that service will cost.

Accepting Payment

When the patient comes to you with the charge slip, you complete the charge slip and ask for payment. There are several effective yet diplomatic ways to request payment. Two examples are, "For today's visit, the total charge is $50. How would you like to pay?" and "The charge for your laboratory work today is $80. Would you like to pay for that now?" Most practices accept several forms of payment, including cash, check, credit card, and insurance. Insurance payment is discussed in detail in Chapter 15.

Cash. If the patient chooses to pay in cash, count the money carefully to be sure you have received the proper amount. Next, record the payment on the patient's ledger card, and give the patient a receipt. (Patient ledger cards are explained in Chapter 18.)

Some practices use a combination charge slip/receipt, which is discussed in Chapter 18. If your practice does not, prepare a cash receipt manually, as shown in Figure 17-3. Then place the money in the cash drawer or cash box.

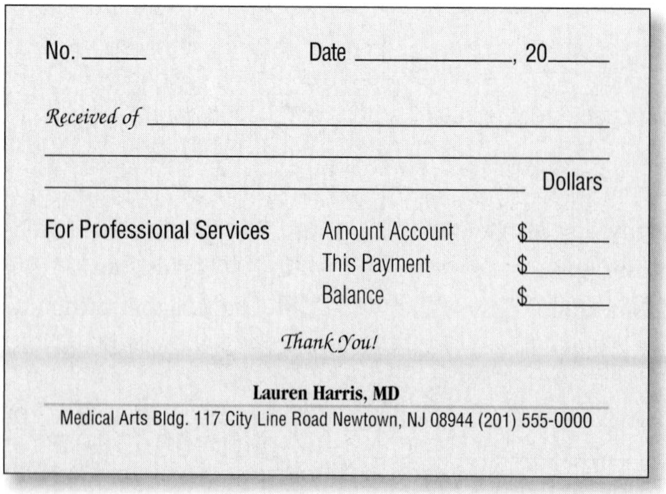
No. ____ Date ________, 20____

Received of ________________

________________ Dollars

For Professional Services Amount Account $____
This Payment $____
Balance $____

Thank You!

Lauren Harris, MD
Medical Arts Bldg. 117 City Line Road Newtown, NJ 08944 (201) 555-0000

Figure 17-3. After writing a receipt for cash, record the payment on the patient's ledger card.

Check. If the patient pays by check, be sure the check is written properly, including the current date. The amount of the check should match the total amount listed on the charge slip, unless the patient has made prior arrangements to pay only part of the amount. The name of the doctor or practice should appear in the "Pay to the Order of" section and should be properly spelled. The check should be signed by the person whose name is printed on the check. After accepting the check, endorse it immediately, and deposit it in the practice bank account.

Credit Card. Many doctors' offices accept credit cards, such as Visa or MasterCard. This payment method offers advantages for both the practice and the patient. For the practice, it provides prompt payment from the credit card company, thus increasing cash flow. It also reduces the amount of time and money spent on preparing and mailing bills, thus decreasing expenses. For the patient, it is convenient and allows a large bill to be paid in several smaller amounts, usually once a month.

Credit cards have one major disadvantage for the practice—cost. The credit card company deducts a percentage of each charge for its collection service, usually between 1% and 5%. If a patient charges $100 in services on a credit card, for example, the practice receives only $95 to $99. The credit card company keeps the difference. A disadvantage for patients is the accrued interest charges on unpaid balances.

If the practice accepts credit card payments, the American Medical Association (AMA) suggests several guidelines.

- Do not set higher fees for patients who pay by credit card.
- Do not encourage patients to use credit cards for payment.
- Do not advertise outside the office that the practice accepts credit cards.

If a patient chooses to pay by credit card, process the transaction carefully to ensure that the credit card company charges the patient correctly. To begin, inform the patient of the amount due, and ask for the credit card.

Check the expiration date on the front of the credit card. If the card has not expired, place it in the credit card machine, and place a credit card voucher on top of it. Slide the imprint arm firmly to the right and back across the machine. Remove the voucher from the machine. Write in the date, and circle the type of credit card, such as Visa or MasterCard, after it is removed from the machine.

Next, obtain the authorization code from the credit card company. Some offices have devices that read the magnetic strip on the credit card and automatically transmit the information to the credit card company by telephone line (Figure 17-4). If your office has such a device, type in the amount to be charged on its keypad. Then, the credit card company issues an authorization code, which appears on the device's screen.

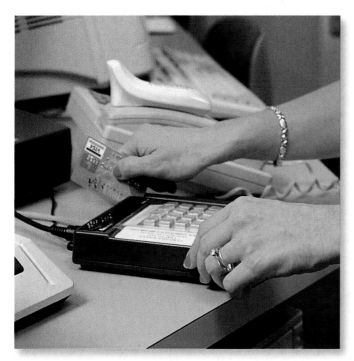

Figure 17-4. Using a device like this one, you can swipe the patient's card through the machine and obtain instant authorization from the credit card company.

If your office does not have such a device, call the credit card company for the authorization code. Give the operator the patient's credit card number and the amount of the payment. The operator then gives you the authorization code.

Write the authorization code in the box marked "Authorization" on the credit card voucher. Initial the voucher in the appropriate box. Then, fill in the services provided and the amount of the charges. Enter the total charges in the box marked "Total."

Give the voucher to the patient to sign. Compare the patient's signature on the voucher with the signature on the back of the credit card (they should, of course, be identical). Keep one copy of the voucher for the office. Give the other copy and the credit card to the patient.

Using the Pegboard System for Posting Payments

Some physicians' offices use the pegboard system to post payments and generate receipts for patients. If your office uses the pegboard system, you may use the pegboard to record the payment on the ledger card and receipt simultaneously. You handle this task in basically the same way, whether the patient pays immediately or later, in response to a bill.

Determining Payment Responsibility

Generally the patient is responsible for payments for medical services. To help promote timely payments, however, you need to know exactly who is responsible for them.

Third-Party Liability. Third-party liability refers to the responsibility of the patient's insurance company to pay for certain medical expenses, which may include doctors' services. Each practice decides how to handle its patients' health insurance claims.

Some practices do not accept any insurance, although these practices are rare. The patient must pay the doctor directly and file an insurance claim for reimbursement. If you work in such a practice, you must give the patient the necessary medical information to fill out the insurance claim. A completed superbill (discussed later in this chapter) provides the information.

Practices increasingly handle all their patients' insurance paperwork to ensure accuracy, timely submission, and prompt payment. Some practices charge a fee for handling patients' insurance claims. Some practices handle paperwork only for patients who find it particularly difficult, such as those who are frail or disabled.

If you work in an office that handles insurance paperwork, you can submit insurance claims manually or electronically. Regardless of which method you use, be sure to use the proper forms, complete them correctly, and submit them within the time limits set by insurers. (Procedures for completing insurance forms and filing claims are discussed in Chapter 15.)

TRICARE, which provides health insurance for dependents of active-duty and retired military personnel, operates differently from other insurers. TRICARE pays the doctor through a local fiscal agent. Patients pay any co-payments and deductible amounts. You must adjust for the difference between the billed fees and the amounts received from TRICARE and the patient. If a TRICARE patient fails to pay the patient's portion, you may take steps to obtain payment just as you would with any other patient.

Responsibility for Minors. When a child's parents are married, either parent may consent (agree) to treatment for the minor child (child under age 18). Both parents are responsible for payment for the minor's treatment. If you must send them a bill, you should address it to both parents to ensure payment. There is one exception to this process. Anyone under the age of 18 who is no longer living at home and is self-supporting is considered an emancipated minor and is responsible for payment. For example, a 16-year-old girl who is pregnant and leaves her parents' home to set up a household with her boyfriend is considered an emancipated minor.

Divorce or separation can create confusion about which parent can consent to the child's treatment and which of the two is responsible for payment. The parent who has **legal custody,** or the court-decreed right to make decisions about a child's upbringing, is the parent who has consent ability and payment responsibility. A divorced couple's legal and financial arrangements are considered private information, however. Therefore, you should assume that the parent who brings the child for treatment has consent ability and payment responsibility. The physician should inform the responsible parent of this assumption before providing treatment.

Professional Courtesy. As a matter of professional courtesy, a doctor may treat some patients free of charge or for just the amount covered by the patient's insurance. These patients often include other doctors and their families, the practice's staff members (including medical assistants) and their families, other health-care professionals (including pharmacists and dentists), clergy members, and hospital employees. If the patient is part of a managed care organization or has Medicare, the provider must collect any co-payment or deductible as part of the contracted agreement with the provider. It may be considered fraud to consistently not collect co-payments or deductibles.

Be sure you know the doctor's policy so that you do not bill these patients in error. If, for example, the doctor agrees to accept only the amount paid by the patient's insurance, note this professional courtesy on the patient's ledger card, and do not request co-payment.

Standard Billing Procedures

If the physician extends credit to patients, you need to know how to prepare invoices. You also have to manage related billing responsibilities, such as establishing and maintaining billing cycles.

Preparing Invoices

As a medical assistant, part of your job is to prepare an invoice to mail to the patient who does not pay when services are rendered or who makes only a partial payment. Figure 17-5 shows an invoice with an itemized list of services. You can obtain most of the information for the invoice from the patient ledger card. The invoice should include the following information:

- Physician's name, address, and telephone number
- Patient's name and address
- Balance (if any) from the previous month(s)
- Itemized list of services and charges, by date, for the current month
- Payments from the patient or insurer during the month
- Total balance due

Whatever invoicing procedure you use, enclose a self-addressed envelope with the invoice to encourage prompt payment.

Using Codes on the Invoice. Write the name of each procedure on the itemized list, or use codes for common procedures, such as OV for office visit. If you use codes, be sure that an explanation of the codes appears with the invoice. (Many practices use invoices with a key to the codes printed at the bottom.) Using an itemized list on invoices is standard procedure in most physicians' offices and is required by all health insurance plans. After completing the invoice, fold it in thirds, and mail it in a typewritten business envelope.

Using the Patient's Ledger Card as an Invoice. As an alternative to writing or typing the invoice, you may photocopy the patient's ledger card and fold the photocopy so that the patient's address shows through the window in a window envelope. If you prepare invoices this way, be sure there are no stray marks or comments written on the card. Also, be sure the photocopy is clean and easy to read.

Generating the Invoice by Computer. In computerized offices, you may print out an invoice for each patient account that has a balance due. Follow the instructions in the software manufacturer's manual. You can then fold the printouts and mail them in window envelopes.

Using an Independent Billing Service. Large practices may have invoices handled by an independent billing service. The billing service may rapidly copy ledger cards for patients with balances due. Then it mails the copies to patients, usually with an envelope for sending payment directly to the physician's office.

Sending Invoices Electronically to Insurance Companies. Invoices to insurance companies may be prepared using one of the methods just described. Physicians' offices that have a computer and modem may bill insurance companies electronically, as discussed in Chapter 15.

Using the Superbill

Some doctors' offices use a **superbill,** which includes the charges for services rendered on that day, an invoice for payment or insurance co-payment, and all the information for submitting an insurance claim. Figure 17-6 shows an example of a superbill. Having all this information on one form saves time and paperwork. These forms are often printed on NCR (no-carbon-required) paper with copies for the practice, patient, and insurance company.

Complete as much of the superbill as possible at the beginning of the patient's visit. (See Procedure 17-1 for specific instructions.) Some practices use a computerized version of the superbill, printing it out instead of completing the initial information by hand. Attach the superbill to the patient's medical record, and give them both to the doctor before he sees the patient.

Managing Billing Cycles

Many practices send out their bills just after the end of each month. You can send out bills at any regular time, however, such as once a week or twice a month. You may also send bills at a particular time of the month at the patient's request.

Cycle billing is a common billing system that bills each patient only once a month but spreads the work of billing over the month. Using this system, you send invoices to groups of patients every few days.

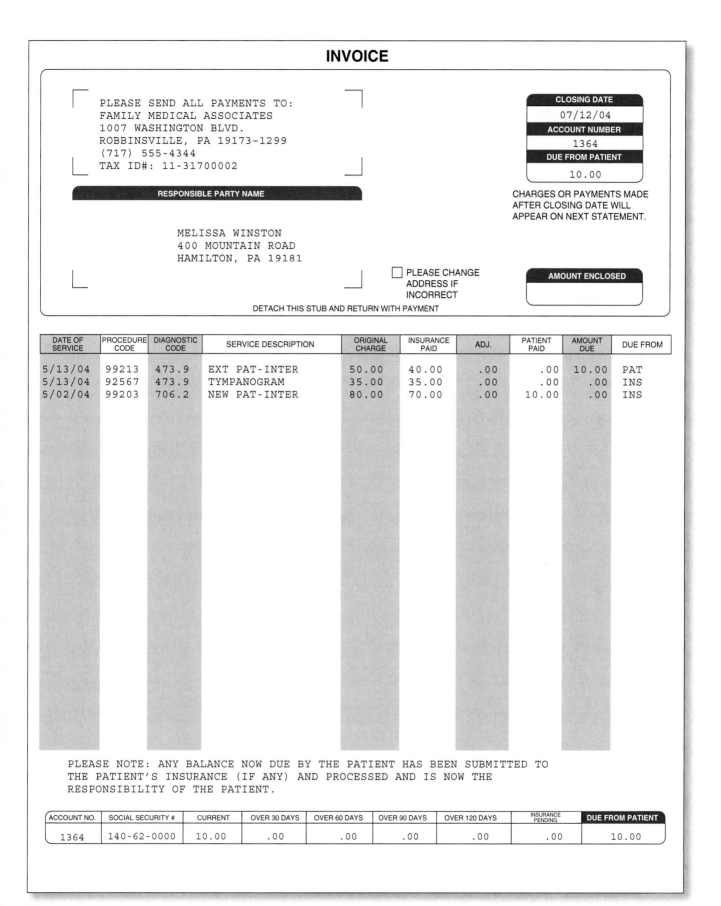

INVOICE

PLEASE SEND ALL PAYMENTS TO:
FAMILY MEDICAL ASSOCIATES
1007 WASHINGTON BLVD.
ROBBINSVILLE, PA 19173-1299
(717) 555-4344
TAX ID#: 11-31700002

CLOSING DATE
07/12/04
ACCOUNT NUMBER
1364
DUE FROM PATIENT
10.00

CHARGES OR PAYMENTS MADE
AFTER CLOSING DATE WILL
APPEAR ON NEXT STATEMENT.

RESPONSIBLE PARTY NAME

MELISSA WINSTON
400 MOUNTAIN ROAD
HAMILTON, PA 19181

☐ PLEASE CHANGE
ADDRESS IF
INCORRECT

AMOUNT ENCLOSED

DETACH THIS STUB AND RETURN WITH PAYMENT

DATE OF SERVICE	PROCEDURE CODE	DIAGNOSTIC CODE	SERVICE DESCRIPTION	ORIGINAL CHARGE	INSURANCE PAID	ADJ.	PATIENT PAID	AMOUNT DUE	DUE FROM
5/13/04	99213	473.9	EXT PAT-INTER	50.00	40.00	.00	.00	10.00	PAT
5/13/04	92567	473.9	TYMPANOGRAM	35.00	35.00	.00	.00	.00	INS
5/02/04	99203	706.2	NEW PAT-INTER	80.00	70.00	.00	10.00	.00	INS

PLEASE NOTE: ANY BALANCE NOW DUE BY THE PATIENT HAS BEEN SUBMITTED TO
THE PATIENT'S INSURANCE (IF ANY) AND PROCESSED AND IS NOW THE
RESPONSIBILITY OF THE PATIENT.

ACCOUNT NO.	SOCIAL SECURITY #	CURRENT	OVER 30 DAYS	OVER 60 DAYS	OVER 90 DAYS	OVER 120 DAYS	INSURANCE PENDING	DUE FROM PATIENT
1364	140-62-0000	10.00	.00	.00	.00	.00	.00	10.00

Figure 17-5. The invoice shows an itemized list of services and charges, organized by date, for the current month.

Lakeridge Medical Group
262 East Pine Street, Suite 100
Lakeridge, NJ 07500

☐ PRIVATE ☐ BLUECROSS ☐ IND. ☐ MEDICARE ☐ MEDI-CAL ☐ HMO ☐ PPO

PATIENT'S LAST NAME	FIRST	ACCOUNT #	BIRTHDATE / /	SEX ☐ MALE ☐ FEMALE	TODAY'S DATE / /
INSURANCE COMPANY	SUBSCRIBER		PLAN #	SUB. #	GROUP

ASSIGNMENT: I hereby assign my insurance benefits to be paid directly to the undersigned physician. I am financially responsible for non-covered services. SIGNED: (Patient, or Parent, if Minor) DATE: / /	RELEASE: I hereby authorize the physician to release to my insurance carrers any information required to process this claim. SIGNED: (Patient, or Parent, if Minor) DATE: / /

✔	DESCRIPTION	M/Care	CPT/Mod	DxRe	FEE	✔	DESCRIPTION	M/Care	CPT/Mod	DxRe	FEE	✔	DESCRIPTION	M/Care	CPT/Mod	DxRe	FEE
	OFFICE CARE						PROCEDURES						INJECTIONS/IMMUNIZATIONS				
	NEW PATIENT						Tread Mill (In Office)		93015				Tetanus		90718		
	Brief		99201				24 Hour Holter		93224				Hypertet	J1670	90782		
	Limited		99202				If Medicare (Set up Fec)		93225				Pneumococcal		90732		
	Intermediate		99203				Physician Interpret		93227				Influenza		90724		
	Extended		99204				EKG w/Interpretation		93000				TB Skin Test (PPD)		86585		
	Comprehensive		99205				EKG (Medicare)		93005				Antigen Injection-Single		95115		
							Sigmoidoscopy		45300				Multiple		95117		
	ESTABLISHED PATIENT						Sigmoidoscopy, Flexible		45330				B12 Injection	J3420	90782		
	Minimal		99211				Sigmoidos. , Flex. w/Bx.		45331				Injection, IM		90782		
	Brief		99212				Spirometry, FEV/FVC		94010				Compazine	J0780	90782		
	Limited		99213				Spirometry, Post-Dilator		94060				Demerol	J2175	90782		
	Intermediate		99214										Vistaril	J3410	90782		
	Extended		99215										Susphrine	J0170	90782		
	Comprehensive		99215				LABORATORY						Decadron	J0890	90782		
							Blood Draw Fee		36415				Estradiol	J1000	90782		
	CONSULTATION-OFFICE						Urinalysis, Chemical		81005				Testosterone	J1080	90782		
	Focused		99241				Throat Culture		87081				Lidocaine	J2000	90782		
	Expanded		99242				Occult Blood		82270				Solumedrol	J2920	90782		
	Detailed		99243				Pap Handling Charge		99000				Solucortef	J1720	90782		
	Comprehensive 1		99244				Pap Life Guard		88150-90				Hydeltra	J1690	90782		
	Comprehensive 2		99245				Gram Stain		87205				Pen Procaine	J2510	90788		
	Dr.						Hanging Drop		87210								
	Case Management		98900				Urine Drug Screen		99000				INJECTIONS - JOINT/BURSA				
													Small Joints		20600		
	Post-op Exam		99024										Intermediate		20605		
							SUPPLIES						Large Joints		20610		
													Trigger Point		20550		
													MISCELLANEOUS				

DIAGNOSIS:

	DIAGNOSIS:	ICD-9											
	Abdominal Pain	789.0		Gout	274.0		C.V.A. - Acute	436.		Electrolyte Dis.	276.9		Herpes Simplex	054.9
	Abscess (Site)	682.9		Asthma	493.90		Cere. Vas. Accid. (Old)	438		Fatigue	780.7		Herpes Zoster	053.9
	Adverse Drug Rx	995.2		Asthmatic Bronchitis	493.90		Cerumen	380.4		Fibrocys. Br. Dis	610.1		Hydrocele	603.9
	Alcohol Detox	291.8		Atrial Fib.	427.31		Chestwall Pain	786.59		Fracture (Site)	829.0		Hyperlipidemia	272.4
	Alcoholism	303.90		Atrial Tachi.	427.0		Cholecystitis	575.0		Open/Close			Hypertension	401.9
	Allergic Rhinitis	477		Bowel Obstruct.	560.9		Cholelithiasis	574.00		Fungal Infect. (Site)	110.8		Hyperthyroidism	242.9
	Allergy	995.3		Breast Mass	611.72		COPD	492.8		Gastric Ulcer	531.90		Hypothyroidism	244.9
	Alzheimer's Dis.	290.1		Bronchitis	490		Cirrhosis	571.5		Gastritis	535.0		Labyrinthitis	386.30
	Anemia	285.9		Bursitis	727.3		Cong. Heart Fail.	428.9		Gastroenteritis	558.9		Lipoma (Site)	214.9
	Anemia - Pernicious	281.0		Cancer, Breast (Site)	174.9		Conjunctivitis	372.30		G.I. Bleeding	578.9		Lymphoma	202.8
	Angina	413.9		Metastatic (Site)	199.1		Contusion (Site)	924.9		Glomerulonephritis	583.9		Mit. Valve Prolapse	424.0
	Anxiety Synd.	300.00		Colon	153.9		Costochondritis	733.99		Headache	784.0		Myocard. Infarction (Area)	410.9
	Appendicitis	541		Cancer, Rectal	154.1		Depression	311.		Headache, Tension	307.81		M.I., Old	412
	Arteriscl. H.D.	414.0		Lung (Site)	162.9		Dermatitis	692.9		Migraine (Type)	346.9		Myositis	729.1
	Arthritis, Osteo.	715.90		Skin (Site)	173.9		Diabetes Mellitus	250.00		Hemorrhoids	455.6		Nausea/Vomiting	787.0
	Rheumatoid	714.0		Card. Arrhythmia (Type)	427.9		Diabetic Ketosis	250.1		Hernia, Hiatal	553.3		Neuralgia	729.2
	Lupus	710.0		Cardiomyopathy	425.4		Diverticulitis	562.11		Inguinal	550.9		Nevus (Site)	216.9
				Cellulitis (Site)	682.9		Diverticulosis	562.10		Hepatitis	573.3		Obesity	278.0

DIAGNOSIS: (IF NOT CHECKED ABOVE)

SERVICES PERFORMED AT: ☐ Office ☐ E.R. ☐ ☐	☐ CLAIM CONTAINS NO ORDERED REFERRING SERVICE	REFERRING PHYSICIAN & I.D. NUMBER

RETURN APPOINTMENT INFORMATION: 5 - 10 - 15 - 20 - 30 - 40 - 60 [DAYS] [WKS.] [MOS.] [PRN]	NEXT APPOINTMENT M - T - W - TH - F - S DATE / / TIME:	AM PM	ACCEPT ASSIGNMENT? ☐ YES ☐ NO	DOCTOR'S SIGNATURE

INSTRUCTIONS TO PATIENT FOR FILING INSURANCE CLAIMS:	☐ CASH	TOTAL TODAY'S FEE	
1. Complete upper portion of this form, sign and date. 2. Attach this form to your own insurance company's form for direct reimbursement. **MEDICARE PATIENTS - DO NOT SEND THIS TO MEDICARE. WE WILL SUBMIT THE CLAIM FOR YOU.**	☐ CHECK #____ ☐ VISA ☐ MC ☐ CO-PAY	OLD BALANCE / TOTAL DUE AMOUNT REC'D. TODAY	

INSUR-A-BILL ® BIBBERO SYSTEMS, INC. • PETALUMA, CA • UP. SUPER. © 6/94 (BIBB/STOCK)

Figure 17-6. A superbill is a form that can also be used as a charge slip and invoice and can be submitted with insurance claims.

PROCEDURE 17.1

How to Bill With the Superbill

Objective: To complete a superbill accurately

Materials: Superbill, patient ledger card, patient information sheet, fee schedule, insurance code list, pen

Method

1. Make sure the doctor's name and address appear on the form.
2. From the patient ledger card and information sheet, fill in the patient data, such as name, sex, date of birth, and insurance information.
3. Fill in the place and date of service.
4. Attach the superbill to the patient's medical record, and give them both to the doctor.
5. Accept the completed superbill from the patient after the patient sees the doctor. Make sure that the doctor has indicated the diagnosis and the procedures performed.

6. If the doctor has not already recorded the charges, refer to the fee schedule for procedures that are marked. Then fill in the charges next to those procedures.
7. In the appropriate blanks, list the total charges for the visit, and the previous balance (if any). Deduct any payments or adjustments received before this visit.
8. Calculate the subtotal.
9. Fill in the amount and type of payment (cash, check, money order, or credit card) made by the patient during this visit.
10. Calculate and enter the new balance.
11. Have the patient sign the authorization-and-release section of the superbill.
12. Keep a copy of the superbill for the practice records. Give the original to the patient along with one copy to file with the insurer.

For example, you may bill on the fifth of the month for patients whose last names begin with A through D. Then, on the tenth of the month, you may bill patients whose names begin with E through H, and so on. In a larger office with more patients, you may prefer to bill more frequently but to smaller groups of patients.

Standard Collection Procedures

Although most patients pay invoices within the standard 30-day period, some do not. When a patient does not pay an invoice during the standard period, you need to take steps to collect the payment. For example, you may need to call or write the patient to determine the reason for nonpayment or to set up a payment arrangement.

Whether you use telephone calls, notes, or letters, there are laws, such as statutes of limitations, and professional standards to guide your efforts to collect overdue payments from patients.

State Statute of Limitations

A **statute of limitations** is a state law that sets a time limit on when a collection suit on a past-due account can legally be filed. The time limit varies with the type of account.

Open-Book Account. An **open-book account** is one that is open to charges made occasionally as needed.

Most of a physician's long-standing patients have this type of account. An open-book account uses the last date of payment or charge for each illness as the starting date for determining the time limit on that specific debt.

Written-Contract Account. A **written-contract account** is one in which the physician and patient sign an agreement stating that the patient will pay the bill in more than four installments. Some states allow longer time limits for these accounts than for open-book accounts. Written-contract accounts are regulated by the Truth in Lending Act, discussed later in this chapter.

Single-Entry Account. A **single-entry account** is an account with only one charge, usually for a small amount. For example, someone vacationing in your area might come in for treatment of a cold. This person's account would list only one office visit. If the vacationer did not become a regular patient, the account would be considered a single-entry account. Some states impose shorter time limits on single-entry accounts than on open-book accounts.

Using Collection Techniques

Individual practices have their own ways of approaching the task of collection. Most begin the process with telephone calls, letters, or statements.

Initial Telephone Calls or Letters. When calling a patient or sending a letter about collections, be friendly and sympathetic. (Do not call a patient at work and leave a message. That type of phone call is an invasion of privacy. Call the patient at home.) Assume that the patient forgot to pay or was temporarily unable to pay. If you do not receive a response to your telephone call or initial collection letter, your next letters may need to be more urgent in tone. Standard collection letters, such as the one shown in Figure 17-7, are available for you to fill in the details, or you can create a letter to reflect the style of the practice.

Preparing Statements. You might send the patient a statement for an account that is 30 days past due. A **statement** is similar to an invoice except that it contains a courteous reminder that payment is due. This reminder can be a typewritten note on the statement, a brightly colored sticker, or a separate handwritten note attached to the statement.

If an account is 60 days past due, you could send a collection letter that says, for example, "If you are unable to pay your account in full this month, please telephone our office at [number] to make payment arrangements."

If an account is 90 days past due, your collection letter can contain stronger wording. For example, it might say, "Please let us know when you plan to pay the $250 past-due balance. We have sent you three monthly reminders. If you cannot pay in full now, please contact us at [number] to make payment arrangements. We want to be understanding but need your cooperation."

If an account is 120 days or more past due, you can send a final letter. It might state, "Every courtesy has been extended to you in arranging for payment of your long overdue account. Unless we hear from you by [date], the account will be given to [name of collection agency] for collection." Be sure to note the cutoff date on the patient's ledger card. By law, you cannot threaten to send an account to a collection agency unless it will actually be sent on that cutoff date. Therefore, you must be sure you are ready to do so before you send such a letter.

If you still cannot collect payment, the physician may indeed choose to hire an outside collection agency. Once an agency has taken over the account, there should not be any more correspondence on this matter between the physician's office and the patient.

Preparing an Age Analysis

Age analysis is the process of classifying and reviewing past-due accounts by age from the first date of billing. A quarterly or more frequent age analysis, such as that shown in Figure 17-8, helps you keep on top of past-due accounts and determine which ones need follow-up.

You can do an age analysis by computer or by hand. An age analysis should list all patient account balances, when the charges originated, the most recent payment date, and any special notes concerning the account.

In a single doctor's office or a small group practice, information for the age analysis may come from the patient

ledger cards. You may place color-coded tags on the patient ledger cards to indicate the number of days past due. For example, a yellow tag might be placed on the ledger card of an account that is 60 days past due. An orange tag might be used for an account that is 90 days past due. A red tag might be used for an account that is 120 days or more past due. In a large practice, however, age analysis is typically done on the computer. The use of patient ledger cards has been phased out as more practices have become computerized.

Following Laws That Govern Debt Collection

Federal and state laws govern debt collection. Table 17-1 outlines the penalties for violating laws that regulate credit and debt.

Fair Debt Collection Practices Act of 1977. This act (also called Public Law 95-109) governs the methods that can be used to collect unpaid debts. It prevents you from threatening to take an action that is either illegal or that you do not actually intend to take. The aim of this law is to eliminate abusive, deceptive, or unfair debt collection practices. For example, the law requires that after you have said you are going to give an account to a collection agency if it is not paid within 1 month, you must actually do so. Not doing what you threaten to do can be construed as harassment, and your practice can be liable for a harassment charge. Following are guidelines for sending letters and making calls requesting payment from patients.

- Do not call the patient before 8 A.M. or after 9 P.M. Calling outside those hours can be considered harassment.

- Do not make threats or use profane language. For example, do not state that an account will be given to a collection agency in 7 days if it will not be.

- Do not discuss the patient's debt with anyone except the person responsible for payment. If the patient is represented by a lawyer, discuss the problem only with the lawyer, unless the lawyer gives you permission to talk to the patient.

- Do not use any form of deception or violence to collect a debt. For example, do not pose as a government employee or other authority figure to try to force a debtor to pay.

Telephone Consumer Protection Act (TCPA) of 1991. This act protects telephone subscribers from unwanted telephone solicitations, commonly known as telemarketing. The act prohibits autodialed calls to emergency service providers, cellular and paging numbers, and patients' hospital rooms. It prohibits prerecorded calls to homes without prior permission of the resident, and it prohibits unsolicited advertising via fax machine.

These regulations do not apply to people who have an established business relationship with the telemarketing

City Medical Group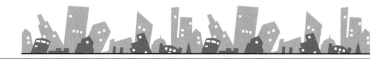

1234 Wayne Street
Smithtown, OR 93689
(503) 555-1217

Internal Medicine
Marianne Harris, MD
Karen Payne-Johnson, MD

May 5, 2004

Mr. J. J. Andrews
1414 First Avenue
Smithtown, OR 93668

Dear Mr. Andrews:

It has been brought to my attention that your account in the amount of <u>$240.00</u> is past due.

Normally at this time the account would be placed with a collection agency. However, we would prefer to hear from you regarding your preference in this matter.

(   )   Payment in full is enclosed.

(   )   Payment will be made in _____ days.

(   )   I would like to make regular weekly/monthly payments of $ _____ until this account is paid in full. My first payment is enclosed.

(   )   I would prefer that you assign this account to a collection agency for enforcement of collection. (Failure to return this letter within 30 days will result in this action.)

(   )   I don't believe I owe this amount for the following reason(s):

Signed: _____

Please indicate your preference and return this letter within 30 days. Please do not hesitate to call if you have any questions regarding this matter.

Sincerely,

Diana Sanchez
Office Manager

Figure 17-7.   Standard collection letters are available for you to fill in the details.

Choosing a Collection Agency

If a patient does not respond to your final collection letter or has twice broken a promise to pay, the doctor may choose to seek the help of a collection agency. This step should be taken carefully, however. Some collection agencies use illegal and unethical tactics to obtain payment. For example, some collectors have made repeated, profane phone calls to frighten debtors. Others have threatened debtors with prison for nonpayment. A good collection agency reflects the humanitarian and ethical standards of the medical profession.

To help select an effective—and ethical—collection agency, ask for a referral from the doctor's colleagues, fellow specialists, or hospital associates. You may also contact one of the following organizations:

American Collectors Association International
P.O. Box 390106
Minneapolis, MN 55439

Medical-Dental-Hospital Bureaus of America
1161 Wayzata Boulevard East
Wayzata, MN 55391

After obtaining a referral, contact the agency and request samples of its letters, reminder notices, and other print material for debtors. Be sure this material is courteous and reflects the way you would handle the collection. Also, be sure the agency uses a persuasive approach rather than simply suing debtors. Ask if the agency reports cases that deserve special consideration to the doctor's office.

Determine what methods the agency uses for out-of-town accounts. For example, it may use out-of-town services to help with those collections. Ask the agency about its collection percentage and fees for large, small, and out-of-town accounts. Be sure the percentages and fees are appropriate for the collection amounts.

After selecting a collection agency, supply all pertinent data to the agency, such as the patient's name, address, and full amount of the debt. Mark the patient's ledger card so that you do not call or write to the patient about the debt. If the patient contacts the office about the account, refer the patient to the collection agency.

If you receive any payments from the debtor, alert the collection agency immediately. (The agency takes a portion of any payments it collects.) Also, contact the agency if you learn anything new about the patient's address or employer.

---

wants to discuss payment, refer the patient to the agency. If the patient sends a payment, forward it to the agency; or, if the agency and the practice agree, keep the payment for the practice, and forward the collection fee to the agency.

The arrangement with the agency should give the doctor the final word on the uncollected account. In other words, the doctor should decide whether to write off the debt or take the matter to court.

Insuring Accounts Receivable

To protect the practice from lost income because of nonpayment, the practice may buy accounts receivable insurance. One type of accounts receivable policy pays when a large number of patients do not pay and the physician must absorb the lost income. It protects the practice's cash flow and helps ensure that the practice will have sufficient income to cover expected expenses.

Credit Arrangements

Sometimes a doctor agrees to extend credit to a patient who is unable to pay immediately. This situation is not uncommon when a patient's medical bills are high. By extending **credit,** the doctor gives the patient time to pay for services, which are provided on trust. If the doctor knows the patient well, she may offer credit without checking the patient's credit history. Otherwise, the doctor may ask you to perform a credit check.

Performing a Credit Check

To perform a credit check, be sure you have the most current information. You will need the patient's address, telephone number, and Social Security number and the patient's employer's name, address, and telephone number. With this information you can verify employment and generate a credit bureau report.

Employment Verification. Explain to the patient that you will be calling his employer to verify employment. Many employers have someone designated to handle such calls. The patient may be able to give you that name before you call the place of employment.

After calling, record the updated information on the patient's registration card, along with any credit references you obtain from the patient.

Credit Bureau Report. A **credit bureau** is a company that provides information about the creditworthiness of a person seeking credit. If a patient's credit history is in

	File No.		
To the Consumer:	Date		
This is a copy of your current credit file. It is being furnished to you based on the information you have provided in accordance with the "Fair Credit Reporting Act." Please use the file number shown on this report on all correspondence. Refer to the reverse side for explanations of codes and abbreviations used in this disclosure.	1/8/04		
	Amount Received		Payment Type
	$15.00		
	Credit Card No.		Exp. Date

In File Since	10/94	

Consumer Name and Address	SSN	Date Rptd.
	Spouse Name SSN	
	Tel.	
Former Address	Date Rptd.	

Present Employer and Address	Position Income	Empl. Date	Date Verif.
Former Employer and Address			
Spouse's Employer and Address			

Subscriber Name	Subscriber Code	Date Opened	High Credit	Date Verif.	Present Status		Payment Pattern	Type Account & MOP
					Balance Owed	Amount Past Due	1–12 Months / 13–24 Months	
Account Number		Terms	Credit Limit	Dated Closed	Maximum Delinquency Date / Amount / MOP		Historical Status No. of Months 25–39 40–59 60+	
Collateral				Remarks	Type Loan			
MIDLANTIC	B382D021	4/92 MIN10	$850	11/98A	$325	$0	111111111111 X11111111111 12 0 0 0	R01
LINCOLN SAV B	B814M006	6/88 360M34	$30.5K	10/94A	$16K	$0	1111X11X1111 111X11111X1X 29 0 0 0	M01
BANK AMER	B196P017	11/89 10M	$5000	10/96A	$1136	$0	111111111111 11111111111X 48 0 0 0	R01
MACY D	D787D008	1/84 MIN20	$475 $1000 *CREDIT LINE CLOSED BY CUSTOMER	11/97A	$0	$0*	111XXXXXXXXX 1111111111XX 48 0 0 0	R01
UJ BK MC	33DB0002	7/91 MIN20	$3000	3/96A	$310	$0	111111111111 111X111111XX 47 0 0 0	R01

Figure 17-9. Credit reports are generated by credit bureaus.

question, you may request a report from a credit bureau. A sample credit report is shown in Figure 17-9. A credit bureau collects information about an individual's payment history on credit cards, student loans, and similar accounts. Three leading national credit bureaus are TRW Inc., Equifax Inc., and Trans Union Credit Information Company.

The physician may decide not to extend credit, based on the credit report. If so, the Fair Credit Reporting Act states that you must inform the patient in writing that credit was denied. You must also provide the name and address of the credit bureau. This information allows the patient to contest the credit report and to correct any incorrect information the credit bureau may have.

Following Laws Governing Extension of Credit

When you help the doctor decide whether to grant credit to a patient, you must comply with certain laws governing extension of credit.

Equal Credit Opportunity Act. This act states that credit arrangements may not be denied based on a patient's sex, race, religion, national origin, marital status, or age. Also, credit cannot be denied because the patient receives public assistance or has exercised rights under the Consumer Credit Protection Act, such as disputing a credit card bill or a credit bureau report.

Under the Equal Credit Opportunity Act, the patient has a right to know the specific reason that credit was denied. Some reasons might include having too little income or not being employed for a certain period of time. Vague reasons about not meeting minimum standards or not receiving enough points on a credit-scoring system are not acceptable.

Truth in Lending Act. This act is Regulation Z of the Consumer Credit Protection Act. The Truth in Lending Act covers credit agreements that involve more than four payments. It requires the physician and patient to discuss, sign, and retain copies of a **disclosure statement** (frequently called a federal Truth in Lending statement), which

Bookkeeping Systems

Three types of manual accounting systems are commonly used in a medical practice: single-entry, double-entry, and pegboard. A computerized system may also be used. All bookkeeping systems record income, charges (money owed to the practice), disbursements (money paid out by the practice), and other financial information. The choice of system is based on the size and complexity of the practice.

Traditional Bookkeeping Methods

Even practices that use computers for many other administrative and clinical functions may still perform bookkeeping methods on paper. This choice is not old-fashioned but simply the preference of the physician/ owner or the office manager. Some people believe that working with numbers on paper forces you to be especially careful and to pay close attention to detail—more so than working on a computer, which has built-in mechanisms for checking arithmetic, decimal alignment, and so on.

Single-Entry System. As the name implies, the single-entry system requires only one entry for each transaction. Therefore, it is the easiest system to learn and use. Unlike the double-entry system, however, the single-entry system is not self-balancing. In addition, it does not detect errors as readily and has fewer accuracy checkpoints. This system is also more likely to produce errors because information must be posted (copied) to the bookkeeping forms.

The single-entry system uses several basic records, as well as auxiliary records:

- A daily log (also called a general ledger, day sheet, or daily journal) to record charges and payments
- Patient ledger cards or an accounts receivable ledger, which shows how much each patient owes
- A checkbook register or cash payment journal, which shows the practice expenses
- Payroll records, which show salaries, wages, and payroll deductions
- Petty cash records, which show disbursements for minor office expenses

The double-entry and pegboard systems, discussed later in this chapter, also use these records.

Daily Log. The daily log is a chronological list of the charges to patients and the payments received from patients each day, as shown in Figure 18-1. In the daily log, you write the name of each patient seen that day. Across from the name, you record the service provided, the fee charged, and the payment received (if any). This process

Hour	Patient	Service Provided	Charge	Paid
	1			
	2			
	3			
	4			
	5			
	6			
	7			
	8			
	9			
	10			
	11			
	12			
	13			
	14			
	15			
	16			
			Totals	

Dr. _____   Date _____

Figure 18-1. A daily log is used to record charges and payments.

is called **journalizing.** You then post (copy) the charges and payments from the daily log to patient ledger cards (described in the next section). Using a daily or monthly cash control sheet, you record checks and cash received as well as deposits made each day.

Some physicians keep a daily log at their desks for entering information after they see each patient. In such cases, it may be helpful to write the name of each scheduled patient in the log to provide an appointment list. You may be responsible for this task.

In other offices, the medical assistants maintain the daily log. You can obtain the information for the log from charge slips and from checks received from patients or insurance companies. (Note: A **charge slip** is the original record of the doctor's services and the charge for those services. Some practices use a combination charge slip/receipt, which automatically creates a receipt to tear off for the patient. Typically, a charge slip/receipt includes a duplicate copy underneath to use for bookkeeping purposes. Remember, you need to track charges *and* receipts for payment, regardless of whether the practice uses separate charge slips and receipts or a combination.) There may also be records of outside visits, such as to nursing homes or hospital emergency rooms.

Be sure to record any night calls or other unscheduled visits in the daily log. Simply check with the physician each morning. If the physician has not noted the charge amount on a charge slip/receipt or record of outside visits, remember to apply the correct fee.

Record in the daily log all payments that come in the mail. If a check from an insurance company includes payment for more than one patient (which frequently is the case), post the appropriate amount to each patient ledger card.

If extra columns are available, you can record additional financial information in the daily log. For example, in addition to showing the total amount charged to the patient, you can show a breakdown of that total into the amounts generated by different physicians in a group practice or by different functions of the office, such as laboratory or x-ray.

At the end of each day, total the charges and receipts in the daily log, and post these totals to the monthly summary of charges and receipts. To double-check your totals, perform the following procedures:

- Ensure that the day's total cash and check receipts are the same as the day's total bank deposit.
- Ensure that the sum of the day's charges for each type of service is the same as the total of the day's charges.

Patient Ledger Cards. Another bookkeeping task is preparing a patient ledger card for each patient. The **patient ledger card** includes the patient's name, address, home and work telephone numbers, and the name of the person who is responsible for the charges (if different from the patient). The ledger card also lists the patient's insurance information, Social Security number, employer's name, and any special billing instructions. Figure 18-2 shows an example of a patient ledger card.

You use the patient ledger card to record charges incurred by the patient, payments received, and the resulting balance owed to the doctor. Because these cards document the financial transactions of the patient account, they are sometimes called account cards. In some practices, they are photocopied for use as monthly statements.

The information for the patient ledger cards comes from the daily log or from charge slips. It is best to complete all the cards at the end of the day. If this is not possible, you may complete them as time permits during the day. To prevent double or omitted postings, put a small check mark next to each entry in the daily log after you post it to the proper ledger card.

Take great care when posting, because errors on ledger cards will be reflected on invoices. To ensure accuracy, add up the total charges and receipts from the ledger cards, and make sure the information matches the total charges and receipts in that day's daily log.

Accounts Receivable. Every day, you must also update the accounts receivable record, which shows the total owed to the practice. Total up the items on the accounts receivable record, and then total up the outstanding balances on the patient ledger cards. The two numbers should match. If they do not, recheck your work to find the cause of the discrepancy.

Accounts Payable. Accounts payable are the amounts the practice owes to vendors. If your responsibilities include accounts payable, keep careful records of equipment and supplies ordered, and compare orders received against the invoices. In the checkbook register, keep detailed and accurate records of accounts paid.

Record of Office Disbursements. The record of office disbursements is a list of the amounts paid for such items as medical supplies, office rent, office utilities, employee wages, postage, and equipment over a certain period of time. It shows the **payee** (the person who will receive the payment), the date, the check number, the amount paid, and the type of expense. Figure 18-3 is an example of a disbursement record.

A checkbook register may be used to record office disbursements. As an alternative, a disbursement journal or the bottom section of the daily log may be used to record office disbursements. For income tax purposes, this record should include only office expenses. The doctor's personal expenses should not be listed here.

Summary of Charges, Receipts, and Disbursements. Charges, receipts, and disbursements are usually summarized at the end of each month, quarter, or year, as shown in Figure 18-4. The summary is used to compare the income and expenses of the current period with the income and expenses from any previous period.

By analyzing summaries, a physician can see which functions of the practice are profitable, the total amount charged for services, the payments received for services, the total cost of running the office, and a breakdown of

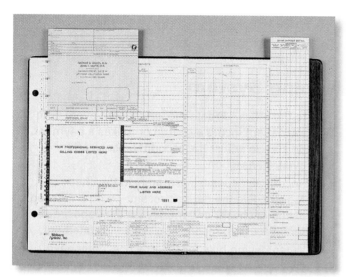

Figure 18-5. A pegboard system allows for simultaneous transfer of information while writing it only once.

Pegboard System. The **pegboard system** lets your write each transaction once while recording it on four different bookkeeping forms. This technique can help to reduce errors and save time. The pegboard system is called the one-write system and used to be the most widely used bookkeeping system in medical practices. This system is now used less commonly in many practices.

A pegboard system usually includes a lightweight board with pegs on the left or right edges (Figure 18-5). The pegs match holes that are punched in daily log sheets, patient ledger cards, charge slips/receipts, and deposit slips. The holes allow the forms to be aligned while stacked on top of each other. Information, entered on only one form, is simultaneously transferred to the form(s) below. Generally these forms are printed on NCR (no-carbon-required) paper. If not, you must place carbon paper between the forms.

Starting the Business Day. Place a daily log sheet on the pegboard at the beginning of each day. Then, place the stack of charge slips/receipts on the pegs, aligning the top line of the first charge slip/receipt with the daily log top line. Because the charge slips/receipts are shingled, or layered one over the other from top to bottom, alignment of the first aligns all the others. The charge slips/receipts are prenumbered. This numbering promotes good cash control and theoretically prevents embezzlement.

Upon Patient Arrival. As each patient comes into the office, place the patient's ledger card under the next available charge slip/receipt. Be sure to align the card's first blank line with the carbon strip on the charge slip/receipt. Write the date, the patient's name, and the patient's previous balance on the charge slip section. The information will automatically be recorded in the daily log and on the patient ledger card.

Attaching the Charge Slip/Receipt to the Patient Chart. Next, remove the charge slip/receipt and attach it to the patient chart so that the doctor will see it. After examining the patient, the doctor fills in the appropriate charges on the charge slip/receipt, indicates when the next appointment is needed, and gives the charge slip/receipt to the patient.

Before the Patient Leaves. The patient comes to you with the completed charge slip/receipt, and you again place the ledger card between the charge slip/receipt and the daily log. Check to be sure you align it properly. On the charge slip/receipt, write the charge slip/receipt number, date, procedure (or code), charges, payments, new balance, and the date and time of the next appointment (if any). As you write this information, it should be automatically transferred onto the ledger card and daily log. Finally, tear off the receipt, and give it to the patient. You can now return the patient ledger card to the file.

Payments After the Patient Visit. If you receive payments sometime after the patient visit, either by mail or in person, record them on the patient ledger card and daily log as you normally would. Record charges for doctor visits to hospitalized patients or other out-of-office visits in the same way. If required, you can use the pegboard system to record bank deposits and petty cash disbursements in the daily log, but you will need the appropriate overlapping forms.

End of the Day. At the end of each day, total and check the arithmetic (addition and subtraction) in all columns. If you find an error, correct it immediately by drawing a line through it and making a new entry on the next available writing line. Remember to make the correction on the patient ledger card also and to issue a new receipt to the patient.

Bookkeeping on the Computer

Physicians or office managers who choose to set up the practice's bookkeeping system on the computer enjoy several important benefits over traditional bookkeeping methods. Computerized bookkeeping saves time; many repetitive tasks are done by the computer. The computer also performs mathematic calculations. Most bookkeeping software programs include built-in tax tables, which can calculate tax liabilities and so on.

As discussed in Chapter 6, many bookkeeping software programs are available on the market. Any bookkeeping software package performs the same tasks described earlier in this chapter under traditional bookkeeping systems. The practice in which you work may already have a computerized bookkeeping program in place. It is a good idea, however, to read current computer software magazines. You may learn about a new software program you might recommend to the physician or office manager, or you may read about a new or more efficient way to use the practice's current software program.

Banking for the Medical Office

Besides bookkeeping, you may be responsible for handling the banking for the practice. Because a practice may use traditional (manual) or electronic (computerized) banking methods, you should be familiar with both. Regardless of which method you use, remember to keep all banking materials secure because they represent the finances of the practice. For example, to prevent theft of checks, always put the checkbook in a securely locked place when it is not in use. Also, file deposit receipts promptly. If they are lost, you have no proof that a deposit was made. Lack of proof could cost the practice thousands of dollars.

Banking Tasks

Banking tasks for the medical practice include:

- Writing checks
- Accepting checks
- Endorsing checks
- Making deposits
- Reconciling bank statements

To perform these tasks properly, you must be familiar with several terms and concepts related to banking.

Checks. A **check** is a bank draft or order for payment. The person who writes the check is called the **payer.** By writing a check, the payer directs the bank to pay a sum of money on demand to the payee. In order to be considered **negotiable** (legally transferable from one person to another), a check must:

- Be written and signed by the payer or maker
- Include the amount of money to be paid, considered a promise to pay a specified sum
- Be made payable to the payee or bearer
- Be made payable on demand or on a specific date
- Include the name of the bank that is directed to make payment

Other Negotiable Papers. You may receive other negotiable paper in addition to standard personal and business checks.

- A **cashier's check** is a check issued on bank paper signed by a bank representative. It is usually purchased by individuals who do not have checking accounts.

- A **certified check** is a payer's check written and signed by the payer and stamped "Certified" by the bank. This certification means that the bank has already drawn money from the payer's account to guarantee that the check will be paid when submitted. (The money is set aside to cover this specific check.) Few banks offer certified checks anymore.
- A **money order** is another kind of certificate of guaranteed payment. Money orders may be purchased from banks (bank money orders) or post offices (postal money orders) or from some convenience stores.

Check Codes. The face (front) of every check contains two important items: the American Banking Association (ABA) number and the magnetic ink character recognition (MICR) code. The **ABA number** appears as a fraction, such as 60-117/310, on the upper edge of all printed checks. It identifies the geographic area and specific bank on which the check is drawn.

Found at the bottom of a check, the MICR code consists of numbers and characters printed in magnetic ink, which can be read by MICR equipment at the bank. This code enables checks to be read, sorted, and recorded by computer.

Types of Checking Accounts. A physician is likely to have three different types of checking accounts: a personal account, a business account for office expenses, and an interest-earning account. The interest-earning account will be used for paying special expenses, such as property taxes and insurance premiums. Most of your work will be with the business checking account. You may sometimes, however, make payments from, or transfer money to, the interest-earning account, as directed.

Accepting Checks. Before accepting any check, review it carefully. First be sure the check has the correct date, amount, and signature and that no corrections have been made. Figure 18-6 shows a correctly written and endorsed check. Do not accept a **third-party check** (one made out to the patient rather than to the practice) unless it is from a health insurance company. Also, do not accept a check marked "Payment in Full" unless it actually does pay the complete outstanding balance. You may accept a check signed by someone other than the payer if the person who signed the check has power of attorney. **Power of attorney** gives a person the legal right to handle financial matters for another person who is unable to do so. Frequently power of attorney is granted to a patient's spouse, son, or daughter.

Be sure to follow the policy of your practice when accepting a check. For example, if a patient is new or unfamiliar, office policy may require you to request patient identification and to compare the signature on the identification with the signature on the check. Policy may also require that you not accept a check for more than the amount due.

PROCEDURE 18.3

Reconciling a Bank Statement

Objective: To ensure that the bank record of deposits and withdrawals agrees with the practice's record of deposits and withdrawals

Materials: Previous bank statement, current bank statement, reconciliation worksheet (if not part of current bank statement), deposit receipts, red pencil, check stubs or checkbook register, returned checks

Method

1. Check the closing balance on the previous statement against the opening balance on the new statement. The balances should match. If they do not, call the bank.

2. Record the closing balance from the new statement on the reconciliation worksheet (Figure 18-9). This worksheet usually appears on the back of the bank statement.

3. Check each deposit receipt against the bank statement. Place a red check mark in the upper right corner of each receipt that is recorded on the statement. Total the amount of deposits that do *not* appear on the statement. Add this amount to the closing balance on the reconciliation worksheet.

4. Put the returned checks in numerical order.

5. Compare each returned check with the bank statement, making sure that the amount on the check agrees with the amount on the statement. Place a red check mark in the upper right corner of each returned check that is recorded on the statement. Also, place a check mark on the check stub or check register entry. Any checks that were written but that do not appear on the statement and were not returned are considered "outstanding" checks. You can find these easily on the check stubs or checkbook register because they have no red check mark.

6. List each outstanding check separately on the worksheet, including its check number and amount. Total the outstanding checks, and

---

HOW TO BALANCE YOUR CHECKING ACCOUNT

1. Subtract any service charges that appear on this statement from your checkbook balance.
2. Add any interest paid on your checking account to your checkbook balance.
3. Check off (✔) in your checkbook register all checks and pre-authorized transactions listed on your statement.
4. Use the worksheet to list checks you have written, ATM withdrawals, and Point of Sale transactions which are not listed on your statement.

5. Enter the closing balance on the statement.	$	.
6. Add any deposits not shown on the statement.	+	.
7. Subtotal	$	.
8. Subtract total transactions outstanding (from worksheet on right).	−	.
9. Account balance (should match balance in your checkbook register).	$	.

IF YOUR ACCOUNT DOES NOT BALANCE

a. Check your addition and subtraction first on this form and then in your checkbook.
b. Be sure the deposit amounts on your statement are the same as those in your checkbook.
c. Be sure all the check amounts on your statement agree with the amounts entered in your checkbook register.
d. Be sure all checks written prior to this reconcilement period but not listed on the statement are listed on the worksheet.
e. Verify that all MAC® ATM, Point of Sale, and other pre-authorized transactions have been recorded in your checkbook register.
f. Review last month's statement to be certain any corrections were entered into your checkbook.

WORKSHEET
Transactions Outstanding

Number or Date	Amount
TOTAL	

Figure 18-9. Use the reconciliation worksheet on the back of the bank statement to reconcile the statement with your checkbook register.

continued ⟶

Reconciling a Bank Statement *(continued)*

subtract this total from the bank statement balance.

7. If the statement shows that the checking account earned interest, add this amount to the checkbook balance.

8. If the statement lists such items as a service charge, check printing charge, or automatic payment, subtract them from the checkbook balance.

9. Compare the new checkbook balance with the new bank statement balance. They should match. If they do not, repeat the process, rechecking all calculations. Double-check the addition and subtraction in the checkbook

register. Review the checkbook register to make sure you did not omit any items. Ensure that you carried the correct balance forward from one register page to the next. Double-check that you made the correct additions or subtractions for all interest earned and charges.

10. If your work is correct, and the balances still do not agree, call the bank to determine if a bank error has been made. Contact the bank promptly because the bank may have a time limit for corrections. The bank may consider the bank statement correct if you do not point out an error within 2 weeks (or other period, according to bank policy).

been entered into the register. Information includes check number, date, payee, and amount. Scrolling up and down reveals all the checks in the register. (Some banks also allow you to access this information by telephone. The Tips for the Office section gives more information about telephone banking.)

Balance Checkbook. The "Balance Checkbook" option electronically reconciles the monthly bank statement. After you enter the appropriate date or dates, the computer screen displays all the checks and deposits that were logged into the register in the order they were posted. Figure 18-10 shows an example of this function.

Tips for the Office

Telephone Banking

Telephone banking is a form of electronic banking that enables you to access your bank's computer system by phone to obtain account information and perform simple banking tasks. To use telephone banking, you should have a push-button telephone, the telephone personal identification number (TPIN) assigned to your practice by the bank, and the telephone number that accesses the telephone banking system.

The telephone banking system prompts you for information. You use the push-button pad on the telephone to provide the information. For example, an automated voice may ask you to press 1 to inquire about deposits or 2 to inquire about withdrawals. Telephone banking is especially useful for the following banking tasks:

- Checking the current balance of an account
- Determining whether deposited funds are available

- Obtaining the date and amount of the last few deposits and the last few checks paid (usually the last three)
- Finding out if a specific check has been paid
- Transferring funds between accounts (if the practice has more than one account)
- Stopping payment on checks

Although this form of electronic banking is especially useful for some services, you cannot use it to manage all banking tasks. For example, you cannot use it to make deposits or reconcile a bank statement. However, it can be quite convenient for the day-to-day banking tasks just listed. If you have a hearing impairment and have a telecommunications device for the deaf (TDD) installed on the telephone, you can bank by phone.

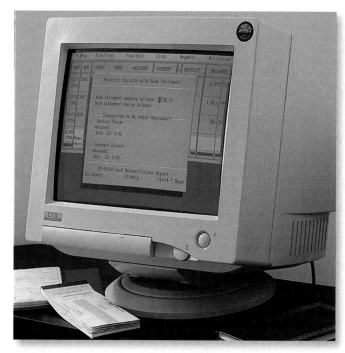

Figure 18-10. Electronic banking will allow you to see the "Balance Checkbook" menu on the screen.

The next screen highlights each check or deposit that has not been seen on a previous bank statement. You are prompted to indicate whether that item appears on the current statement, usually using Y for yes and N for no. After the computer queries these items, it may ask you to enter any items that appear on the current bank statement but are not in the checkbook, such as service charges.

Finally, a message on the screen prompts you to enter the current account balance from the bank statement. Then, the computer reconciles the bank statement. It will alert you if the system balance does not agree with the balance on the bank statement. If the balance does not agree, recheck the information you entered for possible error. If your work is correct, and the balances still do not agree, call the bank to determine if a bank error has been made.

Managing Accounts Payable

As you learned in Chapter 17, accounts payable are the practice's expenses (money leaving the business), and accounts receivable reflect a practice's income (money coming into the business). This section focuses on accounts payable, including payroll. A basic accounting principle to bear in mind is that when a practice's income exceeds its expenses, it has a profit. When a practice's expenses exceed its income, it has a loss.

Because of this relationship between income and expenses, most practices try to reduce expenses by controlling accounts payable. As a medical assistant, you play an important role in helping control accounts payable and maximize profits.

Accounts payable fall into three main groups:

1. Payments for supplies, equipment, and practice-related products and services
2. Payroll, which may be the largest of the accounts payable
3. Taxes owed to federal, state, and local agencies

A practice's accounting system usually consists of several elements. These elements include the daily log, patient ledger cards, the checkbook, the disbursements journal, the petty cash record, and the payroll register.

The daily log and patient ledger cards are used primarily for accounts receivable. The disbursements journal, petty cash record, and payroll register are used primarily in accounts payable. Procedure 18-4 tells you how to set up and use these accounting tools effectively.

Managing Disbursements

A disbursement is any payment the physician's office makes for goods or services. One of the most common disbursements is payment for office supplies. Other disbursements include payments for equipment, dues, rent, taxes, salary, and utilities. No matter what type of disbursement you make on behalf of the practice, you must keep accurate records of the purchase and the payment.

Managing Supplies

In most practices, the physician authorizes one person to handle the purchasing of supplies and other products. This person is usually the office manager or medical assistant.

Guidelines for purchasing supplies are discussed in detail in Chapter 8. When buying clinical or office supplies, keep these six principles in mind to control expenses.

1. Order only the necessary supplies, and order them only in the proper amounts. Buying too much reduces cash flow. Buying too little may cause you to run out of needed items and you may have to reorder too often.
2. Combine orders when possible. You may save money and time by placing a larger order for several items at once rather than placing a smaller order each time an item is needed.
3. Follow your practice's purchasing guidelines, if any. For example, you may have to get the physician's approval for purchases over a specific dollar amount. Employees may have to submit purchase orders (formal requests for goods or services).
4. Buy from reputable suppliers. They are more likely to provide on-time delivery and satisfactory handling of your order. If your office does not already have a list of reliable suppliers, ask for recommendations from other practices.

PROCEDURE 18.4

Setting Up the Accounts Payable System

Objective: To set up an accounts payable system

Materials: Disbursements journal, petty cash record, payroll register, pen

Method

Setting Up the Disbursements Journal

1. Write in column headings for the basic information about each check: date, payee's name, check number, and check amount.
2. Write in column headings for each type of business expense, such as rent and utilities.
3. Write in column headings (if space is available) for deposits and the account balance.
4. Record the data from completed checks under the appropriate column headings.

Setting Up the Petty Cash Record

1. Write in column headings for the date, transaction number, payee, brief description, amount of transaction, and type of expense.
2. Write in a column heading (if space is available) for the petty cash fund balance.

3. Record the data from petty cash vouchers under the appropriate column headings.

Setting Up the Payroll Register

1. Write in column headings for check number, employee name, earnings to date, hourly rate, hours worked, regular earnings, overtime hours worked, and overtime earnings.
2. Write in column headings for total gross earnings for the pay period and gross taxable earnings.
3. Write in column headings for each deduction. These may include federal income tax, Federal Insurance Contributions Act (FICA) tax, state income tax, local income tax, and various voluntary deductions.
4. Write in a column heading for net earnings.
5. Each time you write payroll checks, record earning and deduction data under the appropriate column headings on the payroll register.

---

5. Get the best-quality supplies for the best price.
6. For clinical supplies, consider the amount for which insurance companies will reimburse the practice. For example, if your office does only a few throat cultures a year, it might make more sense to send those patients elsewhere for the test than to stock the supplies required. The small reimbursement amount for a few throat cultures may not justify purchasing the supplies. Also consider shelf life. Do not buy large amounts of clinical supplies that will expire before use.

Writing Checks

Virtually all disbursements are made by check. Paying by check gives the practice complete, accurate records of all financial transactions.

Before writing a check, make sure the checking account balance is up-to-date and large enough to cover the check you want to write. Subtract the amount of each check from the previous balance, enter the new balance, and carry that balance forward to the next stub.

If you use a pegboard system, you will automatically record the date, check number, payee, and check amount

on the check register as you write out the check. You must note the reason for payment and the new balance manually, however. Record that information in the appropriate spaces on the register.

If you make an error when completing a check, write VOID in ink across the front of the check in large letters so that it cannot be used again. Then file the voided check in numerical order with the returned checks.

After filling out the check properly, detach it from the checkbook, and give it to the doctor to sign, along with the invoice to be paid. (With experience, you may be trusted to sign checks under a certain amount.) Mark the date, check number, and amount paid on the invoice. Make a copy of the invoice for your records. Keep these copies with supporting documents, such as order forms or packing slips, in a paid-invoice file. Then, mail the check and the original invoice to the payee in a neatly hand-addressed or typewritten envelope. If you use a window envelope, be sure the payee's address shows through the window.

Commonly Used Checks. Most practices use checks from a standard checkbook, or they use **voucher checks,** business checks with stubs attached. Voucher checks come in several styles. A common style is a large, ring-bound checkbook, with three checks to a page. A perforation divides each check from its matching stub, which the practice retains.

Limited checks are sometimes used for payroll. A **limited check** states that it is void after a certain time limit. Many practices use checks that are void after 90 days.

Other Types of Checks. You or the physician may sometimes need to use other types of checks. The physician may use a cashier's check to pay certain types of taxes. A cashier's check is purchased from a bank, written on the bank's own checking account, and signed by a bank official.

The physician may use a certified check to pay certain taxes or to buy property. A certified check is a standard check that the bank verifies and certifies before it is used. This certification means that funds have been set aside to guarantee payment of the check.

A **counter check** is a special bank check that allows the depositor to withdraw funds from her account only. It states, "Pay to the Order of Myself Only." The physician may use a counter check when she wants to withdraw money but has forgotten her checkbook.

A physician may use **traveler's checks** when attending an out-of-town conference or whenever using a personal check or carrying a lot of cash is not appropriate. Printed in $10, $20, $50, and $100 denominations, these checks must be signed at the location where they are purchased (usually a bank). To use traveler's checks, the physician fills in the payee's name and signs it in a second place. She must sign it in the payee's presence so the payee can ensure that the signatures match.

Recording Disbursements

You may record disbursements in a check register, in a disbursements journal, or on the bottom section of the daily log.

If you use a disbursements journal, follow these steps to record disbursements.

1. When beginning a new journal page, give each column a heading to reflect the type of expense, such as utilities or rent.
2. For each check, fill in the date, payee's name, check number, and check amount in the appropriate columns.
3. Determine the expense category of the check.
4. Record the check amount in the column for that type of business expense.
5. If you must divide a check between two or more expense columns, record the total in the check amount column. Then record the amount that applies to each type of expense in the appropriate column.

Recording disbursements in columns for each type of expense allows you to total and track expenses by category. **Tracking** (watching for changes) is important

because it helps control expenses. Before tracking, check your calculations by performing a trial balance.

1. Total the check amount column.
2. Find the total for each expense column.
3. Add together all the expense column totals. The combined expense column total should match the total in the check amount column.
4. If the amounts do not match, recheck every entry until you find the error. When you find it, draw a line through it, and record the correct information neatly above it or to the side.
5. When the two amounts match (or balance), carry forward all column totals to the disbursements journal for the next month. Remember to prepare summaries and perform balances at the end of every month, quarter, and year.

Managing Petty Cash

Occasionally, you may need to make small (petty) cash disbursements for minor expenses such as postage-due fees or holiday decorations (Figure 18-11). To avoid writing checks for such small amounts, you may pay for them from the **petty cash fund,** cash kept on hand in the office for small purchases. The doctor should determine the amount of the petty cash account (usually $50) and the minimum amount of cash to be kept on hand (such as $15).

Starting and Maintaining a Petty Cash Fund. To start the fund with $50, write a check to "Petty Cash" or "Cash" for that amount. Enter the check in the miscellaneous column of the monthly disbursement record. Then, cash the check. Because this money will be used for small disbursements, be sure to get some of it in pennies, nickels, dimes, quarters, and dollar bills. Put this money in a special petty cash box, along with a stack of petty cash vouchers.

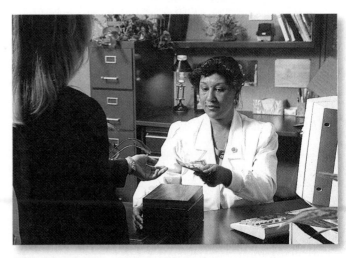

Figure 18-11. You may be in charge of maintaining the practice's petty cash fund. Count cash carefully, and keep accurate records about purchases made.

For each payment from the petty cash fund, obtain a receipt or create a petty cash voucher. The voucher should record the transaction number, date, amount paid, purpose of the expense, your signature (as the person issuing the money), and the signature of the person receiving it. Keep the receipt for any item purchased, along with the completed voucher, in the petty cash box to verify expenses later.

Also, document each petty cash withdrawal on a petty cash record form. Include the transaction number, date, payee, a brief description, amount, and type of expense (such as office expense, auto expense, or miscellaneous expense). If a space is provided, calculate and record the new balance in the petty cash fund.

Replenishing the Petty Cash Fund. At the end of the month (or whenever the fund is low), compare the latest petty cash balance to the money in the petty cash box. If you have not kept a running balance, total the receipts and vouchers, then count the cash on hand. Subtract the total amount on the receipts and vouchers (for example, $35) from the original balance (for example, $50). The difference ($15) should equal the cash on hand in the petty cash box ($15).

To replenish the account, write a check to "Cash" or "Petty Cash" for the amount spent ($35). Cash the check and add the money to the box, bringing the total back up to the original amount of $50. Record the check for $35 on the disbursement record. Also, total the receipts and vouchers by expense category. Record those totals in the appropriate columns on the disbursement record.

Understanding Financial Summaries

The physician may periodically analyze the income and expenses of the practice. Financial summaries provide an easy-to-read report on the business transactions for a given period, such as a month or a year.

An accountant usually prepares financial summaries. Although you will probably not have to create these summaries, you should understand how they are prepared.

Statement of Income and Expense. Also called a profit-and-loss statement, a statement of income and expense highlights the practice's profitability. It shows the physician the practice's total income and then lists and subtracts all expenses.

Cash Flow Statement. A **cash flow statement** shows how much cash is available to cover expenses, to invest, or to take as profits. The cash flow statement begins with the cash on hand at the beginning of the period and shows the income and disbursements made during that period. It concludes with the new amount of cash on hand at the end of the period.

Trial Balance. The doctor may review trial balances periodically to ensure that the books balance. The

combined expense column total should match the total in the check amount column. If the amounts do not match, recheck every entry until you find the error.

Handling Payroll

You may be responsible for handling the office payroll (Table 18-1). If so, your duties may include:

- Obtaining tax identification numbers
- Creating employee payroll information sheets
- Calculating employees' earnings
- Subtracting taxes and other deductions
- Writing paychecks
- Creating employee earnings records
- Preparing a payroll register
- Submitting payroll taxes

Applying for Tax Identification Numbers

Every employer—whether a single physician or a corporate practice—must have an employer identification number (EIN). An EIN is required by law for federal tax accounting purposes. An EIN is obtained by completing Form SS-4 (Application for Employer Identification Number) and submitting it to the Internal Revenue Service (IRS). Some states also require employer tax reports, for which the practice must have a state identification number, obtained from the proper state agency.

Creating Employee Payroll Information Sheets

The practice must maintain up-to-date, accurate payroll information about each employee. You should prepare a payroll information sheet for each employee. Each sheet should have the following information:

- The employee's name, address, Social Security number, and marital status
- An indication that the employee has completed an Employment Eligibility Verification (Form I-9), verifying that the employee is a U.S. citizen, a legally admitted alien, or an alien authorized to work in the United States
- The employee's pay schedule, number of dependents, payroll type, and voluntary deductions

Pay Schedule. On the payroll information sheet, list the employee's **pay schedule,** showing how often the employee is paid. Common pay schedules are weekly, biweekly, and monthly.

Number of Dependents. Record the number of **dependents** (people who depend on the employee for

TABLE 18-1 Payroll Duties

Frequency	Duties
Upon assuming payroll responsibilities	• Apply for an employer identification number (EIN) with Form SS-4 if the physician does not already have an EIN.
Whenever a new employee is hired	• Have the employee complete an Employee's Withholding Allowance Certificate (Form W-4) and Employment Eligibility Verification (Form I-9). • Record the employee's name and Social Security number from the employee's Social Security card.
Every payday	• Withhold federal income tax as well as state and local income taxes (if any). • Withhold the employee's share of FICA taxes (for Social Security and Medicare). Record a matching amount for the employer's share. • Calculate how much the practice must pay for each employee's federal and state unemployment tax.
Monthly or biweekly (depending on your deposit schedule)	• Deposit withheld income taxes, withheld and employer Social Security taxes, and withheld and employer Medicare taxes.
Quarterly (by April 30, July 31, October 31, and January 31)	• File Employer's Quarterly Federal Tax Return (Form 941). With the return, pay any taxes that were not deposited earlier. • Deposit federal unemployment tax, if over $100.
At least once a year	• Have all employees update their W-4 forms.
On or before January 31	• Give employees their Wage and Tax Statements (Form W-2), which show total wages and various withheld taxes. • File Employer's Annual Federal Unemployment (FUTA) Tax Return (Form 940) with tax amount due.
On or before February 28	• File Transmittal of Wage and Tax Statements (Form W-3) along with the government's copies of the W-2 forms.

financial support). Dependents may include a spouse, children, and other family members.

You can find the number of dependents on the Employee's Withholding Allowance Certificate (Form W-4), which should have been completed when the employee was hired (Figure 18-12). Remember to keep the completed W-4 forms in the physician's personnel file, and update them at least annually.

Payroll Type. List the employee's payroll type—hourly wage, salary, or commission—on the payroll information sheet. An hourly wage is a set amount of money per hour of work. A salary is a set amount of money per pay period, regardless of the number of hours worked. A commission is a percentage of the amount an employee earns for the employer. Salespeople, for example, are often paid by commission.

Voluntary Deductions. Finally, document the voluntary deductions to be taken from the employee's check.

These may include additional federal withholding taxes, contributions to a 401(k) retirement plan, or payments to a company health insurance plan. Employees who want additional federal taxes taken out of their paycheck will indicate this deduction on their W-4 form.

Gross Earnings

Gross earnings refers to the total amount of income earned before deductions. Gross earnings must be calculated for each employee as a first step in the payroll process.

Calculating Gross Earnings. For every payroll period, use data from the payroll information sheet to compute each employee's gross earnings. For an hourly employee, use this equation:

Hourly Wage × Hours Worked = Gross Earnings

Form W-4 (2004)

Purpose. Complete Form W-4 so that your employer can withhold the correct Federal income tax from your pay. Because your tax situation may change, you may want to refigure your withholding each year.

Exemption from withholding. If you are exempt, complete only lines 1, 2, 3, 4, and 7 and sign the form to validate it. Your exemption for 2004 expires February 16, 2005. See Pub. 505, Tax Withholding and Estimated Tax.

Note: *You cannot claim exemption from withholding if: (a) your income exceeds $800 and includes more than $250 of unearned income (e.g., interest and dividends) and (b) another person can claim you as a dependent on their tax return.*

Basic instructions. If you are not exempt, complete the **Personal Allowances Worksheet** below. The worksheets on page 2 adjust your withholding allowances based on itemized deductions, certain credits, adjustments to income, or two-earner/two-job situations. Complete all worksheets that apply. **However, you may claim fewer (or zero) allowances.**

Head of household. Generally, you may claim head of household filing status on your tax return only if you are unmarried and pay more than 50% of the costs of keeping up a home for yourself and your dependent(s) or other qualifying individuals. See line **E** below.

Tax credits. You can take projected tax credits into account in figuring your allowable number of withholding allowances. Credits for child or dependent care expenses and the child tax credit may be claimed using the **Personal Allowances Worksheet** below. See Pub. 919, How Do I Adjust My Tax Withholding? for information on converting your other credits into withholding allowances.

Nonwage income. If you have a large amount of nonwage income, such as interest or dividends, consider making estimated tax payments using Form 1040-ES, Estimated Tax for Individuals. Otherwise, you may owe additional tax.

Two earners/two jobs. If you have a working spouse or more than one job, figure the total number of allowances you are entitled to claim on all jobs using worksheets from only one Form W-4. Your withholding usually will be most accurate when all allowances are claimed on the Form W-4 for the highest paying job and zero allowances are claimed on the others.

Nonresident alien. If you are a nonresident alien, see the **Instructions for Form 8233** before completing this Form W-4.

Check your withholding. After your Form W-4 takes effect, use Pub. 919 to see how the dollar amount you are having withheld compares to your projected total tax for 2004. See Pub. 919, especially if your earnings exceed $125,000 (Single) or $175,000 (Married).

Recent name change? If your name on line 1 differs from that shown on your social security card, call 1-800-772-1213 to initiate a name change and obtain a social security card showing your correct name.

Personal Allowances Worksheet (Keep for your records.)

A Enter "1" for **yourself** if no one else can claim you as a dependent . . . . **A** _____

B Enter "1" if:
- You are single and have only one job; or
- You are married, have only one job, and your spouse does not work; or
- Your wages from a second job or your spouse's wages (or the total of both) are $1,000 or less.

. . **B** _____

C Enter "1" for your **spouse**. But, you may choose to enter "-0-" if you are married and have either a working spouse or more than one job. (Entering "-0-" may help you avoid having too little tax withheld.) . . . . **C** _____

D Enter number of **dependents** (other than your spouse or yourself) you will claim on your tax return . . . . **D** _____

E Enter "1" if you will file as **head of household** on your tax return (see conditions under **Head of household** above) . **E** _____

F Enter "1" if you have at least $1,500 of **child or dependent care expenses** for which you plan to claim a credit . . **F** _____

(**Note:** Do **not** include child support payments. See **Pub. 503,** Child and Dependent Care Expenses, for details.)

G **Child Tax Credit** (including additional child tax credit):
- If your total income will be less than $52,000 ($77,000 if married), enter "2" for each eligible child.
- If your total income will be between $52,000 and $84,000 ($77,000 and $119,000 if married), enter "1" for each eligible child plus "1" **additional** if you have four or more eligible children. **G** _____

H Add lines A through G and enter total here. Note: *This may be different from the number of exemptions you claim on your tax return.* ▶ **H** _____

For accuracy, complete all worksheets that apply.
- If you plan to **itemize or claim adjustments to income** and want to reduce your withholding, see the **Deductions and Adjustments Worksheet** on page 2.
- If you have **more than one job** or are **married and you and your spouse both work** and the combined earnings from all jobs exceed $35,000 ($25,000 if married) see the **Two-Earner/Two-Job Worksheet** on page 2 to avoid having too little tax withheld.
- If **neither** of the above situations applies, **stop here** and enter the number from line H on line 5 of Form W-4 below.

- - - - - - - - - - - - - - **Cut here and give Form W-4 to your employer. Keep the top part for your records.** - - - - - - - - - - - -

Form **W-4**	**Employee's Withholding Allowance Certificate**	OMB No. 1545-0010
Department of the Treasury Internal Revenue Service	▶ Your employer must send a copy of this form to the IRS if: (a) you claim more than 10 allowances or (b) you claim "Exempt" and your wages are normally more than $200 per week.	2004

1 Type or print your first name and middle initial	Last name	**2** Your social security number

Home address (number and street or rural route)	**3** ☐ Single ☐ Married ☐ Married, but withhold at higher Single rate.
	Note: *If married, but legally separated, or spouse is a nonresident alien, check the "Single" box.*
City or town, state, and ZIP code	**4** If your last name differs from that shown on your social security card, check here. You must call 1-800-772-1213 for a new card. ▶ ☐

5	Total number of allowances you are claiming (from line **H** above **or** from the applicable worksheet on page 2)	**5**	
6	Additional amount, if any, you want withheld from each paycheck	**6**	$

7 I claim exemption from withholding for 2004, and I certify that I meet **both** of the following conditions for exemption:
- Last year I had a right to a refund of **all** Federal income tax withheld because I had **no** tax liability **and**
- This year I expect a refund of **all** Federal income tax withheld because I expect to have **no** tax liability.

If you meet both conditions, write "Exempt" here . . . . ▶ | **7** |

Under penalties of perjury, I certify that I am entitled to the number of withholding allowances claimed on this certificate, or I am entitled to claim exempt status.

Employee's signature
(Form is not valid unless you sign it.) ▶ _____   **Date** ▶ _____

8 Employer's name and address (Employer: Complete lines 8 and 10 only if sending to the IRS.)	**9** Office code (optional)	**10** Employer identification number (EIN)

For Privacy Act and Paperwork Reduction Act Notice, see page 2.   Cat. No. 10220Q   Form **W-4** (2004)

Figure 18-12. Update all Employee's Withholding Allowance Certificates (W-4 forms) at least once a year.

An employee who earns $8 per hour and works 35 hours, for example, has gross earnings of $280 ($8 × 35 hours) per week.

For a salaried employee, use the salary amount as the gross earnings for the pay period, no matter how many hours the employee worked. An employee who earns a weekly salary of $400, for example, receives that amount whether she worked 30, 40, or 50 hours during that week.

Fair Labor Standards Act. The Fair Labor Standards Act primarily affects employees who earn hourly wages. It limits the number of hours they may work, sets their minimum wage, and regulates their overtime pay. It also requires the employer to record the number of hours they work, usually on a time card or in a time book.

For hourly employees, this act mandates payment of:

- Time and a half (1½ times the normal hourly wage) for all hours worked beyond the normal 8 in a regular workday.
- Time and a half for all hours worked on the sixth consecutive day of the work week.
- Twice the normal wage (double time) for all hours worked on the seventh consecutive workday.
- Double time, plus normal holiday pay, for all hours worked on a company-approved holiday.

The Fair Labor Standards Act also requires overtime payments for part-time hourly employees for every hour worked beyond the normal 8 in a day or 40 in a week.

Making Deductions

The law requires all employers to withhold money from employees' gross earnings to pay federal and state and local (if any) income taxes and certain other taxes. In addition, employees may wish you to make certain voluntary deductions. For example, you might be asked to deduct an amount for child care, if the practice or hospital provides on-site child care. You might also deduct employee contributions to health insurance premiums.

You must deposit all employee deductions and employer payments into separate accounts. Monies from these **tax liability** accounts are used to pay taxes to appropriate government agencies.

Income Taxes. You must withhold enough money to cover the employee's federal income tax for the pay period. You can determine this amount by finding the employee's number of exemptions (from Form W-4) and referring to the tax tables in *Circular E, Employer's Tax Guide,* published by the IRS.

Consult the state and local tax tables for other income taxes. These taxes may be simpler to calculate. For example, they may be 4% and 1% of the employee's gross earnings, respectively.

FICA Taxes. For FICA tax, withhold from the employee's check half of the tax owed for the pay period. Pay the other half from the practice's accounts. The amount of FICA tax that funds Social Security differs from the amount that funds Medicare. Report these two amounts separately. Check IRS *Circular E* for the latest FICA tax percentages and level of taxable earnings.

Unemployment Taxes. Federal unemployment tax is not a deduction from employees' paychecks, but it is based on their earnings. It is paid by the practice. The Federal Unemployment Tax Act (FUTA) requires employers to pay a percentage of each employee's income, up to a certain dollar amount. The percentage may be reduced if the employer also pays state unemployment taxes.

States calculate unemployment taxes differently. Some states tax employers and employees; others tax only employers. State unemployment tax usually varies with the employer's past employment record. Employers with few layoffs, such as physicians, have lower tax rates than those with many layoffs. To compute state unemployment tax, apply the assigned tax rate to each employee's earnings, up to a maximum for the calendar year. For details, consult your state unemployment insurance department.

Workers' Compensation. Some states require employers to insure their employees against possible loss of income resulting from work-related injury, disability, or disease. Although state laws vary, they typically require doctors to carry this insurance with a state insurance fund or state-authorized private insurer. Usually, a medical practice's insurance agent will audit the payroll books annually and then issue a bill for the workers' compensation premium due.

Calculating Net Earnings

Add each employee's required and voluntary deductions together to determine the total deductions. Then, subtract the total deductions from the gross earnings to get the employee's **net earnings,** or take-home pay. Use the following equation:

Gross Earnings − Total Deductions = Net Earnings

Preparing Paychecks

The way you prepare the practice's payroll will depend on the system the practice uses. In a small practice, you may write paychecks manually. In this case, write the check amount for the employee's net earnings, and deduct the check amount from the office checkbook. Payroll may also be handled through electronic banking; see the Tips for the Office section.

If the practice uses a payroll service, you may supply time cards or payroll data to the service by mail or electronically. The service calculates all the deductions, prepares paychecks, and mails them to the practice for distribution.

Tips for the Office

Handling Payroll Through Electronic Banking

An electronic funds transfer system (EFTS) enables you to handle the practice's payroll without writing payroll checks manually. The physician must sign up for EFTS with the bank, and employees must supply their bank account numbers to the employer. Then, the bank electronically deposits employees' paychecks into their bank accounts, as directed.

Most employees like to have their paychecks deposited automatically. The money is available on the day of deposit, and no one has to worry about losing a paycheck, getting to the bank before it closes, or carrying a paycheck around. Also, employees still receive a check stub along with a notification of deposit, so they can track their earnings and deductions.

Contact your bank for more information and specific procedures for setting up EFTS and electronic payroll.

No matter how paychecks are prepared, they should include information about how the check amount was determined. This information usually appears on the check stub. It should match the information on the employee earnings records and payroll register. Procedure 18-5 explains the process for generating payroll.

Maintaining Employee Earnings Records

You need to keep an employee earnings record for each employee (Figure 18-13). When you create the record, list the employee's name, address, phone number, Social Security number, birth date, spouse's name, number of dependents, job title, employment starting date, pay rate, and voluntary deductions.

Then, for each pay period, record the employee's gross earnings, individual deductions, net earnings, and related information. Properly completed earnings records show each employee's earning history.

Maintaining a Payroll Register

A payroll register summarizes vital information about all employees and their earnings (Figure 18-14). At the end of each pay period, record each employee's earnings to date, hourly rate, hours worked, overtime hours, overtime earnings, and total gross earnings. Also, list the gross earnings subject to unemployment taxes and FICA, all required and voluntary deductions, net earnings, and the paycheck number.

Handling Payroll Electronically

Manual payroll preparation and related tasks may take an hour per week for each employee. To save time and to provide the convenience for employees of having their paychecks automatically deposited, some practices handle payroll tasks electronically.

If you work in a relatively small practice, you may handle all payroll tasks in the office, using accounting or payroll software. If you work in a large practice, you may prepare payroll information on the computer and transmit it by modem to an outside payroll service for processing. Depending on which system and software the practice has, you may use the computer to:

- Create, update, and delete employee payroll information files
- Prepare employee paychecks, stubs, and W-2 forms
- Update and print employee earnings records
- Update all appropriate bookkeeping records, such as the payroll ledger and general ledger, with payroll data

To perform these payroll functions electronically, follow the specific instructions in the software manual or get instructions from the payroll service. Generally, you would follow these steps.

Select an option from the "Payroll" menu. Wait for the prompt, then select the appropriate employee from a list of employees.

To create an employee payroll information file for a new employee, input the same information that you would record manually on an employee payroll information sheet: name, address, Social Security number, marital status, pay schedule, number of dependents, payroll type, and voluntary deductions. Print two copies of the employee payroll information file—one for the employee and one for the physician's personnel file.

To update an employee payroll information file when an employee moves, marries, has a child, or wants to change deductions, select "Update Employee File." After making the changes, print out two copies of the file. Show one to the employee to confirm that the information is correct. Then have the employee sign and date it. Keep the signed copy for the physician's personnel file, and give the other to the employee. To ensure that payroll information is always correct and current, you should update it once a year for every employee.

To delete an employee payroll information file when an employee leaves the practice, select "Terminate Employee." Remember to print out and file a copy of this information before deleting it, because the physician is required to keep employees' payroll records for 4 years.

To generate paychecks and stubs, select the employee from the list of employees and choose the "Print Paycheck" option. Then, answer each prompt displayed by the computer (for example, hours worked). The computer has the employee's pay rate, payroll type, and deductions on file and automatically calculates the employee's net earnings, generates a paycheck, and prints a pay stub with the appropriate information.

To create an employee earnings record, select this option and follow the prompts for the needed information. Depending on the software used, each employee's earnings record may be updated automatically every time you generate a paycheck or make changes to other payroll files.

Calculating and Filing Taxes

In many practices, medical assistants set up tax liability accounts for money withheld from paychecks. These accounts are used to submit this money to appropriate agencies.

Setting Up Tax Liability Accounts

You must set up at least two bank accounts to hold the money deducted from paychecks until it can be sent to the appropriate government agencies. One account will hold deductions from employees' paychecks for federal, state, and local income taxes and FICA taxes. Another account will hold employer payments based on payroll, such as federal and state unemployment taxes. For these accounts, choose a bank that is authorized by the IRS to accept federal tax deposits. If the practice makes other paycheck deductions, as for workers' compensation or a 401(k) plan, set up an account for each of these also.

Each time you prepare paychecks, deposit the withheld money into the proper account. Then, record the deposited amounts as debits in the practice's checking account.

Understanding Federal Tax Deposit Schedules

You will probably deposit federal income taxes and FICA taxes (which together are known as employment taxes) on a quarterly, monthly, or biweekly (every-other-week) schedule. Every November IRS personnel decide which deposit schedule your office should use for the next year.

If the IRS does not notify you about this matter, determine your deposit schedule based on the total employment taxes your office reported on the previous year's Employer's Quarterly Federal Tax Returns (Form 941). For example, if your office reported $50,000 or less in employment taxes during the past year, you would make monthly employment tax deposits the present year. If your office reported more than $50,000 during the past year, you would make semimonthly tax deposits.

There are exceptions to the monthly or semimonthly tax deposit schedules: the $500 rule and the $100,000 rule. The $500 rule applies to employers who owe less than $500 in employment taxes during a tax period (such as a quarter). These employers do not have to make a deposit for that period. The $100,000 rule applies to employers who owe $100,000 or more in employment taxes on any one day during a tax period. These employers must deposit the tax by the next banking day after the day that ceiling is reached.

Submitting Federal Income Taxes and FICA Taxes

Some businesses must submit federal income taxes and FICA taxes to the IRS by electronic funds transfer (EFT). The EFT program, known as TAXLINK, began in 1995. Since then, more taxpayers have been required to use it each year. If your practice is not required to use EFT but wishes to do so voluntarily, contact the IRS, Cash Management Site Office, to enroll.

If your practice does not use EFT, you must submit these employment taxes with a Federal Tax Deposit (FTD) Coupon (Form 8109) (see Figure 18-15). FTD Coupons are supplied by the IRS. They are printed with the physician's name, address, and EIN. They have boxes for filling in the type of tax and the tax period for which the deposit is being made.

To make the deposit, write a single check or money order for the total amount of federal income taxes and FICA taxes withheld during the tax period. Make the check payable to the bank where you make the deposit. This must be a Federal Reserve Bank or another bank authorized to make payments to the IRS. Also, complete the FTD Coupon. Then, mail or deliver the check and FTD Coupon to the bank. The bank will give you a deposit receipt.

If you work in a practice with a large payroll, you may need to make deposits every few days. In most practices, however, you will probably make deposits once a month. Then, every 3 months, a more complete accounting is required on a **quarterly return,** called the Employer's Quarterly Federal Tax Return (Form 941).

Submitting FUTA Taxes

FUTA taxes provide money to workers who are unemployed. If the practice owes more than $100 in federal unemployment tax at the end of the quarter, deposit the tax amount with an FTD Coupon (Form 8109). At the end of the year, file an Employer's Annual Federal Unemployment (FUTA) Tax Return (Form 940) with any final taxes owed (Figure 18-16).

Generally, an employer must pay FUTA taxes if employees' wages total more than $1500 in any quarter (3-month period) and if those employees are not seasonal

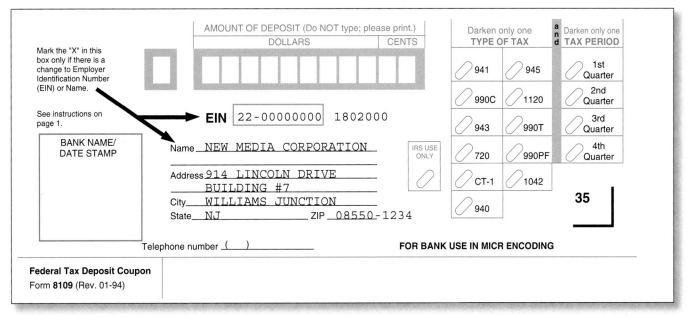

Figure 18-15. Practices that do not use TAXLINK to submit taxes electronically must submit federal income and FICA taxes with a Federal Tax Deposit (FTD) Coupon (Form 8109).

or household workers. The FUTA tax, which is 6.2%, is applied to the first $7000 of income for a year.

Filing an Employer's Quarterly Federal Tax Return

Each quarter, file an Employer's Quarterly Federal Tax Return (Form 941) with the IRS (Figure 18-17). This tax return summarizes the federal income and FICA taxes (employment taxes) withheld from employees' paychecks.

As a general rule, you should file Form 941 at the nearest IRS office by the last day of the first month after the quarter ends. If the practice has deposited all taxes on time, you have an additional 10 days after the due date to file.

Handling State and Local Income Taxes

Send withheld state and local income taxes to the proper agencies, using their forms, procedures, and schedules. If required, prepare quarterly or other tax forms for the state and local governments.

Filing Wage and Tax Statements

After the end of each year, file a Wage and Tax Statement (Form W-2) with the appropriate federal, state, and local government agencies for each employee who had federal income and FICA taxes withheld during the previous year (Figure 18-18). Also, supply copies of Form W-2 to each employee.

Form W-2 shows the employee's total taxable income for the previous year. It also shows the exact amount of federal income taxes and FICA taxes (for Social Security and Medicare) withheld, along with the amounts of state and local taxes withheld (if any).

Along with the W-2 forms, submit Form W-3, a Transmittal of Wage and Tax Statements (Figure 18-19). This form lists the employer's name, address, and EIN and summarizes the amount of all employees' earnings and the federal income taxes and FICA taxes withheld.

Managing Contracts

An **employment contract**—a written agreement of employment terms between employer and employee—may be considered a benefit because it increases employee job security. It also allows the employer to attract and keep the best employees. Although contracts are rarely offered to medical assistants, you should be aware of them because they may be used for doctors and executive management of a practice and because they may be used for medical assistants in the future.

Legal Elements of a Contract

An employment contract is a legal agreement between two or more people to perform an act in exchange for payment. To be binding, the contract must include these main elements:

- An agreement between two or more competent people to do something legal

Form 940

Department of the Treasury
Internal Revenue Service (99)

Employer's Annual Federal Unemployment (FUTA) Tax Return

▶ See separate Instructions for Form 940 for information on completing this form.

OMB No. 1545-0028

2003

T	
FF	
FD	
FP	
I	
T	

You must complete this section. ▶

Name (as distinguished from trade name)   Calendar year

Trade name, if any   Employer identification number (EIN)

Address (number and street)   City, state, and ZIP code

A Are you required to pay unemployment contributions to only one state? (If "No," skip questions B and C.). ☐ Yes ☐ No

B Did you pay all state unemployment contributions by February 2, 2004? ((1) If you deposited your total FUTA tax when due, check "Yes" if you paid all state unemployment contributions by February 10, 2004. (2) If a 0% experience rate is granted, check "Yes." (3) If "No," skip question C.) . . . . ☐ Yes ☐ No

C Were all wages that were taxable for FUTA tax also taxable for your state's unemployment tax? . . . . . ☐ Yes ☐ No

If you answered "No" to any of these questions, you must file Form 940. If you answered "Yes" to all the questions, you may file Form 940-EZ, which is a simplified version of Form 940. (Successor employers, see **Special credit for successor employers** on page 3 of the separate instructions.) You can get Form 940-EZ by calling 1-800-TAX-FORM (1-800-829-3676) or from the IRS website at **www.irs.gov.**

If you will not have to file returns in the future, check here (see **Who Must File** in the separate instructions) **and complete and sign the return** . . . . ▶ ☐

If this is an **Amended Return, check here** (see **Amended Returns** in the separate instructions) . . . . ▶ ☐

Part I Computation of Taxable Wages

1 Total payments (including payments shown on lines 2 and 3) during the calendar year for services of employees **1**

2 Exempt payments. (Explain all exempt payments, attaching additional sheets if necessary.) ▶ _____ **2**

3 Payments of more than $7,000 for services. Enter only amounts over the first $7,000 paid to each employee (see separate instructions). Do not include any exempt payments from line 2. The $7,000 amount is the Federal wage base. Your state wage base may be different. **Do not use your state wage limitation** **3**

4 Add lines 2 and 3 . . . . **4**

5 **Total taxable wages** (subtract line 4 from line 1) . . . . ▶ **5**

Be sure to complete both sides of this form, and sign in the space provided on the back.

For Privacy Act and Paperwork Reduction Act Notice, see separate instructions.   ▼ **DETACH HERE** ▼   Cat. No. 11234O   Form **940** (2003)

Form 940-V

Department of the Treasury
Internal Revenue Service

Payment Voucher

Use this voucher only when making a payment with your return.

OMB No. 1545-0028

2003

Complete boxes 1, 2, and 3. Do not send cash, and do not staple your payment to this voucher. Make your check or money order payable to the "United States Treasury." Be sure to enter your employer identification number (EIN), "Form 940," and "2003" on your payment.

1 Enter your employer identification number (EIN).

2 **Enter the amount of your payment. ▶**   Dollars   Cents

3 Enter your business name (individual name for sole proprietors).

Enter your address.

Enter your city, state, and ZIP code.

Figure 18-16. Tax dollars filed with FUTA tax returns (Form 940) provide money to workers who are unemployed.

Form **941**
(Rev. January 2004)
Department of the Treasury
Internal Revenue Service (99)

Employer's Quarterly Federal Tax Return
▶ See separate instructions revised January 2004 for information on completing this return.
Please type or print.

Enter state code for state in which deposits were made **only** if different from state in address to the right ▶ (see page 2 of separate instructions).

Name (as distinguished from trade name)

Trade name, if any

Address (number and street)

Date quarter ended

Employer identification number

City, state, and ZIP code

OMB No. 1545-0029

T	
FF	
FD	
FP	
I	
T	

If address is different from prior return, check here ▶

IRS Use

1 1 1 1 1 1 1 1 1 1   2   3 3 3 3 3 3 3 3   4 4 4   5 5 5

6   7   8 8 8 8 8 8   9 9 9 9   10 10 10 10 10 10 10 10 10

A If you **do not have to file** returns in the future, check here ▶ ☐ and enter date final wages paid ▶

B If you are a seasonal employer, see **Seasonal employers** on page 1 of the instructions and check here ▶ ☐

1 Number of employees in the pay period that includes March 12th . ▶ | 1 |

2	Total wages and tips, plus other compensation (see separate instructions)	**2**
3	Total income tax withheld from wages, tips, and sick pay . . .	**3**
4	Adjustment of withheld income tax for preceding quarters of **this calendar year**	**4**
5	Adjusted total of income tax withheld (line 3 as adjusted by line 4)	**5**

6	Taxable social security wages	**6a**		× 12.4% (.124) =	**6b**	
	Taxable social security tips	**6c**		× 12.4% (.124) =	**6d**	
7	Taxable Medicare wages and tips . . .	**7a**		× 2.9% (.029) =	**7b**	

8 Total social security and Medicare taxes (add lines 6b, 6d, and 7b). **Check here if wages are not subject to social security and/or Medicare tax** . . . . ▶ ☐ | **8** |

9 Adjustment of social security and Medicare taxes (see instructions for required explanation)
Sick Pay $ _____ ± Fractions of Cents $ _____ ± Other $ _____ = | **9** |

10 Adjusted total of social security and Medicare taxes (line 8 as adjusted by line 9) . . . . | **10** |

11 **Total taxes** (add lines 5 and 10) . . . . | **11** |

12 Advance earned income credit (EIC) payments made to employees (see instructions) . . . | **12** |

13 Net taxes (subtract line 12 from line 11). **If $2,500 or more, this must equal line 17, column (d) below (or line D of Schedule B (Form 941))** . . . . . . | **13** |

14 Total deposits for quarter, including overpayment applied from a prior quarter . . . . . | **14** |

15 **Balance due** (subtract line 14 from line 13). See instructions . . . . | **15** |

16 **Overpayment.** If line 14 is more than line 13, enter excess here ▶ $ _____
and check if to be: ☐ Applied to next return **or** ☐ Refunded.

- **All filers:** If line 13 is less than $2,500, **do not** complete line 17 or Schedule B (Form 941).
- **Semiweekly schedule depositors:** Complete Schedule B (Form 941) and check here . . . . ▶ ☐
- **Monthly schedule depositors:** Complete line 17, columns (a) through (d), and check here . . . . ▶ ☐

17	**Monthly Summary of Federal Tax Liability.** (Complete **Schedule B (Form 941)** instead, if you were a semiweekly schedule depositor.)			
	(a) First month liability	**(b)** Second month liability	**(c)** Third month liability	**(d)** Total liability for quarter

Third Party Designee

Do you want to allow another person to discuss this return with the IRS (see separate instructions)? ☐ **Yes.** Complete the following. ☐ **No**

Designee's name ▶
Phone no. ▶ ( )
Personal identification number (PIN) ▶

Sign Here

Under penalties of perjury, I declare that I have examined this return, including accompanying schedules and statements, and to the best of my knowledge and belief, it is true, correct, and complete.

Signature ▶
Print Your Name and Title ▶
Date ▶

For Privacy Act and Paperwork Reduction Act Notice, see back of Payment Voucher.   Cat. No. 17001Z   Form **941** (Rev. 1-2004)

Figure 18-17. Most practices make tax deposits monthly and then make a more complete accounting once every 3 months on the Employer's Quarterly Federal Tax Return (Form 941), the first page of which is shown here.

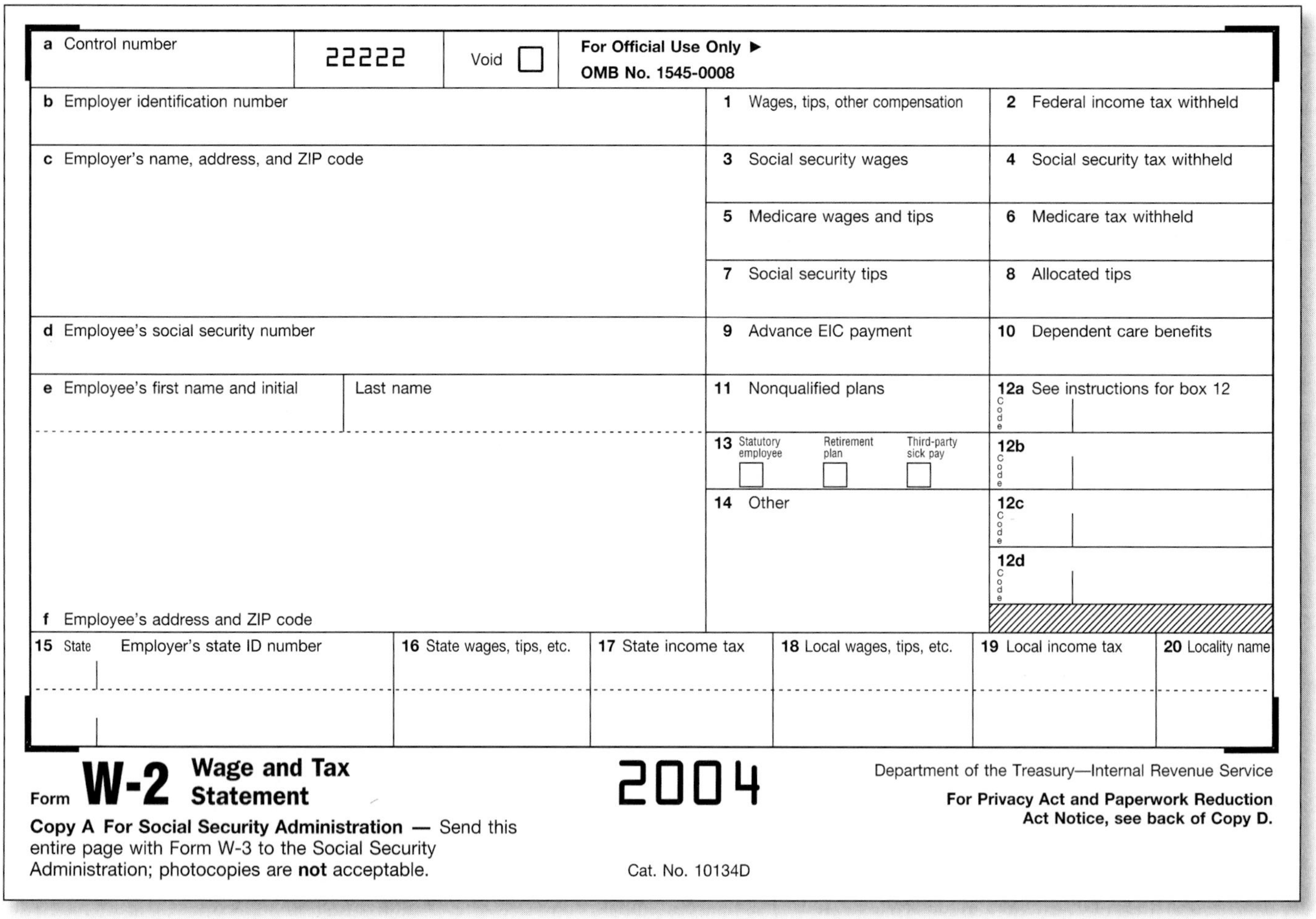

Figure 18-18. A Wage and Tax Statement (Form W-2) records the total amount of taxes withheld during the previous year for each employee.

- Names and addresses of the people involved
- Consideration (whatever is given in exchange, such as money, work, or property)
- Starting and ending dates, as well as date(s) the contract was signed
- Signatures of the employer and employee

A Medical Assistant Contract

Some medical practices use employment contracts for medical assistants. This type of contract would include these elements:

- A description of your duties and your employer's duties
- Plans for handling major changes in job responsibilities
- Salary, bonuses, and other forms of compensation
- Benefits, such as vacation time, sick days, life insurance, and participation in pension plans
- Grievance procedures
- Exceptional situations under which the contract may be terminated by either you or your employer
- Termination procedures and compensation
- Special provisions, such as job sharing, medical examinations, or liability coverage

If you are offered an employment contract, study it closely. Consider any local laws that may apply, and have a lawyer or business adviser review the contract.

Summary

The administrative and accounting duties of the medical assistant may involve several aspects of financial control through the proper understanding and management of accounts receivable and accounts payable. The use of standard bookkeeping and banking procedures is necessary in order to maintain the business of the office in proper form. The tasks involved may include the following:

- Using daily logs of charges and receipts for patient accounts
- Depositing cash and checks in bank accounts
- Summarizing patient charges and receipts
- Reconciling bank accounts to the practice records
- Disbursing funds for petty cash and office purchases
- Managing payroll for employees
- Preparing tax forms for payroll processing
- Assisting with contracts of the practice

DO NOT STAPLE OR FOLD

a Control number	33333	For Official Use Only ▶ OMB No. 1545-0008	

b Kind of Payer ▶	941 ☐ Military ☐ 943 ☐ CT-1 ☐ Hshld. emp. ☐ Medicare govt. emp. ☐ **Third-party sick pay** ☐	**1** Wages, tips, other compensation	**2** Federal income tax withheld
		3 Social security wages	**4** Social security tax withheld
c Total number of Forms W-2	**d** Establishment number	**5** Medicare wages and tips	**6** Medicare tax withheld
e Employer identification number		**7** Social security tips	**8** Allocated tips
f Employer's name		**9** Advance EIC payments	**10** Dependent care benefits
		11 Nonqualified plans	**12** Deferred compensation
		13 For third-party sick pay use only	
		14 Income tax withheld by payer of third-party sick pay	
g Employer's address and ZIP code			
h Other EIN used this year			
15 State Employer's state ID number		**16** State wages, tips, etc.	**17** State income tax
		18 Local wages, tips, etc.	**19** Local income tax
Contact person		Telephone number ( )	For Official Use Only
Email address		Fax number ( )	

Under penalties of perjury, I declare that I have examined this return and accompanying documents, and, to the best of my knowledge and belief, they are true, correct, and complete.

Signature ▶   Title ▶   Date ▶

Form **W-3** Transmittal of Wage and Tax Statements   **2004**   Department of the Treasury
Internal Revenue Service

Send this entire page with the entire Copy A page of Form(s) W-2 to the Social Security Administration. Photocopies are not acceptable.

Do not send any payment (cash, checks, money orders, etc.) with Forms W-2 and W-3.

An Item To Note

Separate instructions. See the **2004 Instructions for Forms W-2 and W-3** for information on completing this form.

Purpose of Form

Use this form to transmit Copy A of **Form(s) W-2,** Wage and Tax Statement. Make a copy of Form W-3, and keep it with Copy D (For Employer) of Form(s) W-2 for your records. Use Form W-3 for the correct year. **File Form W-3 even if only one Form W-2 is being filed.** If you are filing Form(s) W-2 on magnetic media or electronically, **do not** file Form W-3.

When To File

File Form W-3 with Copy A of Form(s) W-2 by February 28, 2005.

Where To File

Send this entire page with the entire Copy A page of Form(s) W-2 to:

**Social Security Administration
Data Operations Center
Wilkes-Barre, PA 18769-0001**

Note: If you use "Certified Mail" to file, change the ZIP code to "18769-0002." If you use an IRS-approved private delivery service, add "ATTN: W-2 Process, 1150 E. Mountain Dr." to the address and change the ZIP code to "18702-7997." See **Circular E (Pub. 15),** Employer's Tax Guide, for a list of IRS approved private delivery services.

Do **not** send magnetic media to the address shown above.

For Privacy Act and Paperwork Reduction Act Notice, see back of Copy D of Form W-2.

Figure 18-19. Submit a Transmittal of Wage and Tax Statements (Form W-3) with the W-2 forms.

REVIEW

CHAPTER 18

CASE STUDY QUESTIONS

Now that you have completed this chapter, review the case study at the beginning of the chapter and answer the following question:

1. What should Ben do to properly record the payment?

Discussion Questions

1. Name three things that are required in a single-entry accounting system.
2. What are the three terms that are used in the double-entry accounting system?
3. Why is the reconciliation of the bank statement so important?
4. Why is a petty cash fund useful?
5. When creating a payroll information sheet, name what it should contain.

Critical Thinking Questions

1. Why is it important for an employer to have an Employer Identification Number?
2. Discuss the importance of having separate accounts for employee deductions.

3. Name some of the banking tasks of the medical practice.
4. Name some of the requirements of the Fair Labor Standards Act.

Application Activities

1. Record the following disbursements made on September 9, 2004, in a disbursements journal:
   - Check no. 1234, payee—Tom Jones (electrician), check amount—$125
   - Check no. 1235, payee—Postmaster (postage), check amount—$32
   - Check no. 1236, payee—Gateway Property Management (rent), check amount—$900
2. Simulate an office petty cash account, using your own personal expenses. Determine a starting amount, and use it for 2 weeks to buy small items. For each purchase, obtain a receipt, or write a petty cash voucher. Record each withdrawal you make from the petty cash account, using a petty cash record. At least once during the 2-week period, write a check to replenish the account.
3. Prepare your personal federal income tax return, using information from the Wage and Tax Statement (Form W-2) and the Employee's Withholding Allowance Certificate (Form W-4) provided by your employer.

PART
Three

Clinical Medical Assisting

"One of the most important things you must remember when assisting with patients is to put yourself in the patient's place. How would you feel if you were told to do something you didn't know how to do? Wouldn't you want to know ahead of time what will be expected of you?

"As a medical assistant, it is your job to anticipate the physician's every need during a physical exam. Compare the process with that of surgery, where the doctor is handed an instrument even before he asks for it. You should try to make as smooth a transition as possible from one step to the next; everyone benefits."

Diane Morlock
Medical Assisting Instructor
Stautzenberger College
Toledo, Ohio

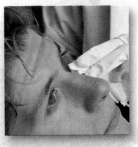

SECTION ONE
The Medical Office Environment

SECTION TWO
Anatomy and Physiology

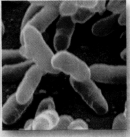

SECTION THREE
Assisting With Patients

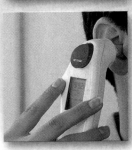

SECTION FOUR
Specialty Practices and Medical Emergencies

SECTION FIVE
Physician's Office Laboratory Procedures

SECTION SIX
Nutrition, Pharmacology, and Diagnostic Equipment

SECTION SEVEN
Externship

These and other contributions to knowledge about infection have evolved into the current techniques for keeping infectious microorganisms out of the medical office and operating room. These techniques are now widely accepted and are legally required in the practice of medicine. You will apply these techniques in your daily work as a medical assistant.

Microorganisms and Disease

Microorganisms live all around us. They are found in and on our bodies, in the air we breathe, in the water we drink, and on almost every surface we touch. Types of microorganisms include:

- Viruses, the smallest infectious agents, many of which cause disease
- Bacteria, single-celled organisms that reproduce quickly and are a major cause of disease
- Protozoans, single-celled organisms found in soil and water, most of which do not cause disease
- Fungi, organisms with a complex cell structure, most of which do not cause disease
- Very small multicellular organisms, a few of which are parasitic (living on or in another organism) and cause disease

Although everyone is surrounded by microorganisms, people are able to escape infection most of the time for the following three reasons:

1. The majority of microorganisms are either beneficial or harmless. **Pathogens,** microorganisms capable of causing disease, comprise only a small portion of the total number of microorganisms that exist in a given environment.
2. The human body has a wide variety of defenses that allow people to resist infection.
3. Conditions must be favorable for a pathogen to grow and to be transmitted to a person who is susceptible (sensitive) to infection.

The Disease Process

Many types of diseases affect humans. An infectious disease is one that is caused by the action of a microorganism. An infection begins when the microorganism finds a human host, that is, a body in which it can survive, multiply, and thrive. To grow, a microorganism requires specific conditions, which include the proper temperature, pH (a measure of the body's acid-base balance), and moisture level. The temperature within the human body (98.6°F, or 37°C), the body's neutral pH, and the body's dark, moist environment are prime conditions for the growth of microorganisms.

Some pathogens nearly always cause disease, whereas others cause disease less often or only under certain circumstances. A microorganism's disease-producing power is called **virulence.** When microorganisms damage the body, they do so in many ways:

- By depleting nutrients or other materials needed by the cells and tissues they invade
- By reproducing themselves within body cells
- By making body cells the targets of the body's own defenses
- By producing toxins, or poisons, that damage cells and tissues

The Body's Defenses

Daily life constantly exposes people to multitudes of pathogens, but the bodies of healthy individuals have built-in defenses against them. The condition of being resistant to pathogens and the diseases they cause is called **immunity.** When these defenses are not functioning properly (as when individuals have poor health, inadequate nutrition, or poor hygiene habits), people become particularly susceptible to invasion, setting the stage for infection to occur.

There are other reasons that a person's defenses may be weak. A break in the skin caused by injury can leave a person especially vulnerable to microorganisms. This type of opening in the body provides the organisms with an unprotected point of entry. Drugs can also weaken the body's ability to fight infection. For example, anticancer drugs may kill healthy cells along with the cancer cells. Disorders of the immune system, such as AIDS, interfere with the body's natural ability to fight infection.

Because people are constantly, and quite literally, surrounded by pathogens, the body's natural defenses against pathogens are crucial to survival. If people do not have these defenses, they are potentially vulnerable to infection by every microorganism they encounter, including those naturally found in the body. Infections by microorganisms that can cause disease only when a host's resistance is low are called **opportunistic infections.** Examples of opportunistic infections are pneumonia caused by *Pneumocystis carinii* (a protozoan) and oral candidiasis, caused by *Candida* (a yeastlike fungus found commonly in the mouth as well as the intestinal tract and vagina). Both of these infections are common in AIDS patients.

The human body has many types of defense mechanisms that work to fight off pathogens. **Normal flora** are beneficial bacteria found in the body that create a barrier against pathogens. These bacteria produce substances that can harm invaders and starve them by using up the resources pathogens need to live. Normal flora colonize the skin, nose, mouth, vagina, rectum, and intestines. For example, some staphylococci bacteria are normally present on the skin and in the upper respiratory tract. The normal flora in any given area are specific (endogenous) to those areas, different from flora in or on other parts of the body.

Intact skin is the best first-line defense people have against disease. Skin secretions also serve as a barrier to

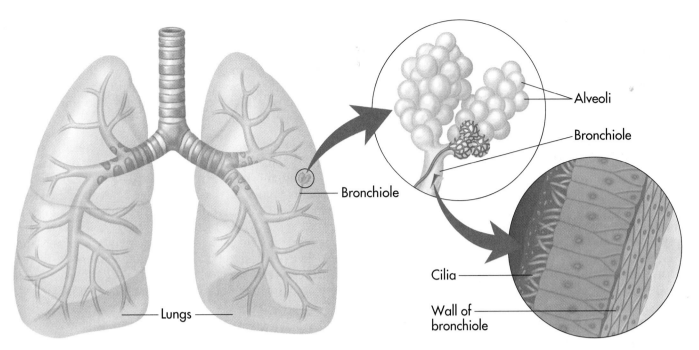

Figure 19-3. The sweeping motion of cilia that line the respiratory tract helps rid the body of foreign particles and some microorganisms.

invaders. Other body fluids and functions protect people from disease as well. Tears, saliva, and internal secretions such as prostatic fluid and cervical mucus have a mild germ-killing acidity. The respiratory tract is lined with cilia, tiny projections that continuously beat upward to expel foreign substances trapped in mucus (Figure 19-3). Coughing and sneezing rid the respiratory tract of excess mucus. Normally high acidic levels of the stomach and urine help to prevent or inhibit bacterial growth. Contractions of smooth muscle along the intestinal tract help rid the body of infectious microorganisms as well.

When microorganisms successfully invade body tissues, the immune system immediately begins to neutralize and destroy them. The immune system includes nonspecific defenses, which are often used in conjunction with the two main types of specific defenses: humoral defenses (fluid mechanisms) and cell-mediated defenses. The immune system also involves the spleen, lymph nodes, tonsils, thymus, lungs, liver, and kidneys, all of which contain lymphatic tissue. Lymphatic tissue is a filtering network of connective tissue containing large numbers of lymphocytes. Lymphocytes are specialized white blood cells that combat infectious agents.

Nonspecific Defense

One type of nonspecific defense is the process known as phagocytosis, which occurs when special white blood cells called **phagocytes** engulf and digest pathogens. (Figure 19-4 shows how a phagocyte "swallows" a pathogen.) A pouch forms around the pathogen as it is engulfed. The phagocyte secretes enzymes and metabolites into the pouch, destroying the trapped material. Phagocytes are the

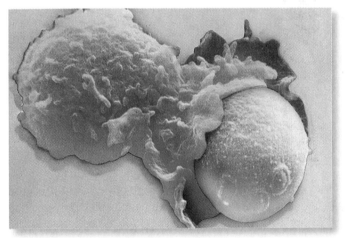

Figure 19-4. Phagocytes protect the body from infection by finding, surrounding, and digesting intruding microorganisms.

cells that form pus as they go to the site of infection to help destroy microorganisms.

There are several varieties of phagocytes, two of which are of particular importance. Neutrophils are phagocytes that move on their own and can act quickly to destroy an invading microorganism. **Macrophages,** which are known as monocytes while in the bloodstream, are phagocytes found in the lymph nodes, liver, spleen, lungs, bone marrow, and connective tissue. They are larger and generally slower-moving than neutrophils, but they live longer. Macrophages also play several roles in humoral and cell-mediated immunity, including presenting the antigens to the lymphocytes involved in these defenses.

Humoral Immunity

One type of humoral protection is provided by **antibodies,** highly specific proteins that attach themselves to foreign substances. This defense involves two types of lymphocytes: B cells (also called B lymphocytes) and T cells (also known as T lymphocytes). When the body is invaded by **antigens** (foreign substances), helper T cells activate B cells to produce antibodies, which combine with the antigens to neutralize them. Although the initial response to a major invasion by an antigen may not be a highly effective defense, memory B cells are produced for the appropriate antibody. A later invasion by the same antigen will be quickly and effectively countered. Specific antibodies are produced in response to specific antigens. These antibodies act as a homing device to attract phagocytes, which then engulf and destroy the antigen.

The formation of antibodies gives the body immunity from a particular disease. Immunity can be natural or artificial, active or passive (Figure 19-5).

- Active immunity is a long-term immunity in which the body produces its own antibodies. Active immunity can be natural or artificial.
- Passive immunity results when antibodies produced outside the body enter the body. Passive immunity can be natural or artificial.
- Natural active immunity results from exposure to organisms that cause a disease, such as mumps. Although the person becomes sick with the disease, the body produces antibodies that prevent the individual from having the disease again if reexposed. A fetus acquires natural passive immunity when the mother's antibodies move across the placenta. Natural passive immunity lasts only a short time, usually a few weeks after birth.
- Artificial active immunity results from administration of an immunization or vaccine with killed or weakened organisms. These organisms induce the formation of antibodies without causing the disease. Artificial passive immunity occurs as a result of some types of immunizations (injections of antibodies) that provide temporary protection for people who have been exposed to serious diseases, such as hepatitis and tetanus. Artificial passive immunity lasts only a short time, usually a few weeks.

The other type of humoral defense is called complement. Complement is a group of proteins that circulates in the blood and body fluids and is always present in low amounts. When it is activated by antibodies, however, complement can multiply rapidly and destroy pathogens. It helps the white blood cells ingest microorganisms, sometimes making a hole in the microorganisms' cells that causes the cells to rupture and consequently be destroyed. The main reason that most bacteria do not cause disease is that these proteins can destroy many species of bacteria.

Cell-Mediated Immunity

In addition to their role in humoral immunity, T cells are instrumental in cell-mediated immunity. Cell-mediated immunity differs from humoral immunity in that T cells do not form antibodies to combat antigens. Instead, they directly attack the invader. Several different types of T cells are involved in the attack process. Helper T cells activate the killer T cells, which bind with the antigen and kill it. Suppressor T cells slow down or stop the attack after the antigen is destroyed. Memory T cells are formed and will respond quickly to another attack by the same antigen.

Cell-mediated defenses against infection often result in inflammation of the affected area. Inflammation occurs when phagocytes enter the area, stick to the lining of the blood vessels, and come out of the vessels to attack the infecting agent. Small blood vessels then dilate and leak fluid, resulting in swelling, redness, and warmth. This process often causes fever, which is a common response to many infections and may play a part in fighting infection.

Immunity

Active Immunity	**Passive Immunity**
Body produces its own antibodies; provides long-term immunity	Antibodies produced outside of the body are introduced into the body; provides only temporary immunity
Natural Active Immunity	**Natural Passive Immunity**
Results from exposure to disease-causing organism	Results when antibodies from the mother cross the placenta to the fetus
Artificial Active Immunity	**Artificial Passive Immunity**
Results from administration of a vaccine with killed or weakened organisms	Results from immunization with antibodies to a disease-causing organism

Figure 19-5. Immunity to a disease can be acquired in a variety of ways: naturally, artificially, actively, and passively.

The fever results when endogenous pyrogen, a product of phagocytic cells, acts on the area of the brain that controls the body's temperature.

The Cycle of Infection

Five elements must be present for infection to occur: a reservoir host, a means of exit, a means of transmission, a means of entrance, and a susceptible host. These elements make up the cycle of infection (Figure 19-6).

Reservoir Host

The cycle of infection begins with establishment of the pathogen in the reservoir host. The **reservoir host** is an animal, insect, or human whose body is susceptible to growth of the pathogen. Most pathogens require a reservoir host to provide nutrition and a place to multiply.

The presence of the pathogen in the reservoir host may cause an infection in the host. At times, however, the host escapes full infection. A human **carrier** is a reservoir host who is unaware of the presence of the pathogen and so spreads the disease. The carrier exhibits no symptoms of infection. A human host also may have a **subclinical case,** which is a manifestation of the infection that is so slight as to be unnoticeable. The host experiences only some of the symptoms of the infection or milder symptoms than in a full case. A wide range of diseases can be manifested subclinically.

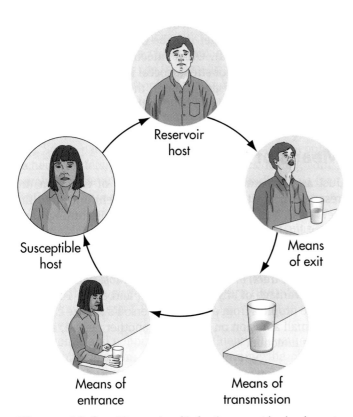

Figure 19-6. The cycle of infection must be broken at some point to prevent the spread of disease.

An infection in the reservoir host may be one of two types. The first is an **endogenous infection,** one in which an abnormality or malfunction in routine body processes has caused normally beneficial or harmless microorganisms to become pathogenic. The second type is an **exogenous infection,** one that is caused by the introduction of a pathogen from outside the body.

Means of Exit

To continue the cycle of infection, the pathogen must exit from the reservoir host. Common routes of exit from this host include the following:

- Through the nose, mouth, eyes, or ears
- In feces or urine
- In semen, vaginal fluid, or other discharge through the reproductive tract
- In blood or blood products from open wounds

Means of Transmission

To reproduce after it has exited from the reservoir host, the pathogen must spread to another host by some means of transmission. The means may be direct or indirect. Direct transmission occurs when the pathogen moves immediately from one host to another. This type of transmission may happen through contact with the infected person or with the discharges of the infected person, such as saliva or blood.

Indirect transmission is possible only if the pathogen is capable of existing independently of the reservoir host. In this case, the pathogen survives until a new host encounters it and the pathogen takes up residence in that new host. Indirect transmission can occur by the following means:

- **Vectors,** which are living organisms, such as insects, that carry microorganisms from an infected person to another person
- **Fomites,** or inanimate objects, such as clothing, body fluids, water, food, or even a stethoscope, that may be contaminated with infectious organisms and thus serve to transmit disease
- Droplets expelled into the air by sneezing, coughing, speaking, or breathing
- Contaminated food or drink

Airborne Transmission. Pathogens can be transmitted to a new host through the air. For example, microorganisms may enter the respiratory tract of a new host by inhalation. Respiratory diseases such as influenza, or flu, are often transmitted this way.

Pathogens may be inhaled from a variety of sources, such as soil particles or secretion droplets. When people inhale contaminated soil particles, fungal diseases may be contracted. If contaminated droplets are inhaled, diseases including influenza, chickenpox or tuberculosis may be

either sterile or not sterile, and if there is any question, you must consider the object or area contaminated. To prevent interruptions in the technique, you must also ensure that when objects touch one another, clean goes against clean, unclean goes against unclean, and sterile goes against sterile.

The surgical scrub is of primary importance in surgical asepsis. Surgical scrub procedures are similar to those for aseptic hand washing, but there are several distinctions. Differences include the following:

- A sterile scrub brush is used instead of a nailbrush.
- Both hands and forearms are washed.
- The hands are kept above the elbows to prevent water from running from the arms onto washed areas.
- Sterile towels are used instead of paper towels.
- Sterile gloves are put on immediately after the hands are dried.

Surgical Asepsis During a Surgical Procedure.
Chapter 42 describes assisting with minor surgery. Several points concerning surgical asepsis, however, are introduced here. Before performing a surgical procedure, the doctor may ask you to help prepare the skin. Your goal is to remove as many microorganisms as possible from around the area that is to undergo surgery so that you reduce the chances of these organisms entering the surgical opening. The skin and body openings, particularly the nose, mouth, and perineum, cannot be considered sterile. Nevertheless, the principles of aseptic technique require that you try to keep the area as contamination-free as possible.

Asepsis also involves keeping instruments and supplies sterile for use during the surgical procedure. After the sterile field has been created, handle items as little as possible to minimize the chance of contamination. Cover items that are not being used immediately with a sterile towel. If you are not wearing sterile gloves during a procedure (as when you are the only medical assistant and you must hand the doctor items from outside the sterile field), you must use transfer forceps to handle a sterile instrument. Transfer forceps look like big scissors or tweezers. Although the handles are not sterile, the tips that touch the instruments are.

If you are wearing sterile gloves, you handle sterile items directly and carefully avoid touching anything that is not sterile. Throughout the procedure, you are responsible for maintaining the sterile field (in this case, the area of surgery).

After the procedure, you continue using aseptic technique in caring for the patient's surgical wound. Typically, you need to apply dressings and keep the wound clean in an aseptic manner to prevent infection. You will also instruct the patient in how to care for the wound.

After you instruct the patient and guide the person out of the room, immediately place any supplies and disposable instruments that were used during the surgery into the appropriate **biohazardous waste containers.** These are leakproof containers that are color-coded red or labeled with a special biohazard symbol to show that they contain **biohazardous materials** (biological agents that can spread disease to living things). These containers are used to store and dispose of contaminated supplies and equipment in a way that preserves aseptic techniques and complies with the law.

Sanitizing, Disinfecting, and Sterilizing Instruments

After disposing of biohazardous waste, you must sanitize, disinfect, and sterilize reusable surgical instruments. **Sanitization** involves reducing the number of microorganisms on an object or a surface to a fairly safe level. To sanitize instruments after surgery, rinse them under warm, running water. If you cannot rinse them with water immediately, soak them in a disinfectant solution that has anticoagulant properties.

After rinsing the instruments, scrub them using hot, soapy water. Use a neutral-pH detergent that does not cause stains, corrosion, scratching, or a high level of suds and that is an effective blood solvent. Always wear utility gloves, use plastic brushes (never steel wool or wire), and keep different types of instruments (sharp, hinged, or of different metals) apart from each other when sanitizing them. After removing all visible stains and residue, rinse the instruments under running water, and roll them in a clean towel to dry them. Examine all instruments closely to make sure that they are in working order.

Disinfection is the destruction of infectious agents on an object or surface by direct application of chemical or physical means. Common disinfectants include chemical germicides, boiling water, and steam. You use disinfectants only on objects and surfaces because they are too strong to use on human tissue. Although disinfection kills a great many pathogens, **bacterial spores** (primitive, thick-walled reproductive bodies capable of developing into new individuals) and some viruses are not eliminated through disinfection.

To kill spores and viruses resistant to disinfection on instruments, you must sterilize them. **Sterilization** is the destruction of all microorganisms, including bacterial spores, by specific means. (For detailed information and procedures on instrument sanitization, disinfection, and sterilization, see Chapter 20.)

Disinfecting Work Surfaces

Another postsurgical aseptic procedure you will perform is disinfecting all work surfaces that were exposed to contamination (Figure 19-12). For this process, you must use bleach or a germ-killing solution approved by the U.S. government's Environmental Protection Agency (EPA). If protective coverings on surfaces or equipment were exposed to contamination during a procedure, they must be replaced.

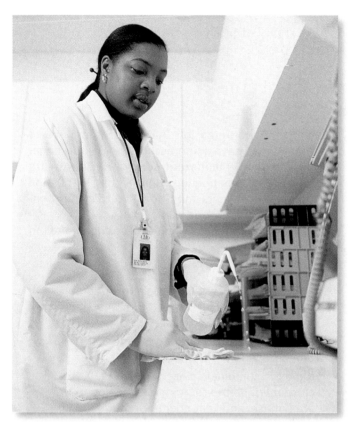

Figure 19-12. Work surfaces must be thoroughly cleaned with an EPA-approved chemical disinfectant.

Medical asepsis and surgical asepsis are required by law. Each individual who works in a medical setting must recognize the importance of asepsis and strictly adhere to aseptic procedures in daily routines.

OSHA Blood-borne Pathogens Standard and Universal Precautions

You must know the laws that require basic practices of infection control in a medical office. You must also know how to apply these laws in your office. Federal regulations related to infection control and asepsis were developed by the Department of Labor's Occupational Safety and Health Administration (OSHA) and described in the OSHA Blood-borne Pathogens Standard of 1991. These laws protect health-care workers from health hazards on the job, particularly from accidentally acquiring infections. They also help protect from health hazards patients and any other people who may come into the medical office.

OSHA Blood-borne Pathogens Standard

To ensure that biohazardous materials do not endanger people or the environment, laws set forth in the OSHA Blood-borne Pathogens Standard of 1991 dictate how you must handle infectious or potentially infectious waste generated during medical or surgical procedures. According to these rules, any potentially infectious waste materials must be discarded or held for processing in biohazardous waste containers. These wastes include the following:

- Blood products
- Body fluids
- Human tissues
- Vaccines
- Table paper, linen, towels, and gauze with body fluids on them
- Used scalpels, needles, sutures with needles attached, and other sharp instruments (known as sharps)
- Used gloves, disposable instruments, cotton swabs, and disposable applicators

Many medical offices today use only disposable paper gowns, drapes, coverings, and towels. Some offices, however, use cloth linens, which must be laundered. Certain rules apply to the laundering of cloth linens that are soiled with potentially infectious materials.

Medical offices use outside, licensed waste management services approved by the EPA to dispose of medical waste. A waste management service can provide instructions for preparing items before they are taken away.

The disposition and handling of contaminated sharps are of special concern because these instruments can easily puncture the skin and expose you to extremely dangerous viruses. Used sharps must never be bent, broken, recapped, or otherwise tampered with. After use, place them in a rigid, leakproof, puncture-resistant biohazardous waste container for sharps. Disposable and reusable sharps are kept in separate containers. Metal basins containing disinfectant are often used to store reusable sharps until they can be processed. The outside waste management company may supply containers for the disposable items, sterilize them on its premises, and discard them in the city trash dump or incinerate them. You may sanitize, disinfect, and sterilize reusable sharps in your office, particularly if the practice is in a rural area without an outside waste management company nearby. See the Caution: Handle With Care section for a discussion of the guidelines you must follow when disposing of biohazardous waste and potentially infectious laundry waste.

OSHA's laws for hazardous waste disposal, as well as other OSHA regulations about measures to prevent the spread of infection, provide a margin of safety, ensuring that medical facilities meet at least the minimal criteria for asepsis. These laws include requirements for training personnel, keeping records, housekeeping, wearing protective gear, and other measures.

Although federal laws exist, individual states have some discretion in applying them. You should become familiar with the laws in your state to ensure that you are helping your medical office comply. Penalties for failing to comply with regulations can be severe (see Table 19-1).

Proper Use of Biohazardous Waste Containers and Handling of Infectious Laundry Waste

Biohazardous waste containers are available in a variety of designs. Frequently, more than one design is used in the clinical setting. These containers are often provided by outside sterilization and waste management companies. Examples of biohazardous waste containers include:

- Bags or containers that are red or have a biohazardous waste label (for any material contaminated with blood or body fluids, such as used dressings or gloves)
- Boxes with biohazardous waste labels (sometimes lined with red bags and used for disposable gowns, examination table covers, and similar items that may be contaminated with blood or body fluids)
- Rigid, leakproof sharps containers that are red or have a biohazardous waste label (for lancets, needles, and other sharp objects)

Every biohazardous waste container has a lid that you must replace immediately after use. In addition, you may not overfill the container, and you must replace it when it is two-thirds full. All biohazardous waste containers must have a fluorescent orange or orange-red label with the biohazard symbol and the word *BIOHAZARD* in a contrasting color (Figure 19-13). Red bags or red containers may be substituted for containers with biohazardous waste labels.

You must follow these guidelines when handling hazardous waste.

- Always wear gloves
- Place hazardous waste in the appropriate biohazardous waste container immediately or as soon as possible
- Keep biohazardous waste containers close to the place where the waste material is generated
- Keep the containers closed when not in use, close them before removing them from the area of use, and keep them upright to avoid any spills

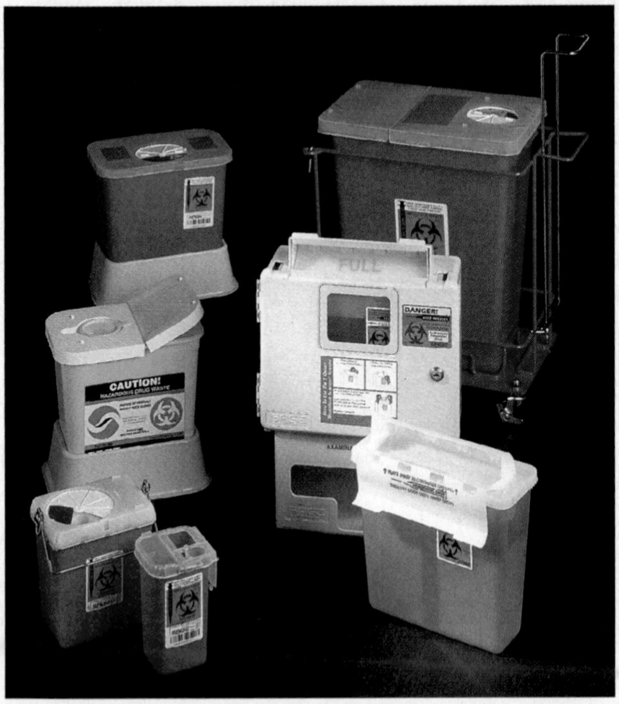

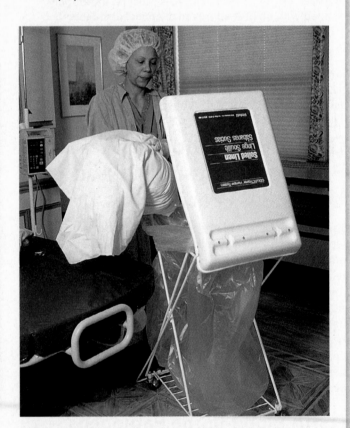

Figure 19-13. All biohazardous sharps containers must be rigid, leakproof, and labeled with the biohazard symbol.

Figure 19-14. Place soiled linens and other laundry in an appropriate bag as soon as possible.

continued ⟶

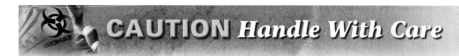

CAUTION *Handle With Care*

Proper Use of Biohazardous Waste Containers and Handling of Infectious Laundry Waste (continued)

- If outside contamination of the primary container occurs, place that container in a secondary container to prevent leakage during handling, processing, storage, and transport
- Drop—do not push—intact contaminated needles into the biohazardous waste container for sharps
- To avoid accidental puncture wounds, never break off, recap, reuse, or handle needles after use
- If there is a danger of hazardous waste puncturing the primary container, place that container in a secondary container
- Do not open, empty, or clean reusable sharps containers by hand
- When they are two-thirds full, discard disposable sharps containers in large biohazardous waste containers

When cleaning up spills, place the resulting contaminated material in a biohazardous waste bag. The bag must be leakproof on the sides and bottom and be closed tightly. Then place the plastic bag in a cardboard box also marked with the biohazard symbol. The outside waste management agency will pick up the box for incineration before disposing of it in a public landfill.

Potentially infectious laundry waste must also be handled in a specific manner. OSHA has issued regulations for handling this type of waste. You must be sure to:

- Place contaminated laundry in a laundry bag that is red, marked with the biohazard symbol, or recognizable to facility employees as contaminated material to be handled using Universal Precautions (Figure 19-14)
- Pack any laundry to be transported so that it does not leak in transit
- Have the laundry washed in a designated area on-site or at a professional laundry facility

Any laundry service the medical office uses should abide by all OSHA regulations. For example, anyone handling laundry must wear gloves and handle contaminated materials as little as possible.

TABLE 19-1	Infectious Waste Disposal: Penalties for Not Following Regulations, as Set Forth by OSHA	
Type of Violation	**Characteristics of Violation**	**Penalties for Violation**
Other than serious violation	Direct relationship to job safety and health but would probably not result in death or serious physical harm	Fine of up to $7,000 (discretionary)
Serious violation	Substantial probability that death or serious physical harm could result; employer knew, or should have known, of the hazard	Fine of up to $7,000 (mandatory)
Willful violation	Violation committed intentionally and knowingly	Fine of up to $70,000, with a $5,000 minimum; if violation resulted in death of employee, additional fine and/or up to 6 months' imprisonment
Repeated violation	Substantially similar (but not the same) violation found upon reinspection; not applicable if initial citation is under contest	Fine of up to $70,000
Failure to correct prior violation	Initial violation was not corrected	Fine of up to $7,000 for each day the violation continues past the date it was supposed to stop

Principles of Asepsis **363**

blood or body fluids penetrate your regular clothes around or through the protective clothing.

OSHA Procedures for Postprocedure Cleanup

After a procedure, personnel in every medical office must follow specific steps to clean and decontaminate the environment. The cleanup steps that OSHA requires are as follows:

1. Decontaminate all exposed work surfaces with bleach or a germ-killing solution approved by the EPA.
2. Replace protective coverings on surfaces or equipment if they have been exposed.
3. Decontaminate receptacles, such as bins, pails, and cans, on a regular basis as part of routine housekeeping procedures.
4. Pick up any broken glass with tongs—never by hand—even when wearing gloves, because the sharp edges may cut the gloves and expose the skin to infecting organisms. Never use a vacuum to pick up broken glass.
5. Discard all potentially infectious waste materials in appropriate biohazardous waste containers.

Applying the Law to Daily Work

In the course of daily work, you and other medical personnel may come in contact with patients who carry dangerous or fatal infectious disease. You are at risk for accidental exposure to these types of disease with every patient. Pathogens may be present in a patient's blood or other body fluids.

A patient or anyone who comes in contact with infectious waste generated by another patient or a health-care worker is at risk for infection. To minimize the risk of cross contamination, you need to become familiar with the OSHA regulations that describe the precautions medical office personnel must take in matters such as clothing, housekeeping, record keeping, and training.

Exposure Incidents

The OSHA Blood-borne Pathogens Standard also specifies what to do in case of an exposure incident. An exposure incident is one in which a worker, despite all precautions, has reason to believe that he has come in contact with a substance that may transmit infection. Contact may occur when a medical worker accidentally sticks himself with a used needle. This "puncture exposure incident" is the most common kind of exposure.

The basic rules covering exposure incidents apply to all serious infections, such as HBV and HIV. The rules covering HBV also include vaccination.

When an exposure incident occurs, the physician or employer must be notified immediately. This prompt action is extremely important because quick and proper treatment can help prevent the development of many diseases, such as hepatitis B. Timely action can also prevent the worker from exposing other people to a potentially acquired infection. Reporting the incident increases the chance of preventing the same type of accident from happening again.

After such an exposure, the employer must offer the exposed employee a free medical evaluation. The employer must refer the employee to a licensed health-care provider who can counsel the employee about what happened as well as about how to prevent the spread of any potential infection. The health-care provider also takes a blood sample and prescribes appropriate treatment. If the employee does not want to participate in the medical evaluation and treatment, he has the right to refuse it. (The employee's refusal should be documented.)

If an employee who has not received the HBV vaccination and is not known to be immune is exposed to any infected person—especially someone who is HBV-positive or at high risk—it is recommended that the employee be tested for HBV and receive the vaccination if necessary. This vaccination may prevent infection. When the source person's HBV status is unknown and the person does not wish to be tested, the employee should be tested. If the source person agrees to be tested, the law requires that the employee be informed of the test results. The employee may agree to give blood but not to be tested. In such a case, the blood sample must be kept for 90 days in case the employee later develops symptoms of HBV or HIV infection and decides to be tested then.

The health-care provider who performs the postexposure evaluation must give the employer a written report stating whether HBV vaccination was recommended and received and that the employee was informed of the results of any blood tests. Any additional information must be kept confidential.

Other OSHA Requirements

OSHA also requires that all health-care workers who have occupational exposure to blood or other potentially infectious materials have the opportunity to receive the HBV vaccine, free of charge, as needed throughout employment. Within 10 days of a medical worker's starting a job, the doctor or employer is required to offer the worker the opportunity to receive this vaccination. The vaccine is recommended for all health-care workers unless:

- They have received it in the past
- A blood test shows them to be immune to the virus
- There are medical reasons for which the vaccine is contraindicated

In most cases, the employee is permitted to decline the vaccination if he signs a form accepting all the conditions. (A few employers require HBV vaccination as a condition for employment.) Even if the health-care worker declines the vaccination when beginning employment, he still has the opportunity to receive the free vaccine and any necessary booster shots throughout his employment.

Transmission From Health-Care Workers to Patients

There may be times when a health-care worker has a serious infection that could be transmitted to a patient. For this reason, OSHA has special recommendations for workers who perform procedures that could result in a patient's exposure to disease. Although the risk of a health-care worker's transmitting an infection to a patient is small if OSHA standards are followed, these additional precautions are advised for high-risk procedures. High-risk procedures include the following:

- Those that are thought to have caused the transmission of infection from a medical worker to a patient in the past
- Those that may carry that risk, such as oral or obstetric or gynecologic procedures
- Those that involve needles, especially if a needle is in a body cavity or a body space that is difficult to see and the health-care worker's fingers are nearby (if the worker's skin was cut, the patient could be exposed to the worker's blood)

Workers who perform high-risk procedures should know their HIV and HBV status. HBV vaccination is strongly recommended. Also, workers who have skin conditions characterized by sores that secrete fluid should forgo direct patient care and the handling of equipment used for exposure-prone procedures until their condition has healed.

A member of the medical staff who is infected with HIV or HBV should not perform procedures that might result in exposure for the patient without the advice of an expert review panel. This panel could include the health-care worker's own physician, someone with expert knowledge about the transmission of infectious disease, a medical professional with expert knowledge about the procedures in question, public health officials, and a member of the infection-control committee of the institution, if applicable.

The panel advises the worker on whether procedures may be performed. The advice includes requiring the worker to inform potential patients of the infection before the procedure. The panel must otherwise protect the health-care worker's confidentiality.

Although great controversy has surrounded the subject of required testing of all health-care workers for HIV or HBV, no recommendations are in place for such testing. The risk of infection transmission from worker to patient is not considered great enough to justify the extensive resources that mandatory testing would require.

Educating Patients About Preventing Disease Transmission

As a medical assistant, you can be influential in educating patients about ways to protect themselves from disease. Whenever you have the opportunity for patient education, you should stress the basic principles of hygiene and disease prevention.

- Wash your hands frequently, especially before eating and after using the toilet, touching dirty objects, coming into contact with bodily fluids (including one's own), and touching doorknobs, railings, and handles
- Take a daily shower or bath, maintain daily dental care, and use clean clothes and bedding
- Thoroughly wash dirty drinking glasses, dishes, and utensils, especially when someone in the household is ill
- Use tissues when coughing or sneezing, and discard them properly after one use
- Maintain adequate light and ventilation in the home
- Routinely use a commercial disinfectant to clean rooms in the home, especially the bathroom and kitchen
- Use condoms if you have sexual intercourse with more than one partner or with people whose HIV or HBV status is unknown
- Adhere to immunization schedules
- Eat nutritious foods and keep physically fit
- Avoid stress
- Protect against exposure to potentially harmful insects or animals

Educating patients about health promotion and disease prevention is an important part of your job. Patients with adequate knowledge can work to keep their defenses functioning properly. They can also avoid exposing themselves to infections and transmitting infections when they are ill. In addition, they are more likely to have a successful recovery from illness. To provide patients with the knowledge they need, you should educate them in the following subjects:

- Nutrition and diet
- Exercise and weight control
- Prevention of sexually transmitted diseases
- Smoking cessation
- Alcohol and drug abuse prevention and treatment
- Proper use of medications and prescribed treatments for an infection already acquired
- Stress-reduction techniques

The goal of patient education is to help patients take care of themselves. In fact, many patients expect this kind of education along with their treatment. Thus, you should

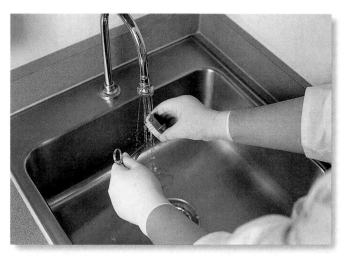

Figure 20-2. Clean all areas of an instrument, using a brush for hard-to-reach surfaces.

storage. Wrap items that require disinfection and sterilization in a clean covering, and set them aside for those processes.

Rubber and Plastic Products

To sanitize rubber and plastic products, you may need to soak them only for a short period or not at all. Some rubber and plastic products fade or discolor if left in a detergent solution. When you sanitize these products, be sure to follow manufacturers' guidelines.

Syringes and Needles

Disposable syringes and needles have replaced reusable ones in medical offices. Using disposable instruments helps reduce the risk of infection to both patients and health-care personnel.

Ultrasonic Cleaning

Delicate instruments or those with moving parts should be sanitized by using ultrasonic cleaners. **Ultrasonic cleaning** involves placing instruments in a special bath. The cleaner generates sound waves through a cleaning solution, loosening contaminants. Ultrasonic cleaning is safe for even very fragile instruments. If your medical office sanitizes instruments with an ultrasonic cleaner, follow the manufacturer's guidelines for operating the device.

Instruments with points or sharp edges and instruments made of different types of metal should be separated from other equipment. The ultrasonic cleaning process can cause one metal to disintegrate and fuse with another metal, rendering all instruments useless. Place all instruments with hinges or ratchets in the ultrasonic cleaner in the open position. If such an instrument is placed in the cleaner in the closed position, contaminated material can become trapped between the two surfaces.

After the instruments have been in the ultrasonic cleaner for the recommended cleaning time, remove them and rinse them under cool running water. Be sure to remove all the ultrasonic cleaning fluid. Then dry the instruments, and wrap them for storage or for disinfection and sterilization.

You can reuse ultrasonic cleaning solution for several cleaning baths. Replace it according to the care and maintenance procedures outlined by the manufacturer of the cleaning device.

Disinfection: The Second Level of Infection Control

Sanitization is often only the beginning of the process of eliminating microorganisms. After sanitization, some instruments and equipment require only disinfection before being used again. Disinfection of other items, however, is merely the second step in infection control, performed before the process of sterilization. You must wear gloves when handling instruments during disinfection procedures because instruments requiring disinfection are considered to be contaminated.

To destroy microorganisms, a disinfectant solution must reach every surface of an instrument; however, disinfection cannot kill all microorganisms. Bacterial spores and certain viruses have been known to survive disinfection with strong chemicals and boiling water. It is essential to understand this limitation of disinfection when you work with instruments and equipment.

Disinfection is usually sufficient for instruments that do not penetrate a patient's skin or that come in contact only with a patient's mucous membranes or other surfaces not considered sterile. Instruments and equipment that you can disinfect and reuse without sterilization include the following:

- Enamelware
- Endotracheal tubes (tubes used to establish an artificial airway through the nose, mouth, or direct tracheal route)
- Glassware
- Laryngoscopes (tubes equipped with lighting and used to examine the interior of the larynx through the mouth)
- Nasal specula (instruments used to enlarge the opening of the nose to permit viewing)

Note that you must sterilize any instrument or piece of equipment—including those just listed—if there is visible contamination with blood or blood products before another use, even if disinfection is commonly considered sufficient. Sterilization is the only reliable measure you can take to eliminate blood-borne pathogens.

Using Disinfectants

Disinfectants are cleaning products applied particularly to instruments and equipment to reduce or eliminate infectious organisms. They are used primarily on inanimate materials. In contrast, cleaning products that are used on human tissues as anti-infection agents are called **antiseptics.**

There are no clear indications that an item has been properly and completely disinfected. To ensure optimum effectiveness of disinfectants, follow the manufacturers' guidelines carefully when using them.

Other factors may also have an impact on the effectiveness of a disinfectant. For example, if the disinfectant solution has been used many times, it may not be as powerful as a fresh solution. When wet items are put in the disinfectant bath, the surface moisture may dilute the solution. Traces of the soap used in the sanitization process can alter the chemical makeup of the disinfectant, making it nonlethal to pathogens. Evaporation can also alter the chemical makeup of the solution.

Choosing the Correct Disinfectant

Manufacturers' guidelines are the most accurate and up-to-date sources of information about the type of disinfectant to use on a given product. Generally, disinfect instruments and equipment by using one or more of the following agents:

- Boiling water
- Germicidal soap products
- Alcohol
- Acid products
- Formaldehyde
- Glutaraldehyde
- Household bleach
- Iodine and iodine compounds

Each of these disinfectants has advantages and disadvantages. Before using any disinfectant product or procedure, it is important to understand some general guidelines about disinfectant use as well as specific concerns with each approach.

Boiling Water. It was long considered sufficient to boil instruments and equipment to achieve sterilization. Research has proved that boiling water is not sufficient to sterilize a surface. Boiling water is, however, an effective means of disinfection. A special unit is used for boiling instruments and equipment for disinfection purposes.

When boiling items, place them in the unit in the open position. Do not preheat the instruments. Place them in the unit at room temperature. Use distilled water in the unit to reduce the formation of mineral deposits on the instruments as well as on the unit itself. Empty the unit, and clean it according to the manufacturer's instructions.

After boiling, allow the instruments to cool. Then remove them, using sterile transfer forceps. Store the instruments carefully according to recommended procedures to prevent contamination.

Germicidal Soap Products. Research has shown that the use of soap in the process of disinfection is less important than the scrubbing and rinsing steps. Germ-killing additives may increase the effectiveness of soap products, however, and a soap-and-water disinfection may be sufficient for items that do not come in contact with a patient's skin or mucous membranes.

Alcohol. Alcohol (70% isopropyl) is commonly used to clean instruments and equipment that would be damaged by immersion in soap and water or other disinfectant solutions. It is a corrosive product, however, and can cause damage to the skin if it is used excessively.

Acid Products. The killing power of concentrated acid products such as phenol (carbolic acid) is quite high. In a concentrated form, acid products are also extremely corrosive and toxic to tissue and should be used with care.

Formaldehyde. Formaldehyde is a corrosive and an irritant to body tissue. It is commonly used as a preservative in a 10% solution, whereas in a 5% solution it can be used as a germicidal agent and a sporicidal agent. Formaldehyde must be used at room temperature because its effectiveness is reduced in cooler environments. After disinfecting items with formaldehyde, rinse them thoroughly with distilled or sterile water before using them on patients.

Glutaraldehyde. Glutaraldehyde (known more commonly by the trade names Cidex, Cidexplus, and Glutarex) is used in chemical sterilization processes, but you can also use it as a disinfectant. Immersing instruments or equipment in a bath of glutaraldehyde for 10 to 30 minutes is sufficient for disinfection. Any chemical used in this "cold disinfection" method must be rated as a sterilant and registered with the EPA.

Household Bleach. Bleach (sodium hypochlorite) is commonly used in laboratory settings to provide a measure of protection against transmission of the human immunodeficiency virus (HIV). It is an effective disinfectant when used in a 10% solution. Bleach is used to disinfect surfaces and to soak rubber equipment before sanitization. Ventilation may be necessary when you use bleach because the fumes should not be inhaled for a prolonged period.

Iodine and Iodine Compounds. Iodine products are used as both disinfectants (solutions stronger than 2%) and antiseptics (solutions weaker than 2%). They are somewhat corrosive, however, and their effectiveness is limited by the presence of blood products, mucus, or soap.

Handling Disinfected Supplies

After disinfecting equipment, handle it with care to prevent contamination of any surface that may later come in contact with a patient. Use sterile transfer forceps, or sterilizing forceps, to remove items from whatever disinfection unit is used. Always wear gloves to handle disinfected items, and make sure you store disinfected equipment in a clean, moisture-free environment.

Tuberculosis

Tuberculosis, also called TB, is an infectious bacterial disease that mainly affects the lungs but can also involve other organs. TB is the leading infectious killer of adults worldwide. A patient infected with tuberculosis may not have any symptoms. The body's immune system often destroys the bacteria, leaving only a scar or spot on the lungs. Sometimes, however, the infection spreads, and the patient exhibits these symptoms:

- Night sweats
- Productive and prolonged cough
- Fever
- Chills
- Fatigue
- Unexplained weight loss
- Diminished appetite
- Bloody sputum

Incidence of Tuberculosis. After a rise in the nationwide number of tuberculosis cases between 1985 and 1992, the incidence in the United States began to decline. Incidence remains high or on the increase in many states, however, particularly in some urban centers. You may encounter patients with tuberculosis, and you can never relax your vigilance when working in environments where there is any risk of infection.

Many factors contribute to the continued high incidence of tuberculosis. You may work with patients who are affected by some or all of these factors:

- Infection with HIV increases the risk for developing tuberculosis after exposure to the pathogen
- The population of the United States is shifting to include a larger percentage of people from countries where there is a higher incidence of tuberculosis
- The number of people living in environments known to pose increased risk, such as long-term institutional settings, homeless centers, and medically underserved neighborhoods, has increased
- The public health-care system is unable to meet the needs of its constituents, resulting in patients who remain untreated
- New drug-resistant strains of the tuberculosis pathogen are appearing, requiring longer and more potent therapy regimens, which are harder to enforce and with which many patients do not comply

Understanding how tuberculosis is transmitted and managed will help you apply the principles of infection control.

Transmission of Tuberculosis. *Mycobacterium tuberculosis,* the microorganism responsible for tuberculosis infection, is spread through droplet transmission. The bacteria can spread through the air near an infected person when the person breathes, coughs, sneezes, or talks.

When another person inhales the bacteria, they travel through that person's respiratory system to lodge in the alveoli. From there, the bacteria can eventually spread throughout the body.

The most effective way to break the growth cycle of the tuberculosis pathogen is to contain the bacteria at the source. Containing the pathogen at this point prevents its entrance into another host. Containment measures include the following:

- Instruct patients in the correct procedure for covering the mouth when sneezing, coughing, laughing, or yawning. Explain that patients should properly dispose of tissues or other materials that have been used to block a sneeze or a cough and should thoroughly wash their hands afterward.
- When you must perform a procedure that induces coughing, conduct the procedure in an area with negative air pressure, such as inside a protective booth. Negative air pressure acts to draw contaminated air out of the immediate area and into a filtration system.
- When you work with a patient who is infectious, wear a personal respirator to prevent inhalation of the bacteria. Be sure also to apply standard sanitization, disinfection, and sterilization techniques to instruments and equipment.

Increasing Resistance to Tuberculosis. Another way to break the pathogenic growth cycle is to decrease the susceptibility of the host. Early diagnosis, prompt treatment, and compliance with the treatment regimen have a positive impact on the outcome of tuberculosis. Risk factors for infection include the following:

- HIV infection or any disease state that weakens the immune system
- Intravenous drug use
- Previous tuberculosis infection
- Diabetes mellitus, a disorder characterized by a deficiency of the hormone insulin
- End-stage renal disease, a type of kidney disease
- Low body weight

Treating Tuberculosis. Tuberculosis infection must be confirmed by a Mantoux tuberculin skin test, in which you administer tuberculin intradermally with a needle and syringe. If the test results are positive, the skin area turns red and becomes raised and hard, which is termed **induration.** A positive test result reveals that a patient has had previous exposure to tuberculosis, either from immunization (common outside the United States) or from coming in contact with the tuberculosis bacteria. If a patient tests positive for tuberculin sensitivity, further tests, including chest x-rays and sputum examination, are performed.

The specific treatment of a patient with active tuberculosis depends on the part of the body affected and the type of tuberculosis involved. In all cases, however, drug therapy must be initiated immediately. Emphasize to patients the importance of completing the entire course of treatment (12 to 18 months on medication). Help patients comply with the treatment by providing education about the disease, the expected course of treatment, the anticipated outcome, and measures patients can take to prevent the spread of the disease.

Patients with active pulmonary tuberculosis should be hospitalized in a facility approved for treating the disease. They should also be placed in an isolation room with negative air pressure. Visitors should be kept to a minimum. Patients may be discharged to their homes after starting TB therapy, even though they may still be infectious. Transmission is less likely to occur after treatment has begun.

Drug-Resistant Microorganisms

Resistance to antimicrobial agents is a severe problem. Drug-resistant pathogens are the cause of many infections. It is the responsibility of physicians, medical staff, and patients to use antibiotics wisely. Becteria and other microorganisms that have developed resistance to antimicrobial drugs include the following:

- **MRSA**—methicillin/oxacillin-resistant *Staphylococcus aureus*
- **VRE**—vancomycin-resistant enterococci
- **VISA**—vancomycin-intermediate *Staphylococcus aureus*
- **VRSA**—vancomycin-resistant *Staphylococcus aureus*
- **ESBLs**—extended-spectrum beta-lactamases, which are resistant to cephalosporins and monobactams
- **PRSP**—penicillin-resistant *Streptococcus pneumoniae*

MRSA and VRE are the most common multidrug-resistant organisms in patients who reside in non-hospital health-care facilities, such as nursing homes and other long-term care facilities. PRSP are more common in patients seeking care in physicians' offices and clinics, especially in pediatric settings.

Risk Factors

There are a number of risk factors for both the development and infection of drug-resistant organisms. These risk factors include the following:

- Advanced age
- Invasive procedures, which include dialysis, the presence of invasive devices, and urinary catheterization
- Previous exposure to antimicrobial agents
- Repeated contact with the health-care system
- Severity of the illness
- Underlying diseases or conditions, especially chronic renal disease, insulin-dependent diabetes mellitus, peripheral vascular disease, and dermatitis or skin lesions.

Reporting Guidelines

The CDC requires reporting of certain diseases to the state or county department of health. This information, which is forwarded to the CDC, helps research epidemiologists control the spread of infection. Figure 20-10 lists diseases that must be reported.

The Notifiable Disease Surveillance System

Acquired immunodeficiency syndrome (AIDS)	Lymphogranuloma venereum
Amebiasis	Malaria
Anthrax	Measles
Aseptic meningitis	Meningococcal infections
Botulism, food-borne	Mumps
Botulism, infant	Pertussis
Botulism, wound	Plague
Botulism, unspecified	Poliomyelitis, paralytic
Brucellosis	Psittacosis
Chancroid	Rabies, animal
Cholera	Rabies, human
Congenital rubella syndrome	Rheumatic fever
Diphtheria	Rocky Mountain spotted fever
Encephalitis, post-chickenpox	Rubella
Encephalitis, postmumps	Salmonellosis
Encephalitis, postother	Shigellosis
Encephalitis, primary	Syphilis, all stages
Gonorrhea	Syphilis, primary and secondary
Granuloma inguinale	Syphilis, congenital
Hansen disease	Tetanus
Hepatitis A	Toxic shock syndrome
Hepatitis B	Trichinosis
Hepatitis C	Tuberculosis
Hepatitis, unspecified	Tularemia
Legionellosis	Typhoid fever
Leptospirosis	Yellow fever
Lyme disease	

Note: The National Notifiable Disease Surveillance System does not require the reporting of varicella (chickenpox) cases. Many state agencies do, however, and the Council of State and Territorial Epidemiologists recommends the reporting of varicella cases to the CDC.

Figure 20-10. These diseases must be reported to the National Notifiable Disease Surveillance System of the CDC, through your state or county health department.

be found in blood, semen, and vaginal secretions and can be transmitted to an uninfected person through mucous membranes in the vagina, rectum, or mouth, especially if there are cuts or open sores in those areas. Some strains of the virus are more likely to infect the cells in the female reproductive tract (Langerhans cells). The HIV strain most common in the United States, however, targets the monocyte or lymphocyte white blood cells and is more prone to being passed along through anal sex and blood-to-blood contact.

The virus can also be spread by the sharing of needles used by intravenous drug users. The minute amount of blood left on a needle after injection provides an ample supply of the virus to transmit the infection to another host. Needles used in tattooing and ear piercing can also pose a risk. In all cases needles should be new and sterile.

The virus can pass from mother to fetus during pregnancy, as well as to an infant during delivery or through breast-feeding. Not every infant born to an infected mother contracts the disease, and some infected infants have cleared the virus from their systems within a year after birth. Scientists are studying these children in an effort to determine how their immune systems allow them to escape infection altogether or to eradicate the virus after infection. Scientists suspect that either the immune systems of the infants in the study fought off an HIV invasion or the infants developed a permanent tolerance for it.

At one time the virus was also being spread through the nation's blood supply. Transmission was occurring through transfusion of HIV-contaminated blood products. This form of transmission has virtually stopped as a result of an aggressive screening program that began in 1985. All blood donations are tested for the virus, and contaminated donations are destroyed. People who received blood prior to 1986 (especially between 1978 and 1985) were at risk for coming down with AIDS. Because of the long incubation period of the virus (8 to 15 years), infected people may not have exhibited any symptoms of infection.

Risk in the Medical Community. Health-care workers have contracted HIV infection as a direct result of occupational activities (see Table 21-1). Investigations showed that infection in most of the cases occurred as a result of **percutaneous exposure,** that is, exposure through a puncture wound or needlestick. **Mucocutaneous exposure,** or exposure through a mucous membrane, resulted in infection in a few cases.

Further analysis identified that in most cases the infecting substance was HIV-infected blood. Concentrated virus cultures in the laboratory and visibly bloody body fluid caused a few of the cases.

Progress of the Infection. Current research has shown that development of AIDS occurs in three main stages:

1. Initial infection
2. Incubation period
3. Full-blown AIDS

Initial infection by the virus can occur years before any symptoms appear to arouse suspicions about HIV infection. In some cases the initial infection is marked by severe flulike symptoms. Identification of the initial infection, however, is almost always through hindsight. The virus attacks helper T cells during this initial phase.

During the initial phase of infection by HIV, the virus enters the cell, and the host cell produces multiple copies of the virus. As a result helper T cells die or are disabled. The body's immune system responds to the attack at this point, cleansing the blood supply of the virus, and the virus enters an inactive phase.

The incubation period begins when the virus incorporates its genetic material into the genetic material of the helper T cells. The virus is trapped within the lymph system, and the host experiences few, if any, symptoms of the disease. Many doctors discover the infection in patients during this period when treating them for other illnesses. This incubation period, in which people are HIV-positive but do not have AIDS, generally lasts 8 to 15 years.

Sometime during the incubation period, HIV becomes active again and continues to attack and destroy helper T cells. As the number of helper T cells dwindles, the patient becomes more prone to opportunistic infections.

The threshold at which a patient is officially diagnosed with AIDS is the point at which there are 200 or fewer helper T cells per milliliter of blood. Once a person has full-blown AIDS—the third phase of infection—opportunistic infections take hold as the overall immune system undergoes deterioration. Neurons are destroyed, resulting in neurological problems, including dementia.

Diagnosis. To know for certain whether a person is infected with HIV, that person must have blood tested specifically for HIV infection. (All HIV testing is anonymous.) The **enzyme-linked immunosorbent assay (ELISA) test** confirms the presence of antibodies developed by the body's immune system in response to an initial HIV infection. ELISA is only about 85% accurate because of cross-reactivity from other viruses. Therefore, positive specimens are confirmed by a different method— the **Western blot test** or the **immunofluorescent antibody (IFA) test.** These tests are more accurate because they are specific to individual viruses.

These HIV tests were first developed for use on blood samples, but the ELISA and Western blot tests can also be run on oral fluid samples obtained in the medical office. Positive results from two of the three HIV tests (ELISA plus one other) yield an accurate diagnosis in almost 100% of patients tested.

Home tests are available that involve an ELISA test followed by either a Western blot test or an IFA test if the ELISA results are positive. These tests are performed on a drop of the patient's blood, which is collected on a specially treated card. Patients are identified only by a number, which they use to obtain their test results. (Keep in mind that people who perform home tests may not report positive results to the proper authorities.)

In all cases involving testing for HIV, you must follow measures to ensure protection of the patient's confidentiality. Knowledge about a patient's test results should be limited to those who will be treating the patient and appropriate authorities as required by law. The patient's decision on whether or not to reveal test results to family and friends should be respected at all times.

Symptoms.　HIV infection can cause a variety of problems as it progresses to AIDS. Patients with AIDS may complain of any of the following symptoms:

- Systemic complaints, such as weight loss, fatigue, fever, chills, and night sweats
- Respiratory complaints, such as sinus fullness, dry cough, shortness of breath, difficulty swallowing, and sinus drainage
- Oral complaints, such as gingivitis, oral lesions, and **hairy leukoplakia,** which is a white lesion on the tongue
- Gastrointestinal complaints, such as diarrhea and bloody stool
- Central nervous system complaints, such as depression, personality changes, concentration difficulties, and confusion or dementia
- Peripheral nervous system complaints, such as tingling, numbness, pain, and weakness in the extremities
- Skin-related complaints, such as rashes, dry skin, and changes in the nail bed
- **Kaposi's sarcoma,** an unusual malignancy occurring in the skin and sometimes in the lymph nodes and organs manifested by reddish purple to dark blue patches or spots on the skin

Because many other diseases can cause these symptoms, the occurrence of any one symptom is not necessarily indicative of AIDS. Be aware, however, that patients exhibiting a combination of symptoms should be tested. The two symptoms most indicative of AIDS are hairy leukoplakia and Kaposi's sarcoma.

Preventive Measures.　The only way to prevent the spread of HIV infection is to avoid specific activities or to take safety precautions when engaging in these activities. Activities requiring preventive measures can be divided into three groups, based on the means of transmission of the disease:

1. Sexual contact
2. Sharing of intravenous needles
3. Medical procedures

Prevention and Sexual Contact.　The most effective method for preventing the spread of AIDS/HIV infection through sexual contact is to avoid high-risk sexual activity. Such high-risk activities or situations include:

- Having unprotected vaginal, oral, or anal sex, either homosexual or heterosexual, *unless* the individuals are involved in a long-term, monogamous relationship,

they both have been tested and received negative results, and they have not engaged in any unsafe sexual activity 6 months before the test or anytime after the test
- Having multiple sexual partners, even when using protection against infection
- Experiencing a concurrent infection with another sexually transmitted disease

In addition, precautions must be taken when using a condom as a means of protection against infection. Proper use of a condom requires adherence to the following guidelines.

- A condom must be used every time the individual has sex and must never be reused.
- Only latex condoms provide protection against spread of the HIV pathogen. Lambskin condoms provide birth control only, not protection against disease.
- If lubrication is required, the lubricant must be water-based, not petroleum-based (such as petroleum jelly). Lubricants other than those specifically formulated for use with latex condoms can damage the condom, rendering it permeable and eliminating its usefulness as a barrier against disease.
- Condoms should be placed on the penis before any risk of leakage of seminal fluid occurs. Space should be left at the tip to act as a reservoir for ejaculated semen.
- Intercourse should not be attempted unless the penis is fully erect, and the penis should be withdrawn while it is still erect.
- The condom must remain in place from the beginning to the end of intercourse and should be held in place during withdrawal to prevent slippage. After withdrawal the condom should be disposed of properly.

Prevention and Intravenous Drug Use.　Intravenous drug users are at risk for infection when they share needles. The most effective means of preventing the spread of the pathogen among drug users is to avoid sharing or reusing needles.

Prevention and Medical Procedures.　Preventing the spread of AIDS/HIV infection in the medical environment involves taking many precautions. You must take precautions to prevent the spread of infection between patients, between yourself and the patient, and when you are working with equipment, supplies, or instruments that may be contaminated.

Strict adherence to Universal Precautions (Standard Precautions in a hospital) when working with patients is the best method for preventing the spread of disease among patients and between the patient and you. You must use gloves whenever there is a risk of contact with blood, tissue, or body fluids, and you must dispose of gloves properly after use. (See Chapter 19 for specific disposal guidelines.)

You must wash your hands carefully and thoroughly between patients. Wear additional personal protective

A rack for the patient's medical records usually hangs on the wall directly outside the examination room or on the outside of the door. A light or other device on the wall or door may be used to signal that the room is occupied.

Furnishings

Furnishings should be arranged for efficiency, the convenience of the physician, and the comfort of the patient. The examining table is the key piece of equipment in the examination room. It should be positioned in the center of the room or coming out from the wall. This arrangement allows the physician and an assistant to attend to the patient on at least three sides. The examining table usually contains a pullout step for the patient to use when getting onto the table. It may also contain drawers for storing instruments and table coverings.

Examining tables are usually adjustable to enable the patient to assume the various positions that the physical examination may require. The physician will probably tell you beforehand if you need to adjust the table in a particular way.

Most examination rooms also have a sink, a countertop, and a writing surface large enough to spread out the patient's records. Shelves, cupboards, and drawers store routine supplies such as dressings, adhesive tape, and bandages.

The examination room may also include the following items:

- One or more chairs
- A rolling stool
- A weight scale with height bar
- A metal wastebasket with a lid
- Biohazardous waste containers for disposal of biohazardous materials (biological agents that can spread disease to living things)
- Puncture-proof containers for disposal of biohazardous sharps
- A high-intensity lamp
- Wall brackets for hanging instruments

Special Features

The Americans With Disabilities Act of 1990 (ADA) requires that businesses, services, and public transportation provide "reasonable accommodations" for the disabled. To comply with this act, the examination room in a medical office must have features that make the area accessible to patients who use wheelchairs or who have visual or other types of physical impairments. **Accessibility** refers to the ease with which people can move in and out of a space. The ADA accessibility guidelines require the following:

- A doorway at least 36 inches (915 mm) wide to allow a person in a wheelchair to pass through

- A clearance space in rooms and hallways that is 60 inches (1525 mm) in diameter to allow a person in a wheelchair to make a 180° turn
- Stable, firm, slip-resistant flooring
- Door-opening hardware that can be grasped with one hand and does not require the twisting of the wrist to use
- Door closers adjusted to allow time for a person in a wheelchair to enter or exit through the door
- Grab bars in the lavatory

Cleanliness in the Examination Room

As you learned in Chapter 19, you can follow specific measures to achieve medical asepsis and prevent the spread of pathogenic microorganisms in the medical office. These measures involve strict housekeeping standards and adherence to government guidelines.

A clean examination room is extremely important in preventing the spread of infectious diseases to patients and health-care workers. Part of your job is to carefully follow infection-control procedures in the medical office and to keep the examination room clean and neat.

Infection Control

People with a variety of contagious diseases visit medical offices every day. The potential for the spread of infection is thus higher in medical offices than in most other places. For that reason, you must be especially careful to follow infection-control procedures at work. You can safeguard the health of staff members and patients by:

- Making hand washing a priority
- Keeping the examining table clean
- Disinfecting all work surfaces

Hand Washing. Clean hands are the first step in preventing infection transmission in the examination room. Wash your hands with disinfectant soap and warm water at the following times:

- At the beginning of the day
- Before and after having contact with each patient
- Before and after using gloves or performing any procedure
- Before handling clean or sterile supplies
- Before and after eating or taking a break
- Before and after using the bathroom
- After blowing your nose, coughing, or sneezing
- Before and after handling specimens or waste
- Before leaving for the day

After washing your hands, use a clean paper towel to handle faucets or doorknobs. The paper towel helps you

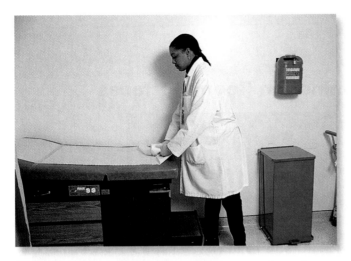

Figure 22-2. When you remove the cover from the examining table, roll it up tightly and quickly. Then carefully prepare it for disposal.

avoid contaminating your clean hands with microorganisms. (See Procedure 19-1 in Chapter 19 for the steps in performing aseptic hand washing.)

Examining Table. The disposable paper that covers the examining table provides a barrier to infection during an examination. Always change the covering after each use (Figure 22-2). Your office might use precut lengths, or you might need to tear off a piece from a roll of paper. Cover pillows with fresh paper. Also, provide paper towels for patients who need to wipe away excess lubricants after certain procedures.

When you remove the used covering from the examining table, roll it up quickly and carefully. You should have a small, tight bundle of paper when you finish. Crumpling the paper haphazardly or shaking it in the air stirs up dust and microorganisms and can spread infection.

Dispose of used paper coverings soiled by body fluids, especially blood, in a biohazardous waste container. (Refer to Chapter 19 for specific guidelines for disposing of hazardous items.) Used coverings with no visible fluids may be disposed of according to the procedures established by your office. Place soiled linen cloths and pillowcases in biohazard-labeled bags for sending to a laundry for cleaning.

Surfaces. You are responsible for disinfecting work surfaces in the examination room, including the examining table, sink, and countertop. As you learned in Chapter 20, disinfection involves exposing all parts of a surface to a disinfectant such as a 10% solution of household bleach in water or a product approved by the Environmental Protection Agency (EPA). Surfaces must be disinfected at the following times:

- After an examination or treatment during which surfaces have become visibly contaminated with tissue, blood, or other body fluids
- Immediately following accidental blood or body fluid spills or splatter
- At the end of your work shift

Clean and disinfect the toilet and sink in the patient lavatory, and inspect and disinfect reusable receptacles such as wastebaskets on a regular basis. In most offices these tasks are performed once a day. You must, however, follow the schedule established by your office. Procedure 22-1 describes how to disinfect work surfaces, floors, and equipment in the examination room. Replace protective coverings on equipment or surfaces that were exposed to blood, other body fluids, or tissue during the examination.

Storage. During the examination, you may need to collect biohazardous specimens, such as blood or urine, from the patient for testing. You are responsible for storing these specimens properly. See the Caution: Handle With Care section for guidelines to follow when storing biohazardous materials.

Storage of testing kits and specimens often involves refrigeration as a means of preservation. Adequate preservation requires maintaining careful control of the temperature in a refrigerator. Read the Caution: Handle With Care section for more information on preventing spoilage by controlling refrigerator temperature.

Putting the Room in Order

After ensuring that the examining table is clean, all surfaces are properly disinfected, and all necessary items are stored, take time to straighten the examination room and put things in order. A neatly arranged room boosts patient confidence and supports the impression of a well-run office. It also contributes to the physical safety of patients and staff. Tasks include the following:

- Putting the rolling stool in its place
- Pushing in the examining-table step
- Returning supplies to containers
- Putting away prescription pads and sample medications that may have been left out

Housekeeping

Medical offices usually contract with a janitorial service for after-hours cleaning. Janitorial services perform general cleaning tasks such as emptying wastebaskets, vacuuming carpets, scrubbing floors, dusting furniture, washing windows, and cleaning blinds. To be sure that the service cleans and sanitizes all areas adequately, you need to work with your employer to develop and implement a cleaning schedule. Take into account the types of surfaces to be cleaned, the type of contamination present, and the tasks or procedures to be performed.

You may be responsible for assigning housekeeping chores to janitorial workers. If so, you will need to monitor their work and let the service know if there are any lapses in cleanliness. You may also do some housekeeping chores yourself, such as damp dusting an open shelf. Because dust harbors bacteria and allergens, it is important to keep the examination rooms as dust-free as possible.

SECTION 2

ANATOMY AND PHYSIOLOGY

CHAPTER 23

Organization of the Body

CHAPTER OUTLINE

- The Study of the Body
- Organization of the Body
- Body Organs and Systems
- Anatomical Terminology
- Body Cavities and Abdominal Regions
- Chemistry of Life
- Cell Characteristics
- Movement Through Cell Membranes
- Cell Division
- Genetic Techniques
- Heredity
- Major Tissue Types

OBJECTIVES

After completing Chapter 23, you will be able to:

23.1 Describe how the body is organized from simple to more complex levels.

23.2 List all body organ systems, their general functions, and the major organs contained in each.

23.3 Define the anatomical position and explain its importance.

23.4 Use anatomical terminology correctly.

23.5 Name the body cavities and the organs contained in each.

23.6 Explain the abdominal regions.

23.7 Explain why a basic understanding of chemistry is important in studying the body.

23.8 Describe important molecules and compounds of the human body.

23.9 Label the parts of a cell and list their functions.

23.10 List and describe the ways substances move across a cell membrane.

23.11 Describe the stages of cell division.

23.12 Describe the uses of the genetic techniques, DNA fingerprinting, and the polymerase chain reaction.

23.13 Explain how mutations occur and what effects they may produce.

23.14 Describe the different patterns of inheritance.

23.15 Describe the signs and symptoms of various genetic conditions.

23.16 Describe the locations and characteristics of the four main tissue types.

KEY TERMS

acids
active transport
allele
anatomical position
anatomy
anterior
atoms
autosome
bases
biochemistry
caudal
cell membrane
cells
chemistry
chromosome
complex inheritance
compound
connective tissue
cranial
cytokinesis
cytoplasm
deep
diaphragm
diffusion
distal
DNA
dorsal
electrolytes
endocrine gland
epithelial tissue
exocrine gland
femoral
filtration
frontal
gene

homologous chromosome	metabolism	organelle	sagittal
inferior	midsagittal	organ	sex chromosome
inorganic	mitosis	organ systems	sex-linked trait
interphase	molecule	organic	superficial
ions	muscle tissue	organism	superior
lateral	mutation	osmosis	tissue
matrix	nervous tissue	physiology	transverse
matter	neuroglial cells	posterior	ventral
medial	neurons	proximal	
meiosis	nucleus	RNA	

Introduction

The human body is complex in its structure and function. This chapter provides an overview of the human body. It introduces you to the way the body is organized from the chemical level all the way up to the organ system level. You will also learn important terminology used in the clinical setting to describe body positions and parts. This chapter also focuses on how diseases develop at the genetic level.

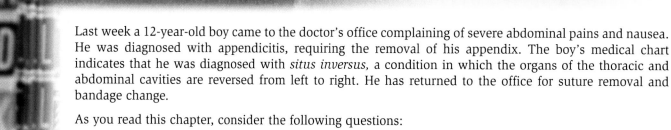

CASE STUDY

Last week a 12-year-old boy came to the doctor's office complaining of severe abdominal pains and nausea. He was diagnosed with appendicitis, requiring the removal of his appendix. The boy's medical chart indicates that he was diagnosed with *situs inversus,* a condition in which the organs of the thoracic and abdominal cavities are reversed from left to right. He has returned to the office for suture removal and bandage change.

As you read this chapter, consider the following questions:

1. On what side of the body is the appendix normally located?
2. If the medical assistant observes the boy's right lower abdominal quadrant for the bandage, is this correct? Why or why not?
3. Where should the bandage be found?
4. What precautions should this patient take given his diagnosis of *situs inversus?*

The Study of the Body

Anatomy is the scientific term for the study of body structure. For example, in discussing the structure or anatomy of the heart, it may be described as a hollow, cone-shaped organ with an average size of 14 centimeters in length and 9 centimeters in width. It is also very important to know the position of normal body structures and how to describe these positions precisely and correctly. **Physiology** is the term used for the study of function. For example, the physiology of the heart can be described by saying that the heart pumps blood into blood vessels for the transportation of nutrients throughout the body. Anatomy and physiology are commonly studied together because they are always related. For example, the anatomy of the heart (a

hollow, muscular organ) allows it to do its function (pump blood into tubular blood vessels). If the heart was not hollow, it could not allow blood to flow into it. If the heart was not muscular, it not could pump blood.

Knowledge of anatomy and physiology will help you grasp the meaning of diagnostic and procedural codes and can help you understand the clinical procedures you will perform as a medical assistant. It will also make it easier to see how and why certain diseases develop. Disease states develop in the body when homeostasis is not maintained. **Homeostasis** is defined as the maintenance of stable internal conditions. Conditions in the body that must remain stable include body temperature, blood pressure, and the concentration of various chemicals within the blood. Individual cells must also maintain homeostasis. For example, if chemicals within a cell change the DNA or genetic make-up of the cell, that cell can become cancerous.

Organization of the Body

The structure of the body can be divided into different levels of organization. The chemical level is the simplest level and refers to the billions of atoms and molecules in the body. **Atoms** are the simplest units of all matter, and many are essential to life. **Matter** is anything that takes up space and has weight. The four most common atoms in the human body are carbon, hydrogen, oxygen, and nitrogen. **Molecules** are made up of atoms that bond together. For example, water is formed when two hydrogen atoms bond to an oxygen atom, which is an example of a small but very important molecule. Proteins and carbohydrates are examples of much larger molecules that consist of hundreds of atoms.

Molecules join together to form **organelles,** which can be thought of as cell parts. Organelles combine to form cells such as leukocytes (white blood cells), erythrocytes (red blood cells), neurons (nerve cells), and adipocytes (fat cells). **Cells** are considered the smallest living units of structure and function in the body. When cells of the same type organize together, they form **tissues.** The four major types of body tissue are epithelia, connective, nervous, and muscle. Two or more tissue types combine to form **organs,** and organs arrange to form **organ systems.** Finally, organ systems combine to form the **organism** called the human body (Figure 23-1).

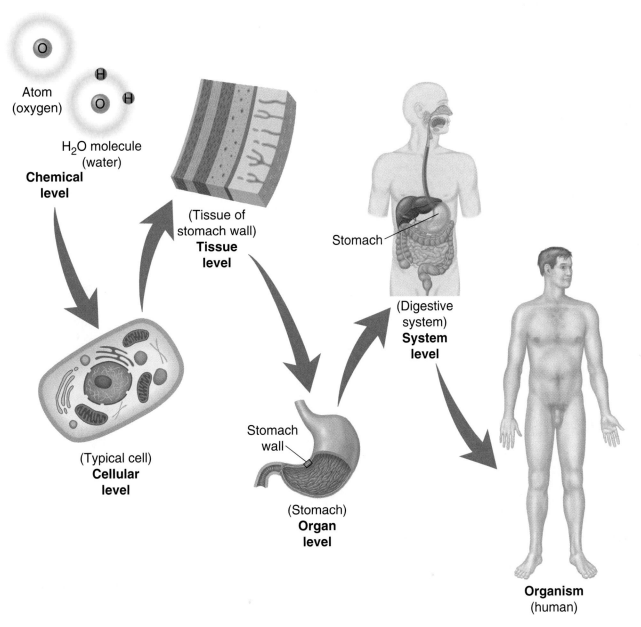

Figure 23-1. The human body is organized in levels, beginning with the chemical level and progressing to the cellular, tissue, organ, system, and organism (whole body) levels.

Body Organs and Systems

Organs can be defined as structures formed by the organization of two or more different tissue types that work together to carry out specific functions. For example, the heart is composed of a wall of cardiac muscle tissue and connective tissue and is lined with an epithelial tissue. These tissues work together to carry out the function of the heart, which is to effectively pump blood into blood vessels. Organ systems are formed when organs join together to carry out vital functions. For example, the heart and blood vessels unite to form the cardiovascular system. The organs of the cardiovascular system function to circulate blood throughout the body to ensure that all body cells receive an adequate supply of nutrients. See Figure 23-2 for a summary of the organ systems of the

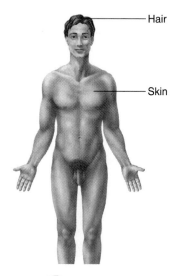

Integumentary System

Provides protection, regulates temperature, prevents water loss, and produces vitamin D precursors. Consists of skin, hair, nails, and sweat glands.

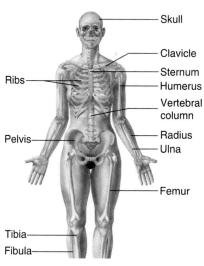

Skeletal System

Provides protection and support, allows body movements, produces blood cells, and stores minerals and fat. Consists of bones, associated cartilages, ligaments, and joints.

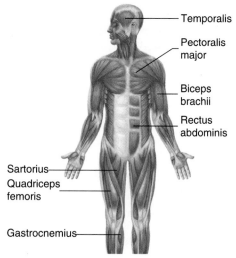

Muscular System

Produces body movements, maintains posture, and produces body heat. Consists of muscles attached to the skeleton by tendons.

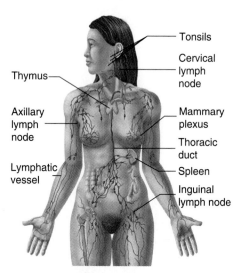

Lymphatic System

Removes foreign substances from the blood and lymph, combats disease, maintains tissue fluid balance, and absorbs fats from the digestive tract. Consists of the lymphatic vessels, lymph nodes, and other lymphatic organs.

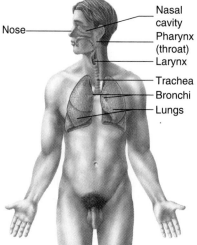

Respiratory System

Exchanges oxygen and carbon dioxide between the blood and air and regulates blood pH. Consists of the lungs and respiratory passages.

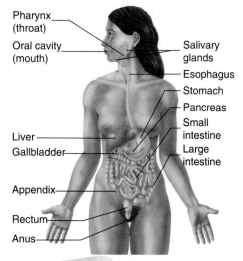

Digestive System

Performs the mechanical and chemical processes of digestion, absorption of nutrients, and elimination of wastes. Consists of the mouth, esophagus, stomach, intestines, and accessory organs.

Figure 23-2. Organ systems of the body.

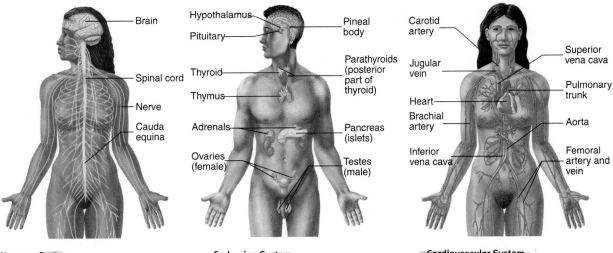

Nervous System

A major regulatory system that detects sensations and controls movements, physiologic processes, and intellectual functions. Consists of the brain, spinal cord, nerves, and sensory receptors.

Labels: Brain, Spinal cord, Nerve, Cauda equina

Endocrine System

A major regulatory system that influences metabolism, growth, reproduction, and many other functions. Consists of glands, such as the pituitary, that secrete hormones.

Labels: Hypothalamus, Pituitary, Thyroid, Thymus, Adrenals, Ovaries (female), Pineal body, Parathyroids (posterior part of thyroid), Pancreas (islets), Testes (male)

Cardiovascular System

Transports nutrients, waste products, gases, and hormones throughout the body; plays a role in the immune response and the regulation of body temperature. Consists of the heart, blood vessels, and blood.

Labels: Carotid artery, Jugular vein, Heart, Brachial artery, Inferior vena cava, Superior vena cava, Pulmonary trunk, Aorta, Femoral artery and vein

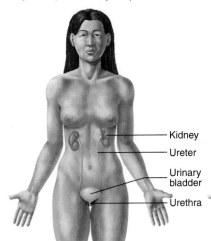
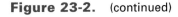

Urinary System

Removes waste products from the blood and regulates blood pH, ion balance, and water balance. Consists of the kidneys, urinary bladder, and ducts that carry urine.

Labels: Kidney, Ureter, Urinary bladder, Urethra

Female Reproductive System

Produces oocytes and is the site of fertilization and fetal development; produces milk for the newborn; produces hormones that influence sexual function and behaviors. Consists of the ovaries, vagina, uterus, mammary glands, and associated structures.

Labels: Mammary gland (in breast), Uterine tube, Ovary, Uterus, Vagina

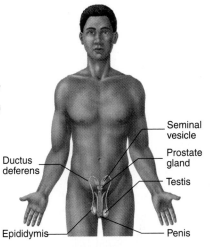

Male Reproductive System

Produces and transfers sperm cells to the female and produces hormones that influence sexual functions and behaviors. Consists of the testes, accessory structures, ducts, and penis.

Labels: Seminal vesicle, Prostate gland, Testis, Penis, Ductus deferens, Epididymis

Figure 23-2. (continued)

body, their general functions, and the organs contained in each.

Anatomical Terminology

Anatomical terms are a group of universal terms used to describe the location of body parts and various body regions. In order to correctly use these terms, it is assumed that the body is in the anatomical position. In the **anatomical position,** a body is standing upright and facing forward with the arms at the sides and the palms of the hands facing forward. Even if patients are lying down, for consistency and correct communication when you use anatomical terms, always refer to patients as if they are in the anatomical position.

Directional Anatomical Terms

The directional anatomical terms are **cranial, caudal, ventral, dorsal, medial, lateral, proximal, distal, superficial,** and **deep.** They are used to identify the position of body structures compared to other body structures. For example, the eyes are medial to the ears but lateral to the nose. See Table 23-1 and Figure 23-3 for an explanation and illustration of these important directional terms.

Organization of the Body 439

TABLE 23-1 Directional Anatomical Terms

Term	Definition	Example
Superior (cranial)	Above or close to the head	The thoracic cavity is superior to the abdominal cavity.
Inferior (caudal)	Below or close to the feet	The neck is inferior to the head.
Anterior (ventral)	Toward the front of the body	The nose is anterior to the ears.
Posterior (dorsal)	Toward the back of the body	The brain is posterior to the eyes.
Medial	Close to the midline of the body	The nose is medial to the ear.
Lateral	Farther away from the midline of the body	The ears are lateral to the nose.
Proximal	Close to a point of attachment or to the trunk of the body	The knee is proximal to the toes.
Distal	Farther away from a point of attachment or from the trunk of the body	The fingers are distal to the elbow.
Superficial	Close to the surface of the body	Skin is superficial to muscles.
Deep	More internal	Bones are deep to skin.

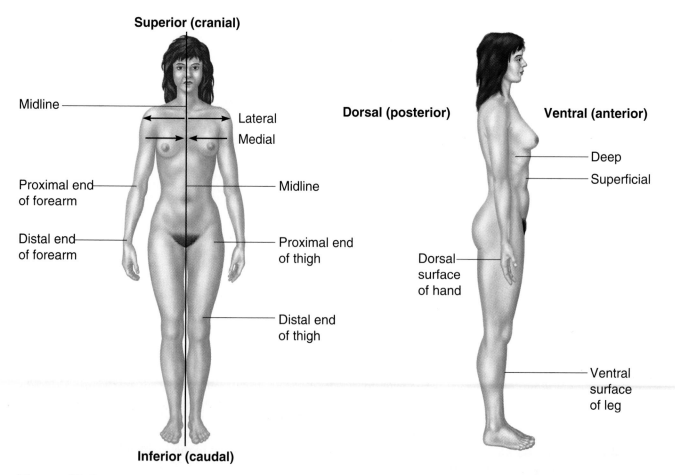

Figure 23-3. Directional terms provide mapping instructions for locating organs and body parts.

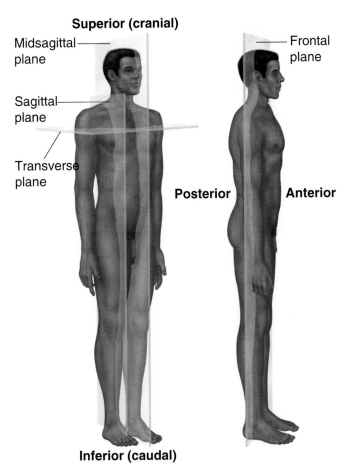

Superior (cranial)

Midsagittal plane

Sagittal plane

Transverse plane

Frontal plane

Posterior   Anterior

Inferior (caudal)

Figure 23-4. Spatial terms are based on imaginary cuts or planes through the body.

Anatomical Terms Used to Describe Body Sections

Sometimes in order to study internal body parts, the body has to be imagined as being divided into sections. It is useful to use the following terms to describe how the body is divided into sections: sagittal, transverse, and frontal (coronal).

A **sagittal** plane divides the body into left and right portions. A **midsagittal** plane runs lengthwise down the midline of the body and divides it into equal left and right halves. A **transverse** plane divides the body into **superior** (upper) and **inferior** (lower) portions. A **frontal,** or coronal, plane divides the body into **anterior** (frontal) and **posterior** (rear) portions. Figure 23-4 illustrates these planes.

Anatomical Terms Used to Describe Body Parts

Many other anatomical terms are used to describe different regions or parts of the body. For example, the term *brachium* refers to the arm and the term **femoral** refers to the thigh. Figure 23-5 illustrates many of the common anatomical terms used to describe body parts.

Body Cavities and Abdominal Regions

The largest body cavities are the dorsal cavity and the ventral cavity. The dorsal cavity is divided into the cranial cavity and the spinal cavity. The cranial cavity houses the brain, and the spinal cavity contains the spinal cord. The ventral cavity is divided into the thoracic cavity and the abdominopelvic cavity. The muscle called the **diaphragm** separates the thoracic and abdominopelvic cavities from each other. The lungs, heart, esophagus, and trachea are contained in the thoracic cavity. The abdominopelvic cavity is divided into a superior abdominal cavity and an inferior pelvic cavity. Most of the organs of digestion are found in the abdominal cavity, and the bladder and internal reproductive organs are located in the pelvic cavity. Figure 23-6 depicts these cavities. The abdominal area is further divided into nine regions or four quadrants, which are illustrated in Figure 23-7.

Chemistry of Life

The lowest level of organization is the chemical level, which includes all the chemical elements that make up matter. Liquids, solids, and gases are all matter. **Chemistry** is the study of what matter is composed of and how matter changes. It is important to have a basic understanding of chemistry when studying anatomy and physiology because body structures and functions result from chemical changes that occur within body cells or fluids.

When two or more atoms are chemically combined, a molecule is formed. Molecules are the basic units of compounds. A **compound** is formed when two or more atoms of more than one element are combined. An example of a molecule is water, which is composed of two hydrogen atoms and one oxygen atom. Water is also an example of a compound because its molecules are made up of atoms of two different elements—hydrogen and oxygen. Water is critical to both chemical and physical processes in human physiology, and it accounts for approximately two-thirds of a person's body weight.

Metabolism is the overall chemical functioning of the body. Metabolism includes all the processes that build small molecules into large ones (anabolism) and break down large molecules into small ones (catabolism).

Electrolytes

When put into water, some substances release **ions,** which are either positively or negatively charged particles; these substances are called **electrolytes.** For example, NaCl (sodium chloride) is an electrolyte. When you put NaCl in water, it releases the sodium ion (Na^+) and the chloride ion (Cl^-). Electrolytes are critical because the movements of ions into and out of body structures regulate or trigger many physiologic states and activities in the body. For

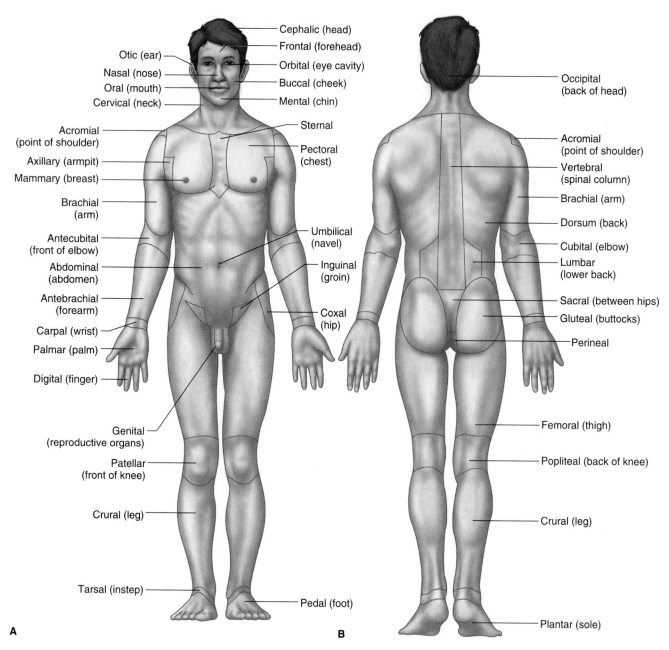

Figure 23-5. Numerous anatomical terms are used to describe regions of the body: (a) anterior view and (b) posterior view.

example, electrolytes are essential to fluid balance, muscle contraction, and nerve impulse conduction.

Acids. **Acids** are a type of electrolytes. They are defined as electrolytes that release hydrogen ions (H^+) in water. For example, hydrochloric acid (HCl) will release hydrogen ions when you put it in water. Therefore, it is acidic. It is also an electrolyte because it releases ions. Many acids, such as lemon juice and vinegar, have a sour taste.

Bases. **Bases** are also a type of electrolytes. They release hydroxyl ions (OH^-) in water. Sodium hydroxide (NaOH) is an example of a base because in water, it releases hydroxyl ions. A basic substance may also be referred to as an alkali. Many basic substances are slippery

and bitter to the taste. Detergents are examples of basic substances.

Testing Acids and Bases. In the clinical setting, litmus paper or a pH meter is often used to determine if a substance is acidic or basic. An acidic substance will turn blue litmus paper red, and a basic substance will turn red litmus paper blue. The pH scale runs from 0 to 14. If a solution has a pH of 7, the solution is neutral, which means that it is neither acidic nor basic. If a solution has a pH less than 7, the solution is acidic. If a solution has a pH greater than 7, it is basic, or alkaline. The more acidic a solution is, the higher the concentration of hydrogen ions it contains. The pH values of some common substances are shown in Figure 23-8.

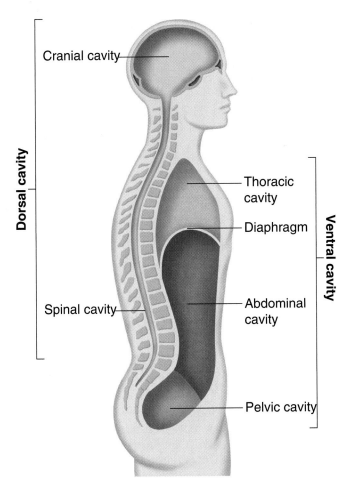

Figure 23-6. The two main body cavities are dorsal and ventral.

Biochemistry

The study of matter and chemical reactions in the body is called **biochemistry.** Matter can be divided into two large categories—organic and inorganic matter. **Organic** matter contains carbon and hydrogen. **Inorganic** matter generally does not contain carbon and hydrogen. Organic molecules tend to be large, whereas inorganic molecules tend to be small. Examples of inorganic substances are water, oxygen, carbon dioxide, and salts such as sodium chloride. Water is the most abundant inorganic compound in the body. The four major classes of organic matter in the body are carbohydrates, lipids, proteins, and nucleic acids.

Carbohydrates. Body cells depend on carbohydrate molecules primarily to make energy. The most common carbohydrate used by body cells is glucose. Glucose can also be stored in the body as a more complex carbohydrate called glycogen. Starches are a type of carbohydrate commonly found in potatoes, pastas, and breads.

Lipids. Three types of lipids found in the body are triglycerides, phospholipids, and steroids. Triglycerides are used to store energy for cells, and phospholipids are primarily used to make cell membranes. Butter and oils are composed of triglycerides, and the body stores these molecules in adipose tissue (fat). Steroids are very large lipid molecules used to make cell membranes and some hormones. Cholesterol is an example of an essential steroid for body cells.

Proteins. Proteins have many functions in the body. Many proteins act as structural materials for the building

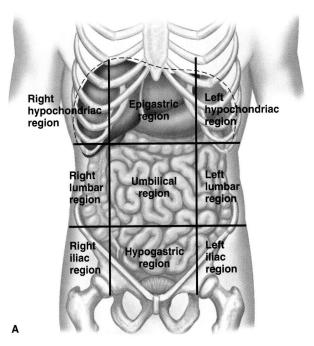

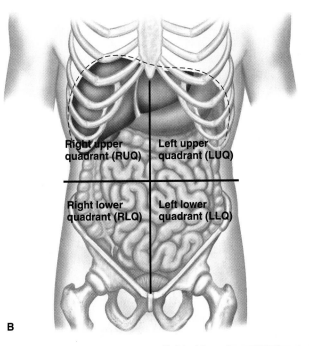

Figure 23-7. (a) The abdominal area divided into nine regions and (b) the abdominal area divided into four quadrants.

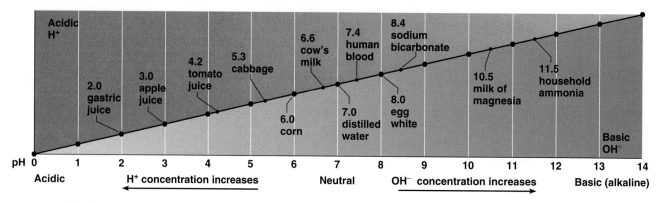

Figure 23-8. pH scale. As the concentration of hydrogen ions (H⁺) increases, a solution becomes more acidic and the pH decreases. As the concentration of hydroxyl ions (OH⁻) increases, a solution becomes more basic and the pH increases.

of solid body parts. Other proteins act as hormones, enzymes, receptors, and antibodies.

Nucleic Acids. **DNA** (deoxyribonucleic acid) and **RNA** (ribonucleic acid) are two examples of nucleic acids. DNA contains the genetic information of cells, and RNA is used to make proteins.

Cell Characteristics

Chemicals react to form the complex substances that make up cells, the basic unit of life. The human body is composed of millions of cells. There are many kinds of cells, and each type has a specific function. Most cells have three main parts: cell membrane, cytoplasm, and nucleus. Figure 23-9 shows the structure of a composite cell.

Cell Membrane

The **cell membrane** is the outer limit of a cell. It is very thin and is described as being selectively permeable, which means that it allows some substances to pass through it while preventing other substances from passing through. The cell membrane is composed of two layers of phospholipids, different types of proteins, cholesterol, and a few carbohydrates.

Cytoplasm

The **cytoplasm** of a cell can be imagined as the "inside" of the cell. It is mostly made up of water, proteins, ions, and nutrients.

Nucleus

The **nucleus** of a cell is typically round in structure and is placed near the center of a cell. It is enclosed by a nuclear membrane that contains nuclear pores so that larger substances can move into and out of the nucleus. It contains

chromosomes, which are threadlike structures made up of DNA.

Movement Through Cell Membranes

The cell membrane controls what moves into and out of cells. Some substances move across the cell membrane without the use of energy. These movements are called passive mechanisms. Sometimes the cell has to use energy to move a substance across its membrane. In this case, the substances move through active mechanisms.

Diffusion

Diffusion is the movement of a substance from an area of high concentration to an area of low concentration—it can be described as the spreading out of a substance. Substances that easily diffuse across the cell membrane include gases such as oxygen and carbon dioxide.

Osmosis

Osmosis refers to the diffusion or movement of water across a semipermeable membrane, such as a cell membrane. You should remember that water will always try to diffuse or move toward the higher concentration of solutes (solids in solution).

Filtration

In **filtration,** some type of pressure, such as gravity or blood pressure, forces substances across a membrane that acts like a filter. Filtration separates substances in solutions. For example, you could separate sand from water by pouring the sand/water mixture through a filter. In the body, capillaries in the kidneys act as filters to separate components in blood.

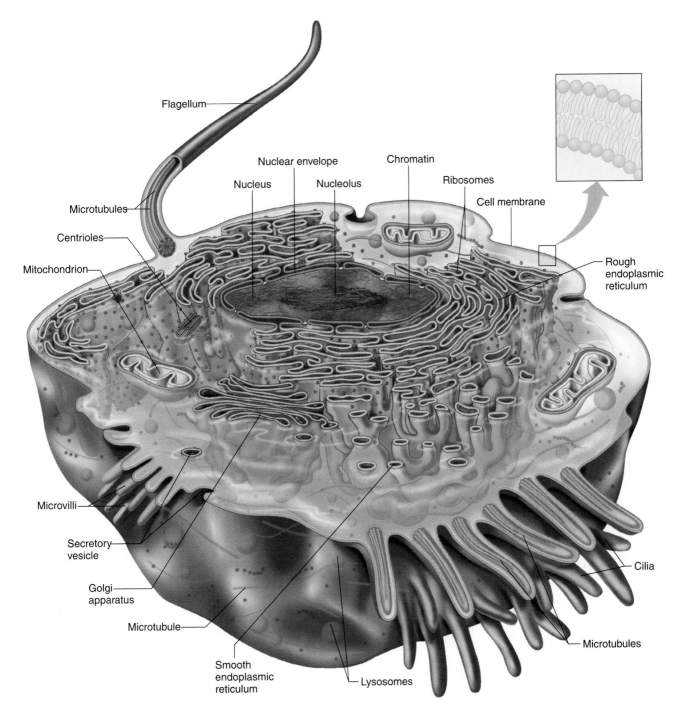

Figure 23-9. Composite cell.

Labels in figure: Flagellum, Microtubules, Centrioles, Mitochondrion, Nuclear envelope, Nucleus, Nucleolus, Chromatin, Ribosomes, Cell membrane, Rough endoplasmic reticulum, Microvilli, Secretory vesicle, Golgi apparatus, Microtubule, Smooth endoplasmic reticulum, Lysosomes, Cilia, Microtubules

Active Transport

In **active transport,** substances move across the cell membrane with the help of carrier molecules from an area of low concentration to an area of high concentration. In other words, substances are gathered together, which is the opposite of diffusion. Some substances that are moved across the cell membrane through active transport include sugars, amino acids, potassium, calcium, and hydrogen ions.

Cell Division

Cells can become damaged, diseased, or worn out, and replacements must be made. Also, new cells are needed for normal growth. Cells reproduce by cell division, a process that involves splitting the nucleus, through **mitosis** or **meiosis,** and splitting the cytoplasm, called **cytokinesis.**

A cell that carries out its normal daily functions and is not dividing is said to be in **interphase.** For example, if a liver cell is in interphase, it is making liver enzymes, detoxifying blood, and processing nutrients. During interphase, a cell prepares for cell division by duplicating its DNA and cytoplasmic organelles. For most body cells, each daughter cell will have the exact same copy of DNA and organelles as the original mother cell. Sometimes when the DNA is duplicated, errors called **mutations** occur. These mutations will be passed on to the descendants (daughter cells) of that cell and may or may not affect the cells in harmful ways.

Mitosis

Following interphase, a cell may enter mitosis, a part of cell division in which the nucleus divides. When mitosis is almost complete, cytoplasmic division (cytokinesis) occurs. During this process, the cell membrane constricts to divide the cytoplasm of the cell. The result is that the organelles of the original cell get distributed almost evenly into the two new cells.

During mitosis, the nucleus makes a complete copy of all 23 of its chromosome pairs (46 chromosomes altogether). As the cell divides, each new cell receives a complete set of chromosome pairs. The resulting cells are identical to each other.

Meiosis

Reproductive cell division, or meiosis, takes place only in the reproductive organs when the male and female sex cells are formed. During meiosis, the nucleus copies all 23 chromosome pairs, but two divisions take place. The four cells that are formed each contain only one of each chromosome pair, for a total of 23 chromosomes. This type of cell division must occur so that when the sex cells combine during fertilization, the resulting cell contains the usual number of chromosomes (46).

Genetic Techniques

DNA is the primary component of genes and is found in the nucleus of most cells within the body. A segment of DNA that determines a body trait is called a **gene**. Genetic techniques involve using or manipulating genes.

DNA molecules are made up of a linear sequence of compounds called nucleotides, and each nucleotide contains one of four different nitrogen bases. The chemical structure of every person's DNA is the same. The only difference among people is the order of the nitrogen bases. The unique sequence of the nucleotides determines the characteristics of an individual. One DNA molecule will contain hundreds or thousands of genes. Each gene occupies a particular location on the DNA molecule, making it possible to compare the same gene in a number of different samples. Two widely used genetic techniques in the clinical setting are the polymerase chain reaction and DNA fingerprinting.

Polymerase Chain Reaction

The polymerase chain reaction, PCR, is a quick, easy method for making millions of copies of any fragment of DNA. This technique has been revolutionary in the study of genetics and has very quickly become a necessary tool for improving human health.

Because PCR can produce millions of gene copies from tiny amounts of DNA, even from just one cell, the method is especially useful for detecting disease-causing organisms that are impossible to culture, such as many kinds of bacteria, fungi, and viruses. It can, for example, detect the AIDS virus sooner—during the first few weeks after infection—than other tests. PCR is also more accurate than standard tests. The technique can detect bacterial DNA in children's middle ear fluid, which indicates an infection, even when culture methods fail to detect bacteria. Other diseases diagnosed through PCR include Lyme disease, stomach ulcers, viral meningitis, hepatitis, tuberculosis, and many sexually transmitted diseases, including herpes and chlamydia.

PCR is also leading to new kinds of genetic testing because it can easily distinguish among the tiny variations in DNA that all people possess. This testing can diagnose people who have inherited disorders or who carry mutations that could be passed to their children. PCR is also used in tests that determine who may develop common disorders such as heart disease and various types of cancer. This knowledge helps individuals take steps to prevent those diseases.

DNA Fingerprinting

A DNA "fingerprint" refers to the unique sequences of nucleotides in a person's DNA and is the same for every cell, tissue, and organ of that person. It cannot be altered by any known method. Consequently, DNA fingerprinting is a reliable method for identifying and distinguishing among human beings, such as in a criminal case.

DNA fingerprinting is also used to diagnosis genetic disorders; it can be used to detect inherited disorders in unborn babies. These disorders include cystic fibrosis, hemophilia, Huntington's disease, familial Alzheimer's, sickle cell anemia, thalassemia, and many others. Detecting genetic diseases early allows patients and medical staff to prepare for proper treatment. Also, studying the DNA fingerprints of groups of individuals with the same disease allow researchers to identify DNA patterns associated with genetic diseases.

Another important use of DNA fingerprints is to establish paternity for custody and child support issues. The biological father has a DNA fingerprint that is very similar to the DNA fingerprint of his child. If the DNA fingerprints are not similar, the paternity test is negative.

Heredity

Heredity is the transfer of genetic traits from parent to child. When a sperm cell and an egg unite, a cell called a zygote forms. The zygote has 46 chromosomes, or 23 chromosomal pairs. One half of each pair came from the sperm, and the other half from the egg. Two chromosomes in each pair are called **homologous chromosomes.** The chromosomes of the first 22 pairs are called **autosomes,** and those of the 23rd pair are called **sex chromosomes.** If the sex chromosomes are an X chromosome and a Y chromosome, the child is a male. If the sex chromosomes are both X chromosomes, the child is a female. Although the sex chromosomes determine the gender of the child, they also determine other body traits. However, the autosomes determine most body traits.

Each chromosome possesses many genes. Homologous chromosomes carry the same genes that code for a particular trait, but the genes may be of different forms, which are called **alleles.** Many times only one allele is actually expressed as a trait even if another allele is present. The allele that is always expressed over the other is called a dominant allele. The one that is not expressed is called recessive. The only way a recessive allele can be expressed is if there is no dominant allele present.

Detached earlobes are an example of a trait that is determine by a dominant allele. If a child inherits a dominant allele for this trait from one parent but inherits the recessive allele from the other parent, the child will have detached earlobes. If the child inherits recessive alleles from both parents, then he will have attached earlobes.

Most traits in the body are determined by multiple alleles. For example, hair color, height, skin tone, eye color, and body build are each determined by many different genes. **Complex inheritance** is the term used to describe inherited traits that are determined by multiple genes. It explains why different children within the same family can each have different characteristics.

Sex-linked traits are carried on the sex chromosomes, X and Y. The Y chromosome is much smaller than the X chromosome and does not carry many genes. Therefore, if the X chromosome carries a recessive allele, it is likely to be expressed because there is usually no corresponding allele on the Y chromosome. For example, red-green color blindness is determined by the presence of a recessive allele that is always found on the X chromosome. This disorder (like most sex-linked disorders) primarily affects males because the corresponding Y chromosome does not have any allele to prevent the expression of the recessive allele.

Genetic influences are known to contribute to many thousands of different health conditions. See the Pathophysiology section for a description of some of the more common genetic disorders.

Pathophysiology

Common Genetic Disorders

Albinism is a condition in which a person is born with little or no pigmentation in the skin, eyes, or hair. Albinism affects all races, and in most cases there is no family history.

- **Causes.** At least six different genes are involved with pigment production. This condition develops when a person inherits one or more faulty genes that do not produce the usual amounts of a pigment.
- **Signs and symptoms.** People with the condition experience visual problems and sun-sensitive skin.
- **Treatment.** Although there is no cure, treatments are available to help the symptoms. Prenatal testing for the condition is available.

Attention deficit hyperactivity disorder (ADHD) is the most common behavioral disorder. It usually begins in childhood.

- **Causes.** Although ADHD is not normally considered a genetic disorder, there is evidence that genetic factors play a role in increasing the susceptibility to this condition. Twin and genetic studies show that several genes are likely to be involved.
- **Signs and symptoms.** People with this disorder have difficulty paying attention without being distracted and find it difficult to control impulsive physical actions. Children with ADHD have normal intelligence but are more likely to be depressed and anxious as well as to have problems with speech and language. Hyperactivity usually improves when the child reaches puberty.
- **Treatment.** There is no cure for ADHD, but treatments such as the drug Ritalin or behavior modification are available.

Cleft lip and *cleft palate* are gaps or depressions in the upper lip or palate (roof of the mouth). These conditions commonly occur together.

- **Causes.** These conditions develop when separate areas of a developing fetus's face and head do not join together during early fetal development. Although genes may play a role in the development of these conditions, other causes include maternal rubella (German measles) or the use of certain medications during pregnancy.
- **Signs and symptoms.** Cleft lip or palate may lead to problems with feeding, recurrent ear infections, aspiration pneumonia, and speech problems later in life.
- **Treatment.** Surgery is usually very successful in repairing these conditions.

continued ⟶

Common Genetic Disorders *(continued)*

Cystic fibrosis is a life-threatening disease that mainly affects the lungs and pancreas. This disease is one of the most common inherited life-threatening disorders among white people in the United States.

- **Causes.** Inheritance is autosomal recessive, so if both parents are carriers, there is a 25% chance that each child born to them will develop cystic fibrosis.
- **Signs and symptoms.** Patients with this disorder have increasing problems with breathing. Thick secretions eventually block passageways in the air, and these secretions may become infected.
- **Treatment.** There is no cure, but treatments are available to help patients live with the complications associated with this disorder. Newborn babies are commonly screened for the disease because the sooner treatment begins, the healthier the child can be. Parents are also commonly screened for the gene to determine the likelihood of having a child with cystic fibrosis.

Down syndrome is a disorder that causes mental retardation and physical abnormalities.

- **Causes.** This disorder occurs when a person has three copies of chromosome 21 instead of two. This condition can be diagnosed through prenatal tests such as amniocentesis. The risk of having a child with Down syndrome increases with the age of the mother.
- **Signs and symptoms.** The signs of Down syndrome include a flat facial profile, protruding tongue, oblique slanting eyes, abundant neck skin, short broad hands, and poor muscle tone. Heart, digestive, hearing, and visual problems are also common in people with this condition. Learning difficulties are common in Down syndrome and can range from moderate to severe.
- **Treatment.** There is no cure, but support programs and the treatment of health problems allow many patients with Down syndrome to live a relatively normal life.

Fragile X syndrome is the most common inherited cause of learning disability. All races and ethnic groups seem to be affected equally by this syndrome.

- **Causes.** In this disorder, one of the genes on the X chromosome is defective and makes the chromosome susceptible to breakage. This sex-linked disorder affects boys more severely than girls. It is estimated that approximately 1 in 300 females are carriers for this disorder.
- **Signs and symptoms.** Mental impairment, learning disabilities, attention deficit disorder, a long face, large ears, and flat feet are some of the signs and symptoms. Fragile X syndrome can be easily diagnosed using prenatal tests such as amniocentesis.
- **Treatment.** There is no cure, but some treatments and support groups are available to patients with this disorder.

Hemophilia is a group of inheritable blood disorders. Each condition may be severe to mild.

- **Causes.** In each type, an essential clotting factor is low or missing. Most types of hemophilia are X-linked recessive disorders; therefore, this disorder primarily affects males. Carriers of the gene can be identified with a blood test, and prenatal tests can diagnose the condition in the fetus.
- **Signs and symptoms.** Symptoms include easy bruising, spontaneous bleeding, and prolonged bleeding. Repeated bleeding in the joints leads to arthritis and permanent joint damage.
- **Treatment.** Treatments include injections of the missing clotting factors.

Klinefelter's syndrome is a chromosomal abnormality that affects males.

- **Causes.** People with this disorder have an extra X chromosome.
- **Signs and symptoms.** Tall stature, pear-shaped fat distribution, small testes, sparse body hair, and infertility are the most common signs and symptoms. Thyroid problems, diabetes, and osteoporosis are also common in patients with this syndrome.
- **Treatment.** There is no cure, but treatments such as testosterone replacement therapy can decrease the risk of osteoporosis and produce more male characteristics.

Muscular dystrophy is a group of genetic disorders that primarily affect the muscular and nervous systems. It most often affects males.

- **Causes.** Most types involve mutations in the genes responsible for producing muscle proteins. Some types of muscular dystrophy are inherited as an X-linked disorder, but some are caused by gene mutations.
- **Signs and symptoms.** In this disorder, muscle cells gradually break down, causing progressive muscle weakness.
- **Treatment.** There is no cure, and few treatments are available to slow down the loss of muscle cells. Prenatal genetic tests are available for some types of muscular dystrophies.

Phenylketonuria (PKU) develops if a person cannot synthesize the enzyme that converts phenylalanine to tyrosine. Phenylalanine is an essential amino acid, but too much of it can be harmful, so the body regularly converts it to tyrosine.

- **Causes.** This condition is inherited as an autosomal recessive disorder.
- **Signs and symptoms.** If phenylalanine builds up in the blood, it can lead to the irreversible damage of organs, including the brain.

continued ⟶

Common Genetic Disorders *(continued)*

- **Treatment.** Phenylalanine is found in many proteins, so meats and other protein-rich foods must be avoided. The early detection of PKU is important in order to prevent developmental delays. There is no cure for PKU, but special diets allow a person to lead a normal life. Most newborns are tested for PKU, and prenatal diagnosis is also available.

Sickle cell anemia is an inheritable genetic condition in which abnormal hemoglobin is produced in red blood cells. Normal hemoglobin carries most of the oxygen in the blood. Patients with sickle cell anemia produce an abnormal type of hemoglobin that cannot carry oxygen and that also causes red blood cells to become rigid and have a sickle shape. These rigid red blood cells are less able to squeeze through small blood vessels, so these blood vessels become blocked. It primarily affects people of African or Caribbean descent.

- **Causes.** This disease is inherited as an autosomal recessive disorder.
- **Signs and symptoms.** Blood vessels can become blocked in organs such as the liver, kidney, lungs, heart, and spleen and can cause severe pain. The red blood cells also break down easily, which leads to anemia.
- **Treatment.** There is no cure for sickle cell anemia, but treatments have been successful in preventing the complications associated with this disease. This condition can be diagnosed with prenatal tests.

Spina bifida occurs when one or more vertebrae do not form properly, leaving a gap in the spinal column and leading to damage of the spinal cord.

- **Causes.** This condition is thought to be caused by a combination of genetic and environmental factors.
- **Signs and symptoms.** Signs and symptoms will vary greatly, depending on the level of the gap in the spinal column. In the most severe forms, paralysis of many body muscles can result. Hydrocephalus (increased pressure in the fluid of the brain) often accompanies spina bifida, which can lead to brain damage. Prenatal tests can sometimes diagnose the condition. Folic acid supplements are believed to reduce the risk of the development of this disorder.
- **Treatment.** The treatment primarily consists of physical therapy, which helps to keep muscles strong.

Turner's syndrome is a disorder that almost exclusively affects females.

- **Causes.** This disease results when an X chromosome is completely or partially missing.
- **Signs and symptoms.** The signs and symptoms may include web neck, broad chest, widely spaced nipples, low hairline, short stature, and infertility. Prenatal tests can diagnose the condition, but most girls are diagnosed in late childhood when they fail to start menstruating.
- **Treatment.** There is no cure for Turner's syndrome, but treatments with growth hormone replacements can increase the height of the patient.

Major Tissue Types

As you learned earlier in the chapter, tissues are groups of cells that have similar structures and functions. The four major tissue types in the body are **epithelial, connective, muscle,** and **nervous.**

Epithelial Tissue

When you think of epithelial tissue, you should think of a covering, lining, or gland. Epithelial tissue covers the body and most organs. Epithelial tissue lines tubes of the body such as blood vessels and the esophagus as well as hollow organs of the body such as the stomach and heart. This type of tissue also lines body cavities (such as the thoracic cavity and the abdominopelvic cavity). Glandular tissue is also classified as a type of epithelial tissue.

Glandular epithelium is composed of cells that make and secrete (give off) substances. If a gland secretes its product into a duct, it is called an **exocrine gland.** If a gland secretes its product directly into tissue fluids or blood, it is called an **endocrine gland.** Endocrine glands do not have ducts, so they have to secrete their products into surrounding tissue fluids or blood.

Epithelial tissues are avascular, which means that they lack blood vessels. However, these tissues have a nerve supply and are very mitotic—they divide constantly. In addition, the cells within epithelial tissues are packed together tightly. Epithelial tissues possess many functions, depending on their location in the body. For example, those covering the body provide protection against invading pathogens and toxins. Those that line the digestive tract secrete a variety of enzymes needed for digestion and often possess microvilli, which allow the body to absorb nutrients. Epithelial tissues lining the respiratory tract have cilia and goblet cells. The goblet cells produce mucus that traps small particles that enter the respiratory tract. The cilia constantly push the mucus and trapped particles away from the lungs (Figure 23-10). Epithelial cells within the kidneys act as filters that help to remove waste products from blood.

Connective Tissue

Connective tissues are the most abundant tissues in the body. The cells of connective tissues do not pack together tightly. Instead, a **matrix** separates the cells. Think of the matrix simply as the matter that is between the cells of

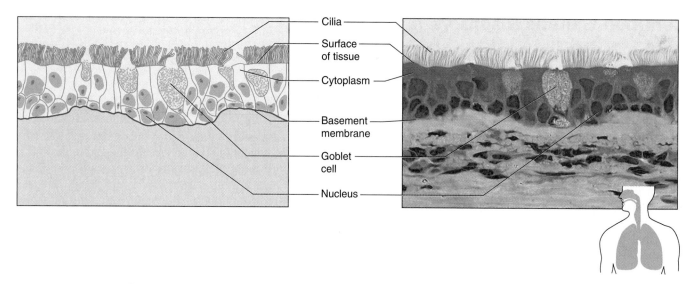

Figure 23-10. Epithelial tissue lining the respiratory tract.

connective tissue. It contains fibers, water, proteins, inorganic salts, and other substances. The components of the matrix vary, depending on the type of connective tissue. Connective tissues generally have a rich blood supply, except for cartilage and some dense connective tissues that contain a very poor blood supply.

There are many different cell types located in connective tissues. The most common cell types are fibroblasts, mast cells, and macrophages. Fibroblasts make fibers, and mast cells secrete substances such as heparin and histamine that promote inflammation during times of tissue damage. Macrophages are cells that destroy unwanted material such as bacteria or toxins.

Blood. This tissue is composed of red blood cells, white blood cells, and plasma. Plasma is the matrix of blood. Unlike other connective tissues, this matrix does not contain fibers. Blood functions to transport substances throughout the body.

Osseous (Bone) Tissue. The matrix of osseous tissue contains mineral salts that make it a very hard tissue. Contrary to popular belief, bone tissue is metabolically active.

Cartilage. The matrix of cartilage is rigid, although it is not as hard as osseous tissue. Cartilage gives shape to structures such as the ears and nose. It also protects the ends of long bones and forms the discs between the vertebrae of the neck and spine.

Dense Connective Tissue. The matrix of dense connective tissue is packed with tough fibers that make it a soft but very strong tissue. Ligaments, tendons, and joint capsules have large amounts of this tissue type. Ligaments

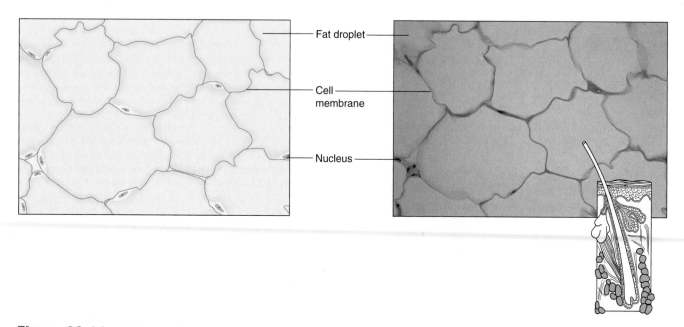

Figure 23-11. Adipose tissue.

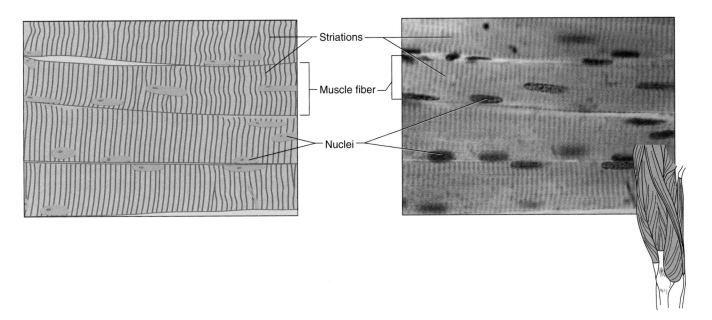

Figure 23-12. Skeletal muscle tissue.

connect bones to bones, tendons connect bones to muscles, and joint capsules surround moveable joints in the body. Dense connective tissues also make up a large part of the dermis of skin. When skin is damaged, this tissue "fills" in the space of damage and forms a scar.

Adipose (Fat) Tissue. Within adipose tissue, unique cells—adipocytes—store fats. The functions of this tissue type include storing energy for cells of the body, cushioning body parts and organs, and insulating the body against excessive heat or cold (Figure 23-11).

Muscle Tissue

Muscle tissue is a specialized type of tissue that shortens and elongates; in other words, it contracts and relaxes. The three types of muscle tissue are skeletal, smooth, and cardiac. Skeletal muscle tissue, as its name suggests, is attached to the skeleton. This type of muscle tissue is described as voluntary because we can consciously control its movement. For example, we can consciously decide to contract the skeletal muscles attached to our arm bones and make them move. It is also referred to as being striated because the cells of this muscle tissue type have striations or stripes in their cytoplasm (Figure 23-12).

Smooth muscle tissue is located in the walls of hollow organs (except the heart), the walls of blood vessels, and the dermis of skin. It is not voluntary because we cannot consciously control its movement. For example, you do not consciously decide when the smooth muscle of your stomach contacts. This tissue is called smooth because its cells do not possess striations in their cytoplasm.

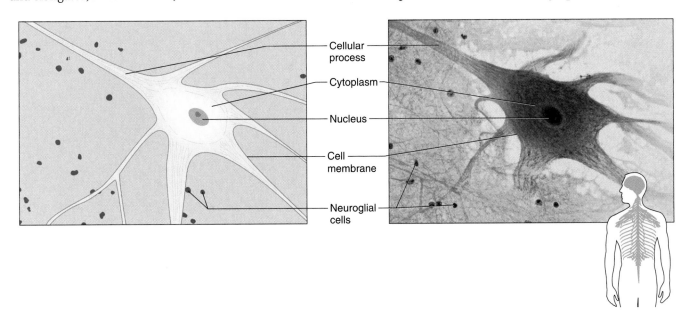

Figure 23-13. Nervous tissue.

Cardiac muscle tissue is located in the wall of the heart. Like skeletal muscle tissue, it is striated and like smooth muscle tissue, it is not under voluntary control.

Nervous Tissue

Nervous tissue is located in the brain, spinal cord, and peripheral nerves. This tissue specializes in sending impulses or electrical messages to the neurons, muscles, and glands in the body. Nervous tissue contains two types of cells: **neurons** and **neuroglial cells.** Neurons are the largest cells and possess characteristic cellular processes. Although neuroglial cells are smaller, they are more abundant and support neurons (Figure 23-13).

Summary

The human body is divided into several levels of organization, from the simplest to the most complex. These levels are chemical, cellular, tissue, organ, organ system, and organism. Anatomy is the study of the structure of the human body. Physiology is the study of its functions. Directional terms are used to describe the location of body parts and regions. These terms always relate to the anatomic position. It is important to understand the basics of the organization of the human body before studying the individual systems.

CHAPTER 23

CASE STUDY QUESTIONS

Now that you have completed this chapter, review the case study at the beginning of the chapter and answer the following questions:

1. On what side of the body is the appendix normally located?
2. If the medical assistant observes the boy's right lower abdominal quadrant for the bandage, is this correct? Why or why not?
3. Where should the bandage be found?
4. What precautions should this patient take given his diagnosis of *situs inversus*?

Discussion Questions

1. Explain the function of the four types of tissues in one of the body systems.
2. Describe the four abdominal quadrants and the nine abdominal regions. What is the importance of knowing these areas in the clinical setting?
3. What are acids and bases? Describe the pH scale.

Critical Thinking Questions

1. Diseases develop when homeostasis is not maintained. What treatments can bring the following conditions back to normal: high body temperature, dehydration, and high blood pressure?
2. What clinical laboratory tests have you encountered that require a knowledge of chemistry to interpret?
3. Moveable joints like elbows and knees always contain cartilage and dense connective tissues. Why are they so slow to heal once they have been injured?

Application Activities

1. Referring to figures in the chapter, name an organ or part of the body that is located:
   a. Distal to the elbow
   b. Proximal to the ankle
   c. In the thoracic cavity
   d. In the pelvic cavity
   e. Medial to the acromial region
2. What organs would you expect to see if you were looking at a transverse plane cut at the level of the umbilicus?

Internet Activity

1. Go to the Web site for the Centers for Disease Control and Prevention (**http:www.cdc.gov**) and answer the following questions:
   a. What are the Centers for Disease Control and Prevention?
   b. Click on Health Topics A–Z, and then click on Spina Bifida. How are spina bifida and folic acid related?
   c. Each year in the United States, about how many infants are born with spina bifida or anencephaly?
   d. What are the annual medical care and surgical costs for persons with spina bifida in the United States?
2. Find an interactive periodic table of elements, and answer the following questions:
   a. Carbon, hydrogen, oxygen, and nitrogen are the four most abundant elements of the human body. What are the atomic symbols for each of these elements?
   b. Who discovered hydrogen?
   c. What is the name origin of oxygen?
   d. When was nitrogen discovered?
   e. How many protons does one carbon atom contain?

CHAPTER 24

The Integumentary System

KEY TERMS

alopecia
apocrine gland
arrector pili
cellulitis
cyanosis
dermatitis
dermis
eccrine gland
eczema
epidermis
follicle
folliculitis
hemoglobin
herpes simplex
herpes zoster
hypodermis
impetigo
keratin
keratinocyte
lunula
melanin
melanocyte
nail bed
psoriasis
rosacea
scabies
sebaceous
sebum
stratum basale
stratum corneum
subcutaneous
warts

CHAPTER OUTLINE

- Functions of the Integumentary System
- Skin Structure
- Skin Color
- Accessory Organs
- Skin Healing

OBJECTIVES

After completing Chapter 24, you will be able to:

24.1 List the functions of skin.

24.2 Explain the role of skin in regulating body temperature.

24.3 Describe the layers of skin and the characteristics of each layer.

24.4 Explain the factors that affect skin color.

24.5 List the accessory organs of skin and describe their structures and functions.

24.6 Describe the appearance, causes, and treatments of various types of skin cancer.

24.7 Describe the appearance, causes, and treatment of common skin disorders.

24.8 Explain the ABCD rule and its use in evaluating melanoma.

24.9 List the different types of burns and describe their appearances and treatments.

24.10 Describe the signs, symptoms, causes, and treatments of other skin disorders and diseases.

Introduction

The integumentary system consists of skin and its accessory organs. The accessory organs of skin are hair follicles, nails, and skin glands. Skin is the body's outer covering and its largest organ.

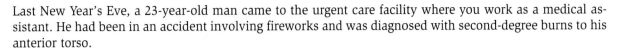
Last New Year's Eve, a 23-year-old man came to the urgent care facility where you work as a medical assistant. He had been in an accident involving fireworks and was diagnosed with second-degree burns to his anterior torso.

As you read this chapter, consider the following questions:

1. Using the rule of nines, estimate the percentage of the patient's body surface that was affected by this burn.
2. What layers of skin has the burn affected?
3. What functions of the skin are lost by this injury?
4. What types of treatments does this burn require?

Functions of the Integumentary System

People are often interested in the appearance of their skin but rarely consider its functions. The integumentary system serves many purposes, including these important functions:

- Protection. As long as skin is intact and not inflamed, it provides very good protection against the entry of bacteria and viruses. It also protects underlying structures from ultraviolet radiation and dehydration.
- Body temperature regulation. Skin plays a major role in regulating body temperature. When a person is hot, dermal blood vessels dilate, which is why a person's skin becomes pinkish. Because the dermal blood vessels are dilated, more blood than normal passes through the skin. This is beneficial because blood carries a lot of the heat in the body. When the blood gets close to the surface of the body (to skin), the heat can escape. Conversely, if a person is cold, the dermal blood vessels constrict, preventing the heat in blood from escaping.
- Vitamin D production. When exposed to sunlight, the skin produces a molecule that is turned into vitamin D. The body needs vitamin D for calcium absorption.
- Sensation. The skin is packed with sensory receptors that can detect touch, heat, cold, and pain.
- Excretion. Small amounts of waste products are lost through skin when a person perspires.

Skin Structure

The skin is a complex organ consisting of two layers, the **epidermis** and the **dermis.** Skin sits on a third layer called the **hypodermis,** also called the **subcutaneous** layer (Figure 24-1).

Epidermis

The epidermis is the most superficial layer of skin. It is made up of many layers of tightly packed cells. The epidermis can be divided into two layers, the stratum corneum and the stratum basale.

The **stratum corneum** is the most superficial layer of the epidermis. Most of the cells in this layer are dead and very flat. Because they have accumulated keratin, the cells in this layer stick together and form an impermeable layer for skin. Most bacteria, viruses, and water cannot penetrate the stratum corneum.

The **stratum basale** is the deepest layer of the epidermis. The cells in this layer are constantly dividing, and older cells are constantly pushed up toward the stratum corneum.

The most common cell type in the epidermis is the **keratinocyte.** This cell makes and accumulates the protein keratin. **Keratin** is a durable protein that makes the epidermis waterproof and resistant to bacteria and viruses. Another cell type of the epidermis is the **melanocyte,** which makes the pigment **melanin.** Melanin is deposited throughout the layers of the epidermis. This pigment traps ultraviolet (UV) radiation from sunlight and prevents the radiation from harming structures in the underlying layers of the skin.

Dermis

The dermis is the deep layer of skin and is the most complex layer. The dermis contains all the major tissue types, including epithelial tissue, connective tissues, muscle tissue, and nervous tissue. The dermis contains sweat glands, sebaceous (oil) glands, hair follicles, the arrector pili muscles, collagen fibers, elastic fibers, nerve fibers, and many blood vessels. The dermis binds the epidermis to the hypodermis.

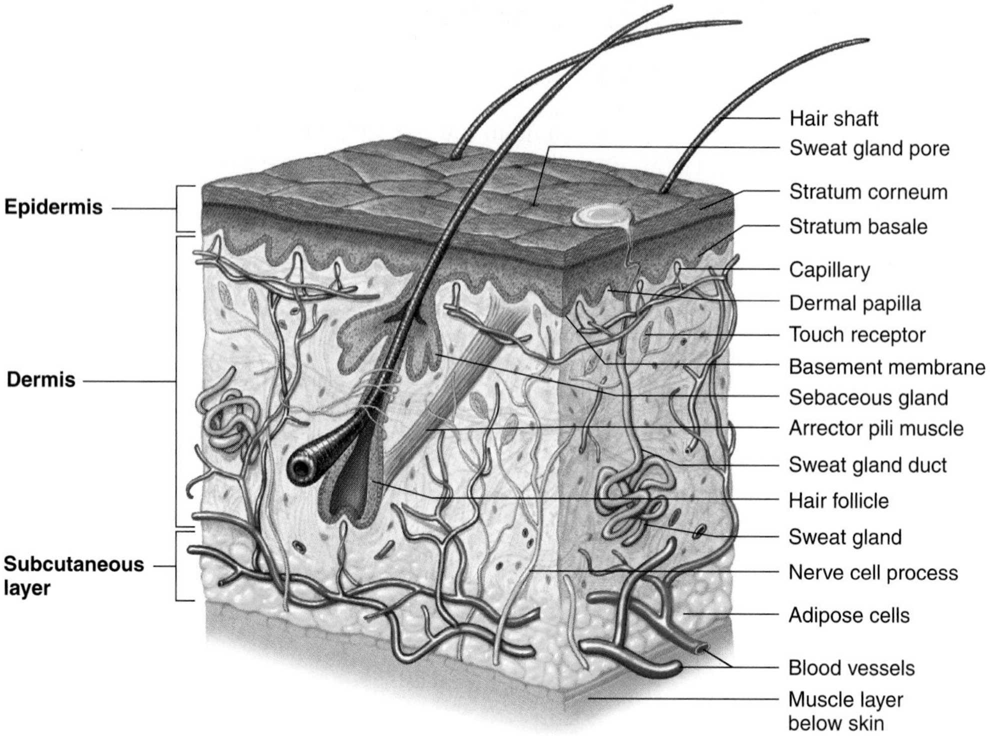

Hair shaft
Sweat gland pore
Epidermis
Stratum corneum
Stratum basale
Capillary
Dermal papilla
Touch receptor
Basement membrane
Dermis
Sebaceous gland
Arrector pili muscle
Sweat gland duct
Hair follicle
Sweat gland
Subcutaneous layer
Nerve cell process
Adipose cells
Blood vessels
Muscle layer below skin

Figure 24-1. Section of skin.

Hypodermis

The subcutaneous layer of skin, the hypodermis, is largely made of adipose tissue. In fact, most adipose tissue in the body is found in your hypodermis. This layer also contains blood vessels and nerves.

Skin Color

Skin color is largely determined by the amount of melanin in the epidermis of skin. Melanin can range in color from yellowish to brownish. The more melanin a person has in the skin, the darker the skin color. All people have about the same number of melanocytes regardless of skin color. What varies from person to person is how active the melanocytes are in producing melanin. A person with dark skin has very active melanocytes.

Another factor that determines skin color is the amount of oxygenated blood in the dermis of skin. **Hemoglobin** is a pigment in blood that is bright red when it is oxygenated. Hemoglobin that is not oxygenated is a dark red color. A person with a rich supply of oxygenated blood will have skin that is a pinkish hue. When the supply of oxygen in the blood is low, the skin looks rather pale or bluish. A bluish color of skin is called **cyanosis.**

Pathophysiology

Skin Cancer and Common Skin Disorders

Skin is vulnerable to many disorders because it is the most exposed of all body organs.

SKIN CANCER

Skin cancer develops from cells in the epidermis of skin. It is more common in people who have light-colored skin and who have had excessive exposure to sunlight. It can occur anywhere on the body but is most likely to appear on skin that is readily exposed to sunlight. The two most common types of skin cancer are basal cell carcinoma and squamous cell carcinoma, but the most deadly type is melanoma (Figure 24-2).

Basal cell carcinoma accounts for approximately 90% of all skin cancers in the United States. Fortunately, it progresses slowly and rarely spreads to other body parts. It is derived from cells of the stratum basale of the epidermis.

continued ⟶

Skin Cancer and Common Skin Disorders *(continued)*

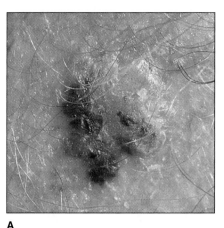
A

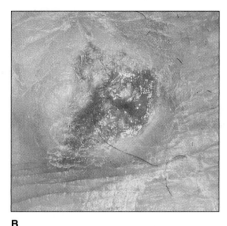
B

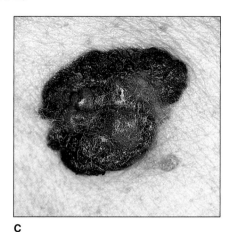
C

Figure 24-2. Types of skin cancer: (a) squamous cell carcinoma, (b) basal cell carcinoma, and (c) malignant melanoma.

- **Signs and symptoms.** Signs and symptoms include changes on the skin and a new growth or sore on the skin that does not heal. Its appearance may be waxy, smooth, red, pale, flat, or lumpy, and it may or may not bleed.
- **Treatment.** Several forms of treatment are available:
  - Curettage and electrodessication. In curettage, a sharp instrument is used to scoop out the cancerous spot. Electrodessication uses electrical currents to minimize bleeding as well as to kill any remaining cancer cells.
  - Mohs' surgery. The cancerous spot is shaved off one layer at a time.
  - Cryosurgery. Freezing is used to kill cancer cells.
  - Laser Therapy. A beam of light destroys cancer cells.

Squamous cell carcinoma is much less common than basal cell carcinoma but is more likely to spread to surrounding tissues. It arises from flat cells of the epidermis. The signs and symptoms and the treatments for this type of cancer are the same as for basal cell carcinoma.

Melanoma is much more aggressive than both basal cell and squamous cell carcinomas. Melanoma can occur anywhere on the body but most often appears on the trunk, head, and neck in men and on the arms and legs in women. Melanoma is cancer that arises from melanocytes.

- **Signs and symptoms.** A mole that itches or bleeds is a common symptom. New moles may develop near it. It may change to have any sign of the ABCD rule:
  - Asymmetry. The mole should not become asymmetrical.
  - Border. The border of the mole should not become irregular.
  - Color. The mole should not change color or become a mixture of colors.
  - Diameter. The mole should not grow larger than the diameter of a pencil eraser.

- **Treatment.** The treatment will depend on the staging of this cancer. Available treatments include the following:
  - Surgery to remove the melanoma
  - Lymph node biopsy to determine if the cancer has spread
  - Removal of cancerous lymph nodes
  - Chemotherapy for advanced stages of cancer
  - Radiation therapy for advanced stages of cancer
  - Immunotherapy to boost the patient's immune system
- **Stages of melanoma.** Melanoma has five different stages, which are described from the least to the most serious:
  - Stage 0. Melanoma is found only in the epidermis
  - Stage I. Melanoma has spread to the epidermis and dermis and has a thickness of 1 to 2 millimeters.
  - Stage II. Melanoma has a thickness of 2 to 4 millimeters and may have ulceration.
  - Stage III. Melanoma has spread to one or more nearby lymph nodes.
  - Stage IV. Melanoma has spread to other body organs or other lymph nodes far away from the original melanoma site.

COMMON SKIN AND HAIR DISORDERS

Alopecia is a disorder that specifically targets hair. This disorder results in hair loss.

- **Causes.** Most of the time, alopecia is inherited. Other common causes include hormonal changes, chemotherapy, stress, burns, and fungal infections of the skin.
- **Signs and symptoms.** Alopecia is more commonly called baldness, but it may occur on areas of skin other than the scalp.

continued ⟶

Skin Cancer and Common Skin Disorders *(continued)*

- **Treatment.** If due to heredity, this disorder is not curable. Hair transplants and some drugs may slow down hair loss. Hair loss caused by other factors is usually temporary.

Cellulitis is an inflammation of connective tissues in skin and primarily occurs on the face and legs.

- **Causes.** This skin disease is caused by staphylococcal and streptococcal bacteria.
- **Signs and symptoms.** Skin appears red and tight and is often painful. The inflammation may trigger a fever.
- **Treatment.** Treatment is with antibiotics.

Dermatitis is a general term defined as inflammation of skin or a rash. It has many causes and is a sign of many types of skin disorders.

Eczema is one type of chronic dermatitis. This condition most commonly occurs in infants but it may also occur in adults.

- **Causes.** Causes of eczema are mostly unknown, but it is thought to be a type of allergy. Environmental irritants, stress, and dry skin can bring about episodes of this disease.
- **Signs and symptoms.** The rashes of eczema are scaly and itchy.
- **Treatment.** Treatments include steroids and other types of anti-inflammatory drugs. Of course, avoiding factors that trigger eczema are also helpful.

Folliculitis, which is a disorder specific to hair, is an inflammation of hair follicles.

- **Causes.** This disorder usually results from shaving or excess rubbing of skin areas. It may also be caused by bacteria and fungi.
- **Signs and symptoms.** Follicles become red and itchy and often look like pimples.
- **Treatment.** Treatments include regular cleansing of skin, topical antibiotics, and use of electric razors instead of razor blades.

Herpes simplex types 1 and 2 are the most common types of herpes simplex.

- **Causes.** Herpes simplex types 1 and 2 are both caused by a virus. Herpes simplex type 1 is very contagious and is spread through saliva. Herpes simplex type 2 is sexually transmitted.
- **Signs and symptoms.** Herpes simplex type 1 causes painful sores on the lips, mouth, and face. Herpes simplex type 2 normally causes painful sores on genital areas.
- **Treatment.** There is no cure for herpes simplex, and its skin lesions usually recur throughout life. However, antiviral drugs prevent frequent outbreaks.

Herpes zoster is a disorder commonly known as shingles.

- **Causes.** Herpes zoster is caused by the same virus that causes chickenpox. After a person has chickenpox, the virus becomes inactive but can become active again later in life to cause shingles.
- **Signs and symptoms.** Herpes zoster causes inflammation that affects the nerves on one side of the body and results in very painful skin blisters.
- **Treatment.** Some antiviral medications shorten the duration of the disease, but normally it is treated only with pain medications. Recovery is usually complete, and reoccurrences of the disease are rare. It is uncertain whether the chickenpox vaccine prevents herpes zoster.

Impetigo causes the formation of oozing skin lesions that eventually crust over.

- **Causes.** This disease is caused by staphylococcal and streptococcal bacteria.
- **Signs and symptoms.** The skin develops oozing lesions that eventually crust over.
- **Treatment.** This condition is treated with antibiotics.

Psoriasis is a common skin problem.

- **Causes.** This skin disorder is most likely an inherited autoimmune disorder.
- **Signs and symptoms.** Patients with psoriasis have frequent episodes of itching and redness and have outbreaks of scaly skin lesions. Some people also have joint pain.
- **Treatment.** Mild cases are treated with anti-inflammatory drugs and special ointments. Severe cases require hospitalization.

Rosacea is a skin disorder that commonly appears as facial redness.

- **Causes.** Rosacea's causes are unknown, but it occurs most frequently in fair-skinned people.
- **Signs and symptoms.** Redness and acne-like symptoms on the face are the most common symptoms.
- **Treatment.** Although it is not curable, rosacea is usually managed well with various medications.

Scabies is a very contagious skin condition.

- **Causes.** Scabies is caused by mites that burrow beneath skin. Sometimes the burrows of the mites, which look like red pencil marks, can be seen.
- **Signs and symptoms.** Redness and severe itching are usually the only symptoms of scabies.
- **Treatment.** Most cases are easily treated with prescription medications. Because scabies is contagious, it is wise to treat an entire family if one member is infected.

continued ⟶

Skin Cancer and Common Skin Disorders *(continued)*

Warts (verrucae) are harmless skin growths that can appear almost anywhere on the body surface but most commonly occur on the hands, feet, and face.

- **Causes.** These growths are caused by a virus.
- **Signs and symptoms.** Warts vary greatly in appearance; they can be smooth, flat, rough, raised, dark, small, or large.

- **Treatment.** Warts are often removed with over-the-counter medications but can also be treated through surgery, lasers, freezing, or burning.

Accessory Organs

The accessory organs of the skin include hair follicles, oil glands, nails, and sweat glands.

Hair Follicles

Hair **follicles** are tube-like depressions in the dermis of skin. Hair follicles are made of epithelial tissue and function to generate hairs (Figure 24-3). Cells called keratinocytes make up most of the hair follicle. As new keratinocytes are produced in the base of the hair follicles, old ones are pushed toward the surface of skin. The old keratinocytes stick together to produce a hair. The portion of the hair embedded in skin is called the root, and the portion of the hair extending from the surface of skin is called the shaft.

Melanocytes are also found in hair follicles. They produce and distribute pigments to create hair color. A person develops gray hair when these melanocytes produce less pigment than normal.

When a hair follicle goes into a resting cycle, the hair falls out. Most of the time, the hair follicle will begin a growing cycle again and produce a new hair. However, sometimes hair follicles completely die, and baldness (alopecia) develops.

Arrector pili muscles are attached to most hair follicles. When a person is cold or nervous, these muscles pull on hair follicles and cause hairs to stand erect. These muscles also pull on fibers in the dermis of skin, causing goose bumps to form (see Figure 24-1).

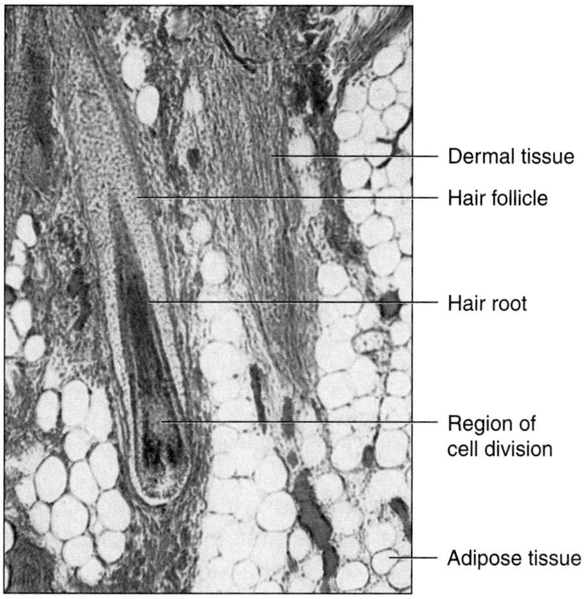

Sebaceous Glands

Sebaceous glands are more commonly called oil glands. They produce an oily substance called **sebum.** Sebum is secreted onto hairs to keep them soft and pliable. Sebum eventually is deposited onto skin to keep it soft as well. Sebum also prevents bacteria from growing on skin (see Figures 24-1 and 24-3).

Nails

Nails function to protect the ends of the fingers and toes. The portion of a nail that you can see is the nail body, and the portion embedded in skin is called the nail root. The nail root contains active keratinocytes that constantly divide to produce nail growth. The white half-moon–shaped area at the base of a nail is called a **lunula.** The lunula also contains very active keratinocytes. Beneath each nail is a layer called the **nail bed.** The nail bed holds the nail down to underlying skin and provides nutrients to the nail (Figure 24-4).

Sweat Glands

Most sweat glands are located in the dermis of skin. However, their ducts open onto the epidermis of skin. There are two types of sweat glands—eccrine and apocrine.

Eccrine sweat glands are the most numerous type. They produce a watery type of sweat and are activated primarily by heat. Once sweat is deposited onto skin, it evaporates and carries heat away from the body. Eccrine sweat glands are most concentrated on the forehead, neck, and back.

Apocrine sweat glands produce a thicker type of sweat that contains more proteins than the type of sweat produced by eccrine sweat glands. Apocrine glands are most concentrated in areas of skin with course hair, such

Dermal tissue

Hair follicle

Hair root

Region of cell division

Adipose tissue

Figure 24-3. Hair follicle.

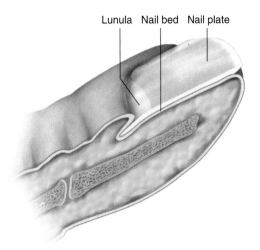

Lunula   Nail bed   Nail plate

Figure 24-4. Section of a nail.

as the armpit and groin areas. They are primarily activated by nervousness or stress but can also be activated by heat. These are the glands responsible for producing a cold sweat. Bacteria often break down the proteins in the sweat produced by apocrine glands. As the proteins are digested, the bacteria release a foul-smelling waste product that is responsible for the smell of body odor.

Skin Healing

When skin is injured, it becomes inflamed. An inflamed area looks red because nearby blood vessels dilate. The inflamed area also swells because the dilated blood vessels "leak" and fluids seep into spaces between cells. Inflamed areas are often painful because the excess fluid activates pain receptors. However, inflammation promotes healing because more blood is delivered to the area. The extra blood carries more nutrients needed for skin repair as well as defensive cells to clear up the cause of inflammation.

When structures and blood vessels of the dermis are injured, a blood clot initially forms. The blood clot is eventually replaced by a scab, which is basically clotted blood and other dried tissue fluids. The scab is normally replaced by collagen fibers that act to bind the edges of the wound together. Collagen fibers are whitish and the major component of scars. Sometimes skin scars are replaced with new skin, but if the wound is extensive, a scar will persist. Scars cannot carry out most functions of skin so their formation leads to the loss of certain functions.

Pathophysiology

Burns

The second leading cause of accidental death in the United States, after motor vehicle accidents, is burn injuries. There are more than 200 special burn care centers in the United States. More than 2 million burn injuries are reported each year, and more than 11,000 patients die annually from burn injuries. This year, about 1 million people will suffer a burn injury that causes a significant or permanent disability.

The extent of the body surface area affected and the severity (degree) of a burn are the most important factors in predicting the risk of death associated with burn injuries. The rule of nines is a quick way to estimate the

continued ⟶

Burns *(continued)*

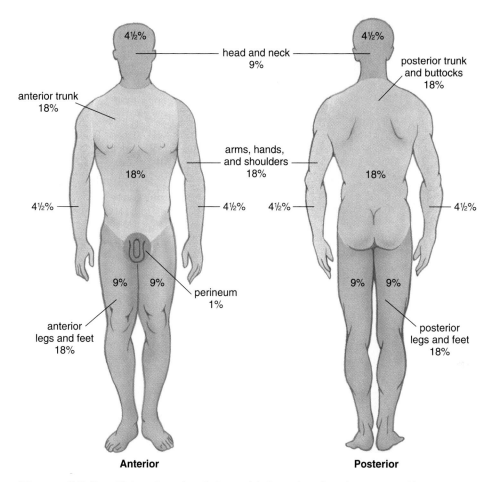

Figure 24-5. Using the rule of nines aids in estimating the extent of burns.

extent of body surface area affected by burns. This method divides the body into 11 areas, each accounting for 9% of the total body surface. The genital area accounts for 1% (Figure 24-5).

- Rule of nines. The 11 body areas of the rule of nines are identified as follows:
  - Head
  - Right arm
  - Left arm
  - Front of right leg
  - Front of left leg
  - Back of right leg
  - Back of left leg
  - Front of body trunk is two areas
  - Back of body trunk is two areas
- Burn severity. The severity of burns indicates the thickness of the injury (Figure 24-6). The following terms are used to report burn severity:
  - *First-degree.* These burns are also called superficial burns. They involve only the epidermis and are characterized by pain, redness, and swelling. Unless they are extensive, they do not require medical attention and usually heal well.

- *Second-degree.* These burns are also called partial-thickness burns and involve the epidermis and dermis. Pain, redness, swelling, and blisters characterize them. Medical staff should treat any second-degree burn that affects 1% or more of the body surface. A body surface area of 1% is about the size of a person's hand. Shock is likely to develop in second-degree burn injuries that affect 9% or more of the body surface. Second-degree burns can be life-threatening, depending on their extent.
- *Third-degree.* These burns are also called full-thickness burns. They involve all layers of skin and often underlying structures such as muscles and bones. The skin often looks black or charred in these burns. They always require medical attention regardless of the extent. A full-thickness burn of any size should always be medically treated.
- General Guidelines for Treating Burns
  - Anything sticking to the burn should not be removed.
  - Butter, lotions, or ointments should not be applied to the burn. Only ointments prescribed by a doctor or recommended by a pharmacist should be used.

continued ⟶

Burns *(continued)*

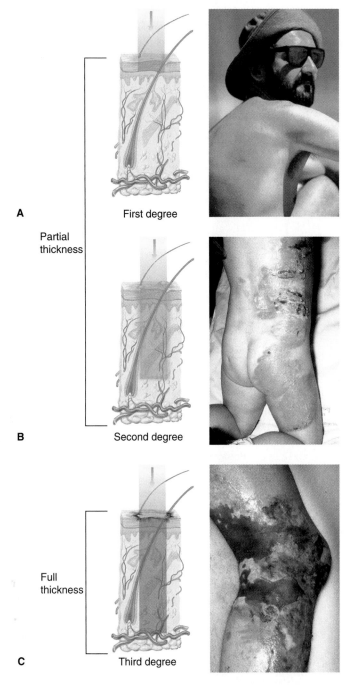

A

Partial
thickness

First degree

B

Second degree

Full
thickness

C

Third degree

Figure 24-6. The degrees of burn severity include
(a) first-degree (superficial burns), (b) second-degree
(partial-thickness burns), and (c) third-degree (full-thickness
burns).

- The burn should be cooled with large amounts of cold water.
- The burn should be covered with a sterile sheet or plastic bag. Burns to the face, however, should not be covered.
- Emergency medical personnel should be contacted for serious burns.
- In burns to the mouth and throat, the airways should be checked to see if there is any swelling. Burns to the head are always more serious than burns to other body parts. They almost always require emergency medical treatment.

Summary

The integumentary system is the first line of defense for the body. The skin covers the surface of the body, protecting it from invading organisms, chemicals, UV light, and water loss. Hair and nails also serve as protective barriers.

In addition, the skin helps regulate body temperature. This system plays an important role in diagnostic testing, including allergy testing and tuberculosis screening. Understanding this system can help you be more effective in your role as a medical assistant.

REVIEW

CASE STUDY QUESTIONS

Now that you have completed this chapter, review the case study at the beginning of the chapter and answer the following questions:

1. Using the rule of nines, estimate the percentage of the patient's body surface that was affected by this burn.
2. What layers of skin has the burn affected?
3. What functions of the skin are lost by this injury?
4. What types of treatments does this burn require?

Discussion Questions

1. Describe the factors that determine skin color.
2. Name the two layers of the epidermis and tell how they differ.
3. Name two types of sweat glands. Where is each located, and how do their secretions differ?

Critical Thinking Questions

1. Why do anti-inflammatory drugs reduce pain? Are these drugs likely to prevent healing or promote healing?

2. Which is more serious, a cat born without arrector pili muscles or a human? Why?
3. Albinos lack melanin. What body structures are affected by this? What precautions must an albino take that non-albinos do not have to worry about?

Application Activities

1. Describe the functions of the following cell types of the epidermis:
   a. Keratinocyte
   b. Melanocyte
2. Describe the role of skin in the following functions:
   a. Protection
   b. Sensation
   c. Body temperature regulation
   d. Excretion
   e. Vitamin D production
3. Describe the following parts of a nail:
   a. Nail root
   b. Lunula
   c. Nail bed
   d. Nail body

The Integumentary System   **463**

CHAPTER 25

The Skeletal System

KEY TERMS

appendicular
articular cartilage
atlas
axial
axis
bursitis
calcaneus
canaliculi
carpal
carpal tunnel syndrome
clavicle
coccyx
condyle
costal
coxal
diaphysis
ear ossicle
endochondral
endosteum
epiphyseal disk
epiphysis
ethmoid
femur
fibula
fontanel
foramen magnum
gout
humerus
hyoid
ilium
intramembranous
ischium
lacunae
lamella
ligament
mandible
marrow
mastoid process

CHAPTER OUTLINE

- Bone Structure
- Functions of Bones
- Bone Growth
- The Skull
- The Spinal Column
- The Rib Cage
- Bones of the Shoulders, Arms, and Hands
- Bones of the Hips, Legs, and Feet
- Bone Fractures
- Joints

OBJECTIVES

After completing Chapter 25, you will be able to:

25.1 Describe the parts of a long bone.

25.2 List the substances that make up bone tissue.

25.3 List the functions of bones.

25.4 Describe how long bones grow.

25.5 List the bones of the skull, spinal column, rib cage, shoulders, arms, hands, hips, legs, and feet. Describe the location of each bone.

25.6 Define fontanels and explain their importance.

25.7 List different types of bone fractures and describe their characteristics.

25.8 Explain how fractures heal.

25.9 Describe the three major types of joints and give examples of each.

25.10 Describe the structure of a synovial joint.

25.11 Describe the characteristics, causes, and treatments of various diseases and disorders of the skeleton.

KEY TERMS (Continued)

maxillae	osteosarcoma	scoliosis
medullary cavity	palatine	sella turcica
metacarpal	parietal	sphenoid
metatarsal	patella	sternum
nasal	pectoral girdle	suture
occipital	pelvic girdle	synovial
ossification	periosteum	tarsal
osteoblast	phalanges	temporal
osteoclast	pubis	tibia
osteocyte	radius	ulna
osteon	sacrum	vomer
osteoporosis	scapula	zygomatic

Introduction

Bones provide the body with structure and support. In this chapter you will learn about the bones of the body, their structure, and how the joints of the body work. The skeletal system is composed of 206 bones as well as joints and related connective tissues. The skeleton has two major divisions—the **axial** skeleton and the **appendicular** skeleton. The axial skeleton contains 80 bones. It includes the bones of the skull, vertebral column, and rib cage. It functions to support the head, neck, and trunk and protects the brain, spinal cord, and the organs in the thorax. The **hyoid** bone, which anchors the tongue, is also included in the axial skeleton. The appendicular skeleton includes the bones of the arms, the legs, the **pectoral girdle** and the **pelvic girdle.** The pectoral girdle attaches the arms to the axial skeleton, and the pelvic girdle attaches the legs to the axial skeleton (Figure 25-1).

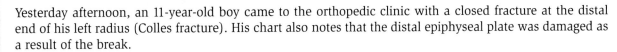

CASE STUDY

Yesterday afternoon, an 11-year-old boy came to the orthopedic clinic with a closed fracture at the distal end of his left radius (Colles fracture). His chart also notes that the distal epiphyseal plate was damaged as a result of the break.

As you read this chapter, consider the following questions:

1. Where is the distal end of the left radius?
2. Will this patient need surgery?
3. Have other tissues been damaged besides bone?
4. Why is the damage to the epiphyseal plate of special concern?

Bone Structure

Bones contain various kinds of tissues, including osseous tissue, blood vessels, and nerves. Osseous tissue can appear compact or spongy (Figure 25-2). At the microscopic level, spongy bone has more spaces within it than compact bone does. These spaces are filled with red marrow. Compact bone looks solid; however, the following structures can be observed with a microscope (Figure 25-3):

- **Osteons.** Osteons are elongated cylinders that run up and down the long axis of the bone. Each osteon has a central canal that contains blood vessels and nerves.
- Bone matrix. The matrix is the substance between bone cells. Bone cells are called **osteocytes.** The components of the matrix are inorganic salts, collagen fibers, and proteins. The primary salt of the matrix is calcium phosphate. This salt makes the matrix of bone very hard.
- **Lamella.** Lamella are layers of bone surrounding the canals of osteons.
- **Lacunae.** Lacunae are holes in the matrix of bone that hold osteocytes.
- **Canaliculi.** These tiny canals connect lacunae to each other. They allow osteocytes to spread nutrients to each other.

All bones are made up of both compact and spongy bone. They are classified according to their shape:

- Long bones. Long bones are located primarily in the arms and legs. Examples include the **femur** (thigh bone) and the **humerus** (upper arm bone). Long bones have the following parts (Figure 25-4):
  - **Diaphysis**—the shaft of a long bone. It is tubular and consists of a thick collar of compact bone that surrounds a central medullary cavity.
  - **Epiphysis**—the expanded end of a long bone. It consists of a thin layer of compact bone surrounding spongy bone. Long bones have an epiphysis at both ends.
  - **Articular cartilage**—the cartilage that covers the epiphyses of long bones. It functions to cushion bones and to absorb stress during bone movements.
  - **Medullary cavity**—a canal that runs through the center of the diaphysis. In adults it contains yellow bone **marrow,** which is mostly fat.
  - **Periosteum**—a membrane that surrounds the diaphysis. It contains bone-forming cells, dense fibrous connective tissue, nerves, and blood vessels.
  - **Endosteum**—a membrane that lines the medullary cavity and the holes of spongy bone. It contains bone-forming cells.

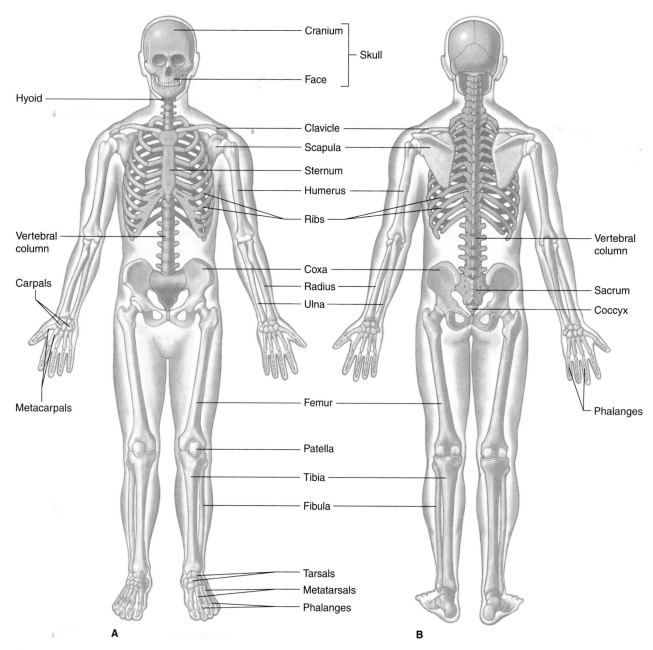

Figure 25-1. Major bones of the skeleton: (a) anterior view and (b) posterior view. The axial skeleton is shown in orange and the appendicular skeleton is shown in yellow.

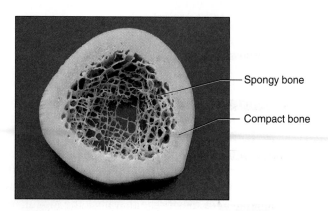

Figure 25-2. Cross section of bone showing compact and spongy bone tissue.

- Short bones. The small bones are located in the wrists and ankles. Examples include the **carpals** (wrist bones) and some of the **tarsals** (ankle bones).
- Flat bones. Flat bones are primarily located in the skull and rib cage. Examples include the ribs and frontal bone.
- Irregular bones. Irregular bones include the vertebrae and the bones of the pelvic girdle.

Functions of Bones

Bones have many functions. They give shape to body parts such as the head, legs, arms, and trunk. Bones also support and protect soft structures in the body. For

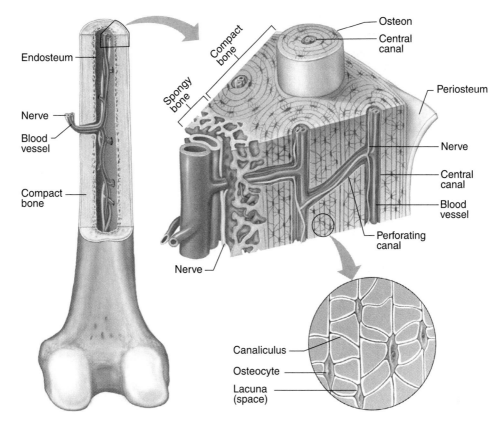

Figure 25-3. Compact bone at the microscopic level.

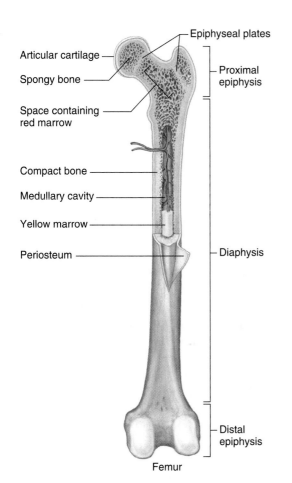

Figure 25-4. Parts of a long bone.

example, the skull protects the brain. Bones also function in body movement because skeletal muscles attach to them.

The red marrow of bone produces new blood cells. Red bone marrow is normally found in spaces of spongy bone. Bones also store calcium for the body. Every cell in the body needs calcium, so the body must have a large supply readily available.

Bone Growth

Bones grow through a process called **ossification.** Two types of ossification are intramembranous and endochondral.

In **intramembranous** ossification, bones begin as tough, fibrous membranes. Eventually, bone-forming cells called **osteoblasts** turn the membrane to bone. Intramembranous bones are found in the skull, except for the lower jawbone.

In **endochondral** ossification, bones start out as cartilage models. Eventually, the osteoblasts form a bone collar around the diaphysis of the cartilage model. Then bone is formed in the diaphysis of the bone. This area is called the primary ossification center. Later, the epiphyses turn to bone (secondary ossification centers), and the medullary cavity and spaces in spongy bone are formed. The cells that form holes in bone are called **osteoclasts.** As long as a bone contains some cartilage between an

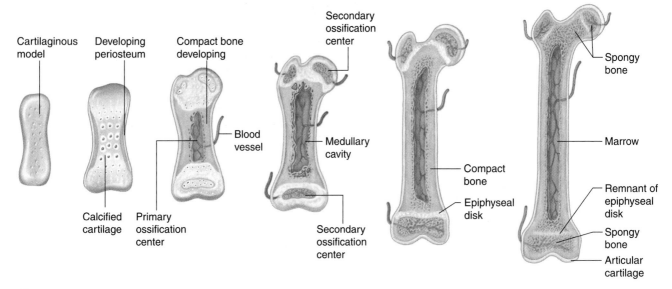

Figure 25-5. Steps in endochondral ossification.

epiphysis and the diaphysis, it can continue to grow in length. This plate of cartilage is called an **epiphyseal disk.** Once the cartilage is gone, bone growth stops. For most people, bone growth stops between the ages of 18 and 25 (Figure 25-5).

Even after bone growth stops, osteoclasts and osteoblasts continually remodel bone tissue. Throughout life, osteoclasts break down bone when the body needs more calcium in the blood, and osteoblasts replace the bone when there is excess calcium in the blood.

Pathophysiology

Common Diseases and Disorders of Bone

Bursitis is inflammation of a bursa, which is a fluid-filled sac that cushions tendons. It occurs most commonly in the elbow, knee, shoulder, and hip.

- **Causes.** Overuse of and trauma to joints are the most common causes of this condition. Bacterial infections can also cause bursitis.
- **Signs and symptoms.** Signs and symptoms include joint pain and swelling as well as tenderness in the structures surrounding the joint.
- **Treatment.** The most common treatments are bed rest, pain medications, steroid injections, aspiration of excess fluid from the bursa, and antibiotics.

Carpal tunnel syndrome occurs when the median nerve in the wrist is excessively compressed. Typists, assembly-line workers, painters, and people who play sports such as racquetball are most likely to develop carpal tunnel syndrome.

- **Causes.** Overuse of the wrist is a common cause of this syndrome.

- **Signs and symptoms.** Weakness and numbness in the hand, and pain in the wrist, hand, or elbow are common symptoms.
- **Treatment.** This condition can be treated with wrist splints, pain medications, and steroid injections and by having the patient change work habits to better position and support the wrists. If these treatments do not improve the patient's condition, surgery to reduce pressure on the nerves may be needed.

Ewing's family of tumors (EFT) is a group of tumors that affect different tissue types. However, the tumors primarily affect bone.

- **Causes.** Causes of EFT are not clear, but it most often affects Caucasians, the long bones of the body, and people between the ages of 10 and 20.
- **Signs and symptoms.** Fever, pain in the tumor location, fractures, and bruises in the tumor location are the primary symptoms.

continued ⟶

Common Diseases and Disorders of Bone *(continued)*

- **Treatment.** Treatment options include surgery, chemotherapy, radiation therapy, a bone marrow transplant, or a stem cell transplant.

Gout is a type of arthritis that usually occurs more frequently with age.

- **Causes.** Gout is caused by deposits of uric acid crystals in the joints. People with gout cannot break down uric acid properly and remove it from their bloodstream.
- **Signs and symptoms.** Symptoms include sudden or chronic joint pain, joint swelling and stiffness, and fever.
- **Treatment.** The most common treatments are pain medications and changes to the patient's diet. Patients should eliminate from their diet certain foods that cause the formation of uric acid (meats, fish, beer, or wine).

Osteogenesis imperfecta is more commonly called brittle-bone disease. People with this disease have decreased amounts of collagen in their bones, which leads to very fragile bones. There are four types of this disease: type 1 is the most common, and type 2 is the most severe.

- **Causes.** The disorder is hereditary and very often runs in a family.
- **Signs and symptoms.** Signs and symptoms include fractures (all types), blue sclera (type 1), dental problems (types 1 and 4), hearing loss (type 1), a triangular face (type 1), abnormal spinal curves (types 1 and 4), very small stature (types 2 and 3), a small chest (type 2), a barrel-shaped chest (type 3), fractures at birth (type 3), loose joints (types 3 and 4), and small muscles (type 3).
- **Treatment.** Because there are many symptoms of this disease, the list of treatments is extensive and includes the following: fractures, surgery to strengthen bones by inserting metal rods into them, dental procedures, physical therapy, braces to prevent bone deformities, wheelchairs and other supportive aids, medications, and counseling. Other surgeries may be required to treat lung and heart problems that sometimes occur with this disease.

Osteoporosis is a condition in which bones become thinned over time. It is a very common disorder in the United States and affects women more than men and Caucasians more than any other race. This condition occurs when bone is broken down to release calcium into the blood but it is not sufficiently replaced.

- **Causes.** The causes include hormone deficiencies (estrogen in women and testosterone in men), a sedentary lifestyle, a lack of calcium and vitamin D in the diet, bone cancers, corticosteroid excess (usually as a result of endocrine diseases), smoking, excess alcohol consumption, and the use of steroids.

- **Signs and symptoms.** There are usually no symptoms in the early stages of this disease. Patients may later experience fractures (usually in spine, wrists, or hips), back and neck pain, a loss of height over time, and an abnormal curving of the spine.
- **Treatment.** The most common treatments include medications to prevent bone loss and relieve bone pain, estrogen replacement therapy, lifestyle changes to prevent bone loss (including regular exercise and diets or supplements that include calcium, phosphorous, and vitamin D), moderation in use of alcohol, and stopping smoking.

Osteosarcoma is a type of bone cancer that originates from osteoblasts, the cells that make bony tissue. It occurs most often in children, teens, and young adults and more often in males than females. Usually this type of cancer affects bones of the legs.

- **Causes.** The causes of this type of cancer are unclear.
- **Signs and symptoms.** Primary symptoms include pain in affected bones (usually the legs), swelling around affected bones, and an increase in pain with movement of the affected bones.
- **Treatment.** Treatments include surgery, chemotherapy, and radiation therapy. Amputation of the affected limb, followed by a prosthesis fitting, may be needed in some cases.

Paget's disease causes bones to enlarge and become deformed and weak. It usually affects people over the age of 40.

- **Causes.** This disease may be caused by a virus or various hereditary factors.
- **Signs and symptoms.** Bone pain, deformed bones, and fractures are common symptoms. Patients may experience headaches and hearing loss if the disease affects skull bones.
- **Treatment.** Treatments include surgery to remodel bones, hip replacements, medications to prevent bone weakening, and physical therapy.

Scoliosis is an abnormal curvature of the spine.

- **Causes.** This disorder can develop prenatally when vertebrae do not fuse together. It can also result from diseases that cause weakness of the muscles that hold vertebrae together. Other causes of scoliosis are unknown but they may be genetic.
- **Signs and symptoms.** A patient with scoliosis usually has a spine that looks bent to one side, with one shoulder or hip appearing to be higher than the other. Patients often experience back pain.
- **Treatment.** Treatment includes different types of back braces, surgery to correct spinal curves, and physical therapy.

Building Better Bones

Bone health is influenced by many factors, including diet, exercise, and a person's overall lifestyle. You can help patients improve or maintain their bone health by teaching them about behaviors that will support bone health.

Bone-Healthy Diet

Good nutrition is essential for proper bone growth during childhood and the teen years. It is equally important in adulthood in order to maintain healthy bones. Bone-building nutrients are found in dairy products, broccoli, kale, spinach, salmon, sardines, egg yolks, whole grains, and fruits—especially bananas and oranges. Calcium and vitamin D are particularly important for healthy bones. Without vitamin D, calcium cannot be absorbed from the digestive tract into the bloodstream. Without calcium, bone tissue will slowly wear away. Supplements can always be taken if a person's diet does not include adequate amounts of calcium and vitamin D.

Bone-Healthy Exercises

Weight-bearing and strength-training exercises are best for bone health. When your muscles contract, they pull on your bones. This tension stimulates

bones to thicken and strengthen. Lifting weights is an effective way to increase the tension on bones. Other activities such as jogging, walking briskly, or playing a sport regularly will also stimulate bones to increase in density.

Bone-Healthy Lifestyle

A person with a bone-healthy lifestyle avoids smoking and alcohol. Smoking rids the body of calcium, which is necessary for bone growth. Alcohol prevents calcium absorption in the digestive tract. People who smoke are almost twice as likely to develop osteoporosis as nonsmokers.

Bone Tests

Bone-density tests and bone scans are currently the most useful tools in determining bone health. Bone-density tests are painless procedures used to determine the density of a person's bones. Because osteoporosis shows no symptoms in early stages, these tests are important to have done when your doctor recommends them. Bone scans help diagnose the causes of bone pain, arthritis, bone infections, and bone cancers. These scans use radioactive dyes that are injected into the patient and that concentrate in bone tissue.

The Skull

Skull bones are divided into two types: cranial and facial bones. Cranial bones form the top, sides, and back of the skull. Facial bones form the face (Figure 25-6). The skull bones of an infant are not completely formed. The "soft spots" felt on an infant's skull are actually **fontanels,** which are tough membranes that connect the incompletely developed bones.

The major cranial bones are the following:

- The frontal bone forms the anterior portion of the cranium. It is also called the forehead bone.

- **Parietal** bones form most of the top and sides of the skull.

- The **occipital** bone forms the back of the skull. A large hole in the occipital bone is called the **foramen magnum.** It allows the brain to connect to the spinal cord. Two bumps called occipital **condyles** are on either side of the foramen magnum. They sit on top of the first vertebra. When you nod your head, your occipital condyles are rocking back and forth on the first vertebra of the spinal column.

- Two **temporal** bones form the lower sides of the skull. A canal called the external auditory meatus runs

through each temporal bone. This canal is commonly called the ear canal. A large bump called the **mastoid process** is located on each temporal bone just behind each ear. Mastoid processes are where major neck muscles attach to your skull.

- A **sphenoid** bone forms part of the floor of the cranium. It is shaped like a butterfly. In the center of this bone is a deep depression called the **sella turcica.** The pituitary gland sits in this deep depression.

- **Ethmoid** bones are between the sphenoid bone and the nasal bones. They also form part of the floor of the cranium.

- **Ear ossicles** are the smallest bones of the body. They are the malleus, incus, and stapes and are in the middle ear cavities of the temporal bones.

The following are major facial bones:

- The **mandible** is the lower jawbone and is the only moveable bone in the skull. It anchors the lower teeth and forms the chin.

- The **maxillae** form the upper jawbone. They anchor the upper teeth to form the central portion of the facial skeleton.

- The **zygomatic** bones form the prominence of the cheeks.

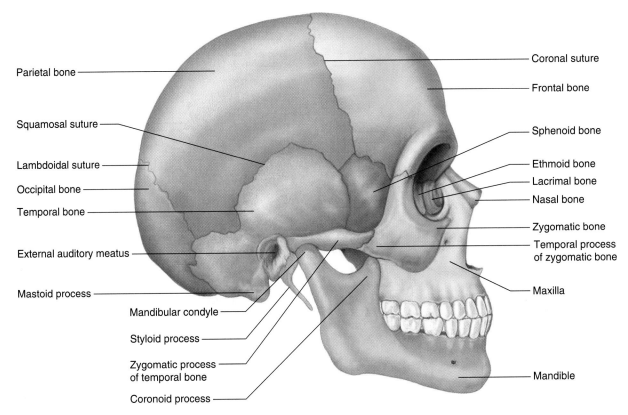

Figure 25-6. Lateral view of the skull.

Parietal bone

Squamosal suture

Lambdoidal suture

Occipital bone

Temporal bone

External auditory meatus

Mastoid process

Mandibular condyle

Styloid process

Zygomatic process of temporal bone

Coronoid process

Coronal suture

Frontal bone

Sphenoid bone

Ethmoid bone

Lacrimal bone

Nasal bone

Zygomatic bone

Temporal process of zygomatic bone

Maxilla

Mandible

- Several thin **nasal** bones fuse together to form the bridge of the nose.
- **Palatine** bones form the anterior portion of the palate, which is the roof of the mouth.
- The **vomer** is a thin bone that divides the nasal cavity.

The Spinal Column

The spinal column consists of 7 cervical vertebrae, 12 thoracic vertebrae, 5 lumbar vertebrae, a sacrum, and a coccyx (Figure 25-7):

- Cervical vertebrae are the smallest and lightest of the vertebrae and are located in the neck region. The first cervical vertebra is called the **atlas** and the second is called the **axis.** When you turn your head from side to side, your atlas is pivoting around your axis.
- Thoracic vertebrae join the 12 pairs of ribs. They have long, sharp, spinous processes that you can feel when you run your finger down someone's spine.
- Lumbar vertebrae have very sturdy structures. They form the small of the back and bear the most weight of all the vertebrae.
- The **sacrum** is a triangular-shaped bone that consists of five fused vertebrae. The **coccyx** is a small, triangular-shaped bone made up of three to five fused vertebrae and is considered unnecessary. It is more commonly called the tailbone.

Cervico- Neck
thoraco- Chest
C-1 — Atlas

The Rib Cage

The rib cage is made of 12 pairs of ribs and the **sternum** (Figure 25-8). The sternum forms the front, middle portion of the rib cage. It is often called the breastplate. The sternum joins with the clavicles and most ribs. All 12 pairs of ribs are attached posteriorly to thoracic vertebrae. Most ribs are also attached to structures anteriorly. Based on what ribs attach to anteriorly, they can be classified as follows:

- True. The first seven pairs of ribs are true ribs. They attach directly to the sternum through pieces of cartilage called **costal** cartilages.
- False. Rib pairs 8, 9 and 10 are called false ribs. They attach to the costal cartilage of rib pair number 7.
- Floating. Rib pairs 11 and 12 are called floating ribs because they do not attach anteriorly to any structure.

Bones of the Shoulders, Arms, and Hands

The bones of the shoulders are called pectoral girdles and include **clavicles** and **scapulae.** They function to attach the arm to the trunk of the body. The clavicles are commonly known as the collarbones. They are slender in shape and each joins with the sternum and a scapula. Clavicles are very commonly broken bones in body.

Falls and Fractures

Falls account for about 50% of all fractures, so it is important to teach patients about preventing falls. Although most fractures are not life-threatening, some are. For example, hip fractures in the elderly can result in complications such as pneumonia. Approximately half of all patients who suffer hip fractures will use some type of walking aid for the rest of their lives.

Persons most at risk for falling are those with the following conditions:

- Muscle weakness
- Difficulty walking
- Poor vision
- Dependence on bifocals
- Hearing loss
- Dependence on medications that cause dizziness or drowsiness
- Alzheimer's disease
- Parkinson's disease

Falls can be prevented through the following steps:

- Awareness. Educate patients to try not to climb or stretch for items that they use regularly. Instead, they should move these items to easy-to-reach places.

- Balance. Patients should stand up gradually, especially from a lying-down position. They should stand for a few seconds before walking. This allows time for blood flow to reach the brain, preventing dizziness.
- Lifestyle. Patients should drink alcohol in moderation in order to prevent falls that result from intoxication. They should also avoid foods high in sugar to prevent dizziness caused by sudden surges of blood sugar. You can also recommend that patients clean up any clutter in their living space so that they are less likely to trip on items.

When a fall can't be prevented, the following steps may be helpful:

- Falling backward, instead of forward or sideways, is less risky.
- Breaking the fall with one's hands is better than not breaking the fall at all. Wrist fractures are painful but are not life-threatening like hip or skull fractures.
- Grabbing onto anything to help break the fall.
- Wearing soft shoes or padded clothing if prone to falls. Hip padding is available from doctors.

The bones of cartilaginous joints are connected together with a disc of cartilage. This type of joint is slightly moveable. The joints between vertebrae are cartilaginous joints.

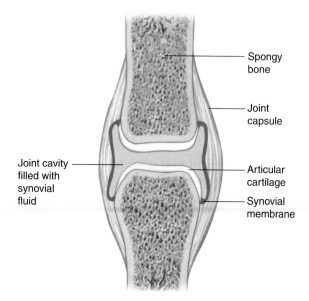

Figure 25-12. Structure of a synovial joint.

Spongy bone

Joint capsule

Joint cavity filled with synovial fluid

Articular cartilage

Synovial membrane

The bones of **synovial** joints are covered with hyaline cartilage and are held together by a fibrous joint capsule (Figure 25-12). The joint capsule is lined with a synovial membrane. The membrane secretes a slippery fluid called synovial fluid, which allows the bones to move easily against each other. Bones are also held together through tough, cord-like structures called **ligaments.** Synovial joints are freely moveable. Examples of synovial joints are the elbows, knees, shoulders, and knuckles.

Summary

The bones of the skeletal system are divided into two major divisions: the axial and the appendicular skeletons. In addition to bones, the skeletal system consists of cartilage, tendons, and ligaments. The skeletal system provides support for the body, protects internal organs, serves as attachments for muscles to produce movement, stores minerals such as calcium, and produces new blood cells. Bones are used as landmarks for procedures such as injections, electrocardiograms, and x-rays. It is important for medical assistants to have knowledge of this system in order to effectively perform their duties.

CHAPTER 25

CASE STUDY QUESTIONS

Now that you have completed this chapter, review the case study at the beginning of the chapter and answer the following questions:

1. Where is the distal end of the left radius?
2. Will this patient need surgery?
3. Have other tissues been damaged besides bone?
4. Why is the damage to the epiphyseal plate of special concern?

Discussion Questions

1. List and describe the functions of bone.
2. Describe how joints are classified. Give examples of each classification.
3. What are the bones and functions of the pectoral and pelvic girdles?

Critical Thinking Questions

1. If a 32-year-old woman developed arthritis, what type is she likely to have? Why?
2. If a physician needed a red bone marrow sample from a patient, from where is he likely to get the sample?
3. Tarsal bones are often called anklebones. Why is this term not entirely correct?

Application Activities

1. State whether each of the following is a bone of the axial skeleton or the appendicular skeleton.
   a. Humerus
   b. Femur
   c. Clavicle
   d. Parietal bone
   e. Nasal bone
   f. Ear ossicles

2. Name the bone that forms the following:
   a. Forehead
   b. Chin
   c. Palms of the hands
   d. Fingers
   e. Hip
   f. Cheekbone
3. Name the bone that contains the following:
   a. External auditory meatus
   b. Foramen magnum
   c. Sella turcica
   d. Mastoid process

Internet Activity

1. Go to the University of Maryland Web site **http://www.umm.edu/bone/** and choose Diagnostic Procedures. Answer the following questions:
   a. What is the role of MRI in diagnosing bone diseases?
   b. What are the two types of biopsy used?
   c. What is bone densitometry and what is it used for?

CHAPTER 26

The Muscular System

CHAPTER OUTLINE

- Functions of Muscle
- Types of Muscle Tissue
- Production of Energy for Muscle
- Structure of Skeletal Muscles
- Attachments and Actions of Skeletal Muscles
- Major Skeletal Muscles

OBJECTIVES

After completing Chapter 26, you will be able to:

26.1 List the functions of muscle.

26.2 Explain how muscle tissue generates energy.

26.3 List the three types of muscle tissue and describe the locations and characteristics of each.

26.4 Describe how smooth muscle produces peristalsis.

26.5 Describe the structure of a skeletal muscle.

26.6 List and define the various types of body movements produced by skeletal muscles.

26.7 Define the terms *origin* and *insertion*.

26.8 List the major skeletal muscles of the body and give the action of each.

26.9 Describe various disorders and diseases of the muscular system.

Introduction

Bones and joints do not themselves produce movement. By alternating between contraction and relaxation, muscles cause bones and supported structures to move. The human body has more than 600 individual muscles. Although each muscle is a distinct structure, muscles act in groups to perform particular movements. This chapter focuses on the differences among three muscle tissue types, the structure of skeletal muscles, muscle actions, and the names of skeletal muscles.

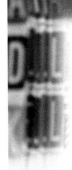

CASE STUDY

Five days ago, a 40-year-old woman came to the doctor's office where you work as a medical assistant. She complained about pain in her back and right leg. Because this patient had a history of disc damage in her spine, she was sent home with pain medication and an order for bed rest for a 24-hour period. Two days later, she returned to the office with nausea, a severe headache, muscle twitching in her legs and arms, severe back pain, and tightness in her chest. The doctor once more asked the patient to elaborate on her activities the day before she fell ill. He was told that she had sprayed her furniture and carpets with an organophosphate insecticide to get rid of fleas in her house. She had also dipped her cats and dogs with the same insecticide. The doctor explained that organophosphates block acetylcholinesterase and immediately transferred her to the hospital for respiratory therapy and medicine to combat the insecticide poisoning.

As you read this chapter, consider the following questions:

1. What is the function of acetylcholinesterase?
2. Why does this patient exhibit muscle twitching and back pain?
3. What type of respiratory therapy will this patient require?
4. What precautions should a person take when using insecticides that contain organophosphates?
5. Why is it important for patients to give their doctor a complete account of their activities prior to an illness?

Functions of Muscle

Muscle tissue is unique because it has the ability to contract. It is this contraction that allows muscles to perform various functions. In addition to allowing the human body to move, muscles provide stability, the control of body openings and passages, and warming of the body.

Movement

Because skeletal muscles are attached to bones, when they contract, the bones attached to them move. This allows for various body motions, such as walking or waving your hand. Facial muscles are attached to the skin of the face, so when they contract, different facial expressions are produced, such as smiling or frowning. Smooth muscle is found in the walls of various organs, such as the stomach, intestines, and uterus. The contraction of smooth muscle in these organs produces movements of their contents, such as the movement of food material through the intestine. Cardiac muscle in the heart produces the pumping of blood into blood vessels.

Stability

You rarely think about it but muscles are holding your bones tightly together so that your joints remain stable. There are also very small muscles holding your vertebrae together to make your spinal column stable.

Control of Body Openings and Passages

Muscles form valve-like structures called **sphincters** around various body openings and passages. These sphincters control the movement of substances into and out of these passages. For example, a urethral sphincter prevents urination, or it can be relaxed to permit urination.

Heat Production

When muscles contract, heat is released, which helps the body maintain a normal temperature. This is why moving your body can make you warmer if you are cold.

Types of Muscle Tissue

There are three types of muscle tissue: skeletal, smooth, and cardiac. Study Table 26-1 to review their locations and features.

Muscle cells are called **muscle fibers** because of their long lengths. The cell membrane of a muscle fiber is called a **sarcolemma**. The cytoplasm of this cell type is called **sarcoplasm**, and the endoplasmic reticulum is called **sarcoplasmic reticulum**. Most of the sarcoplasm is filled with long structures called **myofibrils**. The arrangement of filaments in myofibrils produce the **striations** observed in skeletal and cardiac muscle cells. Muscle fibers are controlled by motor neurons that release neurotransmitters onto the fibers. See Figure 26-1 for an illustration of the structure of a skeletal muscle.

Skeletal Muscle

Skeletal muscle fibers respond only to the neurotransmitter **acetylcholine.** Acetylcholine causes skeletal muscle to contract. Once contraction has occurred, skeletal muscles release an enzyme called **acetylcholinesterase,** which breaks down acetylcholine. This allows the muscle to relax.

Smooth Muscle

There are two types of smooth muscle—multiunit and visceral. **Multiunit smooth muscle** is found in the iris of the eye and the walls of blood vessels. This muscle type contracts in response to neurotransmitters and hormones. **Visceral smooth muscle** contains sheets of muscle cells that closely contact each other. It is found in the walls of hollow organs such as the stomach, intestines, bladder, and uterus. Muscle fibers in visceral smooth muscle respond to neurotransmitters, but they also stimulate each other to contract; therefore, the muscle fibers tend to contract and relax together. This type of muscle produces an action called peristalsis. **Peristalsis** is a rhythmic contraction that pushes substances through tubes of the body.

Two neurotransmitters are involved in smooth muscle contraction—acetylcholine and **norepinephrine.** Depending on the smooth muscle type, these neurotransmitters cause or inhibit contraction.

Cardiac Muscle

Groups of cardiac muscle are connected to each other through **intercalated discs.** These discs allow the fibers in that group to contact and relax together. This design allows the heart to work as a pump. Cardiac muscle is also self-exciting, which means that it does not need nerve stimulation to contract. Nerves only speed up or slow down the contraction of the heart. Like smooth muscle, cardiac muscle responds to two neurotransmitters—acetylcholine and norepinephrine. Acetylcholine slows the heart rate, and norepinephrine speeds it up.

Production of Energy for Muscle

Because a lot of ATP (adenosine triphosphate), which is a type of chemical energy, is needed for sustained or repeated muscle contractions, a muscle cell must have multiple ways to store or make this substance. There are three ways through which muscle cells make this energy:

1. **Creatine phosphate** production. Creatine phosphate is a protein that stores extra phosphate groups. When ATP is used to produce work, it loses a phosphate and energy. Creatine phosphate can then donate a phosphate group to the resulting molecule to restore its energy potential. This is a very rapid way for muscles to produce energy.

2. **Aerobic respiration** of glucose. When a cell wants to make a lot of ATP, it turns to its glucose stores. A cell will break down glucose into pyruvic acid. As long as oxygen is available, the pyruvic acid is converted to a substance called acetyl coenzyme A. Acetyl coenzyme A starts a series of reactions called the **Krebs cycle,** which is also known as the citric acid cycle. This cycle

Muscle Group	Major Location	Major Function	Mode of Control	Rate of Contraction	Intercalated Discs
Skeletal Muscle	Attached to bones and skin of the face	Produces body movements and facial expressions	Voluntary	Fast to contract and relax	No
Smooth Muscle	Walls of hollow organs, blood vessels, and iris	Moves contents through organs; vasoconstriction	Involuntary	Slow to contract and relax	No
Cardiac Muscle	Wall of the heart	Pumps blood through heart	Involuntary	Groups of muscle fibers contract as a unit	Yes

TABLE 26-1 Types of Muscle Tissue

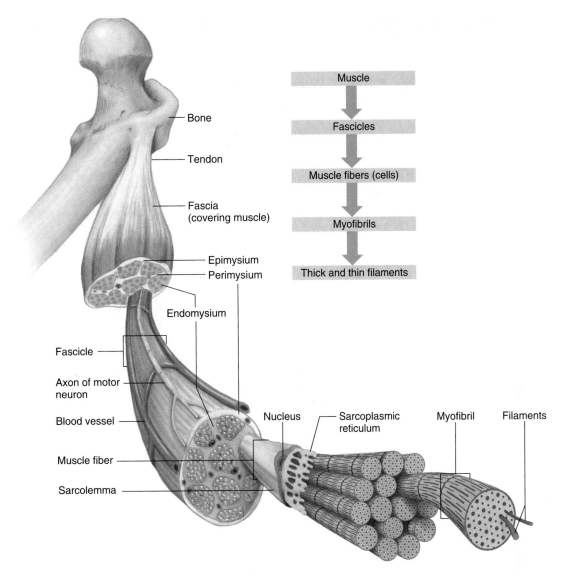

Figure 26-1. Structure of a skeletal muscle.

generates a lot of ATP for the muscle cell. The use of glucose to make ATP is called aerobic respiration because oxygen is required for this production. Because this process requires large amounts of oxygen, muscle cells contain a pigment called **myoglobin,** which stores extra oxygen. This pigment is pinkish in color and is responsible for giving muscles their color.

3. **Lactic acid** production. When a cell is low on oxygen, it must convert pyruvic acid to lactic acid. This reaction generates a small amount of ATP for the cell, but the lactic acid is a waste product that must be released from the cell.

Oxygen Debt

When skeletal muscles are used strenuously for a minute or two, **oxygen debt** develops. This condition occurs when oxygen supplies in the muscle are low and the aerobic respiration of glucose can no longer be used to produce ATP.

When oxygen is low, muscle fibers must convert pyruvic acid to lactic acid to produce energy. The buildup of lactic acid causes muscle fatigue. Lactic acid is then carried by the bloodstream to the liver where it can be converted back into glucose. However, this process requires energy. The oxygen debt is the amount of oxygen the liver cells need to make enough ATP to convert lactic acid into glucose. This process explains why your body still burns energy even after you are done exercising.

Muscle Fatigue

Muscle fatigue is a condition in which a muscle has lost its ability to contract. It usually develops because of an accumulation of lactic acid. It can occur also if the blood supply to a muscle is interrupted or if a motor neuron loses its ability to release acetylcholine onto muscle fibers. Cramps—which are painful, involuntary contractions of muscles—can accompany muscle fatigue.

Structure of Skeletal Muscles

Skeletal muscles are the major organs that make up the muscular system. A skeletal muscle consists of connective tissues, skeletal muscle tissue, blood vessels, and nerves. When you see marbling in a steak, you are actually viewing connective tissues in the steak. The red portion of the steak is the muscle tissue.

The following connective tissue coverings are associated with skeletal muscles (see Figure 26-1):

- **Fascia.** This structure covers entire skeletal muscles and separates them from each other.

- **Tendon.** This tough, cord-like structure is made of fibrous connective tissue that connects muscles to bones.

- **Aponeurosis.** This tough, sheet-like structure is made of fibrous connective tissue. It typically attaches muscles to other muscles.

- **Epimysium.** This tissue is a thin covering that is just deep to the fascia of a muscle. It surrounds the entire muscle.

- **Perimysium.** This connective tissue divides a muscle into sections called **fascicles.**

- **Endomysium.** This covering of connective tissue surrounds individual muscle cells.

Pathophysiology

Common Diseases and Disorders of the Muscular System

Botulism is usually thought of as a disease that affect the gastrointestinal tract, but it can also affect various muscle groups. This disease most commonly affects infants. Although a person can survive this disease, its affects may be long-lasting.

- **Causes.** This disease is a rare but very serious disorder caused by the bacterium *Clostridium botulinum*, which normally lives in soil and water. If this bacterium gets on food, it can produce a toxin that can lead to a type of food poisoning. The foods most likely to contain *Clostridium botulinum* are canned vegetables, cured pork, raw fish, honey, and corn syrup. A person can also acquire this bacterium through open wounds that are not cleaned properly.

- **Signs and symptoms.** This disease causes many symptoms, including difficulty swallowing, paralysis, weak muscles, nausea and vomiting, abdominal cramps, double vision, difficulty breathing, poor feeding and suckling in infants, the inability to urinate, the absence of reflexes, and constipation. The signs and symptoms usually appear 8 to 40 hours after the toxin is ingested. The diagnosis is usually made by either a blood test to identify the toxin or an analysis of the suspected food.

- **Treatment.** Treatment includes emergency hospitalization, intubation to open airways, mechanical ventilation if respiratory muscles are impaired, intravenous fluids or nasogastric feeding if swallowing is impaired, and the administration of an antitoxin. *Antibiotics*

- **Prevention tips.** You can instruct patients to prevent botulism by observing the following guidelines:
  - Never give honey or corn syrup to infants
  - Sterilize home-canned foods properly (250°F for 35 minutes)
  - Do not use foods from bent or bulging cans
  - Never eat foods that smell as if they may have spoiled
  - Cook and store foods properly

Fibromyalgia is a fairly common condition that results in chronic pain primarily in joints, muscles, and tendons. It most commonly affects women between the ages of 20 and 50.

- **Causes.** The causes of this disorder are poorly understood. Fibromyalgia may be caused by sleep disturbance, emotional distress, a decreased blood flow to muscles, a virus, or any combination of these factors.

- **Signs and symptoms.** Symptoms include fatigue, tenderness in different areas of the body, sleep disturbances, and chronic facial pain. The diagnosis is usually made by ruling out other possible diseases. It is not normally diagnosed unless a person has muscle and joint pain for at least three months in certain body areas.

- **Treatment.** Treatment is varied and includes antidepressants, anti-inflammatory medications, physical therapy, lifestyle changes to reduce stress, counseling to improve coping skills, reduction or elimination of caffeine to improve sleeping, and diet supplements to improve nutrition. *Not caused by bacterial infection*

Muscular dystrophy is a group of inherited disorders characterized by muscle weakness and a loss of muscle tissue. There are at least seven types of muscular dystrophy, and they are distinguished from each other by types of symptoms, the age at when symptoms appeared, and the cause.

- **Causes.** The causes of this disorder are primarily hereditary. Genetic fetal testing is available.

continued ⟶

Common Diseases and Disorders of the Muscular System *(continued)*

- **Signs and symptoms.** The signs and symptoms vary widely and depend on the type of muscular dystrophy. The symptoms of Duchenne muscular dystrophy progress steadily and are eventually fatal. Other types cause mild symptoms, and patients usually have normal life expectancies. Specific signs and symptoms include muscle weakness in various muscle groups, depending on the type; difficulty walking; drooling; a delayed development of motor skills; frequent falls; mental retardation in some types; a curved spine; the formation of a claw hand or clubfoot; a loss of muscle mass; the accumulation of fat or fibrous connective tissue in muscles; and arrhythmias in some types. The diagnosis is primarily made through a muscle biopsy. Other tests include DNA testing; an EMG (electromyography) test, which tests muscle weakness; or an ECG (electrocardiogram), which tests cardiac function.
- **Treatment.** Treatment includes physical therapy to maintain muscle function, the use of braces and wheelchairs, various medications based on the type, and spinal surgery.

Myasthenia gravis is a condition in which affected persons experience muscle weakness. In this condition, a person produces antibodies that prevent muscles from receiving neurotransmitters from neurons. It most commonly affects young women and older men, especially if they have other autoimmune disorders.

- **Causes.** This disease is usually considered an autoimmune disorder.
- **Signs and symptoms.** The signs and symptoms usually get better with rest and worsen with activity. They include double vision; muscle weakness; difficulty swallowing, talking, chewing, lifting, or walking; fatigue; drooling; and difficulty breathing. The diagnosis may be difficult, but a single-fiber EMG test is often useful. This test measures the response of a muscle fiber to nervous stimulation. Other tests include acetylcholine receptors antibody tests and the Tensilon test. In a positive Tensilon test, muscle activity increases after medication is given that blocks the breakdown of acetylcholine.
- **Treatment.** Treatments include lifestyle changes to avoid excessive stress and heat, the use of an eye patch to treat double vision, medications to improve communication between nerves and muscles, medications to suppress the immune system, plasmapheresis to remove harmful antibodies from blood, and removal of the thymus.

Rhabdomyolysis is a condition in which the kidneys have been damaged and is related to serious muscle injuries.

- **Causes.** Kidneys become damaged because of toxins released from muscle cells. When muscles are damaged, excessive amounts of the pigment myoglobin are released, which is then broken down into harmful chemicals. Muscles are most often damaged through trauma; excessive use (for example, marathon running); overdoses of cocaine, heroine, and other drugs; alcoholism; and a blockage of the blood supply to the muscles.
- **Signs and symptoms.** Symptoms include dark urine, muscle tenderness, muscle weakness, muscle stiffness, seizures, joint pain, and fatigue. The diagnosis includes urinalysis for the presence of myoglobin, creatine phosphokinase (CPK), and creatinine; blood is also tested for the presence of myoglobin, CPK, or high levels of potassium. CPK is an enzyme released into the blood when muscles are damaged. Creatinine is a protein released by the breakdown of muscle tissue.
- **Treatment.** Treatment includes hydration to rapidly eliminate toxins from the kidneys, diuretics to help flush toxins from the body, medications to flush excess potassium from the body, and therapy for kidney failure.

Tetanus is commonly called lockjaw. This disease has a high mortality rate, especially in infants. Immediate treatment is necessary to prevent death or long-lasting effects. However, this disease is completely preventable through regular vaccinations.

- **Causes.** A toxin produced by the bacterium *Clostridium tetani*, which lives naturally in soil and water, causes this disease. People most commonly acquire this bacterium through open wounds caused by objects contaminated with soil.
- **Signs and symptoms.** Symptoms usually appear between 5 and 10 days after infection. Muscle spasms in the jaw, neck, and facial muscles are usually the first signs. Other signs and symptoms include severe spasms of muscles that spread to other body locations; muscles spasms that may cause bone fractures; breathing difficulties; irritability; fever; profuse sweating; and drooling. The diagnosis is usually based on the type of wound and the characteristic signs and symptoms of the disease. Tetanus antibody tests can also be used in diagnosis, but cultures of the wound site often produce false-negative findings.
- **Treatment.** Administering antitoxin and antibiotics is a key treatment. Others include wound cleaning, muscle relaxants, sedation, and bed rest. The insertion of an endotracheal tube and mechanical ventilation may be needed for patients with severe breathing difficulties.

Trichinosis is an infection caused by parasites (worms).

- **Causes.** This disease is caused by worms that are usually ingested by eating undercooked meat. Once ingested, the worms can leave the digestive tract and infect skeletal muscles, the heart, the lungs, and the brain. This disease is preventable by not eating meat

continued ⟶

from wild animals. Proper cooking will also prevent trichinosis. There is no cure for this disease once the worms leave the digestive tract and infect other tissues.

- **Signs and symptoms.** Common symptoms include abdominal pain, diarrhea, muscle pain, fever, and pneumonia. In more serious cases, arrhythmias (irregular heart rhythms), heart failure, and encephalitis (swelling of the brain) can result. The diagnosis is

usually based on the symptoms, a blood test to determine if there is an increase in eosinophils in blood, or by a muscle biopsy that reveals the presence of the worm.

- **Treatment.** Patients with this disease are treated with medications to kill worms in the digestive tract and with anti-inflammatory drugs to reduce muscle pain and swelling.

Attachments and Actions of Skeletal Muscles

The actions of skeletal muscles depend largely on what the skeletal muscles are attached to. Insertions and origins are sites of attachments for skeletal muscles. An **insertion** is an attachment site that moves when a muscle contracts. An **origin** is an attachment site that does not move when a muscle contracts. For example, the biceps brachii (the muscle on the front of the upper arm) attaches to two places on the scapula and to one site on the radius. When the biceps brachii contracts, the radius moves and the arm bends at the elbow. Therefore, the insertion site of the biceps brachii is its attachment site on the radius. The origin of the biceps brachii is where it attaches to the scapula (Figure 26-2).

Most of the time a body movement is produced not just by one muscle but by a group of muscles. However, one muscle is responsible for most of the movement; this muscle is called the **prime mover**. Other muscles help the prime mover by stabilizing joints; these muscles are called **synergists**. An **antagonist** is a muscle that produces a

movement opposite to the prime mover. When the prime mover contracts, the antagonist must relax in order to produce a smooth body movement. For example, when you bend your arm at the elbow, the prime mover is the biceps brachii. The synergist muscles are the brachialis and brachioradialis. The antagonist is the triceps brachii because its action is to extend the arm at the elbow.

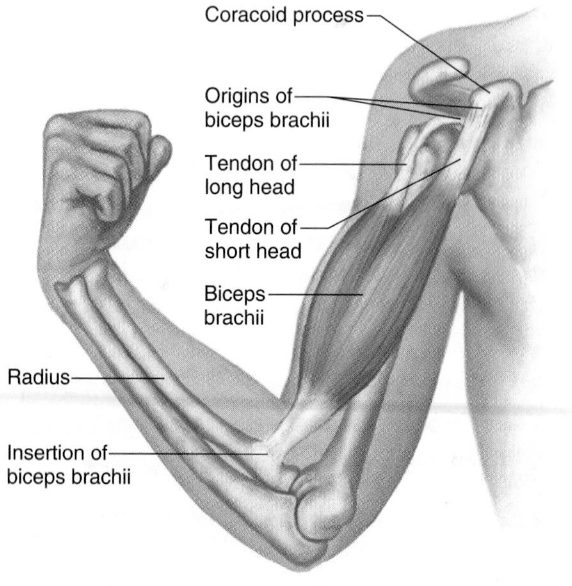

The body movements produced by skeletal muscles include the following:

- **Flexion**—bending a body part
- **Extension**—straightening a body part
- **Hyperextension**—extending a body part past the normal anatomical position
- **Dorsiflexion**—pointing the toes up
- **Plantar flexion**—pointing the toes down
- **Abduction**—moving a body part away from its position in the anatomical position
- **Adduction**—moving a body part toward its position in the anatomical position
- **Rotation**—twisting a body part; for example, turning your head from side to side
- **Circumduction**—moving a body part in a circle; for example, moving your arm in a circular motion
- **Pronation**—turning the palm of the hand down
- **Supination**—turning the palm of the hand up
- **Inversion**—turning the sole of the foot medially
- **Eversion**—turning the sole of the foot laterally
- **Retraction**—moving a body part posteriorly
- **Protraction**—moving a body part anteriorly
- **Elevation**—lifting a body part; for example, elevating your shoulders as in a shrugging expression
- **Depression**—lowering a body part; for example, lowering your shoulders

See Figures 26-3, 26-4, and 26-5 for illustrations of these types of movements.

Figure 26-2. Origins and insertion of biceps brachii.

Major Skeletal Muscles

The name of a skeletal muscle often describes it in some way. Usually the name indicates the location, size, action, shape, or number of attachments of the muscle. For

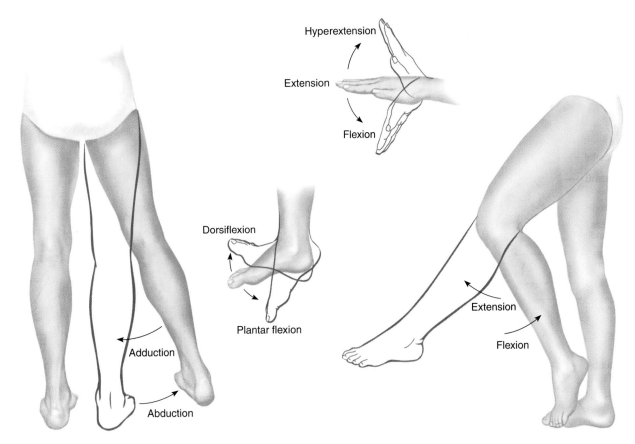

Figure 26-3. Adduction, abduction, dorsiflexion, plantar flexion, hyperextension, extension, and flexion.

example, the pectoralis major is named for its large size (major) and its location (pectoral, or chest, region). The sternocleidomastoid is named for its attachment sites—*sterno* (sternum), *cleido* (clavicle), and *mastoid* (the mastoid process of the temporal bone). As you study muscles, you will find it easier to remember them if you think about what the name describes.

Muscles of the Head

The muscles of the head include those that move the head, provide facial expression, and move the jaw. See Figures 26-6 and 26-7 for illustrations of these various muscles.

Muscles that move the head include the following:

- Sternocleidomastoid. This muscle pulls the head to one side and also pulls the head to the chest.
- Splenius capitis. This muscle rotates the head and allows it to bend to the side.

Muscles of facial expression include the following:

- Frontalis. This muscle raises the eyebrows.
- Orbicularis oris. This muscle allows the lips to pucker.
- Orbicularis oculi. This muscle allows the eyes to close.
- Zygomaticus. This muscle pulls the corners of the mouth up.
- Platysma. This muscle pulls the corners of the mouth down.

The muscles of the jaw allow for mastication (chewing) and include the following:

- Masseter and temporalis. These muscles close the jaw.

Arm Muscles

Muscles that move the arm include muscles of the arm and forearm (see Figures 26-6, 26-7, and 26-8). The muscles of the arm include the following:

- Pectoralis major. This muscle pulls the arm across the chest; it also rotates and adducts the arms.
- Latissimus dorsi. This muscle acts to extend, adduct, and rotate the arm inwardly.
- Deltoid. This muscle acts to abduct and extend the arm at the shoulder.
- Subscapularis. This muscle rotates the arm medially.
- Infraspinatus. This muscle rotates the arm laterally.

Muscles that move the forearm include the following:

- Biceps brachii. This muscle flexes the arm at the elbow and rotates the hand laterally.
- Brachialis. This muscle flexes the arm at the elbow.
- Brachioradialis. This muscle flexes the forearm at the elbow.
- Triceps brachii. This muscle extends the arm at the elbow.

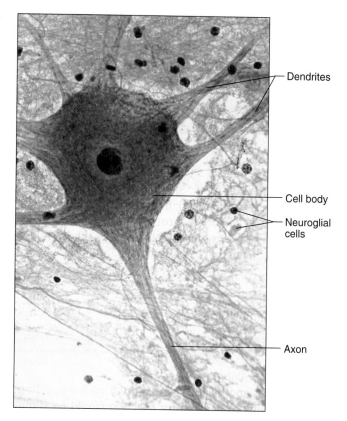

Figure 27-1. A typical neuron surrounded by neuroglial cells.

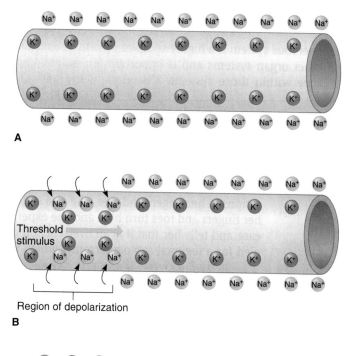

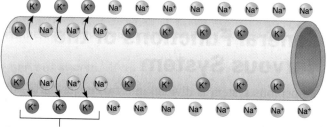

Figure 27-2. Nerve impulse. (a) At rest, or in its polar state, more Na$^+$ is on the outside of the membrane, which makes the outside positive and the inside negative (less positive). (b) When Na$^+$ moves into the cell, the membrane depolarizes, meaning that the inside becomes more positive. (c) The membrane repolarizes when K$^+$ and later Na$^+$ move to the outside of the cell membrane.

Their function is to send information (nerve impulses) away from the cell body.

In the peripheral nervous system, neuroglial cells, called **Schwann cells,** wrap themselves around axons; the axons are coated by the cell membranes of the Schwann cells. The cell membranes contain large amounts of **myelin,** which is a fatty substance. Myelin insulates the axons and allows them to send nerve impulses quickly.

Neurons can be classified as sensory neurons, **interneurons,** or motor neurons based on their functions. Sensory (afferent) neurons carry sensory information from the periphery to the CNS. These neurons pick up sensory information from their receptors, which are usually at the tips of their dendrites. Interneurons are found only in the CNS, and they function to link neurons together. Interneurons also transmit impulses from one part of the spinal cord or brain to another. They are involved in the decision-making function of the nervous system, and they direct information to motor neurons. Motor (efferent) neurons carry information from the CNS to effectors (muscles or glands) in the peripheral nervous system. They are responsible for stimulating muscles to contract or glands to secrete their products.

Nerve Impulse and Synapse

Neuron cell membranes have a cell **membrane potential.** This means the membrane is polarized. Just like a battery is polar—one end is negative and the other end is positive—neuron cell membranes are polar because the inside is negatively charged and the outside is positively charged. In most of the cells in the body, the outside of cell membranes is positively charged because more positive ions are on the outside. The inside of cell membranes is negatively charged because more negative ions are on the inside. This membrane potential is very important for the function of neurons (Figure 27-2).

Potassium and sodium ions are both positively charged and play important roles in generating nerve impulses. When a neuron is at rest or without stimulation, the outside of its membrane is positively charged and the inside is negatively charged because the total of sodium and potassium ions is greater outside the membrane. As long as the neuron is at rest, it remains in this **polarized** state.

However, a neuron will respond to stimuli such as heat, pressure, and chemicals by changing the amount of polarization across its membrane. For example, it can respond to a stimulus by making the outside of its membrane less positive. When this happens, the neuron has **depolarized.** In other words, it has become less polar. To make the outside of the membrane less positive, some of the sodium ions flow to the inside of the cell membrane. If the membrane of an axon becomes depolarized enough, a nerve impulse (**action potential**) is created. A nerve impulse is the flow of electric current along the axon membrane. Eventually, the axon membrane becomes polar again by the return of positively charged ions to the outside of the cell membrane. The return to the original polar (resting) state is called **repolarization.**

An unmyelinated axon does not conduct a nerve impulse as quickly as a myelinated axon does. Also, the speed of the nerve impulse is related to the diameter of the axon. The larger the diameter, the faster the nerve impulse travels to the end of the axon.

When a nerve impulse travels down an axon, the impulse eventually reaches the ends of axon branches, called **synaptic knobs.** These synaptic knobs contact dendrites, cell bodies, and the axons of other neurons. Whatever the synaptic knob is contacting is called a postsynaptic structure. Within synaptic knobs are **vesicles,** or small sacs that contain chemicals called **neurotransmitters.** When the nerve impulse reaches the synaptic knobs, the neurotransmitters are released onto postsynaptic structures (Figure 27-3).

There are about 50 different neurotransmitters. Most neurons release only one type of neurotransmitter but some will release more than one type. Neurotransmitters are released through exocytosis. Their functions include causing muscles to contract or relax, causing glands to secrete products, activating neurons to send nerve impulses, or inhibiting neurons from sending nerve impulses.

Central Nervous System

The central nervous system includes the spinal cord and brain (Figure 27-4). The tissues of the CNS are so delicate that a **blood-brain barrier** and layers of membranes protect them. Tight capillaries form the blood-brain barrier. This barrier prevents certain substances from entering the tissues of the CNS. For example, various waste products and drugs do not cross the blood-brain barrier very well. Inflammation, however, can make this barrier more permeable.

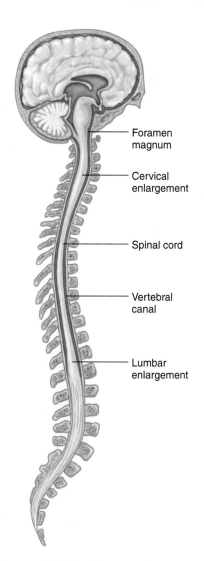

Figure 27-4. The central nervous system(CNS) consists of the brain and spinal cord. The spinal cord ends at the level of third lumbar vertebra.

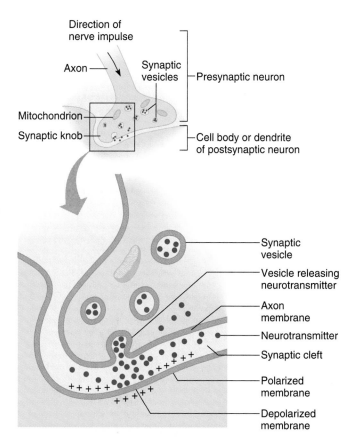

Figure 27-3. Synapse. When a nerve impulse reaches a synaptic knob, it releases a neurotransmitter onto the postsynaptic structure.

Meninges are membranes that protect the brain and spinal cord. The three layers of meninges are dura mater, arachnoid mater, and pia mater. Dura mater is the toughest and outermost layer of the meninges. Arachnoid mater is the middle layer and is wispy in appearance (much like a spider's web—hence the name arachnoid, which means spider). Pia mater is the innermost and most delicate layer. It sits directly on top of the brain and spinal cord and holds blood vessels onto the surface of these structures. Between the arachnoid mater and pia mater is an area called the **sub-arachnoid space.** It contains **cerebrospinal fluid (CSF),** which cushions the CNS.

Spinal Cord

The spinal cord is a slender structure that is continuous with the brain. The spinal cord descends into the vertebral canal and ends around the level of the first or second lumbar vertebra. The spinal cord is divided into 31 spinal segments: 8 cervical segments, 12 thoracic segments, 5 lumbar segments, 5 sacral segments, and 1 coccygeal segment. The thickening of the spinal cord in the neck region is called the **cervical enlargement** and contains the motor neurons that control the muscles of the arms. Another thickening of the spinal cord occurs in the lumbar region. This thickening is called the **lumbar enlargement** and contains the motor neurons that control the muscles of the legs (Figure 27-4).

Gray and White Matter. When you view a cross section of the spinal cord, you observe two differently colored areas. The inner tissue is termed **gray matter** because its color is darker than the outer tissue, which is termed **white matter.** The gray matter contains neuron cell bodies and their dendrites, whereas the white matter contains myelinated axons. The divisions of the gray matter are called horns, and the divisions of the white matter are called columns (funiculi). The columns contain groups of axons called nerve tracts. A canal runs down the entire length of the spinal cord through the center of the gray matter. This canal is called the central canal and contains CSF (Figure 27-5).

Ascending and Descending Tracts. One function of the spinal cord is to carry sensory information up to the brain. The tracts that carry sensory information up to the brain are called **ascending tracts.** Another function of the spinal cord is to carry motor information down from the brain to muscles and glands. These tracts are called **descending tracts.**

Reflexes. Another important function of the spinal cord is to participate in reflexes. A **reflex** is a predictable, automatic response to stimuli. For example, if you touch something very hot, the predictable response is that you will pull your finger away from the hot surface; this type of reflex is called a withdrawal reflex. The information that flows through a typical reflex moves in the following order: from receptors to sensory neurons to interneurons

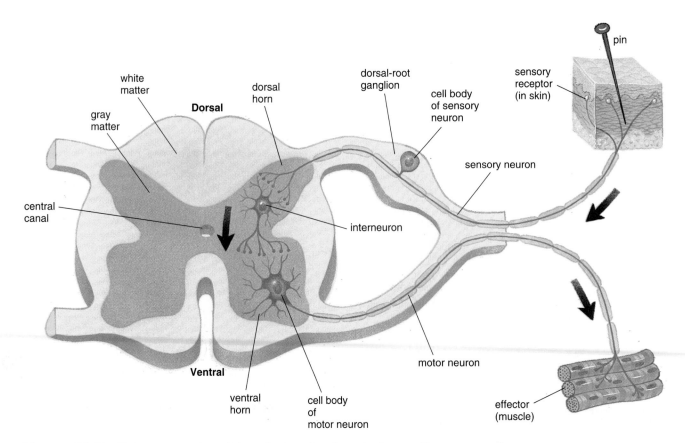

Figure 27-5. This cross section of the spinal cord and a spinal nerve illustrates a reflex arc.

to motor neurons to effectors. In this example of the withdrawal reflex, the receptors are in the skin at the tips of the fingers. These receptors send their information to sensory neurons that relay the information to interneurons in the spinal cord. The interneurons immediately relay the information to motor neurons that activate the muscles (effectors) in the arm. The muscles in the arm coordinate the movement of pulling your finger away from the painful stimulus. A person can consciously inhibit a reflex because the information also goes to the cerebral cortex where a person makes conscious decisions.

Brain

The brain can be divided into four major areas: the cerebrum, the diencephalons, the brain stem, and the cerebellum (Figure 27-6).

Cerebrum.   The **cerebrum** is the largest part of the brain. It is divided into two halves called cerebral hemispheres. A thick bundle of nerve fibers called the **corpus callosum** connects the two hemispheres. The grooves on the surface of the cerebrum are called **sulci.** The "bumps" of brain matter between the sulci are called **gyri,** or **convolutions.** A deep groove called the longitudinal fissure runs between the two longitudinal hemispheres.

Lobes.   Each cerebral hemisphere is divided into **lobes**— frontal, parietal, temporal, and occipital. The frontal lobes contain motor areas that allow a person to consciously decide to produce a body movement such as walking or tapping a pencil. Somatosensory areas are located in parietal lobes. These areas interpret sensations felt on or within the body. For example, if you feel a light touch on your right hand, the somatosensory area interprets the sensation and

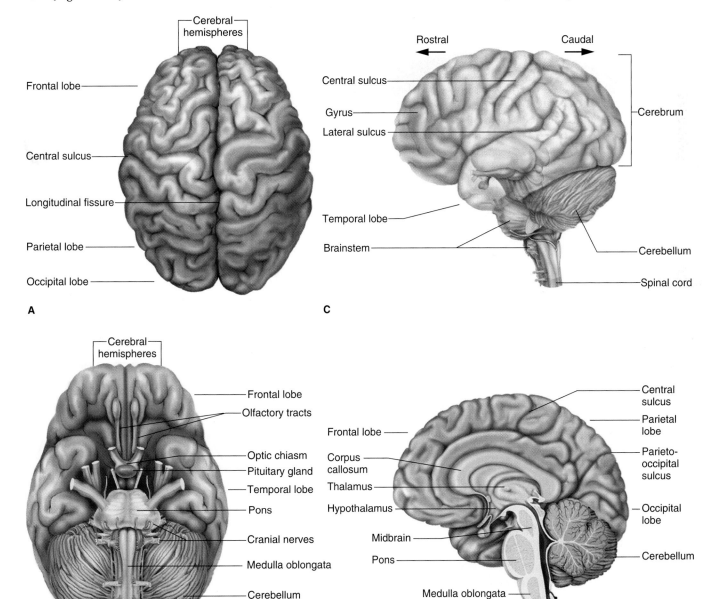

Figure 27-6.   Four views of the brain: (a) superior, (b) inferior, (c) left lateral, and (d) sagittal section.

where it is occurring. The temporal lobes contain auditory areas that interpret sounds. Visual areas are located in the occipital lobes, and they interpret what a person sees.

Cortex. The outermost layer of the cerebrum is called the cerebral **cortex.** It is composed of gray matter and therefore contains neuron cell bodies and dendrites. This layer contains nearly 75% of all neurons in the entire nervous system. Beneath the cerebral cortex is white matter. Besides interpreting sensory information and initiating body movements, the cortex also stores memories and creates emotions.

Ventricles. **Ventricles** are interconnected cavities within the brain. They are filled with CSF. Recall that this fluid is also found in the subarachnoid space of the meninges and the central canal of the spinal cord. Therefore, CSF is located within the brain and spinal cord and also around the brain and spinal cord. This fluid protects and cushions the central nervous system.

Diencephalon. The **diencephalon** is located between the cerebral hemispheres and is superior to the brain stem. The diencephalon includes the thalamus and hypothalamus. The **thalamus** serves as a relay station for sensory information that heads to the cerebral cortex for interpretation. If sensory information does not pass through the thalamus before it reaches the cerebral cortex,

it cannot be interpreted correctly. For example, say you are feeling pain in your left forearm. This information goes up the spinal cord and through the thalamus and then to the cerebral cortex for interpretation. If the information did not go through the thalamus, the cerebral cortex may interpret that you are feeling cold instead of pain in your left forearm. The **hypothalamus** maintains balance by regulating many vital activities such as heart rate, blood pressure, and breathing rate.

Brain Stem. The **brain stem** is a structure that connects the cerebrum to the spinal cord. The three parts of the brain stem are the midbrain, the pons, and the medulla oblongata. The midbrain lies just beneath the diencephalon. It controls both visual and auditory reflexes. An example of a visual reflex is when you see something in your peripheral vision and you automatically turn your head to view it more clearly.

The pons is a rounded bulge on the underside of the brain stem situated between the midbrain and the medulla oblongata. It contains nerve tracts to connect the cerebrum to the cerebellum. The pons also regulates breathing.

The medulla oblongata is the most inferior portion of the brain stem and is directly connected to the spinal cord. It controls many vital activities such as heart rate, blood pressure, and breathing. It also controls reflexes associated with coughing, sneezing, and vomiting.

Educating the Patient

Preventing Brain and Spinal Cord Injuries

In the United States alone, almost half a million people a year suffer brain and spinal cord injuries. The most common causes of these injuries are motor vehicle accidents, sports and recreational accidents—especially diving—and violence. People at the highest risk for spinal cord injuries are children and teens. However, most brain and spinal cord injuries can be prevented. You can use the following tips to educate patients on preventing these types of injuries.

Prevention Tips

- Know the depth of water into which you are diving. More than 90% of diving injuries occur in 5 feet of water or less.
- Explore diving areas before diving. For example, know where rocks are located before you dive.
- Do not drive or do any recreational activity while intoxicated. Alcohol affects good judgment and control. Alcohol-related traffic crashes are the leading cause of disabling brain and spinal cord injuries.

- Always wear a helmet when riding a bike or motorcycle. Your risk of brain injury is 85% greater during a biking accident if you are not wearing a helmet. Make sure your helmet fits properly.
- Always wear appropriate protective gear while playing any sport.
- Avoid surfing headfirst.
- Always wear your safety belt.
- Make sure children use car seats that appropriate for their age and weight.
- Be familiar with ways to get help quickly in emergencies.
- Follow traffic rules and signs while walking, biking, or driving.
- Follow safety rules on playgrounds.
- Store firearms and ammunition in separate and locked places.
- Teach children the safety rules to follow if they find a gun.

Cerebellum. The **cerebellum** is inferior to the occipital lobes of the cerebrum and posterior to the pons and medulla oblongata. It coordinates complex skeletal muscle contractions that are needed for body movements. For example, when you walk, many muscles have to contract and relax at appropriate times. Your cerebellum coordinates these activities. The cerebellum also coordinates fine movements such as threading a needle, playing an instrument, and writing.

Peripheral Nervous System

The peripheral nervous system consists of nerves that branch off the CNS. These nerves are called peripheral nerves and are classified in two types—**cranial nerves** and **spinal nerves.**

Cranial Nerves

Cranial nerves are peripheral nerves that originate from the brain. Roman numerals and names designate the twelve different cranial nerves.

I. *Olfactory nerves* carry smell information to the brain for interpretation.

II. *Optic nerves* carry visual information to the brain for interpretation.

III. *Oculomotor nerves* are found within the muscles that move the eyeball, eyelid, and iris.

IV. *Trochlear nerves* act in the muscles that move the eyeball.

V. *Trigeminal nerves* carry sensory information from the surface of the eye, the scalp, facial skin, the lining of the gums, and the palate to the brain for interpretation. They also are found within the muscles needed for chewing.

VI. *Abducens nerves* act in the muscles that move the eyeball.

VII. *Facial nerves* are found in the muscles of facial expression as well as in the salivary and tear glands. These nerves also carry sensory information from the tongue.

VIII. *Vestibulocochlear nerves* carry hearing and equilibrium information from the inner ear to the brain for interpretation.

IX. *Glossopharyngeal nerves* carry sensory information from the throat and tongue to the brain for interpretation. They also act in the muscles of the throat.

X. *Vagus nerves* carry sensory information from the thoracic and abdominal organs to the brain for interpretation. These nerves are also found within the muscles in the throat, stomach, intestines, and heart.

XI. *Accessory nerves* are found within the muscles of the throat, neck, back, and voice box.

XII. *Hypoglossal nerves* are found within the muscles of the tongue.

Spinal Nerves

Spinal nerves are peripheral nerves that originate from the spinal cord (Figure 27-7). There are 31 pairs of spinal nerves: 8 pairs of cervical nerves (numbered C1 through C8), 12 pairs of thoracic nerves (numbered T1 through T12), 5 pairs of lumbar nerves (numbered L1 through L5), 5 pairs of sacral nerves (numbered S1 through S5), and one pair of coccygeal nerves (Co).

Two roots, a ventral root and a dorsal root, form each spinal nerve (see Figure 27-5). The **ventral root** contains axons of motor neurons only, and the dorsal root contains axons of sensory neurons only. The **dorsal root** also contains a dorsal root ganglion, which contains the cell bodies of sensory neurons.

Except in the thoracic region, the main portions of spinal nerves fuse together to form nerve **plexuses.** The major nerve plexuses are the cervical, brachial, and lumbosacral. Nerves coming off the cervical plexus supply the skin and the muscles of the neck. The phrenic nerve also originates from the plexus. This nerve controls the diaphragm, which is a muscle that is needed for breathing.

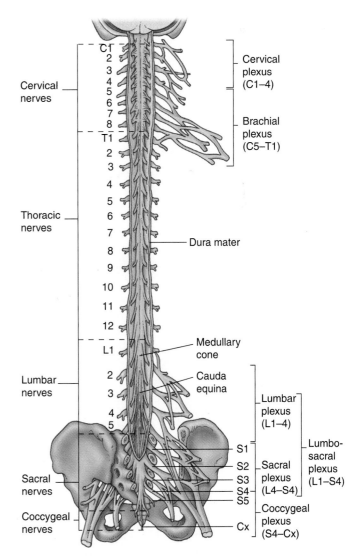

Figure 27-7. Spinal cord, spinal nerves, and plexuses.

The brachial plexus forms nerves that control muscles in the arms. The lumbosacral plexus supplies the lower abdominal wall, external genitalia, buttocks, thighs, legs, and feet. The largest nerve of the body, the sciatic nerve, originates from this plexus. This nerve controls the muscles of the legs.

Somatic and Autonomic Nervous Systems

The peripheral nervous system is divided into a somatic nervous system and an autonomic nervous system. The **somatic** nervous system consists of nerves that connect the CNS to skin and skeletal muscle. The somatic nervous system is often called the "voluntary" nervous system because it controls skeletal muscles, which are under voluntary control. The **autonomic** nervous system consists of nerves that connect the CNS to organs and other structures such as the heart, stomach, intestines, glands, blood vessels, and bladder (among others). The autonomic nervous system controls organs not under voluntary control, so it is often referred to as the "involuntary" nervous system.

In the autonomic nervous system, motor neurons from the brain and spinal cord communicate to other motor neurons that are located in ganglia. **Ganglia** are collections of neuron cell bodies outside the CNS. The motor neurons of ganglia then communicate to various organs and blood vessels.

The two divisions of the autonomic nervous system are the sympathetic and the parasympathetic (Figure 27-8). The **sympathetic** division prepares organs for "fight-or-flight" situations. In other words, it prepares them for stressful or emergency situations. For example, the sympathetic division prepares the heart for a stressful or frightening situation by increasing the heart rate. The **parasympathetic** division prepares the body for resting and digesting. For example, the parasympathetic division prepares the heart for resting by keeping the heart rate relatively low. Notice that sympathetic and parasympathetic actions are antagonistic, meaning that they function in opposite ways. Most of the body's organs are under parasympathetic control.

Many neurons of the sympathetic division are located in the thoracic and lumbar regions of the spinal cord. For this reason, this division is also called the thoracolumbar division. The sympathetic neurons usually release the neurotransmitter norepinephrine into organs and glands. Norepinephrine increases the heart and breathing rates, slows down the activity of the digestive glands, slows down the muscles of the stomach and the intestines, and dilates the pupils. Sympathetic nerves also control the constriction of blood vessels. When blood vessels constrict, blood pressure increases, which is a needed response during an emergency situation.

Many neurons of the parasympathetic division are located in the brain stem and the sacral regions of the spinal

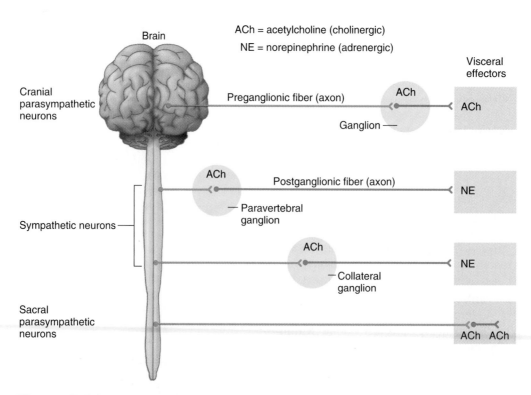

Figure 27-8. Divisions of the autonomic nervous system. Most parasympathetic fibers release acetylcholine onto visceral effectors. Most sympathetic fibers release norepinephrine onto visceral effectors.

cord. For this reason, this division is also referred to as the craniosacral division. All parasympathetic neurons release acetylcholine onto organs and glands. Acetylcholine is a neurotransmitter that slows the heart and breathing rates, constricts the pupils, activates digestive glands, and activates the muscles of the stomach and intestines. Most blood vessels in the body do not receive communication from parasympathetic nerves.

Neurologic Testing

Patients with nervous system disorders may have a wide variety of signs and symptoms, but the most common are headache, muscle weakness, and **paresthesias** (loss of feeling). A typical neurologic examination can determine the following:

- State of consciousness. This state can vary from normal to a state of coma. A patient in a coma cannot respond to stimuli and cannot be awakened. Other terms used to describe states of consciousness include *stupor* (difficulty being awakened), *delirium* (being confused or having hallucinations), *vegetative* (having no cortical function), and *asleep* (can be aroused with normal stimulation).
- Reflex activity. Reflex tests primarily determine the health of the peripheral nervous system.
- Speech patterns. Abnormal speech patterns include a loss of the ability to form words correctly or to form sentences that make sense.
- Motor patterns. Abnormal motor patterns include the loss of balance, abnormal posture, or inappropriate movements of the body. For example, chorea is an exaggerated and sudden jerking of a body part.

Diagnostic Procedures

Common diagnostic procedures to determine neurologic disorders include the following specialized tests:

- Lumbar puncture. Whenever a physician needs to examine CSF, a lumbar puncture is performed. A needle is used to remove CSF from the subarachnoid space usually below the third lumbar vertebra of the spinal column. Analysis of this fluid provides a great deal about the health of a patient. For example, cancer cells in CSF often indicate a brain or spinal cord tumor. White blood cells in this fluid indicate infections such as meningitis. Red blood cells indicate abnormal bleeding.
- Magnetic resonance imaging (MRI). This procedure allows for the brain and spinal cord to be visualized from many angles. It uses powerful magnets to generate images and is useful at detecting tumors, bleeding, or other abnormalities.
- Positron emission tomography (PET) scan. This procedure uses radioactive chemicals that collect in specific areas of the brain. These chemicals allow images of those specific areas to be generated. This test is useful in detecting blood flow to areas of the brain, brain tumors, and the diagnosis of such diseases as Parkinson's and Alzheimer's.
- Cerebral angiography. This procedure uses dyes that can be visualized in the blood vessels of the brain. It is useful in detecting aneurysms (abnormally dilated blood vessels).
- Computerized tomography (CT) scan. This very common procedure produces images that provide more information than a standard x-ray. It is useful in detecting tumors and other abnormal structures.
- Electroencephalogram (EEG). This test detects electrical activity in the brain. It is useful in diagnosing various states of consciousness.
- X-ray. This procedure is useful in detecting skull or vertebral fractures.

Cranial Nerve Tests

Disorders of the cranial nerves can be determined using the following tests:

- The olfactory nerves (I) are tested by asking a patient to smell various substances.
- Cranial nerves III, IV, and VI are tested by asking a patient to track the movement of the physician's finger. If a patient cannot move her eyeballs properly, there may be damage to one of these nerves. Recall that these nerves control the muscles that move the eyeballs.
- Cranial nerve V controls the muscles needed for chewing. To assess this nerve, a patient is asked to clench his teeth. The physician then feels the jaw muscles. If they feel limp or weak, this nerve may be damaged.
- If a person can no longer make facial expressions, then cranial nerve VII may be damaged. This nerve controls the muscles needed to make facial expressions.
- If a patient cannot extend his tongue and move it from side to side, cranial nerve XII may be damaged. This nerve controls tongue movement.

Reflex Testing

Testing a patient's reflexes allows a physician to evaluate the components of a reflex as well as the overall health of the individual's nervous system. The absence of a reflex is called **areflexia. Hyporeflexia** is a decreased reflex, and **hyperreflexia** is a stronger than normal reflex. The following are common reflex tests:

- Biceps reflex. The absence of this reflex may indicate spinal cord damage in the cervical region.
- Knee reflex. The absence of this reflex may indicate damage to lumbar or femoral nerves.
- Abdominal reflexes. These reflexes are used to evaluate damage to thoracic spinal nerves.

Pathophysiology

Common Diseases and Disorders of the Nervous System

Alzheimer's disease is a progressive, degenerative disease that occurs in the brain.

- **Causes.** Fiber tangles within neurons, degenerating nerve fibers, and a decreased production of neurotransmitters cause the symptoms of this disorder. This disease is associated with advanced age, family history, certain genes, and possibly some environmental factors. Many causes have not yet been determined.
- **Signs and symptoms.** Common symptoms include a loss of memory, confusion, personality changes, language deterioration, impaired judgment, and restlessness.
- **Treatment.** There is no cure, but proper nutrition, physical exercise, social activity, and calm environments help to manage the disease.

Amyotrophic lateral sclerosis (ALS) is a fatal disorder characterized by the degeneration of neurons in the spinal cord and brain.

- **Causes.** Most causes are unknown but they are likely to involve hereditary and environmental factors.
- **Signs and symptoms.** Early symptoms include cramping of hand and feet muscles, persistent tripping and falling, chronic fatigue, and slurred speech. Signs and symptoms that appear in later stages include breathing difficulty and muscle paralysis.
- **Treatment.** There is no cure for this disorder; however, physical, speech, and respiratory therapies help to manage the symptoms. Some medications relieve muscle cramping, and one drug that prolongs the life of ALS patients has been approved by the FDA.

Bell's palsy is a disorder in which facial muscles are very weak or totally paralyzed.

- **Causes.** This condition can result from damage to cranial nerve VII (the facial nerve), but many times the cause is unknown. It is more common in people with diabetes, the flu, or a cold.
- **Signs and symptoms.** The most common signs and symptoms are a loss of feeling in the face, the inability to produce facial expressions, headache, and excessive tearing or drooling.
- **Treatment.** Treatments include the use of eyedrops, anti-inflammatory medications, and pain relievers. Symptoms usually diminish or go away within 5 to 10 days.

Brain tumors and cancers are abnormal growths in the brain. A brain tumor with cancer cells is termed malignant. Malignant tumors that start in any tissue of the brain are called primary brain cancers. Those that start in body parts and spread to the brain are classified as secondary brain cancers. The most common primary brain tumors are gliomas that arise from neuroglial cells.

- **Causes.** Like most cancers, the causes are gene mutations. Factors associated with gene mutations include exposure to toxins, an impaired immune system, and hereditary factors.
- **Signs and symptoms.** The signs and symptoms depend on size and location of the tumor. Common symptoms include headache, seizures, nausea, weakness in the arms or legs, fatigue, changes in speech patterns, and a loss of memory.
- **Treatment.** Treatment often includes surgery, radiation therapy, chemotherapy, and gene therapy. The success of the treatment depends on the type of tumor, the extent of the diseases, the location of the tumor, the tumor's response to treatment, and the overall health of the patient.

Epilepsy and **seizures** occur when parts of the brain receive a burst of electrical signals that disrupt normal brain functioning. Seizures may be either partial or generalized. Partial seizures occur on one side of the brain, and generalized seizures occur on both sides. Epilepsy is the condition of having repeated, long-term seizures.

- **Causes.** Causes vary but may include birth trauma, high fevers, alcohol and drug withdrawal, head trauma, infections, brain tumors, and certain medications. Many causes are unknown.
- **Signs and symptoms.** The signs and symptoms may include visual disturbances, nausea, generalized abnormal feelings, a loss of consciousness, and uncontrolled muscle contractions and tremors.
- **Treatment.** The primary treatment is medication to prevent seizures. Surgery is sometimes an option in patients with partial seizures.

Guillain-Barré syndrome is a disorder in which the body's immune system attacks part of the peripheral nervous system. It usually has a sudden and unexpected onset.

- **Causes.** The destruction of myelin by the body's immune system produces the signs and symptoms. Viral infections, immunizations, and pregnancy sometimes trigger the disease.
- **Signs and symptoms.** Symptoms may include weakness or tingling sensations in the legs or arms that can progress to paralysis. Difficulty breathing and an abnormal heart rate are dangerous signs and symptoms. The disease normally runs its course, and with proper medical treatment, it is not fatal.

continued ⟶

Common Diseases and Disorders of the Nervous System *(continued)*

- **Treatment.** Various supportive therapies, such as the use of respirators and heart machines, are necessary until the disease subsides. Physical therapy is used to keep muscles strong.

Headaches affect almost everyone at some point in life. They can affect the very young to the very old. A wide variety of factors produce headaches. Most headaches do not require medical attention, but a physician should evaluate repetitive and severe headaches. Headaches commonly include tension headaches, migraines, and cluster headaches.

Tension headaches are classified as either episodic (occurring randomly) or chronic (occurring frequently):

Episodic tension headaches are the most common type of tension headache.

- **Causes.** This type of headache occurs randomly and is often the result of temporary stress or anger.
- **Signs and symptoms.** Symptoms include pain or soreness in the temples and the contraction of head and neck muscles.
- **Treatment.** Most of these headaches can be managed by taking an over-the-counter (OTC) medicine, and relief usually occurs in 1 or 2 hours. A person who takes medication daily or almost daily for headaches, should see a physician.

Chronic tension headaches occur almost every day and persist for weeks or months.

- **Causes.** This type of headache may be the result of stress or fatigue, but it may also be associated with physical problems, psychological issues, or depression.
- **Signs and symptoms.** As with episodic tension headaches, the symptoms include pain or soreness in the temples and the contraction of head and neck muscles.
- **Treatment.** People who suffer from chronic headaches should seek medical treatment.

Migraines are the most severe type of headache. They are responsible for more "sick days" than any other headache type. Almost 30 million people in the United States suffer from migraines.

- **Causes.** Hormones may influence migraines, which may explain why women experience migraines at least three times more often than men do. Migraine headaches are considered vascular headaches because they are associated with the distension of the arteries of the brain.
- **Signs and symptoms.** Migraines often begin as dull pains that develop into throbbing pains accompanied by nausea and a sensitivity to light and noise. There are many types of migraines but the two most common are *migraine with aura* and *migraine without aura*. Some patients have migraines that begin with an aura. Auras may include the appearance of jagged lines or flashing lights, tunnel vision, hallucinations, or the detection of strange odors. The auras may last up to an hour and usually go away as the headache begins. Most migraine headaches last about 4 hours but some can last up to a week.
- **Treatment.** When treating migraines, a physician will prescribe a drug to relieve the pain but will also try to identify the factors that trigger it. There are many medicines available to treat migraines.

Cluster headaches are so named because the attacks come in groups. They are the most severe type of migraines. More men than women experience these types of headaches.

- **Causes.** Some research indicates that alcohol consumption can bring on attacks of cluster headaches.
- **Signs and symptoms.** Common symptoms include a runny nose, watery eyes, and swelling below the eyes. Cluster headaches normally last about 45 minutes to an hour, although they can last longer. It is common for a patient with this disorder to experience 1 to 4 headaches a day during a cluster time span. Cluster time spans can last weeks or months.
- **Treatment.** Various drugs are available for the treatment of these headaches.

Meningitis is an inflammation of the meninges.

- **Causes.** Causes may include bacterial, viral, and fungal infections. Some types of meningitis can be prevented with vaccines.
- **Signs and symptoms.** Fever, headache, vomiting, stiffness in the neck, sensitivity to light, drowsiness, and joint pain usually accompany this disorder.
- **Treatment.** The treatment varies depending on the type of meningitis. Intravenous antibiotics are used for bacterial meningitis, supportive therapy for viral meningitis, and antifungal drugs for fungal meningitis.

Multiple sclerosis (MS) is a chronic disease of the central nervous system in which myelin is destroyed.

- **Causes.** The causes are mostly unknown, but some known causes are viruses, genetic factors, and immune system abnormalities.
- **Signs and symptoms.** Depending on the type of MS, symptoms can range from mild to severe. In severe cases, a person will lose the ability to walk or speak.
- **Treatment.** There is no cure for MS, but supportive treatments can lessen the symptoms. Some medications are also available to treat symptoms.

Neuralgias are a group of disorders commonly referred to as nerve pain. They most frequently occur in the nerves, of the face.

- **Causes.** There are many causes of neuralgia, including trauma, chemical irritation of the nerves, bacterial

continued ⟶

Common Diseases and Disorders of the Nervous System *(continued)*

infections, and diabetes. Many times the causes are unknown.

- **Signs and symptoms.** Sudden and severe skin pain are the most common symptoms. The pain repeatedly occurs in the same body area. Numbness of skin areas is also common.
- **Treatment.** Many times the disorder goes away by itself, and treatment, other than pain medication, is not needed. Other treatments include injections of anesthetics or surgery to remove the affected nerves.

Parkinson's disease is a motor system disorder. It is slowly progressive and degenerative.

- **Causes.** Most causes are undetermined, although it is known that patients with this disease lack certain chemicals in the brain. Brain tumors, certain drugs, carbon monoxide, or repeated head trauma may produce Parkinson's disease.
- **Signs and symptoms.** The most common signs and symptoms include trembling and stiffness of the arms and legs as well as a lack of coordination and balance.
- **Treatment.** There is no cure, but medications alleviate some symptoms and slow down the progression of this disease. Surgery is useful in some cases of Parkinson's.

Sciatica occurs when the sciatic nerve is damaged.

- **Causes.** The sciatic nerve is commonly damaged by excessive pressure on the nerve from prolonged sitting or lying down. It is also easily damaged from trauma to the pelvis, buttocks, or thighs.
- **Signs and symptoms.** The most usual symptoms include numbness, pain, or tingling sensations on the back of a leg or foot. Weakness of leg and foot muscles can also develop.
- **Treatment.** This disorder is usually treated with pain medication and steroids. Physical therapy is also needed following trauma to the nerve.

Stroke occurs when brain cells die because of an inadequate blood flow. Stroke is sometimes referred to as a "brain attack."

- **Causes.** Most strokes are caused by the blockage of an artery in the neck or brain. They may also be caused by aneurisms that burst.
- **Signs and symptoms.** Signs and symptoms may include paralysis, speech problems, memory and reasoning deficits, coma, and possibly death. Symptoms will vary depending on the location of the stroke within the brain.
- **Treatment.** Because neurons in the brain cannot be replaced, the effects of a stroke can be permanent. However, physical and speech therapy are often very useful in lessening the effects of a stroke.

Summary

The functions of the nervous system include detecting and interpreting sensory information, making decisions about that information, and responding to and carrying out motor functions based on those decisions. The cells responsible for these functions are neurons.

There are two divisions of the nervous system. The CNS consists of the brain and spinal cord. The peripheral nervous system is made up of cranial nerves and spinal nerves. All organs are under the control of the nervous system. Knowledge of this system is essential when assisting the physician during a neurologic exam.

CHAPTER 27

CASE STUDY QUESTIONS

Now that you have completed this chapter, review the case study at the beginning of the chapter and answer the following questions:

1. What effect do sympathetic nerves have on blood vessels?
2. Why does Raynaud's disease produce pain and blue coloration in the fingers and toes?
3. How is a sympathectomy going to help this patient's condition?

Discussion Questions

1. Explain the three general functions of the nervous system.
2. Describe the differences between the ascending and descending tracts of the spinal cord.
3. What are the two divisions of the autonomic nervous system? How do these two divisions differ?

Critical Thinking Questions

1. In some diseases, such as multiple sclerosis, myelin is destroyed. What is the function of myelin in the nervous system, and how can the destruction of myelin contribute to the signs and symptoms of multiple sclerosis?
2. What functional losses would you expect to observe in patients with the following brain injuries?
   a. Stroke in an occipital lobe of the cerebrum
   b. Damage to a temporal lobe of the cerebrum
   c. Stroke in the medulla oblongata
   d. Brain tumor in the primary motor area of the frontal lobe

Application Activities

1. Give the Roman numeral designations and functions of the following cranial nerves:
   a. Facial nerve
   b. Hypoglossal nerve
   c. Trigeminal nerve
   d. Vagus nerve
   e. Optic nerve
2. What are the uses of the following diagnostic procedures?
   a. Lumbar puncture
   b. MRI
   c. CT scan
   d. Cerebral angiography
3. Give the functions of the following neuron types:
   a. Sensory neurons
   b. Motor neurons
   c. Interneurons
4. What parts of a neuron are found in gray matter? In white matter?

Internet Activity

Go to the *MEDLINEplus* Web site at **http://www.nlm.nih.gov/medlineplus/fainting.html,** and answer these questions:
   a. What is the clinical term for fainting?
   b. What are the two major types of fainting?
   c. What tests can be done to determine the causes of fainting?

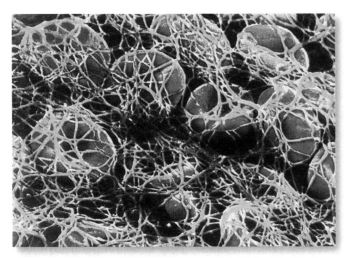

Figure 28-22. Scanning electron micrograph of a blood clot. Yellow fibrin threads are covering red blood cells.

the blood vessel, creating a meshwork that entraps blood cells and platelets. The resulting mass, the blood clot, stops bleeding until the vessel has repaired itself (Figure 28-22).

When a blood vessel is injured, it is normal for a blood clot to form. However, sometimes blood clots form on the side of a blood vessel with no known injury; this abnormal blood clot is called a **thrombus.** The danger of a thrombus is that a portion of it can break off and start moving through the bloodstream. The moving portion of the thrombus is called an **embolus.** An embolus is dangerous because it will eventually block a small artery. An embolus that originates in the vein of a leg travels to the right atrium of the heart through the inferior vena cava and is pumped by the right ventricle to the lungs. Here the embolus gets stuck in a small artery and causes pulmonary embolism, a fatal condition if not treated.

Blood Types

The ABO blood group consists of four different blood types: A, B, AB, and O. They are distinguished from each other in part by their antigens and antibodies.

Agglutination is the clumping of red blood cells following a blood transfusion. This clumping is not desirable because it leads to severe anemia. Agglutination occurs because proteins called *antigens* on the surface of red blood cells bind to antibodies in plasma (Figure 28-23). To prevent agglutination, antigens should not be mixed with antibodies that will bind to them. Fortunately, most antibodies do not bind to antigens on blood cells; only very specific ones bind to them.

Type A. People with type A blood have antigen A on the surface of their red blood cells. They also have antibody B in their plasma. Antibody B will only bind to antigen B.

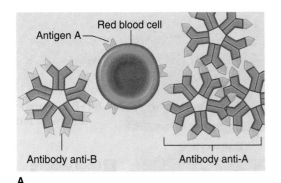

A

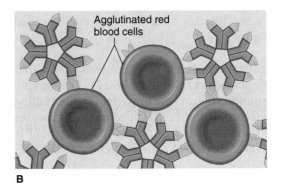

B

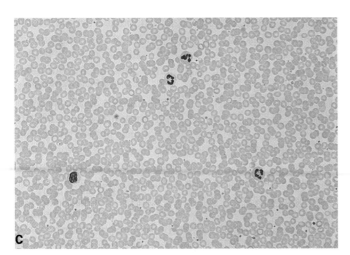

C

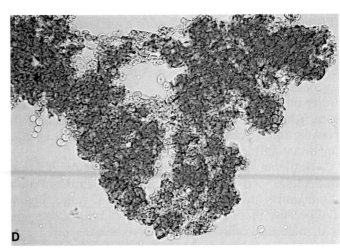

D

Figure 28-23. Agglutination. (a) Red blood cells with antigen A are added to blood that contains antibody anti-A. (b) Antibody anti-A reacts with antigen A, causing the agglutination of blood. (c) Normal blood. (d) Agglutinated blood.

TABLE 28-3 ABO Blood Group

Blood Type	Antigen Present	Antibody Present	Blood That Can Be Received
A	A	B	A and O
B	B	A	B and O
AB	AB	None	A, B, AB, and O
O	None	A and B	O

Type B. People with type B blood have antigen B on the surface of their red blood cells. They also have antibody A in their plasma.

If a person with type A blood is given type B blood, then the antibody B in the recipient's blood will bind with the red blood cells of the donor blood because those cells have antigen B on their surfaces. Therefore, agglutination occurs, and the donated red blood cells are destroyed. This is why a person with type A blood should not be given type B blood (and vice versa).

Type AB. People with type AB blood have both antigen A and antigen B on the surface of their red blood cells. They have neither antibody A nor antibody B in their plasma. People with type AB blood are called universal recipients, because most of them can receive all ABO blood types. They can receive these blood types because they lack antibody A and antibody B in their plasma, so there is no reaction with antigens A and B of the donor blood.

Type O. People with type O blood have neither antigen A nor antigen B on the surface of their red blood cells. However, they do have both antibody A and antibody B in

their plasma. People with type O blood are called universal donors because their blood can be given to most people regardless of recipients' blood type. Type O blood will not agglutinate when given to other people because it does not have the antigens to bind to antibody A or antibody B. Table 28-3 summarizes the ABO blood group. Also see Figure 28-24.

The Rh Factor. The **Rh antigen** is a protein first discovered on red blood cells of the Rhesus monkey, hence the name Rh. People who are Rh-positive have red blood cells that contain the Rh antigen. People who are Rh-negative have red blood cells that do not contain the Rh antigen. If a person who is Rh-negative is given Rh-positive blood, then the Rh-negative person's blood will make antibodies that bind to the Rh antigens. If the Rh-negative person is given Rh-positive blood a second time, the antibodies will bind to the donor cells and agglutination will occur.

Clinically, it is very important for a female to know her Rh type. If an Rh-negative female mates with an Rh-positive male, there is a fifty-fifty chance that her fetus will be Rh-positive. When the blood of a fetus who is Rh-positive mixes with the blood of a mother who is Rh-negative, the

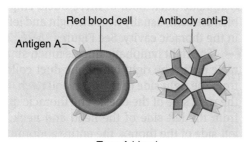

Type A blood

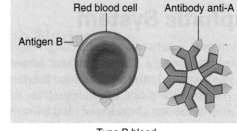

Type B blood

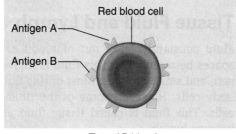

Type AB blood

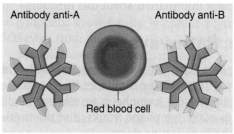

Type O blood

Figure 28-24. A, B, AB, and O blood types.

Antibodies

Antibodies are also called **immunoglobulins.** The following is a list of different types of immunoglobulins (Ig):

- IgG. This antibody primarily recognizes bacteria, viruses, and toxins. It can also activate complements, which are proteins in serum that attack pathogens.
- IgA. This antibody is found in secretions of the body such as breast milk, sweat, tears, saliva, and mucus. It prevents pathogens from entering the body.
- IgM. This antibody is very large and primarily binds to antigens on food, bacteria, or incompatible blood cells. It also activates complements.
- IgE. This antibody is found wherever IgA is located. It is involved in triggering allergic reactions.

When antibodies bind to antigens, they take one of the following actions:

- They allow phagocytes to recognize and destroy antigens.
- They make antigens clump together, causing them to be destroyed by macrophages. This is how incompatible blood cells are destroyed.
- They cover the toxic portions of antigens to make them harmless.
- They activate complements. Complements are proteins in serum that attack pathogens by forming holes in them. Complement proteins also attract macrophages to pathogens and can stimulate inflammation.

Immune Responses and Acquired Immunities

A primary immune response occurs the first time a person is exposed to an antigen. This response is slow and takes several weeks to occur. In this response, memory cells are made. A secondary immune response occurs the next time a person is exposed to the same antigen. This response is very quick and usually prevents a person from developing a disease from the antigen. Memory cells carry out the secondary immune response.

A person is born with very few immunities but normally develops them as long as the person's immune system is healthy. The four types of immunities a person can acquire are: (1) natural acquired active immunity, (2) artificially acquired active immunity, (3) naturally acquired passive immunity, and (4) artificially acquired passive immunity.

Naturally Acquired Active Immunity

A person develops this immunity by being naturally exposed to an antigen and subsequently making antibodies and memory cells against the antigen. Having an infectious disease caused by pathogens leads to the development of this type of immunity. This immunity is usually long lasting.

Artificially Acquired Active Immunity

A person develops this immunity by being injected with a pathogen and then subsequently making antibodies and memory cells against the pathogen. Immunizations or vaccines cause this type of immunity. This type is usually long lasting.

Naturally Acquired Passive Immunity

A person is given this immunity through his mother. When a mother breast-feeds, she passes antibodies to her baby through breast milk. A mother also passes antibodies to her baby across the placenta. This type of immunity is short lived.

Artificially Acquired Passive Immunity

A person is given this immunity when she is injected with antibodies. If a snake bites a person, a physician will inject the patient with antibodies (antivenom) to neutralize the venom. This type of immunity is short lived.

Major Immune System Disorders

A number of diseases and disorders can challenge the immune system. Among them, HIV infection, AIDS, cancer, and allergies are the most significant.

Human Immunodeficiency Virus

Human immunodeficiency virus (HIV) is a viral infection that seriously damages an individual's immunity, primarily by destroying lymphocytes. It causes **acquired immunodeficiency syndrome (AIDS)** and can leave the immune system weak and susceptible to other diseases.

Routes of Transmission. HIV can be located in many body fluids including saliva, tears, blood, semen, vaginal secretions, and breast milk. The most common routes of transmission are through sexual contact, through blood, or from mother to child during pregnancy or breast-feeding. Less common routes of transmission are through accidental needlesticks, artificial insemination, and organ transplants. HIV is not transmitted through casual contact such as holding hands, hugging, and touching objects previously touched by HIV-infected persons. Statistically, persons most likely to get HIV infection are homosexual men, bisexual men, intravenous drug users who share needles, and infants born to HIV-infected mothers.

HIV Testing. A person can have an HIV infection for years before developing any symptoms of this disease. Fortunately, a few tests are available to determine if a person has been infected with HIV. The most sensitive test—but one that is very costly—is polymerase chain reaction (PCR). This test can determine the number of HIV particles in a sample of blood, even if the number is less than 25 viral particles per cubic centimeter of plasma. For this reason, this test is useful for the early diagnosis of HIV infection.

Acquired Immunodeficiency Syndrome

AIDS is the development of severe signs and symptoms caused by HIV. In the United States, AIDS is the fifth leading cause of death in individuals between the ages of 25 and 44. This disease severely suppresses a person's immune system so that what would be minor infections in healthy individuals end up being fatal in patients with AIDS.

AIDS Testing. The most commonly used test to determine the presence of the AIDS virus is called ELISA. This test is considerably less expensive than PCR but is also less reliable. ELISA cannot detect early HIV infections. For this reason, it is preferable to test a high-risk patient three times with ELISA or alternate tests to ensure an accurate diagnosis.

Counts of CD4 cells are used to diagnose the stage of HIV infection. Once CD4 counts fall below 200, a person is diagnosed with AIDS. CD4 cells are types of T cells and are important for the functions of other components of the immune system.

Signs and Symptoms. The signs and symptoms of people who have developed AIDS include low T cell counts, fever, profuse sweating, weakness, weight loss, swollen glands, frequent infections, and some rare types of cancers. Common infections include ulcers of the mouth, skin, or genitals caused by herpes viruses; tuberculosis; yeast infections within the mouth, esophagus, or vagina; pneumonia; meningitis; and encephalitis. Cytomegalovirus (CMV), which is a type of infection caused by the herpes virus, can infect the eyes and other organs. A cancer that commonly appears in AIDS patients is Kaposi's sarcoma. It forms lesions on the skin—usually on the hands and feet first.

Treatment. There is no cure for AIDS, but in the United States, treatments are available that significantly delay the progression of the disease for many patients. Treatments include the use of various antiviral drugs, but many of these drugs have serious side effects. Antibiotics are also used to treat infections.

Cancer

Cancer is defined as the uncontrolled growth of abnormal cells. Healthy cells normally know when to stop reproducing, but cancer cells have lost this ability. Cancer cells often form growths called **malignant** tumors, which are often fatal. In many cases, these cancerous cells or tumors

damage normal cells of tissues and organs, which cause organ systems to fail.

At least 200 different types of cancers are known. In the United States, the three most common cancer types in men are prostate, lung, and colon cancer. The three most common types in women are breast, lung, and colon cancer. Lung cancer is the leading killer of all types of cancer for all people.

Causes. The causes of cancer are mostly unknown but certain risk factors have been identified. These factors include a suppressed immune system, radiation, tobacco, and some viruses. Many other factors are suspected. One of the best ways to prevent cancer is to not smoke and to avoid other known risk factors. A factor that is known to cause the formation of cancer is called a **carcinogen.**

Diagnosis. Most cancers are diagnosed with a **biopsy,** which is a removal of tissues for examination. CT scans are also used to help diagnose most cancer types. Other diagnostic tests include blood counts, an analysis of blood chemistry, and x-rays.

Signs and Symptoms. The symptoms of different types of cancer vary but the following are usually observed in most types: fever, chills, unintended weight loss, fatigue, and a general sense of not feeling well.

Treatment. The treatment of cancer differs depending on the type and stage of cancer. The stage of cancer refers to how large a tumor is and how far cancer cells have spread throughout the body. Table 29-1 provides a summary of cancer staging.

If tumors are localized and have not spread, the cancer can often be successfully treated by surgically removing the tumor. Other treatment options are chemotherapy and radiation therapy. Even if a cancer cannot be cured, its progression can sometimes be slowed, allowing patients to live additional years.

Allergies

An allergic reaction is an immune response to a substance, such as pollen, that is not normally harmful to the body. An allergy can also be an excessive immune response. Substances that trigger allergic responses are called **allergens.**

Allergic reactions involve IgE antibodies and mast cells. When IgE antibodies bind to allergens, they cause mast cells to release histamine and heparin. These chemicals trigger allergic reactions. A patient receiving allergy shots is being injected with tiny amounts of the allergen. This causes the body to produce IgG antibodies that will prevent IgE antibodies from binding to the allergen. IgG antibodies do not trigger immune responses because they do not activate mast cells.

Most allergies do not cause life-threatening conditions, but some do. One life-threatening condition that can result is **anaphylaxis.** In this condition, blood vessels dilate so quickly that blood pressure drops too quickly for organs to adjust.

REVIEW

CHAPTER 30

CASE STUDY QUESTIONS

Now that you have completed this chapter, review the case study at the beginning of the chapter and answer the following questions:

1. Why is the patient wheezing?
2. Is asthma a life-threatening condition?
3. What is the advantage of using a nebulizer to deliver the bronchodilator?
4. Why did the doctor refer the patient for allergy testing?

Discussion Questions

1. Describe the actions of the diaphragm and the rib cage during inspiration and expiration.
2. List the various respiratory volumes that are commonly measured in the clinical setting. What does each volume represent?
3. Describe how the larynx varies the loudness and pitch of the voice. Besides producing sound, what is another function of the larynx?

Critical Thinking Questions

1. Smoking destroys cilia in the respiratory tract. Describe how smoking damages the lungs.
2. What effect would breathing in a paper bag have on oxygen concentrations in the blood? Would this be helpful for a person who is hyperventilating? Why or why not?

Application Activities

1. Describe the locations and functions of the following structures:
   a. pharynx
   b. larynx
   c. primary bronchi
   d. alveoli
   e. epiglottis
2. What carries most oxygen in the blood?
3. How many lobes does the left lung have? The right lung?

CHAPTER 31

The Digestive System

CHAPTER OUTLINE

- Characteristics of the Alimentary Canal
- The Mouth
- The Pharynx
- The Esophagus
- The Stomach
- The Small Intestine
- The Liver
- The Gallbladder
- The Pancreas
- The Large Intestine
- The Rectum and Anal Canal
- The Absorption of Nutrients

OBJECTIVES

After completing Chapter 31, you will be able to:

31.1 List the functions of the digestive system.

31.2 Trace the pathway of food through the alimentary canal.

31.3 Describe the structure and functions of the mouth, teeth, tongue, and salivary glands.

31.4 Describe the structure and function of the pharynx.

31.5 Describe the swallowing process.

31.6 Describe the structure of the esophagus and tell how it propels food into the stomach.

31.7 Describe the structure and functions of the stomach.

31.8 List the substances secreted by the stomach and give their functions.

31.9 Describe the structure and functions of the small intestine.

31.10 List the substances secreted by the small intestine and describe the importance of each.

31.11 Explain the structures and functions of the liver, gallbladder, and pancreas.

31.12 List the substances released by the liver, gallbladder, and pancreas into the small intestine and give the function of each secretion.

31.13 Describe the structure and functions of the large intestine.

31.14 Tell what types of nutrients are absorbed by the digestive system and where they are absorbed.

31.15 Describe the signs, symptoms, causes, and treatments of various disorders and diseases of the digestive system.

KEY TERMS

acinar cells
adenoids
alimentary canal
anal canal
appendicitis
ascending colon
bicuspids
bile
carboxypeptidase
cecum
cellulose
chief cells
chyme
chymotrypsin
cirrhosis
colitis
common bile duct
cuspids
cystic duct
defecation reflex
descending colon
disaccharide
diverticulitis
duodenum
esophageal hiatus
feces
gastric juice
gastritis
gastroesophageal reflux
    disease (GERD)
glycogen
hemorrhoids
hepatic duct
hepatic lobule
hepatic portal vein

hepatitis	lingual tonsil	palatine tonsils	serous cells
hepatocytes	linoleic acid	pancreatic amylase	sigmoid colon
hernia	maltase	pancreatic lipase	sublingual gland
ileocecal sphincter	microvilli	parietal cells	submandibular gland
ileum	molars	parotid glands	submucosa
incisors	monosaccharide	pepsin	sucrase
intestinal lipase	mucosa	pepsinogen	transverse colon
intrinsic factor	mucous cells	peptidases	triglyceride
jejunum	nasopharynx	pharyngeal tonsils	trypsin
lactase	nucleases	polysaccharide	uvula
laryngopharynx	oropharynx	rectum	vermiform appendix
lingual frenulum	palate	serosa	

Introduction

Digestion is the mechanical and chemical breakdown of foods into forms that your body cells can absorb. The organs of the digestive system carry out digestion and can be divided into two categories—those of the alimentary canal and accessory organs. Organs of the alimentary canal extend from the mouth to the anus. They are the mouth, pharynx, esophagus, stomach, small intestine, large intestine, and anal canal. The accessory organs include the teeth, tongue, salivary glands, liver, gallbladder, and pancreas (Figure 31-1).

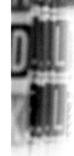

CASE STUDY

Yesterday afternoon, a 55-year-old female came to the gastroenterologist's office complaining of severe pain in her upper right abdomen. She was nauseated and stated that for several months—and especially following meals—she had been having periodic abdominal pain. After several tests, she was diagnosed as having gallstones and was scheduled for the surgical removal of her gallbladder.

As you read this chapter, consider the following questions:
1. What is the function of the gallbladder?
2. How does the gallbladder empty bile into the small intestine?
3. What conditions can result if gallstones are not removed?
4. Will this patient need to change her diet once her gallbladder is removed?

Characteristics of the Alimentary Canal

The wall of the **alimentary canal** consists of four layers:

1. Mucosa. The **mucosa** is the innermost layer of the wall and is mostly made of epithelial tissue that secretes enzymes and mucus into the lumen, or passageway, of the canal. This layer also is very active in absorbing nutrients.
2. Submucosa. The **submucosa** is the layer just deep to the mucosa. It contains loose connective tissue, blood vessels, glands, and nerves. The blood vessels in this layer carry away absorbed nutrients.
3. Muscular layer. This layer is just outside the submucosa. It is made of layers of smooth muscle tissue and contracts to move materials through the canal.
4. Serosa. The **serosa** is the outermost layer of canal and is also known as the visceral peritoneum. It secretes serous fluid to keep the outside of the canal moist and to prevent it from sticking to other organs.

Smooth muscle in the wall of the canal can contract to produce two basic types of movements—churning and

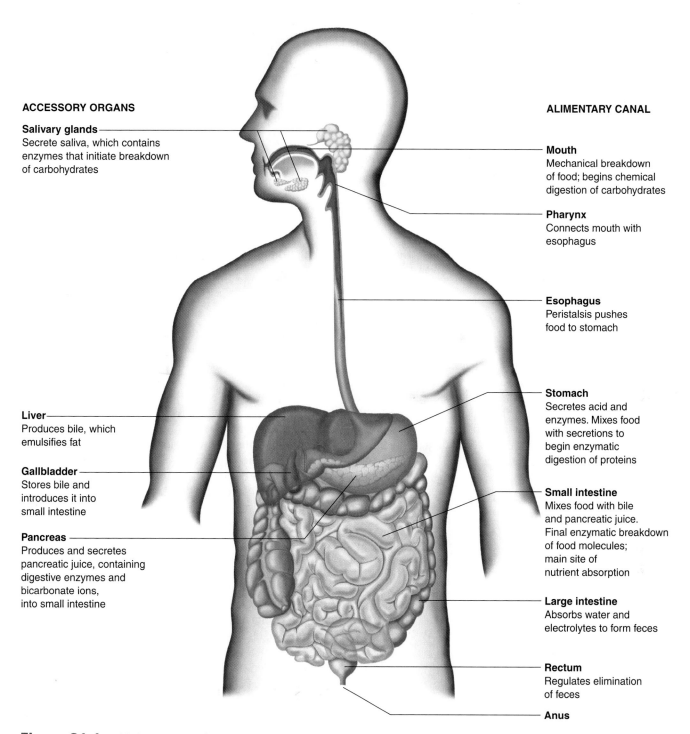

ACCESSORY ORGANS

Salivary glands
Secrete saliva, which contains
enzymes that initiate breakdown
of carbohydrates

Liver
Produces bile, which
emulsifies fat

Gallbladder
Stores bile and
introduces it into
small intestine

Pancreas
Produces and secretes
pancreatic juice, containing
digestive enzymes and
bicarbonate ions,
into small intestine

ALIMENTARY CANAL

Mouth
Mechanical breakdown
of food; begins chemical
digestion of carbohydrates

Pharynx
Connects mouth with
esophagus

Esophagus
Peristalsis pushes
food to stomach

Stomach
Secretes acid and
enzymes. Mixes food
with secretions to
begin enzymatic
digestion of proteins

Small intestine
Mixes food with bile
and pancreatic juice.
Final enzymatic breakdown
of food molecules;
main site of
nutrient absorption

Large intestine
Absorbs water and
electrolytes to form feces

Rectum
Regulates elimination
of feces

Anus

Figure 31-1. Major organs of the digestive system.

peristalsis. Churning mixes substances in the canal. Peristalsis propels substances through the tract (Figure 31-2).

The Mouth

The mouth takes in food and reduces its size through chewing. The mouth also starts to chemically digest food because saliva (spit) contains an enzyme that breaks down carbohydrates.

The cheeks consist of skin, adipose tissue, skeletal muscles, and an inner lining of moist stratified squamous epithelium. The cheeks act to hold food in the mouth. The lips contain a lot of sensory nerve fibers that can judge the temperature of food before it enters the mouth.

The tongue is mostly made of skeletal muscles and is covered by a mucous membrane. The body of the tongue is held to the floor of the oral cavity by a flap of mucous membrane called the **lingual frenulum.** The tongue acts to mix food in the mouth and to hold the food between

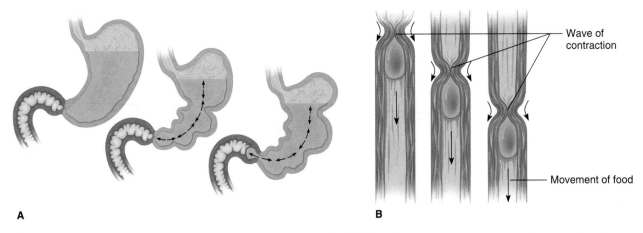

Figure 31-2. Movements through the alimentary canal. (a) Churning movements move substances back and forth to mix them. (b) Peristalsis moves contents along the canal.

teeth. It also contains taste buds. The back of the tongue contains two lumps of lymphatic tissue called **lingual tonsils.** Lingual tonsils act to destroy bacteria and viruses on the back of the tongue.

The **palate** is the roof of the mouth. It functions to separate the oral cavity from the nasal cavity. The front of the palate, the hard palate, is rigid because it has bony plates in it. The back of the palate, soft palate, lacks bony material and therefore is not rigid. The back of the

Lip

Hard palate

Soft palate

Uvula

Palatine tonsils

Tongue

Vestibule

Lip

Figure 31-3. Structures of the mouth.

soft palate hangs down into the throat, and this portion of the soft palate is called the **uvula.** The uvula acts to prevent food and liquids from entering the nose during swallowing.

At the back of the mouth are two masses of lymphatic tissue called **palatine tonsils.** Just above the palatine tonsils are two more masses of lymphatic tissue called the **pharyngeal tonsils (adenoids).** These masses of lymphatic tissue act to protect the area from bacteria and viruses (Figure 31-3).

Teeth act to decrease the size of food particles, and different types of teeth are adapted to handle food in different ways. The most medial teeth, called **incisors,** act as chisels to bite off food pieces. Teeth called **cuspids** are the sharpest teeth and they act to tear tough food (Figure 31-4). The back teeth, called **bicuspids** and **molars,** are flat. They are designed to grind food (Figure 31-5).

Salivary glands secrete saliva, which is a mixture of water, enzymes, and mucus. Salivary glands are made of two types of cells—**serous cells** and **mucous cells.** Serous cells secrete a fluid made mostly of water but the fluid also contains an enzyme called amylase that digests carbohydrates. Mucous cells secrete mucus.

All major salivary glands are paired (Figure 31-6):

- **Parotid glands:** the largest of the salivary glands, located beneath the skin just in front of the ears
- **Submandibular glands:** located in the floor of the mouth just inside the surface of the mandibles (jaws)
- **Sublingual glands:** the smallest of the salivary glands, located in the floor of the mouth beneath the tongue

The Pharynx

The **pharynx** is more commonly called the throat. It is a long, muscular structure that extends from the area behind the nose to the esophagus. It acts to connect the nasal cavity with the oral cavity for breathing through the nose. It

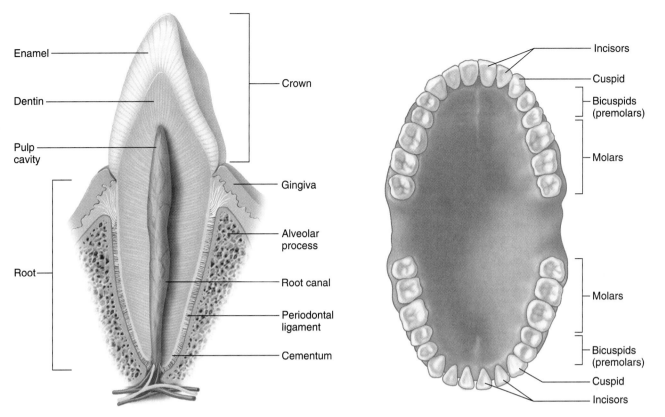

Figure 31-4. Structure of a cuspid tooth.

Figure 31-5. Types of teeth.

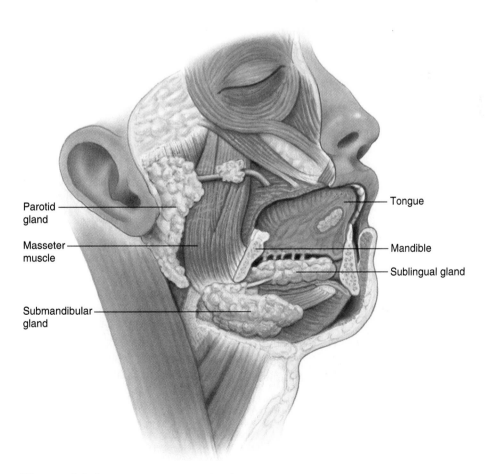

Figure 31-6. Major salivary glands.

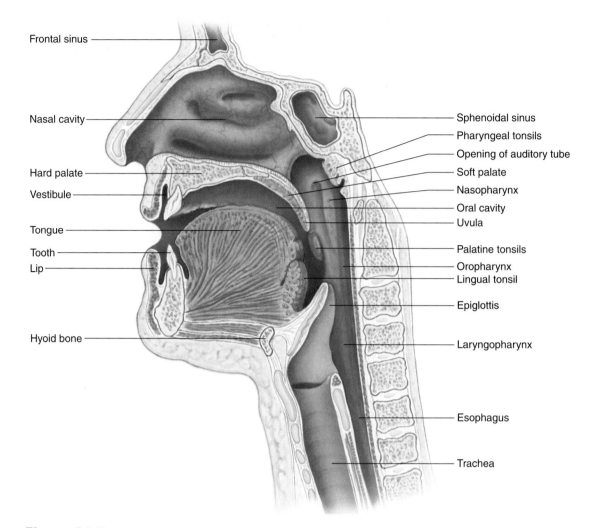

Figure 31-7. Sagittal section of the mouth, nasal cavity, and pharynx.

Frontal sinus

Nasal cavity

Hard palate

Vestibule

Tongue

Tooth

Lip

Hyoid bone

Sphenoidal sinus

Pharyngeal tonsils

Opening of auditory tube

Soft palate

Nasopharynx

Oral cavity

Uvula

Palatine tonsils

Oropharynx

Lingual tonsil

Epiglottis

Laryngopharynx

Esophagus

Trachea

also acts to push food into the esophagus (Figure 31-7). The divisions of the pharynx are:

- **Nasopharynx:** the portion behind the nasal cavity.
- **Oropharynx:** the portion behind the oral cavity.
- **Laryngopharynx:** the portion behind the larynx. The laryngopharynx continues as the esophagus.

Swallowing is largely a reflex. In other words, it is an automatic response that does not require much thought. The following events occur during swallowing:

1. The soft palate rises,causing the uvula to cover the opening between the nasal cavity and the oral cavity.
2. The **epiglottis** covers the opening of the larynx so that food does not enter it (see Figure 31-7).
3. The tongue presses against the roof of the mouth, forcing food into the oropharynx.
4. The muscles in the pharynx contract, forcing food toward the esophagus.
5. The esophagus opens.
6. Food is pushed into the esophagus by the muscles of the pharynx.

The Esophagus

The esophagus is a muscular tube that connects the pharynx to the stomach (Figures 31-7 and 31-8). It descends through the thoracic cavity, through the diaphragm, and into the abdominal cavity where it joins the stomach. The hole in the diaphragm that the esophagus goes through is called the **esophageal hiatus.** This hiatus is a common place for hernias to occur. A **hernia** develops when the stomach gets pushed up into the thoracic cavity through the esophageal hiatus. The esophageal sphincter, also known as the cardiac sphincter, controls the movement of food into the stomach. **Sphincters** are circular bands of muscle located at the openings of many tubes in the body. They open and close to allow or prevent the movement of substances out of a tube.

The Stomach

The stomach lies below the diaphragm in the upper left region of the abdominal cavity. It functions to receive food from the esophagus, mix food with **gastric juice** (secretions

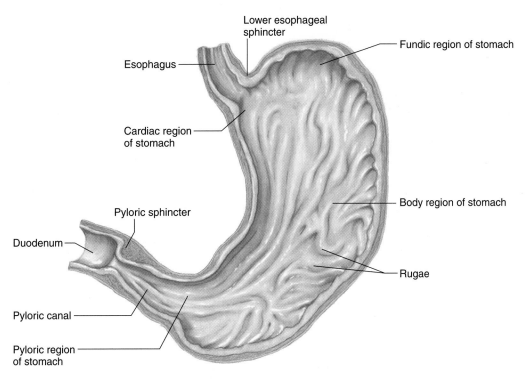

Figure 31-8. Regions of the stomach.

of the stomach lining), start protein digestion, and move food into the small intestine.

The beginning portion of the stomach that is attached to the esophagus is called the cardiac region. The portion of the stomach that balloons over the cardiac portion is called the fundic region, or fundus. The main part of the stomach is called the body, and the narrow portion that is connected to the small intestine is called the pyloric region or pylorus. A sphincter called the pyloric sphincter controls the movement of substances from the pyloric region of the stomach into the small intestine (Figure 31-8).

The lining of the stomach contains gastric glands. These glands are made of the following cell types:

- **Mucous cells.** These cells secrete mucus to protect the lining of the stomach.
- **Chief cells.** These cells secrete **pepsinogen,** which becomes **pepsin** in the presence of acid. Pepsin digests proteins.
- **Parietal cells.** These cells secrete hydrochloric acid, which is necessary to convert pepsinogen to pepsin. They also secrete **intrinsic factor,** which is necessary for vitamin B_{12} absorption.

When a person smells, tastes, or sees appetizing food, the parasympathetic nervous system stimulates the gastric glands to secrete their products. A hormone called gastrin, made by the stomach, also stimulates the gastric glands to become active. A hormone called cholecystokinin (CCK) made by the small intestine inhibits gastric glands. The stomach does not absorb many substances but it can absorb alcohol, water, and some fat-soluble drugs. The mixture of food and gastric juice is called **chyme.** Once chyme

is well mixed, stomach contractions push it into the small intestine a little at a time. It takes 4 to 8 hours for the stomach to empty following a meal.

The Small Intestine

The small intestine is a tubular organ that extends from the stomach to the large intestine. It fills most of the abdominal cavity and is coiled. The small intestine carries out most of the digestion in the body and is responsible for absorbing most of the nutrients into the bloodstream.

The beginning of the small intestine is called the **duodenum.** It is C-shaped and relatively short. The middle portion of the small intestine is called the **jejunum.** It is coiled and forms the majority of the small intestine. The last portion of the small intestine is called the **ileum,** and it is directly attached to the large intestine (Figure 31-9).

The lining of the small intestine contains cells that have **microvilli.** Microvilli greatly increase the surface area of the small intestine so that it can absorb many nutrients. The lining of the small intestine also contains intestinal glands that secrete various substances. The secretions of the small intestine include mucus and water. Water aids in digestion but some toxins cause the secretion of too much water, and this leads to diarrhea—which in turn aids the body in eliminating the toxins. Mucus protects the lining of the small intestine. The following are the major enzymes secreted by the small intestine:

- **Peptidases.** These enzymes digest proteins.
- **Sucrase, maltase,** and **lactase.** These enzymes digest sugars. A person who cannot produce lactase will not be

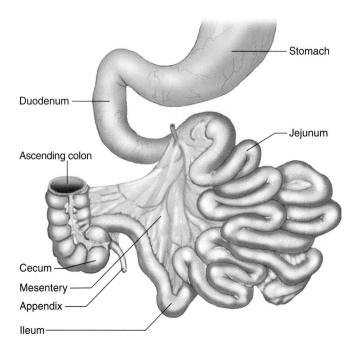

Figure 31-9. Parts of the small intestine.

able to digest lactose, which is the sugar in dairy products. This causes a condition called lactose intolerance.

- **Intestinal lipase.** This enzyme digests fats.

The parasympathetic nervous system and the stretching of the small intestine wall are the primary factors that trigger the small intestine to secrete its products. Almost all nutrients (water, glucose, amino acids, fatty acids, glycerol, and electrolytes) are absorbed by the small intestine. The wall of the small intestine contracts to mix chyme and to propel it toward the large intestine. If chyme moves too quickly through the small intestine, nutrients are not absorbed and diarrhea results. The **ileocecal sphincter** controls the movement of chyme from the ileum to the **cecum,** which is the beginning of the large intestine.

The Liver

The liver is quite large and fills most of the upper right abdominal quadrant. Part of its function is to store vitamins and iron. It is reddish-brown in color and is enclosed by a tough capsule. This capsule divides the liver into a large right lobe and a small left lobe (Figure 31-10). Each lobe is separated into smaller divisions called **hepatic lobules.** Branches of the **hepatic portal vein** carry blood from the digestive organs to the hepatic lobules. The hepatic lobules contain macrophages that destroy bacteria and viruses in the blood. Each lobule contains many cells called **hepatocytes.** Hepatocytes process the nutrients in blood and make **bile,** which is used in the digestion of fats. Bile leaves the liver through the **hepatic duct.** The hepatic duct merges with the **cystic duct** (the duct from the gallbladder) to form the **common bile duct.** This duct delivers bile to the duodenum.

The Gallbladder

The gallbladder is a small, sac-like structure located beneath the liver (Figure 31-10). Its only function is to store bile. Bile leaves the gallbladder through the cystic duct. The hormone cholecystokinin causes the gallbladder to release bile. The salts in bile break large fat globules into smaller ones so that they can be more quickly digested by the digestive enzymes. Bile salts also increase the absorption of fatty acids, cholesterol, and fat-soluble vitamins into the bloodstream.

The Pancreas

The pancreas is located behind the stomach. Pancreatic **acinar cells** produce pancreatic juice, which ultimately flows through the pancreatic duct to the duodenum (Figure 31-11). Pancreatic juice contains the following enzymes:

- **Pancreatic amylase.** This enzyme digests carbohydrates.

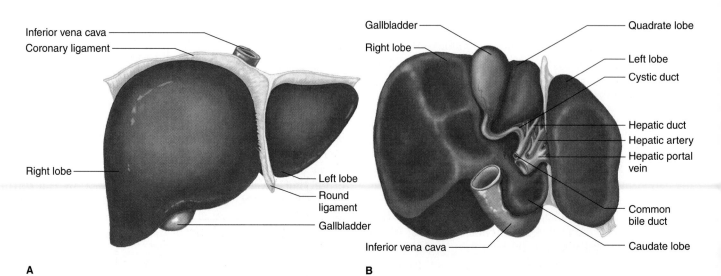

A   **B**

Figure 31-10. Liver and gallbladder: (a) anterior view and (b) inferior view.

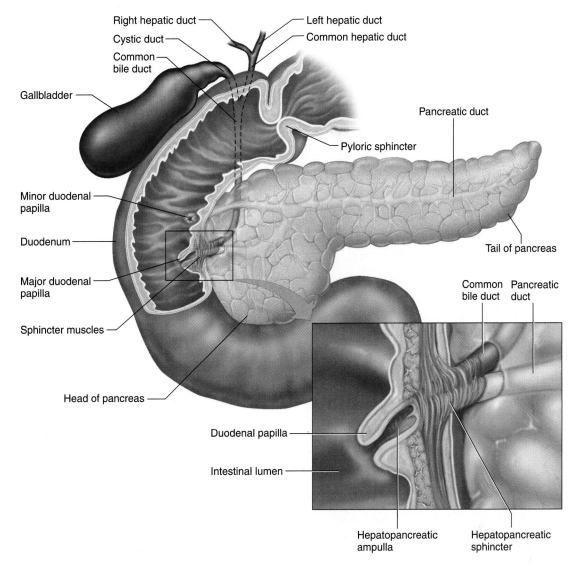

Figure 31-11. Pancreas and its connections to the gallbladder and duodenum.

- **Pancreatic lipase.** This enzyme digests lipids.
- **Nucleases.** These enzymes digest nucleic acids.
- **Trypsin, chymotrypsin,** and **carboxypeptidase.** These enzymes digest proteins.

The pancreas also secretes bicarbonate ions into the duodenum. These ions neutralize the acidic chyme arriving from the stomach. The parasympathetic nervous system stimulates the pancreas to release its enzymes. The hormones secretin and cholecystokinin also stimulate the pancreas to release digestive enzymes. Secretin and cholecystokinin come from the small intestine.

The Large Intestine

The large intestine extends from the ileum of the small intestine to where it opens to the outside world as the anus. The beginning of the large intestine is the cecum. Projecting off the cecum is the **vermiform appendix.** The appendix is mostly made of lymphoid tissue and has no significant function in humans. The cecum eventually gives rise to the **ascending colon,** which is the portion of the large intestine that runs up the right side of the abdominal cavity. The ascending colon becomes the **transverse colon** as it crosses the abdominal cavity; from there it becomes the **descending colon** as it descends the left side of the abdominal cavity. In the pelvic cavity, the descending colon then forms an S-shaped tube called the **sigmoid colon.**

The Rectum and Anal Canal

Eventually the sigmoid colon straightens out to become the **rectum.** The last few centimeters of the rectum is called the **anal canal,** and the opening of the anal canal to the outside world is called the anus (Figure 31-12).

The lining of the large intestine only secretes mucus to aid in the movement of substances. As chyme leaves the small intestine and enters the large intestine, the proximal portion of the large intestine absorbs water and a few electrolytes from it. The leftover chyme is then called **feces.**

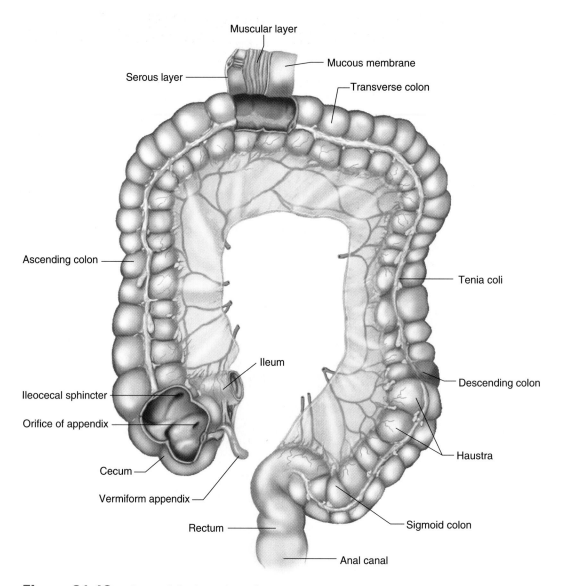

Figure 31-12. Parts of the large intestine.

Feces are made of undigested solid materials, a little water, ions, mucus, cells of the intestinal lining, and bacteria.

The contractions of the large intestine propel feces forward but these contractions normally occur periodically and as mass movements. Mass movements trigger the **defecation reflex,** which allows anal sphincters to relax and feces to move through the anus in the process of elimination. The squeezing actions of the abdominal wall muscles also aid in the emptying of the large intestine.

The Absorption of Nutrients

Nutrients are defined as necessary food substances. They include carbohydrates, proteins, lipids, vitamins, minerals, and water.

Three types of carbohydrates that humans ingest are starches **(polysaccharides),** simple sugars **(monosaccharides** and **disaccharides),** and **cellulose.** Starches come from foods such as pasta, potatoes, rice, and breads. Monosaccharides and disaccharides are obtained from sweet foods and fruits. Cellulose is a type of carbohydrate found in many vegetables that cannot be digested by humans. Therefore, cellulose provides fiber or bulk for the large intestine. This fiber helps the large intestine empty more regularly.

Most body cells use the monosaccharide glucose to make ATP. When a person has an excess of glucose, it can be stored in the liver and skeletal muscle cells as **glycogen.**

Lipids (fats) are obtained through various foods. The most abundant dietary lipids are **triglycerides.** They are found in meats, eggs, milk, and butter. Cholesterol is another common dietary lipid and is found in eggs, whole milk, butter, and cheeses. Lipids are used by the body primarily to make energy when glucose levels are low. Excess triglycerides are stored in adipose tissue. Cholesterol is essential to cell growth and function; cells use it to

TABLE 31-1 Common Vitamins and Their Importance in the Body

Vitamin	Function
Vitamin A	Needed for the production of visual receptors, mucus, the normal growth for bones and teeth, and the repair of epithelial tissues
Vitamin B₁ (thiamine)	Needed for the metabolism of carbohydrates
Vitamin B₂ (riboflavin)	Needed for carbohydrate and fat metabolism and for the growth of cells
Vitamin B₆	Needed for the synthesis of protein, antibodies, and nucleic acid
Vitamin B₁₂ (cyanocobalamin)	Needed for myelin production and the metabolism of carbohydrates and nucleic acids
Biotin	Needed for the metabolism of proteins, fats, and nucleic acids
Folic acid	Needed for the production of amino acids, DNA, and red blood cells
Pantothenic acid	Needed for carbohydrate and fat metabolism
Niacin	Needed for the metabolism of carbohydrates, proteins, fats, and nucleic acids
Vitamin C (ascorbic acid)	Needed for the production of collagen, amino acids, and hormones and for the absorption of iron
Vitamin D	Needed for the absorption of calcium
Vitamin E	Antioxidant that prevents the breakdown of certain tissues
Vitamin K	Needed for blood clotting

make cell membranes and some hormones. People should have the essential fatty acid **linoleic acid** in their diet since the body cannot make it. This fatty acid is found in corn and sunflower oils. People also need a certain amount of fat to absorb fat-soluble vitamins.

Foods rich in protein include meats, eggs, milk, fish, chicken, turkey, nuts, cheese, and beans. Protein requirements vary from individual to individual, but all people must take in proteins that contain certain amino acids (called essential amino acids) because the body cannot make them. Proteins are used by the body for growth and the repair of tissues.

The fat-soluble vitamins are vitamins A, D, E, and K, and the water-soluble vitamins are all the B vitamins and vitamin C. Vitamins have many functions; they are summarized in Table 31-1.

Minerals make up about 4% of total body weight. They are primarily found in bones and teeth. Cells use minerals to make enzymes, cell membranes, and various proteins such as hemoglobin. The most important minerals to the human body are calcium, phosphorus, sulfur, sodium, chlorine, and magnesium. Trace elements are elements needed in very small amounts by the body. They include iron, manganese, copper, iodine, and zinc.

Pathophysiology

Common Diseases and Disorders of the Digestive System

Appendicitis is an inflammation of the appendix. If not treated promptly, it can be life-threatening.

- **Causes.** This disorder is caused by blockage of the appendix with feces or a tumor.

- **Signs and symptoms.** The signs and symptoms include lack of appetite, pain in or around the navel area or in the abdomen, nausea, slight fever, pain in the right leg, and an increased white blood cell count.

continued ⟶

Common Diseases and Disorders of the Digestive System *(continued)*

- **Treatment.** The primary treatments are antibiotics to prevent infection or surgery to remove the appendix.

Cirrhosis is a long-lasting liver disease in which normal liver tissue is replaced with nonfunctional scar tissue.

- **Causes.** This disease is often an autoimmune disease. It may be caused by some medications and alcohol consumption. Hepatitis B and C infections can also contribute to the development of cirrhosis.
- **Signs and symptoms.** There are many symptoms to this disease. They include anemia, fatigue, mental confusion, fever, vomiting, blood in the vomit, an enlarged liver, jaundice, unintended weight loss, swelling of the legs or abdomen, abdominal pain, a decreased urine output, and pale feces.
- **Treatment.** Alcohol consumption should be discontinued. A patient with cirrhosis may be given various medications, including antibiotics and diuretics. A liver transplant may be needed for the most seriously ill patients.

Colitis is defined as inflammation of the large intestine. This condition can be chronic or short-lived, depending on the cause.

- **Causes.** Colitis can be caused by a viral or bacterial infection or the use of antibiotics. Ulcers in the large intestine, Crohn's disease, various other diseases, and stress may also contribute to the development of this disorder.
- **Signs and symptoms.** The primary symptoms are abdominal pain, bloating, and diarrhea.
- **Treatment.** The first goal of therapy is to treat the underlying causes. Changing antibiotics, treating existing ulcers, and drinking plenty of fluids are other treatment options.

Colorectal cancer usually comes from the lining of the rectum or colon. This type of cancer is curable if treated early.

- **Causes.** The causes are mostly unknown. Polyps in the colon or rectum can become cancerous, leading to this disease. Colorectal cancer may be prevented through regular screenings for polyps.
- **Signs and symptoms.** Anemia, unintended weight loss, abdominal pain, blood in the feces, narrow feces, or changes in bowel movement are all common symptoms.
- **Treatment.** Chemotherapy is the first line of treatment. Surgery to remove a cancerous tumor or the affected portions of colon or rectum may be needed in more serious cases.

Constipation is the condition of difficult defecation, which is the elimination of feces.

- **Causes.** The primary causes are a lack of physical activity, a lack of fiber in the diet, the use of certain medications, and thyroid and colon disorders.

- **Signs and symptoms.** Common signs and symptoms include infrequent bowel movements (for example, no bowel movement for 3 days), bloating, abdominal pain and pain during bowel movements, hard feces, and blood on the surface of feces.
- **Treatment.** Treatment includes an increase in fiber intake, regular exercise, and the use of stool softeners, laxatives, and enemas.

Crohn's disease is a common type of disorder called inflammatory bowel disease. It typically affects the end of the small intestine.

- **Causes.** This disease is an autoimmune disorder.
- **Signs and symptoms.** The signs and systems of Crohn's disease include fever, tender gums, joint pain, ulcers, abdominal pain and gas, constipation or diarrhea, abnormal abdominal sounds, weight loss, intestinal bleeding, and blood in the feces.
- **Treatment.** The first treatment is to change the patient's diet. Other treatments include medications to reduce inflammation and antibiotics. For the most serious cases, surgery to remove the affected part of the intestine may be needed.

Diarrhea is the condition of watery and frequent feces. Many cases of diarrhea do not require treatment because they usually stop within a day or two.

- **Causes.** The causes of diarrhea include bacterial, viral, or parasitic infections of the digestive system. It may also be caused by the ingestion of toxins; food allergies, including lactose intolerance; ulcers; Crohn's disease; laxatives; antibiotics; chemotherapy; and radiation therapy. Diarrhea may be prevented by thoroughly washing hands and cooking food properly.
- **Signs and symptoms.** The symptoms include abdominal cramps, watery feces, and the frequent passage of feces.
- **Treatment.** Patients should drink fluids to prevent dehydration. The underlying causes should be treated. Medications and dietary changes are the primary treatment options.

Diverticulitis is inflammation of diverticuli in the intestine. Diverticuli are abnormal dilations in the intestinal wall.

- **Causes.** The causes are mostly unknown. Lack of fiber in the diet and a bacterial infection of the diverticuli can cause this disorder.
- **Signs and symptoms.** Signs and symptoms include fever, nausea, abdominal pain, constipation or diarrhea, blood in the feces, and a high white blood cell count.
- **Treatment.** Treatments include a diet high in fiber, antibiotics, and surgery to remove the affected portion of the intestine.

continued ⟶

Common Diseases and Disorders of the Digestive System *(continued)*

Gastritis is an inflammation of the stomach lining. It is often referred to as an "upset stomach."

- **Causes.** Gastritis can be caused by bacteria or viruses, some medications, the use of alcohol, spicy foods, excessive eating, poisons, and stress. Cooking food properly to kill harmful bacteria and viruses can help to prevent this condition.
- **Signs and symptoms.** Symptoms include nausea, lack of appetite, heartburn, vomiting, and abdominal cramps.
- **Treatment.** Lifestyle changes should be implemented to avoid foods or medications that irritate the stomach lining. Treatment with various medications to reduce the production of stomach acids can provide relief from the symptoms of this disorder.

Heartburn is also called **gastroesophageal reflux disease (GERD)**. It occurs when stomach acids are pushed into the esophagus.

- **Causes.** Alcohol, some foods, a defective esophageal sphincter, pregnancy, obesity, a hiatal hernia, and repeated vomiting can contribute to the development of this disease.
- **Signs and symptoms.** Common symptoms include frequent burping, difficulty swallowing, a sore throat, a burning sensation in the chest following meals, nausea, and blood in the vomit.
- **Treatment.** Treatment includes losing weight, making dietary changes, reducing the consumption of alcohol, taking medications, and not lying down after meals.

Hemorrhoids are varicose veins of the rectum or anus.

- **Causes.** Hemorrhoids are caused by constipation, excessive straining during bowel movements, liver disease, pregnancy, and obesity.
- **Signs and symptoms.** Signs and symptoms include itching in the anal area, painful bowel movements, bright red blood on feces, and veins that protrude from the anus.
- **Treatment.** Constipation can be avoided or improved by eating a high-fiber diet. Other treatments include stool softeners, medications to reduce the inflammation of hemorrhoids, and the surgical removal of hemorrhoids.

Hepatitis is defined as inflammation of the liver. There are many different types of hepatitis.

- **Causes.** Causes include bacteria, viruses, parasites, immune disorders, the use of alcohol and drugs, and an overdose of acetaminophen. Preventive measures include getting vaccinations, practicing safe sex, avoiding undercooked food (especially seafood), and using prescription or over-the-counter drugs at their recommended dosages.

- **Signs and symptoms.** Symptoms include mild fever, bloating, lack of appetite, nausea, vomiting, abdominal pain, weakness, jaundice, the itching of various body parts, an enlarged liver, dark urine, and breast development in males.
- **Treatment.** Patients should avoid using alcohol and drugs. Various medications may be prescribed.

A *hiatal hernia* occurs when a portion of the stomach protrudes into the chest through an opening in the diaphragm.

- **Causes.** The causes are mostly unknown, although obesity and smoking are considered risk factors. Eating small meals can be an effective preventive measure.
- **Signs and symptoms.** Signs and symptoms include excessive burping, difficulty swallowing, chest pain, and heartburn.
- **Treatment.** Treatments are weight reduction, medications to reduce the production of stomach acid, and surgical repair of the hernia.

Inguinal hernias occur when a portion of the large intestine protrudes into the inguinal canal, which is located where the thigh and the body trunk meet. In males, the hernia can also protrude into the scrotum.

- **Causes.** The causes are mostly unknown, although these hernias may be caused by weak muscles in the abdominal walls.
- **Signs and symptoms.** A lump in the groin or scrotum, or pain in the groin area that gets worse when bending or straining are the common symptoms.
- **Treatment.** Pain medications may be prescribed. Surgery to repair the hernia is needed when the large intestine is pushed back into the abdominal cavity.

Oral cancer usually involves the lips or tongue but can occur anywhere in the mouth. This type of cancer tends to spread rapidly to other organs.

- **Causes.** The causes are mostly unknown, although the use of tobacco products and alcohol are known risk factors. Poor oral hygiene and ulcers in the mouth can also cause oral cancer.
- **Signs and symptoms.** Signs and symptoms include difficulty tasting, problems swallowing, and ulcers on the tongue, lip, or other mouth structures.
- **Treatment.** Radiation therapy, chemotherapy, and surgical removal of the tumor are the treatment options.

Pancreatic cancer is the fourth leading cause of cancer death in the United States.

- **Causes.** Causes are mostly unknown, although smoking is considered a risk factor.
- **Signs and symptoms.** Common signs and symptoms include depression, fatigue, lack of appetite, nausea or

continued ⟶

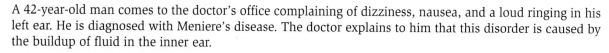
A 42-year-old man comes to the doctor's office complaining of dizziness, nausea, and a loud ringing in his left ear. He is diagnosed with Meniere's disease. The doctor explains to him that this disorder is caused by the buildup of fluid in the inner ear.

As you read this chapter, consider the following questions:

1. Why is the patient experiencing dizziness and difficulty hearing?
2. What is the clinical term for ringing in the ear?
3. What precautions should this patient take because of his dizziness?
4. A diuretic is a drug that decreases fluids in the body. Why might the doctor prescribe a diuretic?

The Nose and the Sense of Smell

Smell receptors are also called **olfactory** receptors and are **chemoreceptors.** This means that they respond to changes in chemical concentrations. Chemicals that activate smell receptors must be dissolved in the mucus of the nose. Therefore, a person who has a "dry nose" has trouble smelling.

Smell receptors are located in the olfactory organ, which is in the upper part of the nasal cavity. Humans have a relatively poor sense of smell compared to animals because chemicals must diffuse all the way up the nasal cavity in order to activate smell receptors.

Once smell receptors are activated, they send their information to the olfactory nerves. The olfactory nerves send the information along olfactory bulbs and tracts to different areas of the cerebrum. The cerebrum interprets the information as a particular type of smell (Figure 33-1).

An interesting fact about smell is that it undergoes **sensory adaptation,** which means that the same chemical can stimulate smell receptors for only a limited amount of time. Eventually, the smell receptors no longer respond to the chemical, and it can no longer be smelled. Sensory adaptation explains why you smell perfume when you first encounter it, but after a few minutes you cannot smell it or may be less aware of it.

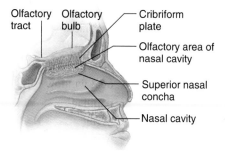

Figure 33-1. The olfactory area (organ) is located in the superior part of the nasal cavity.

Olfactory tract — Olfactory bulb — Cribriform plate — Olfactory area of nasal cavity — Superior nasal concha — Nasal cavity

The Tongue and the Sense of Taste

Taste, or **gustatory,** receptors are located on taste buds. **Taste buds** are found on the "bumps" of the tongue. These bumps are called **papillae,** which many people incorrectly think are the actual taste buds. Taste buds are microscopic and cannot be seen with the naked eye. Some taste buds are also scattered on the roof of the mouth and in the walls of the throat.

Each taste bud is made of taste cells and supporting cells. The taste cells function as taste receptors, and the supporting cells simply fill in the spaces between the taste cells. Taste cells are types of chemoreceptors because they are activated by chemicals that must be dissolved in saliva (Figure 33-2).

There are four types of taste cells, and each type is activated by a particular group of chemicals. Therefore, the following four primary taste sensations are produced:

1. Sweet. Taste cells that respond to "sweet" chemicals are concentrated at the tip of the tongue.
2. Sour. Taste cells that respond to "sour" chemicals are concentrated on the sides of the tongue.
3. Salty. Taste cells that respond to "salty" chemicals are concentrated on the tip and sides of the tongue.
4. Bitter. Taste cells that respond to "bitter" chemicals are concentrated at the back of the tongue.

Eating spicy foods activates pain receptors on the tongue. Once taste cells are activated, they send their information to several cranial nerves. The information eventually reaches the gustatory cortex in the parietal lobe of the cerebrum. The gustatory cortex interprets the information as a particular taste.

The Eye and the Sense of Sight

The sense of sight comes from the eyes and is also supported by visual accessory organs.

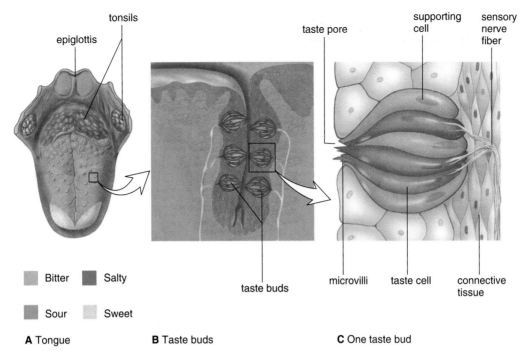

tonsils

epiglottis

taste pore

supporting cell

sensory nerve fiber

- Bitter
- Salty
- Sour
- Sweet

taste buds

microvilli

taste cell

connective tissue

A Tongue   **B** Taste buds   **C** One taste bud

Figure 33-2. Tongue and taste buds. (a) Areas of the tongue are sensitive to different tastes, as indicated. (b) Taste buds are on and in papillae. (c) Taste buds are composed of taste cells and supporting cells.

Structure of the Eye

The eye is hollow and spherical shaped. It consists of cavities, wall layers, and other structures.

The Cavities of the Eye. Each eyeball is divided into two cavities—the anterior and the posterior.

The Anterior Cavity. The anterior cavity is in front of the lens and is filled with a watery fluid called **aqueous humor.** Aqueous humor provides nutrients to structures in the anterior cavity of the eyeball. When too much aqueous humor is produced, a person develops **glaucoma.**

The Posterior Cavity. The posterior cavity of the eyeball is behind the lens and is filled with a very thick fluid called **vitreous humor.** Vitreous humor keeps the retina flat and helps to maintain the shape of the eye.

The Wall of the Eye. In addition to the cavities of the eye, the eye is composed of a wall that has three layers: the outer, middle, and inner (Figure 33-3).

Outer Layer. The outer layer is also called the fibrous layer because it is composed of tough, dense connective tissue. The two divisions of the outer layer are the sclera and cornea. The **sclera** is the "white of the eye" and does not allow light to enter the eye. The **cornea** is anterior to the sclera and allows light to enter the eye. It is often called the "window of the eye." The entire outer layer contains no blood vessels but is supplied with many sensory receptors that can detect even the smallest of particles on the surface of the eyeball.

Middle Layer. The middle layer is also called the vascular and pigmented layer because it is richly supplied with blood vessels and pigments. The middle layer consists of the **choroid, ciliary body,** and **iris.** The choroid lines the sclera and functions to absorb extra light that has entered the eye. The ciliary body functions to hold and move the lens. The lens is moved back and forth to allow the eye to focus on images. The lens is usually transparent but "cloudy" areas called **cataracts** can form, which prevent light from reaching visual receptors. The iris, which is the most anterior structure of this layer, controls the amount of light that enters the eye. The iris also contains the color of a person's eyes. The hole in the iris is called the **pupil.**

Inner Layer. The inner layer is also called the **retina.** This layer contains visual receptors called **rods** and **cones.** Rods allow a person to see images in dim light as well as the general outlines of structures. Rods also detect black, white, and gray shades. A person who suffers from night blindness has defective rods. Cones allow a person to see images in bright light and to see details of structures. Cones also detect colors other than white, black, and gray. A person who has red-green color blindness lacks the cones needed to see reds and greens.

Visual Accessory Organs

Visual accessory organs assist and protect the eyeball. They include eyelids, conjunctivas, the lacrimal apparatus, and extrinsic eye muscles.

REVIEW

CHAPTER 33

CASE STUDY QUESTIONS

Now that you have completed this chapter, review the case study at the beginning of the chapter and answer the following questions:

1. Why is the patient experiencing dizziness and difficulty hearing?
2. What is the clinical term for ringing in the ear?
3. What precautions should this patient take because of his dizziness?
4. A diuretic is a drug that decreases fluids in the body. Why might the doctor prescribe a diuretic?

Discussion Questions

1. Describe how sound waves travel through the ear from the auricle to hearing receptors. Where is sound interpreted?
2. Describe the structures that light must pass through in order to reach the retina. Where is vision interpreted?
3. Identify the four primary taste sensations and tell what part of the tongue is associated with each.
4. Describe how smell receptors are activated.

Critical Thinking Questions

1. Why does a sewage treatment plant have a strong, offensive odor to visitors of the plant but not to regular workers at the plant?

2. How are the signs and symptoms of cataracts, glaucoma, and macular degeneration different?
3. Sudden loud sounds can damage the eardrums. What type of hearing loss will these sounds produce? Chronic loud sounds damage hearing receptors. What type of hearing loss do these sounds produce?

Application Activities

1. Give the functions of the following:
    a. Iris
    b. Cornea
    c. Lens
    d. Retina
    e. Ciliary body
2. State if the following structures are part of the outer, middle, or inner ear. Also give the function of each.
    a. Vestibule
    b. Cochlea
    c. External auditory canal
    e. Ear ossicles
    e. Tympanic membrane
3. What are the two kinds of cells in taste buds?
4. Where is the olfactory organ located?

Internet Activity

Find a Web site that provides information on hearing and balance. Research ways to prevent ear damage that could cause problems with balance.

CHAPTER 34

The Urinary System

CHAPTER OUTLINE

- The Kidneys
- Urine Formation
- The Ureters, Urinary Bladder, and Urethra

OBJECTIVES

After completing Chapter 34, you will be able to:

34.1 Describe the structure, location, and functions of the kidney.

34.2 Define the term *nephron* and describe its structure.

34.3 Explain how nephrons filter blood and form urine.

34.4 List substances normally found in urine.

34.5 Describe the locations, structures, and functions of the ureters, bladder, and urethra.

34.6 Explain how urination is controlled.

34.7 Describe the signs, symptoms, causes, and treatments of various diseases and disorders of the urinary system.

KEY TERMS (Continued)

renin	tubular reabsorption	ureters
retroperitoneal	tubular secretion	urethra
trigone	urea	uric acid

KEY TERMS

afferent arterioles
angiotensin II
calyces
cystitis
detrusor muscle
distal convoluted
    tubule
efferent arterioles
glomerular capsule
glomerular filtrate
glomerular filtration
glomerulonephritis
glomerulus
incontinence
juxtaglomerular
    apparatus
juxtaglomerular
    cells
loop of Henle
macula densa
micturition
nephrons
proximal convoluted
    tubule
pyelonephritis
renal calculi
renal column
renal corpuscle
renal cortex
renal medulla
renal pelvis
renal pyramids
renal sinus
renal tubule

Introduction

The organs of the urinary system are the kidneys, ureters, urinary bladder, and urethra (Figure 34-1). This system functions to remove waste products from the bloodstream. These waste products are excreted from the body in the form of urine. Nephrons are microscopic structures in the kidneys that filter blood and form urine.

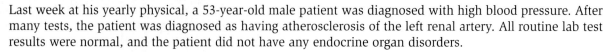

Last week at his yearly physical, a 53-year-old male patient was diagnosed with high blood pressure. After many tests, the patient was diagnosed as having atherosclerosis of the left renal artery. All routine lab test results were normal, and the patient did not have any endocrine organ disorders.

As you read this chapter, consider the following questions:

1. How does atherosclerosis affect blood flow?
2. How does atherosclerosis of a renal artery produce high blood pressure?
3. What lifestyle changes should this patient make?
4. What can happen to the patient's kidney if his atherosclerosis is not treated?

The Kidneys

The kidneys are responsible for removing metabolic waste products from the blood. These metabolic wastes are combined with water and ions to form urine, which is excreted from the body. The kidneys also secrete the hormone erythropoietin, which helps to regulate red blood cell production, and the hormone **renin,** which helps to regulate blood pressure.

The kidneys are bean-shaped organs that are reddish brown in color. Tough, fibrous capsules cover them. The kidneys are **retroperitoneal** in position, which means that they lie behind the peritoneal cavity. They lie on either side of the vertebral column at about the level of the lumbar vertebrae.

The medial depression of a kidney is called a **renal sinus.** The entrance of the sinus is called the hilum and contains the renal artery, renal vein, and ureter. The **ureter** is a tube that carries urine out of a kidney to the urinary bladder. Inside the kidney, the ureter expands as the **renal pelvis.** The renal pelvis divides into small tubes inside the kidney called **calyces.**

The outermost layer of the kidney is called the **renal cortex,** and the middle portion is called the **renal medulla.** The renal medulla is divided into triangular-shaped areas called **renal pyramids.** The renal cortex covers the pyramids and also dips down between the pyramids. The portion of the cortex between pyramids is called a **renal column** (Figure 34-2.)

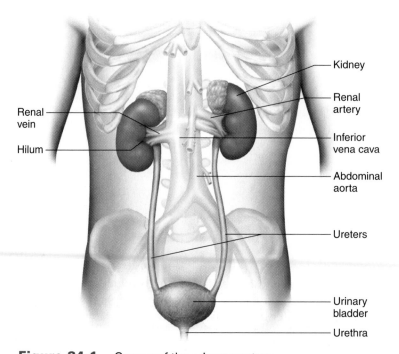

Figure 34-1. Organs of the urinary system.

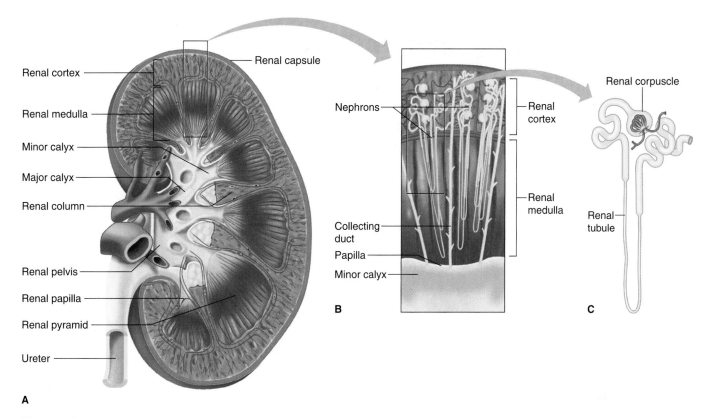

Figure 34-2. (a) Longitudinal section of a kidney, (b) the location of nephrons, and (c) a single nephron.

Blood flows through a kidney by the following pathway:

renal artery → interlobar arteries → arcuate arteries → interlobular arteries → afferent arterioles → nephrons

Blood eventually leaves the kidney through a renal vein.

Nephrons

Waste products are removed from the blood through **nephrons.** Each kidney contains about one million nephrons. Nephrons are made of a **renal corpuscle** and a **renal tubule** (Figure 34-2). A renal corpuscle is composed of a group of capillaries called a **glomerulus,** and the capsule that surrounds the glomerulus is called a **glomerular capsule.** The renal corpuscle is where blood filtration occurs.

Renal tubules extend from the glomerular capsule of a nephron. The three parts of a renal tubule are the **proximal convoluted tubule,** the **loop of Henle,** and the **distal convoluted tubule.** The proximal convoluted tubule is directly attached to the glomerular capsule and eventually straightens out to become the loop of Henle. The loop of Henle curves back toward the renal corpuscle and starts to twist again, becoming the distal convoluted tubule. Distal convoluted tubules from several nephrons merge together to form collecting ducts. These ducts collect urine and deliver it to the renal pelvis, which in turn empties urine into the ureters (Figures 34-2 and 34-3).

Afferent arterioles deliver blood to the glomeruli, and **efferent arterioles** carry blood away from them. Efferent arterioles deliver blood to peritubular capillaries, which are wrapped around the renal tubules of the nephron. Blood leaves the peritubular capillaries through the veins of the kidneys. By the time the blood leaves the peritubular capillaries, it has been cleansed of waste products. Blood flows through a nephron in the following pathway:

afferent arteriole → glomerulus → efferent arteriole → peritubular capillaries → the veins of the kidney

Juxtaglomerular Apparatus. Most nephrons contain a **juxtaglomerular apparatus,** which is made up of two structures—the **macula densa** and **juxtaglomerular cells.** The macula densa is an area of the distal convoluted tubule that touches afferent and efferent arterioles. Juxtaglomerular cells are simply enlarged smooth muscle cells in the walls of either the afferent or efferent arteriole. The juxtaglomerular apparatus secretes the hormone renin, which regulates blood pressure.

Urine Formation

The three processes of urine formation are **glomerular filtration, tubular reabsorption,** and **tubular secretion.**

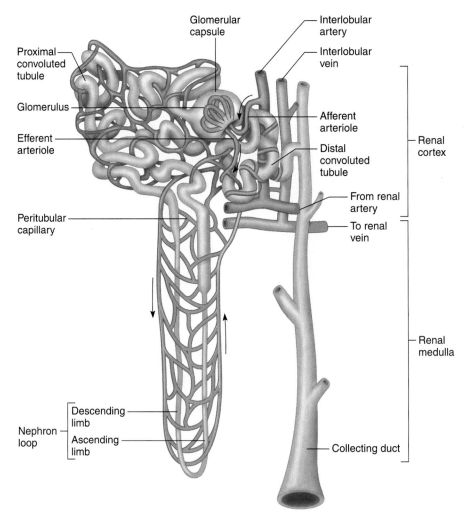

Figure 34-3. Structure of a nephron and its associated blood vessels.

Glomerular Filtration

Glomerular filtration takes place in the renal corpuscles of nephrons. In this process, the fluid part of blood is forced from the glomerulus (the capillaries) into the glomerular capsule (Figure 34-4). The fluid in the glomerular capsule is called the **glomerular filtrate.**

Glomerular filtration depends on filtration pressure, which is the amount of pressure that forces substances out of the glomerulus into the glomerular capsule. It is largely determined by blood pressure. If a person's blood pressure is too low, glomerular filtrate will not form. If filtration pressure increases, the rate of filtration and the amount of glomerular filtrate also increase.

The sympathetic nervous system largely controls the rate of filtration. If blood pressure or blood volume drops, the sympathetic nervous system causes the afferent arterioles in the kidneys to constrict. When afferent arterioles constrict, glomerular filtration pressure decreases and less glomerular filtrate is formed. When less glomerular filtrate is formed, less urine is ultimately formed. This allows the body to retain fluids that are needed to raise blood pressure and blood volume.

The juxtaglomerular apparatus also helps to regulate the filtration rate. When blood pressure drops, juxtaglomerular cells secrete renin. Renin causes the formation of **angiotensin II,** which raises blood pressure and causes the secretion of a hormone called aldosterone. Aldosterone causes the body to retain the fluids needed to maintain blood volume and pressure.

Tubular Reabsorption

Tubular reabsorption is the second process in urine formation. In this process, the glomerular filtrate flows into the proximal convoluted tubule (Figure 34-5a). The body needs to keep many of the substances (nutrients, water, and ions) that are found in glomerular filtrate. In tubular reabsorption, all the necessary substances in the glomerular filtrate pass through the wall of the renal tubule into the blood of the peritubular capillaries.

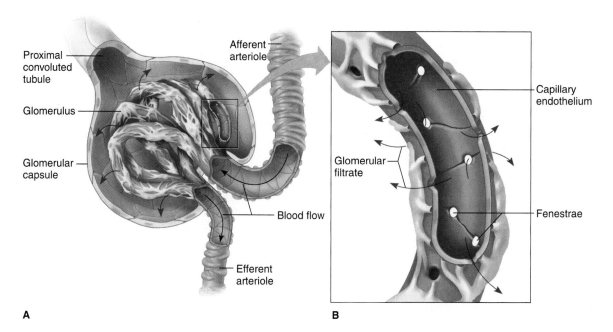

A

B

Figure 34-4. Glomerular filtration. (a) Substances move out of glomerular capillaries and into the glomerular capsule. (b) Glomerular capillaries have large holes called fenestrae that allow substances to move out of them and into a glomerular capsule.

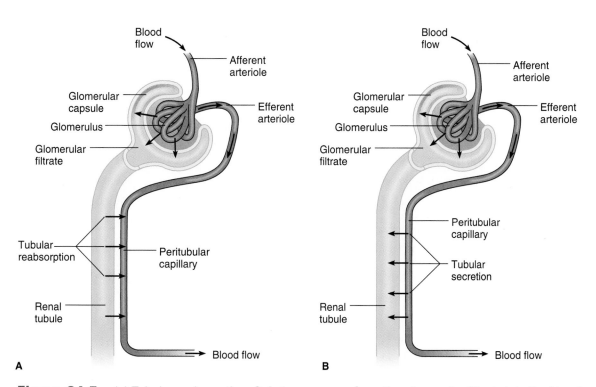

A

B

Figure 34-5. (a) Tubular reabsorption. Substances move from the glomerular filtrate into the blood of peritubular capillaries. (b) Tubular secretion. Substances move out of the blood of the peritubular capillaries into the renal tubule.

Water reabsorption varies depending on the presence of two hormones—antidiuretic hormone and aldosterone. Both of these hormones increase water reabsorption, which decreases urine production.

Tubular Secretion

Tubular secretion is the third process of urine formation. In tubular secretion, substances move out of the blood in the peritubular capillaries and into the renal tubules (Figure 34-5b). Substances that are secreted include drugs, hydrogen ions, and waste products. All of these secreted substances will be excreted in the urine.

Urine Composition

The final solution that reaches the collecting ducts of the kidneys is urine. Urine is mostly made of water but also normally contains **urea, uric acid,** trace amounts of amino acids, and various ions. Urea and uric acid are waste products formed by the breakdown of proteins and nucleic acids.

The Ureters, Urinary Bladder, and Urethra
The Ureters

Ureters are long, muscular tubes that carry urine from the kidneys to the urinary bladder. They propel urine toward the bladder through peristalsis.

Urinary Bladder

The urinary bladder is a distensible (expandable) organ that is located in the pelvic cavity. Its function is to store urine until it is eliminated from the body. The internal floor of the bladder contains three openings—one for the urethra and two for the ureters. These three openings form a triangle called the **trigone** of the bladder. The wall of the bladder contains smooth muscle, called the **detrusor muscle.** This muscle contracts to push urine from the bladder into the urethra (Figure 34-6).

The process of urination is called **micturition.** The stretching of the bladder triggers this process. The major events of micturition are the following:

1. The detrusor muscle contracts.
2. The internal urethral sphincter opens. This sphincter is located just above the opening of the urethra. When this sphincter opens, a person feels the urgency to urinate.
3. The external urethral sphincter opens. This sphincter is located below the internal urethral sphincter. A person can voluntarily keep this sphincter closed.
4. When the external urethral sphincter opens, urine flows out of the bladder through the urethra.

The Urethra

The **urethra** is a tube that moves urine from the bladder to the outside world. In females, the urethra is much shorter than in males. For this reason, females are much more susceptible to urinary tract infections.

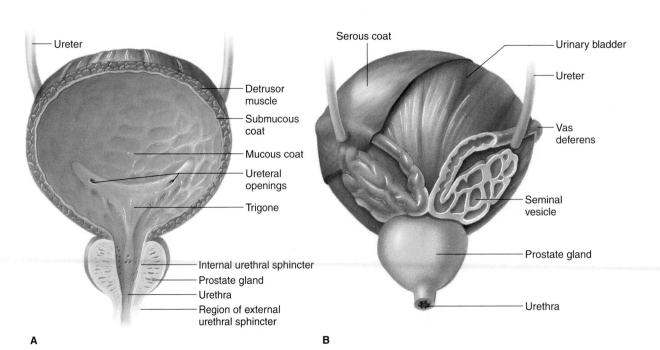

Figure 34-6. Male urinary bladder: (a) anterior view and (b) posterior view.

Pathophysiology

Common Diseases and Disorders of the Urinary System

Acute kidney failure is a sudden loss of kidney function.

- **Causes.** There are many causes and risk factors of kidney failure, including burns, dehydration, low blood pressure, hemorrhaging, allergic reactions, obstruction of the renal artery, various poisons, alcohol abuse, trauma to the kidneys and skeletal muscles, blood disorders, blood transfusion reactions, kidney stones, urinary tract infections, enlarged prostate, childbirth and immune system disorders, and food poisoning involving the bacteria *E. coli*.
- **Signs and symptoms.** The signs and symptoms include decreased urine production or no urine production, excessive urination, swelling of the arms or legs, bloating, mental confusion, coma, seizures, hand tremors, nosebleeds, easy bruising, pain in the back or abdomen, high blood pressure, abnormal heart or lung sounds, abnormal urinalysis, and an increase in potassium levels.
- **Treatment.** The first treatment measure is modifying the diet to decrease the amount of protein consumed. Controlling fluid intake and potassium levels is also recommended. Antibiotics and dialysis may also be needed.

Chronic kidney failure is a condition in which the kidneys slowly lose their ability to function. Sometimes symptoms do not appear until the kidneys have lost about 90% of their function.

- **Causes.** This disorder results from diabetes, high blood pressure, glomerulonephritis, polycystic kidney disease, kidney stones, obstruction of the ureters, and acute kidney failure.
- **Signs and symptoms.** The list of signs and symptoms is extensive and includes headache, mental confusion, coma, seizures, fatigue, frequent hiccups, itching, easy bruising, abnormal bleeding, anemia, excessive thirst, fluid retention, nausea, high blood pressure, abnormal heart or lung sounds, weight loss, white spots on the skin or increased pigmentation, high potassium levels, an increased or decreased urine output, urinary tract infections, and abnormal urinalysis results.
- **Treatment.** This disorder can be treated with antibiotics; blood transfusions; medications to control anemia; restricting the intake of fluids, electrolytes, and protein; controlling high blood pressure; and dialysis. The most serious cases may require surgery to repair an obstruction of the ureters or a kidney transplant.

Cystitis is a urinary bladder infection. Women are much more likely to develop this disorder than men because of the short length of their urethras. The urethral opening in women is also close to the anal opening, allowing bacteria from this area to be more easily introduced into the urinary tract.

- **Causes.** This infection is caused by different types of bacteria (especially those that are found in the rectum) and the placement of a catheter in the bladder. Good hygiene, urinating frequently, and wiping from front to back (for females) can help to prevent this infection.
- **Signs and symptoms.** Common symptoms include fatigue, chills, fever, painful urination, a frequent need to urinate, cloudy urine, and blood in the urine.
- **Treatment.** This infection is treated with antibiotics.

Glomerulonephritis is an inflammation of the glomeruli of the kidney.

- **Causes.** This disorder is caused by renal diseases, immune disorders, and bacterial infections.
- **Signs and symptoms.** The signs and symptoms are hiccups, drowsiness, coma, seizures, nausea, anemia, high blood pressure, increased skin pigmentation, abnormal heart sounds, abnormal urinalysis results, blood in the urine, and a decreased or increased urine output.
- **Treatment.** Treatment begins with a low-sodium, low-protein diet. Medications to control high blood pressure, corticosteroids to reduce inflammation, and dialysis are other treatment options.

Incontinence is a condition in which a person (other than a child) cannot control urination. This condition can be either temporary or long lasting. Women are more likely to develop incontinence than men are.

- **Causes.** This condition can be caused by various medications, excessive coughing (for example, in smokers), urinary tract infections, nervous system disorders, and bladder cancer. In men, prostate problems can lead to the development of this disorder. The weakness of the urinary sphincters from surgery, trauma, or pregnancy can also cause incontinence. It may be prevented by avoiding urinary bladder irritants such as coffee, cigarettes, diuretics, and various medications.
- **Signs and symptoms.** The primary symptom is the involuntary leakage of urine.
- **Treatment.** Treatment includes various medications, incontinence pads, removal of the prostate, Kegel exercises to increase the control of urinary sphincters, and surgery to repair damaged bladders or urethral sphincters.

continued ⟶

Common Diseases and Disorders of the Urinary System *(continued)*

Polycystic kidney disease is a disorder in which the kidneys enlarge because of the presence of many cysts within them. The disease develops relatively slowly, with symptoms worsening over time.

- **Causes.** The causes are hereditary (via an inherited dominant gene from a parent).
- **Signs and symptoms.** Fatigue, high blood pressure, anemia, pain in the back or abdomen, joint pain, heart murmurs, the formation of kidney stones, kidney failure, blood in the urine, and liver disease are the symptoms of this disorder.
- **Treatment.** Treatment includes medications to control anemia and high blood pressure, blood transfusions, draining of the cysts, dialysis, and surgery to remove one or both kidneys.

Pyelonephritis is a type of complicated urinary tract infection. It begins as a bladder infection and spreads to one or both kidneys. This condition can develop suddenly, or it may be long lasting.

- **Causes.** This disorder is caused by bacteria, a bladder infection, kidney stones, or an obstruction of the urinary system ducts.
- **Signs and symptoms.** Signs and symptoms include fatigue, mental confusion, fever, nausea, pain in the back or abdomen, enlarged kidneys, painful urination, and cloudy or bloody urine.
- **Treatment.** Treatment includes intravenous fluids, pain medication, and antibiotics.

Renal calculi are more commonly called kidney stones. These stones can become lodged in the ducts within the kidneys or ureters.

- **Causes.** This condition is caused by gouty arthritis, defects of the ureters, overly concentrated urine, and urinary tract infections.
- **Signs and symptoms.** The signs and symptoms include fever, nausea, severe back or abdominal pain, a frequent urge to urinate, blood in the urine, and abnormal urinalysis results.
- **Treatment.** Treatment includes pain medication, intravenous fluids, medications to decrease stone formation, surgery to remove kidney stones, and lithotripsy (a procedure that uses shock waves to break up stones).

Summary

The kidneys, ureters, bladder, and urethra work together to remove waste products from the blood. The nephrons of the kidneys are involved in urine formation. The ureters, bladder, and urethra are responsible for eliminating urine from the body. The kidneys also play an important role in regulating blood cell production and blood pressure. Knowledge of the anatomy and physiology of the urinary system is important when collecting urine specimens, performing urinary testing, and assisting with cystoscopy.

CASE STUDY QUESTIONS

Now that you have completed this chapter, review the case study at the beginning of the chapter and answer the following questions:

1. How does atherosclerosis affect blood flow?
2. How does atherosclerosis of a renal artery produce high blood pressure?
3. What lifestyle changes should this patient make?
4. What can happen to the patient's kidney if his atherosclerosis is not treated?

Discussion Questions

1. Describe the three steps in the formation of urine.
2. Describe the composition of normal urine.
3. What are the differences between a renal corpuscle and a renal tubule?
4. Explain the functions of the kidneys.

Critical Thinking Questions

1. Why are females more likely than males to develop urinary tract infections?
2. What is the significance of proteins in urine?

3. The position of the kidneys is retroperitoneal. What would be the easiest way for a surgeon to reach a kidney?
4. What effect would vascular shock have on urine production?

Application Activities

1. Define the following parts of a kidney:
   a. Renal pyramid
   b. Renal cortex
   c. Renal medulla
   d. Renal pelvis
2. Name the three openings of the urinary bladder.
3. What is the name of the tubes that carry urine from the kidneys to the bladder?
4. What is the name of the tube that carries urine from the bladder to the outside world?

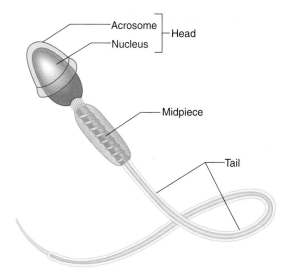

Figure 35-3. Parts of a mature sperm cell.

nutrients and prostaglandins. One milliliter of semen usually contains about 120 million sperm cells.

External Organs of the Male Reproductive System

The two male external reproductive organs are the scrotum and the penis (Figure 35-1).

Scrotum. The scrotum is a pouch of skin that holds the testes. It is lined with a serous membrane that secretes serous fluid to ensure that the testes move freely within it.

Penis. The penis is a cylindrical organ that moves urine and semen to the outside world. The body, or shaft, of the penis contains specialized tissue called **erectile tissue.** The urethra runs the length of the penis. The end of the penis is enlarged into a cone-shaped structure called the **glans penis.** If a male has not been circumcised, a piece of skin, called the **prepuce,** covers the glans penis. The function of the penis is to deliver sperm to the female reproductive tract. The penis also functions in urination because it contains the urethra.

Erection, Orgasm, and Ejaculation

During sexual arousal, the parasympathetic nervous system causes erectile tissue of the penis to become engorged with blood, which produces erection of the penis. During orgasm, sperm cells are propelled out of the testes toward the urethra. The secretions of the prostate, seminal vesicles, and bulbourethral glands are also released into the urethra. The movement of the sperm and secretions into the urethra is called emission. The process of ejaculation occurs when semen is forced out of the urethra. After ejaculation, sympathetic nerve fibers cause the erectile tissue to release blood, and the penis gradually returns to a non-erect state.

Male Reproductive Hormones

The hypothalamus, anterior pituitary gland, and the testes secrete hormones that regulate male reproductive functions. At the onset of puberty, the hypothalamus releases a hormone called **gonadotropin-releasing hormone (GnRH).** GnRH stimulates the anterior pituitary gland to release **follicle-stimulating hormone (FSH)** and **luteinizing hormone (LH).** FSH causes spermatogenesis to begin, and LH stimulates interstitial cells to produce testosterone.

Testosterone stimulates the development of male secondary sex characteristics, which are defined as characteristics that are typically unique to males. Examples of these characteristics are chest hair, thick facial hair, enlarged muscles, enlarged bones, and thickening of vocal cords that produces a deep voice. Testosterone also stimulates the maturation of male reproductive organs.

Testosterone levels in the male are regulated by a negative feedback mechanism. When testosterone levels in the blood increase above normal, the hypothalamus no longer releases GnRH. Therefore, the anterior pituitary gland no longer secretes LH and FSH, which causes testosterone levels to fall. When testosterone levels fall below normal, the hypothalamus begins to secrete GnRH again, which causes the anterior pituitary gland to release LH and FSH again. Testosterone levels begin to rise again, and the cycle repeats itself.

Pathophysiology

Common Diseases and Disorders of the Male Reproductive System

Epididymitis is inflammation of an epididymis. Most cases start out as an infection of the urinary tract that spreads to an epididymis.

- **Causes.** The causes include the use of certain medications, placement of a catheter in the urethra, and bacteria—especially those that cause gonorrhea and chlamydia.

- **Signs and symptoms.** Signs and symptoms include fever, pain in the testes, a lump in the testes, swelling of the scrotum, painful ejaculation, blood in the semen, pain during urination, discharge from the urethra, and enlarged lymph nodes in the pelvic area.

- **Treatment.** Treatment includes pain medication, antibiotics for both the patient and his sexual partner,

continued ⟶

Common Diseases and Disorders of the Male Reproductive System *(continued)*

elevation of the scrotum, and ice packs applied to the scrotum.

Erectile dysfunction is more commonly called **impotence.** It is a disorder in which a male cannot maintain an erect penis to complete sexual intercourse. It is estimated that half of all men between the ages of 40 and 70 have some degree of impotence. Most causes are physical and not psychological.

- **Causes.** Anxiety and depression can cause erectile dysfunction. Common causes include diabetes, high blood pressure, anemia, coronary artery disease, peripheral vascular problems, low testosterone production, various medications, smoking, excessive alcohol consumption, and drugs such as cocaine, marijuana, and heroin.
- **Signs and symptoms.** Signs and symptoms are an inability to achieve an erection and an inability to maintain an erection long enough to complete sexual intercourse.
- **Treatment.** The first treatment step should be lifestyle changes to quit smoking and stop using alcohol or drugs. Counseling to reduce anxiety and depression may also be helpful. Other treatment options include various medications, penile implants, and penile injections of medications if oral medications do not work.

Prostate cancer is the third most common cause of cancer death in men of all ages, although it most frequently occurs in men over the age of 40. In the United States, most cases of prostate cancer are diagnosed before they cause signs or symptoms because most men over age 40 are screened regularly.

- **Causes.** The causes are mostly unknown, although decreased testosterone production may contribute to the development of this disease.
- **Signs and symptoms.** Common symptoms include anemia, weight loss, incontinence, difficult urination, painful urination, pain in the lower back or abdomen, pain during bowel movements, high levels of PSA (a specific type of antigen) in the blood, blood in the urine, and bone pain in advanced cases.
- **Treatment.** Treatments are hormone therapy, chemotherapy, radiation therapy to destroy the tumor, and surgery to remove the prostate.

Prostatitis is an inflammation of the prostate gland. If it develops suddenly, it is called *acute prostatitis.* The slow development of this condition is termed *chronic prostatitis.*

- **Causes.** This condition can be caused by excessive alcohol consumption, a bacterial infection, a catheter in the urethra, trauma to the urethra or urinary bladder, and scarring of the urethra or prostate due to frequent infections. Urinating frequently can help to prevent infection.
- **Signs and symptoms.** Signs and symptoms include fever; pain in the scrotum, pelvic area, or abdomen; difficult urination; frequent urination; painful urination; blood in the urine; painful ejaculation; blood in the semen; discharge from the urethra; a low sperm count; and white blood cells in urine or semen.
- **Treatment.** This condition is treated with antibiotics and may also be treated with surgery to repair damage to the urethra.

The Female Reproductive System
Ovaries and Egg Cell Formation

The ovaries are the primary sex organs of the female because they produce the sex cells (eggs) of the female (Figures 35-4 and 35-5). They also produce **estrogen** and **progesterone.** Most females have two ovaries. They are oval in shape and are located in the pelvic cavity. Each ovary is divided into an inner area called the medulla and an outer area called the cortex. The medulla contains nerves, lymphatic vessels, and many blood vessels. The cortex contains small masses of cells called ovarian follicles. Epithelial tissue and dense connective tissue cover each ovary.

Before a female child is born, **primordial follicles** develop in her ovarian cortex. Each primordial follicle contains a large cell called a primary **oocyte** (immature egg) and smaller cells called **follicular cells.** Unlike males, who make sperm cells throughout their entire life, a female is born with the maximum number of primary oocytes she will ever produce.

Oogenesis is the process of egg cell formation. At the onset of puberty, some primary oocytes are stimulated to continue meiosis. When a primary oocyte divides, it becomes one **polar body** (a nonfunctional cell) and a secondary oocyte. It is the secondary oocyte that is released from an ovary each month during a process called **ovulation.** When the secondary oocyte is fertilized, it divides to form a mature, fertilized egg cell. Therefore, the process of meiosis begins before a female is born and is completed only if a secondary oocyte is fertilized. The mature egg cell contains 23 chromosomes; when it combines with a sperm cell, the resulting cell contains 46 chromosomes.

Internal Accessory Organs of the Female Reproductive System

The female reproductive internal accessory organs are the **fallopian tubes, uterus,** and **vagina.**

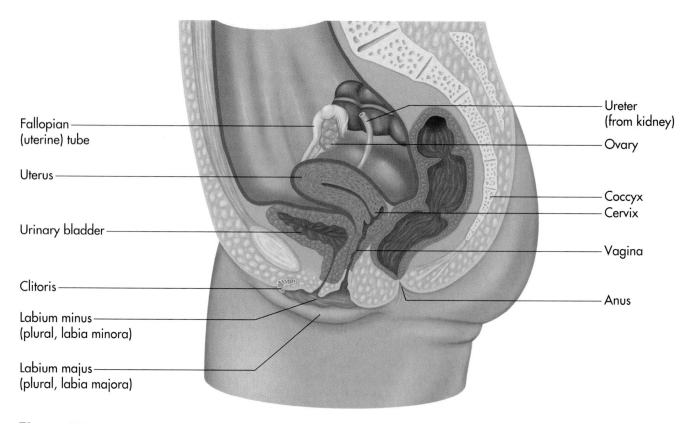

Figure 35-4. Sagittal view of female reproductive organs. The female reproductive system produces eggs for fertilization and provides the place and means for a fertilized egg to develop.

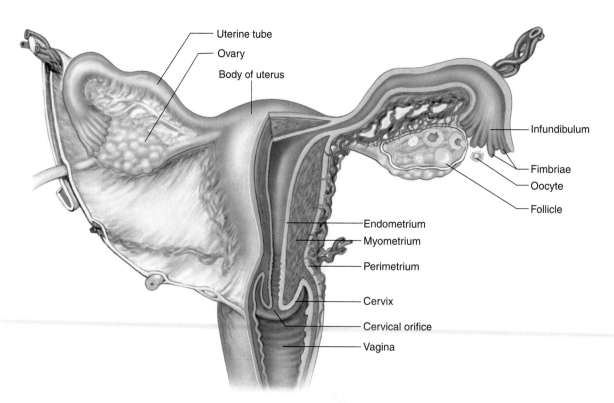

Figure 35-5. Anterior view of internal female reproductive organs. Ovulation of an oocyte is also demonstrated.

Fallopian Tubes. A fallopian tube opens near each ovary and into the uterus. The end of a fallopian tube near an ovary is expanded and is called an **infundibulum** and **fimbriae.** The infundibulum and its fimbriae function to "catch" a secondary oocyte as it leaves an ovary. Fallopian tubes are lined with ciliated cells that sweep the oocyte toward the uterus.

Uterus. The uterus is a hollow, muscular organ that functions to receive an embryo and sustain its development. The upper two-thirds of the uterus is called the body of the uterus, and the narrow, lower portion of the uterus, that extends into the vagina is called the **cervix.** The opening of the cervix is called the **cervical orifice.**

The wall of the uterus has three layers—the **endometrium, myometrium,** and **perimetrium.** The endometrium is the innermost lining of the uterus and contains numerous tubular glands that secrete mucus. The myometrium is the middle, thick, muscular layer. The perimetrium is a thin layer that covers the myometrium. It secretes serous fluid that coats the uterus.

Vagina. The vagina is a tubular organ that extends from the uterus to the outside of the body. It functions to receive an erect penis during sexual intercourse, and it provides an open passageway for uterine secretions and offspring. The opening of the vagina is posterior to the urinary opening and anterior to the anal opening. The wall of the vagina has three layers—an innermost mucosal layer that secretes mucus, a middle muscular layer, and an outermost fibrous layer.

External Accessory Organs of the Female Reproductive System

Mammary glands are the accessory organs of the female reproductive system (Figure 35-6). They secrete milk after pregnancy.

Mammary glands are located beneath the skin in the breast area. A nipple is located near the center of each breast. The pigmented area that surrounds the nipple is called the **areola.** Each gland is made of 15 to 20 lobes and contains **alveolar glands** that make milk under the influence of the hormone prolactin. The hormone oxytocin induces alveolar ducts to deliver milk through openings in the nipples. Therefore, if a woman wants to breast-feed, she must produce adequate amounts of prolactin and oxytocin.

External Organs of the Female Reproductive System

The female external reproductive organs are the **labia majora, labia minora,** and **clitoris.**

Labia Majora. The labia majora are rounded folds of adipose tissue and skin that serve to protect the other external female reproductive organs. At their anterior ends, the labia majora form the **mons pubis,** which is a fatty area that overlies the pubic bones. The labia majora and mons pubis are typically covered in pubic hair in postpubescent females.

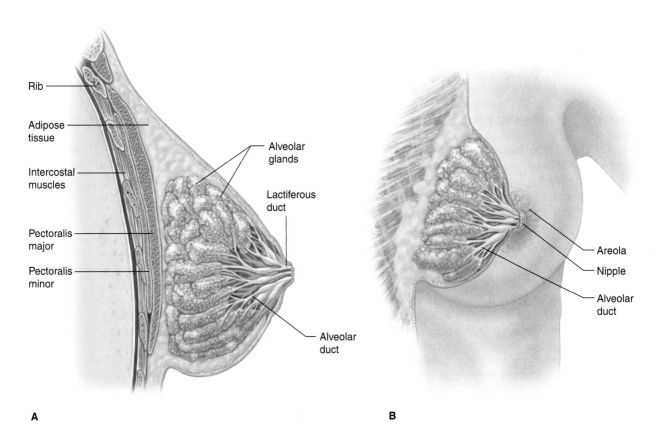

A   B

Figure 35-6. Mammary glands: (a) sagittal view and (b) anterior view.

Labia Minora. The labia minora are folds of skin between the labia majora. They are pinkish in color because of their high degree of vascularity. They merge together anteriorly to form a hood over the clitoris.

The space enclosed by the labia minora is called the vestibule. **Vestibular glands** secrete mucus into this area during sexual arousal. This mucus facilitates insertion of the penis into the vagina.

Clitoris. The clitoris is anterior to the urethral opening. It contains erectile tissue and is rich in sensory nerves.

Erection, Lubrication, and Orgasm

During sexual arousal, nervous stimulation causes the clitoris to become erect and the vestibular glands to become active. At the same time, the vagina elongates. If the clitoris is sufficiently stimulated, an orgasm occurs. During orgasm, the walls of the uterus and fallopian tubes contract to help propel sperm toward the upper ends of the fallopian tubes.

Female Reproductive Hormones

At the onset of puberty, the hypothalamus secretes increasing amounts of GnRH. GnRH causes the anterior pituitary gland to release FSH and LH. FSH and LH then stimulate the ovary to produce estrogen, progesterone, and mature follicles. Estrogen and progesterone also stimulate enlargement of the reproductive organs and the production of female secondary sex characteristics, which are characteristics that are typically unique to females. They include breast development, increased vascularization of the skin, and increased fat deposits in the breasts, thighs, and hips.

Female Reproductive Cycle

The female reproductive cycle is also called the **menstrual cycle.** It consists of regular changes in the uterine lining that leads to a monthly "period," or bleeding. **Menopause** is the termination of the menstrual cycle because of normal aging of the ovaries. The following steps are the major hormonal changes that occur during one reproductive cycle:

1. The anterior pituitary gland releases FSH. FSH stimulates an ovarian follicle to mature.
2. The maturing follicle secretes estrogen. Estrogen causes the uterine lining to thicken.
3. The anterior pituitary gland releases a sudden surge of LH. The LH surge triggers ovulation.
4. Following ovulation, follicular cells of the follicle become a **corpus luteum.**
5. The corpus luteum secretes progesterone, which causes the uterine lining to become more vascular and glandular.
6. If the released oocyte is not fertilized, the corpus luteum degenerates.
7. The degenerating corpus luteum causes estrogen and progesterone levels to fall. The decline in estrogen and progesterone levels causes the uterine lining to break down, and bleeding **(menses)** starts.
8. When the anterior pituitary releases FSH, the reproductive cycle begins again.

Pathophysiology

Common Diseases and Disorders of the Female Reproductive System

Breast cancer affects approximately one in eight women. Depending on tumor size and how far cancer cells have spread, breast cancer is classified in stages from 0 to 4, with stage 4 cancer being the most serious. Early diagnosis through regular mammograms and self-breast examinations greatly increases the success of treatment.

- **Causes.** The causes are largely unknown, although breast cancer may be related to hormonal changes or the presence of certain genes.
- **Signs and symptoms.** Signs and symptoms include a lump in the breast that is usually painless and firm, a lump in the armpit, discharge from the nipples, dimpled skin on the breast or nipple, and breast pain. Swelling of the arm and bone pain may be present in advanced cases.
- **Treatment.** Nonsurgical treatment methods include hormone therapy, radiation therapy, and chemotherapy.

Surgical options include surgery to remove affected lymph nodes, lumpectomy (surgery to remove a lump), and mastectomy (surgery to remove a breast).

Cervical cancer develops slowly and most of the time is treatable without removing the uterus. Early screening for cervical cancer is successful with a yearly Pap smear, which is a test that looks for abnormal cells in the cervix.

- **Causes.** A weak immune system may be a factor in the development of this cancer. It can also be caused by sexual intercourse early in life, multiple sexual partners, and infection with the human papilloma virus.
- **Signs and symptoms.** Primary symptoms include frequent vaginal discharge, sporadic vaginal bleeding, vaginal bleeding after sexual intercourse, and abnormal cells in the cervix. Patients who are in later stages of this disease may experience pain in the pelvic area or legs, or bone fractures.

continued ⟶

Common Diseases and Disorders of the Female Reproductive System (continued)

- **Treatment.** Radiation therapy, chemotherapy, the removal of diseased tissue, and the removal of the uterus (**hysterectomy**) are the treatments for this disease.

Cervicitis is defined as an inflammation of the cervix, which is usually caused by an infection.

- **Causes.** Causes include bacterial or viral infections and allergic reactions to spermicidal creams and latex condoms.
- **Signs and symptoms.** Frequent vaginal discharge, pain during intercourse, and vaginal bleeding after intercourse are common signs and symptoms.
- **Treatment.** This condition is treated with antibiotics and by changing the method of contraception.

Dysmenorrhea is the condition of experiencing severe menstrual cramps that limit normal daily activities. It is a common cause of lost time from work for women.

- **Causes.** Causes include anxiety, endometriosis, pelvic inflammatory disease, fibroid tumors in the uterus, ovarian cysts, abnormally high levels of prostaglandins, and multiple sexual partners.
- **Signs and symptoms.** Common symptoms are abdominal pains, including sharp or dull pain in the pelvic area.
- **Treatment.** Nonsurgical treatments include pain medication, anti-inflammatory drugs, medications that inhibit prostaglandin formation, oral contraceptives, and antibiotics in the case of pelvic inflammatory disease. Surgical treatments include hysterectomy and surgery to remove cysts or fibroids.

Endometriosis is a condition in which tissues that make up the lining of the uterus grow outside the uterus.

- **Causes.** The cause of this disorder is unknown; it may be inherited.
- **Signs and symptoms.** Signs and symptoms include infertility, heavy bleeding from the uterus, pain in the abdomen or pelvis, painful periods, spotting between periods, and pain during sexual intercourse.
- **Treatment.** Oral contraceptives, pain medications, and various hormone therapies may be prescribed. Surgical treatments include laser surgery to remove endometrial tissue outside the uterus, and hysterectomy.

Fibrocystic breast disease is the presence of abnormal tissue in the breasts. It is a common disorder and occurs in more than 60% of women in the United States between the ages of 30 and 50. It is rare in women who have gone through menopause.

- **Causes.** This disorder is caused by hormonal changes associated with the menstrual cycle and various dietary substances (for example, caffeine).

- **Signs and symptoms.** Common symptoms include breasts that feel "bumpy," breast tenderness or pain, itchy nipples, and dense tissues as seen in a mammogram.
- **Treatment.** Treatments are changing one's diet, taking oral contraceptives, and preventing pain by wearing support bras.

Fibroids are benign (noncancerous) tumors that grow in the uterine wall. They are most common in African American women.

- **Causes.** The causes are mostly unknown, although it has been found that tumors enlarge as estrogen levels increase.
- **Signs and symptoms.** The signs and symptoms are pressure in the abdomen, severe menstrual cramps, abdominal gas, heavy menstrual bleeding, and an enlarged uterus.
- **Treatment.** Treatment includes pain medications, hormone treatments to shrink tumors, surgery to remove tumors, hysterectomy, and surgery to decrease the blood supply to the uterus.

Ovarian cancer is more deadly than other types of cancer because its signs and symptoms are usually mild until the disease has spread to other organs. It is the fifth leading cause of cancer death in women.

- **Causes.** The causes are unknown, although the presence of certain genes has been indicated as a risk factor. Some oral contraceptives may lower the risk of developing this disease.
- **Signs and symptoms.** Abdominal and pelvic discomfort, unusual menstrual cycles, indigestion, bloating, nausea, and excessive hair growth are signs and symptoms.
- **Treatment.** Treatments are radiation therapy, chemotherapy, and surgery to remove the ovaries.

Premenstrual syndrome (PMS) is a collection of symptoms that occur just before a menstrual period.

- **Causes.** The causes are mostly unknown.
- **Signs and symptoms.** The signs and symptoms include anxiety, depression, irritability, acne, fatigue, food cravings, bloating, aches in the head or back, abdominal pain, breast tenderness, muscle spasms, diarrhea, weight gain, and loss of sex drive.
- **Treatment.** PMS is commonly treated with pain medications, diuretics, medications to treat depression or anxiety, and oral contraceptives.

Vaginitis is the condition of having abnormal vaginal discharge. Some vaginal discharge is normal for all women,

continued ⟶

Common Diseases and Disorders of the Female Reproductive System (continued)

and it varies throughout the menstrual cycle. Normal vaginal discharge is clear, whitish, or yellowish in color.

- **Causes.** This condition can be caused by yeast infections, tampon use, poor hygiene, bacteria, antibiotics, and sexually transmitted diseases. Vaginitis may be prevented through good hygiene.
- **Signs and symptoms.** Common symptoms include fever, vaginal itching, abnormal increases in the amount of vaginal discharge, decreases in the amount of vaginal discharge, an abnormal color of vaginal discharge (brown or pinkish), and vaginal discharge that has an abnormal odor.
- **Treatment.** The patient may be given medications for fungal or bacterial infections, or the patient and her

sexual partner may be treated for sexually transmitted diseases.

Uterine cancer is most common in women between the ages of 60 and 70. In the United States, it occurs in about 1% of women.

- **Causes.** The causes are mostly unknown, although it may be related to increased levels of estrogen.
- **Signs and symptoms.** Signs and symptoms include abdominal pain, abnormal bleeding from the uterus, pelvic pain, and a thin, white vaginal discharge in postmenopausal women.
- **Treatment.** Treatment includes radiation therapy, chemotherapy, and surgery to remove the uterus, fallopian tubes, and ovaries.

Sexually Transmitted Diseases

Sexually transmitted diseases (STDs) can be caused by bacteria, viruses, or parasites.

Bacterial Causes of STDs

STDs caused by bacteria are chlamydia, syphilis, and gonorrhea. The symptoms of STDs caused by bacterial infections are often absent or too mild to be noticed in both men and women. These symptoms include:

- Discharge from the vagina or penis
- Burning sensations during urination
- Pelvic pain
- Pain in the testes

STDs caused by bacteria are easily and effectively treated with antibiotics. However, both partners must take antibiotics to prevent reinfection. These STDs can lead to complications if left untreated. The most common complication of an untreated bacterial STD is *pelvic inflammatory disease (PID)*. PID is a leading cause of infertility in women because it leads to scarring of the fallopian tubes.

Viral Causes of STDs

STDs caused by viruses are herpes and AIDS. *Herpes simplex 1* usually infects the mouth and causes fever blisters, or cold sores. *Herpes simplex 2* affects the genital area. This virus usually causes only genital ulcers, but it can also infect the eyes, lungs, skin, brain, and a developing fetus. There is no cure for any type of herpes but medication is available to prevent outbreaks. *AIDS* is discussed in Chapter 29.

Parasitic Causes of STDs

Parasites can cause STDs. *Crabs* is an STD caused by bloodsucking insects called lice. Lice that invade hair in the genital region are called pubic lice. They typically attach to pubic hair to lay their eggs. They produce severe itching and can be seen with a magnifying glass and sometimes with the naked eye. They are usually treated with insecticides. It is also important to wash all clothing and linens during treatment.

Trichimonas is caused by a parasitic protozoan. It most often does not produce noticeable symptoms in males. In females, it usually produces a large amount of foul-smelling vaginal discharge. This disease also causes itching and swollen labia. It is easily treated with specific antibiotics.

Pregnancy
Fertilization

Pregnancy is defined as the condition of having a developing offspring in the uterus. Pregnancy results when a sperm cell unites with an egg in a process called **fertilization** (Figure 35-7).

Prior to fertilization, an egg is released from an ovary, and it travels through a fallopian tube. During sexual intercourse, the male deposits semen into the vagina. Sperm cells must travel up through the uterus to the fallopian tubes to fertilize the egg.

Prostaglandins in semen stimulate the flagella of sperm cells to undulate, causing the swimming action of sperm. Prostaglandins also stimulate muscles in the uterus and fallopian tubes to contract. These contractions help the sperm reach the egg. Normally about 10 to 14 days after ovulation, high estrogen levels stimulate the uterus and

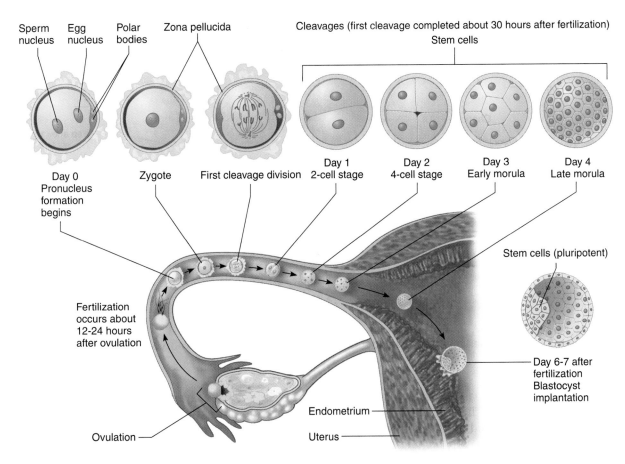

Figure 35-7. Stages of early embryo development.

Image labels: Sperm nucleus, Egg nucleus, Polar bodies, Zona pellucida, Cleavages (first cleavage completed about 30 hours after fertilization), Stem cells, Day 0 Pronucleus formation begins, Zygote, First cleavage division, Day 1 2-cell stage, Day 2 4-cell stage, Day 3 Early morula, Day 4 Late morula, Stem cells (pluripotent), Fertilization occurs about 12-24 hours after ovulation, Day 6-7 after fertilization Blastocyst implantation, Ovulation, Endometrium, Uterus

cervix to secrete a thin watery fluid that also promotes the movement of sperm toward the egg.

Although many sperm cells normally reach an egg, only one unites with the egg to fertilize it. The sperm cell that unites with the egg penetrates the follicular cells and a layer called the **zona pellucida,** which surround the cell membrane of the egg. The acrosome of the sperm releases enzymes to help the sperm penetrate the membrane of the egg. Once a sperm unites with an egg, the egg releases enzymes that prevent other sperm from invading it. The enzymes cause the zona pellucida to become hard and therefore impenetrable to other sperm.

The nucleus of the egg (with 23 chromosomes) and the nucleus of the sperm (with 23 chromosomes) eventually fuse together to make one nucleus that contains 46 chromosomes. The cell that is formed by this union is called a **zygote.**

The Prenatal Period

The **prenatal period** is the time before the offspring is born. The prenatal period is divided into an **embryonic period** (weeks 2 through 8 of pregnancy) and a **fetal period** (week 9 to the delivery of the offspring).

About one day after the zygote forms, it begins to undergo mitosis at a relatively rapid rate. This rapid cell division is called **cleavage.** The resulting ball of cells is called

a **morula.** The morula travels down the fallopian tube to the uterus. Fluid then invades the morula, and this organism is called a **blastocyst.** The blastocyst implants in the wall of the uterus. The process of moving from zygote formation to implantation of the blastocyst takes about one week. Once the blastocyst implants, a group of cells in the blastocyst, called the **inner cell mass,** gives rise to an embryo. Other cells in the blastocyst, along with cells of the uterus, eventually form the **placenta.**

The Embryonic Period. The embryonic period extends from the second week of pregnancy to the end of the eighth week of development. During this stage, the placenta, **amnion, umbilical cord,** and **yolk sac** form along with most of the internal organs and external structures of the embryo (Figure 35-8). The cells of the inner cell mass organize into layers called **primary germ layers.** All organs are formed from the primary germ layers, which include the ectoderm, mesoderm, and endoderm.

- The **ectoderm** gives rise to nervous tissue and some epithelial tissue.
- The **mesoderm,** the middle layer, gives rise to connective tissues and some epithelial tissue.
- The **endoderm** gives rise to epithelial tissues only.

The placenta allows nutrients and oxygen from maternal blood to pass to embryonic blood. It also allows waste

is called active listening. Passive listeners simply sit back and hear. When you are an active listener, you pay attention and provide feedback. For example, you might repeat what the patient says in your own words or ask questions so that you understand details.

Being Aware of Nonverbal Clues and Body Language.
Verbal communication is the asking and answering of questions. To conduct a successful interview, you must also be aware of nonverbal communication. The patient's tone of voice, facial expression, and body language are examples of nonverbal communication. These signs often communicate more than words could ever say. For example, a patient who has difficulty making eye contact may be embarrassed by some symptoms and may need your extra patience and encouragement to report symptoms fully. A child or adolescent may deny or exaggerate pain. Pay attention to the patient's facial expression and how much the patient guards the area in question.

Using a Broad Knowledge Base.
To conduct a successful interview, you must have a broad knowledge base so that you can ask questions that will elicit the most meaningful information about the patient. You must take every opportunity to expand your knowledge base by learning more about medical terminology, symptoms, and diseases.

Summarizing to Form a General Picture.
You will gather a variety of subjective and objective data as you conduct a patient interview. You must consider the relative importance of each piece of information so that you can summarize the data to formulate a general picture of the patient.

Interviewing Successfully

One of the main goals of the patient interview is to give the patient an opportunity to fully explain in her own words the reason for the current office visit. These eight steps will help you conduct a successful interview.

1. Do your research before the patient interview
2. Plan the interview
3. Approach the patient and request the interview
4. Make the patient feel at ease
5. Conduct the interview in private without interruptions
6. Deal with sensitive topics with respect
7. Do not diagnose or give a diagnostic opinion
8. Formulate the general picture

Doing Research Before the Patient Interview.
Before the interview review the patient's medical record for history, medications, and chronic problems (for example, diabetes or high blood pressure). Note whether the patient has family problems that might have an impact on health issues.

Planning the Interview.
Develop a plan for the interview. Have a general idea of the questions you will ask. For example, if a client is being treated for high blood pressure, you might ask about headaches or tinnitus (ringing in the ears), which are common signs of high blood pressure. Planning the interview helps you maintain your focus and ensures that you will obtain all the necessary information.

Approaching the Patient and Requesting the Interview.
Ask the patient whether you may pose some questions about the reason for the visit and the patient's current health situation. You may need to explain that the questions are necessary to plan the most effective care. It is more courteous to seek permission to ask questions than to say that you "need to take a history." Asking permission helps the patient feel more comfortable and emphasizes the importance of the interview process. It also makes the patient feel more like a participant in the medical care being provided.

Making the Patient Feel at Ease.
Using certain words or phrases known as icebreakers can help set the stage for the interview. Icebreakers put the patient at ease and create a relaxed atmosphere. Examples of icebreakers include acknowledging the patient's reason for the visit, introducing yourself, or commenting about the weather. Icebreakers that also convey a sincere and sensitive interest in the patient are asking the patient how she prefers to be addressed or clarifying the pronunciation of a difficult name.

Another way to convey an image of a professional who is sensitive to the patient's needs is to sit with the patient and appear relaxed. By appearing relaxed, you help the patient relax and encourage a more open and comfortable interview.

Conducting the Interview in Private Without Interruptions.
After setting the stage for the interview, ensure privacy by showing the patient to a private room or area or by closing the door if the patient is already in a private room. You can then begin to ask relevant questions. Some approaches are more effective than others, as shown in Table 36-1. Listening carefully to the patient's responses may lead you to ask questions other than those in your interview plan.

Developing a rapport with the patient is essential. Keep the atmosphere relaxed, do not rush, maintain eye contact, and use the patient's name in conversation. Avoid interruptions, such as taking phone calls and letting people walk in and out of the room.

Dealing With Sensitive Topics With Respect.
Sometimes you will have to ask patients questions about sensitive topics. Such topics may be related to sexuality, lifestyle, or behaviors that put a person at risk for diseases, such as those that are sexually transmitted. You must approach these topics gently so that the patient does not feel threatened by the questioning. You can show respect for the patient's rights and privacy by knowing when to stop. Both verbal and nonverbal clues can guide you in this area.

TABLE 36-1 Methods of Collecting Patient Data

Effective Methods	Characteristics
Asking open-ended questions	Requires more than a yes or no answer; allows the patient to more fully explain the situation, resulting in more relevant data. Instead of asking, "Do you have a cough?" ask, "Can you tell me about your symptoms?"
Asking hypothetical questions	Allows you to determine the patient's knowledge of the situation and whether it is accurate. For example, ask a patient who has been prescribed nitroglycerin for chest pain, "What would you do if you have chest pain?"
Mirroring patient's responses and verbalizing the implied	Allows nonthreatening ways for the patient to discuss the situation further and to provide underlying meaning. *Mirroring* means restating what the patient says in your own words. *Verbalizing* the implied means stating what you believe the patient is suggesting by his response. You might say, "So the pain started about three days ago and has been getting worse each day, and today it has not let up at all."
Focusing on patient	Shows the patient that you are really listening to what he is saying. You maintain eye contact (as culturally appropriate), assume a relaxed and open body posture, and use the proper responses.
Encouraging patient to take the lead	Motivates the patient to discuss or describe the situation in his own way. Ask a question such as "Where would you like to begin?"
Encouraging patient to provide additional information	Conveys sincere interest in the patient by continuing to explore topics in more detail when appropriate. You might ask the patient if he has experienced a symptom before or if he associates it with a change in routine.
Encouraging patient to evaluate his situation	Provides an idea of the patient's point of view about the situation; allows you to determine the patient's knowledge of the situation and possible fears. Ask the patient, "What do you think is going on here?"

Ineffective Methods	Characteristics
Asking closed-ended questions	Provides little information because closed-ended questions offer the patient little freedom to explain his answers. Closed-ended questions require only yes or no answers.
Asking leading questions	Leading questions suggest a desired response instead of the patient's true response. The patient tends to agree with such statements instead of elaborating on them. An example of a leading question is "You seem to be making progress, don't you agree?" This type of question limits the patient's response.
Challenging patient	The patient may feel you are disagreeing with what he is saying if you ask an emotional question or use a certain tone of voice. The patient may become defensive, which might block further communication.
Probing	Continuing to question a patient after he appears to have finished giving information can make him feel that you are invading his privacy. The patient may become defensive and withhold information.
Agreeing or disagreeing with patient	When you agree or disagree with a patient, it implies that the patient is either "right" or "wrong." This action can block further communication.

Avoiding Making a Diagnosis or Giving a Diagnostic Opinion. Only the physician can make a diagnosis, based on the patient's symptoms and complaints. If the patient asks for your opinion about a diagnosis, explain that the physician should be asked about diagnoses. If pressed, you may need to say that it is not your place to give opinions about a diagnosis. Never go beyond the scope of your knowledge or job description.

Formulating the General Picture. Summarize the key points of the interview. Ask the patient whether he has questions or other information to add. You will be most successful with the interview process if you remain alert and organized but flexible. Procedure 36-1 demonstrates the proper approach to an interview.

Your Role as an Observer

During the preexamination stage of the office visit, you will gather most of your information through verbal and nonverbal communication. The nonverbal communication that occurs during the interview and history taking, however, sometimes reveals more about a patient than the patient's words. Listening attentively and observing the patient closely may help you detect a problem that might otherwise go unnoted.

Anxiety

Anxiety is a common emotional response in patients. Some patients respond with anxiety to a specific fear, such as fear of pain. Others simply feel anxious when they are in an unfamiliar situation. For example, many patients have what is called "white coat syndrome," which is anxiety related to seeing a physician.

To recognize anxiety, you must understand that its levels vary from mild to severe. A patient with mild anxiety may have a heightened ability to observe and to make connections. A patient with severe anxiety has difficulty focusing on details, feels panicky, and is virtually helpless. A heightened focus or a lack of focus in a patient can hinder your ability to get the information and cooperation you need.

When you observe signs of anxiety in a patient, make every effort to help her relax and release or reduce the anxious feelings. You may be able to help by allowing the patient to describe her feelings. If a patient becomes agitated while discussing a physical complaint, you may need to postpone talking about the matter until the patient is calmer. In either situation, give support in nonverbal ways by trying to make the patient as comfortable as possible. Give the patient time to respond and then wait quietly, provide privacy, make eye contact, and communicate at the level of the patient.

Depression

Some symptoms of depression are the same as those of many common illnesses. Many patients with major depression develop great skill in hiding depression or are unaware they are suffering from it. Thus, depression may be difficult to recognize. Many patients, especially the elderly, have undiagnosed depression.

To recognize depression, you must be aware of common symptoms associated with the condition. Classic symptoms of depression are profound sadness and fatigue. In addition, a depressed person may have difficulty falling asleep at night or getting up in the morning. The depressed patient may suffer from loss of appetite, loss of energy, or both.

Depression seems to occur most frequently during late adolescence, in middle age, and after retirement. It is common in the elderly but is often mistaken for senility. If you observe any signs of depression, indicate them in the patient's chart and alert the physician.

PROCEDURE 36.1

Using Critical Thinking Skills During an Interview

Objective: To be able to use verbal and nonverbal clues to optimize the process of obtaining data for the patient's chart

OSHA Guidelines: This procedure does not involve exposure to blood, body fluids, or tissues.

Materials: Patient chart, pen with black ink

Method
Example 1: Getting at an Underlying Meaning

1. You are interviewing a female patient with type 2 diabetes who has recently started insulin injections. She is in the office for a follow-up visit.
2. You ask her how she is managing her diabetes. (This open-ended questioning allows the patient to explain the situation in her own words and often provides more information than closed-ended questioning.)
3. The patient states that she "just can't get used to the whole idea of injections."
4. To encourage her to verbalize her concerns more clearly, you can **mirror** her response, or restate her comments in your own words. For example, you might say, "You seem to be having some difficulty giving yourself injections." (Your response should encourage her to verbalize the specific area in which she is having problems [for example, loading the syringe, injecting herself, finding the time for the injections, and so on].) Another method you can use is to **verbalize** the implied, which means that you state what

continued ——→

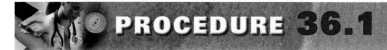
Using Critical Thinking Skills During an Interview *(continued)*

you think the patient is suggesting by her response.

5. After you determine the specific problem, you will be able to address it in the interview or note it in the patient's chart for the doctor's attention.

Example 2: Dealing With a Potentially Violent Patient

1. You are interviewing a 24-year-old male patient who is new to the office. He appears agitated. You ask his reason for seeing the doctor today.

2. The patient explains that he does not want to talk to "some assistant" about his problem. He just wants to see the doctor.

3. You say that you respect his wish not to discuss his symptoms but explain that you need to ask him a few questions so that the doctor can provide the proper medical care. (The patient has the right to refuse to answer a question, even if it is a reasonable one.)

4. The patient begins to yell at you, saying he wants to see the doctor and doesn't "want to answer stupid questions" (Figure 36-2).

5. The fact that the patient appears agitated and begins to raise his voice in anger should be a warning to you that he may become violent. It would be best not to handle this patient by yourself.

6. If you are alone with the patient, leave the room and request assistance from another staff member.

Example 3: Gathering Symptom Information About a Child

1. A parent brings a 6-year-old boy to the office because the child is complaining about stomach pain.

2. To gather the pertinent symptom information, ask the child various types of questions. (Talking to the child first allows him to feel that his view of the problem is important.)

   a. Can he tell you about the pain? (Open-ended questioning allows him to tell you about his problem in his own words.)

   b. Can he tell you exactly where it hurts (Figure 36-3)?

   c. Is there anything else that hurts?

3. To confirm the child's answers, ask the parent to answer similar questions.

4. You should then ask the parent additional questions. Begin with an open-ended question, as above. Follow up with specific questions such as these.

   a. How long has he had the pain?

   b. Is the pain related to any specific event (such as going to school)?

5. Ask the child to confirm the parent's answers. He may be able to provide additional information at this time.

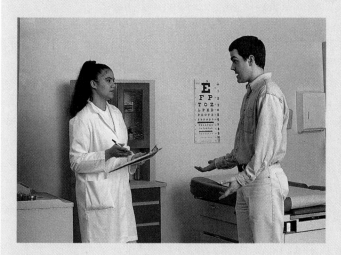

Figure 36-2. Do not try to handle a patient who may become violent by yourself. Ask for help from other staff members.

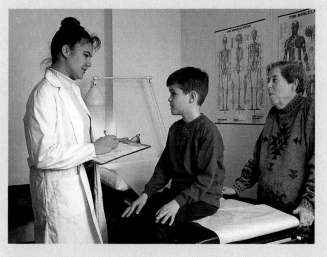

Figure 36-3. Gather any symptom information you can from a child. Then ask the parent or caregiver similar questions.

CAUTION *Handle With Care*

Signs of Depression, Substance Abuse, and Addiction in Adolescents

Signs of depression, substance abuse, and addiction are often hard to distinguish in adolescents. Part of the difficulty is that adolescents are particularly skilled at hiding signs of all three disorders.

Various signs may indicate depression in an adolescent. One teenager may lose interest in or be unable to enjoy everyday activities. Another may sleep for long periods and have difficulty getting up in the morning, whereas yet another may sleep very little. Chronic fatigue or aches and pains may signal depression, as may trouble with concentration or school absenteeism. These signs may also indicate substance abuse or addiction.

It is important to know the difference between substance abuse and addiction. **Substance abuse** refers to the use of a substance, even an over-the-counter drug, in a way that is not medically approved. Inappropriate use includes such practices as using diet pills to stay awake or consuming large quantities of cough syrup that contains codeine. It also includes taking larger-than-prescribed doses of a medication. Substance abusers are not necessarily addicts, however.

Addiction refers to a physical or psychological dependence on a substance. Addiction usually involves a pattern of behavior that includes an obsessive or compulsive preoccupation with a substance and the security of its supply as well as a high rate of relapse after withdrawal.

As a medical assistant, you should not try to make a diagnosis. Quite probably an adolescent with one or more of these disorders will be uncooperative and refuse to answer relevant questions. You must be aware, however, of physical signs or behaviors that may be associated with depression, substance abuse, or addiction in an adolescent patient. The following signs or behaviors are important clues that you should report immediately to the doctor.

- The patient complains of altered eating habits or disturbed sleep patterns (either too much or too little sleep).
- The patient's weight has changed drastically (either up or down) since the previous office visit.
- The patient appears lethargic or sullen or exhibits radical mood changes.
- The patient has slurred speech.
- The patient appears to have illogical thought patterns.
- The patient appears to have needle tracks (anywhere on the body, especially on the arms or legs).
- The patient has pinpoint (highly constricted) pupils.

Signs of depression, addiction, and substance abuse in adolescents can be difficult to distinguish. Signs of substance abuse or addiction can be mistaken for depression. The reverse is also true. Sometimes all three conditions exist simultaneously. If you have any clues that point to one of these conditions in an adolescent patient, notify the physician immediately. For symptoms that may be signs of these disorders, see the Caution: Handle With Care section.

Physical and Psychological Abuse

Abuse can involve people from all walks of life and of all ages. Abuse can be physical, psychological, or both. As a medical assistant, you are in a unique position to detect abuse in the patients you see. (See Chapter 40 for additional information related to child abuse, domestic violence, and elder abuse.)

Although you must not make hasty judgments, you may suspect abuse when a patient speaks in a guarded way. An unlikely explanation for an injury may also be a sign of abuse. There may be no history of the injury, or the history may be suspicious. In either case the following injuries may be signs of physical abuse:

- Head injuries and skull fractures
- Burns (especially those that appear to be deliberate, such as from a cigarette or an iron)
- Broken bones
- Bruises (especially multiple bruises, those that are clearly in the shape of an object, and those in various stages of healing)

Although a patient can recover physically from abuse, the emotional and psychological scars may last a lifetime. Other signs of physical abuse (including sexual abuse and neglect) and signs of psychological abuse include the following:

- A child's failure to thrive
- Severe dehydration or underweight
- Delayed medical attention
- Hair loss

- Drug use
- Genital injuries

Battered Women. Women who are abused by their partners may come to the medical office with bruises or other injuries. Often they are afraid to discuss the problem. A woman may fear that her partner will "get even" if she tells anyone about what happened. The woman may not feel strong enough emotionally to leave an abusing partner. If you suspect abuse, bring it to the physician's attention immediately. You or the physician, or the two of you together, may be able to convince the patient to seek help. Obtain the battered-woman hotline number for your area, and have it available for quick reference.

Abused Children. Children are often the targets of violence, much of which occurs in the home. In addition to being physically, emotionally, or sexually abused, children can be abused by being neglected. If you suspect child abuse, you must report it to the proper authorities. Keep the child abuse hotline number for your area on file.

The Abused Elderly. Physical or mental disabilities can make elderly people dependent on others for care. When such care is perceived as a burden by the caregiver, elder abuse may occur. The disabilities that make an elderly person dependent can also leave him defenseless against abuse. Such a patient may have suspicious injuries or show signs of neglect. Find out whether there is an elder abuse hotline number for your area, and if so keep it available for quick reference.

Drug and Alcohol Abuse

Substance abuse and addiction to drugs or alcohol are serious social problems. Symptoms of substance abuse or addiction differ from drug to drug, as indicated in Table 36-2. Addiction, however, typically causes a gradual decline in

TABLE 36-2 Symptoms Associated With Commonly Abused Drugs

Drug Names/Type	Trade or Other Name	Symptoms, Effects
Amphetamines/stimulants	Benzedrine, Dexedrine, methamphetamine, black beauty, speed, uppers	Altered mental status, from confusion to paranoia; hyperactivity, then exhaustion; insomnia; loss of appetite
Anabolic steroids	Anadrol, Dianabol, Deca-durabotin, Depo-testosterone	Irritability, aggression, nervousness, male-pattern baldness
Barbiturates/sedatives	Amobarbital, phenobarbital, Butisol, secobarbital, yellow jackets, red birds	Slowed thinking, slowed reflexes, slowed respiration, loss of anxiety
Benzodiazepines/sedatives	Ativan, diazepam, Librium, Valium, downers, candy	Poor coordination, drowsiness, increased self-confidence
Cocaine/stimulant	Coke, snow, crack	Alternating euphoria and apprehension, intense craving for more of the drug
Ecstasy/psychoactive	Adam, XTC, MDMA	Confusion, depression, anxiety, paranoia, increase in heart rate and blood pressure
GHB/depressants	G, liquid ecstasy, georgia homeboy	Slow pulse and breathing, lowered blood pressure, drowsiness, poor concentration
Inhalants	Solvents: paint thinner; gases: aerosol, butane or propane	Stimulation, intoxication, hearing loss, arm or leg spasms
LSD (lysergic acid diethylamine)/hallucinogen	Acid, microdot	Heightened sense of awareness, grandiose hallucinations, mystical experiences, flashbacks
Marijuana/cannabinoids/ Hashish	Pot, grass, joint, reefer, weed, bone, buds, hash, boom	Altered thought processes, distorted sense of time and self, impaired short-term memory
Opium, morphine, codeine/ opiate narcotics	Monkey, white stuff	Decreased level of consciousness, detachment, drowsiness, impaired judgment
PCP (phencyclidine)/ hallucinogen	Angel dust	Decreased awareness of surroundings, hallucinations, poor perception of time and distance, possible overdose and death

Morris A. Turner, MD

MEDLAB

266 Line Road
Montclair, Delaware 00956
800-555-4567

C.L.I.A. #21-1862

WELLS, KARLA	09/12/04	09/12/04	09/13/04
Patient Name	Date Drawn	Date Received	Date of Report

F	43	Lisa W. Clark, MD	23341	67294
Sex	Age	22 Landover Lane	ID Number	Account Number

166241809	Newark, Delaware 00964		897211
Patient ID/Soc. Sec. Number			Specimen Number

TEST NAME	RESULT ABNORMAL	RESULT NORMAL	UNITS	REFERENCE RANGE
CHEM-SCREEN PANEL				
GLUCOSE		76.0	MG/DL	65.0–115
SODIUM		139.0	MMOL/L	134–143
POTASSIUM		4.00	MMOL/L	3.60–5.10
CHLORIDE		107.0	MMOL/L	96.0–107
BUN		17.0	MG/DL	6.00–19.0
BUN/CREATININE RATIO		14.2		
URIC ACID		4.30	MG/DL	2.20–6.20
PHOSPHATE		2.40	MG/DL	2.40–4.50
CALCIUM		9.50	MG/DL	8.60–10.0
MAGNESIUM		1.75	MEG/L	1.40–2.00
CHOLESTEROL	237.0		MG/DL	130–200
CHOL. PERCENTILE	90.0		PERCENTILE	1.00–75.0
HDL CHOLESTEROL	41.0		MG/DL	48.0–89.0
CHOL./HDL RATIO		5.80		
LDL CHOL., CALCULATED	175.0		MG/DL	65.5–130
TRIGLYCERIDES		104.0	MG/DL	00.0–200
TOTAL PROTEIN		6.60	GM/DL	6.40–8.00
ALBUMIN		4.10	GM/DL	3.70–4.80
GLOBULIN		2.50	GM/DL	2.20–3.60
ALB/GLOB RATIO		1.64		1.10–2.10
TOTAL BILIRUBIN		0.80	MG/DL	0.20–1.30
DIRECT BILIRUBIN		0.15	MG/DL	0.00–0.20
ALK. PHOSPHATASE		44.0	UNITS/L	25.0–125
G-GLUTAMYL TRANSPEP.		8.00	UNITS/L	1.00–63.0
AST (SGOT)		21.0	IU/L	1.00–40.0
ALT (SGPT)		14.0	IU/L	1.00–50.0
LD		134.0	IU/L	90.0–250
IRON		130.0	MCG/DL	35.0–180

Figure 36-5. Laboratory reports provide physicians with valuable information about patients' health. Test results are accompanied by normal ranges appropriate for the laboratory's testing procedures.

OUTLINE FORMAT PROGRESS NOTES

Patient Name _Hansen_ _Christopher_ _M._ Date of Birth _3_/_1_/_65_ Chart # _H234_
LAST   FIRST   MIDDLE

Prob. No. or Letter	DATE	**S** Subjective	**O** Objective	**A** Assess	**P** Plans	Page _1_
	6/16/04	Patient complaining of pain in lower right quadrant. Has been running fever of between 100.5° F and 101.3° F since Sunday morning. Has queasy feeling in stomach and has been unable to eat since yesterday morning.				
			BP 125/75. Temperature 101.2° F. Abdominal exam revealed rebound tenderness and distension in lower right quadrant.			
				Appendicitis		
					1. Admit to hospital 2. Surgically remove appendix.	

Start each Progress Note (Subjective, Objective, Assessment, and Plans) at the appropriate shaded column to create an outline form. Write through the intervening columns to the right margin of the page.

© 1976 BIBBERO SYSTEMS, INC., PETALUMA, CA   PROGRESS NOTES   TO REORDER CALL TOLL FREE: (800)BIBBERO (800 242-2376)   FORM # 26-7215-01

Figure 36-6. When you use the SOAP approach to documenting patient information, start each progress note at the appropriate shaded column to create an outline form. Write through the intervening columns to the right margin of the page.

if a patient's chief complaint is pain in the left shoulder, you should probe the patient for some pertinent information:

- When did the pain start, and how long have you had the pain? (For example, the type of accident or injury, or the number of days or weeks, etc.)
- When does the pain occur? (For example, on movement, in the morning or evening, etc.)
- Can you describe the pain? (For example, dull, aching, burning, sharp, etc.)
- Rate the pain on a scale of 1 to 10, with 10 being the worst. (A diagram is frequently used for this rating, as shown in Figure 36-8.)

Providing this detailed information is important to the patient's care and treatment. In addition, you will need to chart other information prior to the physician visit. Figure 36-9 shows two types of forms used by the medical assistant and the practitioner when seeing a patient. All information should all be charted completely and accurately. Pay special attention to spelling. If you do not know how to spell a word, look it up or ask someone. Use only approved and recognized abbreviations. Many facilities have a written document identifying these abbreviations. Remember that the chart is a legal document; therefore, special attention to detail is required when charting.

The Health History Form

The medical office usually has a standard medical history form that is used for all patients. The specific arrangement and wording of items vary from office to office. The following sections contain brief descriptions of each of the parts of this form.

Personal Data. This information is obtained from the administrative sheet and includes the patient's name, Social Security number, birth date, and other basic data.

Chief Complaint. Abbreviated as CC, the chief complaint is the reason the patient came to visit the practitioner. It should be short and specific and should cover subjective and objective data.

History of Present Illness. This history includes detailed information about the chief complaint, including when the problem started and what the patient has done to treat the problem (including any medications taken). For example, a chief complaint might be "sore throat" and the history of the present illness would include when the sore throat started (e.g., 3 days ago), how severe the pain is on a scale of 1 to 10 (e.g., pain scale rating of 6 out of 10), and what treatments have been used (e.g., throat lozenges and 4 to 6 aspirin daily).

Past Medical History. The past medical history includes any and all health problems both present and past, including major illnesses and surgery. The past medical history would also include important information about medications and allergies. It should list any medications taken by the patient, including their dosages and the reasons for taking them. Over-the-counter and herbal medications should be considered as well. Known or suspected

HEALTH HISTORY
(Confidential)

Name _____

Age _____ Birthdate _____ Date of last physical examination _____ Today's Date _____

What is your reason for visit? _____

SYMPTOMS Check (✓) symptoms you currently have or have had in the past year.

GENERAL
- Chills
- Depression
- Dizziness
- Fainting
- Fever
- Forgetfulness
- Headache
- Loss of sleep
- Loss of weight
- Nervousness
- Numbness
- Sweats

MUSCLE/JOINT/BONE
Pain, weakness, numbness in:
- Arms
- Back
- Feet
- Hands
- Hips
- Legs
- Neck
- Shoulders

GENITO-URINARY
- Blood in urine
- Frequent urination
- Lack of bladder control
- Painful urination

GASTROINTESTINAL
- Appetite poor
- Bloating
- Bowel changes
- Constipation
- Diarrhea
- Excessive hunger
- Excessive thirst
- Gas
- Hemorrhoids
- Indigestion
- Nausea
- Rectal bleeding
- Stomach pain
- Vomiting
- Vomiting blood

CARDIOVASCULAR
- Chest pain
- High blood pressure
- Irregular heart beat
- Low blood pressure
- Poor circulation
- Rapid heart beat
- Swelling of ankles
- Varicose veins

EYE, EAR, NOSE, THROAT
- Bleeding gums
- Blurred vision
- Crossed eyes
- Difficulty swallowing
- Double vision
- Earache
- Ear discharge
- Hay fever
- Hoarseness
- Loss of hearing
- Nosebleeds
- Persistent cough
- Ringing in ears
- Sinus problems
- Vision – Flashes
- Vision – Halos

SKIN
- Bruise easily
- Hives
- Itching
- Change in moles
- Rash
- Scars
- Sore that won't heal

MEN only
- Breast lump
- Erection difficulties
- Lump in testicles
- Penis discharge
- Sore on penis
- Other

WOMEN only
- Abnormal Pap smear
- Bleeding between periods
- Breast lump
- Extreme menstrual pain
- Hot flashes
- Nipple discharge
- Painful intercourse
- Vaginal discharge
- Other

Date of last menstrual period _____
Date of last Pap smear _____
Have you had a mammogram? _____
Are you pregnant? _____
Number of children _____

CONDITIONS Check (✓) conditions you have or have had in the past.
- AIDS
- Alcoholism
- Anemia
- Anorexia
- Appendicitis
- Arthritis
- Asthma
- Bleeding Disorders
- Breast Lump
- Bronchitis
- Bulimia
- Cancer
- Cataracts
- Chemical Dependency
- Chicken Pox
- Diabetes
- Emphysema
- Epilepsy
- Glaucoma
- Goiter
- Gonorrhea
- Gout
- Heart Disease
- Hepatitis
- Hernia
- Herpes
- High Cholesterol
- HIV Positive
- Kidney Disease
- Liver Disease
- Measles
- Migraine Headaches
- Miscarriage
- Mononucleosis
- Multiple Sclerosis
- Mumps
- Pacemaker
- Pneumonia
- Polio
- Prostate Problem
- Psychiatric Care
- Rheumatic Fever
- Scarlet Fever
- Stroke
- Suicide Attempt
- Thyroid Problems
- Tonsillitis
- Tuberculosis
- Typhoid Fever
- Ulcers
- Vaginal Infections
- Venereal Disease

MEDICATIONS List medications you are currently taking

ALLERGIES To medications or substances

Pharmacy Name _____ Phone _____

(All information is strictly confidential)

FAMILY HISTORY Fill in health information about your family.

Relation	Age	State of Health	Age at Death	Cause of Death	Check (✓) if, your blood relatives had any of the following: Disease	Relationship to you
Father					Arthritis, Gout	
Mother					Asthma, Hay Fever	
Brothers					Cancer	
					Chemical Dependency	
					Diabetes	
Sisters					Heart Disease, Strokes	
					High Blood Pressure	
					Kidney Disease	
					Tuberculosis	
					Other	

HOSPITALIZATIONS

Year	Hospital	Reason for Hospitalization and Outcome

Have you ever had a blood transfusion? ☐ Yes ☐ No
If yes, please give approximate dates.

SERIOUS ILLNESS/INJURIES	DATE	OUTCOME

PREGNANCY HISTORY

Year of Birth	Sex of Birth	Complications if any

HEALTH HABITS Check (✓) which substances you use and describe how much you use.
- Caffeine
- Tobacco
- Drugs
- Other

OCCUPATIONAL CONCERNS Check (✓) if your work exposes you to the following:
- Stress
- Hazardous Substances
- Heavy Lifting
- Other
Your occupation: _____

I certify that the above information is correct to the best of my knowledge. I will not hold my doctor or any members of his/her staff responsible for any errors or omissions that I may have made in the completion of this form.

Signature _____ Date _____

Reviewed By _____ Date _____

Figure 36-7. The health history form must be complete and accurate. This sample form is started by the patient, then checked and completed by the medical assistant.

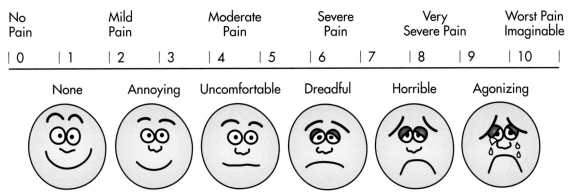

Halifax Regional Medical Center
Pain Management Is Our Concern
e 00964

No Pain		Mild Pain		Moderate Pain		Severe Pain		Very Severe Pain		Worst Pain Imaginable
0	1	2	3	4	5	6	7	8	9	10

None   Annoying   Uncomfortable   Dreadful   Horrible   Agonizing

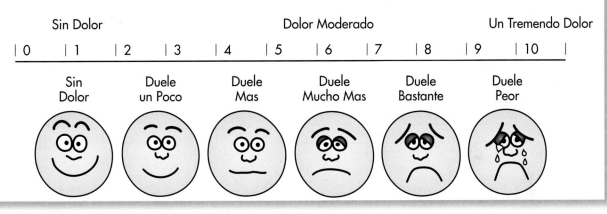

El control del dolor es nuestra responsabilidad

Sin Dolor				Dolor Moderado						Un Tremendo Dolor
0	1	2	3	4	5	6	7	8	9	10

Sin Dolor   Duele un Poco   Duele Mas   Duele Mucho Mas   Duele Bastante   Duele Peor

Figure 36-8. Assessing a patient's pain is part of the interview and history-taking process. This common chart is used to make the process easier for the patient and the medical assistant.

allergies to medications or other substances should be listed and clearly visible. Some facilities use a red sticker or other means on charts to identify allergies immediately.

Family History. This section includes information about the health of the patient's family members. Many times the family history can help lead a practitioner to the cause of a current medical problem. Obtain specific information about family members' current ages and medical conditions or, if deceased, their age at death and the cause. Ask open-ended questions about the siblings, parents, and grandparents. Because the death of a parent or sibling or the limited knowledge of an adopted child can be difficult to discuss, use great care and sensitivity when asking these questions.

Social and Occupational History. Information such as marital status, sexual behaviors and orientation, occupations, hobbies, and the use of chemical substances help determine a patient's risk for disease. Patients should be asked about their use of alcohol, tobacco, recreational drugs, or other chemical substances. Be aware that patients may feel uncomfortable or may refuse to provide certain information. Depending on the circumstances, you may ask the question later in the interview. For example, an adolescent child may not want to answer questions about his sexual behaviors in front of his parents. Occupational information regarding the patient's level of stress, exposure to hazardous substances, and heavy lifting may also be included here.

Review of Systems. Some of this information may be started by the patient but is completed by the practitioner. This systematic review of each of the systems of the body includes questions and an examination by the practitioner. The information is obtained in an orderly fashion but may vary depending on the physician or practitioner.

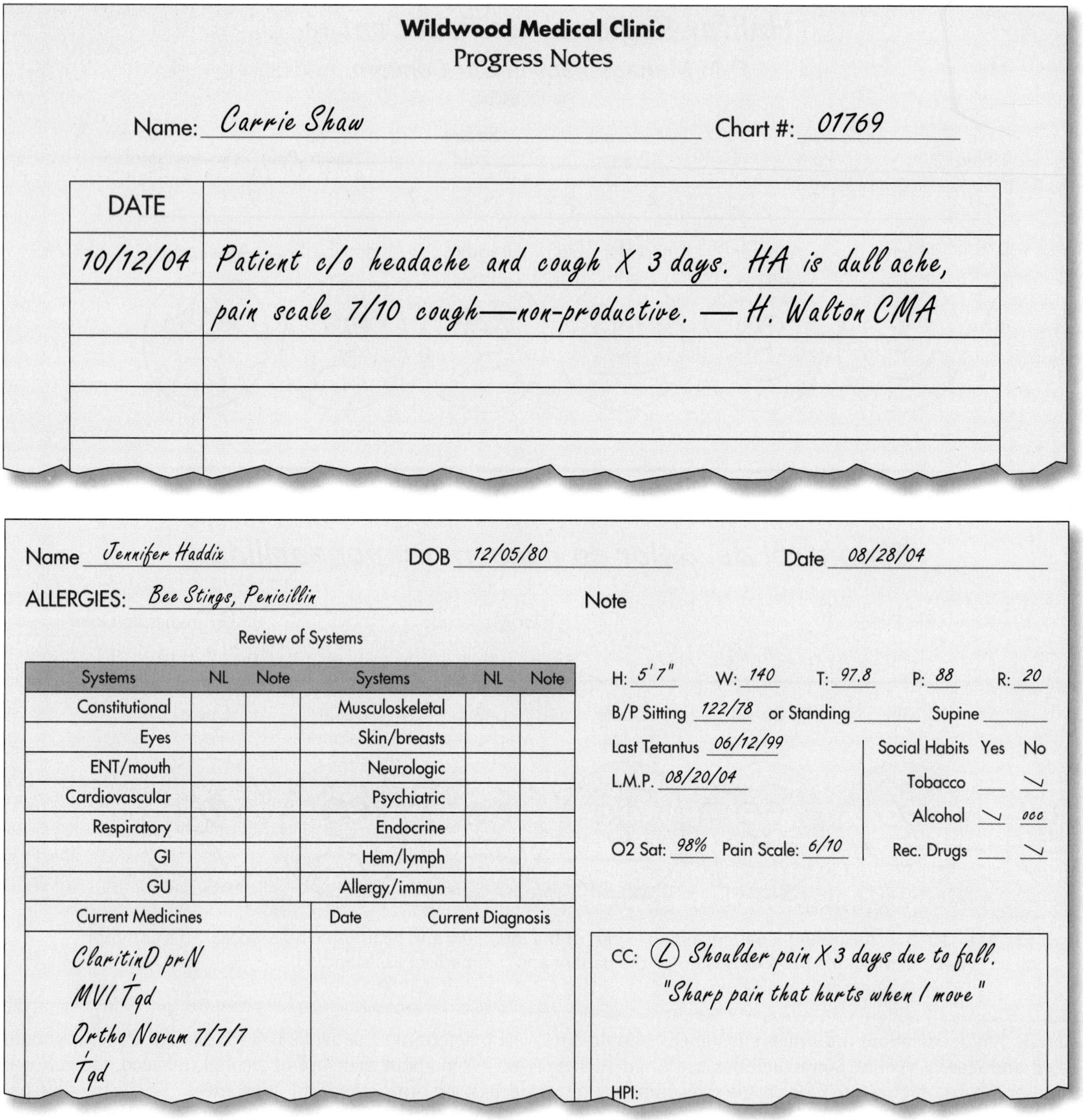

Wildwood Medical Clinic
Progress Notes

Name: _Carrie Shaw_   Chart #: _01769_

DATE	
10/12/04	Patient c/o headache and cough X 3 days. HA is dull ache, pain scale 7/10 cough—non-productive. — H. Walton CMA

Name: _Jennifer Haddix_   DOB _12/05/80_   Date _08/28/04_

ALLERGIES: _Bee Stings, Penicillin_   Note

Review of Systems

Systems	NL	Note	Systems	NL	Note
Constitutional			Musculoskeletal		
Eyes			Skin/breasts		
ENT/mouth			Neurologic		
Cardiovascular			Psychiatric		
Respiratory			Endocrine		
GI			Hem/lymph		
GU			Allergy/immun		

H: _5'7"_   W: _140_   T: _97.8_   P: _88_   R: _20_

B/P Sitting _122/78_ or Standing _____ Supine _____

Last Tetantus _06/12/99_

L.M.P. _08/20/04_

O2 Sat: _98%_ Pain Scale: _6/10_

Social Habits	Yes	No
Tobacco	___	✓
Alcohol	✓	ooo
Rec. Drugs	___	✓

Current Medicines	Date	Current Diagnosis
ClaritinD prN MVI T̄ qd Ortho Novum 7/7/7 T̄ qd		

CC: (L) Shoulder pain X 3 days due to fall. "Sharp pain that hurts when I move"

HPI:

Figure 36-9. These example forms are completed by the medical assistant prior to the physician visit. All information must be complete and accurate as shown.

Summary

As a medical assistant, you will play a key role in a patient's visit to the physician's office. Because you will begin the examination by interviewing the patient, you will set the tone of the visit. Keep in mind that some patients may be nervous or uncomfortable. It is important to make them feel at ease. Using interviewing skills effectively will help make the interview productive as well as comfortable for the patient. Taking a thorough history and using proper documentation methods will also allow you to ensure that patient records are complete and accurate. They will also help the practitioner to diagnose and treat the patient successfully.

CHAPTER 36

CASE STUDY QUESTIONS

Now that you have completed this chapter, review the case study at the beginning of the chapter and answer the following questions:

1. How can you ensure that the interview process goes smoothly?
2. Why is it important that you maintain a positive relationship with this patient?
3. What steps will you take to make sure all the documentation is completed correctly and accurately?

Discussion Questions

1. Explain the difference between subjective and objective data. Give examples of each type.
2. Describe the technique you would use to obtain accurate information from a pediatric patient.
3. What is the significance of each of the parts of the health history form?

Critical Thinking Questions

1. A patient comes into the office with abdominal pain. On her chart is a notation that she is coming in with symptoms of appendicitis. What questions might you ask her to assist the doctor in determining whether her condition is appendicitis?
2. A parent brings in her 3-year-old son, who has chronic diarrhea. You note that the child has a large bruise on the side of his face. He appears very thin and pale. You suspect he may have been abused. What questions might you ask to obtain the information necessary to rule out or confirm abuse?
3. A 31-year-old male patient comes to the clinic after a fall that occurred at work. During the interview, he complains of pain in his left leg and right elbow. He is unable to describe what happened and says he just blacked out. What observations should you make, and what questions should you ask this patient?
4. While interviewing and recording the health history of a patient, you are required to list all the medications the patient is taking. The patient names several medications and provides the dosages; however, you cannot spell one of them and you are not sure about how to write the abbreviations for the dosages. What should you do?

Application Activities

1. Have a partner assume the role of a patient who has come into the office with what appears to be the flu. Conduct an interview and take a patient history.
2. With a partner, practice role-playing both effective and ineffective methods of collecting patient data. Create situations and questions that encourage and discourage communication. Compare and contrast the differences. Use Table 36-1 as a guideline.

Internet Activities

1. Explore the Internet to find resources for charting medical and health information. Find sites for medical abbreviations, medical terminology, and medications, and then create favorites or quick links from the browser on your computer for handy reference when writing in the patient's chart.
2. Research the Internet for a commonly abused drug, and create a brief oral or written report. Include the following information:
   a. The drug's trade and common names
   b. How it affects the body both physically and psychologically
   c. The signs and symptoms of abuse
   d. How you would notice if a patient is abusing this drug

Visit the National Institute of Drug Abuse at **www.nida.nih.gov** to begin your research.

CHAPTER 37

Obtaining Vital Signs and Measurements

KEY TERMS

afebrile
antecubital space
apex
apical
auscultated blood pressure
axilla
brachial artery
calibrate
Celsius (centigrade)
dyspnea
Fahrenheit
febrile
hyperpnea
hypotension
meniscus
palpatory method
radial artery
sphygmomanometer
stethoscope
tachypnea
tympanic thermometer

AREAS OF COMPETENCE

2003 Role Delineation Study

CLINICAL

Patient Care

- Obtain patient history and vital signs

GENERAL

Communication Skills

- Adapt communications to individual's ability to understand
- Recognize and respond effectively to verbal, nonverbal, and written communications
- Utilize electronic technology to receive, organize, prioritize, and transmit information

CHAPTER OUTLINE

- Vital Signs
- Body Measurements

OBJECTIVES

After completing Chapter 37, you will be able to:

37.1 Recognize common terminology and abbreviations used in documenting and discussing vital signs.

37.2 Describe the instruments used to measure vital signs and body measurements.

37.3 Explain the procedure used to measure vital signs and body measurements.

37.4 Demonstrate the procedures for measuring vital signs and body measurements.

Introduction

Vital signs are one of the most important assessments you can make when preparing the patient to be examined by the practitioner. Temperature, pulse, respirations, and blood pressure give information about how a patient will adjust to changes within the body and in the environment. Changes in the vital signs can indicate an abnormality.

Measurements such as height, weight, and head circumference can indicate physical growth and development, especially in infants and children. These measurements are also used to evaluate health problems, such as obesity. You must be accurate when performing and recording vital signs and measurements. The practitioner uses your results when making a diagnosis.

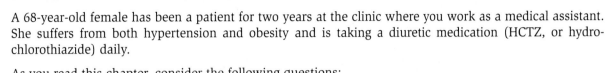

CASE STUDY

A 68-year-old female has been a patient for two years at the clinic where you work as a medical assistant. She suffers from both hypertension and obesity and is taking a diuretic medication (HCTZ, or hydrochlorothiazide) daily.

As you read this chapter, consider the following questions:

1. Why is it essential for you to take accurate measurements of this patient?
2. How can you help ensure the accuracy of these measurements?

Vital Signs

As a medical assistant, you will usually take the vital signs before the doctor examines the patient. Temperature, pulse, respiration, and blood pressure (vital signs) provide the doctor with information about the patient's overall condition.

Preexamination procedures in some offices are performed in a general area outside the patient examination room. In other offices and in most pediatric offices, these measurements are taken in the examination room. In either case you will usually take the measurements before the patient disrobes. Follow the standard procedure used in your office. Also be certain to follow the HIPAA regulations and provide for the privacy of your results.

General Considerations

Vital signs are the primary indicators of a patient's overall general condition. The four vital signs are as follows:

1. Temperature
2. Pulse
3. Respiration
4. Blood pressure

Vital signs are usually measured at every office visit. There is a standard range of values for each measurement, as shown in Table 37-1. Each patient has an individual baseline value that is normal for that patient, however. The difference between a patient's current values and normal values can help the physician in making a diagnosis.

TABLE 37-1 Normal Ranges for Vital Signs

Vital Sign	Age				
	0–1 year	1–6 years	6–11 years	11–16 years	Adult
Temperature					
Oral (°F)	96–99.5 (less than 4 weeks)	98.5–99.5	97.5–99.6	97.6–99.6	97.6–99.6
Rectal (°F)	99.0–100.0	99.0–100.0	98.5–99.6	98.6–100.6	98.6–100.6
Pulse (beats per minute)	80–160	75–130	70–115	55–110	60–100
Respirations (per minute)	26–40	20–30	18–24	16–24	12–20
Blood Pressure (mm Hg)					
Systolic*	74–100	80–112	80–120	88–120	90–120
Diastolic*	50–70	50–80	50–80	58–80	60–80

*According to the American Heart Association, patients with systolic readings from 120 to 139 mm Hg and diastolic readings from 80 to 89 mm Hg are considered prehypertensive.

TABLE 37-2 OSHA Guidelines for Taking Measurements of Vital Signs

Situation	OSHA Guidelines
Before and after all patient contact	Examination area cleaned according to OSHA standards Aseptic hand washing (Procedure 19-1 in Chapter 19)
Temperature by oral or rectal route Contact with patient with lesions Contact with patient suspect for infectious disease	Gloves worn Biohazard bags used for disposal of used thermometer sheaths, otoscope tips, alcohol swabs, dressings, and bandages
In presence of patient suspect for airborne infectious disease (particularly sneezing)	Mask worn Patient weighed, measured, and examined in room away from staff and other patients Protective clothing (laboratory coat, gown, or apron) worn Biohazard bags used as above

You must follow closely the guidelines from the Department of Labor's Occupational Safety and Health Administration (OSHA) for taking measurements of vital signs (Table 37-2). These guidelines are intended to prevent transmission of disease from the patient. They help protect you and keep the workplace safe.

Temperature

When you take a patient's temperature, you will determine whether the patient is **febrile** (has a body temperature above the patient's normal range) or whether the patient is **afebrile** (has a body temperature at about the patient's normal range). A fever is usually a sign of inflammation or infection. You can take a temperature in one of four locations:

1. Mouth (oral)
2. Ear (tympanic)
3. Rectum (rectal)
4. Armpit, or **axilla** (axillary)

Temperature can be measured in degrees **Fahrenheit** (°F) or degrees **Celsius** (**centigrade;** °C). Figure 37-1, gives equivalent values for the two temperature scales. Normal adult oral temperature is considered to be about 98.6°F or 37.0°C. Rectal and tympanic temperatures are normally 1° higher than an oral temperature. The rectal method usually provides the most accurate body temperature; however, the oral method is more commonly used and is accurate when performed properly. Axillary temperatures are normally 1° lower than oral temperatures because the area is outside the body and exposed to air.

Temperature is measured with a thermometer. Thermometers may be one of three types: electronic digital, tympanic, or disposable.

Electronic Digital Thermometers. Electronic digital thermometers are used frequently in medical offices. These thermometers provide a digital readout of the patient's temperature (Figure 37-2). They are accurate, fast, easy to read, and comfortable for the patient.

Fahrenheit and Celsius Equivalents for Temperature

°F	°C	°F	°C	°F	°C	°F	°C
95.0	35.0	98.4	36.9	101.8	38.8	105.2	40.7
95.2	35.1	98.6	37.0	102.0	38.9	105.4	40.8
95.4	35.2	98.8	37.1	102.2	39.0	105.6	40.9
95.6	35.3	99.0	37.2	102.4	39.1	105.8	41.0
95.8	35.4	99.2	37.3	102.6	39.2	106.0	41.1
96.0	35.6	99.4	37.4	102.8	39.3	106.2	41.2
96.2	35.7	99.6	37.6	103.0	39.4	106.4	41.3
96.4	35.8	99.8	37.7	103.2	39.6	106.6	41.4
96.6	35.9	100.0	37.8	103.4	39.7	106.8	41.6
96.8	36.0	100.2	37.9	103.6	39.8	107.0	41.7
97.0	36.1	100.4	38.0	103.8	39.9	107.2	41.8
97.2	36.2	100.6	38.1	104.0	40.0	107.4	41.9
97.4	36.3	100.8	38.2	104.2	40.1	107.6	42.0
97.6	36.4	101.0	38.3	104.4	40.2	107.8	42.1
97.8	36.6	101.2	38.4	104.6	40.3	108.0	42.2
98.0	36.7	101.4	38.6	104.8	40.4		
98.2	36.8	101.6	38.7	105.0	40.6		

Note: °F = (°C × %) + 32; °C = (°F − 32) × %. Conversions are rounded to nearest tenth.

Figure 37-1. Use this chart to convert Fahrenheit temperature readings to Celsius and vice versa.

One type of electronic thermometer is designed for oral, rectal, or axillary use. This type of thermometer has a battery-powered display unit, a wire cord, and a temperature-sensitive probe covered by a disposable plastic tip. Separate probes and tips are available for oral or rectal use. Most units have an audible indicator, such as a beep, to let you know when the temperature has registered and is displayed.

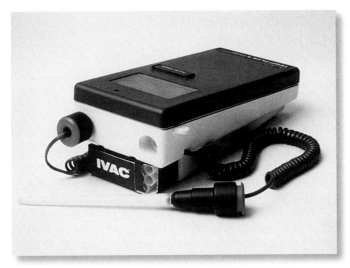

Figure 37-2. The electronic digital thermometer provides a digital readout of the patient's temperature.

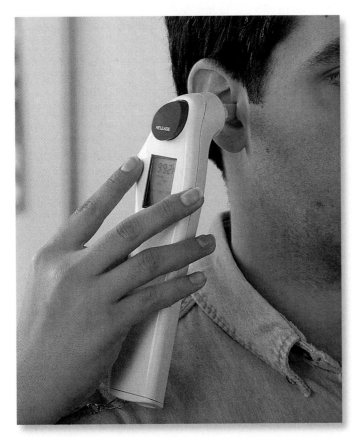

Figure 37-3. The tympanic thermometer measures infrared energy emitted from the tympanic membrane. The result, converted to body temperature, is displayed within seconds of insertion of the shielded tip into the ear.

Tympanic Thermometers. Another type of electronic thermometer, the **tympanic thermometer,** is designed for use in the ear, as shown in Figure 37-3. This thermometer measures infrared energy emitted from the tympanic membrane (eardrum). This energy is converted into a temperature reading. Because of its speed, ease of

use, and comfort for the patient, the tympanic thermometer is popular in pediatric offices. The tip is covered with a disposable sheath to prevent cross-contamination.

Disposable Thermometers. Disposable, single-use thermometers are usually made of thin strips of plastic with specially treated dot or strip indicators. The indicators change color according to the temperature. This type of thermometer is used most commonly for oral and axillary temperature measurements, particularly in children. Typically, it does not give as accurate a reading as other types of thermometers do. However, disposable thermometers are useful for patients in their homes.

Taking Temperatures

Using the proper instrument and technique provides the most accurate temperature readings. Temperatures can vary according to the location used. Thus, you must be sure to indicate the site (oral, rectal, axillary, tympanic) of the temperature measurement when you enter the reading in the patient's chart. If no site is specified, it is presumed to be oral. All temperature measurements should be recorded to the nearest one-tenth of a degree.

Using Tympanic Thermometers. Although accurate when used correctly, tympanic thermometers can give incorrect readings if you do not follow the proper technique exactly. For a description of tympanic thermometers and potential problems with their use, see the Caution: Handle With Care section.

Although you must follow manufacturers' instructions precisely, these thermometers are easy to use. First remove the thermometer from its recharging cradle, then wait for the indicator light to show that the unit is ready. Attach a disposable sheath, and place the thermometer in the opening of the ear so that the fit is snug. Pull the ear up and back for adults and down and back for children. Press the button, and the result will be displayed within seconds. Be certain to press the correct button to read the temperature. Another button on the thermometer releases the sheath. You do not want to release the sheath into the patient's ear.

Measuring Oral Temperatures. To take an oral temperature, make sure the patient is able to hold the thermometer in the mouth. The patient must also be able to breathe through the nose. Place the thermometer under the tongue in either pocket just off-center in the lower jaw. The patient should hold the thermometer with lips closed. Wait at least 15 minutes after a patient has been eating, drinking, or smoking before taking an oral temperature; otherwise, you may obtain an inaccurate result.

Measuring Rectal Temperatures. Temperatures are sometimes measured rectally in infants or adults in whom an oral temperature cannot be taken. When taking rectal temperatures, you must wear gloves to prevent contamination from microorganisms present in the stool.

To take a rectal temperature, use an electronic thermometer with a rectal probe and disposable rectal tip. The

Tympanic Thermometers: What You Need to Know

Tympanic thermometers are popular in medical offices, especially pediatric offices, because they are fast and accurate when used correctly. They are also particularly useful with uncooperative patients and with patients who have been eating, drinking, or smoking, because tympanic temperature readings are not affected by these activities.

If you do not use the proper technique, however, you can get inaccurate temperature readings with a tympanic thermometer. Here is a summary of what you need to know.

Why the Eardrum?

The idea of using the tympanic membrane as a site for temperature measurement originated in the 1960s as a means of measuring temperature in astronauts. The eardrum is an ideal place to measure temperature because it shares the same blood supply with the hypothalamus, the organ that controls body temperature.

How Do Tympanic Thermometers Work?

Tympanic thermometers work by measuring infrared energy, a type of heat energy, emitted from the tympanic membrane (eardrum). The thermometer converts this information into a temperature reading, usually within seconds. Most tympanic thermometers run on a rechargeable battery that must be recharged between uses.

Where Problems Can Occur

The technique for taking a tympanic temperature may vary slightly, depending on which brand of thermometer you use. You must follow the manufacturer's instructions for your instrument to get accurate results.

Most units have an indicator to let you know when the thermometer is ready for use. Some units require taking the temperature within a certain period after removing the thermometer from its charging base. Read the manufacturer's instructions for specific information.

There can be problems with most units if the outer opening of the ear is not sealed completely when the probe is placed at the ear canal. An improper seal may also mean that the thermometer is not aimed at the eardrum and will give an inaccurate reading. You may need to tug gently on the ear to position the thermometer properly and aim it at the eardrum.

If the thermometer has been charging for several hours before use, the initial reading may be inaccurately high. Therefore, some experts believe you should take two measurements on the first patient after charging the unit and record only the second reading.

Even with good technique, errors can sometimes occur. If you do obtain a reading that does not appear to match the patient's general condition, repeat the temperature measurement to be sure.

---

patient should be positioned on one side or on the stomach with the anus exposed. The left side is the preferred position. The bulb of the thermometer should be inserted slowly and gently until it is covered or until you feel resistance, at approximately 1 inch for adults and ½ inch for infants and small children. Hold the thermometer in place while taking the temperature.

Measuring Axillary Temperatures. To take an axillary temperature, first have the patient sit or lie down. Place the tip of the thermometer in the middle of the axilla, with the shaft facing forward. The patient's upper arm should be pressed against his side, and his lower arm should be crossed over the stomach to hold the thermometer in place. Make sure the tip of the thermometer touches skin on all sides of the probe.

Special Considerations in Children. Taking a child's or an infant's temperature can be a challenge. If the infant or child is likely to cry or become agitated, take the temperature last. Measure pulse, respiration, and blood pressure (if ordered) before you take the temperature to avoid having these measurements elevated because of the child's agitation.

Oral thermometers are not appropriate for children under 5 years of age because these children are too young to safely hold the thermometer in their mouths. Instead, take axillary, rectal, or tympanic temperatures. If you use a rectal thermometer, hold it in place until the temperature registers, because the thermometer can be expelled easily. Furthermore, children, especially infants, can injure themselves if they move while having a rectal temperature taken. Tympanic thermometers are especially useful in pediatric offices because of their speed and safety.

Pulse and Respiration

Pulse and respiration are related because the circulatory and respiratory systems work together. Pulse is measured as the number of times the heart beats in 1 minute. Respiration is the number of times a patient breathes in 1 minute.

One breath, or respiration, equals one inhalation and one exhalation. Usually if either the pulse or respiration rate is high or low, the other is also. The usual ratio of the pulse rate to the respiration rate is about 4:1 (for example, a pulse of 80 and a respiration of 20).

Pulse. A pulse rate gives information about the patient's cardiovascular system. It is an indirect measurement of the patient's cardiac output. If the pulse is abnormally fast, slow, weak, or irregular, the patient may have a medical problem.

Measure the pulse of adults at the **radial artery,** where it can be felt in the groove on the thumb side of the inner wrist. Press lightly on this pulse point with your fingers and not your thumb (a pulse is located in your thumb, and you may feel it instead of the patient's pulse), and count the number of beats you feel in 1 minute. Office policy may direct that you count the pulse for 30 seconds and multiply the results by 2 to obtain the beats per minute. If you take a pulse for less than 1 minute and notice irregularities, you must count for 1 full minute and document the irregularities.

In young children the radial artery may be hard to feel. You may instead take the pulse at the **brachial artery,** which is in the bend of the elbow (the **antecubital space**).

You may not be able to feel the brachial artery in an infant. If you cannot, then take the pulse over the **apex** (the left lower corner) of the heart, where the strongest heart sounds can be heard. Count the **apical** pulse while you listen with a **stethoscope,** an instrument that amplifies body sounds. The apex is located in the fifth intercostal space between the ribs on the left side of the chest, directly

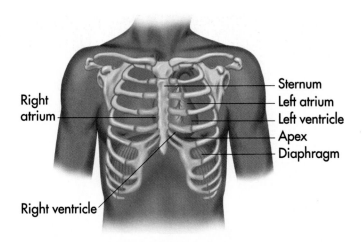

Figure 37-4. A stethoscope is used over the apex of the heart to listen for the pulse in patients in whom pulse is not otherwise detectable.

below the center of the clavicle. Consult Figure 37-4 for placement of the stethoscope.

You may also use other locations to take a pulse. Figure 37-5 shows the location of common pulse points.

Electronic Pulse. The pulse may also be measured electronically using a device attached to the finger or sometimes the earlobe. Figure 37-6 shows one type of device used as part of an electronic blood pressure machine. A pulse oximeter machine, which measures the oxygen level of the blood, can also be used (Figure 37-7). When using these devices, be certain to attach the clip firmly to the finger or lobe. The clip uses an infrared light to measure the pulse and

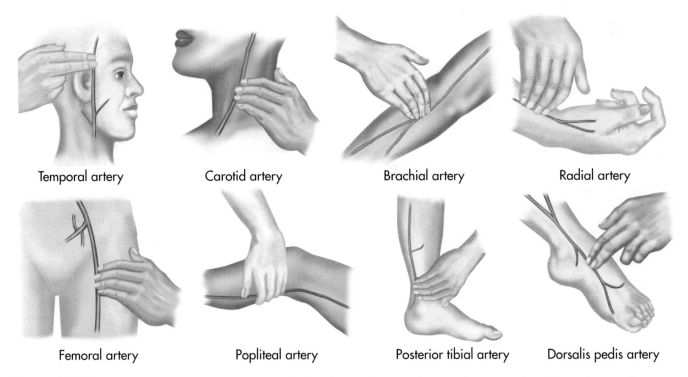

Figure 37-5. There are many locations on the body where major arteries are close enough to the surface to allow a pulse to be felt and counted.

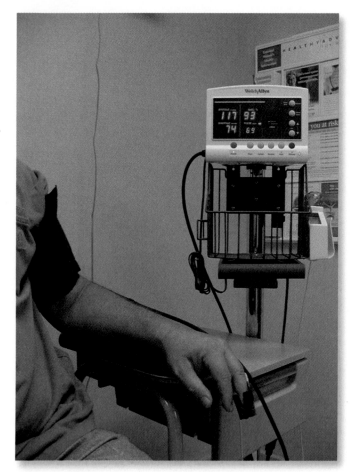

Figure 37-6. Pulse, blood pressure, and oxygen saturation can all be measured with this electronic blood pressure device.
Photo courtesy of Total Care Programming.

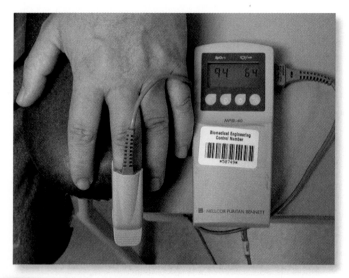

Figure 37-7. A pulse oximeter measures the pulse and oxygen saturation of the blood.
Photo courtesy of Total Care Programming.

oxygen levels, so it works best when no nail polish is present on the patient's finger. The pulse reading and the oxygen saturation of the blood will display on the screen. If the pulse is outside the normal range (see Table 37-1), it should be taken again or performed manually. If the oxygen level is less than 92%, the patient should be asked to take deep breaths during the procedure to increase her oxygen level.

Respiration. Respiration rate indicates how well a patient's body is providing oxygen to tissues. The best way to check respiration is by watching, listening, or feeling the movement at the patient's chest, stomach, back, or shoulders. If you cannot see the chest movement, then place your hand over the patient's chest, shoulder, or abdomen and listen for the movement of air. You may not be able to see or hear the breathing of some patients. Many times the most reliable method for measuring respiration is with a stethoscope. Place the stethoscope on one side of the spine in the middle of the back to count respirations. You need to do this subtly, however, because once the patient is aware that respiration is being measured, he may unintentionally alter his breathing. You may tell the patient that you want to listen to his lungs.

Counting respirations for less than 1 full minute may cause you to miss certain breathing abnormalities. Irregularities such as **dyspnea** (difficult or painful breathing), **tachypnea** (rapid breathing), or **hyperpnea** (deep, rapid breathing) are important indications of possible infection or disease.

Respiration rates are higher in infants and children than in adults. Become familiar with the normal ranges of respiration for each age group, as presented in Table 37-1.

Blood Pressure

Blood pressure (also known as arterial blood pressure) is the force at which blood is pumped against the walls of the arteries. The standard unit for measuring blood pressure is millimeters of mercury (mm Hg). The pressure measured when the left ventricle of the heart contracts is known as the **systolic pressure.** The pressure measured when the heart relaxes is known as the **diastolic pressure.** The diastolic pressure indicates the minimum amount of pressure exerted against the vessel walls at all times.

Expected adult systolic readings range from 100 to 120 mm Hg. Expected adult diastolic readings range from 60 to 80 mm Hg. These values may increase with advancing age. Readings that are higher than these values are considered prehypertensive.

Certain disease states may cause blood pressure to rise above or fall below these ranges. Thus, it is important to recognize these abnormalities. **Hypertension,** or high blood pressure, is a major contributor to heart attack and stroke. The doctor may ask a patient whose blood pressure is elevated to return in 2 months or less for a checkup or blood pressure check. If the blood pressure remains elevated, the patient may be diagnosed with hypertension. **Hypotension,** or low blood pressure, is not generally a chronic health problem. Slightly low blood pressure may be normal for some patients and does not usually require treatment. Severe hypotension may be present with shock, heart failure, severe burns, and excessive bleeding.

Blood Pressure Measuring Equipment. Blood pressure is measured with an instrument called a **sphygmomanometer.** A sphygmomanometer consists of an inflatable cuff, a pressure bulb or automatic device for inflating the cuff, and a manometer to read the pressure. The three basic types of sphygmomanometers differ in how the pressure is displayed.

Aneroid Sphygmomanometers. Aneroid sphygmomanometers have a circular gauge for registering pressure. The needle on the gauge rotates as pressure rises. This type of sphygmomanometer is very accurate. Each measurement line indicates 2 mm Hg (Figure 37-8).

Electronic Sphygmomanometers. Electronic sphygmomanometers provide a digital readout of blood pressure on a lit display (Figure 37-9). Unlike mercury and aneroid sphygmomanometers, these devices do not require use of a stethoscope to determine blood pressure. Although they are easy to use, electronic sphygmomanometers are very costly and may give you an inaccurate reading. However, electronic sphygmomanometers are often used, and newer models have improved accuracy. If you question the results of an electronic blood pressure measurement, take it again with an aneroid cuff.

Mercury Sphygmomanometers. Mercury sphygmomanometers contain a column of mercury. The mercury column rises with an increase in pressure as the cuff is inflated. Mercury sphygmomanometers may be wall-mounted units, tabletop units, or freestanding units on wheels. Mercury instruments are used less frequently because the government has restricted the use of mercury due to its affects on the environment. Consequently, no new mercury sphygmomanometers are being manufactured.

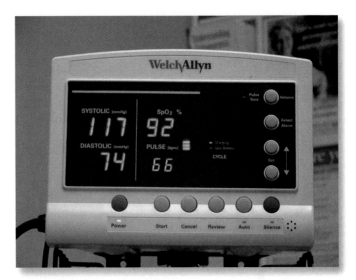

Figure 37-9. This electronic sphygmomanometer displays the patient's blood pressure, pulse, and oxygen saturation. If you question any of the results, repeat the test using a manual method.

Calibrating the Sphygmomanometer. To ensure that sphygmomanometers are working properly, you or a medical supply dealer must calibrate them regularly. To **calibrate** means to standardize a measuring instrument. Mercury sphygmomanometers must be checked for faults, serviced, and calibrated every 6 to 12 months. Aneroid sphygmomanometers must be checked, serviced, and calibrated every 3 to 6 months. Follow the manufacturer's instructions for an electronic sphygmomanometer.

Each time you use a mercury or aneroid sphygmomanometer, you need to ensure that it is correctly calibrated. To do so, follow these steps.

- For a mercury sphygmomanometer, check that the **meniscus** (curve in the air-to-liquid surface of the specimen in the cylinder) of mercury on the mercury column rests at zero when you view it at eye level.
- For an aneroid sphygmomanometer, check that the recording needle on the dial rests within the small square at the bottom of the dial. To calibrate the dial, use a Y connector to attach the dial to a pressure bulb and a calibrated mercury manometer. Use the pressure bulb to elevate both manometer readings to 250 mm Hg. As you let the pressure fall, record both readings at four different points. The difference between paired readings should not exceed 3 mm Hg.

Do not use a sphygmomanometer that is not correctly calibrated. The patient's blood pressure reading will not be accurate.

The Stethoscope. A stethoscope amplifies body sounds, making them louder. It consists of earpieces, binaurals, rubber or plastic tubing, and a chestpiece (Figure 37-10). For best results the earpieces should fit snugly and comfortably in your ears. When placing them in your

ANEROID BLOOD PRESSURE GAUGE

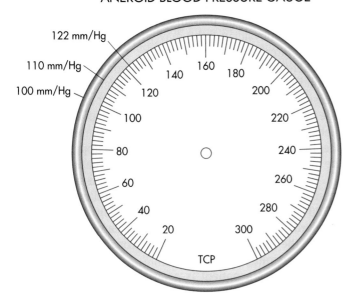

Figure 37-8. Each line on the aneroid gauge indicates 2 mm Hg. To prevent inaccuracies, look directly at this gauge when performing a blood pressure test.

Borrowed from Kathryn Booth, *Health Care Science Technology: Career Technology, 1st ed.,* Peoria, IL: Glencoe/McGraw-Hill, 2004.

38.5 Describe how to position and drape a patient in each of the ten common examination positions.

38.6 Explain ways to assist patients from different cultures, patients with disabilities, children, and pregnant women.

38.7 Identify and describe the six examination methods used in a general physical examination.

38.8 List the components of a general physical examination.

38.9 Explain the special needs of the elderly for patient education.

38.10 Identify ways to help a patient follow up on a doctor's recommendations.

Introduction

Whether a patient comes for a regular checkup or to have a problem diagnosed and treated, the physical examination is the first step in the process for the physician or practitioner. During the physical examination, the medical assistant must make the client comfortable and assist the physician as necessary. A skilled medical assistant who is sensitive to patient needs plus proficient in performing these skills can create an atmosphere that results in a positive outcome for the patient during the physical examination.

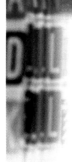

CASE STUDY

A 50-year-old male patient who cannot speak English comes for a general physical examination. You must prepare the patient for the examination, including proper positioning, explain each component of the exam, and assist the physician as necessary.

As you read this chapter, consider the following questions:

1. English is the only language you speak. How can you provide adequate explanation?
2. How can you prevent embarrassment when preparing the patient for the examination?
3. During what parts of the examination do you expect to provide assistance for the physician?

The Purpose of a General Physical Examination

Physicians perform general physical examinations for two purposes. The first is to examine a healthy patient to confirm an overall state of health and to provide baseline values for vital signs and measurements. The second is to examine a patient to diagnose a medical problem.

To confirm a patient's health status, physicians usually perform examinations on a routine basis, such as once a year. Some examinations are done to fulfill a requirement before an individual starts school, begins a new job, or starts an exercise program.

To diagnose medical problems, physicians usually focus on a particular organ system, as indicated by the patient's chief complaint. Because organ systems are so interdependent, however, physicians generally perform an overall physical examination even when a specific medical problem exists.

During a general physical examination, physicians check all the major organs and body systems. They can determine much about a patient's general condition of health from the examination. If appropriate, they also try to make a **clinical diagnosis,** a diagnosis based on the signs and symptoms of a disease.

After forming an initial diagnosis of a patient's problem, physicians may order laboratory or other diagnostic tests. These tests are done to confirm a clinical diagnosis or to rule out other possible disorders. These additional steps are necessary when a patient has symptoms that may indicate more than one condition. Determining the correct diagnosis when two or more diagnoses are possible is called making a **differential diagnosis.**

Laboratory and diagnostic tests may also aid physicians in developing a **prognosis,** or a forecast of the probable course and outcome of the disorder and the prospects of recovery. In addition, such tests help physicians formulate a treatment plan or appropriate drug therapy. Physicians may ask to have these tests repeated as part of the follow-up evaluation of a patient's progress.

The Role of the Medical Assistant

Your job as a medical assistant is to assist both the doctor and the patient during the general physical examination. Your presence enables the doctor to perform his examination as efficiently and professionally as possible. Patients benefit from your positive and caring attention; you contribute to their confidence in the care they receive.

As described in Chapters 36 and 37, the process begins when you first have contact with the patient. You interview the patient, write an accurate history, determine vital signs, and measure weight and height. You then assist the doctor during the examination.

Generally, your responsibilities include ensuring that all instruments and supplies are readily available to the doctor during the examination. You also ensure that the patient is physically and emotionally comfortable during the examination. It is important to observe the patient for signs that indicate distress or the need for assistance. Elderly patients, who may have physical limitations or special needs, often require extra time and attention.

Safety Precautions

As you prepare for and assist with a general physical examination, you will use a variety of safety measures. Some of these are outlined by the Department of Labor's Occupational Safety and Health Administration (OSHA). OSHA standards and guidelines (detailed in Chapter 19) are designed to protect employees and make the workplace safe.

The Department of Health and Human Services' Centers for Disease Control and Prevention (CDC) establishes the guidelines intended to protect both patients and health-care professionals in the medical office and the hospital setting. (These guidelines are also discussed in Chapter 19.) Taken together, these safety measures help protect you, the physician, and the patient from disease transmission.

Safety measures that you must take before, during, and after a general physical examination include the following.

1. Perform a thorough hand washing before and after contact with each patient and before and after each procedure. Procedure 19-1 in Chapter 19 describes how to perform aseptic hand washing. Additionally, according to OSHA standards, you can use an approved waterless, alcohol-based hand cleaner between patients if no gross contamination or visible soilage is on your hands.

2. Wear gloves whenever there is a possibility that you may come in contact with blood, body fluids, nonintact skin, or moist surfaces (during the examination of the patient or when handling specimens). Refer to Chapter 19 for details on personal protective equipment.

3. Wear a mask in the presence of a patient suspected of having an infectious disease that is transmitted by airborne droplets, such as **severe acute respiratory syndrome (SARS)** or tuberculosis (TB) (Table 38-1).

4. Patients with highly contagious infectious diseases, such as diphtheria or chickenpox, must be examined under isolation precautions, such as in a private room. Wear personal protective equipment during contact. For more information on isolation guidelines, see Chapter 20. (Because infectious diseases are common in children, you are most likely to deal with them in a pediatrician's office.)

TABLE 38-1 Infectious Diseases Transmitted by Airborne Droplets

Viral Infections	Bacterial Infections
Chickenpox	Epiglottitis (caused by *Haemophilus influenzae* type B)
Diphtheria	Meningitis
Herpes zoster (shingles)	Pertussis (whooping cough)
Meningitis	Pneumonia
Mumps	Tuberculosis
Pneumonia	
Rabies	
Rubella (German measles)	
Rubeola (measles)	
Severe acute respiratory syndrome (SARS)	

Note: Health-care professionals should use masks when coming in contact with patients suspected of having any of these diseases.

5. Discard in biohazardous waste containers all disposable equipment and supplies that come in contact with a patient's blood or body fluids. See Chapter 19 for guidelines on the proper disposal of biohazardous waste.

6. Clean and disinfect the examination room following the examination of each patient. Refer to Chapter 22 for information on cleanliness in the examination room.

7. Sanitize, disinfect, and sterilize equipment, as appropriate, after the examination of each patient. Chapter 20 describes these procedures in detail.

Preparing the Patient for an Examination

You can help prepare patients for examinations by making sure that they are comfortable and know what to expect. It is easier for the doctor to obtain an accurate assessment of a patient's condition when the patient is emotionally and physically prepared.

Emotional Preparation

To prepare patients, begin by explaining exactly what will occur during the examination. Use simple, direct language that patients can understand. Describe what patients can expect to feel and how their cooperation can contribute to the success of the procedure.

Emotional preparedness is particularly important when dealing with children. They deserve to have the same sort of information and reassurance as adults. To involve children in the examination process, you might allow them to inspect the blunt instruments. Speak to them calmly during the procedure, and praise them when they are cooperative.

Infants and toddlers are likely to be afraid of you because you are a stranger. Approach these children slowly, smile, and use a gentle voice. Children of preschool age are sometimes uncooperative and challenging. In such cases remain calm, perform the procedures quickly, and restrain the child (with assistance from the parent) when appropriate. To prevent children from getting injured, watch them at all times.

If you are a male medical assistant, a female doctor may ask you to remain in the room when she examines a male patient. Likewise, if you are a female medical assistant, a male doctor may ask you to remain in the room when he examines a woman. These measures are for the protection of both the patient and the doctor. Such policies depend on the standard procedures in each medical practice or facility.

Physical Preparation

To ensure that the patient is physically prepared before the doctor enters the examination room, give the patient an opportunity to empty his bladder or bowels. If a urine specimen is needed, it should be collected at this time. That way the patient will be more comfortable during the examination.

When the patient is ready, ask him to disrobe and put on an examination gown or cover himself with a drape. The extent of disrobing depends on the type of examination and the doctor's preference. If the doctor requests a gown for the patient, show the patient how to put on the gown. Include specific instructions on whether the gown should open in the back or front and whether it should be left open or tied. Leave the examination room while the patient disrobes to give him privacy, unless he needs and requests assistance.

Positioning and Draping

During the examination, the patient may need to assume a variety of positions. These positions facilitate the physician's examination of certain areas of the body. The physician will indicate which positions are needed for specific examinations. You will help the patient assume these positions. Some positions are embarrassing or physically uncomfortable for some patients. If you perceive embarrassment, explain the need for the position, and help the patient assume the position when necessary. Help minimize the time a patient spends in any embarrassing or uncomfortable position.

If a patient is physically uncomfortable in a position, you may be able to ease the discomfort by using a small pillow to support part of the body. You may have to help the patient maintain a position during the examination. Always try to make the patient as comfortable as possible.

When you need to make changes in the patient's position, do so gradually. If your office is equipped with an examination table that can be adjusted automatically, learn to use the controls efficiently to maximize patient comfort. Always tell the patient what movement to expect.

When patients have assumed the correct position, cover them with an appropriate drape. Drapes vary in size. Make sure you choose one that will help keep the patient warm and maintain privacy. You will position drapes differently depending on the examination position and the parts of the patient's body that the physician examines.

Examination Positions

The positions commonly used during a medical examination include the following:

- Sitting
- Supine (recumbent)
- Dorsal recumbent
- Lithotomy
- Trendelenburg's
- Fowler's
- Prone

- Sims'
- Knee-chest
- Proctologic

Sitting. In the sitting position, the patient sits at the edge of the examination table without back support (see Figure 38-1a). The physician examines the patient's head, neck, chest, heart, back, and arms. While the patient is in the sitting position, the physician evaluates the patient's ability to fully expand the lungs. She then checks the upper body parts for **symmetry,** the degree to which one side is the same as the other. In this position the drape is placed across the patient's lap for men or across the patient's chest and lap for women.

If a patient is too weak to sit unsupported, another position is necessary. One possible alternative is the supine position.

Supine (Recumbent). In the supine, or recumbent, position, the patient lies flat on the back (Figure 38-1b). (*Supine* means "lying down faceup"; *recumbent* means "lying down." Either term is used to describe this position.) This is the most relaxed position for many patients. A doctor can examine the head, neck, chest, heart, abdomen, arms, and legs when a patient is in the supine position. The patient is normally draped from the neck or underarms down to the feet.

The supine position may not be comfortable for patients who become short of breath easily. Also, patients with a back injury or lower-back pain may find it uncomfortable. You can make these patients more comfortable by placing a pillow under their heads and under their knees. Some patients, however, may need to be placed in the dorsal recumbent position.

Dorsal Recumbent. In the dorsal recumbent position, the patient lies faceup, with his back supporting all his weight. (The term *dorsal* refers to the back.) This position is the same as the supine position, except that the patient's knees are drawn up and the feet are flat on the table, as shown in Figure 38-1c. The physician may examine the head, neck, chest, and heart while a patient is in this position. The patient is normally draped from the neck or underarms down to the feet.

Patients who have leg disabilities may find the dorsal recumbent position uncomfortable or even impossible. On the other hand, patients who are elderly or have painful disorders such as arthritis or back pain may find the dorsal recumbent position more comfortable than the supine position because the knees are bent. This position is sometimes used as an alternative to the lithotomy position when patients have severe arthritis or joint deformities.

Lithotomy. The lithotomy position is used during examination of the female genitalia. In this position, the patient lies on her back with her knees bent and her feet in stirrups attached to the end of the examination table. You may need to help the patient place her feet in the stirrups. She should then slide forward to position her buttocks near the edge of the table, as shown in Figure 38-1d.

Many women are embarrassed and physically uncomfortable in this position, so you should not ask a patient to remain in this position any longer than necessary. Use a large drape that covers the patient from the breasts to the ankles. Placing the drape with one point or corner between the legs will make the examination easier in this position.

A patient with severe arthritis or joint deformities in the hips or knees may have difficulty assuming the lithotomy position. She may be able to place only one leg in the stirrup, or she may need your assistance in separating her thighs. An alternative position for such a patient is the dorsal recumbent position. Other patients who may have difficulty with the lithotomy position are those who are obese or in the late stages of pregnancy.

Trendelenburg's. In Trendelenburg's position, the patient is supine on a tilted table with the head lower than the legs. Some tables have flexible positioning so that the patient's legs can be bent with the feet lower than the knees, as shown in Figure 38-1e. Although physicians do not generally use this position for physical examinations, they use it in certain surgical procedures or emergencies. If this position is necessary on a standard examination table, you can place the patient with the feet at the head of the table and then raise the head. This position may be used for a patient with low blood pressure or a patient experiencing shock. It cannot be used for patients who have a head injury, however. The drape is typically positioned from the neck or underarms down to the knees.

Fowler's. In Fowler's position, the patient lies back on an examination table on which the head is elevated, as shown in Figure 38-1f. Although the head of the table can be raised to a 90° angle, the most common position is a 45° angle. The doctor may examine the head, neck, and chest areas while the patient is in this position. The patient is usually draped from the neck or underarms down to the feet.

Fowler's position is one of the best positions for examining patients who are experiencing shortness of breath or individuals with a lower-back injury.

Prone. In the prone position, the patient is lying flat on the table, facedown. The patient's head is turned to one side, and his arms are placed at his sides or bent at the elbows, as shown in Figure 38-1g. The patient is normally draped from the upper back to the feet.

With the patient in this position, the physician can examine the back, feet, or musculoskeletal system. The prone position is unsuitable for women in advanced stages of pregnancy, obese patients, patients with respiratory difficulties, or the elderly.

Sims'. In Sims' position, the patient lies on the left side. The patient's left leg is slightly bent, and the left arm is placed behind the back so that the patient's weight is resting primarily on the chest. The right knee is bent and raised toward the chest, and the right arm is bent toward

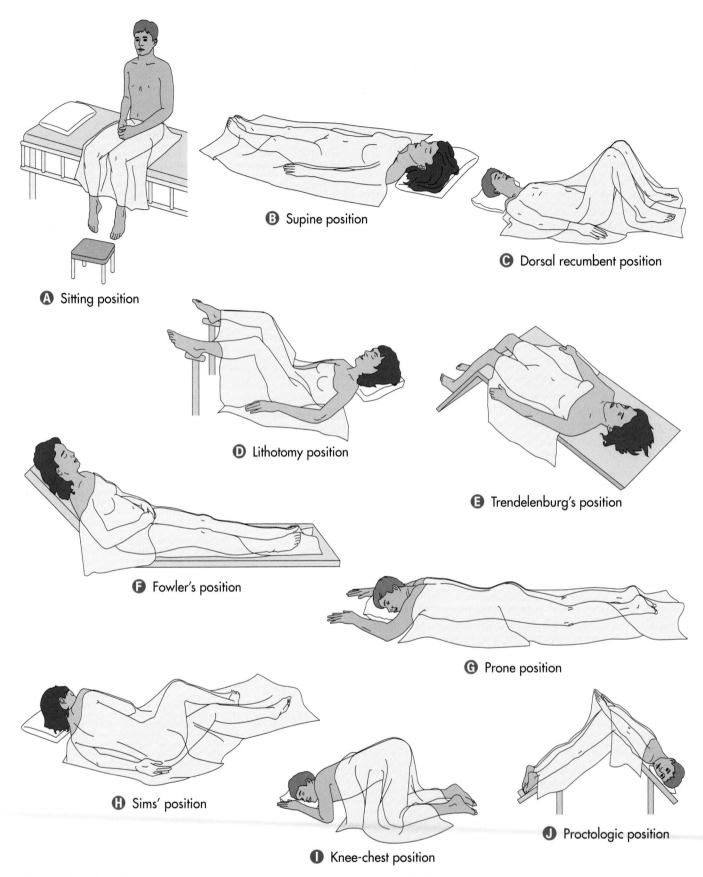

A Sitting position

B Supine position

C Dorsal recumbent position

D Lithotomy position

E Trendelenburg's position

F Fowler's position

G Prone position

H Sims' position

I Knee-chest position

J Proctologic position

Figure 38-1. These positions may be used during the general physical examination.

the head for support, as shown in Figure 38-1h. The patient is draped from the upper back to the feet.

Sims' position is used during anal or rectal examinations and may also be used for perineal and certain pelvic examinations. Patients with joint deformities of the hips and knees may have difficulty assuming this position.

Knee-Chest. In the knee-chest position, the patient is lying on the table facedown, supporting the body with the knees and chest. The patient should have the thighs at a 90° angle to the table and slightly separated. The head is turned to one side, and the arms are placed to the side or above the head, as shown in Figure 38-1i. The patient may need your assistance to assume this position correctly and to maintain it during the examination.

The knee-chest position is used during examinations of the anal and perineal areas and during certain proctologic procedures. Some patients—those who are pregnant, obese, or elderly—have difficulty assuming this position. An alternative that puts less strain on the patient and is easier to maintain is the knee-elbow position. This position is the same as the knee-chest position except that the patient supports body weight with the knees and elbows rather than the knees and chest. In either of these two positions, the patient is commonly covered with a **fenestrated drape,** in which a special opening provides access to the area to be examined.

Proctologic. The proctologic position may be used as an alternative to the Sims' or knee-chest position. In the proctologic position, also called the jackknife position, the patient is bent at the hips at a 90° angle. The patient can assume this position by standing next to the examination table and bending at the waist until the chest rests on the table. If an adjustable examination table is available, the patient can assume the position by lying prone on the table, which is then raised in the middle with both ends pointing down. This places the patient at the correct 90° angle, as shown in Figure 38-1j. In either variation of this position, the patient is draped with a fenestrated drape, as in the knee-chest position.

The steps for placing patients into these positions are described in Procedure 38-1.

PROCEDURE 38.1

Positioning the Patient for an Examination

Objective: To effectively assist a patient in assuming the various positions used in a general physical examination

OSHA Guidelines

Materials: Adjustable examination table or gynecologic table, step stool, examination gown, drape

Method

1. Identify the patient and introduce yourself.
2. Wash your hands.
3. Explain the procedure to the patient.
4. Provide a gown or drape if the physician has requested one, and instruct the patient in the proper way to wear it after disrobing. Allow the patient privacy while disrobing, and assist only if the patient requests help.
5. Explain to the patient the necessary examination and the position required.
6. Ask the patient to step on the stool or the pullout step of the examination table. If necessary, assist the patient onto the examination table.

7. Assist the patient into the required position:
   a. Sitting. Do not use this position for patients who cannot sit unsupported.
   b. Supine (Recumbent). Do not use this position for patients with back injuries, low back pain, or difficulty breathing. Place a pillow or other support under the head and knees for comfort, if needed.
   c. Dorsal Recumbent. This position may be difficult for someone with leg disabilities. It may be used for patients when lithotomy is difficult.
   d. Lithotomy. This position is used to examine the female genitalia, with the patient's feet placed in stirrups. Assist as necessary. The patient's buttocks should be near the edge of the table. Drape the client with a large drape to help prevent embarrassment.
   e. Trendelenburg. This position is a supine position with the patient's head lower than her feet. It is used infrequently in the physician's office but may be necessary for low blood pressure or shock.

continued ⟶

Positioning the Patient for an Examination *(continued)*

f. Fowler's. Adjust the head of the table to the desired angle. Help the patient move toward the head of the table until the patient's buttocks meet the point at which the head of the table begins to incline upward (Figures 38-2 and 38-3).

g. Prone. This position is when the patient lies face down. It is not used for later stages of pregnancy, obese patients, patients with respiratory difficulty, or certain elderly patients.

h. Sims'. In this position, the patient lies on her left side with her left leg slightly bent and her left arm behind her back. Her right knee is bent and raised toward her chest and her right arm is bent toward her head. This position may be difficult for patients with joint deformities.

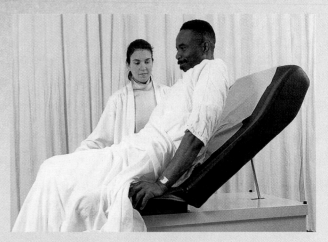

Figure 38-3. Encourage the patient to slide back until the buttocks meet the point at which the head of the table begins to incline upward.

i. Knee-Chest. This position is difficult for patients to assume. The patient is face down, supporting his weight on his knees and chest or an alternative knee-elbow position. This position is used for rectal and perineal exams. Keep the patient in this position for the shortest amount of time as possible.

j. Proctologic. This position is also used for rectal and perineal exams. In this position, the patient bends over the exam table with his chest resting on the table.

8. Drape the client to prevent exposure and avoid embarrassment. Place pillows for comfort as needed.

9. Adjust the drapes during the examination.

10. On completion of the examination, assist the client as necessary out of the position and provide privacy as the client dresses.

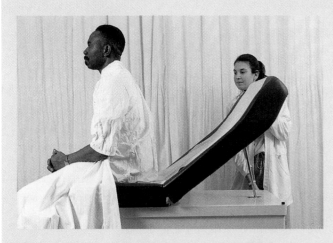

Figure 38-2. Adjust the head of the examination table to a 45° angle.

Special Considerations: Patients From Different Cultures

During your career you will come in contact with patients from many different cultures. A **culture,** in this sociological sense, is defined as a pattern of assumptions, beliefs, and practices that shape the way people think and act. Avoid the temptation to stereotype an individual or group on the basis of a single patient's behavior. Stereotyping can lead to incorrect judgments, which may influence the care you provide to patients. Avoid making judgments about patients or cultural groups on the basis of your experience with other patients or with your own family and friends.

Patients from different cultures may never have had a medical examination by a physician and may not know what to expect. These patients may be more modest than other patients and may have a greater need for privacy. They may not want the physician to examine certain areas of their bodies. Procedure 38-2 describes techniques you can use to ensure effective communication with patients from other cultures while meeting their privacy needs.

Communicating Effectively With Patients From Other Cultures and Meeting Their Needs for Privacy

Objective: To ensure effective communication with patients from other cultures while meeting their needs for privacy

OSHA Guidelines: This procedure does not involve exposure to blood, body fluids, or tissues.

Materials: Examination gown, drapes

Method

Effective Communication

1. When it is necessary to use a translator, direct conversation or instruction to the translator.
2. Direct demonstrations of what to do, such as putting on an examination gown, to the patient.
3. Confirm with the translator that the patient has understood the instruction or demonstration.
4. Allow the translator to be present during the examination if that is the patient's preference.
5. If the patient understands some English, speak slowly, use simple language, and demonstrate instructions whenever possible.

Meeting the Need for Privacy

1. Before the procedure, thoroughly explain to the patient or translator the reason for disrobing. Indicate that you will allow the patient privacy and ample time to undress.
2. If the patient is reluctant, reassure him that the physician respects the need for privacy and will look at only what is necessary for the examination.
3. Provide extra drapes if you think doing so will make the patient feel more comfortable.
4. If the patient is still reluctant, discuss the problem with the physician; the physician may be able to negotiate a compromise with the patient.
5. During the procedure, ensure that the patient is undraped only as much as necessary.
6. Whenever possible, minimize the amount of time the patient remains undraped.

Special Considerations: Patients With Disabilities

As a medical assistant, you will come in contact with patients with physical disabilities. These patients will have different strengths and weaknesses. They will also vary in their ability to ambulate (move from place to place). Many patients with physical disabilities require the use of devices such as wheelchairs, canes, or walkers or other special equipment that permits or enhances mobility.

Depending on the extent of their disability, these patients may require extra assistance in preparing for a general physical examination. You may need to help them disrobe, move from a mobility device to the examination table, and assume certain positions on or off the examination table. At all times you should ask another staff member for assistance if you are not sure whether you can safely move or lift a patient on your own. Procedure 38-3 describes the steps you would take to transfer a patient from a wheelchair to the examination table.

Special Considerations: Children

No matter what type of office you work in, you will probably deal with children at times. You will base your choice of an examination position for children on each child's age and ability to cooperate. Although young infants are usually examined on an examination table, older infants and toddlers may need to be examined while held on a parent's lap. Some toddlers may cooperate while standing on the examination table with a parent nearby. Preschool children can usually be placed on the examination table if a parent is nearby. Regardless of their position, watch children at all times to prevent injury.

When examining young children, doctors typically perform percussion and auscultation first, because children are more likely to be calm and quiet at the outset. Doctors always examine painful areas last. Doctors may examine older children's genitalia last, because after a certain age children tend to find such an examination embarrassing.

Special Considerations: Pregnant Women

When a pregnant patient needs a general physical examination, remember that she has several special needs. Some positions (such as the prone or lithotomy positions) are not recommended for a pregnant patient, especially during late stages of pregnancy. Other positions may be

TABLE 38-2 Components and Materials of a General Physical Examination

Component	Materials Required*
General appearance (skin, nails, hair)	No special materials needed
Head	No special materials needed
Neck	No special materials needed
Eyes and vision**	Penlight, ophthalmoscope, vision and color vision charts
Ears and hearing**	Otoscope, audiometer
Nose and sinuses	Penlight, nasal speculum
Mouth and throat	Gloves, tongue depressor
Chest and lungs	Stethoscope
Heart	Stethoscope
Breasts	No special materials needed
Abdomen	Stethoscope
Genitalia (women)	Gloves, vaginal speculum, lubricant
Genitalia (men)	Gloves
Rectum	Gloves, lubricant
Musculoskeletal system	Tape measure
Neurological system	Reflex hammer, penlight

*Gloves should always be worn if your hands will come in contact with the patient's nonintact skin, blood, body fluids, or moist surfaces or if the patient is suspected of having an infectious disease.

**Procedures performed alone by the medical assistant are described in Chapter 39; all other listed procedures are performed by a physician with help from a medical assistant.

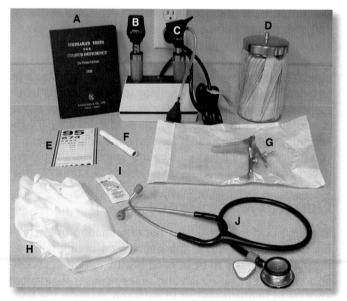

Figure 38-8. Some common instruments and supplies for the general physical examination are (a) color vision chart, (b) ophthalmoscope, (c) otoscope, (d) tongue blades, (e) near vision chart, (f) penlight, (g) vaginal speculum, (h) gloves, (i) lubricant, and (j) stethoscope.

while examining specific body parts. The physician notes the color, texture, moisture level, temperature, and elasticity of the skin. The condition of the skin is a good indicator of overall health. If the physician notices any lesions, she wears gloves to prevent possible transmission of microorganisms. The physician may also request that a specimen be taken from a lesion or wound for later examination to determine the infecting microorganism.

Nails. When the physician examines the patient's nails, he looks at both the nails and the nail beds. The condition of the nails may indicate poor nutrition, disease, infection, or injury. If applicable, remind the patient to remove nail cosmetics prior to the appointment.

Hair. The physician notes the patient's pattern of hair growth and the texture of the hair on the patient's scalp and on the rest of the body. Sudden hair loss or changes in hair growth may be indicators of an underlying disease.

Head

After reviewing the patient's general appearance, the doctor examines the patient's head. He looks for any abnormal condition of the scalp or skin, puffiness around the eyes or lips or in other areas of the face, or any abnormal growths.

Neck

To check the neck, the doctor palpates the patient's lymph nodes, thyroid gland, and major blood vessels. Enlarged lymph nodes may be a sign of infection or a blood cancer. An enlarged thyroid gland may indicate thyroid disease. The doctor also checks the neck for symmetry and range of motion.

Eyes

The physician examines the patient's eyes—particularly the eyelids and conjunctiva—for the presence of disease or abnormalities. She checks eye muscles by observing the patient's ability to follow the movement of a finger. She checks the pupils for their response to light (the pupils should contract—become smaller—when a penlight is directed toward them). Then she uses an ophthalmoscope to examine the patient's retinas and other internal structures of the eyes.

You may be required to perform various vision tests either before or after the general physical examination. (The tests are described in Chapter 39.)

Ears

The doctor checks the patient's outer ears for size, symmetry, and the presence of lesions, redness, or swelling. Using an otoscope, he then examines the inner structures of the patient's ears. The doctor may ask you to assist in keeping the patient's head still during the otoscopic examination, particularly when the patient is a young child. Although this procedure is usually painless, patients with an ear infection may find it uncomfortable or painful.

The doctor checks the patient's ear canals for redness, drainage, lesions, foreign objects, or the presence of excessive **cerumen** (a waxy secretion from the ear, also known as earwax). During the most important part of the examination of the ears, the doctor assesses the color, shape, and reflectiveness of the eardrums. If an eardrum bulges outward or reflects light abnormally, the middle ear could be infected.

One of your responsibilities may be to perform various hearing tests either before or after the general physical examination. (These tests are described in Chapter 39.)

Nose and Sinuses

When examining the nose, the physician checks for the presence of infection or allergy. She uses a penlight to view the color of the **nasal mucosa** (lining of the nose) and notes any discharge, lesions, obstructions, swelling, or inflammation. A mucosa that is red or swollen and is accompanied by a yellowish discharge usually indicates an infection. A pale, swollen mucosa accompanied by a clear discharge indicates an allergy. When examining adults, the physician uses the nasal speculum to view the structures of the nose.

The physician may use palpation to check for tenderness in a patient's sinuses. Tenderness is an indication of inflammation or swelling.

Mouth and Throat

The doctor checks the condition of the patient's mouth to get a general impression of overall health and hygiene. Using a tongue depressor to draw back the patient's cheeks, the doctor examines the lining of the cheeks, the underside of the tongue, and the floor of the mouth. Changes in color or any lesions in these areas may indicate possible infection or oral cancer. The doctor also assesses the condition of the teeth and gums. When examining children, she counts the number of teeth. Most doctors leave this part of the examination of infants and toddlers until last, because children of this age tend to resist opening their mouths.

The doctor examines the patient's throat carefully because it is a common site of infection. She uses a tongue depressor to press the patient's tongue down and out of the way while asking the patient to say "ah." This procedure allows the doctor to view the throat and tonsils more clearly while checking them for redness or swelling, which can indicate the presence of infection.

Chest and Lungs

The physician usually assesses the patient's chest and lungs while the patient sits at the end of the examination table. When the patient is examined in this position, the chest can expand to its maximum capacity. Typically, the physician removes the patient's gown or lowers the drape from the waist up. Then he asks the patient to breathe normally or to take deep breaths. A patient who becomes dizzy during deep breathing may be hyperventilating. **Hyperventilation** is overly deep breathing that leads to a loss of carbon dioxide in the blood. You can help by having the patient breathe into a paper bag. If no bag is available, the patient can breath into cupped hands. With your help the patient should recover quickly.

The physician inspects the patient's chest from the back, side, and front. He checks its shape, symmetry, and postural position and looks for the presence of any type of deformity. Postural abnormalities such as **kyphosis** often occur in the elderly. Frequently, especially in elderly women, these abnormalities are caused by osteoporosis, the loss of bone density. This bone density loss causes the patient to have a rounded back, or "humpback."

The physician also palpates the chest and performs percussion to check for the presence of fluid or a foreign mass in the lungs. The physician then uses a stethoscope to auscultate the chest from the back, side, and front. He listens to the lung sounds during both normal and deep breathing. The stethoscope allows him to hear abnormal breathing that may result from such disorders as bronchitis, asthma, or pneumonia.

Heart

The doctor usually examines the patient's heart and vascular system at the same time as, or immediately after, the lung examination. He may palpate the area first to locate the correct anatomical landmarks for placing the stethoscope. He may use percussion to check the size of the heart. The patient should not speak while the physician auscultates the heart sounds with the stethoscope. The physician notes the rate, rhythm, intensity, and pitch of the heart.

Breasts

During a general physical examination, every woman should have a complete breast examination. Breast cancer is the most common cancer in women. Because growths are also possible in men's breasts, doctors should perform a breast examination on all patients.

The doctor begins the examination with the patient in a sitting position. The doctor asks the patient to hold her arms at her sides while he inspects the breasts for symmetry, contour, masses, and retracted areas. The doctor then asks the patient to raise her arms above her head while he palpates the lymph nodes under her arms.

Next, the doctor asks the patient to lie down and place her hand under her head on the first side to be examined. The doctor may ask you to place a small pillow or folded towel under the patient's shoulder blade on the same side. This procedure allows the breast tissue to flatten evenly against the chest wall, permitting easier palpation. The doctor then palpates the breast in a circular, systematic manner to check for lumps, examines the areola and nipple, and then repeats the procedure on the other side.

When examining male patients, the doctor palpates the patient's breasts and lymph nodes in the same manner that he does with his female patients. The doctor also checks the breasts of his male patients for lesions or swelling.

Abdomen

The physician examines the patient's abdomen while the patient is in a supine position with arms down at the sides. The abdominal muscles should be completely relaxed for this part of the examination. The physician may ask you to place a small pillow under the patient's head or knees (or both) to keep the abdomen relaxed. If the patient is wearing a gown, it is raised to just under the breasts. If the patient is draped, the drape must be lowered to just above the genitalia to allow a complete view of the area. A separate drape should be placed to cover a female patient's breasts.

The order of examination methods for the abdomen is different from the order for other areas. The physician begins with inspection and auscultation, followed by percussion and palpation. Following this order allows the physician to listen to bowel sounds before palpating the abdominal organs. Palpation of this area can change bowel

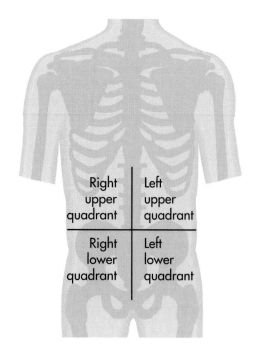

Figure 38-9. The abdomen is typically divided into four equal sections, or quadrants.

sounds in such a way that the physician could misdiagnose a patient's condition.

The physician must assess the abdomen thoroughly, because there are many organs in the abdominal cavity. The physician describes observations based on a system of landmarks that map out the abdominal region. The abdomen is typically divided into four equal sections, or **quadrants,** as shown in Figure 38-9. Some physicians divide the abdomen into nine sections, similar to a tick-tack-toe board, as shown in Figure 38-10.

If the physician has not assessed the skin in this area already, she begins with an inspection of the abdominal skin's color and surface and follows with an inspection of the shape and symmetry of the abdomen. She then uses auscultation to check bowel and vascular sounds and uses percussion to note the size and position of the organs. Lastly, she uses palpation to check muscle tone and to determine the presence of any tenderness or masses.

Female Genitalia

Female patients may feel self-conscious or anxious in the lithotomy position—which is most commonly used during examination of the genitalia. The medical assistant may help the patient relax during this procedure and may assist patients in maintaining the position.

If the doctor who performs the examination is male, a female medical assistant should always be in the room to protect both the patient and doctor from potential lawsuits. This type of examination may be performed by a specialist or by a primary care physician. The procedure for a gynecologic examination is described in detail in Chapter 40.

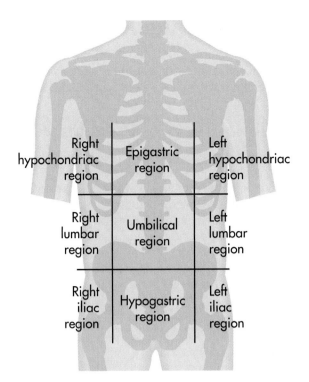

Figure 38-10. Some physicians divide the abdomen into nine sections, similar to a tick-tack-toe board.

Male Genitalia

During the examination of the genitalia, men may be just as embarrassed or uncomfortable as women may be. If the physician who is performing the assessment is female, a male medical assistant should be in the room to protect both the patient and physician from potential lawsuits.

The procedure begins with the patient in the supine position. The physician puts on gloves and visually inspects the patient's penis for signs of infection or structural abnormalities, palpating any lesions. The physician then examines the scrotum in the same manner, palpating the testicles for lumps. The patient is asked to stand while the physician checks for any bulges in the groin that may indicate a hernia. At the same time, the physician palpates the local lymph nodes to check for any abnormality.

Rectum

The doctor usually examines the rectum after examining the genitalia. You may need to assist an adult patient into a dorsal recumbent or Sims' position. The doctor normally examines a child when the child is in the prone position and inspects only the external areas of the rectum.

In adults the doctor uses **digital examination** to palpate the rectum for lesions or irregularities. Doctors recommend that patients older than age 40 have a yearly digital examination for early detection of colorectal cancer. For this examination the doctor puts on a clean pair of gloves. You assist by applying lubricant to the doctor's

gloved index finger before the examination begins. As with examination of the genitalia, patients often find digital examination of the rectum embarrassing and uncomfortable.

After performing the procedure, the doctor may request that any stool found on the glove be tested for the presence of occult blood. The presence of occult blood in the stool is a possible indication of colorectal cancer or gastrointestinal bleeding. This test—often called by its brand name, Hemoccult or Seracult test—involves placing a sample of stool on a special cardboard slide. You assist by presenting the slide to the doctor. To produce an accurate test, three consecutive bowel movements are tested; this sample is usually the first. After the examination you may be responsible for instructing the patient on how to collect the additional two samples. The procedure is outlined on the package of the occult blood-testing kit.

After the rectal examination, offer the patient the opportunity to clean the anal area before you adjust the drape. Dispose of gloves and soiled materials in a biohazardous waste container.

Musculoskeletal System

If the physician did not examine the patient's back during the chest examination, he does so during the musculoskeletal assessment. The physician checks for good posture from the back and side. He may ask the patient to walk so that he can assess her gait. The physician always asks a child to bend at the waist so that he can check for the presence of **scoliosis,** a lateral curvature of the spine. This procedure is discussed further in Chapter 40, Procedure 40-2.

During the musculoskeletal assessment the physician determines range of motion, the strength of various muscle groups, and body measurements. The physician also examines the arms, hands, legs, and feet for any lesions, deformities, or circulatory problems.

The physician checks a patient's range of motion to detect joint deformities and to learn whether the patient has any limitations in movement caused by an injury or other conditions, such as arthritis. Checking a patient's range of motion also allows the physician to follow a patient's progress during recovery from an injury or surgery.

As part of the assessment of a child's health, the physician asks the child to perform certain tasks, such as walking a straight line and balancing or hopping on one foot. The physician uses these tasks to evaluate the child's development and coordination and to provide the physician with information about the functioning of the child's neurological system.

Neurological System

The doctor's neurological assessment includes an evaluation of the patient's reflexes, mental and emotional status (including intelligence, speech, and behavior), and sensory and motor functions. The doctor often performs the neurological assessment at the same time as the musculoskeletal assessment because both systems are involved in movement and coordination.

The doctor may incorporate certain aspects of the neurological assessment into other parts of the examination. For example, testing how a patient's pupils react to light is part of an eye examination, but because this test also examines the patient's light reflex, the test includes a neurological assessment as well.

The doctor checks the patient's reflexes to assess both sensory and motor nerve pathways at different areas of the spinal cord. To check reflexes, the doctor uses a reflex hammer to tap tendons in different areas of the patient's body.

Most examinations of children also include an intellectual assessment, in which the doctor asks the child general questions appropriate to the child's age. Doctors may also test the mental status and memory of older adults to detect disorders such as senility and Alzheimer's disease in patients who show signs of confusion or complain of memory loss.

Completing the Examination

After the physician completes the examination, you should help the patient into a sitting position. Then allow the patient to perform any necessary self-hygiene measures.

Additional Tests or Procedures

Before the patient dresses, check to see whether the physician has ordered any additional tests or procedures that are more conveniently performed while the patient is undressed. These tests might include taking body fat measurements or blood samples or preparing the patient for a diagnostic or therapeutic procedure, such as an x-ray or physical therapy session. The physician may also ask you to perform other procedures. Some of these procedures, which are covered in other chapters, include the following:

- Cold or heat therapy (Chapter 43)
- Applying a bandage (Chapter 44)

CAUTION *Handle With Care*

Helping Patients With Suspected Breast Cancer

If the physician detects a suspicious lump in a patient's breast during the general physical examination, your main concern is to help the patient remain calm. Although most suspicious lumps are not cancerous, the patient is likely to be anxious and upset about the finding. The best thing you can do for her is to schedule her for a mammogram as soon as possible.

Preparing the Patient for a Mammogram

To alleviate some of the patient's fears, explain exactly what a mammogram is. Give the patient the following information.

1. A mammogram is a special type of x-ray of the breast that is used to detect cancer and other abnormalities of the breast.

2. A technician specially trained in performing mammography will position the patient's breast along a flat plastic plate. A second plate will be brought into position and pressure will be applied for about 20 to 30 seconds to flatten the breast (to obtain a clearer x-ray) while the x-ray is taken. This will be done in two directions (planes) for each breast.

3. Mammography is generally not a painful procedure, but some women may find it uncomfortable. Many professionals suggest that patients avoid scheduling a mammogram

during the week prior to a menstrual period to reduce potential discomfort.

4. The mammography appointment normally takes ½ to 1 hour. The actual mammography takes only about 15 minutes.

5. Because the patient will have to undress from the waist up, she should wear a separate top and slacks or a skirt rather than a dress.

6. The patient should have no creams, powders, or deodorants on her breasts or underarms when the mammography is performed because chemicals in these preparations can produce misleading images in the mammogram.

Answer any questions the patient has, and provide patient education materials related to mammography and breast disease. Reassure her that most lumps are not cancerous.

If your office refers patients to a particular facility that you are familiar with, give the patient an idea of how long she can expect to wait for the results. Ensure her that she will be notified as soon as the physician receives the report. You may want to schedule a follow-up visit at this time, based on when results are expected.

Because this is a difficult time for a patient, you should be as supportive as possible. You can help the patient cope by showing your concern and giving her prompt attention. Tell the patient that if she has any questions at all, she should call the physician.

- Collecting culture specimens (Chapters 46, 47, and 48)
- Administering an injection (Chapter 51)
- Applying a topical medication (Chapter 51)

If the physician has not ordered any additional procedures—or if wearing clothing does not interfere with the procedures ordered—the patient may dress. Help the patient get off the examination table, and allow her to dress in privacy. Make sure she knows you are available to assist if she needs help dressing.

The physician may ask you to perform other tests and procedures that can be done after the patient has dressed, including these procedures, which are discussed in detail where noted:

- Vision and hearing tests (Chapter 39)
- Otic or ophthalmic irrigation (Chapter 39)
- Administration of certain medications (Chapter 51)
- Pulmonary function tests (Chapter 52)

Patient Education

The general physical examination provides you with the opportunity to assess the patient's educational needs. Basing your findings on the patient's interview, history, and examination, you can identify areas in which the patient may benefit from additional education.

Pay special attention to educating patients about risk factors for disease. For example, women are often instructed about the risk factors for breast cancer. The risk factors include being older than 50 (many physicians recommend that women older than 40 have a mammogram every 2 years and that women older than 50 have one every year), having a family history of breast cancer, having the first child after age 30, never being pregnant, and beginning to menstruate at an early age.

The physician may also request that you teach patients how to administer certain medications or how to perform self-help or diagnostic techniques, such as a breast

Educating the Patient

How to Perform a Breast Self-Examination

You may be responsible for reinforcing patient education about monthly breast self-examination (BSE), which can be instrumental in the early detection of breast cancer. Figure 38-11 shows the steps suggested by the National Cancer Institute for performing this procedure.

Check the office policy to see which of several methods it recommends for teaching BSE. One approach uses the following steps.

1. Explain the purpose of BSE.
2. Assist the patient to the standing position, and instruct her to use a large mirror to view the breasts during this part of the procedure.
3. Explain to the patient what she should look for when inspecting her breasts while standing.
4. Demonstrate the positioning of arms and hands for this visual inspection: first, her arms at her sides; then, her arms raised and her hands clasped behind her head; finally, her arms lowered with her hands on her hips.
5. Demonstrate, on the patient's breast, how to perform the small rotary motions with the flat pads of the fingers from the outer rim (including the armpit and collarbone area) toward the nipple. (Synthetic breast models are available

that may be helpful in teaching the proper technique.)

6. Demonstrate how to inspect the nipples.
7. Ask the patient to practice the procedure.
8. Observe the patient's self-examination technique. (If the patient is reluctant to examine herself in front of you, have her repeat the highlights of the procedure.)
9. Assist the patient to lie down, with a small pillow or folded towel under the shoulder on the side to be examined.
10. Repeat steps 5 through 8.
11. Suggest that the patient mark her calendar for a monthly reminder to perform the examination 1 week after the onset of menses.
12. Give the patient educational materials that explain how to perform BSE.

Make sure the patient knows that she should perform BSE around the same date of each month—after her period ends, if she is still menstruating. (At this time the breasts are most normal and least swollen and lumpy.) You must also emphasize that BSE is not a substitute for mammograms or regular breast examination by a doctor. Early cancer detection depends on the performance of all three types of breast examination.

continued ⟶

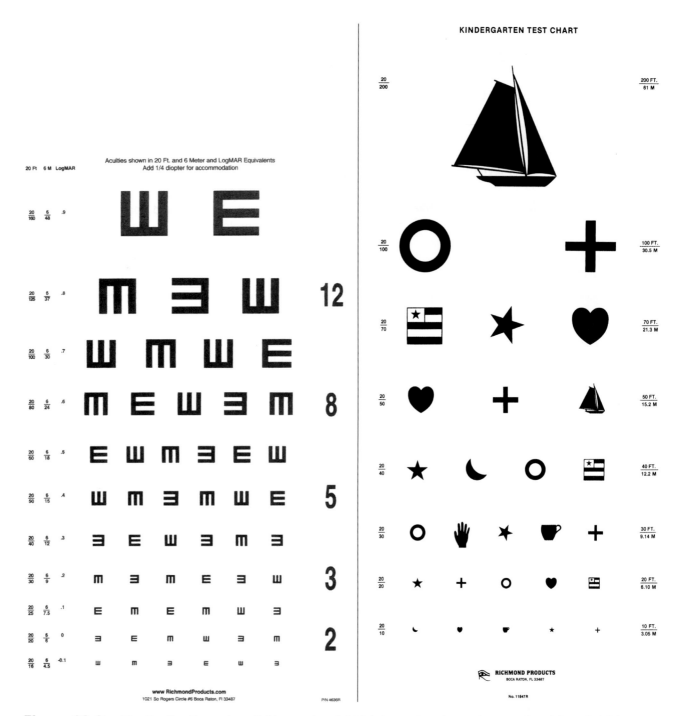

Figure 39-3. The Snellen E eye chart (left) or a pictorial (right) eye chart is used to test the vision of children and nonreading adults. (Courtesy Richmond Products, Inc.)

Near Vision. To test for near vision, special handheld charts are used. These cards contain letters, numbers, or paragraphs in various sizes of print (Figures 39-4 and 39-5). They may be held and read at a normal reading distance or mounted in a plastic and metal frame and read through optical lenses.

Contrast Sensitivity. To test for the ability to distinguish shades of gray (contrast sensitivity), the Pelli-Robson contrast sensitivity chart, the Vistech Consultants vision contrast test system (Figure 39-6), or another testing system is used. Newer systems use special equipment to provide contrast variations in a projected image. These tests can detect cataracts or problems of the retina even before the sharpness of the patient's vision is impaired.

Color Vision. To test color vision, illustrations such as those of the Ishihara color system or the Richmond pseudoisochromatic color test (Figure 39-7) are used. These illustrations contain numbers or symbols made up of colored dots that appear among other colored dots. The

V = .50 D.

The fourteenth of August was the day fixed upon for the sailing of the brig Pilgrim, on her voyage from Boston round Cape Horn, to the western coast of North America. As she was to get under way early in the afternoon, I made my appearance on board at twelve o'clock in full sea-rig, and with my chest, containing an outfit for a two or three years voyage, which I had undertaken from a determination to cure, if possible, by an entire change of life, and by a long absence from books and study, a weakness of the eyes which had obliged me to give up my pursuits, and which no medical aid seemed likely to cure. The change from the tight dress coat, silk cap and kid gloves of an undergraduate at Cambridge, to the

V = .75 D.

loose duck trousers, checked shirt and tarpaulin hat of a sailor, though somewhat of a transformation, was soon made, and I supposed that I should pass very well for a Jack tar. But it is impossible to deceive the practiced eye in these matters; and while I supposed myself to be looking as salt as Neptune himself, I was, no doubt, known for a landsman by every one on board, as soon as I hove in sight. A sailor has a peculiar cut to his clothes, and a way of wear-

V = 1. D.

ing them which a green hand can never get. The trousers, tight around the hips, and thence hanging long and loose around the feet, a superabundance of checked shirt, a low-crowned, well-varnished black hat, worn on the back of the head, with half a fathom of black ribbon hanging over the left eye, and a peculiar tie to the black silk neckerchief, with sundry other *details*, are signs the want of which betray the beginner at once.

V = 1.25 D.

Beside the points in my dress which were out of the way, doubtless my complexion and hands would distinguish me from the regular *salt*, who, with a sun-browned cheek, wide step and rolling gait, swings his bronzed and toughened hands athwartships half open, as though just to ready to grasp a rope. "With all my imperfections

V = 1.50 D.

on my head," I joined the crew, and we hauled out into the stream and came to anchor for the night. The next day we were employed in preparation for sea, reeving and studding-sail gear, crossing royal yards, putting on chafing gear, and taking on board our powder. On the

V = 1.75 D.

following night I stood my first watch. I remained awake nearly all the first part of the night, from fear that I might not hear when I was called; and when I went on deck, so great were my ideas of the importance of my trust, that I

V = 2. D.

walked regularly fore and aft the whole length of the vessel, looking out over the bows and taffrail at each turn, and was not a little surprised at the unconcerned manner in which the billows turned up their

Your glasses are of value to you only as they accurately interpret your prescription and this only as they are fitted and serviced in accordance with these needs. They are a therapeutic device.

 RICHMOND PRODUCTS
BOCA RATON, FL 33487

No. 11974 R

Figure 39-4. This near-vision chart is used to test the ability to see objects at a normal reading distance. (Courtesy Richmond Products, Inc.)

patient is asked to identify what he sees. A patient who is color-blind will not be able to report seeing the numbers or symbols. Color blindness may be inherited; it occurs more commonly in males. Changes in one's ability to see colors, however, may indicate a disease of the retina or optic nerve. For details on how to perform color vision and other vision tests, see Procedure 39-1.

Special Considerations. Certain patients may need special attention when having vision tests. For example, children may be uncooperative or unable to follow directions. To encourage cooperation, show a child the chart you will be using before you begin the test. Point to the symbols and read them aloud once so the child knows the proper term for each symbol. Most physicians use pictorial charts

FOR TESTING AT 40 CM (16 INCHES)

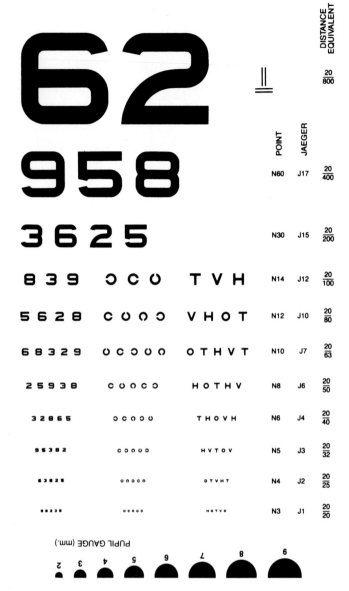

Figure 39-5. The Richmond pocket vision screener is also used to test the ability to see close objects. (Courtesy Richmond Products, Inc.)

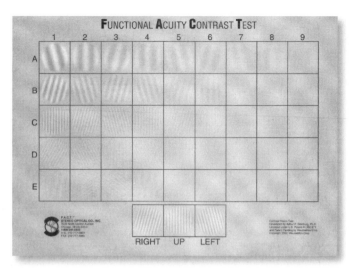

Figure 39-6. The Functional Acuity Contrast Test (FACT™) is used to test the ability to differentiate various shades of gray. (Stereo Optical Co., Inc., Chicago, IL. Copyright Vision Sciences Research Corporation, San Ramon, CA. Developed by Dr. Arthur P. Ginsburg)

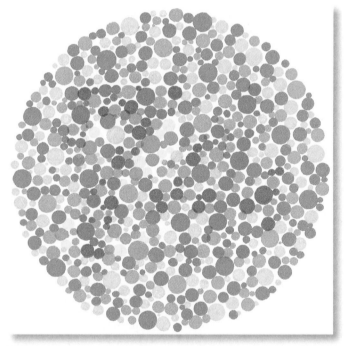

Figure 39-7. The Richmond pseudoisochromatic color chart is used to test a person's ability to see colors. (Courtesy Richmond Products, Inc.)

when they start screening a child's vision at the 4-year or 5-year checkup. You can provide assistance during the test by guiding the child through each step in the procedure or by covering the child's eye. Watch the child closely for signs that she is having difficulty seeing the chart. Examples of signs include straining, blinking or watering of the eyes, and puckering of the face.

If a child has difficulty following directions, enlist the parent's or guardian's help. He may be able to explain or interpret information for the child more effectively than you can. Ask the parent if he has ever observed signs of vision problems in his child. For example, does the child rub her eyes frequently, blink a great deal, or hold books very close to her face? Be sure to note the answers in the child's chart so the physician is aware of them.

A patient with Alzheimer's disease may also require special attention during a vision test. Before the test, encourage a family member to stay with the patient so he is more comfortable. During the test use simple language to explain the procedure and demonstrate whenever possible. Proceed through the examination slowly, one step at a time. Because the patient's memory and language skills may be impaired, you may need to repeat directions many times and help him name a particular object. If he appears to have trouble with one part of the examination, proceed to another part and return later to the part that was difficult for him.

PROCEDURE 39.1

Performing Vision Screening Tests

Objectives: To screen a patient's ability to see distant or close objects, to determine contrast sensitivity, or to detect color blindness

OSHA Guidelines

Materials: Occluder or card, alcohol, gauze squares, appropriate vision charts to test for distance vision, near vision, contrast sensitivity, and color blindness

Method

Distance Vision

1. Wash your hands, identify the patient, introduce yourself, and explain the procedure.
2. Mount one of the following eye charts at eye level: Snellen letter or similar chart (for patients who can read); Snellen E, Landolt C, pictorial, or similar chart (for patients who cannot read). If using the Snellen letter chart, verify that the patient knows the letters of the alphabet. With children or nonreading adults, use demonstration cards to verify that they can identify the pictures or direction of the letters.
3. Make a mark on the floor 20 feet away from the chart.
4. Have the patient stand with the heels at the 20-foot mark or sit with the back of the chair at the mark.
5. Instruct the patient to keep both eyes open and not to squint or lean forward during the test.
6. Test both eyes first, then the right eye, and then the left eye. (Different offices may test in a different order. Follow your office policy.) Refer to Figure 39-8.
7. Have the patient read the lines on the chart (or identify the picture/direction), beginning with the 20-foot line. If the patient cannot read this line, begin with the smallest line the patient can read. (Some offices use a pointer to select one symbol at a time in random order to prevent patients from memorizing the order. It is common to start with children at the 40- or 30-foot line, or larger if low vision is suspected, and proceed to the 20-foot line.)

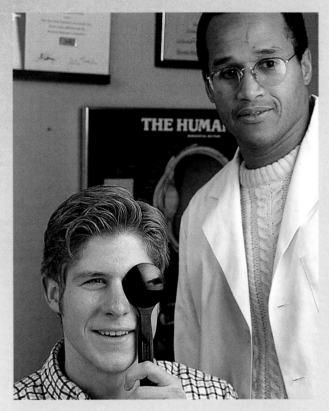

Figure 39-8. Have the patient cover the left eye with the occluder. The patient should keep both eyes open and not squint.

8. Note the smallest line the patient can read or identify. (When testing children, note the smallest line on which they can identify three out of four or four out of six symbols correctly.)
9. Record the results as a fraction (for example, O.U. 20/40 –1 if the patient misses one letter on a line or O.U. 20/40 –2 if the patient misses two letters on a line).
10. Show the patient how to cover the left eye with the occluder or card. Again, instruct the patient to keep both eyes open and not to squint or lean forward during the test.
11. Have the patient read the lines on the chart.
12. Record the results of the right eye (for example, O.D. 20/30).
13. Have the patient cover the right eye and read the lines on the chart.

continued ⟶

Performing Vision Screening Tests (continued)

14. Record the results of the left eye (for example, O.S. 20/20).

15. If the patient wears corrective lenses, record the results using $\overline{cc}$ (if your office uses this abbreviation for "with correction") in front of the abbreviation (for example, $\overline{cc}$ O.U. 20/20).

16. Note and record any observations of squinting, head tilting, or excessive blinking or tearing.

17. Ask the patient to keep both eyes open and to identify the two colored bars, and record the results in the patient's chart.

18. Clean the occluder with a gauze square dampened with alcohol.

19. Properly dispose of the gauze square and wash your hands.

Near Vision

1. Wash your hands, identify the patient, introduce yourself, and explain the procedure.

2. Have the patient hold one of the following at normal reading distance (approximately 14 to 16 inches): Jaeger, Richmond pocket, or similar chart or card.

3. Ask the patient to keep both eyes open and to read or identify the letters, symbols, or paragraphs.

4. Record the smallest line read without error.

5. If the card is laminated, clean it with a gauze square dampened with alcohol.

6. Properly dispose of the gauze square and wash your hands.

Contrast Sensitivity

1. Wash your hands, identify the patient, introduce yourself, and explain the procedure.

2. Mount a contrast sensitivity chart at eye level. (The following steps apply to use of the Vistech Consultants vision contrast test system. The procedures for using other contrast sensitivity charts vary slightly.)

3. Make a mark on the floor 10 feet from the chart.

4. Have the patient stand with the heels at the mark or sit with the back of the chair at the mark.

5. Test both eyes first.

6. Beginning with circle A1, have the patient identify the direction of the stripes in each circle in row A—left, right, up and down, or blank.

7. In column A on the answer grid that accompanies the chart, mark the point for the last circle for which the patient can correctly identify the direction of the stripes. (If the point falls within the shaded area, the patient's vision is within the normal range.)

8. Repeat steps 6 and 7 for rows B through E.

9. Have the patient cover his left eye with an occluder or card, and repeat steps 6 through 8 for the right eye.

10. Have the patient cover his right eye, and repeat steps 6 through 8 for the left eye.

11. Clean the occluder or card with a gauze square dipped in alcohol.

12. Properly dispose of the used gauze square and wash your hands.

Color Vision

1. Wash your hands, identify the patient, introduce yourself, and explain the procedure.

2. Hold one of the following color charts or books at the patient's normal reading distance (approximately 14 to 16 inches): Ishihara, Richmond pseudoisochromatic, or similar color-testing system.

3. Ask the patient to tell you the number or symbol within the colored dots on each chart or page.

4. Proceed through all the charts or pages.

5. Record the number correctly identified and failed with a slash between them (for example, 13 passed/1 failed).

6. If the charts are laminated, clean them with a gauze square dampened with alcohol.

7. Properly dispose of the gauze square and wash your hands.

Treating Eye Problems

Some common eye problems include conjunctivitis (inflammation of the conjunctiva), blepharitis (inflammation of the eyelid), and corneal abrasions (scratching of the cornea).

The eye is an extremely delicate organ. Even what seems to be a minor injury or infection can have lasting consequences. Therefore, you must use the greatest caution as well as proper techniques when treating a patient's eyes. You should also provide patients with information on how

Preventive Eye-Care Tips

You can help patients take care of their eyes and protect their vision by providing them with guidelines to follow. Go over each item slowly and carefully. Ask whether the patient has questions before moving on to the next item. Answer all the patient's questions, and make sure the patient understands the answers. Eye-care tips include the following.

1. Get regular health checkups. Patients may not appreciate the connection between their general health and their eyes. Point out that high blood pressure and diabetes can cause eye problems.

2. Get regular eye examinations. Most people need eye examinations every 1 to 2 years. Patients with diabetes should see their eye-care specialists more frequently.

3. Be alert for the warning signs of eye disease. Tell patients to call their eye-care specialist immediately if they experience any of these signs:
   - Eye pain
   - Loss of vision
   - Double or blurred vision
   - Headache with blurred vision
   - Redness of the eye or eyelid
   - A gritty or sticky feeling around the eye
   - Excessive tearing
   - Difficulty seeing in the dark

   - Flashes of light
   - Halos around lights
   - Sensitivity to light
   - Loss of color perception

4. Wear sunglasses with ultraviolet protection to shield the eyes from bright sunlight, even in the winter. Recommend that patients ask to have ultraviolet protection added when purchasing new distance prescription glasses. Explain to patients that the cornea can get sunburned, which can be painful and damaging. Also tell patients that excessive exposure to the sun is a contributing factor in malignant melanoma of the eye—a dangerous type of skin cancer that may spread through the bloodstream or lymphatic system.

5. Wear protective eye equipment to prevent eye injury. Indicate to patients that they should wear protective eyewear every time they participate in sports, work with chemicals, or encounter a situation in which they may be exposed to flying debris.

6. Use nonprescription eye medications properly. Show patients how to use eyedrops; emphasize that the tip of the dropper should never touch the eye. Explain to patients that medications should be used only as indicated on the label and discarded after the condition has cleared up.

to routinely care for their eyes. See the Educating the Patient section for specific guidelines to follow when presenting preventive eye-care information.

Administration of Medications to the Eye

Your responsibilities as a medical assistant include dispensing medications and explaining their use. Some medications are used to diagnose conditions, whereas others are used to treat conditions. Only medications for ophthalmic use should be used in the eye. You should teach patients to check medication labels carefully before administering them at home. *Optic* medications for use in the eye could easily be confused with *otic* medications for the ear. Medications other than optic medications may be too concentrated or may contain substances that will injure sensitive eye tissue.

If you administer eye medications as part of your job, avoid touching a dropper or ointment tube tip to the eye.

Such touching can injure the eye, cause an infection, and contaminate the medication. Procedure 39-2 describes the proper technique for administering eye medications.

Eye Irrigation

When foreign materials enter the eye, they must be flushed out. Flushing (or irrigation) should be done with a sterile solution especially formulated for this purpose. Someone's eye may also need to be irrigated to relieve discomfort from irritating substances, such as smog, pollen, chemicals, or chlorinated water. The steps involved in irrigating the eye are outlined in Procedure 39-3.

Vision Aids

Vision screening tests may indicate that a patient has a vision problem. Common refractive disorders, such as myopia, hyperopia, presbyopia, and astigmatism, are discussed in detail in Chapter 41. Most of these vision problems

PROCEDURE 39.3

Performing Eye Irrigation

Objective: To flush the eye to remove foreign particles or relieve eye irritation

OSHA Guidelines

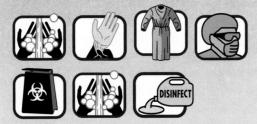

Materials: Sterile irrigating solution, sterile basin, sterile irrigating syringe and kidney-shaped basin, tissues

Method

1. Identify the patient, introduce yourself, and explain the procedure.

2. Review the physician's order. This should include the patient's name, irrigating solution, volume of solution, and for which eye(s) the irrigation is to be performed.

3. Compare the solution with the instructions three times.

4. Wash your hands and put on gloves, a gown, and a face shield (splashing is possible when a syringe is used).

5. Assemble supplies.

6. Ask the patient to lie down or to sit with the head tilted back and to the side that is being irrigated. The solution should not spill over into the other eye.

7. Place a towel over the patient's shoulder (or under the head and shoulder, if the patient is lying down). Have the patient hold the kidney-shaped basin at the side of the head next to the eye to be irrigated.

8. Pour the solution into the sterile basin.

9. Fill the irrigating syringe with solution (approximately 50 mL).

10. Hold a tissue on the patient's cheekbone below the lower eyelid with your nondominant hand, and press downward to expose the eye socket.

11. Holding the tip of the syringe ½ inch away from the eye, direct the solution onto the lower conjunctiva from the inner to the outer aspect of the eye. (Avoid directing the solution against the cornea because it is sensitive; do not use excessive force.)

12. Refill the syringe and continue irrigation until the prescribed volume of solution is used or until the solution is used up.

13. Dry the area around the eye with tissues.

14. Properly dispose of used disposable materials.

15. Remove gloves, gown, and face shield, and wash your hands.

16. Record in the patient's chart the procedure, the amount of solution used, time of administration, and eye(s) irrigated.

17. Put on gloves and clean the equipment and room according to OSHA guidelines.

---

substance also called earwax. The eardrum, or **tympanic membrane,** is a fibrous partition located at the inner end of the canal. The eardrum separates the external ear from the middle ear.

The Middle Ear. The middle ear is a small, air-filled cavity between the eardrum and the inner ear. It contains three small bones: the hammer, the anvil, and the stirrup. The **malleus,** or hammer, is attached to the eardrum, and the **stapes,** or stirrup, is attached to the inner ear. The **incus,** or anvil, lies between them. An opening in the middle ear, the **eustachian tube,** leads to the back of the throat. The eustachian tube helps equalize air pressure on both sides of the eardrum.

The Inner Ear. The inner ear, or **labyrinth,** contains a number of important structures. Among these are the **cochlea,** a spiral-shaped canal that contains the hearing receptors, and three **semicircular canals,** which help a person maintain balance.

The Hearing Process

A sound consists of waves of different frequencies that move through the air. The external ear initiates sound conduction when it collects these waves and channels them to the eardrum. There the waves make the eardrum vibrate. The vibrations, in turn, are amplified by the bones

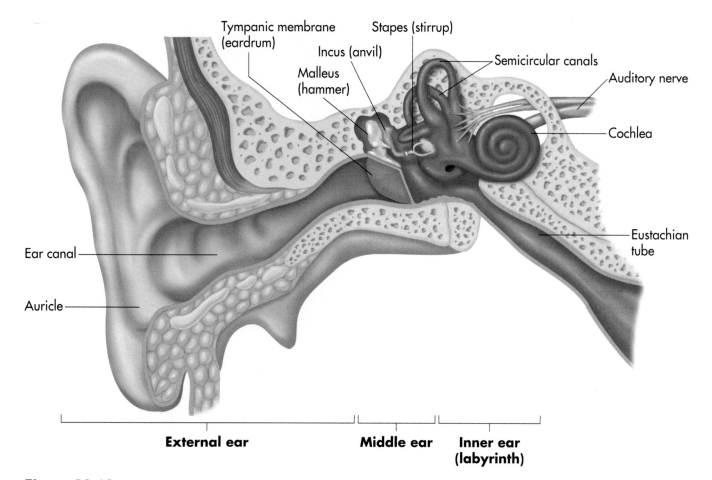

Figure 39-13. The ear is composed of a number of structures that work in harmony to produce hearing and a sense of balance.

of the middle ear. The amplified waves enter the inner ear and the cochlea. These waves cause tiny hairs that line the cochlea to bend. Movements of the hairs trigger nerve impulses. The impulses are transmitted by the auditory nerve to the brain, where they are perceived as sound.

Sound waves are also conducted through the bones of the skull directly to the inner ear, a process called **bone conduction.** This alternative pathway for sound bypasses the external and middle ears. When you hear your own voice, the sound has reached your inner ear mainly through bone conduction. By comparing a person's ability to sense sounds by bone conduction and through the entire ear, doctors can often identify what part of the ear is causing a hearing problem. For example, if bone conduction is normal, a hearing problem likely involves the middle or external ear rather than the inner ear.

The Ear and Balance

The brain constantly monitors the position of one's body on the basis of information it receives from the semicircular canals, eyes, and muscles. Each canal is at a right angle to the other two. In other words, each is oriented in a different dimension or plane: height, depth, and width. Together they detect any change in the position of the body. Such information is passed on to the brain along with data from the eyes and muscles. The brain then uses the information to maintain balance.

The Aging Ear

As a person grows older, a number of changes occur in the ear. The external ear appears larger because of continued growth of cartilage and the loss of skin elasticity. The ear lobe gets longer and may have a wrinkled appearance. The glands that produce cerumen become less efficient, producing earwax that is much drier. The ear canal also becomes narrower.

In the middle ear, changes in the eardrum cause it to shrink and appear dull and gray. The joints between the bones of the middle ear degenerate, so they do not move as freely. In the inner ear, the semicircular canals become less sensitive to changes in position, and this reduced sensitivity affects balance.

Problems with equilibrium make the elderly prone to falls. Some ear disorders are also more common in older individuals.

PROCEDURE 39.4

Measuring Auditory Acuity

Objective: To determine how well a patient hears

OSHA Guidelines

Materials: Audiometer, headset, graph pad (if applicable), alcohol, gauze squares

Method

Adults and Children

1. Wash your hands, identify the patient, introduce yourself, and explain the procedure.
2. Clean the earpieces of the headset with a gauze square dampened with alcohol.
3. Have the patient sit with his back to you.
4. Assist the patient in putting on the headset, and adjust it until it is comfortable.
5. Tell the patient he will hear tones in the right ear.
6. Tell the patient to raise his finger or press the indicator button when he hears a tone.
7. Set the audiometer for the right ear.
8. Set the audiometer for the lowest range of frequencies and the first degree of loudness (usually 15 decibels). (When using automated audiometers, follow the instructions printed in the user's manual.)
9. Press the tone button or switch and observe the patient.
10. If the patient does not hear the first degree of loudness, raise it two or three times to greater degrees, up to 50 or 60 decibels.
11. If the patient indicates that he has heard the tone, record the setting on the graph.
12. Change the setting to the next frequency. Repeat steps 9, 10, and 11.
13. Proceed to the mid-range frequencies. Repeat steps 9, 10, and 11.
14. Proceed to the high-range frequencies. Repeat steps 9, 10, and 11.

15. Set the audiometer for the left ear.
16. Tell the patient that he will hear tones in the left ear, and ask him to raise his finger or press the indicator button when he hears a tone.
17. Repeat steps 8 through 14.
18. Set the audiometer for both ears.
19. Ask the patient to listen with both ears and to raise his finger or press the indicator button when he hears a tone.
20. Repeat steps 8 through 14.
21. Have the patient remove the headset.
22. Clean the earpieces with a gauze square dampened with alcohol.
23. Properly dispose of the used gauze square and wash your hands.

Infants and Toddlers

1. Identify the patient and introduce yourself.
2. Wash your hands.
3. Pick a quiet location.
4. The patient can be sitting, lying down, or held by the parent.
5. Instruct the parent to be silent during the procedure.
6. Position yourself so your hands are behind the child's right ear and out of sight.
7. Clap your hands loudly. Observe the child's response. (Never clap directly in front of the ear because this can damage the eardrum. As an alternative to clapping, use special devices, such as rattles or clickers, that may be available in the office to generate sounds of varying loudness.)
8. Record the child's response as positive or negative for loud noise.
9. Position one hand behind the child's right ear, as before.
10. Snap your fingers. Observe the child's response.
11. Record the response as positive or negative for moderate noise.
12. Repeat steps 6 through 11 for the left ear.

Ear Medications and Irrigation

Part of your job may be to administer ear medications to patients. You may also teach patients how to administer ear medications at home. The proper procedure for administering eardrops is described in Procedure 39-5.

Irrigating the ear may relieve inflammation or irritation of the ear canal and may help loosen and remove impacted cerumen (earwax) or a foreign body. This procedure is performed in the physician's office. The steps used to irrigate the ear are described in Procedure 39-6.

Otitis Media: The Common Ear Infection

Otitis media, commonly referred to as an ear infection, affects almost all children by age 6. This inflammation of the middle ear accounts for 24.5 million doctor visits each year—second only to upper respiratory infections.

Ear infections typically start when fluid becomes trapped in the middle ear. The lining of the middle ear and eustachian tube is blanketed with a layer of fluid similar to that found in the nose. The normal flow of this fluid from the ear into the back of the nose helps keep the middle ear and the eustachian tube free of bacteria. When a child gets a cold or flu, the lining of the eustachian tube and middle ear can become inflamed and can trap the fluid. The child can develop one of the following four types of otitis media.

1. Acute otitis media typically refers to a bacterial infection of the middle ear that comes on suddenly. This type is common in children and typically follows an upper respiratory tract infection. The symptoms include pain, a feeling of fullness in the ear, some loss of hearing, and possible fever. In severe cases the eardrum may rupture because of the fluid pressure. Acute infections are usually treated with oral antibiotics. If not treated, this type of otitis media can cause permanent hearing loss.

2. Recurrent otitis media is diagnosed when a child contracts acute otitis media again and again, perhaps once or twice every month.

3. Otitis media with effusion, also known as OME, involves an accumulation of fluid in the middle ear. Children with OME do not exhibit any symptoms, and they may not experience any discomfort.

4. Chronic otitis media is diagnosed when fluid is present in the ear and fails to clear up after 3 months or more. Infection may or may not be present. Without treatment the undrained fluid thickens, resulting in possible changes in the shape of the eardrum. These changes may cause temporary hearing loss. Antibiotics and reconstructive surgery may be used to treat chronic otitis media.

If a child suffers from recurrent or chronic otitis media, myringotomy, or the surgical insertion of tubes, may be recommended to keep the fluid draining continuously. This procedure usually removes enough fluid so the infection clears up. Depending on the type of tube, it falls out on its own within 3 to 18 months of insertion.

Ear infections may be difficult to identify, especially in a young child who cannot talk. The following symptoms may be indications of a possible ear infection, particularly if more than one is present:

- Tugging or rubbing the ear
- Fever ranging from 100° to 104°F
- Difficulty balancing
- Excessive crankiness
- Difficulty hearing or speaking
- An unwillingness to lie down (The pain may become more severe in a reclining position because of increased pressure against the eardrum.)

Hearing Aids

Hearing aids may be worn inside or outside the ear. If worn outside, they may be located behind the ear, mounted on eyeglasses, or worn on the body. Hearing aids consist of the following parts:

- A tiny microphone to pick up sounds
- An amplifier to increase the volume of sounds
- A tiny speaker to transmit sounds to the ear

You may need to teach patients how to obtain a hearing aid. You can also pass along tips to patients to help them take proper care of their hearing aids and to troubleshoot problems.

Obtaining a Hearing Aid. A patient with signs of hearing loss should be referred to an **otologist,** a medical doctor specializing in the health of the ear, or an **audiologist,** a specialist who focuses on evaluating and correcting hearing problems. Audiologists are not medical doctors and do not treat diseases of the ear. Instead, they evaluate the patient's hearing, fit hearing aids, give instruction in the use of hearing aids, and provide service for hearing aids if necessary. It is important for hearing aids to fit properly. If they do not, sounds may not be transmitted well into the ear.

Care and Use of Hearing Aids. Hearing aids run on batteries that typically last about 2 weeks. Therefore, the patient must keep a fresh supply of batteries on hand. The hearing aid itself must be routinely cleaned, or the microphone, switches, or dials may not work properly. Moisture can damage the aid, so it must not get wet. Hair sprays can clog hearing aid openings or interfere with the operation of moving parts. For these reasons spray should

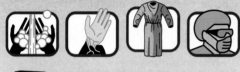

PROCEDURE 39.6

Performing Ear Irrigation

Objective: To wash out the ear canal to remove impacted cerumen, relieve inflammation, or remove a foreign body

OSHA Guidelines

Materials: Fresh irrigating solution, clean basin, clean irrigating syringe, towel or absorbent pad, kidney-shaped basin, cotton balls

Method

1. Identify the patient, introduce yourself, and explain the procedure.
2. Check the doctor's order. It should include the patient's name, irrigating solution, volume of solution, and for which ear(s) the irrigation is to be performed. If the doctor has not specified the volume of solution, use the amount needed to remove the wax.
3. Compare the solution with the instructions three times.
4. Wash your hands and put on gloves, a gown, and a face shield (splashing is possible when a syringe is used).
5. Look into the patient's ear if cerumen or a foreign body needs to be removed so you will know when you have completed the irrigation.
6. Assemble the supplies.
7. If the solution is cold, warm it to room temperature by placing the bottle in a pan of warm water. *Warning:* Internal ear structures

are very sensitive to extreme heat or cold. Administration of cold liquids can result in vertigo or nausea.

8. Have the patient sit or lie on her back with the ear to be treated facing you.
9. Place a towel over the patient's shoulder (or under the head and shoulder if she is lying down), and have her hold the kidney-shaped basin under her ear.
10. Pour the solution into the other basin.
11. If necessary, gently clean the external ear with cotton moistened with the solution.
12. Fill the irrigating syringe with solution (approximately 50 mL).
13. Straighten the ear canal by pulling the auricle upward and outward for adults, down and back for infants and children.
14. Holding the tip of the syringe ½ inch above the opening of the ear, slowly instill the solution into the ear. Allow the fluid to drain out during the process.
15. Refill the syringe and continue irrigation until the canal is cleaned or the solution is used up.
16. Dry the external ear with a cotton ball, and leave a clean cotton ball loosely in place for 5 to 10 minutes.
17. If the patient becomes dizzy or nauseated, allow her time to regain balance before standing up. Then assist her as needed.
18. Properly dispose of used disposable materials.
19. Remove gloves, gown, and face shield, and wash your hands.
20. Record in the patient's chart the procedure and result, amount of solution used, time of administration, and ear(s) irrigated.
21. Put on gloves and clean the equipment and room according to OSHA guidelines.

be applied before a hearing aid is inserted. Cerumen often builds up behind hearing aids that are worn in the ear. Wax buildup reduces sound transmission. If buildup occurs, the earwax plug can be removed by ear irrigation.

Other Devices and Strategies

People whose hearing cannot be substantially improved by hearing aids may need to use other devices or strategies to overcome the problem. These devices include appliances that light up as well as ring, such as telephones, doorbells, smoke detectors, alarm clocks, and burglar alarms. Patients can purchase amplifiers for the telephone, television set, and radio. Many closed-captioned television programs are also available. To benefit from closed captioning, the patient must have a television set with a decoder that translates the captioning and displays the captions on the screen.

Summary

You can help prevent, detect, and treat eye and ear problems in your work as a medical assistant. Because conditions that affect the eyes and ears can have an impact on vision, hearing, and balance, these conditions affect a patient's quality of life. Vision and hearing provide people with information about the world around them; balance allows people to move securely and effectively through their environment.

A basic understanding of the anatomy and physiology of the eyes and ears will help you provide good eye and ear care to patients. You must also become familiar with many health, medication, safety, and hygiene concerns to teach patients to care for their own eyes and ears properly. Take time to comprehend and master the various tests of vision and hearing so you can provide accurate information to the physician about each patient's performance on each test.

Be sensitive to the needs of individual patients as you care for their eyes and ears. Learn all you can about how to meet the special needs of children, elderly patients, and patients with conditions that make preventing, detecting, and treating eye and ear problems a challenge. Practice the administration of eye and ear medications until it becomes second nature to provide the prescribed treatment calmly, accurately, and with the least discomfort to the patient.

The more knowledgeable and proficient you become, the better the eye and ear care you will provide. Knowing just what you are doing and why will make your assistance to the patient and the physician a valuable asset to the office.

and emotional stress. Try to note the interaction between caregiver and patient. If you suspect abuse, inform the doctor. He will then be able to direct the physical examination toward possible internal injuries, malnutrition, or lack of cognitive ability. Signs of neglect include the following:

- Foul odor from the patient's body
- Poor skin color
- Inappropriate clothing for the season
- Soiled clothing
- Extreme concern about money

You can increase your awareness by consulting the guidelines for diagnosis and treatment of elder abuse and neglect published by the American Medical Association (AMA). Most states require doctors who suspect elder abuse or neglect to report their concerns to a designated office. Early intervention usually results in better living arrangements for both the patient and the caregiver.

Diagnostic Testing

Based on a patient's physical examination, an internist may order a number of diagnostic tests. As a medical assistant in an internist's office, you must be familiar with commonly ordered tests. They include urine and blood tests, radiologic tests, bacterial cultures, electrocardiograms (ECGs), and pulmonary function tests, all of which are discussed in later chapters. Descriptions of a few specific diagnostic tests follow.

Measurement of Arterial Blood Gases. The internist may order measurement of **arterial blood gases** to determine the exchange of oxygen and carbon dioxide in

the lungs and to monitor blood chemistry. Blood is drawn from an artery (instead of a vein) for this test, which is usually performed by a respiratory therapist. The oxygen measurement for arterial blood (partial pressure of oxygen) indicates how well the lungs are providing oxygen to body tissues. The carbon dioxide measurement for arterial blood (partial pressure of carbon dioxide) evaluates how well the lungs are eliminating carbon dioxide. These measurements help the physician diagnose and monitor conditions such as central nervous system (CNS) depression, pulmonary disorders, and kidney diseases.

Radiologic Tests. The physician orders a radiologic test to confirm or rule out a diagnosis. The choice of radiologic procedure depends on the suspected problem. Internists order plain films (roentgenograms or x-rays), computed tomography (CT) scans, magnetic resonance imaging (MRI), ultrasound, and radionuclide imaging (also known as nuclear imaging). Radiologic procedures are discussed in detail in Chapter 53.

Although you will not perform radiologic procedures, the physician will expect you to set up appointments and explain procedures to the patient. You may need to explain what kinds of preparations the patient must make prior to the test. Be sure to ask the radiologic facility about the requirements for the specific type of test.

Chest X-Ray. Internists may order a chest x-ray, which can reveal respiratory and cardiac disorders such as pneumonia, tuberculosis, or cardiomegaly (enlarged heart). It may also reveal abnormal masses in the upper thoracic region.

Venography and Venous Ultrasonography. Venography and venous ultrasonography are tests used to rule out deep-vein thrombosis (DVT). A patient has DVT when there is a thrombus, or blood clot, in the veins. If the thrombus becomes dislodged and travels in the bloodstream, it is known as an embolus. This moving blood clot can obstruct a blood vessel, causing an **embolism.** An embolism can be fatal, depending on its location. Risk factors for DVTs are poor circulation, vein injury, prolonged bed rest, recent surgery or childbirth, irregular blood coagulation, and use of oral contraceptives.

For a venogram, a contrast medium is injected into a vein, and x-rays are taken of the veins. Venous ultrasonography uses inaudible sound waves that bounce off liquid (in this case, blood) to form a two-dimensional image. Internists generally prefer venous ultrasonography to venography because it is noninvasive.

Diseases and Disorders

Internists treat a variety of diseases and disorders. Some of the most common include diseases of aging, infectious diseases, and sexually transmitted diseases.

Diseases of Aging. The elderly constitute a large percentage of patients in an internal medicine practice. Many of the serious disorders frequently seen in the elderly are discussed in Chapter 41. They include hypertension, coronary artery disease, and diabetes mellitus. Other disorders, such as constipation, diarrhea, and osteoporosis—while not serious for young and middle-aged adults—can create major problems for the elderly.

Constipation-Diarrhea Cycle. The cycle of constipation followed by diarrhea occurs when people's diets lack the fiber and liquids to maintain healthy bowel function and they use harsh laxatives to treat their constipation. The patient then complains of diarrhea and asks for antidiarrheal medication, which in turn causes constipation again. Encourage elderly patients to eat more high-fiber foods, such as cereals, fruits, and vegetables, and to increase their fluid intake.

Hyperlipidemia. Hyperlipidemia is a condition in which cholesterol levels are above normal. It is not just a disease of the elderly, but it can cause serious problems for older people. High cholesterol levels can lead to atherosclerosis, the accumulation of fatty deposits along the inner walls of arteries (Figure 40-2). These deposits, along with other substances in the blood, can form an atherosclerotic plaque. This plaque can narrow the opening in an artery to the point of obstructing blood flow. Atherosclerosis is a primary cause of cardiovascular disease, including stroke.

Your role as a patient educator is vital to helping people with high cholesterol levels. Take every opportunity to teach patients about eating foods with lower amounts of cholesterol (see Chapter 49). Provide patients with printed materials on cholesterol, available from the AMA and other sources. The doctor may also prescribe medication to lower cholesterol in patients when diet modification and exercise are not adequate.

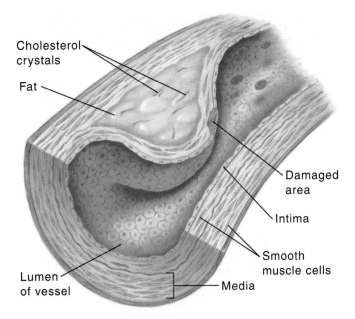

Figure 40-2. High cholesterol can lead to atherosclerosis. Help patients reduce their cholesterol through proper diet and exercise, along with medication, if prescribed.
Source: McGraw-Hill's Digital Asset Library.

Osteoporosis. Osteoporosis is an endocrine and metabolic disorder of the musculoskeletal system. The condition is prevalent in the elderly and is more common in women than men. It is characterized by hunched-over posture (Figure 40-3). The disorder may be caused by inadequate calcium consumption, estrogen deficiency, or alcoholism. Prevention methods include regular exercise, a diet high in calcium (perhaps including supplemental calcium), and hormone replacement therapy in women who are menopausal or postmenopausal.

Alzheimer's Disease. Alzheimer's disease is a severely debilitating brain disorder. Warning signs include changes in personality, mood, or behavior; recent memory loss and an increase in forgetfulness; decreased ability to perform familiar tasks; difficulty with use of language and abstract thinking; decreased powers of judgment; and disorientation to time or place. Because there is no cure, the primary role of caregivers is to provide comfort and safety to the patient.

Infectious Diseases. An internist is usually the primary physician for treating infectious diseases. Most of the infectious diseases discussed in Chapters 20 and 21 are treated by either an internist or a pediatrician. Descriptions of other common infectious diseases follow.

Infectious Mononucleosis. Infectious mononucleosis (mono) is caused by either the cytomegalovirus (CMV) or the Epstein-Barr virus (EBV). Unexplained fever, fatigue, and sore throat are usually the dominant symptoms. If patients have these symptoms without any apparent cause, the doctor orders blood tests to rule out mononucleosis.

or curdlike) on the vagina, and vaginal discharge. The infection is treated with an antimycotic (antifungal) drug.

Chlamydia usually produces symptoms of discharge and uncomfortable urination, although it may be asymptomatic, particularly in women. Untreated, the disease can cause scarring of the fallopian tubes and eventual infertility. Diagnosis is made by aspirating pus from the urethra of men, the endocervix of women, or other infected tissue and having it examined in a laboratory. Chlamydia is treated with antibiotics.

Genital herpes is a type of herpes virus. Symptoms include blisterlike sores on the genitalia, difficult urination, swelling of the legs, fatigue, and a general ill feeling. Because this disease is cyclical, symptoms disappear and reappear periodically. Although there is no cure for genital herpes, an antiviral drug can reduce or suppress the symptoms. Herpes may be transmitted to the fetus during pregnancy or delivery. It is often fatal to an infant.

Genital warts and human papilloma virus (HPV) are found on or in men and women. Patients may generally be asymptomatic, but some have burning and itching in the genital area. There appears to be an increased risk of cancer of the vulva, vagina, and cervix in women with genital warts. There is no treatment for the virus. Its symptoms usually disappear within 6 to 18 months in a person with a normal immune system. However, even though the symptoms subside, the virus remains present in the patient.

Gonorrhea causes inflammation of the genitalia, with a greenish yellow discharge from the cervix, sore throat, anal discharge, swollen glands, and lower abdominal pain. Treatment is with antibiotics such as penicillin or tetracycline.

Trichomoniasis symptoms in women include inflammation of the genital area and an abundant white or yellow vaginal discharge with a foul odor. (It is usually asymptomatic in men.) The infection is diagnosed by inspecting a specimen of the discharge under the microscope. The condition is usually treated with a course of antibiotics.

Other Diseases and Disorders.   Internists may diagnose and treat other diseases and disorders, including anemia, appendicitis, arthritis, gout, and peptic ulcer (Table 40-1). They may also refer patients to a physician in one of the highly specialized areas.

TABLE 40-1 Common Diseases and Disorders Treated by Internists

Condition	Description	Treatment
Anemia	Results from deficiency of iron or vitamins, such as folic acid and vitamin B_{12}; can also result from loss of blood (acute blood loss anemia); body's cells do not get enough oxygen, resulting in fatigue, listlessness, pallor, inability to concentrate, difficulty breathing on exertion	Oral supplements of appropriate vitamin or iron; if caused by acute blood loss, blood transfusion
Appendicitis	Acute inflammation of appendix as result of serious infection, blood clotting, or tissue destruction; inflammation may lead to rupture or perforation of the appendix, which can be fatal; symptoms include general abdominal pain and tenderness often starting at the umbilical area and radiating to lower right quadrant, fever, loss of appetite, gastrointestinal (GI) distress	Surgical removal of appendix
Arthritis	Chronic inflammatory disease of tissues of joints; symptoms include pain and stiffness in joints	Medication to reduce inflammation and pain; surgery in severe cases
Gout	Metabolic disease involving acute joint pain, most commonly in the big toe at night; caused by overproduction or retention of uric acid	Medication and diet restrictions to decrease production of uric acid and promote its excretion
Peptic ulcer	Lesion of mucous membrane of esophagus, stomach, or duodenum (first section of small intestine); symptoms include heartburn, vomiting, and dull, gnawing pain or burning sensation in area	Medication and diet restrictions to reduce amount and acidity of gastric juices; stress reduction; surgery in severe cases

Pediatrics

A pediatrician specializes in the health care of children, monitoring their development and diagnosing and treating their illnesses. Just as with internal medicine, there are subspecialties of pediatrics, such as surgery and oncology. To be a good pediatric medical assistant, you must first like children of all ages. If you do, you will be better able to relate to them and to communicate with them effectively.

Parent or caregiver education, adherence to immunization schedules (see Chapter 20), and child abuse detection are primary areas of responsibility for medical assistants who work in pediatrics. You will also assist with the physical examination and treatment of the pediatric patient. Your role as liaison in these areas between caregiver and physician will be an important one.

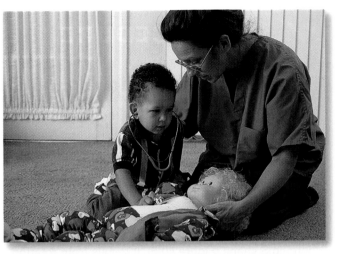

Figure 40-5. Providing a pediatric patient with a diversion may help alleviate the child's fear.

Assisting With a Pediatric Physical Examination

Many of the examination procedures for a pediatric patient are the same as those for an adult. While you prepare the child or adolescent for examination, you might discuss with the parent, caregiver, or child such topics as eating habits, sleep patterns, daily activities, immunization schedules, and toilet training. This discussion will provide important clues to possible abnormal mental, physical, emotional, or social development. Topics such as STDs and drugs and alcohol may be appropriate for you to discuss with an adolescent. Point out potential problems to the doctor.

Be mindful of adolescents' sensitivity toward rapid growth and physical, sexual, and social development when you prepare them for examination. Adolescents and preadolescents often feel awkward and self-conscious about being examined. They may also prefer to dress alone and to be alone with the doctor.

Some children are afraid of going to the doctor's office. You can help relieve a child's fear by calmly explaining procedures before they occur, giving the reason for each procedure, and being cheerful and mindful of a child's feelings. Allowing a child to examine some of the instruments may also alleviate fear (Figure 40-5). If a patient is physically resistant to examination, you may need to call for assistance from the doctor or caregiver, or the child may need to be restrained.

Try to speak in terms aimed at the child's age level, and kneel if necessary to make eye contact with the child. Treat the child with respect and provide positive reinforcement when a child is cooperative. Avoid making light of crying or pain. Make a game out of some aspect of a procedure, and provide a small token reward at the end of a visit. For infants a gentle approach, such as talking quietly and holding them comfortingly, is helpful.

Examining the Well Child. Parents should bring their infants and children to the pediatrician for regular checkups and growth monitoring. The American Academy of Pediatrics recommends the following frequency.

- Infants need seven well-baby examinations during their first year, at these intervals: 2 weeks, 1 month, 2 months, 4 months, 6 months, 9 months, 1 year.
- Children in the second year of life should have checkups at 15 and 18 months.
- From the age of 2, children should have checkups every year.

Follow Universal Precautions and prepare for the physical examination the same way you would for an adult, except for draping and positioning. Ask the parent of an infant or toddler to remove all the child's clothing except the diaper because the child should be nude for the examination. Then keep the child covered until the physician enters the examining room.

An infant or toddler may be crying during the examination. To assist the physician in hearing chest sounds with a stethoscope, ask the parent to allow the child to suck on a pacifier to quiet the crying. Feeding the child during the examination is not encouraged because stomach sounds interfere with clear auscultation.

Parents play a more active role during the examination of infants and toddlers than they play during the examination of older children. You or the parent may assist the child into position during the examination, or the physician may allow the parent to hold the child. Distracting infants and toddlers with mobiles, shiny surfaces, or toys may help the examination go more smoothly.

Examining for Scoliosis. One examination performed frequently in the pediatric office is that for scoliosis, an abnormal lateral curving of the spine into an S curve. It can appear in a child of any age but is more common in adolescent girls during their growth spurt. This condition is undetectable when the child is young. As she grows, however, it can be detected in an examination. Procedure 40-2 explains how to perform a scoliosis examination.

Report any symptoms that you notice during your examination to the pediatrician. If the pediatrician confirms

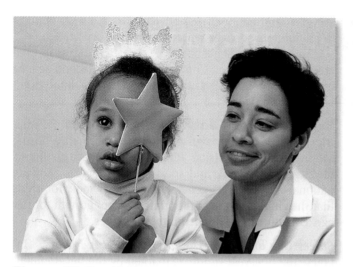

Figure 40-8. Making a game out of the visual acuity test helps put a child at ease.

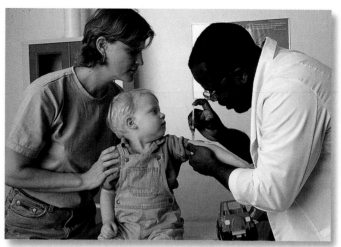

Figure 40-9. Immunizations are part of routine well-child visits in a pediatric practice.

perform the visual acuity test (Figure 40-8). Make a game of covering the child's eye if the child resists this part of the procedure. Watch for signs of visual difficulty during the test, such as tilting the head in a certain direction, blinking, squinting, or frowning. If the caregiver brought the child in specifically for a vision test, record in the child's chart whatever symptoms the caregiver mentions.

General Ear Examination. A pediatric ear examination is important because so many children have ear infections or upper respiratory infections involving the ear. Because children's eustachian tubes are more horizontal than those of adults, fluid collects more easily in the tubes and can promote bacterial growth. The tubes are also short and connected to the throat. Any upper respiratory infections can easily travel to the ear. (The ear examination is described in Chapter 39.)

Diagnostic Testing

Many adult diagnostic procedures are also used for children. The pediatrician uses the same laboratory tests and radiologic tests. He performs some diagnostic tests in the office.

Because streptococcal infection can be especially serious in a child, some pediatricians perform a rapid test for the presence of streptococcal bacteria so they can immediately start the appropriate medical treatment. If the test is positive, the physician begins treatment with antibiotics specifically for this type of bacteria.

Some physicians believe the rapid strep test is not always reliable. To confirm a negative test result, these physicians also do a throat culture. A throat culture can determine which of the streptococcal bacteria is present or whether other organisms are causing the symptoms. The results can indicate a possible change in medication. The method for obtaining a throat culture is outlined in Chapter 46. You may also be required to collect a pediatric urine specimen. This process is described in Procedure 47-2 in Chapter 47. Addi-

tionally, collecting blood may be part of your responsibility. This procedure is discussed in Chapter 48.

Immunizations

Immunizations are usually given during routine office visits (Figure 40-9). Public health authorities recommend a schedule (see Chapter 20) for immunizing children against diseases such as hepatitis B, diphtheria, tetanus, pertussis (whooping cough), poliomyelitis, measles, mumps, rubella (German measles), chickenpox, and *Haemophilus influenzae* type B (Hib). Many vaccines have largely eliminated the threat of these once-prevalent, life-threatening diseases.

The first vaccine, for hepatitis B, is given to a newborn the day after birth. Some vaccines require a series of doses to give immunity. Booster doses may be required for a particular vaccine at a later age. The patient must not have an illness or fever at the time of immunization. If these conditions exist, reschedule the appointment.

Pediatric Diseases and Disorders

If you work in a pediatric office, you should know the signs and symptoms of common childhood diseases. Some diseases, including chickenpox, influenza, measles, mumps, rubella, scarlet fever, and tetanus, are described in Chapter 20. Other common diseases are outlined in Table 40-2. Many common disorders found in children are not specific diseases. Upper respiratory infections, including colds and viral influenza, occur frequently among children.

It is important not to make assumptions regarding diagnosis or treatment. When reported symptoms include fever, sore throat, runny nose, and earache, any number of conditions could be the cause. Encourage the parent to bring the child to the office. You should, however, tell the doctor as soon as possible when a child has an extremely high fever. The doctor may want the child to go to an emergency room. Do not recommend aspirin for fever in

TABLE 40-2	Common Pediatric Diseases and Disorders	
Condition	**Description**	**Treatment**
Head lice	Small insects easily spread among children by head-to-head contact and by sharing objects such as combs and hairbrushes; lice live on scalp and lay eggs strongly attached to hair shafts; symptoms include itchy scalp; identify by locating crawling lice or nits (eggs) attached to hair; examine parted hair carefully at scalp and bottom of hair strands	Antilice shampoo or 1% permethrin cream rinse; removal of eggs with fine-tooth comb; disinfection of clothing, bedding, and washable toys by machine washing and drying in hot cycles or by dry cleaning; tight bagging for 30 days of items that cannot be washed; disinfection of combs and brushes (used for hair) by washing in shampoo
Herpes simplex virus (HSV)	In children virus causes cold-sore blisters on or near mouth; diagnosis made by inspecting lesions; first stage (2–12 days before appearance of blister) involves tingling and itching sensations; later blister ruptures and forms yellow crust; outbreak takes about 3 weeks to heal completely	Application of ice cube to blister, which may promote faster healing; ointments to alleviate cracking and discomfort; avoidance of sun exposure because it may trigger outbreak
Impetigo	Highly contagious dermatologic disease caused by staphylococcal, sometimes streptococcal, bacteria; transmitted by direct contact; causes inflammation and pustules, which are small lymph-filled bumps that rupture and become encrusted before healing; frequently seen around mouth and nostrils	Avoidance of scratching lesions and sharing utensils, towels, bed linens, or bath or pool water that could cause further transmission; careful washing of affected areas two to three times per day to keep lesions clean and dry; topical antibacterial cream
Infectious conjunctivitis ("pink eye")	Highly contagious streptococcal or staphylococcal bacterial infection of conjunctiva of eye; transmitted by direct contact; causes redness, pain, swelling, discharge; usually begins in one eye and spreads to other	Avoidance of scratching eyes and sharing utensils, towels, or bed linens that could cause further transmission; warm compresses to relieve discomfort; antibiotic drops or ointment
Pinworms	Parasites transmitted by swallowing worm eggs, by touching something that infected person has touched, or by putting infested sand or dirt into mouth; when eggs hatch in body, worms attach to intestinal lining; mature females travel to areas just outside rectum to lay eggs, which causes itching	Medication usually given to whole family to treat and prevent further infestation
Ringworm	Contagious fungal infection involving scalp, groin, feet, or other areas of body, causing flat, dry, and scaly or moist and crusty lesions; lesions develop into clear center with outer ring; when scalp is affected, may cause bald patches	Oral and topical antifungal medication; isolation to prevent spreading; frequent changing of towels, bedding, with no sharing with others in family; caution that child not use others' combs or brushes
Streptococcal sore throat ("strep throat")	Contagious disease caused by streptococcal bacteria and spread by droplet; complications include progression to rheumatic fever (with arthritis, nephritis, and inflammation of endocardium, or inner lining of heart); symptoms include headache, high fever, vomiting, and extremely painful, swollen, and red or white sore throat; causes difficulty swallowing	Streptococci-specific antibiotics given as soon as possible; because of potential complications, therapy based on the practitioner's experience is sometimes given without confirmed diagnosis from throat culture; antibiotics are adjusted with confirmation of infecting organism; possible hospitalization in acute cases

and tests. A female medical assistant should be in the examining room during the physical examination to assist a male doctor and to provide legal protection. Your role during the examination is similar to that for the general physical examination.

Ask the patient to empty her bladder; if a urine specimen is needed, it should be collected at this time. Provide the patient with a gown before the examination, and give her privacy while she changes. When you interview her, discuss her gynecologic and general health, and inquire about any changes in appetite, weight, or emotional status. Also find out the date of her last menstrual period. Then have her sit on the examining table while you check her vital signs.

The Physician's Interview. The gynecologic physical examination is more than an internal pelvic examination. It is an evaluation of the patient's total health and a review of factors that could be an indication of possible cancer or STDs. The physician asks questions about the patient's menstrual cycle and about any abnormal discharge or discomfort during sexual intercourse. The physician also listens to the patient's heart and lungs before beginning the gynecologic examination.

Breast Examination. The physician examines the patient's breasts and underarm areas to check for abnormal lumps that could be cancerous. Your role as patient educator is crucial. Patients must understand the need for regular breast examinations. When interviewing the patient and after the examination, emphasize the breast cancer detection guidelines of the American Cancer Society and National Cancer Institute:

1. Beginning at age 40, all women should be encouraged to have a mammogram every year. Mammography should begin earlier in patients with a strong family history of breast cancer.

2. Women should have breast examinations during their annual routine checkups at least every three years for women ages 20 to 39 and yearly for women 40 and older.

3. Women should do breast self-examination (BSE) monthly.

These guidelines emphasize the importance of education and awareness of the patient.

While reviewing the patient's chart, the physician checks to see when the last mammogram was performed. He may also ask the patient whether she knows how to perform a BSE and whether she is performing it monthly. If needed, he may ask you to instruct the patient in performing the BSE. The teaching technique for the BSE is found in the Educating the Patient section on page 663 of Chapter 38.

Pelvic Examination. During the pelvic examination the doctor checks the external genitalia, cervix, vaginal wall, internal reproductive organs, and rectum. Examination methods include palpation and inspection with a **speculum,** an instrument that expands the vaginal opening to permit

viewing of the vagina and cervix. The doctor wears gloves and uses a lubricant for patient comfort.

Your role is to assist the patient into position, with her feet in the stirrups of the examining table and her buttocks at the end of the table. Drape her so that only the area between the thighs is exposed. Assist the doctor by having gloves and instruments ready for use and by applying lubricant to the doctor's gloved fingers. You may also warm the speculum for the patient's comfort. Be prepared to provide reassurance and explanation to a patient who appears to be uncomfortable or nervous. Encourage her to breathe deeply to help relax the pelvic muscles and reduce discomfort. See Procedure 40-3 for further instructions on how to assist with a gynecological examination.

After checking the vagina and cervix and while the speculum is still in place, the doctor will most likely take a Pap smear (Papanicolaou smear) (Figure 40-11). The doctor then removes the speculum and begins the bimanual phase of the examination. She will ask for your assistance in removing the examining gloves, putting on new gloves, and lubricating two fingers. Placing those fingers in the vagina and using the other hand to palpate the abdomen, the doctor assesses the position of the uterus. She may then place a lubricated finger in the rectum and palpate for abnormal growths with the other hand by pressing on the lower abdomen.

When the doctor completes the examination, she usually asks the patient if she has any questions or concerns. Ask the patient whether she has additional questions after the doctor leaves the examining room. You may need to provide written information in addition to answering the patient's questions orally.

The medical assistant in many OB/GYN offices provides handouts describing female anatomy and recommended

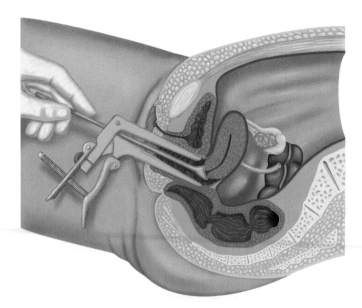

Figure 40-11. A speculum is used to expand the vaginal opening to help view the vagina and cervix.

PROCEDURE 40.3

Assisting with a Gynecological Examination

Objective: To assist the physician and maintain the client's comfort and privacy during a gynecological examination

OSHA Guidelines

Materials: Gown and drape, vaginal speculum, cervical brush and/or scraper, cotton-tipped applicator, examination gloves, tissues, laboratory requisition, water-soluble lubricant, examination table with stirrups, examination light, microscopic slide(s), tissues, spray fixative, pen and pencil

Method

1. Gather equipment and make sure all items are in working order. Write the patient's name and date on the microscopic slide with pencil.

2. Identify the patient and explain the procedure. The patient should remove all clothing, including underwear, and put the gown on with the opening in the front.

3. Ask the patient to sit on the edge of the examination table with the drape until the physician arrives.

4. When the physician is ready, have the patient place her feet into the stirrups and move her buttocks to the edge of the table. This is the lithotomy position.

5. Provide the physician with gloves and an examination lamp as she examines the genitalia by inspection and palpation.

6. Pass the speculum to the physician. For a metal speculum, you may warm it in warm water. For a plastic speculum, a water-soluble lubricant is used. Have this available to the physician as required.

7. For the Pap (Papanicolaou) smear, be prepared to pass a cotton-tipped applicator and cervical brush or scraper for the collection of the specimen. Have the labeled slide available for the physician to place the specimen on the slide. Depending on the physician and the specimen collected, two or more slides may be necessary. They may be labeled based on where the specimen was collected: endocervical = E, vaginal = V, and cervical = C.

8. Once the specimen is on the slide, a cytology fixative must be applied immediately. The **fixative** holds the cells in place until a microscopic examination is performed. A spray fixative is common, and it should be held 6 inches from the slide and sprayed lightly with a back and forth motion. Allow the slide to dry completely.

9. After the physician removes the speculum, a digital examination is performed to check the position of the internal organs. Provide the physician with additional lubricant as needed.

10. Upon completion of the examination, help the patient switch from the lithotomy position to a supine or sitting position.

11. Provide tissues for the patient to remove the lubricant, and ask the patient to get dressed. Assist as necessary or provide for privacy. Explain the procedure for communicating the laboratory results.

12. After the patient has left, don gloves and clean the examination room and equipment. Dispose of the disposable speculum, cervical scraper, and other contaminated waste in a biohazardous waste container.

13. Store the supplies, straighten the room, and discard the used examination paper on the table.

14. Prepare the laboratory slide, and place it and the specimen in the proper place for transport to an outside laboratory.

15. Remove your gloves and wash your hands.

---

female screening procedures. Printed materials are available from a variety of sources, including the AMA, government agencies, and pharmaceutical companies. The Web site of the National Women's Health Information Center, www.4women.gov, is an excellent resource.

Life Cycle Changes

Women experience physical changes as a result of maturation. The two distinct changes that occur as part of the life cycle involve menstruation and menopause.

Menstruation. Menstruation is a woman's normal cycle of preparation for conception (the union of egg and sperm that initiates pregnancy). The normal age range of menarche, the beginning of menstruation, is 10 to 15 years of age. Each month (averaging every 28 days) the endometrium, which lines the uterus, is shed in vaginal bleeding. If the woman becomes pregnant, this shedding does not occur, and the woman misses her menstrual period. Note the last menstrual period (LMP) for each patient in her chart at each visit. A period lasts an average of 5 days, with durations of 3 to 7 days considered normal. Menstrual cycles are prompted by changes in hormonal (estrogen and progesterone) levels.

Menopause. Menopause is the cessation of the menstrual cycle. Menopause is a natural occurrence, not a disease or disorder. Several stages surround menopause. Premenopause is the time period before menopause, during which the menstrual periods may be irregular. The time just before and after menopause is called perimenopause. During perimenopause a woman may experience irregular periods, hot flashes, and vaginal dryness, all caused by changing levels of estrogen. Because hormonal change is occurring, the woman may experience mood swings or other psychological changes.

Menopause can also be brought on by the surgical removal of the uterus and ovaries (see the discussion of hysterectomy in this chapter). The symptoms and treatment are the same as those of naturally occurring menopause.

A woman entering menopause may feel embarrassed to discuss her symptoms with you. Reassure her not only that it is a natural occurrence but also that there are ways to make menopause more comfortable.

Diagnostic Tests and Procedures

The physician uses a number of diagnostic tests, including urine and blood tests (described in Chapters 47 and 48). Many OB/GYN offices have their own small laboratories for immediate results, especially for pregnancy-related tests.

Pregnancy Test. Pregnancy tests are done on a specimen of blood or urine (the patient's first urine of the morning). These tests detect whether or not the hormone human chorionic gonadotropin (HCG), which is produced during pregnancy, is present. A variety of testing kits are available, including over-the-counter urine self-test kits that the patient can use at home.

These tests are not foolproof; false positives and false negatives do occur. An abnormal pregnancy can result in a lower level of HCG, not detectable by the tests. Urine specimens that contain blood, protein, or drugs can also give a false positive result. False negatives may result from testing too early or from a urine specimen that is too dilute. The tests are also subject to human error. The physician confirms pregnancy after taking the patient's history, performing an examination, and ordering a pregnancy test.

Tests for STDs. The doctor diagnoses and treats STDs by taking bacterial and tissue cultures, examining lesions, ordering blood tests, and discussing the patient's history, as appropriate for the specific disease. Some facilities do not permit the release of these results, even to the parents of a minor, without the patient's written consent. Be sure you are familiar with your state's regulations regarding the reporting of STDs to the state epidemiology department.

Radiologic Tests. Several radiologic tests are used in obstetrics and gynecology. The gynecologist uses x-ray, ultrasonography, CT scan, and MRI. X-rays are avoided when a patient is pregnant. If it is crucial for a pregnant woman to have an x-ray, a lead apron must cover her abdomen, and she must be made aware that the x-ray could possibly cause an abnormality in the fetus. You will usually schedule the appointment for radiologic tests. Tell the patient when and where to go for the test, and answer her questions about the procedure. Medical assistants need further training to assist with x-ray procedures.

Hysterosalpingography. Hysterosalpingography is an x-ray examination of the fallopian, or uterine, tubes and the uterus that uses a contrast medium, such as dye or air. Because the procedure is quite uncomfortable, the physician may prescribe a sedative.

Mammogram. A mammogram is a low-dose x-ray of the breast, taken with a special mammogram camera. It can detect cancer about 2 years before it can be palpated with BSE. A first, or baseline, mammogram is taken when a woman is between the ages of 35 and 40 for later comparison.

A patient should schedule mammography for the week after her menstrual period, when the breasts are most normal and least swollen. The procedure involves compressing the breast to obtain a clear x-ray (Figure 40-12). Tell the

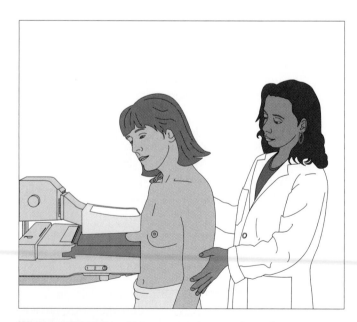

Figure 40-12. Mammography consists of two views of each breast and is achieved by compressing the breast between the radiography plates.

patient that although the procedure is uncomfortable, it is usually not painful. The patient should avoid wearing perfume, deodorant, or body powders on the day of the examination because they can cause false readings.

Fetal Screening.   Tests for determining the health of an unborn child are performed on many women. Some, such as an ultrasound, may be performed routinely. Other tests are used only for women whose unborn babies are at high risk of having birth defects. Fetal screening tests can indicate the presence of several birth defects, including Down syndrome and spina bifida. The doctor will consider the patient's age and medical history and the age of the unborn baby when ordering fetal screening tests.

Alpha Fetoprotein.   Alpha fetoprotein (AFP) is a protein produced by the unborn child that normally passes into the blood of the mother. A blood test determines whether the AFP level in the blood is normal. Too little or too much AFP in the blood can indicate a fetal abnormality. AFP is also measured in amniotic fluid collected by amniocentesis.

Ultrasound.   Ultrasound translates the echoes of sound waves into a picture of an internal part of the body. The picture or image is called a sonogram, and it can help identify and diagnose cysts and tumors in the abdominal cavity or obstructions of the urinary tract. Ultrasound is painless and safe to use on pregnant women to determine fetal size and position. It is also used to guide a physician in performing amniocentesis.

A patient who is going to have an ultrasound examination during early pregnancy should be instructed not to urinate before the test, because a full bladder allows a better view of the uterus. The patient is asked to lie on an examining table, and a gel or lotion is applied to enhance sound wave conduction and reduce friction of the transducer on the skin (Figure 40-13).

Diagnostic and Therapeutic Procedures. Many surgical OB/GYN procedures require the use of needles or other instruments to obtain tissue or amniotic fluid samples. Some procedures are used for obstetric reasons only; others may be used gynecologically and obstetrically.

Amniocentesis.   Amniocentesis is a procedure performed when a genetic or metabolic defect is suspected in a fetus. The test involves removing a small amount of amniotic fluid, which surrounds the fetus, from the uterus. The doctor inserts a needle, which is guided with ultrasonography, through the anesthetized lower abdominal wall. Fetal skin cells obtained from the fluid are then grown in a culture and examined for chromosomal abnormalities. The level of AFP may also be measured in amniotic fluid.

Biopsy.   Biopsy is the surgical removal of tissue for later microscopic examination. It is the most accurate and, in some cases, the only way to diagnose breast and other cancers. Biopsy of the endometrium, which is the mucous membrane lining the uterus, may help the doctor diagnose uterine cancer and show whether ovulation is occurring.

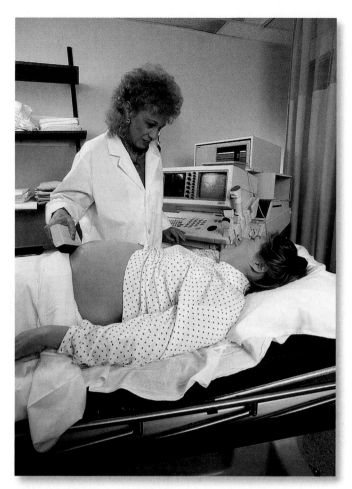

Figure 40-13.   An ultrasound technician lightly rubs the transducer over a pregnant woman's abdomen to reveal the anatomy of her fetus.

It may also indicate whether infection, polyps, or abnormal cells are present. If a patient's Pap smear indicates abnormal cells, a cervical or endocervical biopsy may be performed to rule out or diagnose cervical cancer. Procedure 40-4 explains how to assist with a cervical biopsy.

To assist with these biopsies, you must have knowledge of the female anatomy, the order of procedure, and the instruments used. You will also need to instruct patients about having an escort, appropriate clothing, and any special dietary restrictions. A careful medical history must be obtained to screen for problems such as possible allergic reactions. The day before the biopsy, you might call the patient to confirm the appointment and address any concerns.

A biopsy is considered minor surgery and consequently requires observance of Universal Precautions and sterile technique. Depending on the extent and site of the biopsy, the patient may be given sedation or local anesthesia. During the procedure you may be responsible for clipping excess material from sutures (stitches) and any other special assistance the doctor requests. You must place the biopsy specimen in a sterile, solution-filled container provided by the laboratory. You may assist with or perform the cleaning and bandaging of the site after the procedure.

Assisting With a Cervical Biopsy

Objective: To assist the physician in obtaining a sample of cervical tissue for analysis

OSHA Guidelines

Materials: Gown and drape, tray or Mayo stand, disposable cervical biopsy kit (disposable forceps, curette, and spatula in a sterile pack), transfer forceps, vaginal speculum, biopsy specimen container, clean basin, sterile cotton balls, sterile gauze squares, sanitary napkin

Method

1. Identify the patient and introduce yourself.
2. Look at the patient's chart, and ask the patient to confirm information or explain any changes. Specific patient information you need to ask about and note in the chart includes the following:
   - Date of birth and Social Security number (verify that you have the correct chart for the correct patient)
   - Date of last menstrual period
   - Method of contraception if any
   - Previous gynecologic surgery
   - Use of hormone replacement therapy or other steroids
3. Describe the biopsy procedure to the patient, noting that a piece of tissue will be removed to diagnose the cause of her problem. Explain that it may be painful but only for the brief moment during which tissue is taken.
4. Give the patient a gown, if needed, and a drape. Direct her to undress from the waist down and to wrap the drape around herself. Tell her to sit at the end of the examining table.
5. Wash your hands and put on examination gloves.
6. Using sterile method, open the sterile pack to create a sterile field on the tray or Mayo stand, and arrange the instruments with transfer forceps. Add the vaginal speculum and sterile supplies to the sterile field.
7. When the physician arrives in the examining room, ask the patient to lie back, place her heels in the stirrups of the table, and move her buttocks to the edge of the table.
8. Assist the physician by arranging the drape so that only the genitalia are exposed, and place the light so that the genitalia are illuminated.
9. Use transfer forceps to hand instruments and supplies to the physician as he requests them. When he is ready to obtain the biopsy, tell the patient that it may hurt. If she seems particularly fearful, instruct her to take a deep breath and let it out slowly.
10. When the physician hands you the instrument with the tissue specimen, place the specimen in the specimen container and discard the instrument in the appropriate container.
11. Label the specimen container with the patient's name, the date and time, cervical or endocervical (as indicated by the physician), the physician's name, and your initials.
12. Place the container and the cytology laboratory requisition form in the envelope or bag provided by the laboratory.
13. When the physician has removed the vaginal speculum, place it in the clean basin for later sanitization, disinfection, and sterilization. Properly dispose of used supplies and disposable instruments.
14. Remove the gloves and wash your hands.
15. Tell the patient that she may get dressed. Inform her that she may have some vaginal bleeding for a couple of days, and provide her with a sanitary napkin. Instruct her not to take tub baths or have intercourse and not to use tampons for 2 days. Encourage her to call the office if she experiences problems or has questions.

Colposcopy. **Colposcopy** is the examination of the vagina and cervix with an instrument called a colposcope. Assisting with the colposcopy procedure is similar to assisting with a cervical biopsy. The physician first cleanses the cervix with saline solution. She then cleanses the cervix with acetic acid, which makes abnormal tissue appear white. The physician inserts the colposcope into the vagina and uses the attached magnifying lens to identify abnormal cells, such as cancerous or precancerous cells.

This procedure is often performed prior to a biopsy after results of a Pap smear show the presence of abnormal cells. The abnormal cells may not be cancerous but may be caused by infection or medication.

Dilation and Curettage (D and C). A D and C consists of widening the opening of the cervix (dilation) and scraping the uterine lining (curettage). Reasons for the D and C procedure include assessing the size and shape of the uterus, removing polyps and fibroids from the endometrium, obtaining endometrial specimens for biopsy, performing an abortion, and completing an incomplete miscarriage. Other diagnoses for which a D and C may be performed include abnormal uterine bleeding, abnormal menstrual bleeding, postcoital bleeding, spotting between periods, postmenopausal bleeding, and an imbedded intrauterine device (IUD).

The procedure is usually performed in a hospital or outpatient surgical facility. Tell the patient she will need to have someone take her to and from the facility. Inform the patient that she will have anesthesia before the doctor performs a routine pelvic examination. The doctor then swabs the vagina with an antiseptic and inserts a speculum. After dilating the cervix, the doctor uses a curette to remove a portion of the endometrium to assess the texture. Both cervical and endometrial tissue may be sent to a laboratory for examination. Exploration of the uterine cavity and removal of any abnormal growths complete the procedure.

Instruct the patient not to have intercourse, take tub baths, or use tampons for 1 week after the procedure. She should also avoid strenuous activity.

Fine-Needle Aspiration. During fine-needle aspiration the physician uses a fine needle to remove by vacuum a sample of tissue from a cyst, lump, or tumor of the breast. This procedure may be used instead of mammography to diagnose breast disorders in pregnant patients, thus avoiding the use of radiation. Patients with fibrocystic breast disease (involving multiple cystic lumps within the breast tissue) may have needle aspiration of a cyst followed by replacement of the cystic fluid with a steroid to prevent recurrence.

Hysterectomy. A hysterectomy is the surgical removal of the uterus. If surgery includes removal of one or both fallopian tubes, it is called a hysterosalpingectomy. Surgical removal of the uterus, the fallopian tubes, and the ovaries is called a hysterosalpingo-oophorectomy. A hysterectomy or a related surgery may be performed for the following reasons: cervical or endometrial cancer; severe endometriosis; unusual bleeding; a leiomyoma, or fibroid; defects of pelvic supports; pregnancy-related problems; and pelvic adhesions or other causes of uterine pain not controllable by other methods.

Inform the patient that a procedure of this type is major surgery that requires hospitalization. It also requires preadmission urine and blood tests, cleansing enemas, and shaving of the pelvic area. Normal activities, including sexual intercourse, can usually be resumed within a few weeks.

Premenopausal women who have hysterectomies or hysterosalpingectomies may begin menopause sooner than they otherwise would have. Premenopausal women who have hysterosalpingo-oophorectomies will experience menopause immediately after the surgery. In the past, some doctors prescribed hormone replacement therapy to help alleviate menopausal symptoms.

Laparoscopy. A laparoscope is a long tubular instrument. It contains fiber-optic threads that illuminate the organs and a lens that resembles a small telescope. A physician can use the laparoscope to view the internal female organs. Laparoscopy is used to help determine the cause of infertility, to obtain tissue samples, to remove abnormal growths, and to surgically sterilize a patient. It is also used in the treatment of ectopic pregnancies, endometriosis, and laparoscopy-assisted hysterectomy.

The patient is anesthetized before a tube is inserted into a small incision in or near the navel. Carbon dioxide or another gas is pumped into the abdomen to spread the organs apart and thereby make them easier to see. The patient's body is then tilted with her head lower than her hips to allow the intestines to move away from the lower abdomen. This positioning permits a clearer view of the ovaries, uterus, and fallopian tubes.

Pap Smear. A Pap smear is used to determine the presence of abnormal or precancerous cells. As discussed earlier, during a pelvic examination, cells from the cervix, endocervix, and vagina are smeared on a special, properly labeled slide. They are then sprayed with a fixative and sent to a laboratory for microscopic analysis. The test results are classified according to level of abnormality, using the standardized Bethesda system (Table 40-3).

Pregnancy

Pregnancy progresses in three stages. These stages are referred to as trimesters, and each lasts for 3 months. Figure 40-14 shows the developing fetus during each stage of growth.

First Trimester. After conception, the resulting cell begins to divide. This cluster of cells, the embryo, is implanted in the uterine wall about 36 hours after fertilization. Implantation initiates the embryonic period, during which most of the organ systems develop. The embryonic period lasts 8 weeks, after which the embryo is called a fetus. Week 12 marks the end of the first trimester, or one-third of the pregnancy.

Second Trimester. Fine, soft hair (lanugo) appears on the shoulders, back, and head of the fetus during the fourth month. By the twentieth week fetal movement may be felt, and the pregnant woman begins to show fullness in the abdomen. There are identifiable periods of fetal sleep and wakefulness as the second trimester ends at the completion of the sixth month.

Third Trimester. The last trimester encompasses the most noticeable period of growth, both in the fetus and in the mother. By the end of 30 weeks, the fetus has assumed a head-down position and has a 50% chance of survival if

TABLE 40-3 The Bethesda System for Classification of the Papanicolaou Smear

Classification	What It Means	Tests and Treatments That May Be Included
Negative	No intraepithelial lesion or malignancy	Continue routine Pap smears
ASC—atypical squamous cells, which may present in one of two types:	ASC— abnormalities in the squamous cells, which are the thin, flat cells on the cervix	
ASC-US—atypical squamous cells of undetermined significance	ASC-US—Considered a mild abnormality; may be related to HPV infection	Repeat the Pap smear; sometimes changes can go away without treatment
ASC-H—atypical squamous cells that cannot exclude a high-grade squamous intraepithelial lesion	ASC-H—May be at risk of being precancerous	HPV testing; repeat Pap test; colposcopy and biopsy; administer estrogen cream
AGC—atypical glandular cells (mucus-producing cells)	Glandular cells do not appear normal, but it is uncertain what the changes mean	Colposcopy and biopsy; endocervical curettage
AIS—endocervical adenocarcinoma in situ	Precancerous cells are found in the glandular tissue	Colposcopy and biopsy; endocervical curettage
LSIL—low-grade squamous intraepithelial lesion May also be called mild dysplasia or cervical intraepithelial neoplasia-1 (CIN-1)	Early changes in cells and an area of abnormal tissue; mild abnormalities caused by HPV infection	Colposcopy and biopsy
HSIL—high-grade squamous intraepithelial lesion May also be called moderate dysplasia, severe dysplasia, CIN-2, CIN-3, or carcinoma in situ (CIS)	Marked changes in the size and shape of the abnormal (precancerous) cells; a higher likelihood of progressing to invasive cancer	Colposcopy and biopsy; endocervical curettage; further treatment with cryotherapy, laser therapy, conization, or hysterectomy

it is born at this time. The fetus is said to have come full term after it is approximately 9 months (40 weeks) old.

Nägele's Rule. To estimate the delivery date for a pregnant woman, most doctors use Nägele's rule. Begin with the first day of the patient's last menstrual period, subtract 3 months, and add 7 days plus 1 year. If, for example, the first day of the last menstrual period was June 30, 2004, subtracting 3 months would give you March 30, 2004. After the addition of 7 days plus 1 year, April 6, 2005, would be the estimated delivery date.

Prenatal Care. Pregnant women need to be particularly attentive to nutrition, exercise, medical monitoring, and childbirth classes. They should avoid using tobacco, alcohol, and drugs. Normal manifestations during pregnancy include morning sickness (usually in the first trimester), weight gain, urinary frequency, fatigue, depression, constipation, and swollen hands and feet.

You may perform or assist with routine tests for pregnant women, or you may send them to an outside laboratory. These tests may include the complete blood count (CBC), Rh-antibody determination, blood typing, Pap smear, urinalysis, and hematocrit. Others may include tests for syphilis, hepatitis B antibodies, HIV, and chlamydia.

Assisting With Prenatal Care. You will play an important role in encouraging the obstetric patient to have regular checkups and to take proper care of herself. You will also help teach and support both parents throughout the pregnancy. You must document all information given to or taken from the patient.

Providing information on the effects of using drugs or alcohol during pregnancy is particularly important. Alcohol, for example, crosses the placental barrier and directly affects fetal development. Drinking alcohol during pregnancy can cause fetal alcohol syndrome (FAS). This syndrome may include fetal growth deficiencies, mental retardation or

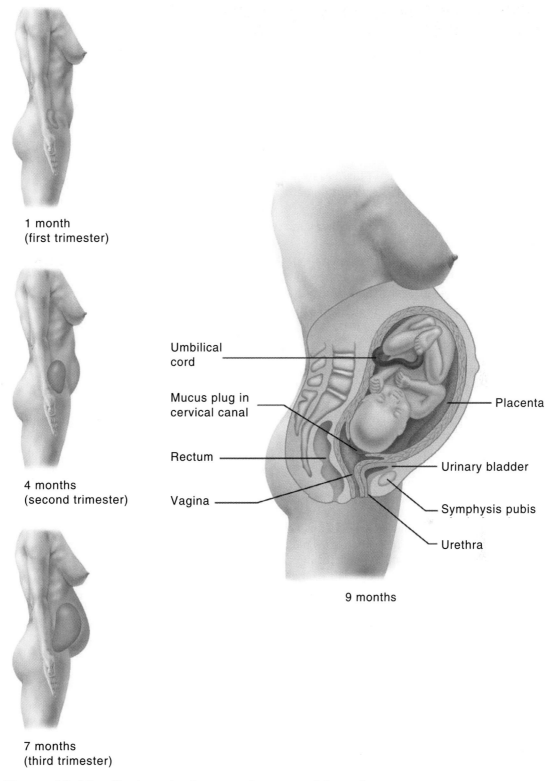

1 month
(first trimester)

4 months
(second trimester)

7 months
(third trimester)

Umbilical cord

Mucus plug in cervical canal

Rectum

Vagina

Placenta

Urinary bladder

Symphysis pubis

Urethra

9 months

Figure 40-14. The fetus develops over the course of three trimesters.
Source: McGraw-Hill's Digital Asset Library.

learning disabilities, heart defects, cleft palate, a small head, a small brain, and deformed limbs. There is no known safe level of alcohol consumption during pregnancy. You can help prevent FAS by teaching all pregnant patients about the potential effects of alcohol on their unborn babies. If a pregnant patient who is an alcoholic expresses a desire to stop drinking, inform the physician, who may wish to discuss admission to an alcoholic rehabilitation program with her. You may also refer the patient to Alcoholics Anonymous or a similar community group for assistance. Drug use during pregnancy poses similar problems for a woman's developing fetus.

When assisting with routine prenatal patient visits, you may:

1. Ask the patient about any problems and record any symptoms she reports.
2. Ask the patient to empty her bladder and obtain a urine specimen in the cup you provide.
3. Weigh the patient and note her weight in the chart.
4. Perform the reagent urine test (chemical analysis) and note the results in her chart.
5. Give the patient a drape and ask her to undress from the waist down if the physician will be performing an internal examination.
6. Assist the patient to the examining table. Take her vital signs. Record them in her chart.
7. Assist the physician as needed with the examination. Provide the flexible centimeter tape measure and Doppler, an instrument used to listen to fetal heartbeat.
8. Assist the patient from the examining table after the examination.

Prenatal Care by the Doctor. The doctor carefully monitors the progress of a pregnancy. She watches blood pressure, weight changes, and urinalysis results for possible signs of preeclampsia. Increased blood pressure (hypertension), unusual weight gain due to edema, and protein in the urine are signs of this serious complication of pregnancy. The doctor examines urine specimens for possible urinary tract infections and occasionally asks for other laboratory tests, such as a complete blood count. She may prescribe special vitamins and iron as dietary supplements.

Labor. Changes occur in the mother's body chemistry when the fetus is ready to be born. These changes signal the release of the hormone oxytocin, which initiates labor. The first stage of labor is marked by regular contractions and cervical dilation. The second stage is characterized by complete cervical dilation and the entrance of the head (or buttocks if it is a breech birth) into the vagina. Further contractions and the mother's bearing down push the baby into the birth canal and out of the mother's body. The last contractions push out the placenta and its membranes (afterbirth), attached to the baby with the umbilical cord. This is the third and final stage of labor.

Delivery. At birth a newborn's average weight and length are 7.5 lb and 20 inches. The baby's mouth and nose are suctioned to clear them of mucus. Crying indicates that the baby is breathing on her own. The lungs inflate, and the color of the skin changes from bluish to normal. The physician clamps, ties, and cuts the umbilical cord and presents the baby to the mother.

If the pregnant woman cannot deliver the baby vaginally, the physician may deliver the baby by performing an operation known as a cesarean section. Several conditions may require a cesarean section, such as a large baby in a breech position. To perform a cesarean section, the physician makes a series of incisions. First the skin, underlying muscles, and abdomen are opened. Then the uterus is opened, and the infant is removed.

Newborn Function Testing. The newborn is assessed at 1 and 5 minutes after delivery for neurological function. This is known as the Apgar test. The tests are repeated until the infant's condition stabilizes. With the Apgar test, the baby's heart rate, respiratory effort, muscle tone, reflex irritability, and color are each evaluated with a score of 0, 1, or 2. The best possible Apgar rating is 10 (five evaluations with a score of 2). A score of 7 to 9 is adequate; 4 to 6 indicates that treatment and close observation are warranted; below 4 requires immediate treatment.

Breast-Feeding. Human milk is the preferred form of nutrition for an infant. Colostrum, the first milk the mother produces after delivery, is rich in antibodies that provide passive natural immunity to the baby as well. Breast-feeding is economical and convenient. There is no need to buy or make formula or wash bottles and nipples. Breast milk is always available to the baby at the correct temperature.

A woman's success at breast-feeding depends largely on her desire to breast-feed, her satisfaction with it, and her available support systems. You can support patients who choose to breast-feed by providing them with pamphlets and other written materials. Emphasize how essential the mother's nutritional intake is, and explain that she needs to follow a high-protein, high-calorie diet. Patients who need help may be referred to lactation consultants or support groups such as the La Leche League.

Contraception

Couples who want to prevent pregnancy practice contraception. The type of contraception chosen is based on variables such as price, convenience, effectiveness, and side effects. The only method that is 100% effective is abstinence. Contraceptive methods include the following:

- The birth control pill is a daily oral contraceptive. Synthetic hormones in the pills inhibit ovulation.
- The birth control patch is placed on the lower abdomen or buttocks. It is replaced once a week for 3 weeks, then no patch is used the 4th week.
- Subdermal implants consist of 6 capsules of synthetic hormone that are surgically implanted under the skin of the arm. They provide 5 years of contraception and are reversible.
- Injection is a method in which a synthetic hormone is administered every 3 months to inhibit ovulation.
- A condom is worn on the penis or inserted into the vagina to serve as a barrier to sperm.
- Spermicidal foam, cream, jelly, and vaginal suppositories contain spermicides (sperm-killing chemicals). They are inserted into the woman's vagina.
- A diaphragm is a dome-shaped rubber cup prescribed to fit over the patient's cervix and used with spermicide to provide a barrier to sperm.

- A vaginal contraceptive ring is inserted by the woman for 3 weeks and then removed for 1 week.
- A cervical cap is similar to a diaphragm, except that it covers a smaller area of the woman's cervix.
- An IUD is a small piece of plastic or metal that fits inside the uterus and inhibits fertilization or implantation. Insertion of an IUD is performed by a doctor.
- Sterilization is a surgical procedure. A man can have a vasectomy, in which the doctor removes a section of each tube that carries sperm from each testicle to the penis. A female can have her fallopian tubes cut or blocked.
- Periodic abstinence (sometimes called the rhythm method) involves refraining from sexual intercourse when a woman is fertile and likely to become pregnant.
- Withdrawal consists of withdrawing the penis from the vagina before ejaculation occurs.
- Postcoital pills taken to prevent implantation of the embryo in the uterus must be taken within 72 hours of having unprotected sex.

Contraception information should be obtained and provided to patients as required. The Planned Parenthood Federation, the National Library of Medicine, and the FDA are valuable resources.

Infertility

Infertility is the inability of a couple to conceive a child. Physicians usually test both the man and woman for infertility. Depending on the cause of the problem, the physician may treat the man, the woman, or both.

If you work in an OB/GYN office, the physicians may test couples for fertility and provide them with treatments or options so they can have children. In such an office you should be familiar with basic infertility tests and treatments. You may need to explain procedures to couples, assist with tests or treatments, and provide emotional support and encouragement.

Tests to determine the cause of infertility in a woman examine whether ovulation occurs, whether the fallopian tubes are clear of obstruction, whether the uterus is healthy enough to support the implantation and growth of a fetus, and whether the woman is healthy enough to maintain pregnancy. Tests to determine the cause of infertility in a man examine whether the sperm are healthy and numerous enough to fertilize an egg.

TABLE 40-4 Common Obstetric and Gynecologic Diseases and Disorders		
Condition	**Description**	**Treatment**
Cancer	Common occurrence in cervix, endometrium (uterus), ovaries; cells divide uncontrollably, eventually forming tumor or other growth of abnormal tissue; most often seen in women between the ages of 50 and 60; symptoms differ for each type of cancer	Surgery (hysterectomy), radiation, chemotherapy, hormones; for ovarian cancer, surgical removal of all reproductive organs, affected lymph nodes, appendix, and some muscle tissue, followed by chemotherapy (to extend survival time)
Ectopic pregnancy	Fertilized egg unable to move out of fallopian tube into uterus for implantation; patient experiences pain within a few weeks of conception; can be fatal	Surgery to remove embryo from fallopian tube before tube ruptures
Endometriosis	Endometrial tissue present outside uterus, usually in pelvic area; not life-threatening but may cause sterility; symptoms include abnormal menstruation and pain (sometimes severe) in lower abdominal area and back	Hormone therapy, hysterectomy for severe cases, endometrial ablation (1-day surgery, alternative to hysterectomy), leuprolide acetate injection
Fibroids, or leiomyomas	Common, benign, smooth tumors of muscle cells (not fibrous tissue) grouped in uterus; symptoms include excessive menstruation and bloating; diagnosis by bimanual examination and ultrasound	Surgery for severe cases
Fibrocystic breast disease	Benign, fluid-filled cysts or nodules in breast; sometimes confused with malignant growths in breast until complete diagnostic tests performed; symptoms include pain and tenderness	Depending on severity, vitamin E supplements, hormones, compresses, analgesics, aspiration, biopsy; restricted caffeine intake

continued ⟶

41.4 Describe the medical assistant's duties in performing a scratch test.

41.5 Describe the medical assistant's role in assisting with a sigmoidoscopy.

41.6 Outline the medical assistant's responsibilities in preparing the ophthalmoscope for use.

41.7 Describe the medical assistant's role in assisting with a needle biopsy.

Introduction

Many physicians choose to specialize within various fields. As a medical assistant, you may be employed in a role to assist with specialized examinations. This chapter introduces you to many of the specialties, their diseases and disorders, the types of examinations involved, and how the medical assistant can assist with diagnostic testing by collecting and processing specimens. Certain specialized tests and how to correctly administer them are also included in this chapter.

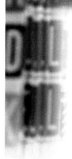

CASE STUDY

A young, apparently healthy 35-year-old male has a consultation appointment with a cardiologist today in the office where you work as a medical assistant. When he presents to the office, he is complaining of a recent onset of shortness of breath and an unexplained swelling (edema) of the lower extremities. As part of the screening process, the physician orders an electrocardiogram (EKG), which shows abnormalities. The patient states that he had some dental work done approximately two weeks before the symptoms of shortness of breath and edema began. Because the EKG was abnormal, the physician asks you to schedule a stress test with Doppler studies for later in the week. The diagnosis on the chart is to rule out a suspected cardiomyopathy.

As you read this chapter, consider the following questions:

1. What was the purpose of the EKG?
2. What special instructions should be provided to the patient when scheduling him for the stress test and Doppler studies?
3. What educational requirements should you meet in order to conduct these tests with the physician present?

The Medical Assistant's Role in Specialty Examinations

You learned about examinations in a number of basic medical specialties in Chapter 40. This chapter discusses examinations that are highly specialized. Physicians working in these areas focus on one body system (such as the skin) or even on a single type of disease (such as cancer) or medical intervention (such as surgery).

Although the examinations and procedures differ from specialty to specialty, as a medical assistant you will be expected to perform certain tasks wherever you are employed. You will, for example, perform general administrative and clinical tasks. You will assist with examinations and procedures and perform certain procedures on your own. It is important that you understand the anatomy and physiology of various body systems as well as the specific examination and procedural steps for each specialty area.

Another responsibility will be communicating with and educating patients. Certain concerns and questions are common to patients within a specialty area. Being prepared to address these concerns and questions will allow you to help patients effectively and fulfill a vital role on the medical team.

Allergy

An allergist specializes in diagnosing and treating allergies. Allergies involve inappropriate immune system responses to substances that are normally harmless. During an allergic reaction, inflammation and tissue damage occur. The substances that cause allergic reactions are called allergens. Common allergens include certain foods (such as eggs and nuts), pollens, medications, insect venom, and animal saliva or dander. Allergic reactions may show themselves locally—with a skin rash or nasal congestion—or may manifest themselves throughout the body.

The most severe kind of allergic reaction is anaphylaxis, or anaphylactic shock, which is life-threatening. Symptoms of anaphylaxis include respiratory distress, difficulty in swallowing, pallor, and a drastic drop in blood pressure that can lead to circulatory collapse. When anaphylaxis occurs, immediate medical intervention is needed to save the patient's life. Chapter 44 addresses emergency medical intervention in anaphylaxis.

Allergy Examinations

An allergy examination involves a medical history and, usually, several diagnostic tests. You may assist with these tests or perform them yourself under a physician's supervision. Skin tests, for example, involve introducing solutions containing suspected allergens onto or just below the skin. Any reaction is observed and assessed.

As an allergist's medical assistant, you will need to understand the function of the immune system and how allergies are commonly treated. Allergy treatments include allergen avoidance, medications, and desensitization to a substance by means of injections. Part of your job will be to encourage patients to make necessary lifestyle changes to avoid allergens. You will also help them adhere to regimens of injections or medication.

Allergy Testing

Three tests are commonly performed in the allergist's office. They are the scratch test, the intradermal test, and the patch test. The radioallergosorbent test is performed in a laboratory.

Scratch Test.   A **scratch test** is performed to test the patient for specific allergies. Extracts of suspected allergens are applied to the patient's skin, usually on the arms or back. One site is always a negative control— a solution like the one used to carry the allergens but containing no allergen is applied. Then the skin is scratched to allow the extracts to penetrate. Procedure 41-1 describes how to

PROCEDURE 41.1

Performing a Scratch Test

Objective: To determine substances to which a patient has an allergic reaction

OSHA Guidelines

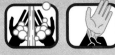

Materials: Disposable sterile needles or lancets, allergen extracts, control solution, cotton balls, alcohol, timer, adhesive tape, ruler, cold packs or ice bag

Method

1. Wash your hands and assemble the necessary materials.
2. Identify the patient and introduce yourself.
3. Show the patient into the treatment area. Explain the procedure and discuss any concerns.
4. Put on examination gloves and assist the patient into a comfortable position.
5. Swab the test site, usually the upper arm or back, with an alcohol-soaked cotton ball. Allow the test site to air-dry.

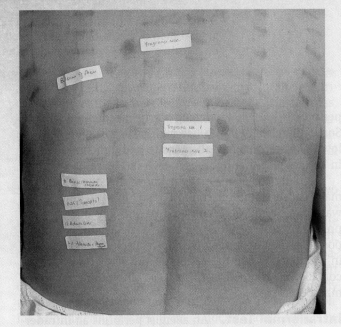

Figure 41-1. Label each site with the name of the allergen or an accepted abbreviation.

6. Apply small drops of the allergen extracts and control solution onto the test site at evenly spaced intervals, about 1½ to 2 inches apart.

continued ⟶

reflected back through a mechanical device. The echoes, which are recorded on paper, can indicate conditions such as structural defects and fluid accumulation (Figure 41-6).

Cardiac catheterization is a diagnostic method in which a catheter (a slender, hollow tube) is inserted into a vein or artery in the right or left arm or leg and passed through the blood vessels into the heart. The cardiologist can use this method to take blood samples for analysis, measure the pressure in the heart's chambers, and view the heart's motions with the aid of fluoroscopy. The procedure is performed in the hospital and is often combined with angiography.

Cardiac Diseases and Disorders

All of these diagnostic tests are used to reveal heart diseases and disorders. Table 41-1 lists the types of diseases and disorders you may encounter in a cardiologist's office.

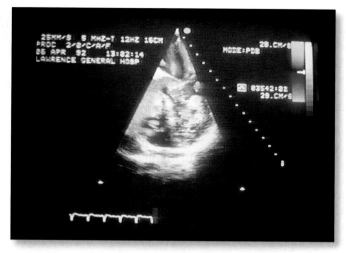

Figure 41-6. An echocardiograph shows the structures and function of the heart.

TABLE 41-1 Types of Cardiovascular Diseases and Disorders

Category of Disease/Disorder	Common Conditions	Treatment
Arterial/vascular disorders	Aneurysms: abnormal dilation of artery wall caused by area of weakness	Medication, surgery
	Arteriosclerosis: thickening or hardening of arterial wall	Medication, lifestyle and diet management, surgery
	Atherosclerosis: accumulation of deposits along inner walls of arteries, obstructing blood flow	Medication, lifestyle and diet management, surgery
	Hypertension: persistent high blood pressure; systolic pressure greater than 120 mm Hg, diastolic pressure greater than 80 mm Hg	Medication, lifestyle and diet management, stress management
	Varicose veins: distended veins in the legs caused by weakening of vein walls and failure of one-way valves inside veins	Wearing of elastic stockings, weight loss, elevation of legs, weight control, surgery
Cardiomyopathy: disease of heart muscle causing fatigue, breathing problems, and leading to heart failure	Dilated cardiomyopathy: dilated heart chambers	Medication, heart transplant surgery
	Hypertrophic cardiomyopathy: thickening of heart walls and narrowing of chambers	Medication, heart transplant surgery
	Restrictive cardiomyopathy: decrease in elasticity and narrowing of heart chambers	Medication, heart transplant surgery
Coronary artery disease: condition involving partial or complete blockage of major coronary arteries that surround heart	Angina pectoris: disorder caused by reduced blood supply to heart muscle	Medication, rest, lifestyle management
	Myocardial infarction: death of heart tissue because of oxygen deprivation	Medication, oxygen administration, rest, lifestyle management

continued ⟶

TABLE 41-1 Types of Cardiovascular Diseases and Disorders *(continued)*

Category of Disease/Disorder	Common Conditions	Treatment
Dysrhythmias: disorders of heartbeat	Atrial fibrillation: uncoordinated atrial contractions, resulting in diminished cardiac output	Medication, cardioversion (delivery of electric shock to myocardium, or heart muscle)
	Conduction delays or blocks: problems with transmission of electrical impulses in heart	Medication, implantation of pacemaker
	Tachycardia: rapid heartbeat (more than 100 beats per minute)	Medication, diet management
Heart failure	Congestive heart failure: inability of heart to pump blood effectively, causing fluid to build up in tissues and lungs	Medication, diet management, rest
Inflammations: infections of heart tissue, often caused by systemic infections	Endocarditis: inflammation of heart lining, including valves	Medication, surgery to repair or replace valves
	Myocarditis: inflammation of myocardium, or heart muscle	Specific treatment for underlying cause, medication, rest
	Pericarditis: inflammation of pericardium (tissue sac covering heart)	Medication, rest
Valvular diseases: disorders in which heart valves do not open or close fully	Aortic stenosis: narrowing of aortic valve opening, restricting blood flow	Surgical replacement of valve
	Mitral stenosis: narrowing of mitral valve opening, restricting blood flow	Medication, rest, surgical repair or replacement of valve
	Mitral valve prolapse: condition in which a portion of mitral valve falls into left atrium during systole	Medication (usually antibiotic prophylaxis to prevent subacute bacterial endocarditis)

Dermatology

Dermatologists diagnose and treat skin diseases and disorders such as acne, eczema, and skin cancer. Some skin conditions involve only the skin itself; others are a sign of disease elsewhere in the body.

To assist in a dermatologist's office, you must understand the basic elements of dermatologic examinations and procedures. You should develop familiarity with skin disorders and their treatments. You also need to understand the terminology used to describe skin lesions, as outlined in Table 41-2.

Assisting with positioning and draping during a skin examination and taking skin scrapings or wound cultures might be among your duties in a dermatologist's office. You might also perform procedures such as administering sunlamp treatments and applying topical medications. You will also instruct patients about caring for a skin condition or wound site at home.

Dermatology Examinations

During a **whole-body skin examination,** the dermatologist examines the visible top layer of the entire surface of the skin, including the scalp, the genital area, and the areas between the toes. The physician uses a magnifying lens and a bright light to look for lesions, especially suspicious moles or precancerous growths. The physician may photograph or sketch a lesion to aid in detecting future changes.

Your role in this examination includes preparing patients and helping them into the proper position before examination of each skin area. During the examination, drape patients to protect their privacy as much as possible while exposing the area to be examined. The physician may also ask you to take photographs or make sketches of lesions.

Another type of dermatologic examination is the **Wood's light examination,** in which the physician inspects the patient's skin under an ultraviolet lamp in a darkened room. This examination highlights certain abnormal skin characteristics and aids in diagnosis. The dermatologist may also perform more limited, focused examinations to evaluate specific skin conditions or disorders.

Dermatologic Conditions and Disorders

The condition of the skin plays a large part in a person's appearance. Patients with skin disorders, therefore, may worry about their attractiveness to and acceptance by

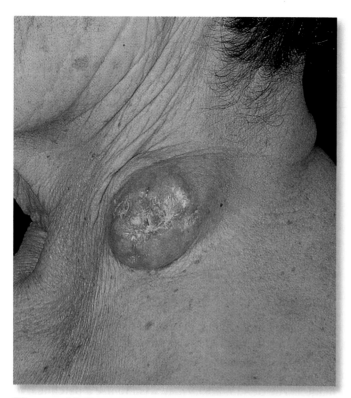

Figure 41-7. Left untreated, basal cell carcinomas can damage bones or blood vessels.

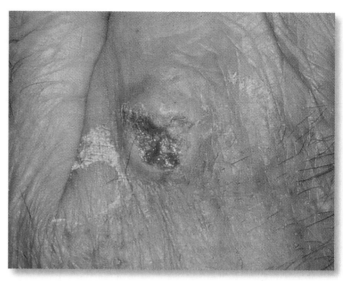

Figure 41-8. Repeated injury to an area, as well as sun exposure, is a risk factor for squamous cell carcinoma.

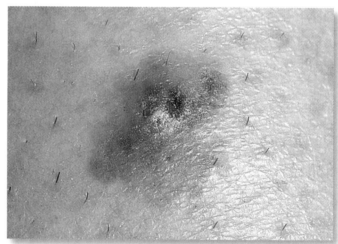

Figure 41-9. Early diagnosis is critical in successfully treating malignant melanoma.

can appear in the form of basal cell carcinomas, squamous cell carcinomas, and malignant melanomas. Overexposure to the sun is a risk factor for all these types of skin cancer. Other triggers include x-rays, irritants, various chemical carcinogens, and the presence of premalignant lesions. The following people have a higher-than-average risk of developing skin cancer: those who have had severe, blistering sunburns in their teens or 20s; those who have fair skin and hair and light-colored eyes; and those who work outdoors.

Basal cell carcinomas are malignant lesions that occur most often on areas exposed to the sun, such as the face and neck. Basal cell carcinomas are the most common malignant tumor in Caucasians. The lesions look like small, waxy craters with rolled borders (Figure 41-7).

Squamous cell carcinomas also appear on sun-exposed areas. The lesions often look ulcerated or have a crust (Figure 41-8). They invade deeper into the skin and have a greater tendency to spread to other areas of the body than do basal cell carcinomas.

Malignant melanomas, which originate in cells that produce the pigment melanin, are the most dangerous type of skin cancer (Figure 41-9). Malignant cells may spread through the bloodstream or lymphatic system to the liver, lungs, and other parts of the body. A sudden or continuous change in the appearance of a mole may signal melanoma. Early diagnosis is critical for successful treatment.

Treatments for skin cancer vary with the type of cancer and its extent. Treatments include surgery, electrosurgery, cryosurgery, radiation therapy, and chemotherapy.

Warts. Warts (verrucae) are benign skin tumors that result from a viral skin infection. If a wart is scratched open,

the virus may spread by contact to another part of the body or to another person. There are several kinds of warts. Common warts are raised, rounded, flesh-colored lesions that usually occur on the hands and fingers. Plantar warts appear on the soles of the feet. Venereal warts appear on the genitalia and anus and are transmitted through sexual contact.

Treatment depends on the type of wart. Some warts go away without treatment. Physicians often remove warts by burning or freezing the wart tissue. Instruct the patient to keep the wart removal site clean and dry until a scab forms or the wart falls off in a few days.

Other Conditions and Disorders. The following conditions may also be diagnosed and treated in a dermatologist's office:

- Eczema: skin inflammation that may be an allergic response to allergens, such as chemicals or foods

- Impetigo: highly contagious bacterial skin infection
- Psoriasis: chronic noninfectious disease that manifests itself in itching lesions covered with scales
- Herpes zoster: acute viral infection of nerves under the skin, often called shingles; causes painful skin eruptions
- Scabies: contagious skin disease caused by a mite; causes intense itching

Endocrinology

Endocrinologists treat diseases and disorders of the endocrine system, which includes glands that regulate and coordinate the systems of the body. Hormonal imbalances can affect the basic processes of growth, metabolism, and reproduction. In the endocrinologist's office you will assist with examinations as well as collect specimens for analysis.

Endocrine Examinations

Before an examination you will take a thorough medical history. The physician will assess the patient's skin condition, weight, and cardiac functioning for clues about illness. Most of the endocrine glands are located deep within the body; only the thyroid, the testes and, to some extent, the ovaries can be examined with palpation or auscultation. Therefore, diagnostic urine and blood tests are essential. You may be asked to collect a urine specimen or draw blood (see Chapters 47 and 48). Other diagnostic tools used in endocrinology include radiologic tests such as x-rays and iodine scans.

An endocrinologist will perform a complete physical examination, including palpation of the thyroid gland. In a thyroid scan the patient receives an oral or intravenous (IV) dose of radioactive iodine, and the thyroid is x-rayed as the material is absorbed. Ultrasound can also be employed to view glands or detect tumors. Urine and blood may be tested for the presence of glucose or hormones.

Endocrine Diseases and Disorders

An endocrine disorder commonly treated by endocrinologists is diabetes mellitus. This name is used for several related disorders characterized by hyperglycemia, an elevated level of glucose in the blood. When blood sugar is abnormally low, the condition is called hypoglycemia. Normally, the glucose level is regulated by insulin, a hormone secreted by the pancreas. A deficiency of insulin interferes with the metabolism of carbohydrates, proteins, and fats, raising the glucose level in the blood.

One form of diabetes, insulin-dependent diabetes mellitus (IDDM), may appear before age 30. Non-insulin-dependent diabetes mellitus (NIDDM) usually appears after age 40. Other forms of diabetes can occur during pregnancy (gestational diabetes) or as a result of other disorders. Symptoms include excessive thirst, hunger, excessive urination, and fatigue. Diabetes is treated through diet

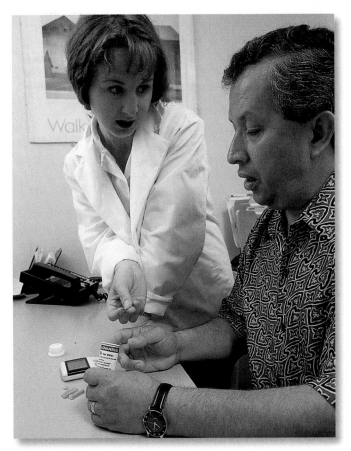

Figure 41-10. Patients with diabetes can use a glucometer to monitor their own blood glucose levels.

and weight control, oral medications, and insulin injections. Special, thorough patient education is necessary for the patient to cope successfully with the blood glucose monitoring, dietary restrictions, and self-care measures associated with this disorder (Figure 41-10). Physicians must pay special attention to certain secondary conditions, such as eye and foot problems, in patients with diabetes.

Thyroid Gland Dysfunctions. Several of the most common endocrine system disorders occur when there is a dysfunction of the thyroid gland. These disorders include hypothyroidism, hyperthyroidism, and goiter.

Hypothyroidism. Hypothyroidism is characterized by decreased activity of the thyroid gland and underproduction of the hormone thyroxine. This shortage can cause cretinism in children, with resulting mental and physical retardation. Underproduction of thyroxine in adults results in myxedema. Patients with this condition have fatigue, low blood pressure, dry skin and hair, facial puffiness, and goiter. Treatment for hypothyroidism consists of thyroid hormone supplements.

Hyperthyroidism. Hyperthyroidism, also called Graves' disease, is characterized by increased thyroid gland activity. Too much thyroxine is produced, and the patient has anxiety, irritability, elevated heart rate and blood pressure, tremors, and weight loss despite an increased appetite. Sometimes hyperthyroidism causes the patient's eyes to protrude, a condition known as exophthalmos. Treatment includes the administration of radioactive iodine, antithyroid drugs, or surgery to remove part or all of the thyroid gland. Many patients require supplemental thyroid hormones following treatment for a hyperactive thyroid.

Goiter. An enlarged thyroid gland, commonly called a goiter, is usually caused by a deficiency of iodine in the diet. Iodine is found in seafood, iodized salt, and vegetables grown in soil containing iodine. Without this mineral the thyroid gland enlarges in an attempt to produce more thyroid hormones. Treatment usually involves the administration of iodine.

Cushing's Syndrome.
Cushing's syndrome results from overproduction of hormones by the adrenal cortex. This overproduction may be caused by a tumor of the pituitary gland or adrenal cortex. Cushing's syndrome may be a side effect of certain prescription medications. Symptoms include high blood pressure, muscle weakness, easily bruised skin with purple streaks, a rounded face, a fatty hump between the shoulders, and rapidly deposited fat that causes obesity in the trunk while the arms and legs remain slender. Some diabetic symptoms, such as hyperglycemia, may also appear. Treatments include medications to suppress adrenal function and surgical removal of tumors causing the disorder.

Gastroenterology

Gastroenterologists diagnose and treat disorders of the entire gastrointestinal (GI) tract, from the mouth to the anus, as well as the liver and pancreas. (Proctologists treat disorders of the rectum and anus only.)

A patient who sees a GI specialist has usually been referred by a family doctor, internist, or pediatrician who suspects a GI problem requiring additional expertise. You will need to understand the basic elements of GI examinations and procedures to assist in a gastroenterologist's office. You must also be familiar with common GI disorders, their treatments, and the terminology used to describe them.

In a gastroenterologist's office you will tell patients how to prepare for examinations, whether in the office, a radiology facility, or a hospital. You will order informational brochures and make them available to patients. You will also be prepared to answer patient questions.

Gastrointestinal Examinations

The gastroenterologist's examination of the patient's GI tract covers the mouth (lips, oral cavity, and tongue), the abdomen and lower thorax, the lower sigmoid colon, the rectum, and the anus. Your role as a medical assistant will be to prepare the equipment and the patient.

Depending on the patient's symptoms, the physician may perform an invasive examination procedure during the patient's first visit. Formerly, such procedures were performed only in hospitals or special medical facilities. Now many GI specialists' offices are equipped for these procedures and the management of possible resulting emergencies.

You must provide reassurance during examinations and help patients be as comfortable as possible. Your duties during the procedures will vary according to your state's scope of practice and the physician for whom you work. Instruct patients in advance to arrange for someone to drive them to and from the examination. After a procedure in which patients have had a local anesthetic at the back of the throat, caution them to avoid eating until the drug has been eliminated from the body. Otherwise, they could choke or aspirate food particles into the trachea.

Gastric Lavage.
Gastric lavage involves obtaining a sample of stomach contents by inserting an orogastric tube into the mouth (or nasogastric tube through the nose) and passing it down through the esophagus into the stomach. The patient is usually sedated. You will spray the back of the throat with a local anesthetic to inhibit the gag reflex. The patient should be awake, however, to assist in swallowing the tube. The gastric sample is suctioned up through the tube and sent to a laboratory for analysis.

Endoscopy.
Endoscopy generally refers to any procedure in which a scope is used to visually inspect a canal or cavity within the body. Several endoscopic examinations are performed with a flexible fiber-optic tube that has a lighted instrument on the end. These examinations provide direct visualization of a body cavity and provide a means for collecting tissue biopsies and removing polyps, as in the colon. Endoscopy helps diagnose tumors, ulcers, structural abnormalities, and other problems. It is particularly useful in performing procedures that formerly would have required an incision, such as removing stones from the bile duct.

Peroral Endoscopy. Peroral endoscopy involves inserting the scope by way of the mouth (Figure 41-11). The patient is sedated, and the gag reflex is inhibited with a local anesthetic. The peroral endoscopic procedures include panendoscopy (esophagus, stomach, and duodenum), esophagoscopy (esophagus only), gastroscopy (stomach only), and duodenoscopy (duodenum only).

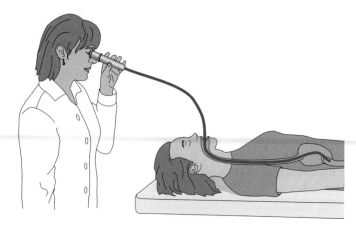

Figure 41-11. To perform peroral endoscopy, the physician inserts a scope into the patient's mouth.

Colonoscopy. **Colonoscopy,** which is performed by inserting a colonoscope through the anus, can provide direct visualization of the large intestine. The gastroenterologist uses this procedure to determine the cause of diarrhea, constipation, bleeding, or lower abdominal pain.

Patient preparation is designed to clear the colon of fecal material so that the colon can be seen clearly. Instruct patients to follow a liquid diet for 24 to 48 hours before the procedure. Patients should take a prescribed cathartic on the two evenings prior to the colonoscopy. Instruct patients to use one or more prepackaged enema preparations on the night before and the day of the procedure. (Alternatively, provide patients with 4 liters of a prepared electrolyte solution to consume over a 2- to 4-hour period. During this time patients should keep a record of their intake, output, and symptoms. Tell patients to expect diarrhea and possibly mild cramps.)

Immediately before the procedure instruct patients to empty the bladder. Patients should be given a sedative or an analgesic before undergoing the procedure. Patients lie in the Sims' position as the scope is guided through the large intestine. The doctor may manipulate the abdomen to facilitate passage of the scope.

Proctoscopy. **Proctoscopy** is an examination of the lower rectum and anal canal. After an initial digital examination, the proctoscopy is performed with a 3-inch instrument called a proctoscope. This examination can detect hemorrhoids, polyps, fissures, fistulas, and abscesses.

Sigmoidoscopy. **Sigmoidoscopy** is similar to colonoscopy, except that only the sigmoid area of the large intestine (the S-shaped segment between the descending colon and the rectum) is examined. Sigmoidoscopy is an important part of many complete physical examinations and is performed by many general practitioners and internists. It aids in diagnosing colon cancer, ulcerations, polyps, tumors, bleeding, and other lower intestinal problems.

Patient preparation involves using one or two prepackaged enemas either the night before or the morning of the procedure, depending on the doctor's instructions. The method for assisting the doctor during a sigmoidoscopy is described in Procedure 41-2. The sigmoidoscope, a lighted

PROCEDURE 41.2

Assisting With a Sigmoidoscopy

Objective: To assist the doctor during the examination of the rectum, anus, and sigmoid colon using a sigmoidoscope

OSHA Guidelines

Materials: Sigmoidoscope, suction pump, lubricating jelly, drape, patient gown, tissues

Method

1. Wash your hands and assemble and position materials and equipment according to the preference of the doctor.
2. Test the suction pump.
3. Identify the patient and introduce yourself.
4. Show the patient into the treatment room. Explain the procedure and discuss any concerns the patient may have.
5. Instruct the patient to empty the bladder, take off all clothing from the waist down, and put on the gown with the opening in the back.

6. Put on examination gloves and assist the patient into the knee-chest or Sims' position. Immediately cover the patient with a drape.
7. Use warm water to bring the sigmoidoscope to slightly above body temperature; lubricate the tip.
8. Assist as needed, including handing the doctor the necessary instruments and equipment.
9. Monitor the patient's reactions during the procedure, and relay any signs of pain to the doctor.
10. Clean the anal area with tissues after the examination.
11. Properly dispose of used materials and disposable instruments.
12. Remove the gloves and wash your hands.
13. Help the patient gradually assume a comfortable position.
14. Instruct the patient to dress.
15. Put on clean gloves.
16. Sanitize reusable instruments and prepare them for disinfection and/or sterilization, as necessary.
17. Clean and disinfect the equipment and the room according to OSHA guidelines.
18. Remove the gloves and wash your hands.

medium or air into the spinal subarachnoid space (between the second and innermost of three membranes that cover the spinal cord). This test can reveal tumors, cysts, spinal stenosis, or herniated disks.

Skull X-Ray. Skull x-rays may be used to detect breaks in the skull. They can also be used to locate tumors.

Other Tests. Other diagnostic tests do not involve imaging techniques. They include lumbar puncture and electromyography. A lumbar puncture, or spinal tap, involves collecting a sample of cerebrospinal fluid. A needle is inserted between two lumbar vertebrae and into the subarachnoid space. The collected fluid is sent to a laboratory for analysis. This test is used to diagnose infection, to measure cerebrospinal fluid pressure, and to check for blood cells and proteins in the fluid.

Electromyography is used to detect neuromuscular disorders or nerve damage. Needle electrodes are inserted into some of the patient's skeletal muscles. When the muscles contract, a monitor records the nerve impulses and measures conduction time.

Neurological Diseases and Disorders

Common diseases of the neurological system are described in Table 41-4. Trauma can also cause damage to the nervous system. Traumatic injuries can result in loss of sensation

TABLE 41-4 Common Diseases of the Neurological System

Condition	Description	Treatment
Alzheimer's disease	Disabling disease that usually affects elderly people; involves dementia and deterioration of physical function	Frequent stimulation to possibly help slow deterioration, medications that may slow progression of some symptoms
Bell's palsy	Suddenly occurring cranial nerve disease that causes weakness or paralysis on one side of face	Usually resolves without treatment in 1 to 8 weeks
Encephalitis	Inflammation of brain tissue usually caused by viral infection; symptoms include fever, headache, vomiting, stiff neck, drowsiness	Medication, rest
Epilepsy	Disease caused by misfiring of nerve groups in brain, resulting in seizures	Medication
Herpes zoster	Disease caused by virus that causes chickenpox; symptoms include painful blisters that form along path of one or more nerves	Medication to relieve pain
Meningitis	Inflammation of meninges (membranes covering brain and spinal cord) caused by bacterial or viral infection; symptoms include fever, chills, stiff neck, headache, vomiting	Medication such as antibiotics and drugs to reduce swelling
Migraine headaches	Severe headaches caused by vascular disturbance and characterized by pain, nausea, and sometimes visual disturbances	Medication
Multiple sclerosis	Degenerative disease of central nervous system that results in visual problems, muscle weakness, paralysis	Anti-inflammatory medications used during attacks
Neuritis	Inflammation of one or more nerves; symptoms include severe pain and discomfort or paralysis of affected area	Medication and rest
Parkinson's disease	Progressive neurological disease, causing symptoms of muscular rigidity and tremors	Medication to relieve symptoms
Sciatica	Inflammation of sciatic nerve causing pain in back of thigh and down leg	Medication to relieve pain, rest, heat applications

and voluntary motion. Paralysis on one side of the body, as a result of damage to the opposite side of the brain, is called hemiplegia. Paraplegia involves motor or sensory loss in the lower extremities. Paralysis of the arms, legs, and muscles below the place where the spinal cord is damaged is called quadriplegia.

Patients with acquired immunodeficiency syndrome (AIDS) may exhibit specific neurological symptoms related to their disease. These include:

- Meningitis caused by a fungal infection
- Encephalopathy (degenerative effect on the brain), resulting in headaches, difficulty concentrating, and apathy
- Peripheral neuropathies (disorders of the peripheral nerves) that result in pain or changes in gait

Oncology

An oncologist specializes in the detection and treatment of tumors and cancerous growths. The term *cancer* refers to a number of oncologic diseases that affect different body systems. All cancers are characterized by the uncontrolled growth and spread of abnormal cells.

A tumor is a lump of abnormal cells. Tumors are classified as benign or malignant. Benign tumors contain abnormal cells, but the cells do not invade and actively destroy surrounding tissue. Malignant tumors contain cells

that grow uncontrollably, invading and actively destroying the tissue around them. Malignant, or cancerous, growths are capable of **metastasis,** the transfer of abnormal cells to body sites far removed from the original tumor. When cells become malignant, the process is called carcinogenesis.

You will encounter patients with a variety of medical conditions in an oncologist's office. You must be aware of the various types of cancer, what their symptoms are, and how they are treated (Table 41-5). Part of your job will involve preparing patients for the side effects of cancer treatment and helping patients deal with them. Patient and family education and support are essential.

Diagnostic Testing

Cancer is detected and diagnosed through a variety of procedures. You will schedule some of these tests and provide pretest instructions and explanations to patients. You may obtain blood specimens for some tests and assist in other diagnostic procedures, including:

- X-rays
- CT scan
- MRI
- Blood tests, especially those to detect tumor markers, such as carcinoembryonic antigen (CEA) (increased levels of CEA indicate a variety of cancers), CA125, and CA15-3

TABLE 41-5 Common Cancers by Body System

Body System	Symptoms	Treatment
Skeletal System		
Osteosarcoma: malignant lesion, usually in femur, tibia, or humerus	Pain and swelling, central hardened portion with softer edges, possible pathologic fracture	Radiation and chemotherapy to minimize tumor, surgery
Chondrosarcomas: malignant tumors of cartilage	Dull pain and swelling	Radiation and chemotherapy to minimize tumor, surgery
Nervous System		
Malignant gliomas: tumors of brain and brainstem	Headache, vomiting, changes in sensation or personality	Surgery, radiation, chemotherapy
Endocrine System		
Thyroid cancer	Nodules on thyroid gland	Surgery, radiation
Pancreatic cancer	Weight loss, abdominal pain, jaundice; very lethal form of cancer	Surgery, chemotherapy with radiation
Circulatory System		
Leukemia: several diseases involving abnormal overproduction of cells in bone marrow	Fatigue, paleness, repeated infections	Chemotherapy, bone marrow transplants

continued ——→

lines to appear out of focus. It can occur along with either nearsightedness or farsightedness. Astigmatism is treated with lenses that correct the unevenness of the cornea.

A surgical vision-correcting treatment for myopia and astigmatism is radial keratotomy. The procedure, which is done on an outpatient basis under local anesthesia, involves making corneal incisions in a wheel-spoke configuration. The incisions allow the eye to return to a normal or almost normal shape. This procedure has been very successful for some patients. Others, however, have experienced complications, including worsening of vision. Newer techniques that use lasers to correct vision are largely replacing the radial keratotomy method.

Orthopedics

Orthopedics is the medical specialty focusing on disorders, injuries, and diseases of the muscular and skeletal systems. The two systems are so interdependent that they are sometimes referred to as the musculoskeletal system, especially by orthopedists. In the office of an orthopedist, you will be asked to assist with general examinations. Other responsibilities may include assisting with x-rays, helping with casting, applying hot or cold treatments (discussed in Chapter 43), and educating patients about therapy regimens. You must be knowledgeable about the musculoskeletal system and its common disorders and treatments.

Orthopedic Examinations

An orthopedist uses inspection, palpation, and a variety of diagnostic tests to assess the structure and function of the musculoskeletal system. The patient is asked to stand, walk, and perform several range-of-motion exercises. In these maneuvers the patient moves a joint in a variety of ways; the doctor usually measures the degree of mobility with a device called a goniometer. A complete examination takes some time, and you may need to help drape, position, or physically support the patient, especially if the patient is elderly or incapacitated. You may also be responsible for instructing the patient about care for a musculoskeletal condition, including how to perform therapeutic exercises.

Orthopedists use a variety of diagnostic tests. As in most other specialties, x-rays play a vital role in diagnosis. They are especially useful in determining the nature and extent of a bone injury. Other common radiographic examinations in the orthopedic specialty include the following:

- CT scan
- MRI
- Angiography (for affected vascular structures)
- Myelography (for spinal disorders)
- Diskography (for intervertebral disk disorders)
- Arthrography (for joint disorders)
- Bone scans

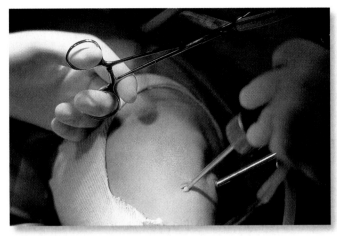

Figure 41-20. Arthroscopy can be used for diagnosis as well as biopsy and surgical repair.

Arthroscopy enables the orthopedist to see inside a joint, usually the knee or shoulder, with an arthroscope. This tubular instrument includes an optical system; when the tube is inserted into the joint, it can be visualized (Figure 41-20). Arthroscopy is used to give the physician a closer look at conditions such as injuries and degenerative joint diseases and to guide surgical procedures.

Bone and muscle biopsies may be performed to detect disorders such as bone infection and muscle atrophy. Electromyography is another diagnostic tool used in this specialty. An orthopedist may also order urine and blood tests to detect levels of substances such as calcium or phosphorus.

Orthopedic Diseases and Disorders

Table 41-6 lists many of the diseases and disorders you will encounter in an orthopedic specialty. Back pain, especially lower-back pain, is a common disorder. It can have many causes, including muscle strain, osteoarthritis, and the presence of a tumor. The orthopedist determines the nature of the problem based on the symptoms and diagnostic x-rays and CT scans. Treatments include the application of heat, administration of analgesics or muscle relaxants, exercise therapy, special braces, and traction.

Another condition that is commonly encountered in the orthopedist's office is a **fracture,** or break in a bone. Fractures and their treatment are discussed in Chapter 44.

Otology

An otologist treats diseases and disorders of the ears. Procedures common to this specialty are sometimes performed by other physicians as well, especially general practitioners, internists, and allergists. Chapters 33 and 39 cover the anatomy of the ear and the types of ear examinations and procedures that might be done in a general practitioner's office. Some of these are performed in an otologist's office too. You may assist with or perform

TABLE 41-6 Common Diseases and Disorders of the Musculoskeletal System

Condition	Description	Treatment
Arthritis	Inflammation of joints—rheumatoid or degenerative (osteoarthritis); rheumatoid arthritis causes joint stiffness and soreness, pain, and swelling and may lead to deformity; osteoarthritis produces pain, stiffness, and possible enlargement of bones, without deformity	Anti-inflammatory medications, application of heat, rest, exercise, occupational and physical therapy, surgery such as joint replacement (arthroplasty)
Bursitis	Inflammation of one or more bursae (sacs surrounding joints); symptoms include pain (especially on movement), restricted motion, and swelling	Anti-inflammatory medications
Carpal tunnel syndrome	Compression of median nerve, causing wrist pain and numbness	Rest and occupational adjustments, splinting of wrists, injection of corticosteroids, surgical decompression of nerve
Dislocation	Displacement of bones at joint so that parts that are supposed to make contact no longer come together; occurs most often to fingers, shoulder, knee, and hip	Relocation, or shifting bones back into place; anti-inflammatory medications
Herniated intervertebral disk (HID)	Protruding contents of disk compress nerve roots and cause severe pain	Rest, traction, physical therapy, muscle relaxants, surgery
Osteomyelitis	Infection of bone; principal symptom is pain	Antibiotics and analgesics, surgery
Osteoporosis	Metabolic disorder that causes decreased bone mass; bones become brittle and fracture easily	Exercise, dietary supplements, hormone therapy, drug therapy (alendronate)
Paget's disease	Chronic condition that causes bone deformities and affects 2% to 3% of people over age 50	Exercise, dietary supplements, hormone therapy, drug therapy (alendronate)
Scoliosis	Abnormal curving of spine	Back brace, surgery
Sprain	Injury to ligament caused by joint overextension; symptoms include pain, swelling, and discoloration	Rest, support, application of cold, anti-inflammatory medications
Tendonitis	Inflammation of tendon	Rest, support, anti-inflammatory medications

auditory screening, and you may help with diagnostic tests such as tympanometry. Otology specialists whose practices include problems affecting the nose and throat are called otorhinolaryngologists.

Common Disorders of the Outer Ear

Several disorders affect the external parts of the ear. These include cerumen impaction, otitis externa, and pruritus.

Cerumen Impaction. A condition called cerumen impaction occurs when the ear canal becomes blocked by a buildup of cerumen (earwax). The symptoms include a feeling that the ear is stopped up, partial hearing loss, ringing in the ear, and occasionally, pain. The wax can be softened with special eardrops, and irrigation can be performed to remove the wax.

Otitis Externa. Otitis externa is an infection of the outer ear, usually caused by bacteria or fungi. The infection can be localized, as with a boil or abscess, or the entire ear

Testicular Self-Examination

Testicular cancer is rare, but when it occurs, it usually affects men between the ages of 29 and 35. The American Cancer Society recommends that all men perform a monthly testicular self-examination (TSE) from age 15 onward to increase the chances of early detection. Although testicular cancer is one of the most curable cancers, early detection is vital to its treatment.

A man who perceives an abnormality during TSE should be examined by a physician right away. TSE should be performed after a warm shower or bath, when scrotal skin is relaxed.

1. The man first observes the testes for changes in appearance, such as swelling. He then manually examines each testicle, gently rolling it between the fingers and thumbs of both hands to feel for hard lumps (see Figure 41-21).
2. After examining each testicle, the man should locate the area of the epididymis and spermatic

cord. This area can be felt as a cordlike structure originating at the top back of each testicle.

Warning signs of testicular cancer include a heavy or dragging feeling in the groin, enlargement of one testicle, and a dull ache in the groin.

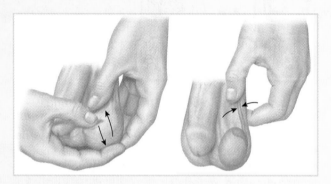

Figure 41-21. Males from age 15 onward should perform a monthly testicular self-examination.

---

urination (dysuria), and incontinence. The physical examination usually includes palpation of the kidneys and bladder and visual inspection of the external genitalia. Women are examined in the lithotomy position, and men are usually seated when the examination begins.

During examination of the male reproductive system, the urologist inspects and palpates the patient's penis and scrotum. The genitalia are usually examined with the patient standing and the chest and abdomen draped. The doctor usually examines the inguinal region for a hernia and, in men over 40, checks the prostate gland. This gland is examined by digital insertion into the rectum.

The doctor instructs the patient as needed in performing regular testicular self-examination (TSE). This instruction, discussed in the Educating the Patient section, may also be your responsibility.

Diagnostic Testing

Urologists sometimes use imaging techniques, such as CT scans and MRIs. Pyelography is an x-ray of the kidney area with an iodine-based contrast agent. It is used to diagnose renal (kidney-related) disorders. Urologists also use several other diagnostic techniques.

Urine and Blood Tests. Urinalysis is the most common test ordered in a urology practice. Urine can be tested for the presence of bacteria, blood, and other substances.

Blood testing is also done for a variety of reasons, including monitoring for dysfunctions of the prostate gland and for certain sexually transmitted diseases (STDs). The Leydig's cell test is a blood test used to assess testosterone levels.

Semen Analysis and Smears. Semen samples may be obtained to determine fertility or to evaluate the success of a vasectomy. The patient usually collects these samples at home, but you may be required to provide a container, written instructions, and laboratory paperwork. Smears are used in diagnosing infections.

Cystometry. Cystometry is used to measure urinary bladder capacity and pressure. Using a catheter passed through the urethra, the doctor fills the bladder with carbon dioxide gas. The test results are examined to diagnose disorders of bladder function.

Cystoscopy. In cystoscopy the physician examines the walls of the bladder and urethra by visualization and inspection. A special viewing instrument, called a cystoscope, is used for this procedure. The cystoscope is inserted into the bladder through the urethra.

Testicular Biopsy. Testicular biopsy, a hospital procedure, involves obtaining a tissue sample of a mass for laboratory examination. The patient will need your emotional support because he will most likely be very anxious about the nature of the lump.

Urologic Diseases and Disorders

Diagnostic tests are used to identify a variety of urologic diseases and disorders. If you work in a urologist's office, you will probably encounter many of these conditions.

Cystitis. Cystitis is an inflammation of the urinary bladder resulting from a bacterial infection. Among women, who are more prone to this disorder than are men, the most common cause is the bacterium *Escherichia coli*. In men the infection is usually related to a separate condition such as prostatitis or epididymitis. The symptoms of cystitis are bladder spasms, fever, nausea and vomiting, chills, lower-back pain, and pain on voiding (dysuria). Diagnosis of cystitis is confirmed through urinalysis, and the condition is treated with antibiotics. Female patients should be taught to wipe and cleanse the perineal area from front to back to prevent bacteria from the rectum from infecting the urethra.

Epididymitis. Epididymitis is a bacterial infection of the epididymis. It causes pain, swelling, and sometimes fever. It is treated with rest and antibiotic medications.

Hydrocele. Hydrocele is the name for excess fluid in the scrotum. It is usually caused by infection of the epididymis or testes. In other cases it results from a congenital defect or occurs after injury. The fluid may be aspirated to relieve discomfort.

Impotence. Impotence is the inability either to achieve or to maintain an erection. The cause may be physical, as when it results from cardiovascular or endocrine disease, or it may be a side effect of some medication such as certain diuretics and chemotherapy agents. The cause may also be psychological or emotional. In at least half the cases, a combination of physical and emotional factors is involved. Treatment depends on the cause or causes and may include medication, counseling, or surgical procedures.

Kidney Stones. Kidney stones occur when chemical substances in the urine form crystals in the kidney, ureter, or bladder. If kidney stones cannot pass through the ureter, they can cause excruciating pain. Although some stones pass, large stones often must be removed surgically or broken up by means of sound waves (lithotripsy) or laser techniques.

Prostatic Hypertrophy. Prostatic hypertrophy, or enlargement of the prostate gland, occurs most commonly in men over 50. Hypertrophy may constrict the urethra, causing difficulty in urinating and repeated urinary infections. Medications to reduce the hypertrophy and surgery are common treatments.

Prostatitis. Prostatitis is an inflammation of the prostate, usually bacterial. Symptoms are pain on urination and, often, fever. Patients are instructed to avoid sitting for long periods. Treatments include antibiotic medications and sitz baths.

Prostate Cancer. Prostate cancer is the most common type of cancer among men. Often no symptoms are evident. Sometimes a nodule may be felt on palpation of the prostate; if the growth is large enough, problems with urination may occur. A blood test known as a prostate-specific antigen (PSA) is used for screening in men over 50 years of age; an abnomal elevation of the PSA could indicate prostate cancer. Treatment options include radiation therapy and removal of the prostate.

STDs. Urologists also diagnose and treat STDs. These diseases are discussed in Chapter 40.

Urethritis. Urethritis is an inflammation of the urethra. Like cystitis, it is usually caused by bacterial infection and requires similar, if not the same, treatment. Urethritis frequently accompanies cystitis.

Summary

As a medical assistant, you will find interesting and stimulating work in a specialty medical practice. Each specialty has precise requirements for knowledge and skills that are particular to that field of practice. All medical specialties require that you have a firm foundation in and understanding of basic principles and procedures.

You will need to familiarize yourself with the anatomy and physiology relevant to the specialty in which you work. You will assist with highly specialized examinations, diagnostic testing, and modes of treatment. By working to understand the diseases and disorders common to the specialty you choose, you will develop the ability to better educate patients and respond to their concerns.

PROCEDURE 42.1

Creating a Sterile Field

Objective: To create a sterile field for a minor surgical procedure

OSHA Guidelines: This procedure does not involve exposure to blood, body fluids, or tissues.

Materials: Tray or Mayo stand, sterile instrument pack, sterile transfer forceps, cleaning solution, sterile drape, additionally packaged sterile items as required

Method

1. Clean and disinfect the tray or Mayo stand.
2. Wash your hands and assemble the necessary materials.
3. Check the label on the instrument pack to make sure it is the correct pack for the procedure.

4. Check the date and sterilization indicator on the instrument pack to make sure the pack is still sterile (Figure 42-8).
5. Place the sterile pack on the tray or stand, and unfold the outermost fold away from yourself.
6. Unfold the sides of the pack outward, touching only the areas that will become the underside of the sterile field.
7. Open the final flap toward yourself, stepping back and away from the sterile field (Figure 42-9).
8. Place additional packaged sterile items on the sterile field.
   - Ensure that you have the correct item or instrument and that the package is still sterile.

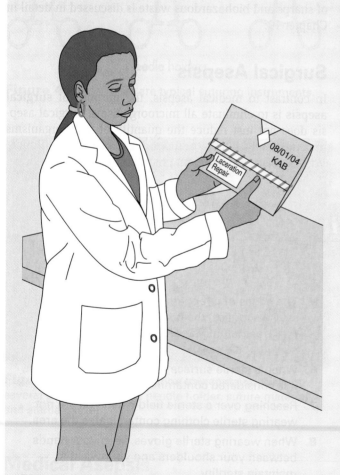

Figure 42-8. Before you open it, confirm that you have the correct instrument pack and that it has not expired.

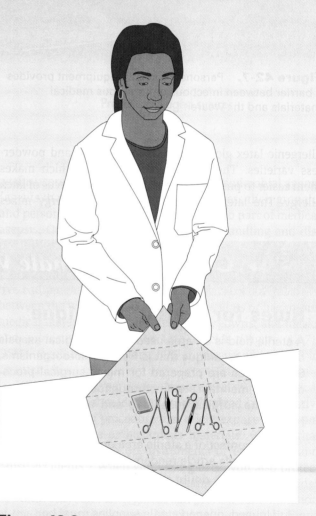

Figure 42-9. The fully open instrument pack constitutes a sterile field.

continued ⟶

Creating a Sterile Field (continued)

- Stand away from the sterile field.
- Grasp the package flaps and pull apart about halfway. Bring the corners of the wrapping beneath the package, paying attention not to contaminate the inner package or item.
- Hold the package over the sterile field with the opening down; with a quick movement, pull the flap completely open and snap the sterile item onto the field.

9. Place basins and bowls near the edge of the sterile field so you can port liquids without reaching over the field (Figure 42-10).

10. Use sterile transfer forceps if necessary to add additional items to the sterile field (Figure 42-11).

11. If necessary, don sterile gloves after a sterile scrub to arrange items on the sterile field.

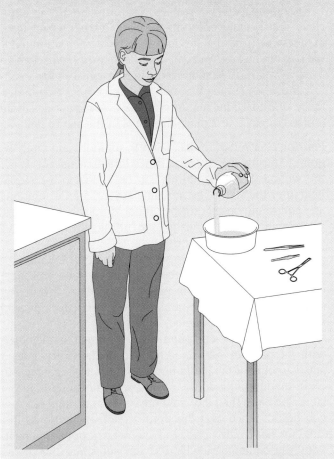

Figure 42-10. Pour a sterile solution into a sterile bowl near the edge of the sterile field without touching the rim of the bowl, splashing the solution, or reaching over the field.

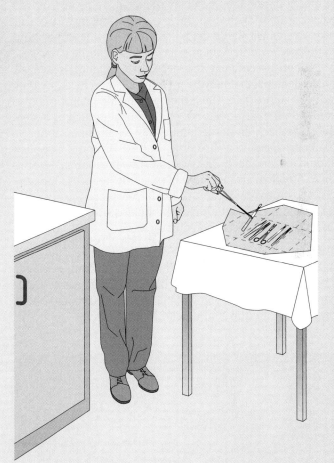

Figure 42-11. You can place sterile items on the sterile field by using transfer forceps.

Common procedures involving sterile technique that you will be expected to perform include the following:

- Creating a sterile field
- Adding sterile items to the sterile field
- Performing a surgical scrub
- Putting on sterile gloves
- Sanitizing, disinfecting, and sterilizing equipment

Creating a Sterile Field. A **sterile field** is an area free of microorganisms that will be used as a work area during a surgical procedure. Always be aware that in the following instances the sterile field is considered to become contaminated and must be redone:

- An unsterile item touches the field
- Someone reaches across the field
- The field becomes wet

The sterile field is often set up on a **Mayo stand,** a movable stainless steel instrument tray on a stand. You should adjust the stand so the tray is above waist level. Remember, items placed below waist level are considered contaminated. Before beginning, disinfect the Mayo stand with 70% isopropyl alcohol, and allow it to dry.

To create the sterile field, cover the stand with two layers of sterile material. This material can be sterile disposable drapes, separately sterilized muslin towels, or the muslin towels that the surgical instruments are wrapped in before autoclaving to produce office-sterilized sterile instrument packs. Commercially prepared sterile instrument packs, usually with disposable paper wrappings, are also used to create a sterile field. Procedure 42-1 describes how to prepare a sterile field and how to open sterile packages.

When assembling the necessary supplies, place all unsterile items that may be used during the procedure outside the sterile field. Unsterile items include items that are sterile on the inside but not on the outside, such as a sterile gauze pack or sterile liquid such as alcohol, saline, or peroxide inside an unsterile bottle. Unsterile supplies should be arranged on a counter away from the sterile field. A typical arrangement of unsterile items used in surgery is shown in Figure 42-12. If you place an unsterile item within the sterile field, the field is no longer sterile, and you must repeat the entire process.

Adding Sterile Items to the Sterile Field. The outer 1 inch of the sterile field is considered contaminated. Therefore, before you add sterile items to the sterile field, carefully plan where you will place the instruments so that they are within the sterile field.

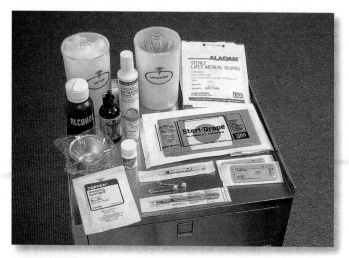

Figure 42-12. For each surgical procedure, unsterile surgical supplies must be gathered and arranged in an area separate from the sterile field.

Instruments and Supplies. If you have used sterile disposable drapes or separately sterilized muslin towels to create the sterile field, you will need to add the necessary instruments. Stand away from the sterile field, and open the sterile instrument pack in the manner described in Procedure 42-1. Place the pack on a counter or hold it open in your hand. Transfer and arrange the instruments on the sterile field with sterile transfer forceps (see Figure 42-11). Avoid reaching across the sterile field.

If you must add other items to the field, open them using the same method. Stand away from the sterile field. As you unwrap the item, gather the corners of the wrapping beneath it. You can place the contents on the sterile field by using sterile transfer forceps or by using the sterile inside of the wrapping to prevent your hands from touching the item. Place basins or bowls near the edge of the sterile field so you can pour liquids without reaching over the field.

Some instruments are sterilized individually in autoclave bags, and sterile supplies are often prepackaged. Stand away from the sterile field as you open an individual bag or package. You can pull the flaps of the packaging partway apart, then snap (remove from position by a sudden movement) the item onto the sterile field from a distance of 8 to 12 inches. Alternatively, you can use sterile forceps to grasp and place the items in the sterile field.

Pouring Sterile Solutions. Sterile solutions are often required during the surgical procedure to rinse or wash the wound. Sterile solutions can be added to the sterile field after the sterile instruments. Several sterile solutions are commonly used during minor surgical procedures. These include sterile water and physiological (normal) saline (0.9% sodium chloride).

Bottles of these sterile solutions come in a variety of sizes. You should choose the smallest size that will meet the solutions needed during the procedure. Using the smallest size possible minimizes the cost because unused solutions must be discarded.

When pouring a solution, cover the label on the bottle with the palm of your hand to keep the label dry. Pour a small amount of the liquid into a liquid waste receptacle to clean the lip of the bottle. As you pour the solution into a sterile bowl on the field, hold the bottle at an angle so that you do not reach over the sterile area (see Figure 42-10). Hold the bottle fairly close to the bowl without touching it. Pour the contents slowly to avoid splashing the drape, which would contaminate the field.

When a sterile solution bottle is opened and may be used again during the procedure, do not let any unsterile object touch the inside of its cap. To accomplish this, place the cap on a clean location in the same position it was in on the bottle (the sterile inside of the cap facing down).

Performing a Surgical Scrub and Donning Sterile Gloves. If you assist in a surgical procedure, you must perform a surgical scrub and wear sterile surgical gloves. You may wonder why a surgical scrub is necessary if you are planning to wear sterile gloves. The answer is that there is always the possibility that a glove may be punctured. If the skin is as clean as possible, the risk of contamination from a punctured glove is minimized. Nevertheless, if a glove is damaged during a sterile procedure, you must consider anything touched by that glove to be contaminated. Contaminated items must be resterilized or replaced before you continue.

A surgical scrub removes microorganisms more effectively than does routine hand washing. Routine hand washing removes bacteria present on the skin's surface, whereas the surgical scrub removes bacteria in deeper layers of the skin—where the hair follicles and oil-producing glands are. Procedure 42-2 describes the process.

Sterile gloves are required for many procedures. You don sterile gloves after you perform the surgical scrub. The process is described in Procedure 42-3.

Remember that once you are wearing sterile gloves, you may touch only the items in the sterile field. Therefore, you must remove any drape covering the sterile instrument tray before you glove. Sterile gloves provide a small margin of safety in preventing contamination. You must keep your movements controlled and precise to work within that margin to protect the sterile area.

Sanitizing, Disinfecting, and Sterilizing Equipment.

Many supplies used in a doctor's office are disposable. Most surgical instruments, however, are made of steel and are reusable. Preparing surgical instruments for reuse involves cleaning them with soap and water (a process called sanitization), then disinfecting and/or sterilizing them, depending on how the equipment will be used. (These procedures are described more fully in Chapter 20.)

Wearing gloves, first clean surgical instruments with soap and water to remove dirt and debris. Then rinse and dry them. After you have sanitized the instruments, disinfect them. If you cannot wash surgical instruments immediately after use, place them directly in disinfectant.

The most common disinfecting agents are chemicals and boiling water. Remember that disinfection kills many microorganisms but does not kill bacterial spores and some viruses. For this reason instruments used in surgical procedures are always sterilized. It is also common to sterilize surgical instruments, even when they will be used in nonsurgical procedures, to reduce the possibility of infection.

Autoclaving is the most common method of sterilization. The autoclave kills microorganisms and spores by means of steam under pressure. The dry heat oven provides another method of sterilization. This technique is preferred for sterilizing sharp instruments, because the moist heat in the autoclave may damage cutting edges.

The Chemiclave is another type of sterilization equipment. It uses alcohol under pressure rather than steam. Cold sterilization methods involve lengthy periods of soaking in sterilizing chemicals. Gas sterilization with ethylene oxide is sometimes used for equipment that might be damaged by heat or moisture. The drawback with ethylene oxide gas is that it is highly toxic to humans and the environment. Because of this potential danger, gas sterilization is generally used only in hospital and manufacturing environments.

Preoperative Procedures

You must complete a number of steps before a surgical procedure. The steps include performing various preliminary duties, preparing the surgical room, and physically preparing the patient for surgery.

Preliminary Duties

You will perform several preliminary tasks before the surgery. They include providing **preoperative** (prior to surgery or "preop") instructions to the patient, completing various administrative tasks, and easing the patient's fears.

Preoperative Instructions. When a patient is scheduled for a minor surgical procedure in the doctor's office, you must explain the preoperative instructions. You should also be prepared to answer the patient's questions about the procedure and about possible risks. The patient may ask you, rather than the doctor, such questions or may need clarification of information provided by the doctor.

A patient may need to follow certain dietary and fluid restrictions before a minor surgical procedure. Not eating or drinking for a specific period of time is a common restriction. There may also be restrictions on what medications a patient may take, because of the administration of an anesthetic during the procedure. You will need to tell non-English-speaking patients to bring along a family member or other interpreter who can help them understand the forms they must sign and their instructions.

You should instruct the patient to wear either comfortable, loose-fitting clothes that will not interfere with the procedure or clothing that can be removed easily. In most cases patients also need to arrange for someone to drive them home after a procedure.

Administrative and Legal Tasks. You must ensure that all the necessary paperwork is completed before surgery. Routine administrative tasks include completing the required insurance forms and obtaining prior authorization from the patient's insurance company.

Make absolutely certain that the patient reads, understands, and signs the surgical consent form. The patient needs a clear understanding of what to expect during and after the surgery to give informed consent as required by law. Sometimes surgery is performed on a child or a patient with limited understanding of legal documents. In such cases the consent form must be signed by the patient's parent or legal guardian.

Failure to obtain the necessary paperwork prior to a surgical procedure can cause serious legal problems. The doctor and other staff members could be held legally liable if problems were to develop during or after the procedure.

PROCEDURE 42.2

Performing a Surgical Scrub

Objective: To remove dirt and microorganisms from under the fingernails and from the surface of the skin, hair follicles, and oil glands of the hands and forearms

OSHA Guidelines: This procedure does not involve exposure to blood, body fluids, or tissues.

Materials: Dispenser with surgical soap, sterile surgical scrub brush, orange stick, sterile towels

Method

1. Remove all jewelry and roll up your sleeves to above the elbow.

2. Assemble the necessary materials.

3. Turn the water on and adjust it so that it is warm.

4. Wet your hands from the fingertips to the elbows. You must keep your hands higher than your elbows to prevent water from running down your arms and contaminating the washed area.

5. Apply surgical soap, and for 2 minutes scrub your hands, fingers, areas between the fingers, wrists, and forearms with the scrub brush, using a firm circular motion (Figure 42-13).

6. Rinse from fingers to elbows, always keeping your hands higher than your elbows (Figure 42-14).

7. Use the orange stick to clean under your fingernails, and rinse your hands again.

8. Apply more surgical soap, and again use the brush to completely scrub your hands, fingers, areas between the fingers, wrists, and forearms. Scrub for at least 3 minutes, and then rinse from fingers to elbows again.

9. Thoroughly dry your hands and forearms with sterile towels, working from the hands to the elbows (Figure 42-15).

10. Turn off the faucet with the foot or knee pedal. Use a clean paper towel if a foot or knee pedal is not used.

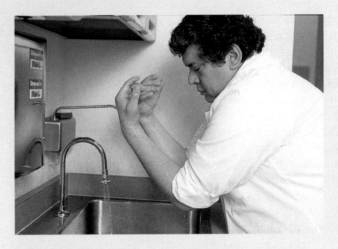

Figure 42-14. Keep your hands above your elbows while rinsing from fingertips to elbows.

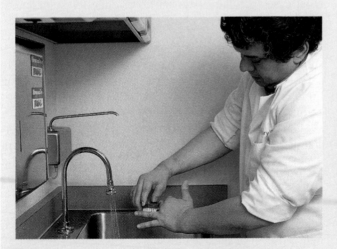

Figure 42-13. Use the scrub brush to work the surgical soap into your fingers, then your wrists, and then your forearms with a firm, circular motion.

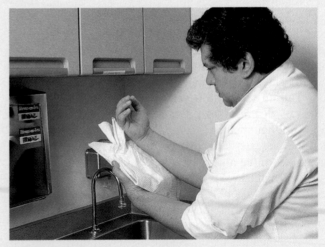

Figure 42-15. Dry your hands thoroughly before carefully drying your forearms.

PROCEDURE 42.3

Donning Sterile Gloves

Objective: To don sterile gloves without compromising the sterility of the outer surface of the gloves

OSHA Guidelines: This procedure does not involve exposure to blood, body fluids, or tissues.

Materials: Correctly sized, prepackaged, double-wrapped sterile gloves

Method

1. Obtain the correct size gloves.
2. Check the package for tears, and ensure that the expiration date has not passed.
3. Perform a surgical scrub.
4. Peel the outer wrap from gloves and place the inner wrapper on a clean surface above waist level (Figure 42-16).
5. Position gloves so the cuff end is closest to your body.
6. Touch only the flaps as you open the package.
7. Use instructions provided on inner package, if available.
8. Do not reach over the sterile inside of the inner package.
9. Follow these steps if there are no instructions:
   a. Open the package so the first flap is opened away from you.
   b. Pinch the corner and pull to one side.
   c. Put your fingertips under the side flaps and gently pull until the package is completely open.
10. Use your nondominant hand to grasp the inside cuff of the opposite glove (the folded edge). Do not touch the outside of the glove. If you are right-handed, use your left hand to put on the right glove first, and vice versa.
11. Holding the glove at arm's length and waist level, insert the dominant hand into the glove with the palm facing up. Don't let the outside of the glove touch any other surface (Figure 42-17).
12. With your sterile gloved hand, slip the gloved fingers into the cuff of the other glove.
13. Pick up the other glove, touching only the outside. Don't touch any other surfaces (Figure 42-18).
14. Pull the glove up and onto your hand. Ensure that the sterile gloved hand does not touch skin (Figure 42-19).
15. Adjust your fingers as necessary, touching only glove to glove.
16. Do not adjust the cuffs because your forearms may contaminate the gloves.
17. Keep your hands in front of you, between your shoulders and waist. If you move your hands out of this area, they are considered contaminated.

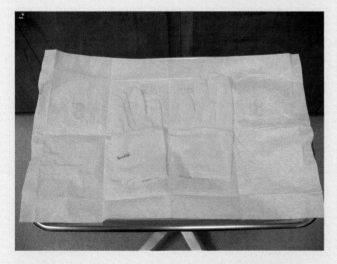

Figure 42-16. You must put these sterile gloves on without reaching across the sterile surfaces of the gloves or the sterile inner wrap of the pack.

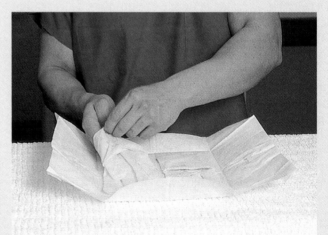

Figure 42-17. Your palm should face up as you slide your dominant hand into the first glove.

continued ⟶

Donning Sterile Gloves *(continued)*

18. If contamination or the possibility of contamination occurs, change gloves.

19. Remove gloves the same way you remove clean gloves, by touching only the inside.

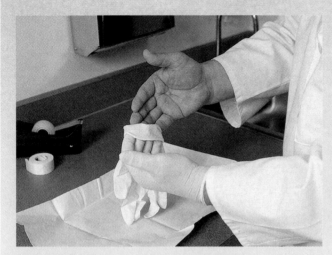

Figure 42-18. Your gloved fingers secure the remaining glove while you slip it over your nondominant hand.

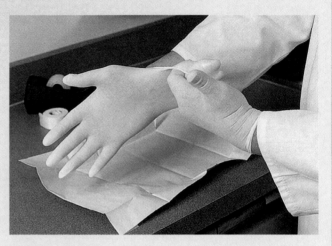

Figure 42-19. Unfold the cuff over your arm while touching only the sterile surface of the glove.

It is common practice to call the patient the day before the surgery to confirm the appointment. This call also provides a chance to ensure that the patient follows the preoperative instructions. You may be responsible for making this call.

Easing the Patient's Fears. Knowing what to expect during and after a surgical procedure will ease patients' fears. This information allows them to plan their daily activities and, if necessary, to arrange for help at home during the recovery period.

Some offices may have educational materials such as brochures, fact sheets, or videotapes about the procedure the patient will undergo. The availability of such materials varies with the practice specialty and the frequency with which the procedure is performed. You may assist in preparing or acquiring these materials if your office's policy includes such participation for medical assistants. This type of information is extremely helpful to the patient. It may increase patient compliance with the pre- and post-operative instructions.

Much of a patient's fear about a surgical procedure can be overcome if you spend sufficient time before the procedure explaining what to expect. Be prepared to answer the patient's questions honestly, calmly, and confidently. Your calm and knowledgeable manner will reassure the patient. If the answer to a question requires experience or knowledge beyond your own, pass the question on to the doctor.

Preparing the Surgical Room

Prior to surgery the doctor should inform you of specific instructions concerning patient preparation. He will also tell you what special equipment or supplies are necessary for the procedure.

Because patients are likely to feel anxious before a procedure, it is best to have everything ready in the surgical room before you escort the patient into the room. Make sure the room is clean, neat, and free of waste from previous procedures. The examining table should have been cleaned and disinfected, and surface barriers (table paper and pillow covers) should have been changed.

Check to see that there is adequate lighting. Make sure that all equipment and supplies necessary for the procedure are available. Check the date and sterilization indicator on sterilized packs and supplies. Sterile packs are typically considered unsterile if more than 1 month has passed since they were originally sterilized.

You will then wash your hands, put on examination gloves, and prepare the sterile field as outlined in Procedure 42-1. The sterile field and the instruments should be draped with a sterile towel.

Preparing the Patient

Just before the surgery, various concerns must be addressed and procedures completed in sequence. The initial tasks are followed by gowning and positioning the patient and preparing the patient's skin for surgery.

Initial Tasks. Before leading the patient into the surgical room, find out whether he has followed the presurgical instructions. Restrictions on food and fluid intake are of particular concern. It is also important to ask what medications the patient is taking and whether he has taken that day's dosage.

Measure the patient's vital signs. Ask if there are any symptoms or problems the doctor should know about before the surgery. If any unusual signs or symptoms are present, notify the doctor. The doctor will want to examine the patient before proceeding.

Check the chart for medication orders, such as pain medication or a tranquilizer to calm the patient. Medications should be administered at this time so that they will take effect before surgery.

Gowning and Positioning the Patient. Some procedures require the patient to disrobe and put on a gown to expose the surgical site. If this is the case, you should offer to assist, if appropriate, or leave the room while the patient changes. You should then help the patient onto the table and into the position required for the procedure. You may use one or more small pillows to make the patient as comfortable as possible. Then adequately drape the patient to retain body heat and preserve personal dignity.

Sterile drapes are also used to create a sterile field on a patient's body around the surgical site. Drapes come in a variety of sizes and styles. A fenestrated drape has a round or slitlike opening cut out in the center to provide access to the surgical site.

Surgical Skin Preparation. Proper preparation of the patient's skin before surgery reduces the number of microorganisms and the risk of infection. The prepared area should extend 2 inches beyond the surgical field—the area exposed in the center of the fenestrated drape. This extra margin allows for draping without contaminating the field.

Cleaning the Area. Before proceeding with the surgical skin preparation, wash your hands and put on examination gloves. Place a plastic-backed drape under the surgical site to absorb any liquids. Clean the site first with antiseptic soap and sterile water, using forceps and gauze sponges dipped in the solution. Begin at the center of the surgical site, and work outward in a firm, circular motion (Figure 42-20). Discard the gauze sponge after each complete pass. Clean in concentric circles until you cover the full preparation area. Continue the process, repeating as necessary, for at least 2 minutes or the amount of time specified in the office's procedure manual. Cleaning takes more time if a wound is dirty or contains foreign materials. When procedures are performed on a hand or foot, clean the entire hand or foot.

Shaving the Area. Depending on office policy, you may be required to shave the surgical site to remove hair. Shaving often causes many small wounds on the skin, however, and may increase the risk of infection. Because of this fact some experts feel that hair should not be removed unless it

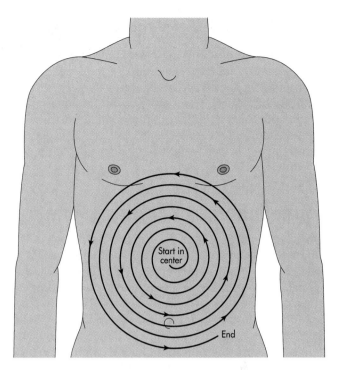

Figure 42-20. Use concentric circles to clean the surgical site and apply antiseptic solution.
From Medical Assisting, Administrative & Clinical Competencies 4th edition by KEIR/WISE/KREBS. © 1998. Reprinted with permission of Delmar Learning, a division of Thomson Learning: www. thomsonrights.com. Fax 800-730-2215.

is thick enough to interfere with surgery. Alternatively, hair may be trimmed with scissors or smoothed out of the way.

When shaving is indicated, use a disposable razor and soap for lubrication. Shave in the direction in which the hair grows, and include the same area you cleaned beforehand. When you finish, rinse the area with sterile water and allow it to air-dry. You may also pat the area dry with sterile gauze, starting at the surgical site and moving outward in a circular motion.

Applying the Antiseptic. Next apply antiseptic solution to the area. Antiseptics are agents that are applied to the skin to limit the growth of microorganisms and to help prevent infection. Povidone iodine (Betadine) is most commonly used, but chlorhexidine gluconate (Hibiclens) or benzalkonium chloride (Zephiran Chloride) may also be used, particularly if the patient is allergic to iodine. Swab an area 2 inches larger than the surgical field with the antiseptic solution in a circular outward motion, starting at the surgical site. This is the same motion that is used for cleaning the surgical site. For surgery on a hand or foot, swab the entire hand or foot. Allow the antiseptic to air-dry; do not pat it dry—that would remove some of the solution's antiseptic properties.

When the area is dry, treat it as a sterile field. Instruct the patient not to touch the area. Cover the area with a sterile fenestrated drape, from front to back. Avoid reaching over the field.

At this point notify the physician that the patient is ready. Then prepare yourself to assist with the surgery.

Intraoperative Procedures

Intraoperative procedures are procedures that take place during surgery. You may be asked to perform a wide variety of unsterile and sterile tasks during surgery, such as preparing local anesthetic for the doctor, monitoring the patient, processing specimens, and handing instruments to the doctor. The doctor may also ask you to explain to the patient step by step what will be done next during the procedure.

Administering a Local Anesthetic

Before beginning the surgical procedure, the physician will administer a local anesthetic. Some local anesthetics are injected. An injected anesthetic is packaged in a sterile **vial** (a small glass bottle with a self-sealing rubber stopper). Other local anesthetics come in a cream, gel, or spray form. These anesthetics are **topical** (applied directly to the skin) and affect only the area to which they are applied.

Lidocaine (Xylocaine) is the most commonly used anesthetic. It is often used as a topical gel anesthetic. Tetracaine hydrochloride (Pontocaine), a long-acting anesthetic, is injected.

The physician administers the local anesthetic by injection or by applying it directly to the skin. The choice of administration methods depends on how invasive or painful the procedure is likely to be.

Topical Application. Anesthetic gels, creams, and sprays may be used topically in certain surgical procedures. A topical anesthetic is useful when the pain will be mild or when only the upper layers of the skin are affected. It is common to use such agents to anesthetize the area of a small laceration prior to suturing. Sometimes an anesthetic cream is applied before a local anesthetic is injected. This application reduces or eliminates the pain caused by the injection. A topical anesthetic must usually remain on the skin for 10 to 15 minutes for the area to become sufficiently anesthetized.

Injections. If a local anesthetic is to be injected, it is typically administered after the skin is prepared but before the patient is draped. In some cases, however, the anesthetic is injected prior to skin preparation to allow time for it to take effect. In either case it is important to note the time of anesthetic administration in the patient's chart.

If the doctor is already wearing sterile gloves, you may be asked to assist in administering the anesthetic. Administering anesthetic is an unsterile task because the outside of the vial is unsterile. When performing this task, follow proper procedure to protect the sterility of the doctor's gloves and the anesthetic solution.

First check the label of the anesthetic vial three times to confirm that it is the correct solution. Clean the vial's rubber stopper with 70% isopropyl alcohol, and leave the cotton or gauze on top of the stopper. Present the requested needle and syringe to the doctor by peeling half

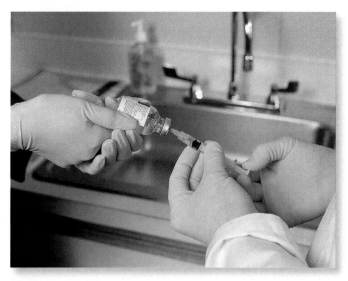

Figure 42-21. You must hold the anesthetic vial firmly to allow the physician to puncture the rubber stopper with the needle.

the outer wrapper away and allowing the doctor to remove them from the wrapper.

Remove the cotton or gauze from the rubber stopper, and hold the vial so the doctor can verify that it is the proper medication. Turn the vial upside down, and hold it securely around the base, without touching the sterile stopper. Be sure to hold the vial in front of you at shoulder height. Because significant force will be necessary to push the needle through the rubber stopper, you should brace the wrist of the hand holding the vial with your free hand. Hold the vial firmly so the doctor can withdraw the anesthetic from it (Figure 42-21).

Potential Side Effects of the Anesthetic. You should inform the patient of possible reactions to the anesthetic medication. Although rare, reactions may include dizziness, loss of consciousness, seizures, or cardiac arrest. Adverse reactions can occur if the anesthetic dose is too high or if it is absorbed too quickly. They can also occur if the patient is taking other medications that should not be mixed with the anesthetic. It is vital to document all medications (including over-the-counter ones) that the patient is taking at the time of the surgery.

Use of Epinephrine. Epinephrine is a sterile solution that is sometimes injected along with an anesthetic. Epinephrine constricts the blood vessels, making them narrower. This constriction reduces bleeding and prolongs the action of the local anesthetic. Epinephrine is used if the site of surgery is an area with many small blood vessels that are expected to bleed profusely (such as the head). Reducing bleeding makes it easier to see and to repair the wound. (Epinephrine should be used with caution, however, in patients with heart disease or respiratory disease.)

When epinephrine is combined with the anesthetic to reduce bleeding, it prolongs the anesthesia because epinephrine slows the rate at which anesthetic spreads into the tissue. This effect may or may not be desirable. Epinephrine should not be used in areas such as the fingers, toes, nose, or ears, where it could also compromise the local blood supply. There is some concern that epinephrine may increase wound infection rates.

Assisting the Physician During Surgery

Your role in surgical assisting depends on the type of surgery and the physician's preference. You may assist the physician in one of two capacities. You may serve as a **floater,** an unsterile assistant who is free to move about the room and attend to unsterile needs. Alternatively, you may serve as a **sterile scrub assistant,** who assists in handling sterile equipment during the procedure. The duties are different for the two functions. Procedure 42-4 outlines the tasks performed by both sterile and unsterile assistants.

The Floater. First the surgical room is set up and the patient is prepared. If you are assisting as a floater (sometimes called a circulator), you will perform a routine scrub and put on examination gloves. Remember that you cannot touch sterile items in the sterile field because you have not performed a surgical scrub and are not wearing sterile gloves.

Monitoring and Recording. One of the most important duties of a floater is to monitor the patient during the procedure. You must measure vital signs regularly and observe the patient for reactions to the anesthetic. Record all observations in the patient's chart. Also write down any information or notes the doctor requests. You must keep a record of time, including when the anesthetic is administered, when the procedure begins, and when the procedure is completed.

Processing Specimens. When you serve as a floater during surgery, the doctor may ask you to receive and process specimens for laboratory examination. Most tissues are placed in a 10% formalin solution to preserve them before they are sent to the laboratory. Half-fill the specimen container with the formalin solution ahead of time. Remove the lid of the specimen container without touching the rim. Hold the container out toward the doctor so she can place the tissue directly into it without contaminating the sample (Figure 42-22).

The container should be labeled with the following information:

- The patient's name and the doctor's name
- The date and time of collection
- The body site from which the specimen was obtained
- Your initials

If more than one specimen is obtained from a patient, place each specimen in a separate container. Label each container with the necessary information, along with a number to indicate the order in which the specimens are

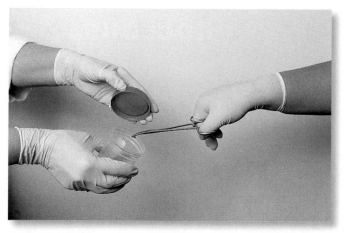

Figure 42-22. Be sure to hold the specimen container so that the doctor can place the tissue in it without touching the rim or the outside of the container with the tissue.

obtained (no. 1, no. 2, and so on). You will also fill out a laboratory requisition slip to send along with the specimen(s). Specimen containers should be red in color or labeled with the biohazard symbol. Specimen containers should be placed in specially designed bags for transport.

Other Duties. As a floater you may also be asked to perform a number of other duties, including these:

- Assisting with the injection of additional anesthetic
- Adding additional sterile items to the sterile tray
- Pouring sterile solutions
- Keeping the surgical area clean and neat during the procedure
- Repositioning the patient as necessary
- Adjusting lighting

The Sterile Scrub Assistant. When you serve as a sterile scrub assistant, you perform a surgical scrub and wear sterile gloves. You may be asked to perform a variety of tasks under sterile conditions. Remember not to touch unsterile items after putting on sterile gloves.

Handling Instruments. Your first duty as a sterile scrub assistant is, typically, to close the instruments on the sterile tray because they are normally left in the open position during sterilization. Your next duty is to rearrange the instruments on the tray. Instruments should be arranged in the order in which they will be used or according to the doctor's preference. Instruments are generally used in the following sequence:

- Cutting instruments
- Grasping instruments
- Retractors
- Probes
- Suture materials
- Needle holders and scissors

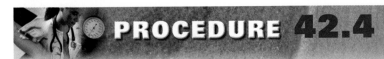

PROCEDURE 42.4

General Assisting Procedures for Minor Surgery

Objective: To provide assistance to the doctor during minor surgery while maintaining clean or sterile technique as appropriate

OSHA Guidelines

Materials: Sterile towel, tray or Mayo stand, appropriate instrument pack(s), needles and syringes, anesthetic, antiseptic, sterile water or normal saline, small sterile bowl, sterile gauze squares or cotton balls, specimen containers half-filled with preservative, suture materials, sterile dressings and tape

Method

Floater (Unsterile Assistant)

1. Perform routine hand washing and put on examination gloves.
2. Monitor the patient during the procedure; record the results in the patient's chart.
3. During the surgery assist as needed.
4. Add sterile items to the tray as necessary.
5. Pour sterile solution into a sterile bowl as needed.
6. Assist in administering additional anesthetic.
   a. Check the medication vial three times.
   b. Clean the rubber stopper with alcohol (write the date opened when using a new bottle); leave cotton or gauze on top.
   c. Present the needle and syringe to the doctor.
   d. Remove the cotton or gauze from the vial, and show the label to the doctor.
   e. Hold the vial upside down, and grasp the lower edge firmly; brace your wrist with your free hand. (This firmly supports the vial to

sustain the force of the needle being inserted into the rubber stopper.)
   f. Allow the doctor to fill the syringe.
7. Receive specimens for laboratory examination.
   a. Uncap the specimen container; present it to the doctor for the introduction of the specimen.
   b. Replace the cap and label the container.
   c. Treat all specimens as infectious.
   d. Place the specimen container in a transport bag or other container.
   e. Complete the requisition form to send the specimen to the laboratory.

Sterile Scrub Assistant

1. Perform a surgical scrub and put on sterile gloves. (Remember to remove the sterile towel covering the sterile field and instruments before gloving.)
2. Close and arrange the surgical instruments on the tray.
3. Prepare for swabbing by inserting gauze squares into the sterile dressing forceps.
4. Pass the instruments as necessary.
5. Swab the wound as requested.
6. Retract the wound as requested.
7. Cut the sutures as requested.

Floater or Sterile Scrub Assistant (After Surgery)

1. Monitor the patient.
2. Put on clean examination gloves, and clean the wound with antiseptic.
3. Dress the wound.
4. Remove the gloves and wash your hands.
5. Give the patient oral postoperative instructions in addition to the release packet.
6. Discharge the patient.
7. Put on clean examination gloves.
8. Properly dispose of used materials and disposable instruments.
9. Sanitize reusable instruments and prepare them for disinfection and/or sterilization as needed.
10. Clean equipment and the examination room according to OSHA guidelines.
11. Remove the gloves and wash your hands.

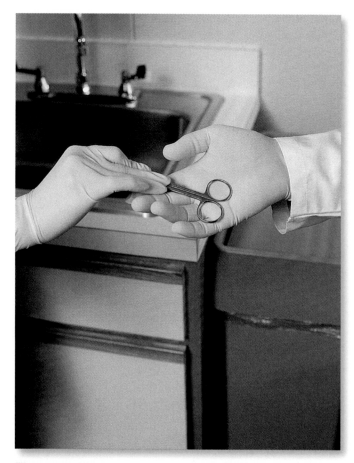

Figure 42-23. Holding the scissors by the hinge, slap the handles into the doctor's hand.

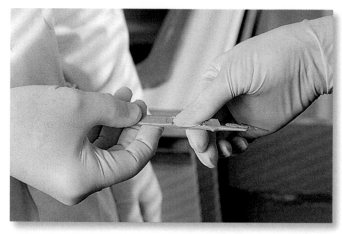

Figure 42-24. Hold a scalpel above and just behind the cutting edge as you pass the handle into the palm of the doctor's hand.

Prepare for swabbing by placing several sterile gauze squares in the dressing forceps. They will then be ready when needed. As the sterile scrub assistant, you will be asked to pass instruments to the doctor during the procedure. You must hold instruments so that the doctor can grasp them securely and will not need to reposition them in her hands. At the same time, the instruments must be handled properly to maintain their sterility.

When passing scissors and clamps, hold them by the hinge (Figure 42-23). You will have a clear view of the tip of the instrument, and the doctor will have full use of the handles. Firmly slap the instrument handles into the doctor's extended palm. The doctor's hand will close around the handles as a reflex action to the slapping. This technique reduces the risk of dropping an instrument. If the scissors or clamp is curved, the curve should follow the same curve as the doctor's hand.

When passing a scalpel, hold it above and just behind the cutting edge of the blade so the doctor can grasp the entire handle (Figure 42-24). Pass a needle holder with suture material so that the needle is pointing up, and hold the end of the suture material with your other hand to prevent the material from becoming tangled in the handles.

Other Duties. As a sterile scrub assistant, you may also be asked to swab fluids from a wound or to retract the edges of a wound to help the doctor view the area. While the doctor is closing the wound, you may be required to cut the suture material after each stitch. The doctor may not verbalize every request to you. With practice and after experience with a particular doctor, you will learn how to respond to the doctor's actions.

When cutting suture materials, leave ⅛ inch of the material above the knot. This excess material prevents the suture from coming untied. It also leaves the material short enough so that it does not bother the patient.

Postoperative Procedures

You will be responsible for the patient's **postoperative** ("postop") follow-up after the surgical procedure. Your duties may include immediate care of the patient, proper cleaning of the surgical room, and follow-up care of the patient.

Immediate Patient Care

Patient care is your top priority as a medical assistant. Except for intravenous medications, you will administer postoperative medications that the physician requests for the patient. You will also ensure that the patient remains lying down on the examining table for the prescribed length of time after the procedure. During this period continue to monitor the patient's vital signs, and watch for adverse reactions. It is important to document your observations in the patient's chart.

Dressing the Wound. You may also dress the wound during the monitoring period. **Dressings** are sterile materials used to cover an incision. They serve a number of functions. They protect the wound from further injury and keep the wound clean, thus preventing infection. Dressings also reduce bleeding, absorb fluid drainage, reduce discomfort to the patient, speed healing, and reduce the possibility of scarring. Gauze dressings are the most common type of dressings and come in a variety of sizes and shapes.

Before dressing the wound, put on clean examination gloves. Clean the site with povidone iodine (Betadine), and allow it to dry. If ordered by the physician, apply antibiotic ointment over the wound. Place the sterile dressing over the site, and secure it appropriately.

Bandaging the Wound. It may be necessary to apply a bandage (a clean strip of gauze or elastic material) over the dressing to help hold it in place. Bandages may also be used to improve circulation, to provide support or reduce tension on a wound or suture and prevent it from reopening, or to prevent movement of that area of the body. Adhesive tape may also be used for these purposes. Some patients are allergic to the adhesive, but most tapes are now hypoallergenic. The patient is usually more comfortable after a bandage or adhesive tape has been applied.

Postoperative Instructions. After the procedure, provide oral postoperative instructions to the patient. You may do this during the monitoring part of the postoperative period or afterward. These instructions include guidelines for pain management and instructions for wound care. Postoperative information also includes dietary or activity restrictions, if any, and when to come in for a follow-up appointment. It is a good idea to ask patients to repeat what you say so that you know they understand the information.

Instructions are often also provided in writing and may be part of a complete postoperative information packet. You may be asked to help prepare or update packet materials, especially if you routinely assist patients as they recover from minor surgery. A postoperative information packet might include the following information:

- Proper wound-care instructions
- Suggestions for pain relief and reduction of swelling, such as medications and hot or cold packs
- Dietary restrictions
- Activity restrictions
- Timing for a follow-up appointment or an appointment card

Wound-care instructions include details on dressing changes, which will vary depending on the depth and size of the wound. Generally a patient should clean the wound daily with soap and water or dilute hydrogen peroxide (3%) and allow it to air-dry. The patient should then apply an antibiotic cream and place a dry, sterile dressing over the wound. Except when cleansing the wound, the patient should keep it dry. The dressing should be replaced if it gets wet. Although cleansing aids wound healing, a wet dressing provides bacteria and other contaminants with access to the wound.

Descriptions, and often illustrations, of normal and infected incisions are an important part of wound-care instructions. The patient should call the physician if any signs of infection are noted. The instructions should also encourage the patient to protect the incision from exposure to the sun. This guideline is advisable for as long as 3 to 6 months to prevent the incision line from becoming darker than surrounding skin.

The length of time it takes for a wound to heal varies with the site, the patient's age, and the severity of the wound. Each patient therefore needs specific instructions on how long to continue with the dressings and when to return for suture or staple removal.

Patient Release. Notify the doctor when the patient is stabilized and ready to leave. The doctor may want to further observe and instruct the patient. Be sure to offer assistance if the patient needs help getting dressed.

Then help the patient check out. Schedule the next appointment for the patient. Make sure the patient has the correct discharge packet. Confirm arrangements to transport the patient home. Finally, assist the patient to the car or other transport if this is part of office procedure.

If a patient insists on driving himself home, enter this information on the chart. Indicate the time and have the patient initial the entry. This documentation is important for legal reasons. It would clarify liability should an accident occur as a result of a reaction to the surgery or the anesthetic.

Surgical Room Cleanup

If there is time during the monitoring period, begin to clean up the surgical area. If time is not available then, perform the cleanup routine after the patient has been released.

Until the reusable instruments can be cleaned, place them in a disinfectant soak that has anticoagulant properties. A reusable sharps container is generally used for this purpose for surgical instruments. Place disposable waste in the sharps or biohazardous waste container. Clean the counters, examining table, and trays according to OSHA guidelines by disinfecting them. A 10% chlorine bleach solution, which is one part household bleach to nine parts water, is commonly used. Disinfect small pieces of nonsurgical equipment (stethoscopes, thermometers, and so on) with 70% isopropyl alcohol. Replace paper table and pillow covers at this time, along with necessary supplies.

Follow-Up Care

During a follow-up appointment the physician examines the patient's surgical wound. You may be asked to change the dressing or remove the wound closures.

Typically, suture or staple removal takes place 5 to 10 days after minor surgery. The sutures or staples are ready for removal when a clean, unbroken suture line is observed. There should be no scabs, no seepage from the wound, and no visible opening. Any of these signs may indicate unhealed areas. Suture removal is described in Procedure 42-5. Staple removal is similar, except that staple removal forceps, rather than forceps and scissors, are used to remove the staples.

PROCEDURE 42.5

Suture Removal

Objective: To remove sutures from a healing wound while maintaining sterile technique and protecting the integrity of the closed wound

OSHA Guidelines

Materials: Tray or Mayo stand, suture removal pack (suture scissors and thumb forceps), sterile towel, antiseptic solution, hydrogen peroxide (3%), two small sterile bowls, sterile gauze squares, sterile strips or butterfly closures, sterile dressings and tape

Method

1. Clean and disinfect the tray or Mayo stand.
2. Wash your hands and assemble the necessary materials.
3. Check the date and sterilization indicator on the suture removal pack.
4. Unwrap the suture removal pack, and place it on the tray or stand to create a sterile field.
5. Unwrap the sterile bowls and add them to the sterile field.
6. Pour a small amount of antiseptic solution into one bowl, and pour a small amount of hydrogen peroxide into the other bowl.
7. Cover the tray with a sterile towel to protect the sterile field while you are out of the room.
8. Escort the patient to the examination room and explain the procedure.
9. Perform a routine scrub, remove the towel from the tray, and put on examination gloves.
10. Remove the old dressing.
    a. Lift the tape toward the middle of the dressing to avoid pulling on the wound.
    b. If the dressing adheres to the wound, cover the dressing with gauze squares soaked in hydrogen peroxide. Leave the wet gauze in place for several seconds to loosen the dressing.

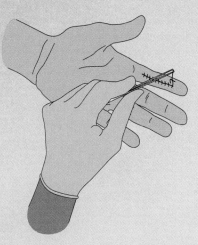

Figure 42-25. Without pulling on the wound, lift the suture knot away from the skin to make room for the suture scissors.

    c. Save the old dressing for the doctor to inspect.
11. Inspect the wound for signs of infection.
12. Clean the wound with gauze pads soaked in antiseptic, and pat it dry with clean gauze pads.
13. Remove the gloves and wash your hands.
14. Notify the doctor that the wound is ready for examination.
15. Once the doctor indicates that the wound is sufficiently healed to proceed, put on clean examination gloves.
16. Place a square of gauze next to the wound for collecting the sutures as they are removed.
17. Grasp the first suture knot with forceps.
18. Gently lift the knot away from the skin to allow room for the suture scissors (Figure 42-25).
19. Slide the suture scissors under the suture material, and cut the suture where it enters the skin (Figure 42-26).
20. Gently lift the knot up and toward the wound to remove the suture without opening the wound (Figure 42-27).
21. Place the suture on the gauze pad, and inspect to ensure that the entire suture is present.
22. Repeat the removal process until all sutures have been removed.

continued ⟶

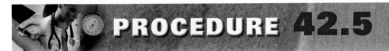
Suture Removal *(continued)*

23. Count the sutures and compare the number with the number indicated in the patient's record (Figure 42-28).

24. Clean the wound with antiseptic, and allow the wound to air-dry.

25. Dress the wound as ordered, or notify the doctor if the sterile strips or butterfly closures are to be applied.

26. Observe the patient for signs of distress, such as wincing or grimacing.

27. Properly dispose of used materials and disposable instruments.

28. Remove the gloves and wash your hands.

29. Instruct the patient on wound care.

30. In the patient's chart, record pertinent information, such as the condition of the wound and the type of closures used, if any.

31. Escort the patient to the checkout area.

32. Put on clean gloves.

33. Sanitize resuable instruments and prepare them for disinfection and/or sterilization as needed.

34. Clean the equipment and examination room according to OSHA guidelines.

35. Remove the gloves and wash your hands.

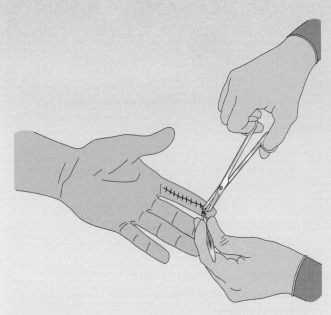

Figure 42-26. Cut the suture material as close as possible to its entry point in the skin.

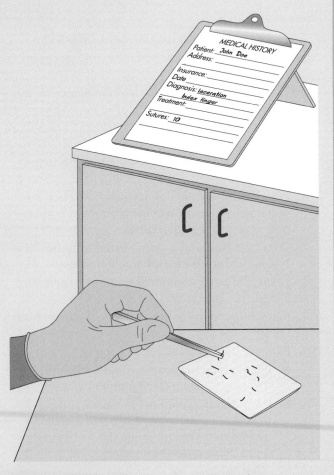

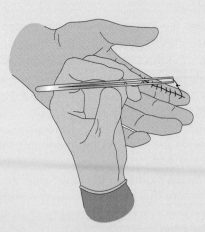

Figure 42-27. Remove the suture by lifting the knot up and toward the wound.

Figure 42-28. Compare the number of sutures removed with the recorded number of sutures placed.

Summary

As the doctor's assistant in minor surgical procedures, you perform many functions. Your responsibilities during the patient's preoperative and postoperative care, however, are just as important.

Before surgery you provide the patient with preoperative instructions, make sure the necessary administrative and legal forms are completed, help prepare the patient emotionally, and set up the surgical room. You then confirm that the patient has followed all preoperative instructions and physically prepare the patient for surgery.

During the procedure you follow proper medical and surgical aseptic techniques. Your actual responsibilities vary with the role you play as a floater or a sterile scrub assistant for a particular surgery. At all times you ensure the safety and comfort of the patient and are knowledgeable enough to function as the doctor's "right hand" during the procedure.

After the surgery you provide the postoperative patient with care and instruction that will help ensure prompt healing. Then you clean the surgical room and prepare it for the next procedure.

REVIEW

CHAPTER 42

CASE STUDY QUESTIONS

Now that you have completed this chapter, review the case study at the beginning of the chapter and answer the following questions:

1. How could you reduce the patient's apprehension?
2. What would you say to her before the physician arrives to perform the minor surgery?

Discussion Questions

1. Explain the stages of wound healing and the benefit of approximation.
2. List five different categories of surgical instruments by function, give an example of each, and describe how instruments in each category are used.
3. List three minor surgical procedures you may assist with in the doctor's office. Name one procedure you may perform on your own.

Critical Thinking Questions

1. What might you say to ease the fears of an anxious patient who is about to undergo a laceration repair?
2. Explain the procedure you would follow if you were functioning as a sterile scrub assistant and your glove was punctured while you were handling instruments during a surgical procedure.
3. Explain how to make sure that a patient has understood the postoperative instructions for wound care.
4. A patient arrives at the clinic with a laceration to the left thumb that occurred while she was washing dishes. She is holding a bloody paper towel on the thumb. She states, "I cannot take this towel off—the blood will gush right out of the cut. It just would not stop bleeding." What should you do?
5. A patient will need to have a minor surgical procedure done next week at your clinic. What administrative tasks must you perform before the procedure?

Application Activities

1. Using instrument flash cards or actual instruments, choose and list the types of instruments you would need during a procedure to clean and repair a laceration.
2. Working with one or two classmates, practice opening a sterile pack and creating a sterile field. Practice adding additional instruments and a sterile bowl to the sterile field. Offer suggestions to each other for improving your techniques.
3. With a partner, practice handing surgical instruments to each other. The receiver should look the other way while receiving the instrument. This approach simulates actual conditions in which the doctor may be concentrating on a procedure rather than looking at the instrument. This approach also tests the ability of the person handing the instrument to use proper technique.
4. With a partner, practice preparing a site for surgery. Obtain the necessary equipment to clean the site, apply antiseptic, and drape. Follow the procedure steps carefully, paying close attention to your cleaning technique. Be certain to use concentric circles. Practice various surgical sites, and evaluate each other's technique. Note: You may choose not to use actual soap and antiseptic for practice in order to avoid irritation.

Internet Activities

Use the Internet to learn more about surgical instruments and to create your own personal flash cards. Use picture search engines such as **www.google.com** and **www.ixquick.com** to search for pictures of various instruments used in different procedures. Once you find a picture you would like to print, right-click on it and save it in a folder for later printing.

CHAPTER 43

Assisting With Cold and Heat Therapy and Ambulation

AREAS OF COMPETENCE

2003 Role Delineation Study

ADMINISTRATIVE

Administrative Procedures
- Schedule, coordinate, and monitor appointments
- Schedule inpatient/outpatient admissions and procedures

CLINICAL

Fundamental Principles
- Screen and follow up patient test results

GENERAL

Professionalism
- Work as a member of the health-care team

Communication Skills
- Serve as liaison

Instruction
- Instruct individuals according to their needs
- Explain office policies and procedures

KEY TERMS

cryotherapy
diathermy
erythema
fluidotherapy
gait
goniometer
hydrotherapy
mobility aid
physical therapy
posture
range of motion (ROM)
therapeutic team
thermotherapy
traction

CHAPTER OUTLINE

- General Principles of Physical Therapy
- Cryotherapy and Thermotherapy
- Hydrotherapy
- Exercise Therapy
- Traction
- Mobility Aids
- Referral to a Physical Therapist

OBJECTIVES

After completing Chapter 43, you will be able to:

43.1 Explain how medical assistants might assist with some forms of physical therapy.

43.2 Describe ways to test joint mobility, muscle strength, gait, and posture.

43.3 Discuss the benefits of cold and heat therapies.

43.4 List contraindications to cold and heat therapies.

43.5 Identify various cold and heat therapies.

43.6 Demonstrate how to perform cold and heat therapies.

43.7 Describe hydrotherapy methods.

43.8 Identify several methods of exercise therapy.

43.9 Compare different methods of traction.

43.10 Demonstrate how to teach a patient to use a cane, a walker, crutches, and a wheelchair.

Introduction

Applying cold and heat therapy and assisting patients with ambulation are common responsibilities of a medical assistant. These activities are part of the field of physical therapy. For a full program of physical therapy, a physician generally refers a patient to a licensed physical therapist. However, a physician may request that you assist with some forms of physical therapy, including:

- Applying cold and heat
- Teaching basic exercises
- Demonstrating how to use a cane, walker, and crutches
- Demonstrating how to use a wheelchair
- Discussing with the patient specific therapies for use at home

CASE STUDY

While on vacation, a 28-year-old male had a mountain biking accident that resulted in a broken leg and other injuries. He went to the local emergency room for treatment and was instructed to follow up with his primary care physician on arriving home. Three days after the accident, he presents in your office with crutches and a cast on his left leg. Using the crutches, he stumbles and almost falls as you ask him back to the examination area. You also notice a dry, crusted, bloody injury on his left forearm.

As you read this chapter, consider the following questions:

1. What type of teaching do you think this patient will need?

2. What type of therapy may be necessary for the crusted bloody injury on his forearm, and how would you perform it?

General Principles of Physical Therapy

Physical therapy is a medical specialty for the treatment of musculoskeletal, nervous, and cardiopulmonary disorders. A physical therapist uses a variety of treatments, including cold, heat, water, exercise, massage, and traction. Some physical therapy regimens combine two or more treatments. Exercising in a pool, for example, combines the use of water and exercise. In addition, the physical therapist actively promotes patient education and rehabilitation programs.

Physical therapy benefits patients in several ways. It restores and improves muscle function, builds strength, increases joint mobility, relieves pain, and increases circulation. Physical therapy is used to treat various disorders, including arthritis, stroke, lower-back pain, muscle spasms, muscle injuries or diseases, pressure sores, skin disorders, and burns.

Assisting Within a Therapeutic Team

Many people who require physical therapy are recovering from traumatic injuries or dealing with chronic illnesses. They may therefore be receiving therapeutic attention from several different specialists. Physicians, nurses, medical assistants, and other specialists who work with patients dealing with chronic illness or recovery from major injuries make up a **therapeutic team.** When you work with such patients, your responsibilities may include:

- Coordinating the patient's schedule of sessions with different specialists
- Making referrals, as directed by the physician
- Explaining a specialist's treatment approach to the patient
- Communicating the physician's findings to the specialist

Educating the Patient

Specialized Therapies and Their Benefits

Health-care professionals recognize the contribution of specialized therapies to a patient's recovery. Because many people do not know about these specialized therapies, you may be called on to explain them to patients. You can educate patients about potential benefits of art therapy or other specialized therapies. When specialized therapies are ordered, patients will be more at ease if they know what to expect. You can help when necessary by explaining the following types of therapies and their advantages.

- In art therapy, patients learn to express themselves visually through drawing, painting, and sculpture. Art therapy aids both physical and mental healing; provides a recreational outlet; improves mobility and fine motor coordination; provides an outlet for expressing fears or other emotions that patients may be unaware of or unable or unwilling to express verbally; helps relieve anxiety; allows patients to focus on something other than their physical condition; and encourages patients to take better care of themselves. To aid in the art therapy process, encourage patients to relax and give this approach time to work. Although the benefits of art therapy may be evident immediately, they are just as likely to be perceived only after the course of therapy is well under way.

- In music therapy, patients listen to and create music to calm themselves and to alleviate anxiety. This therapy is often used with surgical patients and patients with chronic pain.

- In dance therapy, patients participate in dance to improve balance, flexibility, strength, and quality of life.

- In writing therapy, patients express themselves through a chosen form of writing such as poetry or a journal.

- In crafts therapy, patients express themselves by using a variety of media to create handiworks.

- In pet therapy, patients play with, groom, or walk a pet. Pets provide companionship and the opportunity to nurture.

- In aquatic therapy, patients swim in a therapeutic pool equipped with a ramp and a lift so that it is accessible to all. Many patients who cannot walk when on land can move their legs remarkably well in water.

- In horticultural therapy, patients work with plants and flowers to bring beauty into their daily lives and to help improve their balance, strength, memory, and socialization skills.

- In equestrian therapy, patients ride horses to help develop strength, coordination, and muscle tone and to improve balance.

- Documenting the specialist's treatments and findings for the physician
- Reinforcing the specialist's instructions for the patient
- Answering the patient's questions

To fulfill these responsibilities, you must have a working knowledge of therapy techniques. If, for example, the physician refers a patient to an art therapist, you would set up an art therapy appointment and explain in general terms what the patient can expect. The Educating the Patient section offers basic information about various specialized therapies.

Besides learning the basic information you need to know about physical therapy, you will want to keep up-to-date on emerging techniques. You may want to become proficient in some of these new techniques. By expanding your knowledge and skills, you increase your value as a member of the therapeutic team.

Assisting With Patient Assessment

Before the doctor prescribes physical therapy, she assesses the patient's physical abilities and condition. She inspects and palpates the patient's joints and muscles and tests the patient's joint mobility, muscle strength, gait, and posture. You will typically assist with these tests. In some cases the doctor may direct you to perform them.

Joint Mobility Testing. People usually assume that their joints are mobile until stiffness or injury limits them. When a patient complains of these difficulties, the doctor may ask you to assist in testing range of motion. **Range of motion (ROM)** is the degree to which a joint is able to move, measured in degrees with a protractor device called a universal **goniometer** (Figure 43-1). The measurement of joint mobility is known as goniometry, a noninvasive test that is frequently performed in doctors'

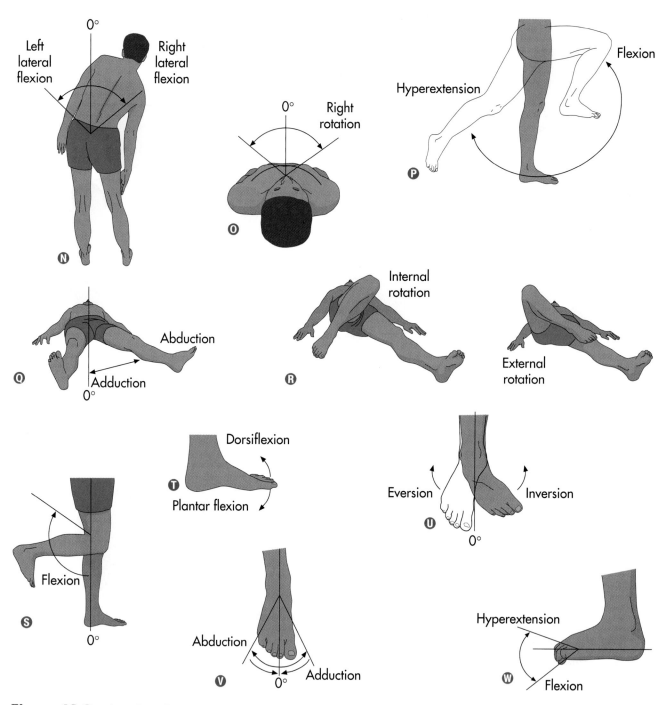

Figure 43-2. (continued)

it passes the left foot. At the end of the swing, the right foot slows, and heel strike occurs again.

Generally, a physician or physical therapist assesses a patient's gait. To do so, the physician asks the patient to walk away, turn around, and walk back. Assessment of gait includes an appraisal of the patient's length of stride, balance, coordination, direction of knees (inward or outward), and direction of feet (inward or outward).

Posture Testing. **Posture** is body position and alignment. The doctor assesses posture by looking at the patient's spinal curve from the sides, back, and front. Normally, the thoracic spine has a convex (outward) curve, and the lumbar spine has a concave (inward) curve. The doctor also notes the symmetry of alignment of the shoulders, knees, and hips.

To assess alignment and degree of straightness of the spine, the doctor asks the patient to bend at the waist and let the arms dangle freely. To assess knee position, the doctor asks the patient to stand with both feet together to determine whether the knees are at the same height, facing forward, and symmetrical.

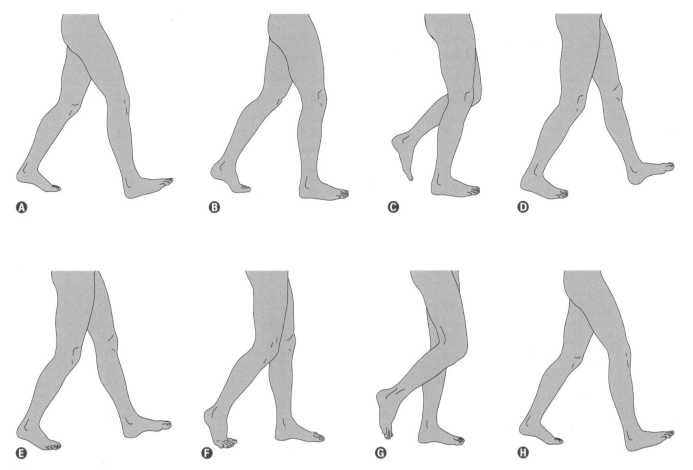

Figure 43-3. These are the two phases of gait. Illustrations (a) through (d) show the movements of the stance phase; illustrations (e) through (h) show the movements of the swing phase: (a) right heel strike, (b) flat right foot, (c) midstance, (d) push off with right foot, (e) right foot poised, (f) left heel strike, (g) midswing, (h) right heel strike.

Cryotherapy and Thermotherapy

Applying cold to a patient's body for therapeutic reasons is called **cryotherapy.** This type of therapy can be administered in a number of ways. Treatments may be dry or wet, and they may be chemical or natural. Examples of dry cold applications are ice bags and ice packs. Wet cold applications include cold compresses and ice massage.

Applying heat to a patient's body for therapeutic reasons is called **thermotherapy.** As with cryotherapy, thermotherapy can be administered in a variety of ways. Examples of devices used in dry heat treatments are electric heating pads, hot-water bottles, and heat lamps. Moist heat treatments include hot soaks and the use of hot compresses and hot packs.

Factors Affecting the Use of Cryotherapy and Thermotherapy

To choose a cold or heat therapy for a patient, the physician considers the therapy's purpose, the location and condition of the affected area, and the patient's age and general health. After choosing a therapy, the physician may direct you to apply the cold or heat treatment and to teach the patient and family how to continue the therapy at home.

Performed correctly, cold and heat therapies generally promote healing. These therapies can, however, cause side effects in some patients. Therefore, you need to exercise caution when applying the therapies. You also need to be aware of conditions that contraindicate (make inadvisable) cold or heat therapies. Table 43-2 summarizes circumstances that warrant precautions or contraindications for the therapies as well as possible side effects. When performing any cold or heat therapy, you should consider the age of the patient, treatment location, patient problems with circulation or sensation, and individual temperature tolerance.

Age. Age is an important consideration because young children and elderly patients usually are more sensitive than others to cold and heat. When administering cryotherapy or thermotherapy, stay with the patient during its application to check the patient's skin frequently for excessive paleness or redness.

Treatment Location. Thin-skinned areas that are usually covered with clothing (such as the back, chest, and

TABLE 43-2	Contraindications, Precautions, and Side Effects Related to Cold and Heat		
Therapy	**Precautions**	**Contraindications**	**Side Effects**
Dry and moist cold applications	Poor circulation, extreme age or youth, arthritis, impaired sensation (insensitivity to cold)	Inability to tolerate weight of device, pain caused by application (more common with moist cold)	Numbness, pain, very pale or bluish skin, blood clots (rare)
Dry and moist heat applications	Impaired kidney, heart, or lung function; arteriosclerosis and atherosclerosis; impaired sensation (insensitivity to heat); extreme age or youth; pregnancy	Possibility of hemorrhage; malignancy; acute inflammation, such as appendicitis; severe circulation problems; pain caused by weight of device	Burns (especially with heat lamps), increased respiratory rate, lowered blood pressure

abdomen) are more sensitive to cold and heat therapies than other areas, such as the face and hands. Use caution around any broken skin (as with a wound), because it is susceptible to further tissue damage from cryotherapy or thermotherapy.

Circulation or Sensation Impairment.   Patients with diabetes or cardiovascular disease may have impaired circulation or sensory perception. These impairments may prevent such patients from sensing that a treatment is too cold or too hot. These patients require close monitoring during cryotherapy or thermotherapy. Carefully observe their skin to determine the treatment's therapeutic effect.

Temperature Tolerance.   Tolerance of temperature extremes varies greatly from person to person. Some people are unusually sensitive to cold or to heat. Listen carefully to patients for any indication of temperature intolerance during treatment. Cases of intolerance should be reported to the physician, who may decide to change the treatment.

Principles of Cryotherapy

The application of cryotherapy causes blood vessels to constrict and involuntary muscles of the skin to contract. These physiologic responses can have the following results:

- Prevention of swelling by limiting edema, or fluid accumulation in body tissue
- Control of bleeding by constricting blood vessels
- Reduction of inflammation by slowing blood and fluid movement in the affected area
- Provision of an anesthetic effect for pain by reducing inflammation
- Reduction of pus formation by inhibiting microorganism activity
- Lowering of body temperature

Administering Cryotherapy

Cryotherapy is highly effective in alleviating swelling, pain, inflammation, and bleeding caused by various types of injuries. For best results, cryotherapy should be used frequently (about 20 minutes every hour) for the first 48 hours after an injury. As cold is applied, the skin becomes cool and pale because blood vessels constrict, decreasing the blood supply to the area. The decreased blood supply also reduces tissue metabolism, oxygen use, and waste accumulation.

Dry Cold Applications.   Dry cold applications include ice bags, ice collars, and chemical ice packs. An ice bag is a rubber or plastic bag with a locking lid. An ice collar is a rubber or plastic kidney-shaped bag that is specially curved to fit around the back of the neck.

A chemical ice pack is usually a flat plastic bag containing a semifluid chemical (Figure 43-4). Ice packs come in various sizes and types. Some are disposable, whereas others can be stored in a freezer and reused. The chemical prevents them from freezing solid, allowing them to be

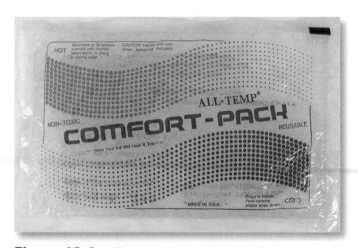

Figure 43-4.   This chemical pack can be frozen, boiled, or microwaved for cold or heat therapy.

molded to the area to be treated. Chemical ice packs may require squeezing or shaking to activate the cooling action. Most packs remain cold for 30 to 60 minutes. Some ice packs come with a soft covering; others must be wrapped in a cloth before they are applied to the skin.

Wet Cold Applications. Wet cold applications include cold compresses and ice massage. A cold compress is a cloth or gauze pad moistened with ice water. It may be used to treat the pain associated with a toothache, tooth extraction, eye injury, or headache. The ice used in ice massage may be a cube wrapped in a plastic bag or water frozen in a paper cup. The combination of the cold temperature and the motion of the massage can provide therapeutic relief for the localized pain resulting from a sprain or strain. Although cold causes muscles to contract, the pain-relieving effect can help a patient relax. The procedure for administering cryotherapy is outlined in Procedure 43-1.

Principles of Thermotherapy

The application of thermotherapy causes blood vessels to dilate (expand), which increases the blood supply to the area. Increased blood supply brings about an increased tissue metabolism that carries oxygen and nutrients to the cells of the area being treated. Increased metabolism carries toxins and wastes away from the cells. During thermotherapy, the treated skin becomes warm and develops **erythema** (redness) as the capillaries in the deep layers of the skin fill with blood. These physiologic responses can have the following results:

- Relief of pain and congestion
- Reduction of muscle spasms
- Muscle relaxation
- Reduction of inflammation
- Reduction of swelling by increasing the fluid absorption from the tissues

Administering Thermotherapy

Thermotherapy is highly effective in relieving pain, congestion, muscle spasms, and inflammation and promoting muscle relaxation. However, if heat is applied for too long, it may increase skin secretions that soften the skin and lower resistance. Heat that is too extreme can burn the skin or increase edema. Always monitor patients receiving thermotherapy, particularly children and elderly patients. The three basic types of thermotherapy are dry heat, moist heat, and diathermy. The general principles for administering the following types of thermotherapy are outlined in Procedure 43-2.

Dry Heat Therapies. There are several types of dry heat therapy. They include the use of chemical hot packs, heating pads, hot-water bottles, heat lamps with infrared or ultraviolet bulbs, and fluidotherapy.

Chemical Hot Pack. A chemical hot pack is a disposable, flexible pack of chemicals that becomes hot when you activate it by kneading or slapping it. After activating the pack, cover it with a cloth, and place it on the patient's skin in the area being treated. Chemical hot packs are pliable and conform to body contours. For best results, follow the manufacturer's directions.

Heating Pad. A heating pad is a flat pad with electrical coils between layers of soft fabric. When turned on, the coils provide localized heat. The physician should specify the heating pad temperature (low, medium, or high) and the length of time the pad should be applied.

Before applying a heating pad, cover it with a pillowcase or towel, check to be sure the cord is not frayed, and plug it into an electrical outlet. Make sure the patient's skin is dry. Then turn on the pad, and set the temperature selector switch to the specified temperature. The patient should never lie on top of a heating pad.

Hot-Water Bottle. A hot-water bottle is a flat, flexible, plastic or rubber bottle with a stopper. Fill the bottle with hot water, using a thermometer to make sure the water temperature does not exceed 125°F. For children under the age of 2 years and for elderly patients, the temperature should range from 105° to 115°F. For older children, a safe temperature is 115° to 125°F. Fill the bottle halfway; then compress it to expel air. The half-filled bottle can conform to the area to be treated. A half-filled bottle is also lighter than a full one and therefore more comfortable for the patient. Cover the bottle with a cloth or pillowcase before you apply it.

After you apply the hot-water bottle, check with the patient to make sure the temperature is not too hot. Check the temperature frequently, and replace the hot water as needed. Each time you remove the bottle, check the patient's skin to make sure that it is merely warm to the touch.

Heat Lamp. A heat lamp uses an infrared or ultraviolet bulb to provide heat. When the lamp is turned on, infrared rays heat and penetrate the skin's surface to a depth of 3 to 5 millimeters. To avoid burning the skin, place an infrared heat lamp 2 to 4 feet from the area being treated. Treatment usually lasts for 20 to 30 minutes or as directed by the physician.

Although ultraviolet rays produce little heat, they can burn the skin and damage the eyes. They are used to kill bacteria and to promote vitamin D formation. Ultraviolet rays stimulate epithelial cells and cause blood vessels to overfill, increasing the skin's defenses against bacterial infections. Ultraviolet lamps are used to treat acne, psoriasis, pressure sores, and wound infections.

Before recommending the use of an ultraviolet lamp, the physician assesses the patient's sensitivity and determines the treatment duration. Treatments typically range from 30 seconds to a few minutes. The duration is usually increased in 10-second intervals. Because ultraviolet rays can burn the skin, monitor the patient closely. Do not leave the room during the treatment. Both you and the patient must wear goggles to prevent harm to the eyes.

Fluidotherapy. **Fluidotherapy** is a relatively new technique for stimulating healing, particularly in the hands

Admi

Objecti

OSHA

Materi
applicati
hot pack,
containe
gauze fo

Metho

1. Dou
   kno
   tem
   it sl

2. Ide
   anc
   que

3. Hav
   req
   nee

4. Wa
   glo
   dep
   tre

5. Po

6. Re
   pla

7. Ch
   an
   de
   ter

8. Pr
   •

   •

Adı

Obje
admir

OSH

Mate
requi
pack,

Metl

1. [

2. |

3. |

4. '

5. |

6. |

7. |

8. |

- Avoid indenting the cast until it is completely dry
- Check the movement and sensation of the visible extremities frequently
- Restrict strenuous activities for the first few days
- Avoid allowing the affected limb to hang down for any length of time
- Do not put anything inside the cast
- Keep the cast dry
- Follow the physician's orders regarding restrictions of activities

Sprains and strains often result from sports injuries and accidents. A **sprain** is an injury characterized by partial tearing of a ligament that supports a joint, such as the ankle. A sprain may also involve injuries to tendons, muscles, and local blood vessels and contusions of the surrounding soft tissue. A **strain** is a muscle injury that results from overexertion. For example, back strain may occur when a person carries a heavy load.

Symptoms of a sprain include swelling, tenderness, pain during movement, and local discoloration. If you suspect a sprain, splint the joint, apply ice, and call the EMS system if needed. Inform the patient that an x-ray may be required to confirm that there is no fracture. A strain causes pain on motion. In most cases it should be examined by a physician, who may prescribe rest, application of heat, and a muscle relaxant.

Head Injuries

Head injuries include concussions, contusions, fractures, intracranial bleeding, and scalp hematomas and lacerations. Some head injuries can be life-threatening and require immediate medical attention.

Concussion. A **concussion** is a jarring injury to the brain. It is the most common type of head injury. Someone who has a concussion may lose consciousness. Temporary loss of vision, pallor (paleness), listlessness, memory loss, or vomiting can also occur. Symptoms may disappear rapidly or last up to 24 hours. A concussion may produce slow intracranial bleeding. Teach the patient and the patient's family basic precautions after this type of injury. See the Educating the Patient section for more information on concussions.

Severe Head Injuries. Contusions, fractures, and intracranial bleeding cause symptoms similar to, but more profound than, symptoms of concussions. Symptoms to look for are leakage of clear or bloody fluid from the ears or nose, seizures, and respiratory arrest. A patient with a severe head injury requires immediate hospitalization. Your priority is to maintain the patient's airway and to begin rescue breathing or CPR if needed.

Scalp Hematomas and Lacerations. A **hematoma** is a swelling caused by blood under the skin. A scalp hematoma causes a bump on the head. This swelling can

Educating the Patient

Concussion

Because a concussion can cause intracranial bleeding, handle gently a patient who is being treated for this type of injury. If bleeding is slow, it might take up to 24 hours to produce symptoms. Because intracranial bleeding may require brain surgery, use the following patient education guidelines to help ensure patient safety after a concussion.

- Inform the patient that the first 24 hours after the injury are the most critical.
- Tell the patient to refrain from strenuous activity, to rest, and to return to regular activity gradually.
- Instruct the patient to avoid using pain medicines other than acetaminophen, unless the drugs are approved by the physician.
- Advise the patient to eat lightly, especially if nausea and vomiting occur.
- Tell a family member to check on the patient every few hours. The family member should make sure the patient knows his own name, his location, and the name of the family member.

- Instruct the family member to call for medical assistance immediately if the patient exhibits any of these warning signs:
  - Any symptom that is getting worse, such as headaches, sleepiness, or nausea, including nausea that doesn't go away
  - Changes in behavior, such as irritability or confusion
  - Dilated pupils (pupils that are bigger than normal) or pupils of different sizes
  - Trouble walking or speaking
  - Drainage of bloody or clear fluids from ears or nose
  - Vomiting
  - Seizures
  - Weakness or numbness in the arms or legs
  - A less serious head injury in a patient taking blood thinners or who has a bleeding disorder such as hemophilia

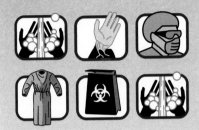

PROCEDURE 44.5

Controlling Bleeding

Objective: To control bleeding and minimize blood loss

OSHA Guidelines

Materials: Clean or sterile dressings

Method

1. If you have time, wash your hands and put on examination gloves, face protection, and a gown to protect yourself from splatters, splashes, and sprays.

2. Using a clean or sterile dressing, apply direct pressure over the wound.

3. If blood soaks through the dressing, do not remove it. Apply an additional dressing over the original one.

4. Elevate the body part that is bleeding.

5. If direct pressure and elevation do not stop the bleeding, apply pressure over the nearest pressure point between the bleeding and the heart (Figure 44-11). For example, if the wound is on the lower arm, apply pressure on the brachial artery. For a lower-leg wound, apply pressure on the femoral artery in the groin.

6. When the doctor or EMT arrives, assist as requested.

7. After the patient has been transferred to a hospital, properly dispose of contaminated materials.

8. Remove the gloves and wash your hands.

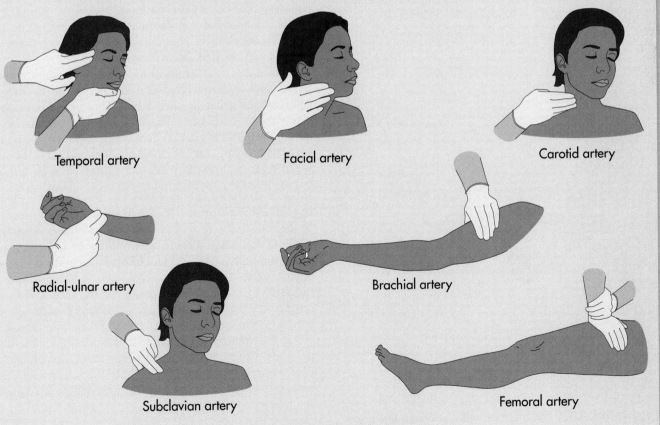

Temporal artery

Facial artery

Carotid artery

Radial-ulnar artery

Brachial artery

Subclavian artery

Femoral artery

Figure 44-11. Apply pressure on these pressure points to stop bleeding.

be reduced by applying ice immediately after the injury. Because blood vessels in the scalp are close to the skin, scalp lacerations often bleed profusely and look worse than they really are. Apply direct pressure to stop bleeding from a scalp laceration, wash the area with soap and water, and apply a dry, sterile dressing over the area.

Hemorrhaging

Hemorrhaging (heavy or uncontrollable bleeding) is generally the result of an injury. It may also be caused by an illness. The first-aid treatment remains the same in both cases. Bleeding can be internal or external. When administering first aid to a patient who may have internal bleeding, cover the patient with a blanket for warmth, keep the patient quiet and calm, and get medical help immediately.

Control external bleeding to prevent rapid blood loss and shock. Use direct pressure, apply additional dressings as needed, elevate the bleeding body part, and put pressure over a pressure point, as described in Procedure 44-5 and as illustrated in Figure 44-11. Then transport the patient to an emergency care facility.

As a last resort, if medical help is more than an hour away, you may need to use a tourniquet (Figure 44-12) to save a person's life. You apply a tourniquet over the main pressure point just above the wound and tighten the tourniquet until the bleeding stops. Many people do not recommend applying a tourniquet in any situation because it may be difficult to judge when a person's life is at stake. Keep in mind that application of a tourniquet to a person's limb almost surely leads to loss of the limb.

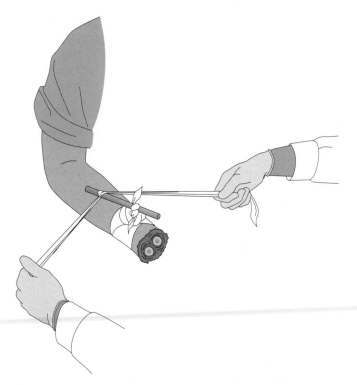

Figure 44-12. Apply a tourniquet only as a last resort, that is, if bleeding cannot be stopped and the patient is likely to die as a result.

Multiple Injuries

Sometimes a patient sustains more than one type of injury—for example, an arm fracture, head injury, lacerations, and internal bleeding. Multiple injuries often result from a car accident or a fall. If you need to assist a patient with multiple injuries, assess the ABCs and perform CPR if needed. Then call (or have someone else call) the EMS system or the physician. Once you have ensured an open airway, breathing, and circulation, perform first aid for the most life-threatening injuries first.

Poisoning

A poison is a substance that produces harmful effects if it enters the body. Poisoning is serious and it can result in death or permanent injury if immediate medical care is not provided.

In addition to being able to handle a poisoning emergency, you need to educate patients in how to do the same. You should teach them about the symptoms of and treatment for the different types of poisoning. Provide them with pamphlets that describe the procedures to follow and stickers with the telephone number of the regional poison control center.

The majority of accidental poisonings happen to children under the age of 5. Young children are not necessarily put off by strong smells or burning sensations when they swallow something. Common causes of poisoning in children are household cleaning products, household plants, and medications. Poisons can also be caused by improperly prepared or contaminated food. These types of poisons are ingested, or swallowed.

Poisoning that results from coming in contact with plants, such as poison ivy, poison sumac, and poison oak, is common and generally fairly minor. This type of poisoning is referred to as absorbed poisoning. It can be serious, however, if the poisoning occurs over a large surface of the body.

Poisons can also be inhaled. This situation occurs when a person inhales a poisonous gas such as carbon monoxide or the fumes from burning poisonous plants.

Ingested Poisons. Poison that is swallowed remains in the stomach only a short time. Most of it is absorbed while in the small intestine. Symptoms of poisoning include abdominal pain and cramping; nausea; vomiting; diarrhea; odor, stains, or burns around or in the mouth; drowsiness; and unconsciousness. You should also suspect poisoning if packages containing poisonous substances are near a person who has one or more of these symptoms.

It is extremely important to call a poison control center (if available), hospital emergency room, doctor, or the EMS system for instructions if you think a patient has swallowed a poison. When you call, you will need to know the following:

- The patient's age
- The name of the poison

- The amount of poison swallowed
- When the poison was swallowed
- Whether or not the person has vomited
- How much time it will take to get the patient to a medical facility

Poisons vary in their toxicity. Some cause damage right away, whereas others cause damage several hours later. If the patient is alert and not having convulsions, follow these steps.

1. Call the regional poison control center.
2. Induce vomiting with ipecac syrup if directed by the poison control center.
3. Seek immediate medical attention.

Do not induce vomiting unless directed by a medical authority. The patient may have ingested a strong acid, alkali, or petroleum product, such as chlorine bleach or gasoline. These products may cause further damage to the throat and esophagus during vomiting. If you do not know what the patient ingested, never induce vomiting.

Turn the patient on her left side. This position delays stomach emptying by several hours and prevents aspiration if the patient vomits. Take both poison container and vomited material to the hospital for inspection.

Food poisoning, another type of ingested poisoning, can occur when bacteria produce toxins in food. Botulism, for example, results from eating improperly canned or preserved foods that have been contaminated with the bacterium *Clostridium botulinum*. Symptoms appear within 12 to 36 hours after eating contaminated food. Initial symptoms include dry mouth, sore throat, weakness, vomiting, and diarrhea.

Food poisoning is often difficult to detect because the signs and symptoms vary greatly. A patient with food poisoning usually has abdominal pain, nausea, vomiting, gas, frequent bowel sounds, and diarrhea. Chills, joint pain, and excessive sweating may also occur. If you suspect that a patient has food poisoning, call the poison control center, and arrange for immediate transport to the hospital.

Absorbed Poisons. Most people have had the red, itchy rash that results from contact with poison ivy, poison sumac, or poison oak. In some people, however, the rash may be accompanied by a generalized swelling, burning eyes, headache, fever, and abnormal pulse or respirations.

To treat a patient who has come in contact with an absorbed poison, call the regional poison control center. Have the patient immediately remove all contaminated clothing. Then wash the affected skin thoroughly with soap and water, drench it with alcohol, and rinse well. To help relieve symptoms, apply wet compresses soaked with calamine lotion. Also suggest baths in colloidal oatmeal or applications of a paste made from 3 teaspoons baking soda and 1 teaspoon water to soothe the itching. If the rash is severe, the doctor may prescribe a corticosteroid ointment. Tell the patient to seek medical assistance if a fever or swelling develops.

Inhaled Poisons. A patient may inhale poisons by breathing air contaminated by chemicals in the workplace or by a malfunctioning stove or furnace in the home. The patient may not realize she has been exposed to a poisonous gas until symptoms arise. Even then, a patient may merely suspect the flu, because some symptoms of inhalation poisoning mimic those of influenza. Common symptoms include headache, tinnitus (ringing in the ears), angina (chest pain), shortness of breath, muscle weakness, nausea, vomiting, confusion, and dizziness, followed by blurred or double vision, difficulty breathing, unconsciousness, and cardiac arrest. Also, a patient who has facial burns may have sustained an inhalation injury.

To treat poisoning by inhalation, first get the patient into fresh air. Have someone call the EMS system or the regional poison control center. Loosen tight-fitting clothing and wrap the patient in a blanket to prevent shock. Check the patient's ABCs and begin CPR if needed. Expect the EMS team to treat the patient with 100% oxygen.

Carbon monoxide is a major cause of inhalation poisoning in the home. It is a colorless and odorless natural gas produced by incomplete combustion of organic fuels, such as coal, wood, or gasoline. Carbon monoxide is especially dangerous in closed spaces because, when inhaled, it replaces oxygen in the blood. If you suspect carbon monoxide poisoning, look for clues in the environment such as a malfunctioning furnace or a car engine left running in a closed space such as a garage.

Mild carbon monoxide poisoning can cause headache and flulike symptoms without fever. Moderate poisoning may cause tinnitus, drowsiness, severe seizures, coma, and cardiopulmonary problems. Because the gas is odorless, people are often unaware they are being poisoned. They may fall asleep, lapse into unconsciousness, and die.

Weather-Related Injuries

Exposure to extreme cold, extreme heat, and the sun's damaging rays can cause weather-related injuries. These injuries may require emergency medical attention.

Frostbite. When body tissues are exposed to below-freezing temperatures, frostbite can occur. Frostbite causes ice crystals to form between tissue cells, and these crystals enlarge as they extract water from the cells. Frostbite also causes obstruction to the blood supply in the form of blood clots. This aspect of frostbite prevents blood from flowing to the tissues and causes additional, severe damage to cells.

Symptoms of frostbite include white, waxy, or grayish yellow skin. The affected body part feels cold, tingling, and painful. The skin surface may feel crusty and the underlying tissue soft in comparison. If the frostbite is deep, the body part may feel cold and hard and not be sensitive to pain. Blisters may appear after rewarming.

Treat frostbite by wrapping warm clothing or blankets around the affected body part or placing it in contact with another body part that is warm. Do not rub or massage the affected area, or you may cause further damage to the frozen tissue. Call for medical assistance. If you are in a remote area, use the wet rapid rewarming method. This method involves placing the affected part in warm (100° to 104°F) water. Hot water should be added at regular intervals to keep the temperature of the bath stable. As an alternative method, you can heat the affected area with warm compresses. Because warming may cause pain, administer aspirin or acetaminophen. Continue rewarming for 20 to 40 minutes. After the affected area becomes soft, place dry, sterile gauze between skin surfaces, such as between the toes or the fingers or between the ear and the side of the head. Do not massage the skin or break blisters.

Heatstroke. Heatstroke results from prolonged exposure to high temperatures and humidity. This condition may lead to excessive loss of fluids (dehydration) and insufficient blood in the circulatory system (hypovolemic shock). High body temperature can damage tissues and organs throughout the body. If untreated, the patient will die. People most susceptible to heatstroke are children, the elderly, athletes, and patients who are obese, are diabetic, or have circulatory problems or other chronic illnesses.

Symptoms of heatstroke include hot, dry skin; high body temperature; altered mental state; rapid pulse; rapid breathing; dizziness; and weakness. If you suspect that a patient has heatstroke, check the patient's ABCs, and call the EMS system. Move the patient to a cool place, and remove outer clothing unless it is made of light cotton or other light fabric. Also, cool the patient with any means available, such as gentle spraying with a hose, movement to an air-conditioned place, vigorous fanning, or application of a wet sheet. If the humidity is above 75%, place ice packs on the patient's groin and armpits. Stop cooling when the patient's mental state improves. Keep the patient's head and shoulders slightly elevated.

Sunburn. Do not dismiss a sunburn as trivial. It is a burn that can cause redness, tenderness, pain, swelling, blisters, and peeling skin. It can lead to skin damage or cancer later in life.

Soak sunburned skin in cool water to help reduce the heat. Apply cold compresses, and later calamine lotion, to bring relief from the burning sensation. Have the patient elevate the legs and arms to prevent swelling. The patient should also drink plenty of water and take a pain reliever.

Educate the patient about the importance of using sunscreen and reapplying it every 2 to 3 hours when outdoors. Advise the patient to stay out of direct sunlight between 10:00 A.M. and 2:00 P.M., because the sun's rays are strongest during that period.

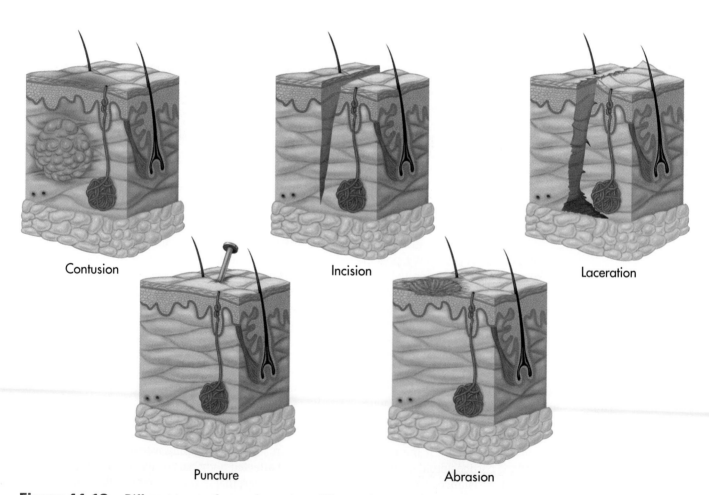

Contusion

Incision

Laceration

Puncture

Abrasion

Figure 44-13. Different types of wounds produce different degrees of tissue damage.

Wounds

A wound is an injury in which the skin or tissues under the skin are damaged. Wounds can be either open or closed. Figure 44-13 shows the various types of wounds.

Open Wounds. An open wound is a break in the skin or mucous membrane. Types of open wounds include incisions, lacerations, abrasions, and punctures.

Incisions and Lacerations. An incision is a clean and smooth cut, such as that from a kitchen knife. A laceration has jagged edges, as may result when a child steps on a piece of broken glass in the sand at the beach. Care of minor incisions and lacerations involves controlling bleeding by covering the wound with a clean or sterile dressing and applying direct pressure. After the bleeding stops, clean and dress the wound. Procedure 44-6 explains how to clean minor wounds. Teach the patient the importance of keeping the wound clean and checking for signs of infection, such as heat, redness, pain, and swelling.

If the wound is deep and involves muscle, tendons, the face, the genitals, the mouth, or the tongue, control the bleeding with direct pressure to the wound (with a sterile dressing or clean cloth held against its surface), elevation,

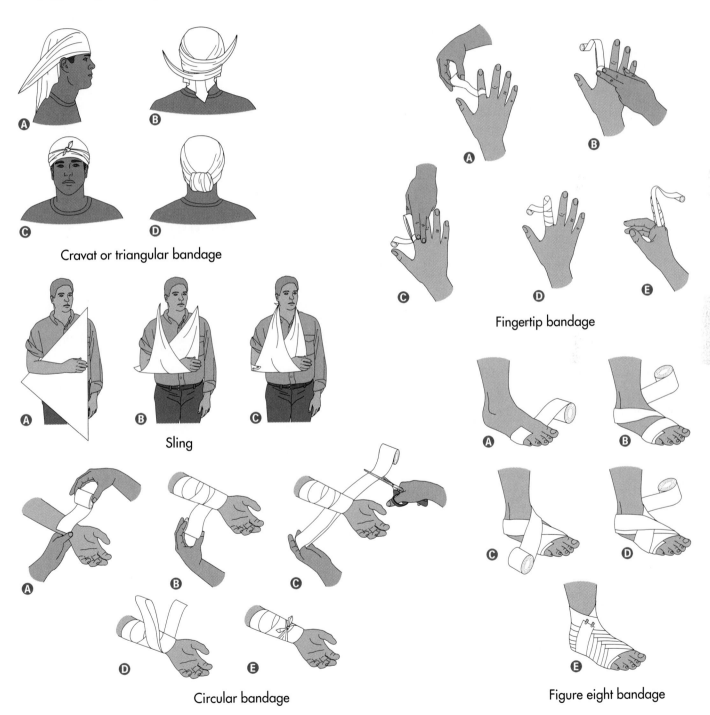

Cravat or triangular bandage

Sling

Circular bandage

Fingertip bandage

Figure eight bandage

Figure 44-14. Apply a bandage, as needed, to a wound.

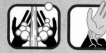

PROCEDURE 44.6

Cleaning Minor Wounds

Objective: To clean and dress minor wounds

OSHA Guidelines

Materials: Sterile gauze squares, basin, antiseptic soap, warm water, sterile dressing

Method

1. Wash your hands and put on examination gloves.
2. Dip several gauze squares in a basin of warm, soapy water.
3. Wash the wound from the center outward to avoid bringing contaminants from the surrounding skin into the wound. Use a new gauze square for each cleansing motion.
4. As you wash, remove debris that could cause infection.
5. Rinse the area thoroughly, preferably by placing the wound under warm, running water.
6. Pat the wound dry with sterile gauze squares.
7. Cover the wound with a dry, sterile dressing. Bandage the dressing in place.
8. Properly dispose of contaminated materials.
9. Remove the gloves and wash your hands.
10. Instruct the patient on wound care.
11. Record the procedure in the patient's chart.

and use of pressure points. Contact the doctor and, if necessary, the EMS system.

Abrasions. An abrasion is a scraping of the skin, as when someone slides across gravel during a softball game. Abrasions require washing with soap and water. Be sure to remove all the dirt and debris to prevent tattooing (dark discoloration under the skin). Minor abrasions do not need a dressing or bandage, but large ones do. Various types of bandaging are shown in Figure 44-14. As with any wound, teach the patient to watch for signs of infection.

Punctures. A puncture wound is a small hole created by a piercing object, such as a bullet, knife, nail, or animal tooth. Puncture wounds are a potential breeding ground for tetanus bacteria, because the bacteria can live and thrive in the absence of oxygen. Allow the wound to bleed freely for a few minutes to help wash out bacteria. Then clean the wound with soap and water, and apply a dry, sterile dressing. If the patient has not had a tetanus toxoid immunization in the past 7 to 10 years, inform the physician so that one can be ordered.

Closed Wounds. A closed wound is an injury that occurs inside the body without breaking the skin. Closed wounds, which are usually called **contusions** (bruises), are caused by a blunt object striking the tissue. This action produces broken blood vessels and internal, localized bleeding (hematoma) below the area that has been struck. Treat such a wound with cold compresses to reduce swelling. The affected area will turn from black and blue to green to yellow as blood pigments oxidize. Inform the patient that these color changes are part of the normal healing process.

Common Illnesses

A variety of common illnesses frequently call for emergency medical intervention. As a patient educator, you can help ensure that patients recognize the symptoms of these illnesses and know when to call for medical assistance. Teaching patients the importance of following physician's orders for follow-up care is also your responsibility. Common illnesses include the following:

- Abdominal pain
- Asthma
- Dehydration
- Diarrhea
- Fainting
- Fever
- Hyperventilation
- Nosebleed
- Tachycardia
- Vomiting

Abdominal Pain

Acute abdominal pain that occurs suddenly and is accompanied by fever may indicate an emergency that requires surgery. The pain may involve spasmodic contractions. It may feel knifelike or ache dully, and it may be localized or may radiate. The location of the pain gives clues to its cause. Acute pain in the right upper quadrant, for example, may signal a gallbladder attack. Pain in the right lower quadrant may indicate appendicitis.

Other causes include internal hemorrhage, intestinal perforation or obstruction, peptic ulcer, and hernia. In women, pelvic pain can indicate a gynecologic problem. Obviously, trauma to the area, such as wounds or blows, can produce acute abdominal pain.

While waiting for patient transport, have the patient lie on his back with his knees flexed (unless there is a wound or swelling in the abdomen). This position lets the abdominal muscles relax. Keep the patient quiet and warm, and act calm and concerned. Do not give anything by mouth, and keep an emesis basin handy in case the patient vomits. Do not apply heat to the abdomen because heat may exacerbate inflammation. Monitor the patient's pulse and consciousness, and check for signs of shock.

Asthma

Asthma is a common disorder caused by spasmodic narrowing of the bronchi. It is often an inherited tendency—that is, several members of one family may suffer from it. A patient who is having an acute attack wheezes, coughs, and is short of breath. She may become frightened and feel as if she cannot get enough air. If you spot an asthma attack, check the patient's ABCs, and notify the doctor at once. You may assist the patient in using a respiratory inhaler if she carries one with her. If directed, administer a mininebulizer treatment with a bronchodilator (drug that opens the bronchi), such as albuterol (Proventil) or epinephrine.

Dehydration

Dehydration results from a lack of adequate water in the body. The body's fluid intake is not sufficient to meet its fluid needs. Severe dehydration can result from vomiting, excessive heat and sweating, diarrhea, or lack of food or fluid intake. The following are symptoms of dehydration:

- Extreme thirst
- Tiredness
- Light-headedness
- Abdominal or muscle cramping
- Confusion (especially in elderly people)

Perform the following steps to administer first aid to a dehydrated person.

1. Move the victim into the shade or to a cool area.
2. To replace lost fluids, give the victim water, tea, fruit juice, a commercial electrolyte replacement fluid, or clear broth.
3. If symptoms persist or are accompanied by nausea, diarrhea, or convulsions, call for the EMS system or a physician.

Diarrhea (Acute)

Acute diarrhea can be caused by an intestinal infection, food poisoning, a bowel disorder, or the side effects of medication. Severe diarrhea causes dehydration and dangerous electrolyte imbalances that can lead to shock. Symptoms of shock include rapid pulse, low blood pressure, and pale, clammy skin.

Help the patient lie on his back and elevate his legs. Report the patient's condition to the doctor. As directed, prepare to assist in administering intravenous fluids to correct dehydration and restore electrolytes and to draw blood for testing.

Fainting (Syncope)

Fainting, or syncope, is a partial or complete loss of consciousness. It usually follows a decrease in the amount of blood flow to the brain. Before fainting, patients may feel weak, dizzy, cold, or nauseated. They may perspire or look pale and anxious.

If you are with a patient who feels as if she is going to faint, tell her to lower her head between her legs and to breathe deeply. Stay with her until the feeling passes. If the patient is having difficulty breathing or faints, lay her flat on her back with her feet slightly elevated. Loosen tight clothing and apply a cold cloth to her face. Observe the patient carefully, monitoring her breathing and level of consciousness. Observe for weakness in her arms and legs. Let her rest for at least 10 minutes after she regains full consciousness. Notify the physician that the patient fainted.

If your efforts do not revive a patient who has fainted, call the physician and the EMS system. The patient may be slipping into a coma.

Fever

Fever is a common clinical sign that often indicates infection. Mild or moderate fever can accompany a cold or an upset stomach. It can usually be managed with aspirin or acetaminophen. A fever of 106°F or higher (hyperthermia) is dangerous, however, because irreversible brain damage can occur if the fever is not lowered immediately.

If a patient's temperature is dangerously high, you must proceed at once to check the other vital signs and the level of consciousness. Notify the doctor and be prepared to start rapid cooling measures. Place ice packs on the groin and axilla, or give the patient a tepid sponge bath. If the patient is a child, be prepared to manage seizures (discussed later in this chapter).

Hyperventilation

Some patients who are under a great deal of stress lack the skills to deal with the stress effectively. They may seem anxious, frazzled, and more emotional than average patients. Patients under stress may begin to hyperventilate, or breathe too rapidly and too deeply. This breathing disturbs the normal balance of oxygen and carbon dioxide in the blood, and the carbon dioxide concentration falls below normal levels. Patients who are hyperventilating may also feel light-headed and as if they cannot get enough air. In addition, they may have chest pain and feel apprehensive.

Move a hyperventilating patient to a quiet area. Have the patient sit quietly and visualize a calm and serene environment, such as a beach or the mountains. With a calm and soothing voice, coach the patient to take slow, normal breaths.

Nosebleed

Nosebleed, or **epistaxis,** can occur for a variety of reasons. They include blowing the nose too hard, local irritation or dryness, frequent sneezing, fragile or superficial blood vessels, high blood pressure, a blow to the nose, and a foreign body in the nose. Nosebleeds are common in children, especially at night.

Treat a nosebleed by having the patient sit up with the head tilted forward to prevent blood from running down the back of the throat. Next, have the patient gently pinch the nostrils shut at the bottom for at least 5 minutes. If that does not stop the bleeding, apply an ice pack or cold compress to the nose and face, and continue to pinch the nostrils. If the bleeding cannot be controlled, arrange for transport to the office or to a hospital for cauterization or nasal packing.

Tachycardia

Tachycardia is a rapid heart rate, generally in excess of 100 beats per minute. A patient with tachycardia may report having **palpitations,** unusually rapid, strong, or irregular pulsations of the heart. He may feel as if his heart is pounding. Help the patient lie down, take his vital signs, and if instructed, obtain an electrocardiogram (ECG). (Electrocardiography is discussed in Chapter 52.) If tachycardia is accompanied by low blood pressure and light-headedness, notify the physician immediately. These symptoms indicate that the patient could faint or go into shock. Remain with the patient and keep him calm. If directed, obtain another ECG.

Vomiting

Vomiting is a symptom common to many disorders, ranging from food poisoning to various infections. When severe, it can lead to dehydration and dangerous changes in electrolyte levels, especially in patients who are very young, very old, or diabetic or who also have diarrhea. Because these problems can be severe, notify the doctor and provide appropriate care. Procedure 44-7 describes how to provide emergency care for a patient who is vomiting.

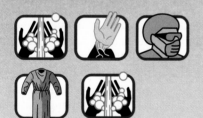

PROCEDURE 44.7

Caring for a Patient Who Is Vomiting

Objective: To increase comfort and minimize complications, such as aspiration, for a patient who is vomiting

OSHA Guidelines

Materials: Emesis basin, cool compress, cup of cool water, paper tissues or a towel, and (if ordered) intravenous fluids and electrolytes and an antinausea drug

Method

1. Wash your hands and put on examination gloves and other PPE.
2. Ask the patient when and how the vomiting started and how frequently it occurs. Find out whether she is nauseated or in pain.

3. Give the patient an emesis basin to collect vomit. Observe and document its amount, color, odor, and consistency. Particularly note blood, bile, undigested food, or feces in the vomit.
4. Place a cool compress on the patient's forehead to make her more comfortable. Offer water and paper tissues or a towel to clean her mouth.
5. Monitor for signs of dehydration, such as confusion, irritability, and flushed, dry skin. Also monitor for signs of electrolyte imbalances, such as leg cramps or an irregular pulse.
6. If requested, assist by laying out supplies and equipment for the physician to use in administering intravenous fluids and electrolytes. Administer an antinausea drug if prescribed.
7. Prepare the patient for diagnostic tests if instructed.
8. Remove the gloves and wash your hands.

Less Common Illnesses

Even though some illnesses are less common than those previously discussed, you should still be familiar enough with them so that you can handle them effectively if a physician or EMT is not immediately available. Educate patients about symptoms they may encounter that require emergency medical intervention as well as about the importance of follow-up care when they are recovering from such illnesses. Less common illnesses that may require emergency medical intervention include the following:

- Anaphylaxis
- Bacterial meningitis
- Diabetic emergencies
- Gallbladder attack
- Heart attack
- Hematemesis
- Obstetric emergencies
- Respiratory arrest
- Seizures
- Shock
- Stroke
- Toxic shock syndrome
- Viral encephalitis

Anaphylaxis

Anaphylaxis, or anaphylactic shock, is a severe, often life-threatening allergic reaction. The reaction can be immediate or delayed up to 2 hours. It happens to people who have become sensitized to certain substances. For example, it can result from eating a type of food, being stung by an insect, or taking a particular type of medication, such as penicillin.

The first sign of anaphylaxis usually comes from the patient's skin. It becomes itchy, turns red, feels hot, and develops hives. The face may also become puffy. The throat may swell so that the patient has trouble breathing and swallowing and feels as if he has a "lump in the throat." Other symptoms include pallor, perspiration, and a weak, rapid, irregular pulse. If you detect these symptoms or if the patient becomes restless, has a headache, or says that his throat feels as if it is closing up, take the following steps immediately.

Check the patient's ABCs and then notify the doctor. As directed, administer epinephrine, oral antihistamines, and oxygen, and help the patient sit up. After the patient receives epinephrine, monitor his vital signs every 2 to 3 minutes. Note skin color and monitor the airway. If he does not recover quickly, arrange for immediate transport to the hospital.

When severely allergic patients stabilize, the doctor prescribes an epinephrine autoinjector for patients to carry with them. You are responsible for teaching patients how to use this device. See the Educating the Patient section in Chapter 51 for directions.

Because of the possibility of anaphylaxis, a patient who has just received any type of injection should routinely be kept in the office for 20 to 30 minutes of observation. This procedure reduces the possibility that an allergic reaction to the medication will occur while the patient is unattended.

A less severe allergic reaction to drugs or certain foods may cause sneezing, itching, slight swelling of the skin, rash, or hives. This type of reaction can usually be controlled with diphenhydramine hydrochloride (Benadryl) or another antihistamine. The patient should be monitored closely, however, to make sure the condition does not progress to anaphylaxis.

Bacterial Meningitis

Bacterial meningitis is almost always a complication of another bacterial infection, such as otitis media (middle ear infection) or pneumonia. Therefore, first find out whether the patient currently has or recently has had a bacterial infection. The signs of bacterial meningitis are fever, chills, headache, neck stiffness, and vomiting. If the patient has these signs and then develops a fever of 102°F, becomes less alert, has altered respirations, or experiences seizures, the infection has progressed to a dangerous state.

If these signs are present, assess the patient's ABCs and notify the physician of the change in the patient's condition. Expect to arrange for transport to the hospital, where the patient will be treated with intravenous antibiotics.

Diabetic Emergencies

Diabetes is a fairly common disorder of carbohydrate metabolism (see Chapter 41). The body needs insulin, a hormone secreted by the pancreas, to use blood sugar to fuel body cells. Insulin secretion is impaired in patients with diabetes.

You can teach patients who have diabetes or who are at risk for diabetes how to recognize early signs of **hypoglycemia** (low blood sugar) and **hyperglycemia** (high blood sugar) before these conditions become medical emergencies. Symptoms of hypoglycemia include dizziness; headache; hunger; weakness; full, rapid pulse; and pallor. Symptoms of hyperglycemia include dry mouth, intense thirst, muscle weakness, and blurred vision. You should also be familiar with the signs and symptoms of the two most common diabetic emergencies you will encounter: insulin shock and diabetic coma.

Insulin Shock. Insulin shock is basically very severe hypoglycemia, in which a patient has too little sugar in the blood. Insulin shock occurs when insulin levels are so high that they move too much sugar from the blood into cells. Symptoms include rapid pulse; shallow respiration; hunger; profuse sweating; pale, cool, clammy skin; double vision; tremors; restlessness; confusion; and possibly fainting. Insulin shock can usually be corrected with administration of some form of sugar (candy, juice, or regular soda for a conscious patient or a sprinkle of table sugar

CPR Instructor

To gain medical assistant credentials, you must fulfill the requirements of either the American Association of Medical Assistants (for a Certified Medical Assistant) or the American Medical Technologists (for a Registered Medical Assistant). After obtaining your medical assistant certification or registration, you may wish to acquire additional skills in specialty areas through course work or on-the-job training. Although this course work or training may not lead to an additional certification or degree, it will enable you to expand your role in the medical office and advance your career as the demand for skilled health professionals increases.

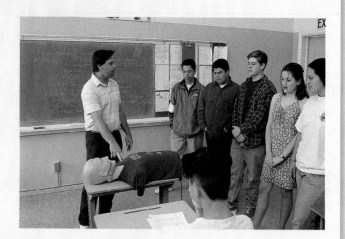

Skills and Duties

A CPR (cardiopulmonary resuscitation) instructor provides people with the knowledge and skills necessary to help save a person's life in an emergency. He teaches his students how to:

- Call for help.
- Help sustain life.
- Reduce pain.
- Minimize the consequences of injury or sudden illness until professional medical help arrives.

To teach a CPR class, an instructor must plan and coordinate the course in conjunction with a local American Red Cross unit or American Heart Association affiliate. He demonstrates the appropriate skills to his students and observes their technique. He then provides constructive feedback as they learn skills and make decisions regarding the appropriate action to take in an emergency.

The instructor is responsible for identifying participants who are having difficulty with the skills. He must develop effective strategies to help these students meet the course objectives. At the end of the course, the CPR instructor submits completed course records to the local American Red Cross chapter or American Heart Association affiliate.

Workplace Settings

CPR instructors teach classes in a variety of settings, including schools and universities, community rooms, camps, religious institutions, and medical clinics. Some employers, such as operators of swimming pools, camps, and day-care facilities, may require CPR instruction as a condition of employment.

Education

To be certified as a CPR instructor by the Red Cross, you must be at least 17 years old. In addition, you must complete two Red Cross courses. The first, the instructor candidate training course, provides instruction in teaching methods, evaluation, and reporting. After completing this course, you will be awarded an instructor candidate training certificate, which qualifies you to take the first aid and CPR instructor course. You must then pass a written test with a grade of 80% or better to gain certification. CPR instructors must teach one class every 2 years for recertification from the Red Cross.

The American Heart Association also provides training for CPR instructors. You must first pass the basic life support course for health-care providers, which teaches CPR skills. You then must take the instructor course, which covers teaching methods. After passing the instructor course, you must coteach a CPR class with an experienced instructor, who will monitor your performance. You will then become an approved instructor. CPR instructors affiliated with the American Heart Association are required to teach a minimum of two classes a year. The association has no minimum age to become an instructor.

CPR instructors may be paid or work as volunteers. There is no specific salary range for the job.

Where to Go for More Information

American Heart Association
National Center
7272 Greenville Avenue
Dallas, TX 75231-4596
(800) 242-8721, or call your local center

American Red Cross
17th and D Streets, NW
Washington, DC 20006
(202) 728-6400, or call your local chapter

on the tongue for an unconscious patient). If the cause of a diabetic emergency is unknown, give sugar. Patients will improve quickly if the cause is insulin shock and will not be harmed if the cause is diabetic coma, provided they are then transported to the hospital.

Diabetic Coma. Diabetic coma is the end result of severe hyperglycemia, in which a patient has too much sugar in the blood. It occurs when insulin levels are insufficient to move blood sugar into body cells. Its symptoms include rapid, deep gulping breaths; flushed, warm, dry skin; thirst; acetone breath (a sweet or fruity odor from the mouth); and disorientation or confusion. If you suspect diabetic coma, notify the doctor at once, and expect to arrange transport to the hospital.

Gallbladder Attack (Acute)

A classic acute gallbladder attack occurs after a person eats a high-fat meal rich in cholesterol. The patient may wake up in the night with acute abdominal pain (gallbladder colic) in the right upper quadrant. The pain is caused by inflammation of the gallbladder, usually related to gallstones obstructing the cystic duct, through which bile is secreted by the gallbladder. The pain may radiate to the back between the shoulder blades or be localized in the epigastric region (the upper central region of the abdomen) and the front chest area. The attack may be accompanied by nausea and vomiting. The pain is usually so severe that the patient seeks medical attention; many patients think they are having a heart attack.

Gallbladder attacks caused by gallstones are more common among women who are over age 40 and obese, and the frequency of attacks increases with age (especially after age 65). Diagnosis is usually made with the help of ultrasonography. The patient may require surgery to remove the gallstones.

Heart Attack

A heart attack, or **myocardial infarction (MI),** occurs when the blood flow to the heart is reduced as a result of blockage in the coronary arteries or their branches. Chest pain is the cardinal symptom of a heart attack. The patient may describe the pain as crushing, burning, heavy, aching, or like that of indigestion. The pain may radiate down the left arm or into the jaw, throat, or both shoulders. It may be accompanied by shortness of breath, sweating, nausea, and vomiting. The patient may be pale and have a feeling of doom. If you cannot easily detect pallor (paleness) because the patient has dark skin, check the patient's inner lip for paleness. Elderly patients may experience atypical symptoms of a heart attack, such as jaw pain, because responses to pain diminish during the aging process. The pain of a heart attack is not relieved by nitroglycerin.

If you think a patient is having a heart attack, notify the physician and EMS system immediately. Do not let the patient walk. Loosen tight clothing and have the patient sit up to aid breathing. The physician may order you to administer oxygen at 4 to 6 liters per minute; make sure that no one in the area is smoking. Stay with the patient, observe the ABCs, and begin CPR if required (Procedure 44-8). If directed, obtain an ECG. Take apical and radial pulses, as instructed by the physician. Be prepared to obtain medication from the crash cart or use a defibrillator if required.

Ventricular fibrillation (VF) is an abnormal heart rhythm. It is the most common cause of cardiac arrest. During VF the heart's rhythm becomes chaotic and the heart does not pump blood. The treatment for VF is defibrillation using a medical device called a defibrillator. This device works by delivering an electrical shock to the heart, which interrupts the chaotic rhythm. Defibrillators are effective only if used within minutes of the patient's collapse. An **automated external defibrillator (AED)** is a computerized defibrillator programmed to recognize VF and other lethal heart rhythms (Figure 44-15). These devices are found in many public places, including airports, but may also be used at the clinic where you are employed.

To use an AED, attach the adhesive electrode pads to the client's chest in a specific arrangement as determined by the manufacturer. Look at the illustration on the electrode's packing or machine. Activate the AED, and it will analyze the rhythm of the heart and determine if a shock is required. Pressing the "Shock" button will deliver an electrical charge to the patient's heart by way of the AED's electrode wires, which are attached to the chest.

In order to use an AED, you must be properly trained. Training is included as part of the CPR courses of the American Red Cross and the American Heart Association. Obtaining CPR and first aid certification will be an asset to you as a medical assistant.

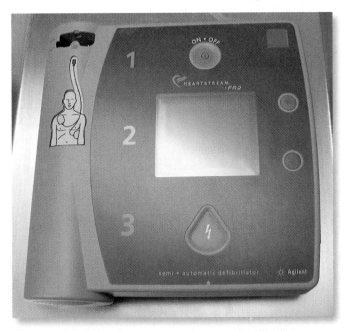

Figure 44-15. An automated external defibrillator delivers an electric current to the heart to stop a chaotic rhythm such as ventricular defibrillation.

CHAIN OF CUSTODY FORM

MADISON CLINICAL LABORATORY

195 North Parkway
Madison, WA 90869
(608) 555-3030

SPECIMEN I.D. NO:

STEP 1—TO BE COMPLETED BY COLLECTOR OR EMPLOYER REPRESENTATIVE.

Employer Name, Address, and I.D. No.:   OR   Medical Review Officer Name and Address:

_____   _____

_____   _____

_____   _____

Donor Social Security No. or Employee I.D. No.: _____

Donor I.D. verified: ❏ Photo I.D.   ❏ Employer Representative _____
                                                                                                    Signature

Reason for test: (check one)   ❏ Preemployment   ❏ Random   ❏ Postaccident

                                                      ❏ Periodic   ❏ Reasonable suspicion/cause

                                                      ❏ Return to duty   ❏ Other (specify)

Test(s) to be performed: _____   Total tests ordered: ☐

Type of specimen obtained: ❏ Urine   ❏ Blood   ❏ Semen   ❏ Other (specify)

Submit only one specimen with each requisition.

STEP 2—TO BE COMPLETED BY COLLECTOR.

For urine specimens, read temperature within 4 minutes of collection.
Check here if specimen temperature is within range.   ❏ Yes, 90°–100°F/32°–38°C
Or record actual temperature here: _____

STEP 3—TO BE COMPLETED BY COLLECTOR.

Collection site: _____   Address _____

City _____   State _____   Zip _____   Phone _____

Collection date: _____   Time: _____   ❏ a.m.   ❏ p.m.

I certify that the specimen identified on this form is the specimen presented to me by the donor identified in step 1 above, and that it was collected, labeled, and sealed in the donor's presence.

Collector's name: _____   Signature of collector _____

STEP 4—TO BE INITIATED BY DONOR AND COMPLETED AS NECESSARY THEREAFTER.

Purpose of change	Released by Signature	Received by Signature	Date
A. Provide specimen for testing			
B. Shipment to Laboratory			
C.			

Comments:

STEP 5—TO BE COMPLETED BY THE LABORATORY:

Specimen package seal(s) intact when received in lab?   ❏ Yes   ❏ No. If no, explain.
Laboratory receiver's initials _____

Copy 1 - Original - Must accompany specimen to laboratory.

Figure 44-26. The chain of custody form provides documentation that specific specimen collection safeguards have been followed.

The first link in the chain of custody is collecting the specimen. Semen specimens are commonly collected for typing in a rape examination. Other samples collected from the victim's body and clothing may include hair and skin that can help identify the offender.

Proper specimen identification is important. Without it, the chain of custody is broken at the beginning. If you are responsible for collecting the specimen, you must be sure the specimen is collected from the correct patient and that no one tampers with it. The chain of custody form (see Figure 44-26) must be completed correctly, and the patient may be required to sign or initial the form as well.

Multiple copies of the form are used as a safeguard system. One copy, usually the original, accompanies the specimen in a sealed envelope. Another copy is attached to the outside of the envelope so that each person who handles the specimen can initial the form. A third copy is usually retained in the patient's file.

These general procedures help maintain an intact chain of custody. Always refer to your office's procedures to make sure you are meeting all relevant requirements.

The Patient Under Stress

In emergency situations patients and family members are under a great deal of stress. You must realize that people react differently to emergency situations. You can learn how to detect signs of extreme stress by being alert for patients whose behavior varies from that previously observed or who cannot focus or follow directions.

Your role during many emergency situations may be to keep victims and their families and friends calm. You can promote calmness by listening carefully and giving your full attention. Your first priority, at all times, is the victim's well-being. If he is very distraught, for example, hold his hand while the doctor examines him. If one of his relatives is crying and causing him to become emotional, suggest that the relative do something to help—for example, fill out paperwork in another room.

You may face special challenges when communicating with victims during emergencies. Victims may not speak your language, or they may have a visual or hearing impairment. In such instances, follow these guidelines.

- Use gestures throughout the process for non-English-speaking victims. Continue to speak, however, because they may be able to understand some English.
- Tell patients who have visual impairments what you are going to do before you do it, and maintain voice and touch contact while caring for them.
- Ask patients who have hearing impairments whether they can read lips. If they can, speak slowly to them and never turn away while you are speaking. If they cannot read lips, communicate by writing and using gestures. At all times try to remain face-to-face and keep direct physical contact.

Educating the Patient

During minor medical emergencies, after major emergencies have been resolved, and during routine office visits, you can educate patients about ways to prevent and handle various medical emergencies. For example, you might tell them how to contact the local American Red Cross office, post notices of upcoming classes that the Red Cross offers, and encourage patients and family members to learn basic first aid. You might also develop a first-aid kit checklist and make it available to patients and families.

Make sure that all family members, including children, are familiar with the local EMS system and know how to contact it in an emergency. Suggest that families keep emergency numbers by the telephone. In addition, teach parents how to childproof their home for children of various ages. Remember that childproofing differs for different children—for example, for children who can crawl as opposed to children who can walk.

Provide brief, easy-to-read handouts to reinforce the information you present to patients. Prepare handouts in multiple languages if you provide care for non-English-speaking patients. Find and use patient education resources for the types of patients seen by the practice. For example, if you work in an obstetric office, obtain educational materials for pregnant and postpartum patients from companies that provide pregnancy-related products. Ask company representatives what materials are available. Many companies provide free videos and booklets.

Disasters

Your skills in dealing with emergencies, including first-aid and CPR training, will be an enormous help to your community in the event of a disaster. To be fully effective, you must also be familiar with standard protocols for responding to disasters. Table 44-3 shows ways that you can help in certain types of disasters. You may even want to participate in fire or other disaster drills to familiarize yourself with emergency procedures.

Disasters can occur in any community. Two of the most common types of disasters are floods and hurricanes. One of the biggest floods in the United States occurred in the Midwest in the summer of 1993. Even before national disaster relief personnel could respond, local medical personnel were called to the scene to triage injured and displaced residents. In this type of disaster, many people suffer from emotional shock (which often results in physical problems), injuries, and illnesses. These people require skilled medical assistance.

Bioterrorism

Bioterrorism is the intentional release of a biologic agent with the intent to harm individuals. The CDC defines a biologic agent as a weapon when it is easy to disseminate,

TABLE 44-3 Assisting in Disasters

Type of Disaster	Action to Take
Weather disaster, such as flood or hurricane	Report to the community command post. Have your credentials with you. Receive an identifying tag or vest and assignment. Accept only an assignment that is appropriate for your abilities. Expect to be part of a team. Document what medical care each victim receives on each person's disaster tag.
Office fire	Activate the alarm system. Use a fire extinguisher if the fire is confined to a small container, such as a trash can. Turn off oxygen. Shut windows and doors. Seal doors with wet cloths to prevent smoke from entering. If evacuation is necessary, proceed quietly and calmly. Direct ambulatory patients and family members to the appropriate exit route. Assist patients who need help leaving the building.

has a high potential for mortality, can cause a public panic or social disruption, and requires public health preparedness. There are numerous biologic agents identified as weapons, including anthrax, tularemia, smallpox, plague, and botulism. The CDC maintains an Internet site with current information about identified biologic agents at www.bt.cdc.gov.

Physicians' offices will be on the front lines should a biologic agent be intentionally released. It will be up to physicians and their staff to sound the alarm to public

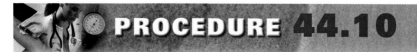

PROCEDURE 44.10

Performing Triage in a Disaster

Objective: To prioritize disaster victims

OSHA Guidelines

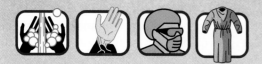

Materials: Disaster tag and pen

Method

1. Wash your hands and put on examination gloves and other PPE if available.
2. Quickly assess each victim.
3. Sort victims by type of injury and need for care, classifying them as emergent, urgent, nonurgent, or dead.
4. Label the emergent patients no. 1, and send them to appropriate treatment stations immediately. Emergent patients, such as those who are in shock or who are hemorrhaging, need immediate care.
5. Label the urgent patients no. 2, and send them to basic first-aid stations. Urgent patients need care within the next several hours. Such patients may have lacerations that can be dressed quickly to stop the bleeding but can wait for suturing.
6. Label nonurgent patients no. 3, and send them to volunteers who will be empathic and provide refreshments. Nonurgent patients are those for whom timing of treatment is not critical, such as patients who have no physical injuries but who are emotionally upset.
7. Label patients who are dead no. 4. Ensure that the bodies are moved to an area where they will be safe until they can be identified and proper action can be taken.

officials that something may be amiss. Physicians and medical assistants should be vigilant about cases that present themselves as well as common trends in syndromes. Be on the lookout for unusual patterns in affected patients. Indications of a bioterrorist attack might include many patients having been in the same place at the same time or an unusual distribution for common illnesses, such as an increase in chickenpox-like illness in adults that might be smallpox.

If you suspect that bioterrorism is responsible for an illness, report your suspicians to the physician. It is the responsibility of your facility to immediately contact the local public health department. The information about the patient should be recorded, and appropriate tests should be performed. The laboratory should be notified of the potential for bioterrorism. Additionally, consultations with specialists and discussions of all findings are necessary when bioterrorism is suspected. The following is a list of clues of a bioterroristic attack as defined by the American College of Physicians—American Society of Internal Medicine.

- Unusual temporal or geographic clustering of illness
- Unusual age distribution of common disease, such as an illness that appears to be chickenpox in adults but is really smallpox
- A large epidemic with greater caseloads than expected, especially in a discrete population
- More severe disease than expected
- Unusual route of exposure
- A disease that is outside its normal transmission season or is impossible to transmit naturally in the absence of its normal vector
- Multiple simultaneous epidemics of different diseases
- A disease outbreak with health consequences to humans and animals
- Unusual strains or variants of organisms or antimicrobial resistance patterns

In any disaster, you may be asked to perform triage. When you perform triage, you give each injured victim a tag that classifies the person as emergent (needing immediate care), urgent (needing care within several hours), nonurgent (needing care when time is not critical), or dead. The triage process is outlined in Procedure 44-10.

Summary

A medical emergency can occur anywhere—in a doctor's office, at home, in a restaurant, or on the street. The more you learn about handling each type of medical emergency, the more valuable your contributions to the situation become. You can make a substantial, positive difference in the health and lives of people who face medical emergencies to which you respond.

Always notify the doctor or the local EMS system when you encounter a medical emergency. Do not, at any time, perform procedures you have not been trained to do. Use common sense, assess the situation and the patient's condition, and provide first aid until a doctor or EMT arrives.

Patients having a medical emergency are often under extreme stress. Remember to stay calm and communicate clearly. Communicating with non-English-speaking patients and those with visual or hearing impairments requires special skills. You can develop these skills through educational and training programs you seek out or during routine office visits with these patients.

You may not be present when medical emergencies occur, so patients need to know how to respond to emergency circumstances. Take every opportunity to educate patients about preventing and responding to medical emergencies. Remember to draw on community resources when you provide information or support to patients and their families. There will always be opportunities to expand your knowledge, skills, and network for dealing with medical emergencies in your medical assisting work.

using an approved solution such as 10% bleach, before beginning any other procedure.

- Dispose of waste products carefully and correctly.
- Be sure to remove protective gear before leaving the laboratory.

Hazard Communication Standard. The Hazard Communication Standard requires that employees receive training regarding workplace hazards, including how to interpret documentation about hazardous substances that pose an exposure threat. Hazardous materials must be correctly labeled, and employees must have access to information about the materials. The information must include the measures that employees can take to protect themselves against harm from these substances.

Biohazard Labels. All containers used to store waste products, blood, blood products, or other specimens that may be contaminated with blood-borne pathogens are considered biohazardous. They must be clearly marked with the **biohazard symbol,** as shown in Figure 45-9. The biohazard symbol label must be bright orange-red and clearly lettered so that no one can mistake the meaning of the warning. Labels should be securely attached to containers.

In addition to individual biohazard labels that identify particular containers, warning signs must be posted in the

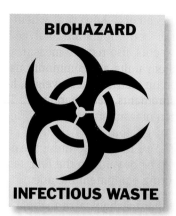

Figure 45-9. The biohazard symbol identifies material that has been exposed to potentially contaminated substances such as blood, blood products, or other body fluids.

laboratory itself. These signs, such as the one shown in Figure 45-10, identify the presence of biohazardous material and list important safeguards to follow.

Material Safety Data Sheets. Material Safety Data Sheets (MSDSs) contain information about hazardous chemicals or other substances. A sample MSDS is shown in Figure 45-11. Each MSDS must contain the following

BIOHAZARDS PRESENT!!!

- **NO** EATING.
- **NO** DRINKING.
- **NO** SMOKING.
- **NO** MOUTH PIPETTING.
- DO **NOT** APPLY COSMETICS OR LIP BALM.
- DO **NOT** MANIPULATE CONTACT LENSES.

Figure 45-10. The biohazard warning sign alerts personnel to the presence of potentially contaminated substances and advises them about safety guidelines.

860   **CHAPTER 45**

WAVICIDE-01

MATERIAL SAFETY DATA SHEET

Date Issued:

SECTION 1   IDENTIFICATION

Manufacturers Name and Address: Wave Energy Systems, Inc.
25 Mansard Court
Wayne, NJ 07470

Phone: 1-800-252-1125
Fax: (201) 633-1023

Hazardous Chemicals: Glutaraldehyde
Routes of entry: Inhalation ✓ Skin/Eye ✓ Ingestion ✓

Product Name: WAVICIDE-01 (2.5% aqueous glutaraldehyde solution)

Product Code: 0104 (case of 4 gallons) or 0112 (case of 12 quarts)

Product Type/General Information: Chemical Sterilant/Disinfectant

EPA Registration Number: 15136-1

Chemical Name: (active ingredient) 2.5% glutaraldehyde

PRECAUTIONARY LABELING
(HMIS Rating System)

Health	3
Flammability	0
Reactivity:	0
Physical Hazard:	None

The New Jersey Poison Control Center has been provided information for use in medical emergencies involving this product. Call 1-800-962-1253.

SECTION 2   HAZARDOUS INGREDIENTS/IDENTITY INFORMATION

WAVICIDE-01 contains the following hazardous ingredients at concentrations greater than 1.0%:

CHEMICAL COMPONENTS	CAS%	% w/v	OSHA PEL	ACGIH TLV
Glutaraldehyde (active ingredient)	111-30-8	2.5	0.2 ppm[1]	0.2 ppm

WAVICIDE-01 contains no hazardous ingredients listed as carcinogens or potential carcinogens by the National Toxicology Program (NTP), International Agency on Cancer (IARC) or OSHA, and present at a concentration greater than 0.1%.

[1] The OSHA Permissible Exposure Level (PEL) for glutaraldehyde was invalidated in 1992 by court order. However, the PEL may remain valid in some OSHA approved state plans, and also can be enforced by federal OSHA under its General Duty Clause.

SECTION 3   PHYSICAL/CHEMICAL CHARACTERISTICS

Boiling Point:	100°C/212°F	**Evaporation Rate:**	0.81 (Butyl Acetate = 1)
Specific Gravity:	1.005 - 1.013	**Solubility (H₂O):**	Complete
Vapor Pressure:	16.9 mm Hg	**Appearance & Color:**	A clear, slightly yellow liquid with typical aldehyde odor and added lemon scent.
Melting point:	N/A	**pH:**	Approximately 6.30
Vapor Density:	1.1 (air = 1)	**Molecular Weight:**	100.11 (glutaraldehyde)
Freezing Point:	0°C/32°F (same as water)	**Odor Threshold:**	0.04 ppm, detectable (ACGIH)

SECTION 4   FIRE AND EXPLOSION HAZARD DATA

Flash Point (Test Method): None (Tag Closed Cup ASTM D 56)

Special Fire Fighting Procedures: Self-Contained Breathing Apparatus (SCBA) and protective clothing should be worn when fighting chemical fires.

Unusual Fire and Explosion Hazards: None known   **Extinguishing Media:** Carbon dioxide, foam, dry chemical.

SECTION 5   REACTIVITY DATA

Stability: Unstable _____ Stable ✓   **Hazardous Polymerization:** May Occur _____ Will Not Occur ✓

Hazardous Decomposition Products: Thermal decomposition may produce carbon dioxide and or carbon monoxide.

Conditions and Materials to Avoid: Alkaline (pH > 10) and acidic (pH < 3) materials catalyze an aldol-type condensation (exothermic but not expected to be violent). Avoid High temperatures above 40°C/104°F and or evaporation of H₂O.

Figure 45-11. This two-page Material Safety Data Sheet (MSDS), as required by OSHA, contains important information about each hazardous substance used in the POL. (Courtesy of Wave Energy Systems, Inc., Wayne, NJ.) (continued)

Date Issued:

SECTION 6	HEALTH HAZARD DATA

Routes of Entry: *Inhalation.* ✓ *Skin.* ✓ *Ingestion:* ✓ *Eyes:* ✓

Signs and Symptoms Associated With Overexposure (one-time or repeated):

Ingestion: May cause irritation and possibly chemical burns of the mouth, throat, stomach and esophagus. May produce discomfort in the mouth, throat, chest and abdomen, nausea, vomiting, diarrhea, dizziness, faintness, drowsiness, thirst and weakness.

Eyes: Solution contact may cause damage, including severe corneal injury, which could permanently impair vision if prompt first-aid and medical treatment are not obtained. Vapors may cause stinging sensation in the eye with excess tear production, blinking, and redness of the conjuntiva.

Skin: Direct solution contact may cause skin irritation or aggravation of an existing dermatitis. May also cause skin to turn a harmless yellow or brown color.

Inhalation: Vapor is irritating to the respiratory tract. May cause stinging sensations in the nose and throat, chest discomfort and tightening, difficulty with breathing and headache. May also aggravate pre-existing asthma and pulmonary disease.

Emergency and First Aid Procedure:

Ingestion: DO NOT INDUCE VOMITING. Drink large quantities of water and call a physician immediately
NOTE TO PHYSICIAN: Probable mucosal damage from oral exposure may contraindicate the use of gastric lavage.

Eyes: Immediately flush eyes with water and continue washing for at least 15 minutes. Obtain medical attention immediately, and follow up with an ophthalmologist.

Skin: Immediately remove contaminated clothing and flush skin with soap and water for a minimum of 15 minutes. If irritation persists, seek medical attention. Wash or discard contaminated clothing.

Inhalation: Remove to fresh air. Give artificial respiration if not breathing. If breathing is difficult, oxygen may be given by qualified personnel. If irritation persists, seek medical help.

Medical Conditions Generally Aggravated by Overexposure: See above.

SECTION 7	PRECAUTIONS FOR SAFE HANDLING AND USE

Steps to be Taken if Material is Released or Spilled: Wear suitable protective equipment, including nitrile gloves, chemically resistant gown or apron, and protective eyewear (safety glasses or shield). A full face respirator, or half-face respirator with gas proof goggles, both worn with organic vapor cartridges, is recommended for small spills. A respirator is essential for large spills, or if you experience discomfort watery eyes, nasal or respiratory irritation) due to inadequate ventilation. For small spills of 1 gallon or less, gather up a bucket, household ammonia, and a sponge or mop. Don protective equipment and mix approximately 1 cup of ammonia with 1 cup of water in the bucket. Mop or sponge the ammonia mixture into the spill until thoroughly combined (about 2 minutes). Wipe or mop up resulting mixture and discard down the drain with a copious amount of water. Rinse bucket, mop or sponge with water, and give spill area a final wipe or mop with fresh water. Re-rinse all equipment, and allow spill area to dry. For large spills of more than 1 gallon, remove people from immediate spill area, and isolate until cleaned up. Don protective equipment including a respirator with organic vapor cartridges. Contain spill with absorbent material, ie. towels. Add approximately 228 grams of sodium bisulfite powder per gallon of WAVICIDE-01 spilled (aqueous sodium hydroxide and ammonium will also neutralize glutaraldehyde). With a sponge, mix neutralizing chemical into spill, and allow 5 minutes for deactivation to occur. Discard resulting mixture according to your facility's waste disposal guidelines. Mop spill area with fresh water. Rinse out all equipment (bucket, mop, towels) with large amounts of water. If paper towels were used, dispose of in a tightly closed trash bag. Let spill area dry, and if possible increase ventilation. Once glutaraldehyde odor is below allowable levels (TLV), the area may be released from isolation.

Waste Disposal Method: Dispose of WAVICIDE-01 after 30 days of re-use, or the MEC Indicator shows the solution is below it's minimum effective concentration (1.7% w/v), which ever is sooner. This may be accomplished by pouring solution down drain in accordance with state and local regulations. Flush with a large quantity of water. Do not reuse empty containers. Rinse thoroughly with water and dispose of in trash.

Precautions to be Taken in Handling and Storing: WAVICIDE-01 should be stored in it's original sealed container at controlled room temperature (15°C/50°F to 30°C/85°F).

Precautionary Labeling: Avoid contact with eyes, prolonged and repeated contact with skin, and contamination with food.

SECTION 8	TRANSPORTATION DATA & ADDITIONAL INFORMATION			

| Proper Shipping Name: | 2.5% Glutaraldehyde Solution | DOT (ground): Not regulated | IATA (air): Not Regulated | IMO (ocean): Not Regulated |
| Hazard Class: None | Labels: None needed | Packaging: None | ID#: None | Special Instructions: None | Reportable Quantity: None |

SECTION 9	CONTROL MEASURES

Eye Protection: Safety glasses, goggles or face shield recommended when working with WAVICIDE-01. An eye wash, and full face respirator with organic vapor cartridges or half face respirator with gas proof goggles and organic vapor cartridges should be available for emergency situations.

Ventilation: WAVICIDE-01 should be used in closed containers with tight fitting lids. The working area should be large enough with ventilation necessary to keep the level of atmospheric glutaraldehyde below the Threshold Limit Value (TLV). If the solution vapors are irritating to eyes and nose, the TLV is probably being exceeded, and additional ventilation may be necessary. A fume hood or self contained fume absorber may be appropriate for this purpose. Any ventilation should pull fumes away from worker and towards the floor.

Skin Protection: Nitrile gloves and a chemical resistant gown or apron should be worn when working with WAVICIDE-01. Rubber boots may be needed to contain large spills.

Respiratory Protection: None required if glutaraldehyde vapor levels are below the TLV. A full face respirator with organic vapor cartridges or SCBA should be available for emergencies.

SECTION 10	SPECIAL REQUIREMENTS

None

Figure 45-11. Material Safety Data Sheet (continued)

information about the product it describes:

- Substance name, as it appears on the container label
- Chemical name(s) of each ingredient
- Common name(s) of each ingredient
- Chemical characteristics of the product (boiling point, specific gravity, melting point, appearance, odor)
- Physical hazards posed by the product (fire, vapor pressure)
- Health hazards posed by the product (carcinogenicity [ability to cause cancer], routes and methods of entry, signs and symptoms of exposure)
- Guidelines for safe handling of the substance
- Emergency and first-aid procedures to be followed in the event of exposure

Hazard Labels. In addition to the MSDS, each hazardous substance must be identified with a hazard label. A **hazard label** is a shortened version of the MSDS that is permanently affixed to the substance container. A sample hazard label is shown in Figure 45-12.

OSHA Bloodborne Pathogens Standard. The

OSHA Bloodborne Pathogens Standard identifies methods for reducing the risk of transmission of blood-borne pathogens, specifically the hepatitis B virus (HBV) and the human immunodeficiency virus (HIV). HIV is the virus that causes acquired immunodeficiency syndrome (AIDS). The standard identifies laboratory procedures that must be followed to prevent occupational exposure. It also describes the procedure that must be followed in the event of exposure to one of these viruses. To be in compliance with this standard, an employer must meet the following requirements.

- A written OSHA Exposure Control Plan must be created and updated annually or whenever procedures that require exposure to potentially contaminated material are added or changed. The plan must be available to all employees and to authorized OSHA authorities.
- Training must be provided to all employees describing the documentation mandated by the standard. This documentation includes the symptoms, methods of transmission, and epidemiology of infectious diseases caused by blood-borne pathogens. Employees must also be instructed in the use of personal protective equipment, Universal Precautions, and engineering controls designed to prevent exposure. Procedures to follow in the event of exposure or emergency situations must also be part of the training.
- The employer must make hepatitis B vaccine available at no charge to all employees who are at risk for occupational exposure. Employees must either receive the vaccination or decline it in writing. The employer must maintain documentation of vaccinations and refusals. Employees who initially decline the vaccine are free to reverse their decision at any point during their employment.

Hazardous Waste Operations and Emergency Response Final Rule. OSHA regulations also extend

to the disposal of waste products generated during laboratory procedures. Hazardous waste products include the following:

- Blood
- Blood products
- Body fluids
- Body tissues
- Cultures
- Vaccines, killed or attenuated (live but weakened)
- Sharps
- Gloves
- Specula
- Inoculating loops
- Paper products contaminated with body fluids

Hazardous waste must be disposed of in properly constructed and labeled containers. Containers for sharps must be puncture-proof, leak-resistant, and rigid

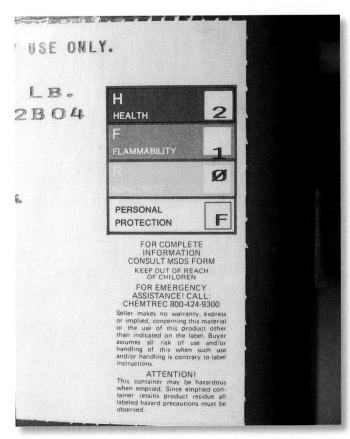

Figure 45-12. A hazard label is a condensed version of the MSDS and displays important information about a substance. It must be permanently affixed to the substance container.

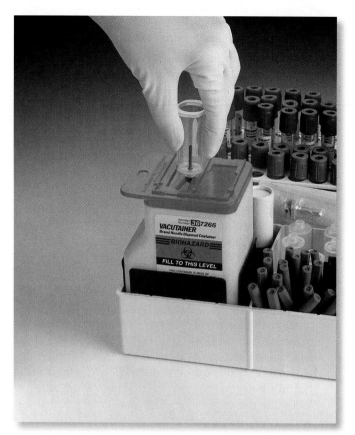

Figure 45-13. A sharps disposal container is a receptacle for used needles, lancets, specimen slides, and other disposable pointed or edged instruments, supplies, and equipment.

(Figure 45-13). Needles should be dropped into the sharps container without bending, breaking, or recapping them and with as little extra handling as possible. Other waste must be placed in plastic bags clearly labeled to identify the infectious contents. All biohazardous waste containers should be placed as close as possible to the area in which the waste is generated. This last procedure is followed to reduce the risk of spillage on the way to the disposal container.

Needlestick Safety and Prevention Act. In response to the Needlestick Safety and Prevention Act, which was signed into law in November 2000, OSHA revised the Bloodborne Pathogens Standard. The additional provisions to the standard are:

- Health-care employers must evaluate new safety-engineered control devices on an annual basis and implement the use of devices that reasonably reduce the risk of needlestick injuries
- Health-care facilities must maintain a detailed log of sharps injuries that are incurred from contaminated sharps
- Health-care employers must solicit input from employees involved in direct patient care to identify, evaluate, and implement engineering and work practice controls

Accident Prevention Guidelines

Work in the POL exposes you to hazards of four main types: physical, fire and electrical, chemical, and biologic. The following safeguards reduce the risk in one or more of these hazard categories. For example, by handling chemical containers carefully and correctly, you protect yourself from harmful chemical exposure as well as from physical injury from broken glass or other materials.

Physical Safety. There are many ways to ensure physical safety in the laboratory. You must understand and apply all the appropriate safeguards. Because accidents can happen, however, post emergency numbers in multiple locations throughout the laboratory. Once each quarter, make sure the numbers are accurate and up-to-date.

Some safeguards come under the heading of common sense. Their application requires no special knowledge.

- Walk, do not run, in the laboratory. Be careful when carrying objects through the laboratory, especially when approaching blind corners.
- Close all cabinet and closet doors and all desk and worktable drawers.
- Never use damaged equipment or supplies, such as cracked or chipped glassware.
- Do not overextend your reach when attempting to grasp supplies. Use only approved equipment, such as stepladders or stools, to reach high shelves. Do not climb onto chairs, desks, or tables to reach anything.
- When lifting an object, squat close to the object. Keep your back straight but not rigid. Lift the item by pushing up with your legs, not by pulling with your back. Hold the load firmly with both hands, close to your body. If necessary, put on a back-support belt before attempting to move heavy loads.

Being aware of the laboratory environment will help you protect your health and well-being. For example:

- Adjust your seat to the correct position to prevent back strain.
- If you are using a computer, take frequent breaks to reduce eyestrain and hand cramping.
- Do not eat or drink in the laboratory, and do not store food there. Never use laboratory supplies, such as beakers or flasks, for eating or drinking.
- Do not put anything in your mouth while working in the laboratory. (Some people have a habit of chewing on the end of their pencils, for example.)
- Do not apply makeup or lip balm or insert contact lenses in the laboratory.
- Familiarize yourself with the location of the first-aid kit. If you are responsible for the kit in your area, check it weekly to make sure that it is adequately stocked with supplies and that expiration dates on medications have not passed.
- Familiarize yourself with the location and operation of the emergency eyewash and shower stations.

Wear appropriate protective gear and clothing in the laboratory. Use heat-resistant mitts or gloves to prevent burns. Wear sturdy, low-heeled, closed-toe shoes with rubber soles to prevent injury if you drop or spill something and to avoid slipping. Do not wear dangling jewelry or loose clothing that could get caught in laboratory equipment. Keep hair pulled back or covered for the same reason.

When you work with laboratory equipment, always follow manufacturers' guidelines. For example, wait for centrifuges to stop spinning before you open them.

Many laboratory materials and supplies require special handling and precautions.

- Store caustic chemicals and other hazardous substances below eye level to reduce the risk of upsetting the container and spilling the substance into your eyes.
- Do not attempt to grasp bottles, jars, or other containers if your hands or the containers are wet.
- Close containers immediately after use.
- Clean up spills immediately. If the floor is wet, either dry it or use appropriate warning devices to alert others to the hazard.
- Clean up broken glass with a broom. Do not handle the debris. If the material is biohazardous, use tongs or forceps to pick up the glass. Package the pieces in a sturdy container with a label identifying the contents.

Fire and Electrical Safety. The equipment and materials used in the POL make it especially vulnerable to fire and electrical hazards. It is critical for you to know how to respond to a fire or electrical accident.

- Familiarize yourself with the location of all fire extinguishers and fire blankets in the laboratory. Review the floor plan, noting the location of fire exits.
- Make sure you know how to operate the fire extinguishers.
- Participate in all office fire drills.
- Familiarize yourself with the location of circuit breakers and emergency power shutoffs.

It is, of course, never acceptable to smoke in the laboratory. Keep your area clear of clutter such as boxes or empty storage containers. Such materials can feed, or even start, a fire. The following safeguards reduce electrical hazards.

- Avoid using extension cords. If they must be used, be sure the circuit is not overloaded. Tape extension cords to the floor to avoid tripping.
- Repair or replace equipment that has a broken or frayed cord.
- Dry your hands before working with electrical devices.
- Do not position electrical devices near sinks, faucets, or other sources of water. Be sure electrical cords do not run through water.

Work in the laboratory may sometimes require that you use a flame. Special precautions are essential in such circumstances.

- If you must use an open flame, extinguish it immediately after use.
- When using an open flame, be careful to keep your hair, clothing, and jewelry away from the flame source.
- If you must use a chemical in a procedure that requires an open flame, double-check the MSDS to identify the level of risk of fire for that chemical. If necessary, bring a fire extinguisher to the area in which you will be working.
- Never lean over an open flame.
- Never leave an open flame unattended.
- Turn off gas valves immediately after use. If you must use an open flame in the vicinity of a gas valve, always double-check to be sure the gas is off. Make sure there is adequate ventilation.

Chemical Safety. Familiarize yourself with the MSDS and hazard label of every chemical you will use during a procedure. If the MSDS indicates the need for special equipment or conditions to use a chemical safely, be sure you meet the requirements before beginning to work with the substance. General precautions as you prepare include the following.

- Wear protective gear to prevent harm to your skin or damage to your clothing. (Be sure to remove the protective gear before leaving the laboratory.)
- Always carry chemical containers with both hands as you gather supplies.
- Make sure you work in an area that is properly ventilated.

When you are ready to begin work, adhere to these guidelines.

- If you must smell the chemicals you are using, do not hold them directly under your nose. Instead, hold them a few inches away, and fan air across them and toward your nose.
- Work inside a fume hood if the chemical vapor is hazardous.
- Wear a personal ventilation device when working with certain chemicals, as specified by the MSDS.
- Never combine chemicals in ways not specifically required in test procedures.
- Mouth pipetting is prohibited at all times.
- If you are combining acids with other substances, always add the acid to the other substance. Adding substances to acid increases the risk of splashing.
- If you encounter a spill of an unknown chemical substance, do not pour any other chemicals on it. Clean it up following strict hazardous waste control procedures. Never touch an unknown substance with your bare hands.

Biologic Safety.   You will work with test specimens that may be contaminated with blood-borne or other pathogens. Treat every specimen as if it were contaminated.

- Follow Universal Precautions.
- If you have any cuts, lesions, or sores, do not expose yourself to potentially contaminated material. Consult your supervisor if you have any doubt about whether you can safely perform test procedures.
- Wash your hands before and after every procedure and whenever you come in contact with a potentially contaminated substance.
- Wear gloves at all times. Use other protective gear as appropriate to prevent exposing your eyes, nose, and mouth to potentially contaminated material.
- Mouth pipetting is prohibited at all times. Use specially made rubber suction bulbs to draw specimens mechanically.
- Work in a biologic safety cabinet (similar to a fume hood) when completing procedures that are likely to generate droplet sprays or splashes of potentially contaminated material.
- When transferring a blood specimen from a collection tube to another container, cover the tube stopper with an absorbent pad or a commercial stopper remover to prevent spray or splatter from the tube. Do not rock the stopper back and forth, because this could cause the tube to break. Always remove the stopper by opening it away from your face so that the vapor pressure flows away from you. Place the stopper on a sterile gauze pad while you work with the collection tube. Do not allow the stopper to come in contact with other work surfaces. Keep the collection tube stoppered unless you are actively using it.
- Establish clean and dirty areas in the laboratory. Place all used instruments and equipment in the dirty area for sanitization, disinfection, and sterilization.
- Disinfect your work area at least once a day with a 10% bleach solution or a germ-killing solution approved by the Environmental Protection Agency (EPA). If a spill occurs, immediately disinfect the work area.
- Dispose of waste products immediately.
- Dispose of needles in the appropriate sharps container. Do not bend, break, or recap a used needle, and never reuse a disposable needle.
- If an instrument or piece of equipment must be serviced, be sure it has been decontaminated first.
- If you use a bleach solution for disinfection, change it daily.

Accident Reporting.   Despite all precautions, accidents still occur in the laboratory. Armed with an understanding of the materials with which you are working and basic first-aid procedures, you should be able to deal with most emergencies. Your office should also have written procedures to follow in the event of an accident. Familiarize yourself with the procedures beforehand so that you will know what to do if an accident occurs.

Your first responsibility is to ensure your safety and that of your colleagues and patients. If someone is injured as a result of an accident, administer first aid if required, and take steps to ensure that appropriate health-care personnel take charge of the injured person.

If exposure to spilled chemicals or other substances does not pose a threat, clean up the spill. Take precautions to prevent any of the spilled substances from coming in contact with your skin or clothes. Use appropriate cleaning products for spilled chemicals. Do not touch broken pieces of glass with your hands. Use tongs or a broom and dustpan to pick up the pieces.

Disinfect the surfaces on which the substance spilled. Soaking surfaces with a 10% bleach solution, made fresh each day, is usually sufficient to remove any contamination from blood, blood products, or body fluids.

Report the accident to your supervisor or other personnel as required by your office's policies. If the accident involves exposure to blood or blood products, OSHA regulations require that several steps be followed:

1. Immediate cleaning of the area, including disinfection of contaminated surfaces and sterilization of contaminated instruments and equipment
2. Notification of a designated emergency contact, as identified in your office's safety manual
3. Documentation of the incident on a form similar to that shown in Figure 45-14, including the names of all parties involved, the names of witnesses, a description of the incident, and a record of medical treatments given to those involved
4. Medical evaluation and follow-up examination of the employees involved
5. Written evaluation of the medical condition of the involved individuals as well as testing for infection, provided that such testing does not violate confidentiality regulations

Housekeeping

There is a high risk of serious contamination in the laboratory. Laboratory housekeeping duties are designed to reduce the risk of disease transmission. Great care must be taken to ensure that these duties are done correctly and regularly. Guidelines to ensure good operating procedures and to reduce the risk of infection are as follows:

- Refer to your office's written policies and procedures to ensure that you are performing housekeeping duties correctly and according to schedule.
- Immediately clean up spills or splashes of potentially contaminated material. Depending on the material,

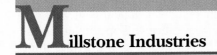

Millstone Industries

Central State Division
Incident Report

Name of Injured Employee _____

Department _____ Job Title _____

Supervisor _____

Date of Accident _____ Time _____

Nature of Injury _____

Was injured acting in a regular line of duty? _____

Was first aid given? _____ By whom? _____

Was designated emergency contact notified? _____

Did injured receive medical treatment? _____

Was injured tested for infection? _____ If no, why not? _____

Did injured go to ER? _____ Other? _____

Did injured leave work? _____ Date _____ Hour _____ A.M. P.M.

Did injured return to work? _____ Date _____ Hour _____ A.M. P.M.

Other Parties Involved _____

Names of Witnesses _____

Describe where and how accident occurred. _____

_____

_____

What, in your opinion, caused the accident? _____

_____

Has anything been done to prevent a similar accident? _____

_____

Has the hazard causing the injury been reported by telephone or in writing? _____

_____   _____
Date   Employee's Signature

_____   _____
Date   Supervisor's Signature

IF TREATMENT IS NEEDED, TAKE THE ORIGINAL AND DUPLICATE OF THIS FORM TO THE EMERGENCY ROOM.

....

This part for Employee Health Office use only

Was incident investigated? _____

Has injured had follow-up medical care? _____

Comments _____

Original copy to Employee Health Office   *Duplicate copy to supervisor*

Figure 45-14. In the event of an accident or exposure incident in the POL, OSHA regulations require completion of an incident report form.

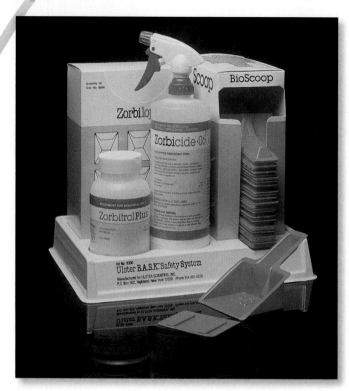

Figure 45-15. Certain substances require cleanup with specially formulated products such as these.

you may need to use special hazardous waste control products, such as those shown in Figure 45-15. Be sure to dry the area if appropriate, or clearly indicate that the area is still wet.

- Clean laboratory equipment immediately after use. Contaminants often become hard to remove if they are left on for a long time.
- Dispose of waste products carefully and correctly. Use extreme caution when handling and disposing of sharps. Procedure 45-2 describes how to dispose of biohazardous waste properly.

Quality Assurance Programs

The operation of a POL can have a significant impact on the health of the patients who depend on the medical practice for care. Accurate testing of specimens from patients is a primary concern. A **quality assurance program** is designed to monitor the quality of the patient care that a medical laboratory provides.

Clinical Laboratory Improvement Amendments

In response to public concern over the accuracy of laboratory tests, Congress enacted the **Clinical Laboratory Improvement Amendments of 1988 (CLIA '88).** This law placed all laboratory facilities that conduct tests for diagnosing, preventing, or treating human disease or for assessing human health under federal regulations

administered by the Health Care Financing Administration (HCFA) and the CDC. State governments have the ability to implement their own standards, which must be at least as stringent as federal standards. If your state has its own standards, your office will operate under those standards. The state health department provides information about which standards to follow in a given locale.

CLIA '88 has had a major impact on office laboratories. Because of the complexity of the regulations and the expense required to meet them, many doctors have closed their laboratories or sharply reduced the number of tests they perform. Several attempts have been made to change the federal legislation, including an effort to exempt POLs from the regulations. As the health-care debate continues, you may see changes in laboratory operations as a result of changes in CLIA '88 regulations.

As updated and implemented in 1992, CLIA '88 standards apply to four areas of laboratory operation: standards, fees, enforcement, and accreditation programs. Most of the regulations relate to laboratory standards. The specific standards that must be met depend on the test. Tests have been divided into three categories, based on complexity. They are Certificate of Waiver tests; Level I tests, of moderate complexity; and Level II tests, of high complexity.

Certificate of Waiver Tests. The **Certificate of Waiver tests,** as listed in Figure 45-16, are laboratory tests defined as follows.

- The tests pose an insignificant risk to the patient if they are performed or interpreted incorrectly

Certificate of Waiver Tests

Urine tests
- Urinalysis by dipstick (reagent strip) or tablet reagent (nonautomated) for bilirubin, glucose, hemoglobin, ketone, leukocytes, nitrite, pH, protein, specific gravity, and urobilinogen
- Ovulation (visual color comparison tests)
- Pregnancy (visual color comparison tests)

Blood tests
- Erythrocyte sedimentation rate (ESR), nonautomated
- Hemoglobin by copper sulfate, nonautomated
- Spun microhematocrit
- Blood glucose (using devices approved by the FDA for home use)
- Fecal occult blood
- Hemoglobin by single analyte instruments automated

Figure 45-16. A POL that performs only these tests is exempt from CLIA '88 standards once the POL has been granted a Certificate of Waiver.

PROCEDURE 45.2

Disposing of Biohazardous Waste

Objective: To correctly dispose of contaminated waste products, including sharps and contaminated cleaning and paper products

OSHA Guidelines

Materials: Biohazardous waste containers, gloves, waste materials

Method

To dispose of sharps or other materials that pose a danger of cutting, slicing, or puncturing the skin:

1. While wearing gloves, hold the article by the unpointed or blunt end.

2. Drop the object directly into an approved container. (If you are using an evacuation system, unscrew the needle and allow it to drop into the receptacle.) The container should be puncture-proof, with rigid sides and a tight-fitting lid.

3. If you are disposing of a needle, do not bend, break, or attempt to recap the needle before disposal. If the needle is equipped with a safety shield, slide the shield over the needle, and drop the entire assembly into the sharps container.

4. When the container is two-thirds full, replace it with an empty container. Depending on your office's procedures, the container and its contents may be sterilized before further disposal, or they may be collected by an authorized waste management agency.

5. Remove the gloves and wash your hands.

To dispose of contaminated paper waste:

1. While wearing gloves deposit the materials in a properly marked biohazardous waste container. A standard biohazardous waste container has an inner plastic liner, either red or orange and marked with the biohazard symbol, and a puncture-proof outer shell, also marked with the biohazard symbol.

2. If the container is full, secure the inner liner and place it in the appropriate area for biohazardous waste. (Biohazardous waste must be held in an area separate from regular waste and trash.)

3. Remove the gloves and wash your hands.

- The procedures involved are simple and accurate to such a degree that the risk of obtaining incorrect results is minimal
- The tests have been approved by the Food and Drug Administration (FDA) for use by patients at home

If laboratory management decides to perform these tests only, the office may apply for a Certificate of Waiver. When the certificate is granted, the laboratory is exempt from meeting various CLIA '88 standards that apply to the other two test categories. Such laboratories, however, are subject to the following: (1) random inspections to ensure that laboratories operating under a Certificate of Waiver are performing only those tests that qualify for the waiver and (2) investigation of the laboratory if there is any reason to believe the laboratory is not operating safely or if there have been complaints against the laboratory.

Level I Tests. Level I tests are moderately complex and make up approximately 75% of all tests performed in the laboratory. Among these tests are blood cell counts and cholesterol screening. Test procedures falling into the Level I category include studies involving

bacteriology, mycobacteriology, mycology, parasitology, virology, immunology, chemistry, hematology, and immunohematology.

A laboratory that performs Level I tests must be run by a pathologist who has an MD or PhD degree. Technicians performing the tests must have training beyond the high school level as defined by CLIA '88 regulations. All personnel must participate in a quality assurance program for laboratory procedures, and the laboratory is subject to periodic unannounced inspections and proficiency testing.

Level II Tests. Level II tests are considered high-complexity procedures. They include more complicated tests in the specialties and subspecialties included in Level I; any test in clinical cytogenics, histopathology, histocompatibility, and cytology; and any test not yet categorized by the CMS. Manufacturers' guidelines for testing products are often the best source for discovering the CMS determination for a test. The CMS publishes a directory of all Level I and Level II tests.

Like a laboratory that conducts Level I tests, a laboratory that conducts Level II tests is subject to inspection, proficiency testing, and participation in a quality assurance program, and it must be headed by a medical doctor or a scientist who has a PhD degree. Testing procedures can be performed only by qualified laboratory personnel, whose training exceeds that provided by high schools and is defined by CLIA '88 regulations.

Components of Quality Assurance

Every quality assurance program must include the following components, in a measurable and structured system, to satisfy CLIA '88 requirements:

- Quality control
- Instrument and equipment maintenance
- Proficiency testing
- Training and continuing education
- Standard operating procedures documentation

Quality Control and Maintenance

A **quality control program** is one component of a quality assurance program. The focus of the quality control program is to ensure accuracy in test results through careful monitoring of test procedures. To be in compliance with quality control standards, a laboratory must follow certain procedures.

Calibration. Testing equipment must be calibrated regularly, in accordance with manufacturers' guidelines. Calibration ensures that the equipment is operating correctly. Each calibration must be recorded in a quality control log, such as the one shown in Figure 45-17. Calibration routines are performed on a set of standards. A **standard** is a specimen, like the patient specimens you would normally process with the equipment except that the value for each standard is already known. The calibration procedure requires that the test equipment yield the correct results

for the standards supplied. Calibration routines are run on the standards alone, never with patient samples. They are used exclusively to ensure that the equipment is performing according to manufacturers' specifications.

Control Samples. **Control samples** are similar to standards in that they are specimens like those taken from a patient and have known values. Unlike standards, however, control samples are used every time before a patient sample is processed. Using a control sample serves as a check on the accuracy of the test. If the control tests do not fall within the manufacturer's prescribed ranges, patient samples are not analyzed, which prevents erroneous results.

The control samples for certain laboratory procedures show normal (negative) and abnormal (positive) results. Generally, positive and negative control samples are used with tests that yield a **qualitative test response** (the substance being tested for is either present or absent).

Other control samples are formulated to show when results fall within a normal range. These samples are used for tests that yield **quantitative test results** (the concentration of a test substance in a specimen). At least two control samples containing different concentrations of the test substance should be run for quantitative tests.

Reagent Control. Control samples or standards are also run every time you open a new supply of testing products, such as staining materials, culture media, and reagents. **Reagents** are chemicals or chemically treated substances used in test procedures. A reagent is formulated to react in specific ways when exposed under specific conditions. One example of a reagent is the chemically coated strip used in blood glucose monitoring. A visual change on the reagent strip (also called a dipstick) occurs in the presence of glucose in a blood sample. To ensure

Quality Control Daily Log								
Name of Unit	Glucose Control Solution	Strip Lot No./ Exp. Date	Low Control Value 35–65 mg/dL	High Control Value 175–235 mg/dL	Analyzed By	Date	Remedial Action Taken If Control Values Abnormal	Retest After Remedial Action Taken
XYZ Glucometer	Check-strip control solution	Lot 851 10/15/99	39 mg/dL	230 mg/dL	MSM	1/17/99		
Mitchell Drugs Glucometer	Check-strip control solution	Lot 851 10/15/99	50 mg/dL	267 mg/dL	MSM	1/17/99	Machine cleaned	220 mg/dL high value
XYZ Glucometer	Check-strip control solution	Lot 851 10/15/99	Unable to read	Unable to read	LMC	1/18/99	Battery changed	38 mg/dL low 198 mg/dL high
Mitchell Drugs Glucometer	Check-strip control solution	Lot 851 10/15/99	45 mg/dL	226 mg/dL	LMC	1/18/99		

Figure 45-17. The quality control log shows the completion of every quality control check conducted on a piece of equipment.

Reagent Strip / Lot # & Exp. Date	Test	Specific Gravity	pH	Protein	Glucose	Ketone	Bilirubin	Blood	Nitrite	Urobi-linogen	Control Test Date	Remedial Action Taken If Reading Is Abnormal	Retest Date	Technician Initials
	Reagent Strip Expected Range													
	Test Results													
	Reagent Strip Expected Range													
	Test Results													

Control Solution Exp. Date _____ Lot # _____

Figure 45-18. The reagent control log shows the quality testing performed on every batch or lot of reagent products.

the quality of reagents, you should keep a reagent control log. If a defective reagent test is identified, it can be tracked to its source. A sample reagent control log is shown in Figure 45-18.

Maintenance. Testing instruments and equipment must be properly maintained, and all maintenance procedures must be documented. Follow manufacturers' guidelines for performing instrument and equipment maintenance. A maintenance log provides a complete record of all work performed on an instrument or a piece of equipment (Figure 45-19).

Documentation. A quality control program depends first on careful adherence to procedures designed to identify problems with equipment calibration, errors in testing procedures, and defective testing supplies. The second component of a quality control program is the careful documentation of all procedures. Besides maintaining the quality control log, the reagent control log, and the equipment maintenance log, you will also complete the following records as part of a quality control program:

- Reference laboratory log, which lists specimens sent to another laboratory for testing
- Daily workload log, which shows all procedures completed during the workday

Proficiency Testing

All laboratories that perform Level I and Level II tests as identified by CLIA '88 must participate in a proficiency testing program. **Proficiency testing programs** measure the accuracy of test results and adherence to standard operating procedures. Generally, proficiency tests include two parts: (1) a control sample from the proficiency testing

Acme Medical Supplies
Equipment Maintenance Record

Practice Russo and Russo Medical Associates
Name of Equipment Acme Microscope Model ABC-123
Location Lab   **Purchase Date** 12/1/04

Date	Cleaning	Maintenance/Repair	Technician Initials
6/5	Microscope	Cleaned	CJC
6/11	Microscope high objective	Cleaned	DWM
6/14	Microscope	Changed bulb	CJC
6/16	Microscope eyepiece	Lens cover replaced	CJC
6/17	Microscope high objective	Cleaned	CJC

Figure 45-19. A maintenance log must be kept for every piece of laboratory equipment. All work done on the equipment must be recorded in the log.

organization engaged by your laboratory and (2) forms that must be completed to record the steps in the testing procedure. The control sample is processed normally, under the same conditions as any patient sample. The results, the forms, and sometimes the control samples are returned to the proficiency testing organization, which then informs your office of whether it has passed or failed the test. A passing mark means that your laboratory can continue to perform that particular test. A failing mark can mean that your laboratory must discontinue that test and possibly other tests as well.

Training, Continuing Education, and Documentation

One of your employer's responsibilities is to provide opportunities for employee training and continuing education. Another is to provide written reference materials and documentation for all procedures conducted in the POL. Your responsibility is to consult reference materials and take part in available training to keep your skills sharpened and up to date.

It may seem unnecessary to refer to written instructions for procedures that you do many times a day. Changes can be made in a procedure for many reasons, however, and you must be aware of these changes. Here are some reference materials with which you should be familiar:

- Material Safety Data Sheets
- Standard operating procedures
- Safety manuals
- Equipment manufacturers' user or reference guides
- Clinical Laboratory Technical Procedure Manuals
- Regulatory documentation (OSHA standards, CLIA '88 requirements)
- Maintenance and housekeeping schedules

Filling Out a Laboratory Requisition Form

As a medical assistant, it is your responsibility to ensure that the laboratory requisition form is properly completed. Missing information can lead to improper testing or lost results. The completed form should be included with the specimen collected or sent with the patient to the laboratory. Be sure to include the following information on all requisitions:

- Patient's full name, sex, date of birth, and address
- Patient's insurance information
- Physician's name, address, and phone number
- Source of the specimen
- Date and time of the specimen collection
- Test(s) requested

- Preliminary diagnosis
- Any current treatment that might affect the results

See Figure 45-20 for a sample laboratory requisitions form.

Communicating With the Patient

In your job as a medical assistant, you will be involved with patients before they submit samples for laboratory testing, during the specimen collection procedure, and after the physician has interpreted the test results. It is your responsibility to ensure that patients understand what is expected of them every step of the way.

Before the Test

Certain tests require patients to prepare by fasting or restricting fluid intake. It is your duty to explain test preparations. Use simple, nontechnical language and check with patients to be sure they understand the information. In some cases providing a written instruction sheet may be helpful.

Explaining the reason for the preparation can help ensure compliance or unearth potential problems. For example, if you explain to a patient that he is to refrain from drinking anything for a particular period, he might ask whether that includes the water he uses to take a certain medication. You can then make sure the patient receives the answers he will need for carrying out the physician's orders in light of his own circumstances.

If you are the person who collects specimens, you need to determine whether patients have correctly completed the required test preparations. Test results are invalid in some cases if patients fail to follow test preparation guidelines. When preparations have not been completed correctly, discuss the situation with the physician or other appropriate staff member as required by your office to determine whether the specimen should still be collected. If the specimen is not collected, document the reason the test was not carried out as requested. Review the guidelines for specimen collection with the patient, and schedule another appointment if appropriate.

During Specimen Collection

The instructions you deliver to patients during specimen collection vary with the nature of the specimen. Always deliver instructions clearly and in language patients can understand. Do not assume that patients do not need to hear the instructions, even if they have had the test before. Explain what you must do and what patients must do before moving to each new step in the process.

Patients are understandably nervous during many collection procedures. In addition to communicating technical information, you should provide any helpful advice

<table>
<tr><td colspan="2">LAB USE ONLY</td><td rowspan="2">Laboratory
Name & Address</td><td colspan="2">Requesting Physician
Information</td></tr>
<tr><td>Acct #</td><td></td><td rowspan="2">Address</td></tr>
<tr><td>DATE</td><td></td><td></td></tr>
<tr><td>TIME</td><td></td></tr>
</table>

Patient Information Patient Name (Last)	(First)		(MI)	Date of Birth / /	Phone Number
Address	City, State		Zip	Phone Number	
Patient I.D. Number	Responsible Party (Last)	(First) (Phone)	□ Male □ Female		
Social Security Number	Physician		Date Time Specimen Collection		

Bill: Check One
□ Our account   □ Medicare
□ Insurance Co./Patient

Complete the Following Information for Billing a Patient and/or a Third Party Agency

Policy Holder Name	Policy Holder Address: Policy Holder Phone Number:	Relation □ Self □ Spouse □ Child □ Other _____
Insurance Co. Name	Address Insurance Co.	City , State, Zip
Employer		
Policy Group #	PATIENT or GUARDIAN SIGNATURE:	DATE:

CHECK DESIRED TESTS   PLEASE PROVIDE ICD=9-CM#

√	ORGAN DISEASE PANELS, BLOOD	ICD-9	√	TEST, BLOOD	ICD-9	√	TEST, BLOOD	ICD-9	√	TEST, URINE	ICD-9
	ACUTE HEP. A,B,C			ESR			WBC with diff			U/A Routine	
	BASIC METABOLIC			EBV			PT				
	THYROID			FBS			PTT				
	ELECTROLYTES	A β-Kemp strep			Bleeding time						
	HEPATIC FUNCTION			Hgb			PCO_2				
	LIPID PROFILE			Hct			PO_2				
	RENAL FUNCTION			HgbA1c			CO_2				
	TEST, BLOOD			HIV antibodies			HCO_3			**MICROBIOLOGY**	
	ACE			Insulin			Ca^{++}			AFB culture	
	ADH			Iron			Cl^-			C & S	
	ALT			Ketone bodies						Chlamydia screen	
	AFP			LD						Endocervical culture	
	Amylase			pH						GC screen	
	Acetone			Phenylalanine						Gram stain	
	AST			K^+ and Na^+			**TEST, URINE**			O & P	
	Bilirubin			Proteins, Albumin			Cys			Strep A culture	
	BUN			Proteins, Fibrinogen			CrCl			Throat culture	
	CEA			PSA			Glucose			Urine culture	
	Calcium, total			RBC			HCG			Viral culture	
	Carbon dioxide, total			Sickle cells			UBG			Wound culture	
	Cholesterol, total			TSH			UFC				
	Cholesterol, HDLs			T3			UK				
	Cholesterol, LDLs			T4			UNA				
	CK			Uric Acid			Uosm				
	CMV			WBC			UUN				

Figure 45-20. The laboratory requisition form must be accurately completed.

that may make the test easier. Also provide reassurance as appropriate. For example, if a patient asks whether the blood-drawing procedure is painful, explain that a sharp stick or stinging sensation may be experienced when the needle is inserted but that no pain should be felt after that. Let the patient be your guide in determining how much information to provide. Some people want to know every detail, whereas others prefer to know as little as possible.

One important aspect of communicating with patients about testing procedures is your nonverbal communication skills. Even if you deliver accurate technical information and answer every question patients have, there can still be a breakdown in communication if your nonverbal signals do not support your verbal message. Follow these guidelines to ensure that your nonverbal actions are helping, not hindering, the communication process.

- Strike a balance between a strict, businesslike attitude and overly familiar friendliness. Your actions must impress on the patient that you are well informed about the procedure involved and that you care about the patient's understanding of it.
- Treat the patient with respect. Address the patient by name, using the appropriate courtesy title unless you have been invited to use the patient's first name or the patient is a child. Provide privacy during specimen collection. Privacy needs may be met by using a separate room or contained area for drawing blood, for example; a private bathroom is best for collecting urine specimens.
- Recognize that the patient may be under stress because of the test procedure or the pending results. Some patients may be familiar with the test procedures, but others may not know what to expect. You may need to repeat instructions or explain what you are doing more than one time. Remain calm and patient—never be abrupt or condescending.
- Direct your attention to the patient, particularly during a procedure that might be uncomfortable, such as drawing blood. Unless an emergency develops, pay attention to nothing else at that time.

After Specimen Collection

If the patient must follow particular guidelines after you collect the specimen, explain them. Commonly, posttest instructions deal with care of venipuncture sites, signs and symptoms of infection, additional or continuing dietary restrictions, and the schedule for further testing if it is necessary.

When the Test Results Return

When you receive the tests results, do not communicate them to the patient but to the doctor. Only the doctor is qualified to interpret test results for the patient. Your role in reporting results comes after the doctor examines the test information and prepares a report. Sometimes the doctor discusses the results with the patient. At other times you will be asked to convey the test results to the patient along with instructions from the doctor. Answer only those patient questions that are within the range of your knowledge and experience. If the patient needs more information than you can provide, refer the patient to the doctor.

Record Keeping

The importance of accurate and complete record keeping can be summed up in one statement: If it is not written down, it was not done. This motto applies to all your duties as a medical assistant. Besides recording information about quality control and equipment maintenance, you may be called on to handle inventory control, record test results in patient records, and keep track of every specimen that passes through your hands. You may need to use standard abbreviations for measures when recording test results. Figure 45-21 provides a list of common abbreviations used in the laboratory.

Inventory Control

You will be responsible for taking inventory of equipment and supplies to ensure that the POL never runs out of them. To do so, you will keep a list of items that are used routinely and reordered systematically. Establish a regular

Abbreviations for Common Laboratory Measures

cm = centimeter
cm^3 = cubic centimeter
dL = deciliter
fl oz = fluid ounce
g = gram
L = liter
lb = pound
m = meter
mg = milligram
mL = milliliter
mm = millimeter
mm Hg = millimeters of mercury
oz = ounce
pt = pint
QNS = quantity not sufficient
qt = quart
U = unit
wt = weight

Figure 45-21. You may encounter these common abbreviations when recording patients' test results.

schedule for counting items in the POL, perhaps every week or so. Then estimate when you will probably need to reorder an item—and put the date on your calendar.

Patient Records

When recording test results, it is your responsibility to identify unusual findings. Many offices require that out-of-range test results be circled or underlined in red. Follow the procedure established by your office. Test results are not communicated to the patient until the physician has had the opportunity to review the information. The physician usually initials or otherwise marks the records after examining them.

Specimen Identification

All specimens must be clearly identified with the patient's name, the patient's identification code if your office uses one, the date and time the specimen was collected, the initials of the person who collected the specimen, the physician's name, and other information as required by the test procedure or your office. If you encounter an unidentified or incorrectly identified specimen, you must make an effort to track it to its source. The specimen will probably be discarded or destroyed, however, because there is no guarantee that it was identified correctly. Even if you do manage to identify it, it may have been compromised in some way.

Summary

The physician's office laboratory offers many opportunities for interesting and satisfying work in your role as a medical assistant. Those opportunities carry with them the responsibility to maintain and improve your technical skills; to stay abreast of technological, legislative, and regulatory developments; to take every precaution to prevent the transmission of disease and the occurrence of accidents or emergency situations; and to seek ways to improve the quality of patient care.

Keeping a level head and applying common sense will go a long way toward making your work in the laboratory efficient and accurate. Take time to do a procedure correctly the first time. Avoid shortcuts—they lead to mistakes and lost time.

The quantity of information you will need to learn, integrate, and convey to the patient through your actions and educational efforts may be daunting at first. As you gain understanding and confidence in your skills, however, much of it will become routine.

REVIEW

CHAPTER 45

CASE STUDY QUESTIONS

Now that you have completed this chapter, review the case study at the beginning of the chapter and answer the following questions:

1. What is a POL?
2. What enactment regulates laboratories, personnel, and the testing they perform?
3. What is the difference between waived testing and Level I testing?
4. Does quality control have an impact on laboratories? If so, how?
5. Should you perform the testing as requested? Why or why not?

Discussion Questions

1. Identify five common physical hazards in the laboratory and the steps you can take to eliminate them.
2. What responsibilities does an employer have under the OSHA Bloodborne Pathogens Standard?
3. A common instrument used in laboratories is a microscope. Identify the component parts of a microscope.
4. What information must be included on MSOSs for chemicals?
5. When laboratory results return for a patient, how should the report be routed?

Critical Thinking Questions

1. While you are holding a vial of blood, it slips out of your hand and breaks. What should you do?
2. How could a physician's office laboratory be more advantageous than a reference laboratory? What advantages does a reference laboratory afford?

3. What types of accident prevention guidelines fall under a commonsense heading?
4. What nonverbal communication techniques can you use when you are instructing patients during the specimen collection process?

Application Activities

1. Examine a prepared slide under a microscope. With a partner, practice bringing the slide specimen into focus with each objective. Partners should check each other's work.
2. Obtain a Material Safety Data Sheet, and review the information on it. Explain to another student what hazards the substance poses, what measures can be taken to avoid injury from the substance, and what steps should be taken in the event of an accident.
3. With another student acting as your patient, explain the preparations necessary for a common blood test. Prepare a set of written instructions, but before giving them to the "patient," ask him to repeat the oral instructions you gave. Compare the patient's version to your written instructions to see how clearly you conveyed the preparation information.

Internet Activity

Use the Internet to access the Web site for the American Society of Clinical Pathologists and American Medical Technologists. Provide a description of the educational requirements that you need in order to take their examinations and become a medical laboratory assistant.

CHAPTER 46

Introduction to Microbiology

AREAS OF COMPETENCE

2003 Role Delineation Study

CLINICAL

Fundamental Principles

- Apply principles of aseptic technique and infection control
- Comply with quality assurance practices

Diagnostic Orders

- Collect and process specimens
- Perform diagnostic tests

Patient Care

- Obtain patient history and vital signs

GENERAL

Legal Concepts

- Document accurately

CHAPTER OUTLINE

- Microbiology and the Role of the Medical Assistant
- How Microorganisms Cause Disease
- Classification and Naming of Microorganisms
- Viruses
- Bacteria
- Protozoans
- Fungi
- Multicellular Parasites
- How Infections Are Diagnosed
- Specimen Collection
- Transporting Specimens to an Outside Laboratory
- Direct Examination of Specimens
- Preparation and Examination of Stained Specimens
- Culturing Specimens in the Medical Office
- Determining Antimicrobial Sensitivity
- Quality Control in the Medical Office

OBJECTIVES

After completing Chapter 46, you will be able to:

46.1 Define microbiology.

46.2 Describe how microorganisms cause disease.

46.3 Describe how microorganisms are classified and named.

46.4 Explain how viruses, bacteria, protozoans, fungi, and parasites differ and give examples of each.

KEY TERMS

- acid-fast stain
- aerobe
- agar
- anaerobe
- antimicrobial
- bacillus
- coccus
- colony
- culture
- culture and sensitivity (C and S)
- culture medium
- etiologic agent
- facultative
- fungus
- gram-negative
- gram-positive
- Gram's stain
- KOH mount
- microbiology
- mold
- mordant
- O and P specimen
- parasite
- protozoan
- qualitative analysis
- quality control (QC)
- quantitative analysis
- smear
- spirillum
- stain
- vibrio
- virus
- wet mount
- yeast

46.5 Describe the process involved in diagnosing an infection.

46.6 List general guidelines for obtaining specimens.

46.7 Describe how throat culture, urine, sputum, wound, and stool specimens are obtained.

46.8 Explain how to transport specimens to outside laboratories.

46.9 Describe two techniques used in the direct examination of culture specimens.

46.10 Explain how to prepare and examine stained specimens.

46.11 Describe how to culture specimens in the medical office.

46.12 Explain how cultures are interpreted.

46.13 Describe how to perform an antimicrobial sensitivity determination.

46.14 Explain how to implement quality control measures in the microbiology laboratory.

Introduction

Humans are surrounded by tiny living organisms invisible to the naked eye. For the most part, these microorganisms cause no problems; however, when they are pathogenic in nature or are displaced from their natural environment, they can cause infections and disease. This chapter addresses the different life forms of microorganisms and how they may be identified; it also teaches you the proper collection technique for common types of specimens. You will learn about the processes involved in identifying microorganisms, the types of culture media used for these processes, how antimicrobial testing is done, and how quality control fits into ensuring reliable patient results.

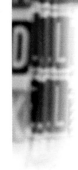

CASE STUDY

You awoke this morning with a scratchy sore throat and slight fever. You decide to go to work at the doctor's office because you don't really feel that bad, but as the morning progresses, so do your symptoms. You ask the doctor for permission to have a throat culture obtained, and with approval, you ask another medical assistant to collect the specimen. While the specimen is being collected, you can't help but notice that the swab touches your lips and tongue, but not the back of your throat. The rapid strep test is negative, so the doctor does not prescribe any medication for you. The next morning when you arise, you feel much worse and have a temperature of 102.8°. When you return to the office, the doctor briefly examines you and decides to repeat the test; this one is properly collected and the results come back as positive for strep throat. You are then prescribed antibiotics and sent home to rest.

As you read this chapter, consider the following questions:

1. What is the proper technique for collecting a throat specimen?
2. Why do you think the first test result came back as negative?
3. What organism is responsible for causing strep throat?
4. What complications may have developed if you had not had another throat culture obtained and been prescribed antibiotics?

Microbiology and the Role of the Medical Assistant

Microbiology is the study of microorganisms—simple forms of life that are microscopic (visible only through a microscope) and are commonly made up of a single cell. Microorganisms are found everywhere. Some microorganisms are normally found on the skin and within the human body; they are called normal flora. They do not typically cause disease. Instead, they perform a number of important functions. For example, microorganisms in the intestines produce vitamins and help digest food. They also help protect the body from infection.

Many microorganisms cause infections. These microorganisms are referred to as pathogenic, or disease-causing. Infections can be mild, as in the case of the common cold. Infections can, however, sometimes lead to serious conditions. The proper diagnosis and treatment of infections are essential to restoring good health.

You may assist the physician in performing a number of microbiologic procedures that aid in diagnosing and treating infectious diseases. The types of microbiologic procedures you may be required to perform in the medical office include obtaining specimens or assisting the physician in doing so, preparing specimens for direct examination by the physician, and preparing specimens for transportation to a microbiology laboratory for identification.

Some physicians' offices have their own laboratories and are equipped to perform certain microbiology procedures. If you work in such an office, you may be required to perform additional microbiologic procedures.

How Microorganisms Cause Disease

Anton van Leeuwenhoek first observed single-celled organisms through a microscope more than 300 years ago. It was not until much later, however, that microorganisms were identified as the cause of disease, through the works of scientists such as Louis Pasteur and Robert Koch.

Microorganisms can cause disease in a variety of ways. They may use up nutrients or other materials needed by the cells and tissues they invade. Microorganisms may damage body cells directly by reproducing themselves within cells, or the presence of microorgan-isms may make body cells the targets of the body's own defenses. Some microorganisms produce toxins, or poisons, that damage cells and tissues. Infecting microorganisms, or toxins they produce, may remain localized or may travel throughout the body, damaging or killing cells and tissues. The resulting symptoms include local swelling, pain, warmth, and redness along with generalized symptoms of fever, tiredness, aches, and weakness. Infection by certain organisms may also cause skin reactions, gastrointestinal upset, or other symptoms.

Pathogenic organisms can be transmitted from one person to another in one of two ways:

1. Through direct person-to-person contact, such as touching
2. Through indirect contact, as with vectors, contaminated objects, droplets expelled in the air, or contaminated food or drink

The microorganisms that make up normal flora, in addition to intact skin and mucous membranes, act as a barrier against infection by certain pathogens. Even these protective microorganisms, however, can cause infection if they invade other areas of the body.

Classification and Naming of Microorganisms

There are many different types of microorganisms, several of which can cause disease. Scientists classify microorganisms on the basis of their structure. Common classifications of microorganisms include the following:

- Subcellular, which consist of hereditary material, either deoxyribonucleic acid (DNA) or ribonucleic acid (RNA), surrounded by a protein coat
- Prokaryotic, which have a simple cell structure with no nucleus and no organelles in the cytoplasm
- Eukaryotic, which have a complex cell structure containing a nucleus and specialized organelles in the cytoplasm

Table 46-1 lists the characteristics that distinguish these classifications as well as the types of microorganisms found in the classifications. Types of microorganisms include the following:

- Viruses
- Bacteria
- Protozoans
- Fungi
- Multicellular parasites

These types may be further divided into special groups that share certain characteristics. For example, within the bacteria are the special groups mycobacteria and rickettsiae, within each of which the members share distinct characteristics.

Specific microorganisms are named in a standard way, using two words. The first word refers to the genus (a category of biologic classification between the family and the species) to which the microorganism belongs. The second word refers to the particular species of the organism. Each species represents a distinct kind of microorganism. For

TABLE 46-1 Classifications of Microorganisms		
Classification	**Characteristics**	**Examples**
Subcellular	Noncellular Nucleic acid surrounded by protein coat	Viruses
Prokaryotic cells	Simple structure Single chromosome No organelles	Bacteria
Eukaryotic cells	Highly structured Nucleus and cytoplasm Organelles	Protozoans, fungi, parasites

example, within the bacteria is the *Staphylococcus* genus. Then within that genus are various species such as *Staphylococcus aureus* and *Staphylococcus epidermidis*. Although the two bacteria belong to the same genus, they differ greatly in their ability to cause disease. The first letter of the genus is always capitalized, and the species name is always written in all lowercase letters.

Viruses

Viruses are among the smallest known infectious agents. They cannot be seen with a regular microscope. Viruses are a simpler life form than the cell, consisting only of nucleic acid surrounded by a protein coat, as shown in Figure 46-1. Because of this fact, viruses can live and grow only within the living cells of other organisms.

Many viruses cause disease in people. Viruses are the cause of many of the common illnesses and conditions seen frequently in the medical office, including the common cold, influenza, chickenpox, croup, hepatitis, mononucleosis, and warts. Other illnesses caused by viruses are acquired immunodeficiency syndrome (AIDS), mumps, rubella, measles, encephalitis, and herpes. Vaccines are available to protect people from many of these viruses.

Bacteria

Bacteria are single-celled prokaryotic organisms that reproduce very quickly and are one of the major causes of disease. Under the right conditions—the right temperature, the right nutrients, and moisture—bacterial cells can double in number in 15 to 30 minutes. This rapid reproduction is one reason why untreated infections can be dangerous.

Classification and Identification

There are many different kinds of bacteria and many ways to identify them. Bacteria can be classified according to their shape, their ability to retain certain dyes, their ability to grow with or without air, and certain biochemical reactions. Table 46-2 lists some of the major groups of bacteria, with distinguishing characteristics and a few examples.

Shape. The most common way to classify bacteria is according to their shape. A **coccus** (plural, cocci) is spherical, round, or ovoid; a **bacillus** (plural, bacilli) is rod-shaped;

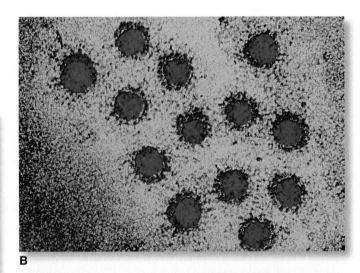

B

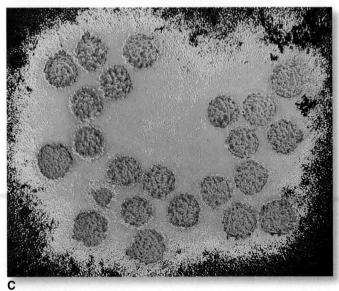

A

C

Figure 46-1. Three types of viral diseases often seen in medical offices are (a) influenza, (b) hepatitis, and (c) warts.

TABLE 46-2 Some Major Groups of Bacteria

Gram-Positive Bacteria

Shape	Characteristic	Genus	Species
Spherical, round, or ovoid	Grow in clusters Grow in chains	Staphylococcus Streptococcus	aureus epidermidis pyogenes pneumoniae
Straight rod	Are aerobic Are anaerobic	Bacillus Clostridium	subtilis botulinum tetani

Gram-Negative Bacteria

Shape	Characteristic	Genus	Species
Spherical, round, or ovoid	Are aerobic	Neisseria	meningitidis gonorrhoeae
Straight rod	Are aerobic	Pseudomonas Haemophilus	aeruginosa influenzae
	Are facultative	Escherichia Salmonella Shigella	coli typhi dysenteriae
Comma	Are facultative	Vibrio	cholerae
Spiral	Move by undulating	Treponema	pallidum

Other Groups

Shape	Characteristic	Genus	Species
Straight, curved, or branched rod	Are acid-fast	Mycobacterium	tuberculosis
Variable	Have no rigid cell wall Are intracellular parasites	Mycoplasma Rickettsia	pneumoniae rickettsii
Spherical, round, or ovoid	Are intracellular parasites	Chlamydia	trachomatis

a **spirillum** (plural, spirilla) is spiral-shaped; and a **vibrio** (plural, vibrios) is comma-shaped. Figure 46-2 illustrates the four shapes.

- Cocci can be further divided into three types. Staphylococci are grapelike clusters of cocci commonly found on the skin. One species of this microorganism causes a variety of infections, including boils, acne, abscesses, food poisoning, and a type of pneumonia. Diplococci are pairs of cocci. The causative agents for gonorrhea and some forms of meningitis are diplococci. Streptococci are cocci that grow in chains. These microorganisms are responsible for infections such as strep throat, certain types of pneumonia, and rheumatic fever.
- Bacilli, or rod-shaped bacteria, are responsible for a wide variety of infections, including gastroenteritis, tuberculosis, pneumonia, whooping cough, urinary tract infections, botulism, and tetanus.
- Spirilla, or spiral-shaped bacteria, are responsible for infections such as syphilis and Lyme disease.
- Vibrios, or comma-shaped bacteria, are responsible for diseases such as cholera and some cases of food poisoning.

Ability to Retain Certain Dyes. In addition to their shape, bacteria are commonly classified by how they react to certain stains. A **stain** is a solution of a dye or group of dyes that imparts a color to microorganisms. The most common staining procedure in use today is the **Gram's stain,** a method of staining that differentiates bacteria according to the chemical composition of their cell walls. This procedure is often performed in the medical office. Another important stain is the **acid-fast stain,** a staining procedure for identifying bacteria with a waxy cell wall. The bacteria that cause tuberculosis can be stained with this procedure.

Ability to Grow in the Presence or Absence of Air. Bacteria that grow best in the presence of oxygen are referred to as **aerobes.** Those that grow best in the absence of oxygen are referred to as **anaerobes.** Organisms that can grow in either environment are referred to as being **facultative.** Although most common bacteria are aerobes, many of the bacteria that make up the normal flora of the body are anaerobes. Not surprisingly, anaerobes are often responsible for infections within the body.

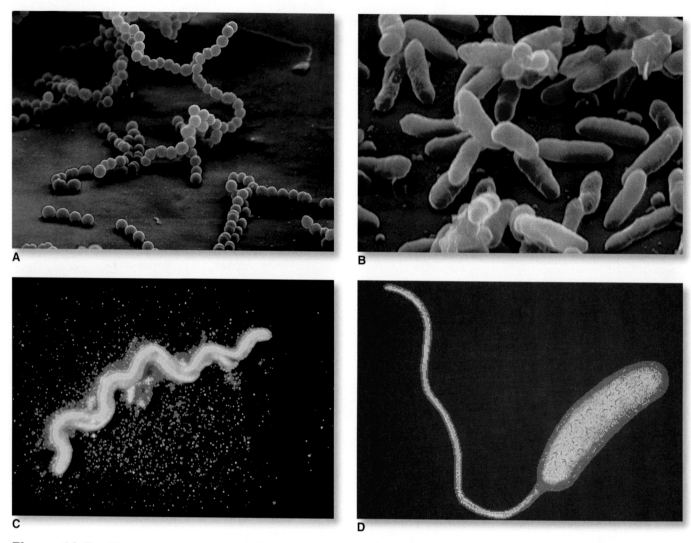

Figure 46-2. The four bacterial classifications by shape are (a) coccus, (b) bacillus, (c) spirillum, and (d) vibrio.

Biochemical Reactions. Many closely related bacteria can be differentiated from one another only by certain biochemical reactions that occur within the bacterial cell. One way to identify a particular bacterial strain is to look at what type of sugars the bacteria can use as food.

Special Groups of Bacteria

Several groups of bacteria have certain characteristics that set them apart from most other bacteria. These include the mycobacteria, rickettsiae, chlamydiae, and mycoplasmas.

Mycobacteria. Mycobacteria are rod-shaped bacilli with a distinct cell wall that differs from that of most bacteria. Certain types of mycobacteria cause disease in humans. For example, *Mycobacterium tuberculosis* causes the respiratory disease tuberculosis, and *Mycobacterium leprae* causes leprosy.

Rickettsiae. Rickettsiae are very small bacteria that can live and grow only within other living cells. Rickettsiae are commonly found in insects such as ticks and mites but

may be transmitted to humans through bites. Rickettsiae are responsible for diseases such as Rocky Mountain spotted fever and typhus.

Chlamydiae. Chlamydiae are organisms that differ from other bacteria in the structure of their cell walls. Like rickettsiae, they can live and grow only within other living cells. In humans, chlamydiae can cause venereal disease, eye disease, certain types of pneumonia, and certain types of heart disease.

Mycoplasmas. Mycoplasmas are small bacteria that completely lack the rigid cell wall of other bacteria. These bacteria cause a variety of human diseases, including venereal disease and a form of pneumonia.

Protozoans

Protozoans are single-celled eukaryotic organisms that are generally much larger than bacteria. Protozoans are found in soil and water, and most do not cause disease in people. Certain protozoans are pathogenic, however, and cause diseases such as malaria (see Figure 46-3), amebic dysentery (a type of diarrhea), and trichomoniasis vaginitis (a type of venereal disease). Protozoal diseases are a leading cause of death in developing countries because the lack of proper sanitation in some areas promotes their spread. These diseases are also common in patients with depressed immune systems.

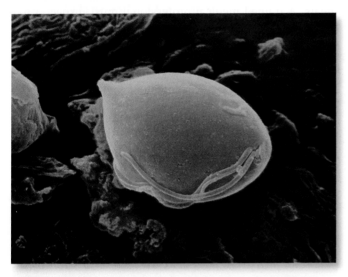

Figure 46-3. The protozoan *Trichomonus vaginalis* causes a venereal disease in humans.

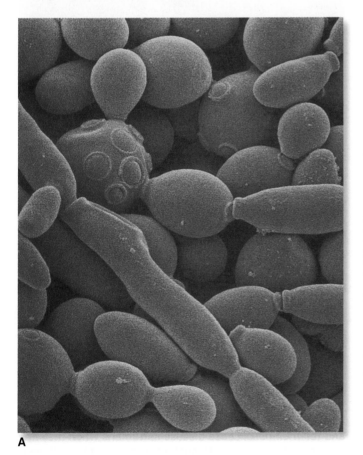

Fungi

A **fungus** (plural, fungi) is a eukaryotic organism that has a rigid cell wall at some stage in the life cycle. Fungi that grow mainly as single-celled organisms that reproduce by budding are referred to as **yeasts,** whereas fungi that grow into large, fuzzy, multicelled organisms that produce spores are called **molds.** Figure 46-4 shows the differences between these two types of fungi.

Most fungi do not cause disease in humans. Of those that do, the majority produce superficial infections such as athlete's foot (tinea pedis), ringworm, thrush, and vaginal yeast infections. Fungi can produce serious, life-threatening illness, however, when they infect the body's internal tissues. This kind of infection can occur when patients have a depressed immune system, as in patients who are undergoing treatment for cancer and patients with AIDS.

Multicellular Parasites

A **parasite** is an organism that lives on or in another organism and uses that other organism for its own nourishment, or for some other advantage, to the detriment of the host organism. Viruses, rickettsiae, chlamydiae, and some protozoans are parasitic. Multicellular organisms can also be parasitic, and some of these organisms are microscopic during all or part of their lives. An infection caused by a parasite is called an infestation. Multicellular parasites that cause human disease include certain worms and insects, as illustrated in Figure 46-5.

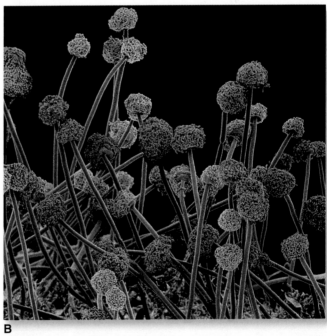

A   B

Figure 46-4. Because fungi lack the ability to make their own food, they depend on other life forms. (a) Single-celled fungi are called yeasts. (b) Multicelled fungi are called molds.

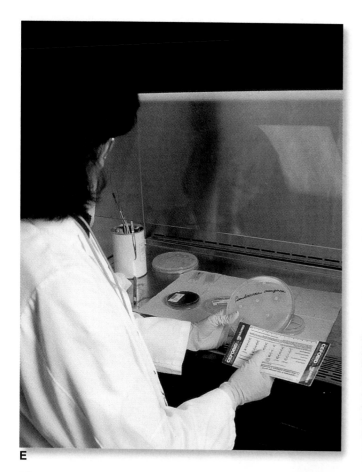

E

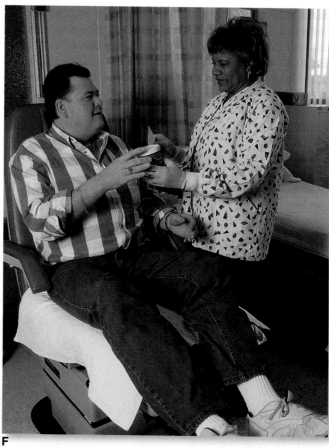

F

Figure 46-6. (continued)
(e) Determine the culture's antibiotic sensitivity. (f) Treat the patient as ordered by the physician.

Step 2. Obtain One or More Specimens

To determine the cause of an infection, you may need to obtain material from one or more areas of the patient's body. Label each specimen properly and include with it the physician's presumptive diagnosis. If the sample is to be transported to an outside laboratory, ensure that it is transported in such a way that any pathogenic organisms remain alive (and safely contained) during transit.

Step 3. Examine the Specimen Directly

You must sometimes obtain more than one specimen from each site. The doctor or specially trained laboratory or microbiology personnel will then directly examine one specimen under the microscope. The specimen may be viewed in one of two ways:

1. As a **wet mount,** a preparation of a specimen in a liquid that allows the organisms to remain alive and mobile while they are being identified
2. As a **smear,** in which a specimen is spread thinly and unevenly across a slide

If you make a smear, allow it to dry, and stain or treat it as ordered before it is examined microscopically. In some cases direct examination allows the doctor to make a presumptive diagnosis of the offending microorganism.

Step 4. Culture the Specimen

If the physician still needs a more definitive identification of the microorganism, you may perform a **culture,** in which a sample of the specimen is placed in or on a substance that allows microorganisms to grow. A **culture medium** is a substance that contains all the nutrients a particular type of microorganism needs. Most media come in the form of a semisolid gel. The particular medium is chosen according to the site from which the specimen was obtained and the suspected cause of infection. After you inoculate (place a sample of the specimen in or on) the medium, place it in an incubator (a chamber that can be set to a specific temperature and humidity) to allow the microorganism to grow.

The culture is examined visually and microscopically after a specified time, and a preliminary identification is made. The physician sets up additional tests to confirm the identification of the microorganism that has been isolated from the specimen. See Table 46-3 for information on specific microbial diseases and the body systems they

TABLE 46-3 Microbial Diseases

System	Disease	Causative Organism	Route of Transmission	Signs and Symptoms
Integumentary System	Anthrax	*Bacillus anthracis*	Inhalation or ingestion of spores; consumption of contaminated food	Fever, chills, night sweats, cough, shortness of breath, fatigue, muscle aches, sore throat
	Skin infections	*Staphylococcus aureus*	Direct contact of individuals colonized or infected with this bacteria; hand hygiene is the single most important step in controlling spread of these bacteria	Minor: pimples, boils Major: septicemia, surgical wound infection, necrotizing fasciitis
	Chickenpox	*Varicella-zoster virus*	Droplets spread through coughing and sneezing	Skin rash of blister-like lesions, usually on the face, scalp, or trunk
Respiratory System	Pneumonia	*Haemophilus influenzae Streptococcus pneumoniae Mycoplasma pneumoniae*	Direct contact with respiratory droplets	Fever, decreased breath sounds, shortness of breath, increased heart rate (tachycardia), increased respiratory rate (tachypnea)
	Legionellosis • Legionnaire's disease (severe form) • Pontiac fever (mild form)	*Legionella pneumophila*	Breathing water mists contaminated with *Legionella* bacteria (spa, air conditioner, shower)	Fever, chills, and a cough; muscle aches, headache, tiredness, loss of appetite, and occasionally diarrhea
	Tuberculosis	*Mycobacterium tuberculosis*	Respiratory droplet spread	Bad cough that lasts longer than 2 weeks, pain in the chest, coughing up blood or sputum (phlegm from deep inside the lungs), weakness, fatigue, weight loss, no appetite, chills, fever, and night sweats
	Pertussis	*Bordetella pertussis*	Contact with respiratory droplets	Typically manifested in children with paroxysmal spasms of severe coughing, whooping, and post-tussive vomiting
	Diphtheria	*Corynebacterium diphtheriae*	Person-to-person spread through respiratory tract secretions	Sore throat; low-grade fever; adherent membrane of the tonsils, pharynx, or nose; neck swelling

continued ⟶

TABLE 46-3 Microbial Diseases *(continued)*

System	Disease	Causative Organism	Route of Transmission	Signs and Symptoms
Blood and Immune System	Plague	*Yersinia pestis*	Flea-borne from infected rodents to humans; respiratory droplets from cats and humans with pneumonic plague	Bubonic plague: enlarged, tender lymph nodes, fever, chills, and prostration. Septicemic plague: fever, chills, prostration, abdominal pain, shock, and bleeding into skin and other organs. Pneumonic plague: fever, chills, cough, and difficulty breathing; rapid shock
	Rocky Mountain spotted fever	*Rickettsia rickettsii*	Tick-borne ixodid ticks infected with *R. rickettsii*	Fever, nausea, vomiting, severe headache, muscle pain, lack of appetite, rash, abdominal pain, joint pain, and diarrhea
	Lyme disease	*Borrelia burgdorferi*	Tick-borne deer ticks infected with *Borrelia burgdorferi*	Fever, headache, fatigue, and myalgia
	Mononucleosis	Epstein-Barr virus	Contact with saliva of infected person	Fever, sore throat, and swollen lymph glands
	HIV/AIDS	Human immunodeficiency virus	Blood and body fluids	The following *may be* warning signs of infection with HIV: rapid weight loss; dry cough; recurring fever or profuse night sweats; profound and unexplained fatigue; swollen lymph glands in the armpits, groin, or neck; diarrhea that lasts for more than a week; white spots or unusual blemishes on the tongue, in the mouth, or in the throat; pneumonia; red, brown, pink, or purplish blotches on or under the skin or inside the mouth, nose, or eyelids; memory loss, depression, and other neurological disorders
	Malaria	*Plasmodium:* *P. falciparum,* *P. vivax, P. ovale,* or *P. malariae*	Mosquito-borne from Anopheles mosquito infected with *P. malariae*	Fever and influenza-like symptoms, including chills, headache, myalgias, and malaise

Source: Centers for Disease Control, Health Topics A to Z. Atlanta, Georgia, 2003. http://www.cdc.gov/health/default.htm

affect. Most microbiology laboratories and some physicians' office laboratories are equipped to grow routine bacterial cultures and some fungal cultures. Physicians' office laboratories, in particular, may have to send out other types of cultures, such as virus cultures, to a specialized laboratory for identification.

Step 5. Determine the Culture's Antibiotic Sensitivity

In many cases of bacterial infection, a **culture and sensitivity (C and S)** is performed. This procedure involves culturing a specimen and then testing the isolated bacterium's susceptibility (sensitivity) to certain antibiotics. The results help the doctor determine which antibiotics might be most effective in treating the infection.

Step 6. Treat the Patient as Ordered by the Physician

On the basis of identification of the microorganism and antibiotic sensitivity, if determined, the physician can prescribe an **antimicrobial.** This agent, which kills microorganisms or suppresses their growth, should help clear up the patient's infection.

Specimen Collection

Perhaps the most important step in isolating and identifying a microorganism as the cause of an infection is collecting the specimen. If you do not collect the specimen properly, the organism may not grow in culture so that it can be identified. The result may be an untreated infection. Furthermore, if the specimen becomes contaminated during collection and the contaminant is mistakenly identified as the cause of the infection, the patient may receive incorrect or even harmful therapy.

In addition to vaginal specimens (discussed in detail in Chapter 40), the most common types of culture specimens involve the following:

- Throat
- Urine
- Sputum
- Wound
- Stool

Specimen-Collection Devices

To help ensure optimal recovery of microorganisms, you must use the appropriate collection device or specimen container. This container is usually provided by the laboratory where the specimen is going to be analyzed. Special collection devices are available for the collection of sputum, urine, and stool specimens, as shown in Figure 46-7. These containers are designed with large openings to allow collection of the specimen with minimal chance of

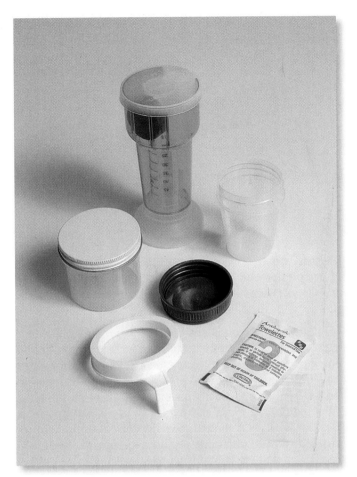

Figure 46-7. You may use specially designed collection containers to collect sputum, urine, and stool specimens.

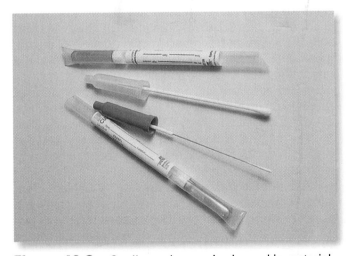

Figure 46-8. Sterile swabs vary in size and in material.

contamination. They also have tight-fitting caps to prevent leakage and contamination.

Sterile Swabs. The most common device for obtaining cultures is the sterile swab. They vary in the absorbent material at the tip and in the composition of the shaft (Figure 46-8).

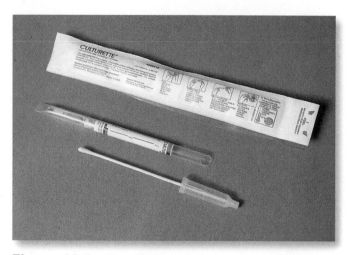

Figure 46-9. The CULTURETTE is used to obtain and transport microbiologic specimens to outside laboratories. (Courtesy of Becton Dickinson Microbiology Systems)

Although cotton is absorbent, it is no longer used for culture swabs because natural chemicals in cotton inhibit the growth of certain microorganisms. Polyester, rayon, or calcium alginate fibers are preferred. Most swabs used to collect routine specimens have a wooden or plastic shaft for rigidity. There are also swabs with a small tip and a flexible wire shaft made especially for culturing hard-to-reach areas and obtaining pediatric specimens. Some collection containers contain two swabs—one for a culture and one for a smear.

Collection and Transport Systems. Sterile, self-contained systems for obtaining and transporting specimens are commercially available from many suppliers. The CULTURETTE Collection and Transport System, manufactured by Becton Dickinson Microbiology Systems of Sparks, Maryland, is a well-known example. The unit, shown in Figure 46-9, contains a polyester swab and a small, thin-walled vial of transport medium in a plastic sleeve. If a specimen will not be tested within 30 minutes after it is obtained, the swab is replaced in the sleeve, and the vial is crushed between the thumb and the index finger. The moisture and nutrients provided by the transport medium help keep the bacteria alive during transport to the laboratory.

Several collection systems are also available for culturing anaerobic organisms. These systems provide a means of generating an oxygen-free environment so that the anaerobic organisms remain viable (alive and able to reproduce) during transport.

Specimen-Collection Guidelines

To collect specimens properly, you should follow a number of general guidelines.

- Obtain the specimen with great care to avoid causing the patient harm, discomfort, or undue embarrassment. If patients are to collect specimens on their own,

give them clear, detailed instructions along with the proper container.

- Collect the material from a site where the organism is most likely to be found and where contamination is least likely to occur. For example, the best location to obtain a specimen for diagnosing strep throat is at the back of the throat in the area of the tonsils. A properly collected sputum specimen should contain mucus that is coughed up from the respiratory tract, but it should not contain saliva, which is a contaminant.

- Obtain the specimen at a time that allows optimal chance of recovery of the microorganism. Knowledge of the infectious disease process allows the doctor to determine the best time to collect a specimen. For example, certain viruses are more readily isolated during the early, symptomatic stage of an illness.

- Use appropriate collection devices, specimen containers, transport systems, and culture media to ensure optimal recovery of microorganisms. The purpose of such equipment and materials is to preserve the viability of any microorganisms so that they will grow in culture. Special collection devices are available for certain body areas or suspected pathogens.

- Obtain a sufficient quantity of the specimen for performing the requested procedures. If, for example, both a culture and a direct examination of a swabbed specimen will be done, you must collect two specimens. Each procedure requires its own sample.

- Obtain the specimen before antimicrobial therapy begins. If the patient is already taking an antibiotic, note this fact on the laboratory request form, or ask the doctor whether you should obtain the specimen.

After correctly collecting the specimen, you must label the container and include the appropriate requisition form. The label should contain the following information:

- Patient's name and identification number (if appropriate)
- Source (collection site) of the specimen
- Date and time of collection
- Doctor's name
- Your initials (if you obtained the specimen)

The requisition form should include the following information:

- Patient's name, address, and identification number
- Patient's age and gender
- Patient's insurance billing information
- Type and source of the microbiologic specimen (for example, discharge from wound, big toe)
- Date and time of microbiologic specimen collection
- Test requested
- Medications the patient is currently receiving
- Doctor's presumptive diagnosis
- Doctor's name, address, and phone number
- Special instructions or orders

Throat Culture Specimens

A microbiologic procedure frequently performed in a medical office is obtaining a throat culture. The doctor may request a culture on patients with signs or symptoms of an upper respiratory, throat, or sinus infection. Identification of the microorganism responsible for the infection allows the doctor to treat the patient as effectively as possible.

In most cases the doctor wants to determine whether the patient has strep throat, an infection caused by the bacterium *Streptococcus pyogenes*. It is particularly important to diagnose and treat this infection because, left untreated, strep throat can lead to complications such as rheumatic fever. Rheumatic fever is an inflammation of the heart tissue that occurs more frequently in school-age children than in any other population.

When you obtain a throat culture specimen, you must avoid touching any structures inside the mouth, because this will contaminate the specimen. The correct technique for obtaining a throat culture specimen is outlined in Procedure 46-1.

Many doctors order rapid strep tests done if strep is suspected. Antigen-antibody test kits for strep are available in a variety of brands. They provide immediate indications of the presence of the strep antigen on a throat swab, sparing the patient the expense and waiting period associated with having a culture done.

If your office does not culture microbiologic specimens, you need to use a sterile collection system to obtain the specimen. If your office has the equipment to perform its own cultures, use a sterile swab and inoculate a culture plate directly with the swab. Specimens to be evaluated in the office should be cultured immediately after collection.

Urine Specimens

To minimize contaminants in urine specimens, it is important to obtain a clean-catch midstream specimen. You must process urine specimens within an hour of collection or refrigerate them to prevent continued bacterial growth. (Collection of urine specimens for culturing is discussed in detail in Chapter 47.)

Sputum Specimens

To obtain sputum specimens, have the patient expectorate (cough up) mucus from the lungs into a wide-mouthed specimen container. Beforehand, instruct the patient to avoid contaminating the specimen with saliva. If sputum specimens are not cultured right away, they should be refrigerated.

Observe Universal Precautions whenever you handle sputum samples. Wear a face shield or mask and goggles when collecting such a specimen, especially if the patient is coughing. Even when tuberculosis is not suspected, the potential for transmission of this type of bacteria always exists.

Wound Specimens

You usually obtain specimens from infected wounds and lesions by swabbing. The procedure is similar to that of a throat culture. Be sure you obtain representative material from a deep area and a surface area of the wound without contaminating the swab by touching areas outside the site.

Stool Specimens

If the physician suspects that the patient has certain diseases, such as cancer or colitis or bacterial, protozoal, or parasitic infections, you may need to obtain stool specimens. The collection technique varies with the suspected microorganism. Although both you and the patient may be embarrassed to discuss instructions for collecting stool specimens, do not let this interfere with proper specimen collection.

Patients must collect stool specimens properly so they are not contaminated with urine or water from the toilet, both of which can lead to inaccurate results. Patients can collect stool specimens on a clean paper plate, in a clean waxed-paper carton, or in a container or on collection tissue that you provide. Another way to collect a stool specimen is to place plastic wrap loosely over the toilet seat with enough material to form a collection pocket in the middle. Patients then use a tongue depressor to place a portion of the sample in a specimen container with a tight-fitting lid.

Suspected Bacterial Infection. Bacterial infections caused by species of the *Shigella* or *Salmonella* genus can cause loose, bloody, or mucus-tinged stools. A doctor who suspects that a patient has one of these types of infections may request that a stool specimen be obtained for culture.

Successful recovery of these pathogenic bacteria from a stool specimen depends on timely inoculation of special culture media. The doctor may request obtaining a sample in the office whenever possible to avoid delay in processing the specimen. Several types of culture media promote the growth of intestinal pathogens while suppressing the growth of other microorganisms.

Suspected Protozoal or Parasitic Infection. In cases of a suspected protozoal or parasitic infection, the physician may request what is known as an **O and P specimen,** short for an ova and parasites specimen. This type of stool sample is examined for the presence of certain forms of protozoans or parasites, including their eggs (ova).

When a physician requests an O and P test, obtain both a fresh and a preserved stool specimen. A fresh specimen is examined both macroscopically and microscopically for the presence of microorganisms. A preserved specimen is also necessary because certain forms of these organisms are destroyed within a short time after leaving the body and may not be detected in the fresh specimen. You must always obtain a preserved specimen when stool samples are sent to an outside laboratory.

Special stool collection kits are available. They contain a specimen container for a fresh sample along with vials

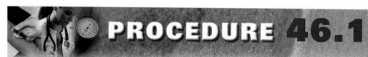

PROCEDURE 46.1

Obtaining a Throat Culture Specimen

Objective: To isolate a pathogenic microorganism from the throat or to rule out strep throat

OSHA Guidelines

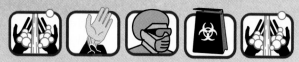

Materials: Tongue depressor, sterile collection system or sterile swab plus blood agar culture plate

Method

1. Identify the patient, introduce yourself, and explain the procedure.

2. Assemble the necessary supplies; label the culture plate if used.

3. Wash your hands and put on examination gloves and goggles and a mask or a face shield. (The patient may cough while you swab the throat.)

4. Have the patient assume a sitting position. (Having a small child lie down rather than sit may make the process easier. If the child refuses to open the mouth, gently squeeze the nostrils shut. The child will eventually open the mouth to breathe. Enlist the help of the parent to restrain the child's hands if necessary.)

5. Open the collection system or sterile swab package by peeling the wrapper halfway down; remove the swab with your dominant hand.

6. Ask the patient to tilt back her head and open her mouth as wide as possible.

7. With your other hand, depress the patient's tongue with the tongue depressor.

8. Ask the patient to say "Ah."

9. Insert the swab and quickly swab the back of the throat in the area of the tonsils (Figure 46-10), twirling the swab over representative areas on both sides of the throat. (Avoid touching the uvula, the soft tissue hanging from the roof of the mouth, because touching it will make the patient gag and will contaminate the specimen.)

10. Remove the swab and then the tongue depressor from the patient's mouth.

11. Discard the tongue depressor in a biohazardous waste container.

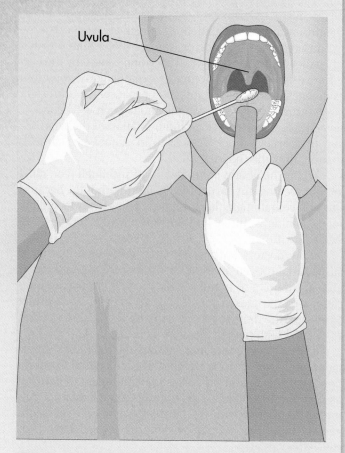

Uvula

Figure 46-10. When obtaining a throat culture specimen, swab the back of the throat in the area of the tonsils on each side, taking care to avoid touching the uvula.

To transport the specimen to a reference laboratory:

12. Immediately insert the swab back into the plastic sleeve, being careful not to touch the outside of the sleeve with the swab.

13. Crush the vial of transport medium to moisten the tip of the swab (Figure 46-11).

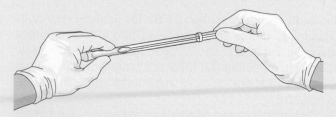

Figure 46-11. The transport medium released from the crushed capsule keeps microorganisms alive while in transit to the laboratory for culturing.

continued ⟶

PROCEDURE 46.1

Obtaining a Throat Culture Specimen (continued)

14. Label the collection system and arrange for transport to the laboratory.

To prepare the specimen for evaluation in the physician's office laboratory:

12. Immediately inoculate the culture plate with the swab, using a back-and-forth motion.

13. Discard the swab in a biohazardous waste container.

14. Place the culture plate in the incubator.

When finished with all specimens:

15. Remove the gloves and wash your hands.

16. Document the procedure in the patient's chart.

---

of two types of preservatives, formalin (a dilute solution of formaldehyde) and polyvinyl alcohol (PVA). Instruct the patient to place the stool sample in the specimen container and to mix portions of the specimen in each of the preservative vials. The laboratory will examine all specimens for the presence of microorganisms.

When a physician suspects that a patient has a protozoal or parasitic infection, he will request that a series of

at least three stool specimens be examined. Three specimens are required because different diagnostic forms of the microorganism may be present in the stool at different times. The presence of the microorganism could be missed with only one sample. Because certain medications can interfere with detection of these microorganisms, the patient may be asked to refrain from using medications such as antidiarrheal compounds, antacids,

---

PROCEDURE 46.2

Preparing Microbiologic Specimens for Transport to an Outside Laboratory

Objective: To properly prepare a microbiologic specimen for transport to an outside laboratory

OSHA Guidelines

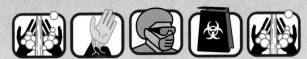

Materials: Specimen-collection device, requisition form, secondary container or zipper-type plastic bag

Method

1. Wash your hands and put on examination gloves (and goggles and a mask or a face shield if you are collecting a microbiologic throat culture specimen).

2. Obtain the microbiologic culture specimen.

   a. Use the collection system specified by the outside laboratory for the test requested.

   b. Label the microbiologic specimen-collection device at the time of collection.

   c. Collect the microbiologic specimen according to the guidelines provided by the laboratory and office procedure.

3. Remove the gloves and wash your hands.

4. Complete the test requisition form.

5. Place the microbiologic specimen container in a secondary container or zipper-type plastic bag.

6. Attach the test requisition form to the outside of the secondary container or bag, per laboratory policy.

7. Log the microbiologic specimen in the list of outgoing specimens.

8. Store the microbiologic specimen according to guidelines provided by the laboratory for that type of specimen (for example, refrigerated, frozen, or 37°C).

9. Call the laboratory for pickup of the microbiologic specimen, or hold it until the next scheduled pickup.

10. At the time of pickup ensure that the carrier takes all microbiologic specimens that are logged and scheduled to be picked up.

11. If you are ever unsure about collection or transportation details, call the laboratory.

and mineral oil laxatives for at least a week before samples are obtained.

Transporting Specimens to an Outside Laboratory

Many physicians' offices do not perform microbiologic testing. They choose to send their culture specimens to an outside laboratory. In addition, many specialized microbiologic procedures cannot be performed routinely in the office laboratory and must be sent out. One example of a specialized procedure is a virus culture. Culturing and identifying viruses require special techniques and equipment that are almost never found in a physician's office laboratory. Culturing a specimen for bacteria such as chlamydia is also a procedure that requires special techniques.

Your Main Objectives

When you collect and transport a microbiologic specimen to an outside laboratory, you have three main objectives:

1. To be sure you follow the proper collection procedures and use the proper collection device. Most laboratories have specific directions for sample collection and packaging that you must follow. A laboratory may even provide specific containers in which to collect and transport samples. If you collect or package any specimens improperly, the laboratory may not accept them for testing.
2. To maintain the samples in a state as close to their original as possible. You must take specific steps to prevent them from deteriorating.

3. To protect anyone who handles a specimen container from exposure to potentially infectious material. To do so, ensure that the specimen container has a tight-fitting lid. As extra protection against leakage, place the specimen container in a secondary container or zipper-type plastic bag. The laboratory usually provides such a bag.

Methods of Transportation

Specimens that are to be tested by an outside laboratory may be transported there in one of three ways:

1. During regularly scheduled daily pickups by the laboratory
2. During an as-needed pickup by the laboratory
3. Through the mail

Pickup by the laboratory is the most reliable and timely method of transporting microbiologic specimens. Although each laboratory has its own procedure, the general steps for preparing specimens for transport to a laboratory are outlined in Procedure 46-2.

Sending Specimens by Mail

There may be times when you must send a specimen through the mail to a special reference laboratory for a test that is not normally done by a local laboratory. The U.S. Postal Service accepts a package containing microbiologic specimens as long as the total volume of specimen material is less than 50 milliliters and it is packaged under strict regulations specified by the U.S. Public Health Service.

When sending specimens through the mail, pack them securely with adequate cushioning material to prevent

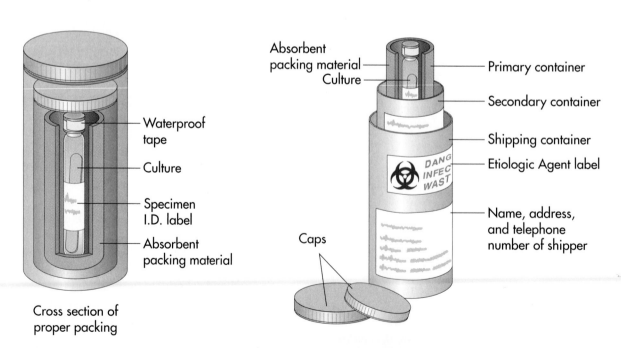

Figure 46-12. When packaging and labeling a specimen for mail delivery, you must follow the procedures set by the CDC, based on U.S. Public Health Service regulations.

breakage and leakage. Leakage can not only contaminate the specimen but also put mail handlers at risk of contamination with infectious materials. The proper technique for packaging and labeling microbiologic specimens is outlined by the CDC and shown in Figure 46-12.

Securely close the primary culture container, and surround it with enough absorbent packing material to absorb the entire fluid contents if the container were to leak. Place these items together in a secondary container, commonly a metal container with a screw-top or snap-on lid. Then place the secondary container in an outer shipping carton made of cardboard or Styrofoam.

In addition to the address label, microbiologic specimens sent through the mail must have an Etiologic Agent label affixed to the package, as shown in Figure 46-12. This label uses the biohazard symbol to alert the mail carrier as to the nature of the contents. The term **etiologic agent** refers to a living microorganism or its toxin that may cause human disease.

Direct Examination of Specimens

At times, the physician may directly examine the specimen under a microscope to detect the presence of microorganisms or to identify them. The physician may perform this procedure in the office to get the information needed to initiate treatment immediately.

Two types of procedures that allow direct examination of microbiologic specimens are preparing wet mounts and preparing potassium hydroxide (KOH) mounts. You may be required to perform these procedures as part of your duties.

PROCEDURE 46.3

Preparing a Microbiologic Specimen Smear

Objective: To prepare a smear of a microbiologic specimen for staining

OSHA Guidelines

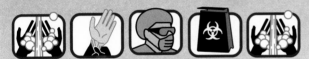

Materials: Glass slide with frosted end, pencil, specimen swab, Bunsen burner, forceps

Method

1. Wash your hands and put on examination gloves.
2. Assemble all the necessary items.
3. Use a pencil to label the frosted end of the slide with the patient's name.
4. Roll the specimen swab evenly over the smooth part of the slide, making sure that all areas of the swab touch the slide (Figure 46-13).
5. Discard the swab in a biohazardous waste container. (Retain the microbiologic specimen for culture as necessary or according to office policy.)
6. Allow the smear to air-dry. Do not wave the slide to dry it, because this may spread pathogens or contaminate the slide.
7. Heat-fix the slide by holding the frosted end with forceps and passing the clear part of the slide, with the smear side up, through the flame of a Bunsen burner three or four times. (Your

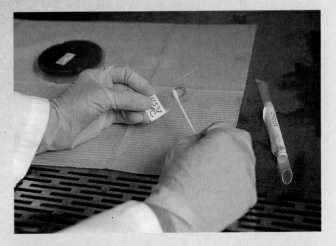

Figure 46-13. Rolling the swab ensures that representative microorganisms collected on it are deposited on the slide.

office may use an alternate procedure for fixing the slide, such as flooding the smear with alcohol, allowing it to sit for a few minutes, and either pouring off the remaining liquid or allowing the smear to air-dry. Pap smear slides must be fixed with a chemical spray within 10 seconds. Chlamydia slides come with their own fixative.)

8. Allow the slide to cool before the smear is stained.
9. Return the materials to their proper location.
10. Remove the gloves and wash your hands.

Wet Mounts

A wet mount permits quick identification of many microorganisms. Wet mounts are easy to prepare.

1. Wearing examination gloves, mix a small amount of the specimen with a drop of normal saline (0.9% sodium chloride [NaCl] solution) on a glass slide.
2. Apply a coverslip over the mixture.
3. Provide the doctor with the slide for direct examination under the microscope.

If you obtain a specimen from a body site that is normally sterile, detection of microorganisms on a wet mount immediately tells the doctor whether there is infection. Wet mounts are also useful in determining whether a microorganism is motile, or able to move, which helps in identifying the microorganisms.

Potassium Hydroxide (KOH) Mounts

A **KOH mount** is a type of mount used when a physician suspects that a patient has a fungal infection of the skin, nails, or hair. It is difficult to visualize a fungus directly in these types of specimens because the body produces a tough, hard protein called keratin that often masks any fungus present. The chemical potassium hydroxide (KOH) is added to the specimen to dissolve the keratin and allow visualization of any fungus.

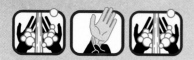

PROCEDURE 46.4

Performing a Gram's Stain

Objective: To make bacteria present in a specimen smear visible for microscopic identification

OSHA Guidelines

Materials: Heat-fixed smear, slide staining rack and tray, crystal violet dye, iodine solution, alcohol or acetone-alcohol decolorizer, safranin dye, wash bottle filled with water, forceps, blotting paper or paper towels (optional)

Method

1. Assemble all the necessary supplies.
2. Wash your hands and put on examination gloves.
3. Place the heat-fixed smear on a level staining rack and tray, with the smear side up.
4. Completely cover the specimen area of the slide with the crystal violet stain (Figure 46-14a). (Many commercially available Gram's stain solutions have flip-up bottle caps that allow you to dispense stain by the drop. If the stain bottle you are using does not have an attached dropper cap, use an eyedropper.)
5. Allow the stain to sit for 1 minute; wash the slide thoroughly with water from the wash bottle (Figure 46-14b).
6. Use the forceps to hold the slide at the frosted end, tilting the slide to remove excess water.
7. Place the slide flat on the rack again, and completely cover the specimen area with iodine solution (Figure 46-14c).
8. Allow the iodine to remain for 1 minute; wash the slide thoroughly with water (Figure 46-14d).
9. Use the forceps to hold and tilt the slide to remove excess water.
10. While still tilting the slide, apply the alcohol or decolorizer drop by drop until no more purple color washes off (Figure 46-14e). (This step usually takes no more than 10 seconds.)
11. Wash the slide thoroughly with water (Figure 46-14f); use the forceps to hold and tip the slide to remove excess water.
12. Completely cover the specimen with safranin dye (Figure 46-14g).
13. Allow the safranin to remain for 1 minute; wash the slide thoroughly with water (Figure 46-14h).
14. Use the forceps to hold the stained smear by the frosted end, and carefully wipe the back of the slide to remove excess stain.
15. Place the smear in a vertical position and allow it to air-dry. (The smear may be blotted lightly between blotting paper or paper towels to hasten drying [Figure 46-14i]. Take care not to rub the slide, or the specimen may be damaged.)
16. Sanitize and disinfect the work area.
17. Remove the gloves and wash your hands.

continued ⟶

Performing a Gram's Stain *(continued)*

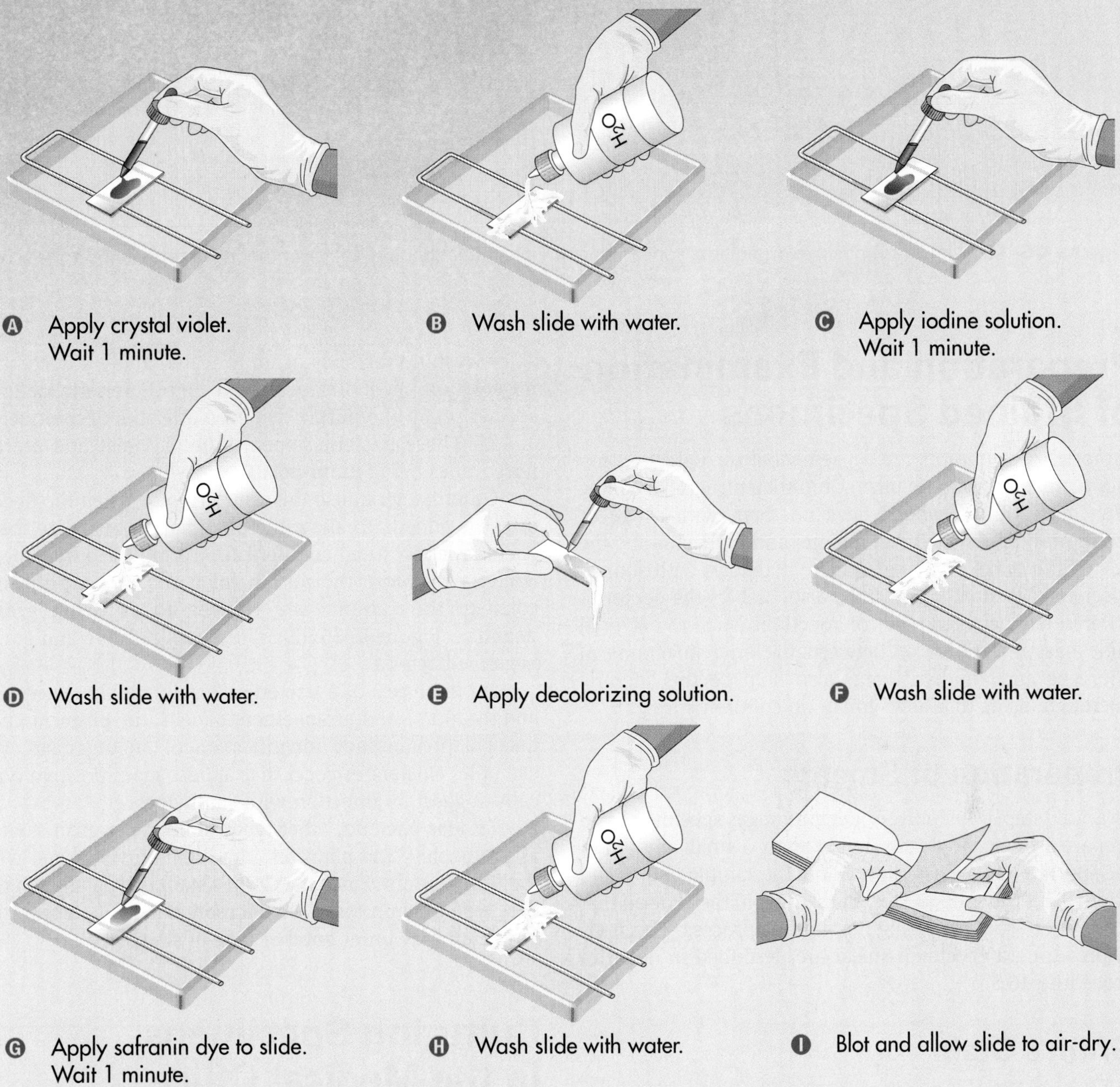

A   Apply crystal violet. Wait 1 minute.

B   Wash slide with water.

C   Apply iodine solution. Wait 1 minute.

D   Wash slide with water.

E   Apply decolorizing solution.

F   Wash slide with water.

G   Apply safranin dye to slide. Wait 1 minute.

H   Wash slide with water.

I   Blot and allow slide to air-dry.

Figure 46-14. The procedure for performing a Gram's stain on a microbiologic specimen involves covering the specimen with a series of stains, water washes, and alcohol in a specific order, for precise periods of time.

To prepare a KOH mount, follow these steps.

1. Wearing examination gloves, suspend the specimen of skin, hair, or nails in a drop of 10% KOH on a glass slide.

2. Apply a coverslip.

3. Allow the specimen to sit at room temperature for 30 minutes to dissolve the keratin. To speed up this process, gently heat (do not boil) the slide in the flame of a Bunsen burner.

4. Provide the physician with the slide to examine for microscopic evidence of fungal structures.

Introduction to Microbiology   **899**

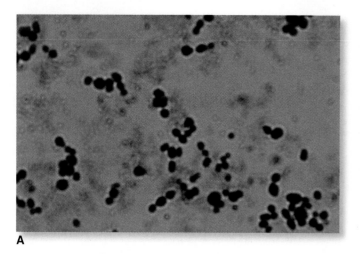

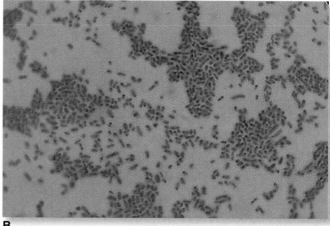

Figure 46-15. (a) Gram-positive organisms appear blue or violet after staining. (b) Gram-negative organisms appear red.

Preparation and Examination of Stained Specimens

Although wet mounts are a useful tool for detecting microorganisms, microorganisms and their structures can be seen more clearly when you stain them with a dye or group of dyes. As with wet mounts and KOH mounts, the doctor can make a quick, tentative diagnosis with stained specimens. A stained specimen also enables the doctor to differentiate between types of infections, such as bacterial and yeast infections, or between bacterial infections of one type and another. Stains also help doctors identify microorganisms that have grown on culture plates.

Preparation of Smears

The first step in staining a microbiologic specimen is to prepare a smear. To do so, simply apply a small amount of the specimen to a glass slide. Allow the sample to dry, and briefly heat the slide to "fix" the sample to the slide so that it does not wash off during the staining process. The steps in preparing a specimen smear are described in detail in Procedure 46-3.

Gram's Stain

The stain that is most frequently used for microscopic examination of bacteriologic specimens is the Gram's stain. A Gram's stain is a simple procedure that you can easily perform in the medical office. The steps for performing a Gram's stain are outlined in Procedure 46-4.

A Gram's stain involves performing a series of staining and washing steps on the heat-fixed smear. First, apply a purple stain called crystal violet (also known as gentian violet) to the smear. After washing the slide in water, apply iodine. The iodine acts as a **mordant,** a substance that can intensify or deepen the response of a specimen to a stain. Iodine helps bind the dye to the bacterial cell wall.

After washing the slide again in water, apply a decolorizing solution (alcohol or acetone-alcohol). Certain bacterial species retain the purple dye even after the decolorizer is added. These bacteria appear blue or violet and are referred to as being **gram-positive.**

Other bacteria lose their purple color when the decolorizer is added. To allow the physician to visualize these bacteria, apply a red counterstain (safranin) to the smear. Bacteria that lose the purple color and pick up the red color of the safranin are referred to as being **gram-negative.** Figure 46-15 illustrates gram-positive and gram-negative bacteria.

On the bases of a bacterium's staining characteristics and the shape and arrangement of cells, the physician can make a presumptive identification of an organism. For example, clusters of cocci that appear gram-positive typically suggest an infection with staphylococci.

Besides bacteria, other types of microorganisms, such as protozoans and parasites, can often be visualized with the Gram's stain. Since the Gram's stain is typically not the best type of stain for these microorganisms, however, the physician may order another type of stain.

Culturing Specimens in the Medical Office

If your medical office is equipped with a laboratory and if you have the necessary on-the-job training or additional courses, you may be required to culture certain specimens. It is, however, becoming more common for doctors' offices to send specimens to outside laboratories because of Clinical Laboratory Improvement Amendments of 1988 (CLIA '88) guidelines and the additional requirements concerning personnel and administrative work.

Culturing involves placing a sample of the specimen on or in a specialized culture medium. This medium contains nutrients that enable microorganisms such as bacteria and fungi to grow. The medium is placed in an incubator set at 37°C (body temperature), the optimal temperature for growth. As the microorganism multiplies, a **colony**—a distinct group of the organisms—can be seen on the surface of the culture medium. The microorganism is identified according to the colony appearance, its staining characteristics, and certain biochemical reactions.

Culture Media

Culture media come in liquid, semisolid, and solid forms. In the medical office you will most likely work with a semisolid. The medium contains **agar,** a gelatin-like substance derived from seaweed that gives the medium its consistency. This form of medium comes commercially prepared in culture plates—round, covered glass or plastic dishes also called petri dishes.

When using petri dishes, handle them only on the outside, so that they do not become contaminated. You can avoid introducing contaminants by storing the petri dishes with the agar side up. Use the palm of your hand to pick up the agar-containing part of the dish when you are ready to inoculate it with a specimen.

Types of Media. Many different types of semisolid media are commercially available. The type of medium used for culturing depends on the type of suspected organism and the site from which the specimen is obtained. Some types allow the growth of only certain kinds of bacteria while inhibiting the growth of others. These types are referred to as selective media. Selective media are commonly used for specimens that normally contain bacteria, such as stool or vaginal samples.

Other types of media support the growth of most organisms and are referred to as nonselective media. The most common type of culture medium used in the laboratory is blood agar, a nonselective medium. Blood agar gets its red color from sheep's blood. Comparing the growth of a specimen on selective and nonselective media often provides important information about the microorganisms present.

You will typically use a blood agar plate when you culture a throat swab specimen. The organism that causes strep throat (*Streptococcus pyogenes*) can be identified when it grows on blood agar because it destroys the blood cells in the agar, leaving a clear zone surrounding each colony. This process of red blood cell destruction is referred to as hemolysis.

Special Culture Units. Small physicians' office laboratories often use commercial culture units with specific culturing purposes. Units for performing rapid urine culture, such as Uricult (manufactured by Orion Diagnostica, Somerset, New Jersey), are typical. Uricult consists of a small vial that has a double-sided paddle attached to a screw-on top (Figure 46-16). Each side of the paddle contains a different type of medium on its surface. To culture a urine specimen, simply dip the media paddle into the clean-catch midstream urine specimen or catheterized

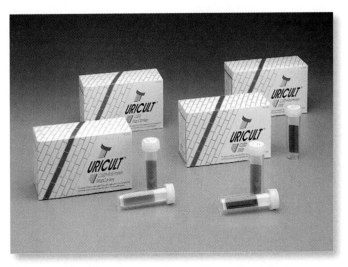

Figure 46-16. One common urine culture device consists of a lid and attached double-sided paddle that screws into a vial.

specimen, coating both sides of the paddle. Then remove the paddle from the specimen, screw it into the vial, and place it upright in the incubator for 18 to 24 hours. If bacteria are present, they will grow on the surfaces of the media. Other units for culturing urine, throat specimens, vaginal specimens, and blood are also simple to use. These units usually enable you to obtain an estimate of the number of bacteria in the sample in addition to identifying the bacteria.

Inoculating a Culture Plate

Inoculating a culture plate involves transferring some or all of the specimen onto the plate. Before inoculating a plate, label it on the bottom (agar side) rather than the lid, because the lid can be lost or switched. Label the plate with the patient's name, doctor's name, source of the sample, date and time of inoculation, and your initials. You can apply a label or write the information with a grease pencil or permanent marker.

In the case of a specimen swab, inoculate the plate by streaking the swab across the plate. Bacterial colonies can be identified by their appearance. This determination of the type of pathogen is referred to as a **qualitative analysis** of the specimen.

To perform a qualitative analysis of a specimen such as urine, introduce only a small portion of the specimen onto the plate. A calibrated inoculating loop is used for this purpose. A loop is a small circle of wire or plastic attached to a long handle. When this loop is dipped into the specimen, a small amount of liquid can be transferred to the plate.

In addition, you may need to perform a separate determination of the number of bacteria present in specimens such as urine. This determination is referred to as a **quantitative analysis.** A quantitative analysis is important

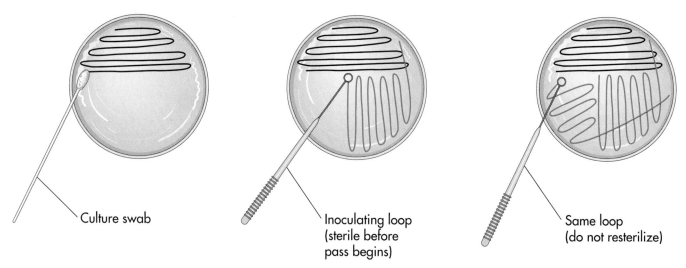

Figure 46-17. When inoculating a plate for qualitative analysis, roll and streak the culture swab or inoculating loop of specimen material across one-third of the surface of the culture plate. Begin the next pass with a sterile loop.

Culture swab

Inoculating loop (sterile before pass begins)

Same loop (do not resterilize)

with a specimen such as urine because a few bacteria may contaminate a urine sample during collection. A true infection is confirmed by the presence of a certain number of bacteria; any number beneath this level is typically considered contamination.

Inoculating for Qualitative Analysis.

To inoculate an agar plate for qualitative analysis, perform the first pass with a culture swab (as with a throat culture) or an inoculating loop (as with a urine culture). If you use a culture swab, roll and streak it back and forth across an area covering roughly one-third of the culture plate to deposit the microorganisms. When using an inoculating loop, spread the material by streaking the loop across one-third of the plate in the same back-and-forth pattern. Figure 46-17 shows the correct pattern for inoculating a plate.

Because there may be a great many microorganisms in the specimen, you need to streak the inoculated (first-pass) area with a sterile loop to separate out individual colonies that can be identified on the remaining areas of the culture plate. Unless you use a sterile disposable loop, first sterilize the loop by heating it in a bacterial loop incinerator until it glows red. Allow the loop to cool, and pass it once across the inoculated area of the plate to pick up a small number of microorganisms. Then streak it in a back-and-forth pattern over the second one-third of the plate. Next pass it once across the second inoculated area of the plate, and streak it back and forth over the last one-third of the plate. Each successive pass serves to reduce the concentration of the microorganisms. This procedure allows isolated colonies, or colony-forming units, to be observed in the area of the last pass of the loop, as Figure 46-18 shows.

For throat cultures, the physician may simply want you to screen the sample to see whether streptococcal organisms are present. You may not need to use a loop to spread the microorganisms; the swab will be sufficient, as described in Procedure 46-1, when preparing the specimen for screening.

Inoculating for Quantitative Analysis.

To perform a quantitative analysis of a urine specimen, use a calibrated loop to withdraw a portion of urine from the sample. The circle on a calibrated loop is a precise size that picks up an exact volume of liquid when it is dipped into the specimen. For example, calibrated loops may allow you to pick up either 0.01 or 0.001 milliliter of liquid.

When you perform a quantitative analysis, be sure the urine specimen is well mixed before taking the sample. Mixing is required because the microorganisms may settle to the bottom of the specimen cup. Sterilize, cool, and dip the calibrated loop into the sample. Transfer the entire volume to the surface of an agar plate by making a single streak down the center of the plate. Next spread the specimen evenly across the plate at a right angle to the initial streak, using the same loop (without sterilizing it). Turn the plate and spread the material again, at a right angle to the

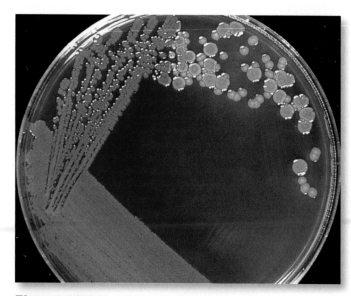

Figure 46-18. You can see individual colony-forming units in the last third of an inoculated culture plate.

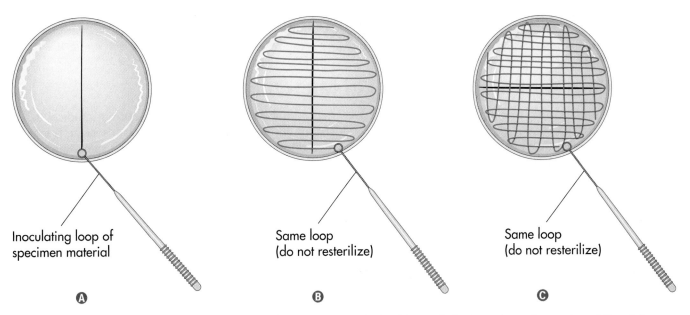

Figure 46-19. When inoculating a plate for quantitative analysis, (a) streak the loop down the center of the plate. Next (b) streak the loop at right angles to the first inoculation. Then (c) turn the plate 90°, and streak the entire surface once more.

last streak, over the entire surface. Figure 46-19 illustrates this technique.

After the microorganisms are allowed to grow for 24 hours, estimate the number of microorganisms by counting the number of colonies that appear on the surface of the plate. For example, if you use a 0.001 milliliter loop to streak the plate and 50 colonies grow, multiply the 50 colonies by 1000 to obtain the number of colonies per milliliter. In this case you would estimate that there are 50,000 colony-forming units per milliliter of urine. You must be especially careful that your counts and calculations are correct so that the doctor has accurate information on which to base a diagnosis.

Incubating Culture Plates

After inoculating a plate, place it in an incubator set at 35° to 37°C (human body temperature) to allow the bacteria to grow. Plates are always incubated with the agar side up, so that any moisture that collects in the plate will fall on the inside of the lid and not on the growing surface of the agar. How long plates are allowed to grow varies with the type of culture. Most bacteria grow sufficiently within 24 hours, but some require 48 hours. Fungi typically take longer to grow than bacteria and may grow at a slightly lower temperature (35° to 36°C).

Interpreting Cultures

After incubation, cultures are assessed for growth and are interpreted. Pathogens may be identified at this time. This process requires considerable skill and practice because pathogens must often be differentiated from normal flora. This step may be performed by the physician, a

microbiologist, or a technician who has been properly trained to do so through on-the-job training or additional course work. The Tips for the Office section discusses the types of qualifications and training you need to interpret cultures.

The process of interpreting a culture typically involves several determinations. The characteristics of the colonies growing on the agar are noted, along with their relative numbers. In addition, any changes in the media surrounding the colonies are noted, because these changes may reflect certain characteristics of the microorganism.

The physician decides at this point whether additional procedures are required. In the case of a throat culture, the presence of colonies of a characteristic shape, size, and color, surrounded by areas of hemolysis, suggests strep throat, as shown in Figure 46-20. A Gram's stain and

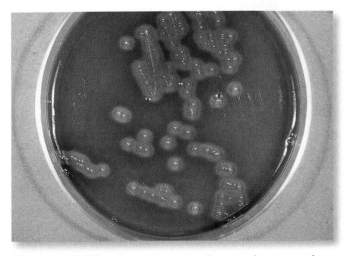

Figure 46-20. A positive strep throat culture contains distinctive colonies surrounded by areas of hemolysis.

Obtaining Additional Training in Microbiology

Identifying microorganisms in culture specimens requires considerable skill and practice. In a microbiology laboratory, these tests may be performed by medical technologists (MTs), medical laboratory technicians (MLTs), or other health professionals, including medical assistants who have received special training.

These classifications differ in the amount of education and training required. Medical technologists, also called clinical laboratory scientists, must earn a bachelor's degree and undergo 1 year of clinical training. Medical laboratory technicians must have completed a 2-year program at an accredited college (or the equivalent amount of course work), be a graduate of an accredited professional school or armed forces school, or hold certification in another related field while completing specific on-the-job training. Certification for both MTs and MLTs requires successful completion of a national certifying examination. In addition to certification, some states require MTs and MLTs to obtain a state license to work in a laboratory.

As part of their training, MTs and MLTs routinely receive instruction in microbiology. They also learn the clinical laboratory skills involved in identifying microorganisms. As part of your current medical assistant curriculum, you are learning the basic principles of microbiology and some of the techniques of specimen collection and processing. To be able to perform microbiologic tests, such as sensitivity tests, and interpret cultures of specimens, however, you would need additional training.

You can learn these types of skills and advance your career by taking part in the continuing education programs your office has to offer. Local colleges or schools of allied health may also offer clinical microbiology courses. Such a course will enable you to become proficient in performing microbiologic identification. All laboratories, including those in the doctor's office, require employees to participate in a proficiency testing program, according to guidelines set forth by the Clinical Laboratory Improvement Amendments of 1988 (CLIA '88).

Developing clinical skills in the area of microbiology can be challenging and satisfying. These skills will contribute to your office's efficiency and ability to provide high-quality patient care. Additional training in microbiology will also enhance your career by making you more valuable to any medical practice or facility.

---

determination of bacterial shape may be all that is necessary for a confirmed diagnosis. Many cultures, however, require additional biochemical and, in some cases, serologic tests for definitive identification of the pathogen.

Determining Antimicrobial Sensitivity

After a particular bacterial (or sometimes fungal) pathogen is identified, the organism's sensitivity (also called susceptibility) to several different antimicrobial agents must be determined. This information enables the doctor to choose an agent for treating the infection that is likely to be effective in curing it. If your office does not perform antimicrobial sensitivity tests but, instead, receives reports on them from reference laboratories, the results are reported as sensitive (no growth), intermediate (little growth), or resistant (overgrown).

Performing an antimicrobial sensitivity test involves taking a sample of the isolated pathogen, suspending it in a small amount of liquid medium, and streaking it evenly on the surface of a culture plate. Small disks of filter paper containing various antimicrobial agents are placed on top of the inoculated agar plate. Although this step can be done manually using sterile forceps, a special dispenser that is often used places all the disks down at once (Figure 46-21).

The plate is then incubated at 37°C, and the results are evaluated the following day. If a particular antimicrobial

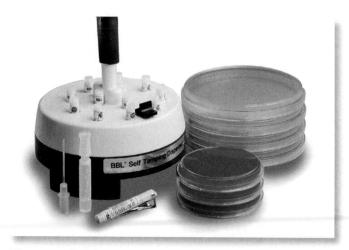

Figure 46-21. Antimicrobial disk dispensers simplify placement of antimicrobial disks, help ensure that each disk contains a single antimicrobial agent, and reduce the probability of contaminating the culture.

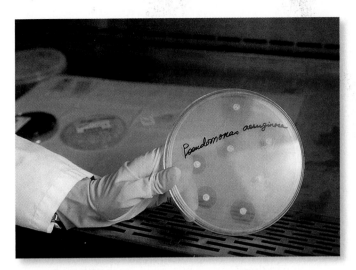

Figure 46-22. The effectiveness of different antimicrobial agents against an organism is apparent when an antimicrobial sensitivity test is performed.

agent is effective against the microorganism, there will be a clear zone around the disk, indicating that the growth was inhibited in the area of the agent, as seen in Figure 46-22. If there is growth right up to the disk, it means that the agent is not effective against the organism. Each zone is measured in millimeters and compared to a standard chart to determine the degree of effectiveness of the antimicrobial agent. The doctor uses these results to choose an effective antimicrobial agent to treat the patient.

Many bacterial identification systems are now available as automated systems. These systems are used at most larger institutions and reference laboratories. They require special instrumentation that has the capability to identify the organism. This instrumentation also determines the antibiotic susceptibility, a procedure known as MIC (minimum inhibitory concentration). This susceptibility testing is performed in special welled plates that test the organism against an antibiotic dilution to determine the minimum antibiotic concentration that is required to inhibit bacterial growth.

Quality Control in the Medical Office

Medical offices are required to have a **quality control (QC)** system in place, which is an ongoing system to evaluate the quality of medical care being provided. Although quality is sometimes difficult to define, most people would agree that high-quality care involves achieving the best possible medical outcome for each patient while attending to both the patient's and the family's needs. Quality control in the medical office provides an objective means of defining, monitoring, and correcting potential problems that affect the quality of care.

Part of quality control in the medical office includes risk management, which is the development of strategies for helping to minimize the chances of accidents or the risk of infection. These strategies include following general safety rules and regulations and Universal Precautions. Keep in mind that, in practice, medical offices use Universal Precautions when obtaining and handling all types of specimens, not only those capable of transmitting blood-borne pathogens.

Quality control involves an ongoing assessment of the reliability and quality of the work performed. As with all laboratory procedures, quality control in the microbiology laboratory of a medical office is particularly important in achieving quality assurance.

Quality Control in the Microbiology Laboratory

Quality control is necessary in several areas in a microbiology laboratory. All media, staining solutions, and reagents (chemicals and chemically treated substances used in test procedures) should be evaluated frequently for effectiveness. Media must also be evaluated for sterility. Equipment such as refrigerators, freezers, and incubators should be properly maintained, cleaned, and checked for accuracy of temperature. The essential components of a quality control program as established by the College of American Pathologists are outlined in the Tips for the Office section.

The Impact of CLIA '88

In addition to an internal quality control program, all laboratories must incorporate the appropriate policies and procedures to comply with CLIA '88. (See Chapter 45 for a full discussion of CLIA '88.) A substantial part of these requirements involves proper documentation of laboratory policies and procedures, materials, and personnel qualifications and training. If a laboratory has a good quality control program in place, it is likely that the required guidelines are already being followed.

In addition, any laboratory that performs certain procedures must enroll and participate in an approved proficiency testing program. A proficiency testing program monitors the quality of a laboratory's test results. The procedures in a microbiology laboratory that require proficiency testing include those classified as moderately complex or highly complex. An example of a moderately complex procedure is performing a culture and sensitivity test.

Proficiency testing involves culturing, identifying, and determining the sensitivity of blind specimen samples, that is, samples that are unknown to laboratory personnel. The results are then checked for accuracy. If you perform these types of procedures in the medical office, you may be asked to participate in the proficiency testing program.

Tips for the Office

Guidelines for a Quality Control Program in a Microbiology Laboratory

To maintain the highest possible standards of patient care and safety, all facets of a medical laboratory must be checked and monitored. The essential components of a quality control program in a microbiology laboratory include the following:

- Developing an up-to-date procedures manual. This manual is one of the most important documents in the laboratory. The procedures manual directs day-to-day activities and ensures that proper procedures are followed. It should include all general policies, regulations, and procedures, including those involving quality control and the transport of specimens to outside laboratories. The manual should be placed in a binder and kept in a location where all employees can refer to it. At least once a year, the laboratory director or supervisor should update and revise the manual.

- Monitoring laboratory equipment. A quality control program should include a preventive maintenance program for all laboratory equipment to ensure proper functioning. All equipment should be checked and cleaned at regular intervals. Temperatures of refrigerators, freezers, heating blocks, water baths, and incubators should be checked daily with an accurate standardized thermometer. Autoclaves should be tested each week with a spore strip to check sterility, and pH meters must be tested for accuracy using pH-calibrating solutions. A tachometer should be used to check the revolutions per minute of serology rotators and

centrifuges. (All centrifuges must have lids.) Safety hoods should be checked two to four times per year to make certain that they permit adequate air flow. The results of all quality control tests should be documented each time a test is performed.

- Monitoring media, supplies, and reagents. Media should be periodically checked for sterility and the ability to grow certain strains of stock organisms. Stains and reagents should also be checked with control organisms to ensure accurate results. Each culture tube, plate of medium, and reagent should be labeled as to its content and its preparation and expiration dates.

- Ensuring qualified personnel. Only qualified personnel should be hired, and employees should be offered an effective continuing education program. All personnel should be given the opportunity to learn new skills. This procedure benefits the laboratory and can also help advance employees' careers. Proficiency testing of blind samples may be used as teaching exercises and should be made available to all interested personnel.

- Ensuring adequate space. One issue of quality control and safety in the laboratory that is often overlooked is the allocation of sufficient work space for personnel. A minimum of 100 square feet of work space for each full-time equivalent employee is recommended. Safety and high-quality performance are enhanced when there is sufficient space to perform each task.

Summary

A variety of microorganisms can cause infection. They are a major cause of disease in humans. As a medical assistant, you play an important role in the diagnosis and treatment of infection.

Collecting a microbiologic specimen is the most important step in diagnosing an infection. To ensure accurate results, you must use the correct collection device and technique. Then you must process the specimen or transport it to the laboratory in a timely manner to enable recovery of microorganisms.

The process of identification often begins when the doctor examines the fresh or stained specimen. Most specimens

are cultured and incubated, and the resultant growth is evaluated. The antibiotic sensitivity of an isolated pathogen can then be determined to aid the doctor in making treatment decisions.

Quality control in the microbiology laboratory is an important factor in ensuring high-quality medical care. The focus and attention you bring to this part of your work will pay handsome dividends in terms of patient care, laboratory safety, and personal satisfaction. Developing your clinical skills will be an asset to the office and will allow you to advance in your career.

CASE STUDY *QUESTIONS*

Now that you have completed this chapter, review the case study at the beginning of the chapter and answer the following questions:

1. What is the proper technique for collecting a throat specimen?
2. Why do you think the first test result came back as negative?
3. What organism is responsible for causing strep throat?
4. What complications may have developed if you had not had another throat culture obtained and been prescribed antibiotics?

Discussion Questions

1. What are the different classifications of microorganisms, and how do the classifications differ?
2. List the common sites from which cultures may be obtained.
3. What information should be included on a laboratory requisition form when sending a specimen to an outside laboratory?

Critical Thinking Questions

1. Gram's stain is a procedure performed to stain bacteria for microscopic examination. What are the reagents used to perform this test? Identify the staining characteristics of gram-positive and gram-negative organisms.
2. What are the basic steps for diagnosing and treating infections?
3. Why are cotton-tipped swabs no longer used as sterile specimen collection devices?

Application Activities

1. With your instructor's approval, practice performing a throat culture on a partner.
2. Use one of your throat culture specimens to inoculate a blood agar plate. Incubate the culture and observe the appearance of normal throat flora.
3. Fill out a laboratory request form for a microbiology test being sent to a reference laboratory.

CHAPTER 47

Collecting, Processing, and Testing Urine Specimens

KEY TERMS

anuria

bilirubinuria

cast

catheterization

clean-catch midstream
  urine specimen

crystal

drainage catheter

enzyme immunoassay
  (EIA)

first morning urine
  specimen

glycosuria

hematuria

hemoglobinuria

myoglobinuria

nocturia

oliguria

phenylketonuria (PKU)

proteinuria

random urine specimen

refractometer

splinting catheter

supernatant

timed urine specimen

24-hour urine specimen

urinalysis

urinary catheter

urinary pH

urine specific gravity

urobilinogen

AREAS OF COMPETENCE

2003 Role Delineation Study

CLINICAL

Fundamental Principles

- Apply principles of aseptic technique and infection control

Diagnostic Orders

- Collect and process specimens
- Perform diagnostic tests

GENERAL

Communication Skills

- Adapt communications to individual's ability to understand

CHAPTER OUTLINE

- The Role of the Medical Assistant
- Anatomy and Physiology of the
  Urinary System
- Obtaining Specimens
- Urinalysis

OBJECTIVES

After completing Chapter 47, you will be able to:

47.1 Describe the characteristics of urine, including its formation, physical
  composition, and chemical properties.

47.2 Explain how to instruct patients in specimen collection.

47.3 Identify guidelines to follow when collecting urine specimens.

47.4 Describe proper procedures for collecting various urine specimens.

47.5 Explain the process of urinary catheterization.

47.6 List special considerations that may require you to alter guidelines when
  collecting urine specimens.

47.7 Explain how to maintain the chain of custody when processing urine
  specimens.

47.8 Explain how to preserve and store urine specimens.

47.9 Describe the process of urinalysis and its purpose.

47.10 Identify the physical characteristics present in normal urine specimens.

47.11 Identify the chemicals that may be found in urine specimens.

47.12 Identify the elements categorized and counted as a result of microscopic examination of urine specimens.

Introduction

The routine analysis of a urine specimen is a simple, noninvasive diagnostic test that provides a health-care provider with a window to a patient's health. Many significant conditions may be noted with the assessment of the physical, chemical, and microscopic examinations of a patient's specimen. This chapter reviews the function of the urinary system and the formation of urine. You will learn about various types of urine specimens and how to properly instruct or assist patients with the collection of these specimens. Additionally, you will learn how to correctly process a specimen, including a random specimen and a chain of custody drug screen. You will learn to identify normal and abnormal constituents of urine samples and what may cause these abnormal elements to be present in a specimen.

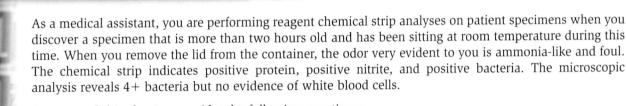

CASE STUDY

As a medical assistant, you are performing reagent chemical strip analyses on patient specimens when you discover a specimen that is more than two hours old and has been sitting at room temperature during this time. When you remove the lid from the container, the odor very evident to you is ammonia-like and foul. The chemical strip indicates positive protein, positive nitrite, and positive bacteria. The microscopic analysis reveals 4+ bacteria but no evidence of white blood cells.

As you read this chapter, consider the following questions:

1. What is the maximum length of time that a urine specimen should be left at room temperature? If analysis cannot be performed within that maximum length of time, how should the specimen be handled?
2. An ammonia-like or foul odor associated with a specimen ordinarily indicates what condition or disease?
3. Does the chemical analysis confirm your suspicion associated with the odor?
4. Given the circumstances, can you trust the results on this specimen?

The Role of the Medical Assistant

You will help collect, process, and test urine specimens. To perform your duties, you need to know about the anatomy and physiology of the kidneys, how urine is formed, and what its normal contents are. This information will help you collect various specimen types, process them, and perform urinalysis on them. Dealing with a variety of patient groups who require special care, including elderly patients and pediatric patients, will also be an important part of your job as a medical assistant.

Although you will not generally be dealing with bloodborne pathogens when obtaining and processing urine specimens, you will deal with potentially infectious body waste. For this reason you must take precautions to protect yourself, the patient, and others in the environment from transmitting disease-causing microorganisms. Most medical offices use Universal Precautions when dealing with urine. (See Chapters 19, 20, and 21 for detailed information on these precautions.) During all procedures you must be sure to wear adequate personal protective equipment (PPE), handle and dispose of specimens properly, dispose of used supplies and equipment properly, and sanitize, disinfect, and/or sterilize all reusable equipment.

Anatomy and Physiology of the Urinary System

The urinary system comprises two kidneys, two ureters, a bladder, and a urethra. The kidneys are located behind the peritoneum on either side of the lumbar spine. They remove excess water from the body and waste products from the

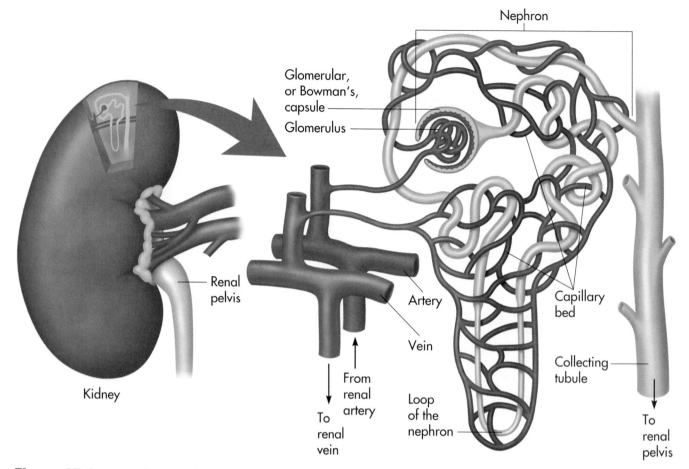

Figure 47-1. Urine is formed in the nephron, a long tubular structure, during a complex filtering process.

blood in the form of urine. The urine then drains through the ureters and into the urinary bladder. The urinary bladder stores urine until it leaves the body through the urethra. The ureters, bladder, and urethra make up the urinary tract.

Formation of Urine in the Kidney

Urine formation is essentially a filtering process that occurs in the nephrons. Nephrons are the structural and functional units of the kidney (Figure 47-1). Each kidney contains about a million nephrons, each of which is capable of forming urine.

Glomerular filtration occurs as blood moves through a tight ball of capillaries called the glomerulus. The glomerular capsule (Bowman's capsule) surrounds the glomerulus. Filtered fluid collects in this capsule, which is the functional beginning of the nephron. A capillary bed surrounds the winding tubule that makes up the rest of the nephron structure. Reabsorption of water, nutrients, and some electrolytes returns these substances to the blood as the filtered fluid passes through the long tubule. Other electrolytes and some additional substances are secreted from the blood into the tubule. Urine is the fluid that flows out of the nephron into the collecting tubule, passes through the funnel-shaped renal pelvis, leaves the kidney, and is carried down the ureter to the bladder.

The specific function of the nephron is to remove certain end products of metabolism from the blood plasma. Because the nephron allows for reabsorption of water and some electrolytes back into the blood, the nephron also plays a vital role in maintaining normal fluid balance in the body.

Physical Composition and Chemical Properties

Urine is made up of 95% water and 5% waste products and other dissolved chemicals. Components other than water include urea, uric acid, ammonia, calcium, creatinine, sodium, chloride, potassium, sulfates, phosphates, bicarbonates, hydrogen ions, urochrome, urobilinogen, a few red blood cells, and a few white blood cells. If a patient is taking any drugs that are excreted renally, the drugs may also show up in the urine. Urine in males may contain a few sperm cells. Table 47-1 provides a list of abbreviations commonly used in urine analysis and testing.

Obtaining Specimens

It is essential to collect, store, and preserve urine specimens in ways that do not alter their physical, chemical, or microscopic properties. You must follow guidelines each

TABLE 47-1 Abbreviations Common to Urine Analysis and Testing

Abbr.	Meaning	Abbr.	Meaning
ADH	antidiuretic hormone	RBCs	red blood cells
BIL; bili; BR	bilirubin	SPG; sp gr; sp.gr.	specific gravity
BJP	Bence Jones proteins	U/A	urinalysis
Ca	calcium	UBG	urobilinogen
CC	clean catch (urine)	U/C	urine culture
CCMS	clean catch, midstream (urine)	UC	urinary catheter
CL VOID	clean voided specimen (urine)	UC&S	urine culture and sensitivity
CrCl	creatinine clearance	UcaV	urinary calcium volume
CSU	catheter specimen (urine)	UCRE	urine creatinine
Cys	cysteine	UFC	urinary free cortisol
CYS	cystoscopy	UK	urine potassium
EMU	early morning urine(s)	Una	urinary sodium
HCG; hcg; hCG	human chorionic gonadotropin	Uosm	urine osmolarity
IVP	intravenous pyelogram	UTI	urinary tract infection
K	potassium	UUN	urinary urea nitrogen
pH	hydrogen ion concentration	UV	urinary volume
PKD	polycystic kidney disease	Vol	volume
PKU	phenylketonuria	WBCs	white blood cells

time you obtain specimens and instruct patients in the proper guidelines to follow.

General Collection Guidelines

When you collect urine specimens from patients, follow these guidelines.

- Make sure you are following the procedure that is specified for the urine test that will be performed.
- Use the type of specimen container indicated by the laboratory. If a patient must bring in a specimen, be sure that the container is provided by the physician's office or that the container is appropriate for the testing protocol.
- Label the specimen container before giving it to the patient or on receipt of a container that the patient provides. Include the patient's name, the physician's name, the date and time of collection, and the initials of the person collecting the sample. Label the side of the specimen container, not the lid, because lids may be lost or switched.
- If the patient is having an invasive test, such as catheterization, always explain the procedure to the patient completely, using simple, clear language.
- If you are assisting in the collection process, wash your hands before and after the procedure, and wear gloves during the procedure.

- Complete all necessary paperwork, recording the collection in the patient's chart and making sure you use the correct request slip for the test that has been ordered.

In many instances, patients need to collect a urine specimen at home. It is your responsibility to give patients instructions for obtaining the specific type of specimen. In addition, provide them with the following general instructions.

- Urinate into the container indicated by the laboratory. In most instances urinate into a widemouthed, throw-away, spouted specimen container as instructed. Do not add anything to the container except the urine.
- If the collection container contains liquid or powdered preservative, do not pour it out.
- If any of the preservative spills on you, wash the area immediately and contact the physician's office.
- Always refrigerate the labeled collection container or keep it in a cooler or pail filled with ice.
- Be sure to keep the lid on the container.

Specimen Types

Many different tests are performed on urine. You may need to obtain different types of specimens for different tests. Specimens vary in two ways: in the method used to collect them and in the time frame in which they are collected.

Whenever you collect a specimen, you must follow the steps in the procedure exactly—or have the patient follow them exactly. Quality assurance is essential in the physician's office laboratory. As discussed in Chapter 45, control samples must be used every time you test patient specimens. These are the types of urine specimens:

- Random
- First morning
- Clean-catch midstream
- Timed
- 24-hour

Random Urine Specimen. The **random urine specimen** is the most common type of sample. It is a single urine specimen taken at any time of the day. A random urine specimen is collected in a clean, dry container. If the doctor is requesting that a culture be done on the specimen, provide the patient with a sterile container.

If the collection of a random urine specimen is to be done at the doctor's office, supply the patient with a urine specimen container. Show the patient to the bathroom, and ask the patient to void a few ounces of urine into the specimen cup and to leave the cup on the sink. Retrieve the specimen when the patient leaves the bathroom and attach a properly completed label and requisition slip. Transport the specimen to the laboratory immediately. Urine specimens should be processed within 1 hour of collection. If this is not possible, refrigerate the specimens. Before processing refrigerated specimens, however, allow them to come to room temperature. If specimens will be shipped to an outside laboratory, chemical preservatives are added.

If patients are to collect a random urine specimen at home, have them use the container indicated by the laboratory. Either provide patients with a urine specimen container or instruct them to use a clean, widemouthed glass jar with a tight-fitting lid. Explain that a household dishwasher provides hot enough water to disinfect a jar adequately. Tell patients to refrigerate specimens until they bring them to the doctor's office and to keep them cool during transport.

First Morning Urine Specimen. The **first morning urine specimen** is collected after a night's sleep. This type of specimen contains greater concentrations of substances that collect over time than do specimens taken during the day. A urine specimen container or clean, dry jar is used to collect the urine as per the laboratory's request.

Clean-Catch Midstream Urine Specimen. The **clean-catch midstream urine specimen,** sometimes referred to as midvoid, may be collected and submitted for culturing to identify the number and the types of pathogens present. The presence of clinical symptoms or unexplained bacteria in a urinalysis specimen is an indication for urine culture. This method is not like other urine tests in which urine is simply voided into a specimen container. Instead, the clean-catch midstream method requires special cleansing of the external genitalia to avoid contamination by organisms residing near the urethral meatus (the external opening of the urethra). Voiding a small amount of urine into the toilet prior to collecting the midstream specimen flushes the normal flora out of the distal urethra to prevent possible contamination of the specimen. The only other way to obtain a specimen without this type of contamination is through catheterization, a procedure not routinely recommended because of the risk of infection. Procedure 47-1 describes how to collect a clean-catch midstream urine specimen and how to instruct patients to perform this technique.

Timed Urine Specimen. A physician may order a **timed urine specimen** to measure a patient's urinary output or to analyze substances (see also the discussion of the 24-hour urine specimen). First determine whether the required time period means that the patient must collect the specimen at home. If so, provide the patient with the proper collection container; written instructions on the process, including preservation of the specimen; and the following oral instructions.

- Discard the first specimen
- Then collect *all* urine for the specified time (2 to 24 hours)
- Be sure the urine does not mix with stool or toilet paper
- Keep the sample refrigerated until returning it to the physician's office or laboratory

24-Hour Urine Specimen. A **24-hour urine specimen** is collected over a 24-hour period and is used to complete a quantitative and qualitative analysis of one or more substances, such as sodium, chloride, and calcium. You need to instruct the patient in the proper collection process. If an outside laboratory will be testing the specimen, you will receive protocols for collection, preservation, and transport. See the Educating the Patient section for specific information on the 24-hour collection process.

Catheterization

A **urinary catheter** is a sterile plastic tube inserted to provide urinary drainage. Such a catheter may be inserted into the kidney, the ureter, or the bladder. **Catheterization** is the procedure during which the catheter is inserted. Catheterization is performed for various reasons, including to:

- Relieve urinary retention
- Obtain a sterile urine specimen from a patient
- Measure the amount of residual urine in the bladder to determine how much urine remains after normal voiding (Patient voids and is then catheterized; more than 50 milliliters is considered abnormal.)
- Obtain a urine specimen if the patient cannot void naturally
- Instill chemotherapy as a treatment for bladder cancer
- Empty the bladder before and during surgery and before some diagnostic examinations

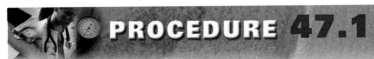

PROCEDURE 47.1

Collecting a Clean-Catch Midstream Urine Specimen

Objective: To collect a urine specimen that is free from contamination

OSHA Guidelines

Materials: Dry, sterile urine container with lid; label; written instructions (if the patient is to perform procedure independently); antiseptic towelettes

Method

1. Confirm the patient's identity and be sure all forms are correctly completed.

2. Label the sterile urine specimen container with the patient's name, the physician's name, the date and time of collection, and the initials of the person collecting the specimen.

When the patient will be completing the procedure independently:

3. Explain the procedure in detail. Provide the patient with written instructions and the labeled sterile specimen container.

4. Confirm that the patient understands the instructions, especially not to touch the inside of the specimen container and to refrigerate the specimen until bringing it to the physician's office.

When you are assisting a patient:

3. Explain the procedure and how you will be assisting in the collection.

4. Wash your hands and put on examination gloves.

When you are assisting in the collection for female patients:

5. Remove the lid from the specimen container, and place the lid upside down on a flat surface.

6. Use three antiseptic towelettes to clean the perineal area by spreading the labia and wiping from front to back. Wipe with the first towelette on one side and discard it. Wipe with the second towelette on the other side and discard it. Wipe with the third towelette down the middle and discard it. To remove soap residue that could cause a higher pH and affect chemical test results, rinse the area once from front to back with water.

7. Keeping the patient's labia spread to avoid contamination, tell her to urinate into the toilet. After she has expressed a small amount of urine, instruct her to stop the flow.

8. Position the specimen container close to but not touching the patient.

9. Tell the patient to start urinating again. Collect the necessary amount of urine in the container. (If the patient cannot stop her urine flow, move the container into the urine flow and collect the specimen anyway.)

10. Allow the patient to finish urinating. Place the lid back on the collection container.

11. Remove the gloves and wash your hands.

12. Complete the test request slip, and record the collection in the patient's chart.

When you are assisting in the collection for male patients:

5. Remove the lid from the specimen container, and place the lid upside down on a flat surface.

6. If the patient is circumcised, use an antiseptic towelette to clean the head of the penis. Wipe with a second towelette directly across the urethral opening. If the patient is uncircumcised, retract the foreskin before cleaning the penis. To remove soap residue that could cause a higher pH and affect chemical test results, rinse the area once from front to back with water.

7. Keeping an uncircumcised patient's foreskin retracted, tell the patient to urinate into the toilet. After he has expressed a small amount of urine, instruct him to stop the flow.

8. Position the specimen container close to but not touching the patient.

9. Tell the patient to start urinating again. Collect the necessary amount of urine in the container. (If the patient cannot stop his urine flow, move the container into the urine flow and collect the specimen anyway.)

10. Allow the patient to finish urinating. Place the lid back on the collection container.

11. Remove the gloves and wash your hands.

12. Complete the test request slip, and record the collection in the patient's chart.

How to Collect a 24-Hour Urine Specimen

When a patient needs to collect a 24-hour urine specimen, you must explain the procedure thoroughly and provide explicit written instructions. Be sure the patient understands that she must collect all her urine over the 24-hour period.

Provide the patient with a labeled sterile urine container with a lid. Tell her that at the start of the observation period (usually early in the morning), she should void and discard that specimen. Then every time she voids for the next 24 hours, she must collect the entire amount in the sterile container.

Tell the patient that the urine will be tested for substances that are released sporadically into the urine. Thus, it is extremely important to avoid using a bedpan, urinal, or toilet tissue, which could retain the substances for which the test is being done. Instead, the patient should urinate directly into a small collection container and then pour the urine into the large urine specimen container. Explain that the small container must be sanitized between uses with soap and warm water.

Explain that the large specimen container may have a preservative in it to prevent contamination and other alterations in the specimen. Instruct the patient to keep the specimen covered and in the refrigerator when not in use during the collection period. Emphasize the need to deliver the specimen to the doctor's office or laboratory as soon as possible after the 24-hour period is over, keeping the specimen cool during transport.

There are two primary types of urinary catheters:

- **Drainage catheters,** which are used to withdraw fluids and include an indwelling urethral (Foley) catheter placed in the bladder, a retention catheter in the renal pelvis, a ureteral catheter, a catheter for drainage through a wound that leads to the bladder (cystostomy tube), and a straight catheter to collect specimens or instill medications
- **Splinting catheters,** which are inserted after plastic repair of the ureter and must remain in place for at least a week after surgery

Catheterization is not routinely recommended because it can introduce infection. Some states do not permit medical assistants to perform catheterization, and in most health-care institutions, only a physician or nurse can insert or withdraw a catheter. Check the protocol in your state. If you cannot perform the procedure, you may be asked to assemble the necessary supplies and to assist the physician during it.

Catheterization performed in a physician's office is usually done for diagnostic purposes. Specially prepared catheterization kits are available that contain all necessary instruments and supplies. These kits include a sterile instrument pack that is used to create a sterile field for the procedure.

If a patient is incontinent, the physician may use a bladder-drainage catheter to help drain the bladder and keep the patient dry. Another type of drainage catheter, the ureteral, is inserted into the ureter to help drain urine.

The indwelling urethral (Foley) catheter is designed to stay in place within the bladder (Figure 47-2). It consists of two tubes, one inside the other. The inside tube is connected to a balloon, which is filled with water or air to keep the catheter from slipping out of the bladder. Urine travels through the bladder and drains from the outside tube into a soft plastic container. The physician may order a leg bag to attach to the patient's thigh. To prevent backflow into the patient's bladder, the container must always be lower than the bladder.

Special Considerations

When you obtain a urine specimen from a patient or take a history of a patient who may have a urinary problem, you need to consider the patient's sex, condition, and age. Some patients may require special care during collection procedures.

Special Considerations in Male and Female Patients. Depending on the test, you may need to alter guidelines for collecting urine specimens from a male or female patient. For example, Procedure 47-1 describes how to assist in collecting a clean-catch urine specimen from a female patient and from a male patient. In addition, when you take a medical history on a male or female patient, you will need to ask particular questions as part of your assessment. For example, if a female patient leaks urine when laughing or coughing, she may have bladder dysfunction, which would affect collecting a 24-hour urine specimen.

Special Considerations in Pregnant Patients. Pregnant women normally have increased urinary frequency. They may also be prone to urinary tract infections. At each prenatal visit pregnant women must have their urine checked for abnormal levels of glucose (a screening test for diabetes) and abnormal levels of protein (a screening test for preeclampsia or renal problems).

Ask a pregnant patient whether she has any pain during urination or in the kidney area. A positive response may indicate a urinary tract infection or kidney stones.

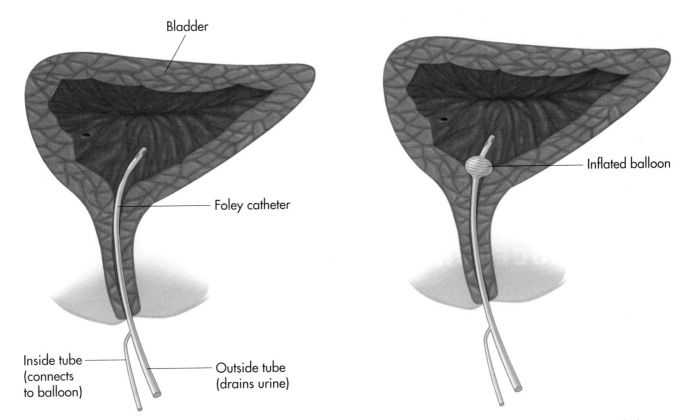

Figure 47-2. A Foley catheter stays in place within the bladder and has a collection container that is emptied periodically.

Also ask about urine leakage and whether she has previously been pregnant. Leakage may occur in a woman who has had multiple births, because the pressure of the fetus on the bladder or delivery of the baby may have weakened the patient's bladder control. Additionally, ask whether any of the babies were delivered by forceps, which can injure urinary and genital structures.

Special Considerations in Elderly Patients. When you collect urine specimens from elderly patients, you must consider several points.

- Bladder muscles weaken with age, often leading to incomplete bladder emptying and chronic urine retention, which can cause urinary tract infection, **nocturia** (excessive nighttime urination), and incontinence. Incontinence can interfere with collecting a 24-hour urine specimen.
- Weakening of the supports of the uterus may cause it to prolapse (work its way down the vaginal canal). The uterus pulls with it the vaginal walls, bladder, and rectum. This weakening, which is often the result of several childbirths, may not occur until a woman is postmenopausal. Symptoms include pressure, incontinence, and urinary retention. Normal activities, such as walking up the stairs, can aggravate the problem. This condition can interfere with collecting a 24-hour specimen.
- Find out whether the patient ever loses bladder control. If so, ask whether it occurs suddenly or whether a

feeling of intense pressure precedes it. These symptoms can be a sign of weakening of the bladder muscles, which can interfere with collecting a 24-hour specimen.
- Keep in mind that some elderly patients need assistance in providing a urine specimen. For example, you may have to accompany the patient to the bathroom and hold the specimen container. (Wash your hands before and after doing so, and wear gloves while providing this help.)
- If necessary, offer repeated explanations or reminders about the procedure or the specimens that need to be provided.

Special Considerations in Pediatric Patients. When you collect a urine specimen from a pediatric patient, involve the child (if age-appropriate) and the parents or guardians. Explain the procedure thoroughly and ask specific questions, including the following.

- If the child is in diapers, ask whether there is a problem of persistent diaper rash. (Rash may indicate a change in urine composition because of renal dysfunction.)
- Is the child excessively thirsty? (In this case the patient may not be taking in enough fluids for the amount of urine being excreted. Excessive thirst, combined with increased urinary frequency and volume, is symptomatic of diabetes.)
- Has the child experienced any difficulty urinating or a urine stream change? (These signs may suggest an obstruction in the urinary tract.)

PROCEDURE 47.3

Establishing Chain of Custody for a Urine Specimen

Objective: To collect a urine specimen for drug testing, maintaining a chain of custody

OSHA Guidelines

   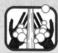

Materials: Dry, sterile urine container with lid; chain of custody form (CCF); two additional specimen containers

Method

1. Positively identify the patient. (Complete the top part of CCF with the name and address of the drug testing laboratory, the name and address of requesting company, and the Social Security number of the patient. Make a note on the form if the patient refuses to give her Social Security number). Ensure that the number on the printed label matches the number at the top of the form.

2. Ensure that the patient removes any outer clothing and empties her pockets, displaying all items.

3. Instruct the patient to wash and dry her hands.

4. Instruct the patient that no water is to be running while the specimen is being collected.

5. Instruct the patient to provide the specimen as soon as it is collected so that you may record the temperature of the specimen.

6. Remain by the door of the restroom.

7. Measure and record the temperature of the urine specimen within 4 minutes of collection. Make a note if its temperature is out of acceptable range.

8. Examine the specimen for signs of adulteration (unusual color or odor).

9. *In the presence of the patient*, check the "single specimen" or "split specimen" box. The patient should witness you transferring the specimen into the transport specimen bottle(s), capping the bottle(s), and affixing the label on the bottle(s).

10. The patient should initial the specimen bottle label(s) *after* it is placed on the bottle(s).

11. Complete any additional information requested on the form, including the authorization for drug screening. This information will include:
    - Patient's daytime telephone number
    - Patient's evening telephone number
    - Test requested
    - Patient's name
    - Patient's signature
    - Date

12. Sign the CCF; print your full name, note the date and time of the collection, and the name of the courier service.

13. Give the patient a copy of the CCF.

14. Place the specimen in a leakproof bag with the appropriate copy of the form.

15. Release the specimen to the courier service.

16. Distribute additional copies as required.

Urinalysis

Urinalysis is the evaluation of urine by various types of testing methods to obtain information about body health and disease. Urinalysis consists of three types of testing:

- Physical
- Chemical
- Microscopic

There are normal values for all tests done on urine. The normal value for a specific substance may be negative or none, or it may be a range in concentration. Urine test results within normal ranges indicate health and normality. Table 47-2 identifies normal values for a variety of urine tests. Because a urine test is a screening test, all abnormal values must be followed up with a confirmatory test.

Urinalysis is done as part of a general physical examination to screen for certain substances or to diagnose various medical conditions (Table 47-3). For example, daily urine output provides a picture of renal function. With adequate fluid intake, the average adult daily urine output is 1250 milliliters per 24 hours. When total intake and output measurements are not approximately equal, urinary tract dysfunction may be the cause.

The urinary system works with other body systems to help the body function normally. Therefore, a disorder in another body system can affect urinary function. For example, the kidneys interact with the nervous system to help regulate blood pressure and control urination. Thus, a nervous system disorder can affect the circulatory and urinary systems. The cardiovascular system delivers blood to the kidneys for filtration, and the kidneys regulate fluid balance, which helps maintain circulation of blood and

TABLE 47-2 Standard Urine Values

Acetoacetate	None		Glucose, qualitative	Negative
Acetone	None		Glucose, quantitative	50–500 mg/24 hours
Albumin, qualitative	Negative		Ketones	Negative
Albumin, quantitative	10–140 mg/L (24 hours)		Lead	0.021–0.038 mg/L
Ammonia	140–1500 mg/24 hours		Odor	Distinctly aromatic
Bacteria (culture)	<10,000 colonies/mL		pH	4.5–8.0
Bilirubin	Negative		Phenylpyruvic acid	Negative
Blood, occult	Negative		Phosphorus	0.4–1.3 g/24 hours
Calcium, quantitative	100–300 mg/24 hours		Potassium	40–80 mEq/24 hours
Casts	Rare/high-power field		Protein (Bence Jones protein/free light chains)	Negative
Catecholamines, total	<100 µg/24 hours			
Chloride	110–120 mEq/24 hours		Red blood cells	0–3/high-power field
Chorionic gonadotropin	Negative		Sodium	80–180 mEq/24 hours
Color	Pale yellow to dark amber		Specific gravity, single specimen	1.005–1.030
Creatine, nonpregnant women/men	<100 mg/24 hours (or <6% of creatinine)		Specific gravity, 24-hour specimen	1.015–1.025
Creatine, pregnant women	≤12% of creatinine		Turbidity	Clear
Creatinine, men	1.0–1.9 g/24 hours		Urea nitrogen	12–20 g/24 hours
Creatinine, women	0.8–1.7 g/24 hours		Uric acid	0.25–0.75 g/24 hours
Crystals	Negative		Urobilinogen, quantitative	1.0–4.0 mg/24 hours
Cystine and cysteine	<38.1 mg/24 hours		Urobilinogen, semiquantitative	≤1 E. U./2 hours
Estrogens, men	4–25 µg/g creatinine/ 24 hours			
			White blood cells	0–8/high-power field
Estrogens, women Follicular	7–65 µg/g creatinine/ 24 hours		Volume, adult females	600–1600 mL/24 hours
			Volume, adult males	800–1800 mL/24 hours
Midcycle	32–104 µg/g creatinine/ 24 hours		Volume, children	3–4 times adult rate/kg
Luteal	8–135 µg/g creatinine/ 24 hours			

myocardial function. A cardiovascular system disorder can allow blood to be delivered to the kidneys at a pressure inadequate for filtration, which would affect urinary system function.

Physical Examination and Testing of Urine Specimens

The first step in urinalysis is the visual examination of physical characteristics. Prior to starting the physical examination, it is essential to check the specimen for proper labeling. As part of quality assurance, examine it to make sure there is no visible contamination and that no more than 1 hour has passed since collection (or since the sample was refrigerated and brought back to room temperature). These physical characteristics are examined:

- Color and turbidity
- Volume
- Odor
- Specific gravity

TABLE 47-3 Common Urine Tests According to Clinical Condition

Clinical Condition or Suspected Disease	Types of Urine Testing
Acidosis	Reagent strip* for pH Specific gravity
Alkalosis (metabolic, respiratory)	Reagent strip* for pH Specific gravity
Diabetes mellitus	Odor (fruity) Microscopic examination for fatty, waxy casts Reagent strip* for ketonuria, glycosuria Specific gravity
Drug abuse	Gas chromatography; mass spectrometry**
Genitourinary infections (prostatitis, urethritis, vaginitis)	Cultures for bacteria, yeasts, parasites Microscopic examination for bacteria, RBCs
Human immunodeficiency virus (HIV)	Culture for virus (antibiotic added to kill bacteria) Other tests as indicated by specific symptoms
Hypercalcemia	Microscopic examination for calcium oxalate crystals Specific gravity
Hypertension	Microscopic examination for casts (hyaline, RBC) Specific gravity
Infectious diseases (bacterial) or other inflammatory diseases	Color and odor Cultures for bacteria, yeasts, viruses Microscopic examination for bacteria, WBCs, RBC casts (in severe cases) Reagent strip* for bacteria Turbidity
Metabolic disorders (except diabetes mellitus)	Color Microscopic examination for cystine crystals Reagent strip* for ketonuria, fructosuria, galactosuria, pentosuria, pH
Nephron disorders (nephrotic syndrome, glomerulonephritis, nephrosis, nephrolithiasis, pyelonephritis)	Color Microscopic examination for casts (epithelial, fatty, waxy, RBC), RBCs Reagent strip* for proteinuria Specific gravity Turbidity
Phenylketonuria	Color Reagent strip* for pH
Poisoning (arsenic, cadmium, lead, mercury)	Color Mass spectrometry**
Polycystic kidney disease	Proteinuria Urinary volume
Pregnancy	Reagent strip* for human chorionic gonadotropin (HCG)

continued ⟶

Clinical Condition or Suspected Disease	Types of Urine Testing
Renal infections (acute glomerulonephritis, nephrotic syndrome, pyelonephritis, pyogenic infection)	Color Microscopic examination for epithelial cells (especially with tubular degeneration), numerous casts (granular, hyaline, WBC), RBCs, WBCs Radioimmunoassay (RIA)** Reagent strip* for bacteria, albumin Specific gravity Turbidity Urinary volume
Renal disease, renal failure, severe renal damage, acute renal failure, renal tubular degeneration	Microscopic examination for epithelial cells (especially with tubular degeneration), numerous casts (hyaline, fatty, waxy, RBC) Reagent strip* for proteinuria (albumin), pH Specific gravity Turbidity Urinary volume
Sickle cell anemia	RBC casts
Starvation, dietary imbalance, extreme change in diet, dehydration	Color Odor (fruity) Reagent strip* for ketonuria Specific gravity
Urinary tract infection or mild inflammation (cystitis, pyelonephritis)	Color and odor Cultures for bacteria, yeasts, viruses Microscopic examination for bacteria, WBC casts, RBCs, WBCs Reagent strip* for bacteria, albumin, pH Specific gravity Turbidity
Urinary obstruction (tumor, trauma, inflammation)	Color Microscopic examination for RBCs Specific gravity Urinary volume

*Federal listings of waived tests refer to these as dipstick tests.

**Drug screening and some other common urine tests must be performed by a forensic laboratory or other laboratory capable of performing gas chromatography, mass spectrometry, and radioimmunoassay.

Color and Turbidity. Normal urine ranges from pale yellow (straw-colored) to dark amber. The color, which comes from a yellow pigment called urochrome, depends on food or fluid intake, medications (including vitamin supplements), and waste products present in the urine. In general, a pale color indicates dilute urine, and a dark color indicates concentrated urine.

You will assess urine for turbidity, or cloudiness, by noting whether the urine is clear, slightly cloudy, cloudy, or very cloudy. Typically, urine is clear, although cloudy urine does not always indicate an abnormal condition.

The color of urine and any turbidity that is present can reveal medical conditions that require treatment. Table 47-4 provides more information on variations in urine color and turbidity and the possible causes or sources of these variations. Both pathologic (resulting from disease) and nonpathologic causes are noted.

Volume. Normal urine volume, or output, varies according to the patient's age. Normal adult urine volume is 600 to 1800 milliliters per 24 hours (average of 1250 millileters per 24 hours). Infants and children have smaller

TABLE 47-4 Urine Color and Turbidity: Possible Causes

Color and Turbidity	Pathologic Causes	Other Causes
Colorless or pale straw color (dilute)	Diabetes, anxiety, chronic renal disease	Diuretic therapy, excessive fluid intake (water, beer, coffee)
Cloudy	Infection, inflammation, glomerular nephritis	Vegetarian diet
Milky white	Fats, pus	Amorphous phosphates, spermatozoa
Dark yellow, dark amber (concentrated)	Acute febrile disease, vomiting or diarrhea (fluid loss or dehydration)	Low fluid intake, excessive sweating
Yellow-brown	Excessive RBC destruction, bile duct obstruction, diminished liver-cell function, bilirubin	
Orange-yellow, orange-red, orange-brown	Excessive RBC destruction, diminished liver-cell function, bile, hepatitis, urobilinuria, obstructive jaundice, hematuria	Drugs (such as pyridium, rifampin), dyes
Salmon pink		Amorphous urates
Cloudy red	RBCs, excessive destruction of skeletal or cardiac muscle	
Bright yellow or red	RBCs (hemorrhage, myoglobin, hemoglobin), excessive destruction of skeletal or cardiac muscle, porphyria	Beets, drugs (such as phenazopyridine hydrochloride), dyes (such as food coloring and contrast media)
Dark red, red-brown	Porphyria, RBCs (menstrual contamination, hemorrhage, hemoglobin), blood from previous hemorrhage	
Green, blue-green	Biliverdin, *Pseudomonas* organisms, oxidation of bilirubin	Vitamin B, methylene blue, asparagus (for green)
Green-brown	Bile duct obstruction	
Brownish black	Methemoglobin, melanin	Drugs (levodopa)
Dark brown or black	Acute glomerulonephritis	Drugs (nitrofurantoin, chlorpromazine, iron preparations)

total urine volumes, although they produce more urine per unit of body weight. Urine volume is typically measured on a timed specimen (such as a 24-hour urine specimen) rather than a random specimen.

Oliguria, insufficient production (or volume) of urine, occurs in such conditions as dehydration, decreased fluid intake, shock, and renal disease. The absence of urine production is called **anuria.** Renal or urethral obstruction and renal failure can cause anuria.

Odor. Although the odor of urine is not typically recorded or considered a significant indicator of disease, it can provide clues about the body's condition. The odor of normal, freshly voided urine is distinct but not unpleasant and is sometimes characterized as aromatic. After urine has been standing for a while, bacteria in the specimen decompose the urea, which causes an odor similar to ammonia.

Diseases, the presence of bacteria, and particular foods (such as asparagus and garlic) can cause changes in urine odor. For example, in the presence of urinary tract infections, urine is foul-smelling, and in patients with uncontrolled diabetes, the smell is characterized as fruity (because of the presence of ketones). Phenylketonuria, a congenital metabolic disease, produces a strange, "mousy" odor in an infant's wet diaper.

Specific Gravity. **Urine specific gravity** is a measure of the concentration or amount of substances dissolved in urine. Because the kidneys remove metabolic wastes and other substances from the blood, the specific gravity of the urine they produce is an indicator of kidney function. The physician's office laboratory uses any of three methods to determine specific gravity:

1. Urinometer
2. Refractometer
3. Reagent strip (dipstick)

Specific gravity is a relative measure that is always compared to a standard. The standard for liquids is distilled water, which contains no dissolved substances.

$$\text{Specific gravity} = \frac{\text{weight of sample}}{\text{weight of distilled water}}$$

The specific gravity of distilled water is 1.000. You use special equipment to test for specific gravity (Figure 47-5).

The normal range of urine specific gravity is 1.005 to 1.030. Specific gravity fluctuates throughout the day in response to fluid intake. A first morning urine specimen normally has a higher specific gravity than a specimen provided later in the day. An increase in urine specific gravity indicates that the kidneys cannot properly dilute the urine. The urine then becomes more concentrated, causing it to darken. Increased specific gravity may indicate such conditions as a urinary tract infection, dehydration (for example, from fever, vomiting, or diarrhea), adrenal insufficiency,

hepatic disease, or congestive heart failure. A decrease in the specific gravity of urine causes a lighter than normal urine color, may indicate that the kidneys cannot properly concentrate the urine, and may suggest such conditions as overhydration (excess fluid in the body), diabetes insipidus, chronic renal disease, or systemic lupus erythematosus.

Refractometer Measurement. A **refractometer** is an optical instrument that measures the refraction, or bending, of light as it passes through a liquid. The degree of refraction, or refractive index, is proportional to the amount of dissolved material in the liquid. You must calibrate a refractometer each day with distilled water by setting the instrument at 1.000 with the set screw. Two standard solutions (solutions of known specific gravity) are also used to ensure accuracy. Advantages of using a refractometer to measure urine specific gravity are that the process takes little time and requires little urine. Only a drop of urine is used for this determination. Procedure 47-4 describes how to measure specific gravity with a refractometer.

Reagent Strip Measurement. You may use special reagent strips, or dipsticks, to test for specific gravity. Test pads along these plastic strips contain chemicals that react with substances in the urine and change color in precise ways. The reagent strip container includes a color chart for interpreting color changes on the test pads. When you evaluate urine specific gravity in this way, keep in mind that this type of test depends on precisely timed intervals identified by the manufacturer. Follow all directions exactly. The general steps for using reagent strips are as follows.

1. Wash your hands and put on examination gloves.
2. Identify the specimen.
3. After checking the expiration date on the reagent strip container (never use expired strips), remove a reagent strip from the container, holding the strip in your hand or placing it on a clean paper towel. Immediately replace the cap on the container.
4. Swirl the specimen to mix it thoroughly.
5. Note the time and simultaneously dip the strip into the urine and quickly remove it.
6. Draw the reagent strip across the specimen container's lip to remove excess urine.
7. Hold the strip horizontally and, after waiting for the specified time interval, compare the strip to the color chart on the container.
8. Read the value that corresponds to the matching color (for specific gravity in this case), and record the value on the laboratory report form.
9. Remove the gloves and wash your hands.
10. Place the laboratory report form in the patient's chart.

Chemical Testing of Urine Specimens

As a medical assistant, you may be asked to perform chemical tests on urine. Prior to performing chemical tests,

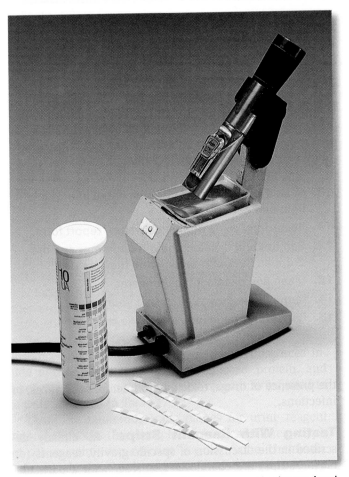

Figure 47-5. Specific gravity is commonly determined using a refractometer or reagent strips.

PROCEDURE 47.5

Performing a Reagent Strip Test

Objective: To perform chemical testing on urine specimens (This test is used to screen for the presence of leukocytes, nitrite, urobilinogen, protein, pH, blood, specific gravity, ketones, bilirubin, and glucose.)

OSHA Guidelines

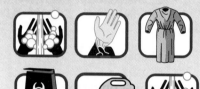

Materials: Urine specimen, laboratory report form, reagent strips, paper towel, timer

Method

1. Wash your hands and put on personal protective equipment.
2. Check the specimen for proper labeling and examine it to make sure that there is no visible contamination. Perform the test as soon as possible after collection. Refrigerate the specimen if testing will take place more than 1 hour later. Bring the refrigerated specimen back to room temperature prior to testing.
3. Check the expiration date on the reagent strip container and check the strip for damaged or discolored pads.
4. Swirl the specimen to mix it thoroughly.
5. Dip a urine strip into the specimen, making sure each pad is completely covered. Briefly tap the strip sideways on a paper towel. *Do not blot* the test pads.
6. Read each test pad against the chart on the bottle at the designated time. Note: It is important to read each pad at the appropriate time. Most reagent strip results are invalid after 2 minutes.
7. Record the values on the laboratory report form.
8. Discard the used disposable supplies.
9. Clean and disinfect the work area.
10. Remove your gloves and wash your hands.
11. Record the result in the patient's chart.

Ketone Bodies. Ketone bodies (or ketones) are intermediary products of fat and protein metabolism in the body. They include acetone, acetoacetic acid, and beta-hydroxybutyric acid. Only the first two substances can be determined by a reagent strip test. Normally, there are no ketones in urine. The presence of ketones in the urine may indicate that a patient is following a low-carbohydrate diet, or it may indicate that the patient has a condition such as starvation, excessive vomiting, or diabetes mellitus. Because ketones evaporate at room temperature, be sure to test urine immediately or cover the specimen tightly and refrigerate it until testing can be done.

pH. Urinary pH is a measure of the degree of acidity or alkalinity of the urine. Determination of pH can provide information about a patient's metabolic status, diet, medications being taken, and several conditions. The normal pH of freshly voided urine ranges from 5.0 to 8.0. The average urine pH is 6.0, which is slightly acidic. A pH of 7.0 is neutral, a lower pH is acidic, and a higher one is alkaline. Patients with alkaline urine may have such conditions as urinary tract infection or metabolic or respiratory alkalosis. Those with acidic urine may have such conditions as phenylketonuria or acidosis. Reagent strip, or dipstick, tests on both urine and blood are used to measure pH in the body. (See Chapter 48 for information on blood tests for pH.)

Blood. A patient who has blood in the urine may be menstruating, have a urinary tract infection, or have trauma or bleeding in the kidneys. To test for blood in urine, use a reagent strip that reacts with hemoglobin. There are two indicators on the strip. One is for nonhemolyzed blood, the other for hemolyzed blood.

Colors on the strip range from orange through green to dark blue and may indicate **hematuria** (the presence of blood in the urine) caused by cystitis; kidney stones; menstruation; or ureteral, bladder, or urethral irritation. The presence of free hemoglobin in the urine is known as **hemoglobinuria,** a rare condition caused by transfusion reactions, malaria, drug reactions, snakebites, or severe burns. Injured or damaged muscle tissue—such as occurs in crushing injuries, myocardial infarction, muscular dystrophy, or injuries during contact sports—can cause **myoglobinuria** (the presence of myoglobin in the urine). Reagent strip testing does not distinguish between these two conditions.

Bilirubin and Urobilinogen. When hemoglobin breaks down, it converts into conjugated bilirubin in the liver and then to urobilinogen in the intestines. Presence of the bile pigment **bilirubin** in the urine (**bilirubinuria**) is one of the first signs of liver disease or conditions that involve the liver. When bilirubin is present, urine turns yellow-brown to greenish orange. You usually use a reagent strip to test for bilirubin.

Although **urobilinogen** is present in the urine in small amounts, elevated levels of this colorless compound formed in the intestines may indicate increased red blood cell destruction or liver disease. Lack of urobilinogen in the urine may suggest total bile duct obstruction, as a result of which urobilinogen is not formed in the intestines or reabsorbed in the circulation. To test for urobilinogen, you use reagent strips.

Testing for either bilirubin or urobilinogen must be performed on a fresh urine specimen. Bilirubin decomposes rapidly in bright light to form biliverdin, which is not detected by the reagent strip test for bilirubin. Urobilinogen breaks down to urobilin on standing.

Glucose. Glucose is present in patients with normal urine, but only in small quantities not detectable by the reagent strip test for glucose. **Glycosuria** (the presence of significant glucose in the urine) is common in patients with diabetes. Blood is more commonly tested for glucose than urine is, because reagent strip tests may show false-negative results when used for testing urine.

Protein. Although a small amount of protein is excreted in the urine every day, an excess of protein in the urine **(proteinuria)** usually indicates renal disease. Proteinuria is also common in pregnant patients or after heavy exercise.

Nitrite. The presence of nitrite in the urine suggests a bacterial infection of the urinary tract. The test is not definitive, however, because some bacteria cannot convert nitrate to nitrite. Also, if an insufficient number of bacteria are present in the urine or if the urine has not incubated long enough in the bladder for a reaction to take place, a negative nitrite test can occur. The best urine specimen to test for nitrites is the first morning specimen.

When testing for urinary nitrite, you must test the urine immediately or refrigerate the specimen. Bacteria can multiply in a specimen that is allowed to sit at room temperature, thus causing a false-positive test result. Bacteria can also further metabolize the nitrite already produced, thus causing a false-negative result.

Leukocytes. Leukocytes appear in the urine in urinary tract or renal infections. Use strip tests for leukocyte esterase, a chemical seen when leukocytes are present, to test for leukocytes.

Phenylketones. The presence of phenylketones in a patient's urine indicates **phenylketonuria (PKU),** a genetically inherited disorder in which the body cannot properly metabolize the nutrient phenylalanine. This disorder causes phenylketones to accumulate in the bloodstream, resulting in mental retardation. PKU can be treated successfully by limiting dietary intake of phenylalanine, which makes up 5% of all natural protein, from early infancy. Although urine can be tested for the presence of phenylketones, blood testing is routine for newborns before discharge, at least 24 hours after birth.

Other Types of Chemical Testing. There are other types of chemical tests that may be performed on urine specimens. They generally involve testing for electrolytes and osmolality. Because these tests are performed in an outside laboratory rather than in a physician's office laboratory, you do not need to know the steps in each procedure.

Pregnancy Tests. Pregnancy testing is based on detecting the hormone secreted by the placenta. The name of the hormone is human chorionic gonadotropin, or HCG. The levels of HCG vary throughout pregnancy: they usually peak at about eight weeks; they drop to lower levels in the second trimester; and then detectable levels recur in the last trimester. Many commercial pregnancy tests are manufactured for use in the clinical setting and at home. These tests are sensitive, easy to perform and interpret, and give quick results. Most tests are now designed as an **enzyme immunoassay (EIA)** test, which always involves an antigen, an antibody specific for the antigen, and a second antibody conjugated to an enzyme. Newer technologies have been developed that are called membrane EIAs; in these tests, most of the reagents are incorporated into an absorbent membrane in a plastic case. Using either urine or serum, a sample is added through a chamber window where it migrates through the membrane and combines with the reagents to produce a reaction. Although the technology used in the design of these tests is quite complex, the actual test itself is easy to set up and interpret (Procedure 47-6). The tests are all designed with a control feature incorporated into the reagent pack for quality assurance of the test results.

Urine Tests for the Presence of STDs. In response to increasing numbers of sexually transmitted diseases, the CDC recommends that all sexually active females between the ages of 15 and 25 be screened annually for chlamydia. To accomplish this, several tests called nucleic acid amplification tests (NAATs) have recently been developed. These tests utilize urine samples to detect the presence of nucleic acid. Patients infected with either *Chlamydia trachomatis* or *Neisseria gonorrhoeae* will have nucleic acid in their urine. By amplifying nucleic acids specific to chlamydia and gonorrhea, the test can detect the presence of very small numbers of bacteria.

These tests have several advantages:

- Sample collection is noninvasive and easily collected.
- The tests are highly specific.
- The tests are highly sensitive. As little as one copy of bacterial nucleic acids can be detected in a urine specimen.
- Organisms do not have to be living to be detected.
- The tests are good screening tools for asymptomatic patients.

The tests also have some disadvantages:

- The tests are expensive.
- No living organisms remain for use in a follow-up culture. Therefore, positive tests must be confirmed by culture from an endocervical or urethral swab.

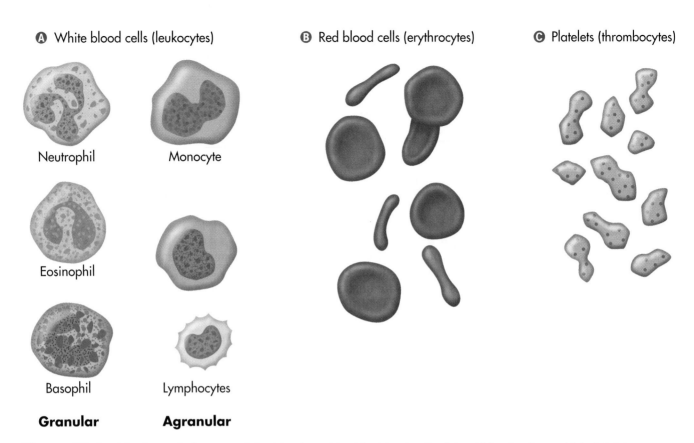

A White blood cells (leukocytes) **B** Red blood cells (erythrocytes) **C** Platelets (thrombocytes)

Neutrophil   Monocyte

Eosinophil

Basophil   Lymphocytes

Granular   **Agranular**

Figure 48-1. The formed elements of the blood are (a) white blood cells, (b) red blood cells, and (c) platelets.

plasma, or fluid part of blood, forms 55% of blood volume. The red blood cells, white blood cells, and platelets comprise the other 45% of blood volume, which is known as the **formed elements** (Figure 48-1). **Whole blood** is the total volume of plasma and formed elements.

Red Blood Cells

Red blood cells (RBCs), or **erythrocytes,** play a vital role in internal respiration (the exchange of gases between blood and body cells). Blood transports oxygen to body cells in two forms. About 98% of the oxygen is bound to **hemoglobin,** the main component of erythrocytes. The other 2% to 3% of the oxygen is dissolved in plasma. In addition, erythrocytes transport carbon dioxide from body cells to the lungs, although most carbon dioxide is carried in plasma. Healthy RBCs are disk-shaped and have concave sides (biconcave). Hemoglobin, a protein that contains iron, gives RBCs their rusty red color. A mature erythrocyte contains no nucleus.

White Blood Cells

White blood cells (WBCs), or **leukocytes,** protect the body against infection. (The function of WBCs as part of the body's defense against disease is discussed in Chapter 19.) Leukocytes are divided into two primary groups: **granular leukocytes** (also known as polymorphonuclear leukocytes) and **agranular leukocytes** (also known as mononuclear leukocytes). The division is based on the type of nucleus and cytoplasm in the cell. Each type of leukocyte performs a specific defense function, and the shape of each is suited to its role.

Granular Leukocytes. Granular, or polymorphonuclear, leukocytes have segmented nuclei and granulated cytoplasm. The three types of granular leukocytes are **basophils, eosinophils,** and **neutrophils.** Basophils produce the chemical histamine, which aids the body in controlling allergic reactions and other exaggerated immunologic responses. Eosinophils capture invading bacteria and antigen-antibody complexes through **phagocytosis,** or the engulfing of the invader. The number of eosinophils increases during allergic reactions and in response to parasitic infections. Neutrophils aid in phagocytosis by attacking bacterial invaders. They are also responsible for the release of **pyrogens,** which cause fever.

Agranular Leukocytes. Agranular leukocytes have solid nuclei and clear cytoplasm. The two types of agranular leukocytes are lymphocytes and monocytes. Lymphocytes are divided into two groups: B lymphocytes and T lymphocytes. **B lymphocytes** produce antibodies to combat specific pathogens. **T lymphocytes** regulate immunologic response. T lymphocytes are further classified as helper T cells and suppressor T cells. T cells are the cells attacked by human immunodeficiency virus (HIV), the virus that causes acquired immunodeficiency syndrome (AIDS). **Monocytes** are large white blood cells with oval or

Phlebotomist

To gain medical assistant credentials, you must fulfill the requirements of either the American Association of Medical Assistants (for a Certified Medical Assistant) or the American Medical Technologists (for a Registered Medical Assistant). After obtaining your medical assistant certification or registration, you may wish to acquire additional skills in specialty areas through course work or on-the-job training. Although this course work or training may not lead to an additional certification or degree, it will enable you to expand your role in the medical office and advance your career as the demand for skilled health professionals increases.

Skills and Duties

Traditionally, a phlebotomist's job has been to draw blood from patients for analysis. Today, however, phlebotomists perform many additional duties. Many phlebotomists now perform simple tests on blood samples at the patient's hospital bedside or in close proximity to the patient. This "point of care" testing speeds physician diagnoses, often reducing the length of a patient's stay in the hospital.

Other phlebotomists are trained to perform patient care functions, which differ from hospital to hospital. For example, they may run electrocardiogram equipment, change beds, deliver trays, or transport patients. While phlebotomists in the past worked primarily in the hospital laboratory, today's phlebotomists work closely with the nursing department and have more direct contact with patients.

Blood collection remains the mainstay of a phlebotomist's job. As part of this process, a phlebotomist performs administrative duties such as documenting the collected blood samples and labeling specimens. A phlebotomist may also administer a health-related questionnaire to the patient if one is required by the physician or an insurance company.

Workplace Settings

Most phlebotomists work in a hospital setting. Others are employed in laboratories, physicians' offices, and health departments. Some phlebotomists work with homebound individuals in nursing homes or private residences.

The job market for phlebotomists is good, provided that they are cross-trained in other specialties. Most institutions prefer phlebotomists who have additional training in areas such as performing blood tests.

Education

Most states require phlebotomists to be certified. The American Society of Phlebotomy Technicians (ASPT) is one of the bodies that provides certification.

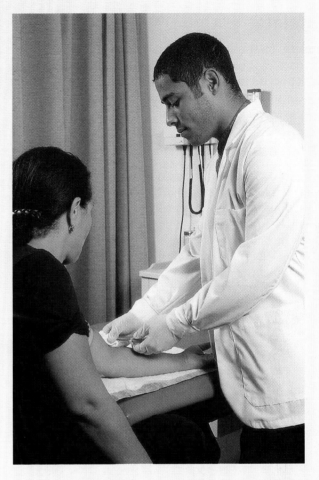

To take the ASPT's national phlebotomy examination, you must either have 6 months of full-time work experience (or 1 year of part-time work experience), or graduate from an accredited phlebotomy training program. A high school diploma or general equivalency diploma (GED) is needed to enroll in such a program. To receive full certification, candidates must have at least 100 successful, documented vein punctures and 25 successful, documented skin punctures.

Where to Go for More Information

American Society of Clinical Pathologists
2100 West Harrison
Chicago, IL 60612
(312) 738-1336

American Society of Phlebotomy Technicians
P.O. Box 1831
Hickory, NC 28603
(704) 322-1334

National Phlebotomy Association
5615 Landover Road
Hyattsville, MD 20784
(301) 386-4200

horseshoe-shaped nuclei. They also defend the body by phagocytosis, recognizing and destroying foreign organisms and particles. Monocytes have a unique ability to pass through capillary walls into the body's tissues, where they perform phagocytosis.

Platelets

Platelets, or **thrombocytes,** are fragments of cytoplasm (the part of the cell that surrounds the nucleus) of megakarocytes that are smaller than either RBCs or WBCs. Platelets are irregular in shape and have no nucleus. These cell fragments are crucial to clot formation.

Plasma and Serum

Plasma is a clear, yellow liquid in which the formed elements of blood are suspended. Plasma is nearly 90% water; it also contains about 9% protein and 1% other substances in suspension (Figure 48-2). These other substances include carbohydrates, fats, gases, mineral salts, protective substances, and waste products.

Serum is the clear, yellow liquid that remains after a blood clot forms. It differs from plasma in that it does not contain fibrinogen, a protein involved in clotting. The fibrinogen converts into fibrin (a sticky protein) and traps formed elements of the blood in a clot. The process of clotting is called **coagulation.**

Blood Types or Groups

An individual's RBCs may carry one or both of two major antigens on their surface. These antigens are known as A and B. The presence or absence of these antigens determines the blood type or group to which that person's blood belongs. Blood that contains neither A nor B antigen is designated O.

In addition to antigens, an individual's blood may contain certain antibodies. Blood that carries only the A antigen contains anti-B antibodies, and blood that carries only the B antigen contains anti-A antibodies. Blood that carries neither antigen contains both anti-A and anti-B antibodies, whereas blood that carries both antigens contains neither anti-A nor anti-B antibodies.

Blood is carefully matched before a blood transfusion. If a patient is given incompatible blood, the antibodies in the patient's blood will combine with the antigens in the transfused blood. This reaction leads to clumping of the

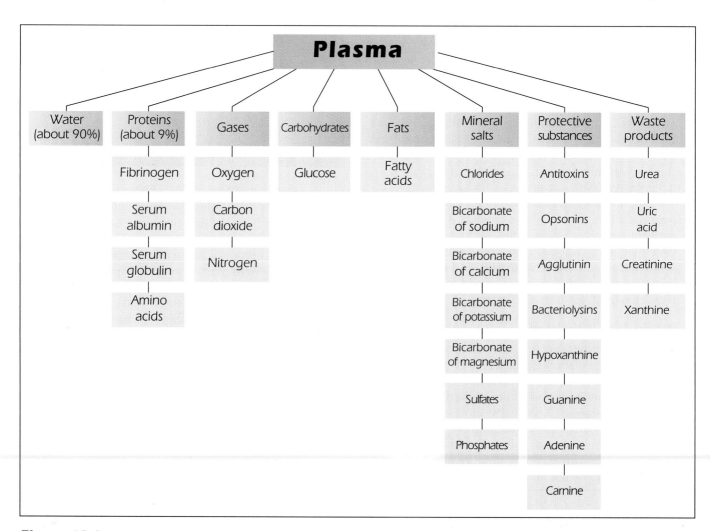

Figure 48-2. A wide variety of substances account for about 10% of plasma by volume. The remainder is water.

RBCs and possible **hemolysis** (the rupturing of red blood cells, which releases hemoglobin). The released hemoglobin can block the renal tubules and cause kidney failure and death.

Technologists can determine blood type by mixing a blood specimen with serum containing different antibodies and noting the clumping reactions that occur. The most common system for identifying blood types is the ABO system. The ABO system designates the two major antigens A and B and consists of four groups:

- A: only the A antigen (and anti-B antibodies) present
- B: only the B antigen (and anti-A antibodies) present
- AB: both A and B antigens (and neither antibodies) present
- O: neither A nor B antigen (but both antibodies) present

In addition to the ABO classification, another important blood identifier is the Rh factor. The Rh factor, so named because it was discovered through research on the rhesus monkey, is another antigen found on the surface of the RBC. Approximately 85% of people have the Rh factor in their blood, and their blood type is considered to be Rh positive (Rh+). The other 15% are Rh negative (Rh−). Like the antigens that identify the main group to which a sample belongs, the Rh antigen is also capable of generating a similar, potentially fatal, antigen-antibody reaction.

In these two classification systems, blood is identified by type and Rh factor. The following list identifies eight combinations and the approximate percentage of the population with each type, according to the American Red Cross:

- Type A+: 34%
- Type A−: 6%
- Type B+: 8%
- Type B−: 2%
- Type AB+: 3%
- Type AB−: 1%
- Type O+: 39%
- Type O−: 7%

Type O negative (O−) is considered the universal donor blood because it lacks the A, B, and Rh antigens. Type AB positive (AB+) is considered the universal recipient blood because it will not react with donated blood from any blood group. Note that recipient and donor must be compatible with regard to A and B antigens as well as the Rh factor for transfusion to be safe.

Collecting Blood Specimens

There is a standard process for drawing blood specimens. Following these steps will enable you to perform the procedure smoothly, accurately, and safely and ensure that documentation is completed properly.

Reading and Interpreting the Test Order

The first steps in preparing to draw blood for testing are to review the written testing request and to assemble the equipment and supplies. The patient should arrive with a laboratory request form if you are working in a physician's office laboratory or a laboratory drawing station. You will probably receive a test order from your supervisor if you are working in a hospital.

Reviewing the Test Order. It is essential to first review the patient's blood-collection order to determine what tests will be run. Many tests require expedited or special handling to ensure accurate results.

Your office will have specific collection procedures for each type of test. If you have any questions about these procedures, ask your supervisor. If you will be sending the blood specimen to a reference laboratory for testing, make sure you know its requirements. The cost of reprocessing a test far surpasses the extra time needed to be sure of the process requirements.

When reviewing the test order, you will need to know the meaning of certain abbreviations. Many abbreviations used in laboratory work and their meanings are presented in Figure 48-3. If you are ever in doubt or if the resources in your office or laboratory do not provide the answers you need, ask the doctor or your supervisor.

Assembling the Equipment and Supplies. Specific blood-drawing equipment and collection devices vary with the type of test. Make sure you have the appropriate equipment to collect all necessary samples if more than one test is ordered. All specimen-collection tubes, slides, and other containers should be labeled immediately after collection with the patient's name, the date and time of collection, the initials of the person collecting the specimen, and other information as required by the test procedure or your office. Some offices use an identification code for each patient.

Alcohol and cotton balls or alcohol wipes, sterile gauze, and adhesive bandages are standard supplies for procedures during which blood is drawn from a vein or capillaries. Alcohol causes inaccurate results for certain tests, however, so for these tests, povidone iodine or benzalkonium chloride is used. You will need a tourniquet (a flat, broad length of vinyl or rubber or a piece of fabric with a Velcro closure) for **venipuncture,** the puncture of a vein—performed with a needle for the purpose of drawing blood.

Preparing Patients

After you review the test order and assemble the necessary equipment and supplies, take a moment to relax, gather your thoughts, and consider your purpose. This may strike you as odd advice, but your calm and positive demeanor helps establish the best possible relationship with a patient who may be uneasy about having blood drawn. The moment you use to relax and focus may save you time and

Common Abbreviations Used in Blood Tests

Ab	antibody		CT	calcitonin
ABO	classification system for four blood groups		DAF	decay accelerating factor
AcAc	acetoacetate		DHEA	dehydroepiandrosterone, unconjugated
ACE	angiotensin-converting enzyme		Diff	differential (blood cell count)
ACT	activated coagulation time		EBNA	Epstein-Barr virus nuclear antigen
ACTH	adrenocorticotropic hormone		EBV	Epstein-Barr virus
ADH	antidiuretic hormone		EDTA	ethylenediaminetetraacetic acid
AFB	acid-fast bacillus		Eos	eosinophil
AFP	alpha-fetoprotein		EP	electrophoresis
Ag	antigen		Eq	equivalent
AG	anion gap		ERP	estrogen receptor protein
A/G R	albumin-globulin ratio		ESR	erythrocyte sedimentation rate
AHF	antihemolytic factor		FBS	fasting blood sugar
Alb	albumin		FFA	free fatty acids
Alc	alcohol		FSH	follicle-stimulating hormone (follitropin)
ALG	antilymphocyte globulin			
ALP; alk phos	alkaline phosphatase		FT_4	free thyroxine
ALT	alanine aminotransferase		FT_4I	free thyroxine index
ANA	antinuclear antibody		GFR	glomerular filtration rate
APAP	acetaminophen		GH	growth hormone
APTT	activated partial thromboplastin time		GHRH	growth hormone–releasing hormone
ASA	acetylsalicylic acid (aspirin)		GnRH	gonadotropin-releasing hormone
AST	aspartate aminotransferase		GTT	glucose tolerance test
AT-III	antithrombin III		HA	hemagglutination
B	blood (whole blood)		HAI	hemagglutination inhibition test
Baso	basophil		HAV	hepatitis A virus
BCA	breast cancer antigen		Hb; Hgb	hemoglobin
BJP	Bence Jones protein		HbCO	carboxyhemoglobin
BT	bleeding time		HBV	hepatitis B virus
BUN	blood urea nitrogen		HCG; hCG	human chorionic gonadotropin
Ca; Ca^{++}	calcium		Hct	hematocrit
CA	cancer antigen		HCV	hepatitis C virus
CBC	complete blood (cell) count		HDL	high-density lipoprotein
CEA	carcinoembryonic antigen		HDV	hepatitis delta virus
CHE	cholinesterase		HGH; hGH	human growth hormone
CK	creatine kinase		HIV	human immunodeficiency virus
CMV	cytomegalovirus		HLA	human leukocyte antigen
CN-	cyanide anion		HPV	human papilloma virus
CO	carbon monoxide		HSV	herpes simplex virus
CO_2	carbon dioxide		HTLV	human T-cell lymphotrophic virus
COHb	carboxyhemoglobin		Ig	immunoglobulin
Cr	creatinine		IgE	immunoglobulin E
CrCl	creatinine clearance		INH	inhibitor

continued ⟶

Figure 48-3. These abbreviations are routinely used in blood tests.

Source: Adapted from Norbert W. Tietz, ed., *Clinical Guide to Laboratory Tests,* 3d ed. (Philadelphia: W. B. Saunders, 1995).

Common Abbreviations Used in Blood Tests (continued)

IV	intravenous	PV	plasma volume
L	liver	PZP	pregnancy zone protein
LD; LDH	lactate dehydrogenase	RAIU	thyroid uptake of radioactive iodine
LDL	low-density lipoprotein	RBC	red blood cell; red blood (cell) count
LH	luteinizing hormone	RBP	retinol-binding protein
LMWH	low-molecular-weight heparin	RCM	red cell mass
Lytes	electrolytes	RCV	red cell volume
MCV	mean cell volume	RDW	red cell distribution of width
MetHb	methemoglobin	Retic	reticulocyte
MLC	mixed lymphocyte culture	RF	rheumatoid factor; relative fluorescence unit
MONO	monocyte	Rh	rhesus factor
MPV	mean platelet volume	RIA	radioimmunoassay
MSAFP	maternal serum alpha-fetoprotein	rT_3	reverse triiodothyronine
NE	norepinephrine	S	serum
NPN	nonprotein nitrogen	Segs	segmented polymorphonuclear leukocyte
OGTT	oral glucose tolerance test	SPE	serum protein electrophoresis
P	plasma	T_3	triiodothyronine
PAP	prostatic acid phosphatase	T_4	thyroxine
PB	protein binding	TBG	thyroxine-binding globulin
PBG	porphobilinogen	TBV	total blood volume
PCT	prothrombin consumption time	TG	triglyceride
PCV	packed cell volume (hematocrit)	TRH	thyrotropin-releasing hormone
P_i	inorganic phosphate	TSH	thyroid-stimulating hormone
PKU	phenylketonuria	VDRL	Venereal Disease Research Laboratory (test for syphilis)
PLT	platelet	VLDL	very-low-density lipoprotein
PMN	polymorphonuclear (leukocyte; neutrophil)	WB	Western blot
PRL	prolactin	WBC	white blood cell; white blood (cell) count
PSA	prostate-specific antigen		
PT	prothrombin time		
PTH	parathyroid hormone		
PTT	partial thromboplastin time		

Figure 48-3. (continued)

save patients unnecessary discomfort by contributing to a quick, efficient procedure.

Greeting and Identifying Patients. Greet patients pleasantly, introduce yourself, and explain that you will be drawing some blood. It is essential to identify patients correctly before you begin the procedure. Ask patients to state their full name, and be sure you hear both the first and last names correctly. Verify that the name the patient gives is the name on the order. (In some facilities, the phlebotomist may ask for a Social Security number or a patient ID or chart number to further identify the patient.)

Confirming Pretest Preparation. The presence and level of certain substances in blood are affected by food and fluid intake or by other activities in daily life.

Some tests require that the patient follow certain pretest restrictions. The purpose behind these restrictions is either to minimize the influence of the restricted food on the blood or to stress the body to see how it responds, as indicated by the blood.

One test that requires patients to follow pretest instructions closely is the glucose tolerance test, which measures a patient's ability to metabolize carbohydrates. This test is used to detect hypoglycemia and diabetes mellitus. You instruct the patient to eat a diet high in carbohydrates for the 3 days before the test and to fast for the 8 to 12 hours before the appointment. After initial blood and urine samples are taken, the patient ingests a measured dose of glucose solution. Blood and urine samples are then taken at prescribed intervals as ordered by the physician.

The glucose levels in the samples are often graphed for the physician's review.

Before you draw blood for any test, determine whether the patient has complied with pretest instructions. If the patient has not followed pretest instructions, explain that the test cannot be performed. Make a note on the order, and report the information to the physician or your supervisor.

Explaining the Procedure and Safety Precautions. Explain to the patient the procedure you will use to obtain the blood specimen for testing. Be clear and brief when you describe what you will do; too much detail leaves some patients queasy. You must follow Universal Precautions during all phlebotomy procedures, as described in the Caution: Handle With Care section. These precautions may be second nature to you, but they may raise concerns in the patient. Explain the need for each of the preventive measures you are taking in language the patient can understand. Assure the patient that these measures protect against exposure to infection.

Establishing a Chain of Custody. You will need to follow specific guidelines to establish a chain of custody

for blood samples drawn for drug and alcohol analysis. (Chapter 44 explains general chain of custody procedures.) Because donating a specimen for drug and alcohol testing is potentially self-incriminating, the patient must sign a consent form for the testing. (This form is discussed in Chapter 47.) Although the clerical procedures for blood tests for drug and alcohol analysis are similar to those for urine tests, blood tests differ because you can confirm by direct observation that a blood specimen has been taken from the patient in question.

Handling an Exposure Incident. When you adhere to Universal Precautions, the risk of exposure to blood-borne pathogens is very small. Accidents can occur, however. If you suffer a needlestick or other injury that results in exposure to blood or blood products from another person, you must report the incident to the appropriate staff members immediately. Wash the injured area carefully and apply a sterile bandage. Record the time and date of the incident, the names of the people involved, and the nature of the exposure. Depending on the situation, you may receive medications. You and the other person involved will be asked to undergo blood testing and be

CAUTION *Handle With Care*

Phlebotomy and Personal Protective Equipment

The Centers for Disease Control and Prevention (CDC) has classified all phlebotomy procedures as a risk for exposure to contaminated blood or blood products. You must use appropriate protective equipment during all phlebotomy procedures. Remember, it is up to you to protect yourself and the patient.

Gloves

Gloves are the first line of defense during a phlebotomy procedure. They protect against spills and splashing of contaminated blood. Wash your hands and put on clean examination gloves that fit snugly before you work with each patient. Remove the gloves, dispose of them in a biohazardous waste container, and wash your hands after working with each patient.

Garments

Garments such as laboratory coats and aprons can protect your clothing from spills and splashes and provide a measure of protection from contaminated materials. Some garments are designed to resist penetration by blood or blood products. You may find it necessary to wear such garments when drawing blood or performing blood tests.

Masks and Protective Eyewear

Mucous membranes are especially vulnerable to invasion by infectious agents. Use masks and protective

eyewear to help safeguard mucous membranes in your mouth, nose, and eyes from infection.

Masks help protect your mouth and nose from splashes or sprays of blood or blood products. You cannot predict when exposure to blood may occur. Accidental puncture of an artery during a phlebotomy procedure could result in a spray of blood. Blood may also spray or splash accidentally during some testing protocols. Most medical assistants do not routinely wear masks for phlebotomy procedures, however, once they have achieved proficiency in performing them.

Goggles can protect your eyes from splashing and spraying during blood drawing or testing. Health-care workers in dental offices often wear goggles because patient treatments can easily expose workers to contaminated blood or bloody saliva.

Clear plastic face shields combine the protection of masks and goggles. They are often used during major surgical procedures. You may use a face shield if you do extensive testing on blood specimens. Face shields are not usually worn when drawing blood.

Personal protective equipment works two ways: it protects you from a patient's contaminated blood, and it also protects the patient from infectious agents you may be carrying. By using PPE correctly, you will make your workplace a safer place for you and the patients.

PROCEDURE 48.1

Quality Control Procedures for Blood Specimen Collection

Objective: To follow proper quality control procedures when taking a blood specimen

Materials: Necessary sterile equipment, specimen-collection container, paperwork related to the type of blood test the specimen is being drawn for, requisition form, marker, proper packing materials for transport

Method

1. Review the request form for the test ordered, verify the procedure, prepare the necessary equipment and paperwork, and prepare the work area.

2. Identify the patient and explain the procedure. Confirm the patient's identification. Ask the patient to spell her name. Make sure the patient understands the procedure that is to be performed, even if she has had it done before.

3. Confirm that the patient has followed any pretest preparation requirements such as fasting, taking any necessary medication, or stopping a medication. For example, if a fasting specimen is being taken, the patient should not have eaten anything after midnight of the day before. Some doctors' offices will let the patient drink water or black coffee, however. It often depends on the type of specimen being taken.

4. Collect the specimen properly. Collect it at the right time intervals if that applies. Use sterile equipment and proper technique.

5. Use the correct specimen-collection containers and the right preservatives, if required. For example, blood collected into a test tube with additives should be mixed immediately, or it will clot.

6. Immediately label the specimens. The label should include the patient's name, the date and time of collection, the test's name, and the name of the person collecting the specimen. Do not label the containers before collecting the specimen.

7. Follow correct procedures for disposing of hazardous specimen waste and decontaminating the work area. Used needles, for instance, should immediately be placed in a biohazard sharps container.

8. Thank the patient. Keep the patient in the office if any follow-up observation is necessary.

9. If the specimen is to be transported to an outside laboratory, prepare it for transport in the proper container for that type of specimen, according to OSHA regulations. Place the container in a clear plastic bag with a zip closure and dual pockets with the international biohazard label imprinted in red or orange. The requisition form should be placed in the outside pocket of the bag. This ensures protection from contamination if the specimen leaks. Have a courier pick up the specimen and place it in an appropriate carrier (such as an insulated cooler) with the biohazard label. Place specimens to be sent by mail in appropriate plastic containers, and then place the containers inside a heavy-duty plastic container with a screw-down, nonleaking lid. Then place this container in either a heavy-duty cardboard box or nylon bag. The words *Human Specimen* or *Body Fluids* should be imprinted on the box or bag. Seal with a strong tape strip.

---

involved in follow-up studies. The Occupational Safety and Health Administration (OSHA) requires every employer to have an established procedure for handling exposure incidents.

Drawing Blood

Some, but not all, states permit medical assistants to obtain blood samples. Your office will clarify which duties, if any, you may perform related to phlebotomy procedures. If your duties include collecting blood samples, you will obtain them either through venipuncture or capillary puncture. You must understand when these techniques are used and

know how to perform them. Procedure 48-1 details quality control procedures for collecting blood specimens.

Venipuncture. Venipuncture requires puncturing a vein with a needle and collecting blood into either a tube or a syringe. The most common sites for venipuncture are the median cubital and cephalic veins of the forearm, although other sites may be used if the primary site is unacceptable. Figure 48-4 shows the veins in the antecubital fossa (the small depression inside the bend of the elbow) and the forearm that are used for venipuncture.

Various instruments are used to perform venipuncture. Practice using the devices so that your technique is smooth, steady, and competent.

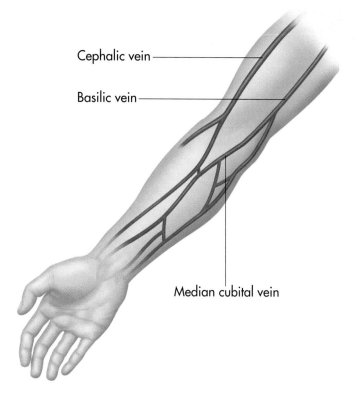

Figure 48-4. Veins commonly used for venipuncture include the cephalic vein, the basilic vein, and the median cubital vein.

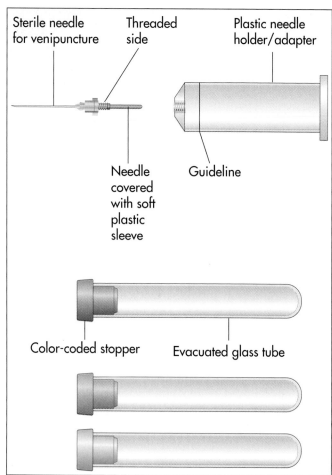

Figure 48-5. The VACUTAINER system uses interchangeable collection tubes that allow you to draw several blood specimens from the same venipuncture site.

Evacuation Systems. Evacuation systems, the most common of which is the VACUTAINER system (manufactured by Becton Dickinson VACUTAINER Systems, Franklin Lakes, New Jersey), use a special double-pointed needle, a plastic needle holder/adapter, and collection tubes (Figure 48-5). The collection tubes are sealed to create a slight vacuum. You insert the covered inner point of the needle into one end of the holder/adapter and the first collection tube into the other end. Remove the plastic cap from the outer needle of the assembled system. Hold the needle at a 15° angle to the patient's arm, and puncture the patient's vein with the needle. Then press the collection tube fully onto the covered needle tip, piercing the stopper and allowing the vacuum to help draw blood into the collection tube. Procedure 48-2 explains how to use an evacuation system to draw a blood sample.

An evacuation system has several advantages over other methods of blood collection. It is easy to collect several samples from one venipuncture site using the interchangeable vacuum collection tubes. Tubes are calibrated by evacuation to collect the exact amount of blood required. Some collection tubes are prepared with additives needed to correctly process the blood sample for testing, such as anticoagulants. Finally, because there is no need to transfer blood from a collection syringe to a sample tube, the potential for exposure to contaminated blood is reduced.

Needle and Syringe Systems. An evacuation system is not the best choice for drawing blood in every case. For example, if the patient has small or fragile veins, the vacuum created when the collection tube is pressed over the needle point can cause the veins to collapse. You may collect blood using a sterile needle and syringe assembly when an evacuation system is not suitable, such as when the patient is difficult to stick. You can use a smaller needle and control the vacuum in the syringe by pulling the plunger back slowly. Other aspects of the procedure are essentially the same, except that the blood sample is collected in the syringe and must immediately be transferred to a collection tube.

Butterfly Systems. You may also use a butterfly system, or winged infusion set, when you work with patients who have small or fragile veins. Flexible wings attached to the needle simplify needle insertion. A length of flexible tubing (either 5 or 12 inches, approximately) connects the needle to the collection device. The inserted needle remains completely undisturbed while the collection device is manipulated. Because it is motionless, the needle causes less trauma to the vein and surrounding tissue than do other systems for venipuncture. A butterfly system generally uses a smaller needle (23 gauge) than other venipuncture

Performing Venipuncture Using an Evacuation System

Objective: To collect a venous blood sample using an evacuation system

OSHA Guidelines

Materials: VACUTAINER components (needle, needle holder/adapter, collection tubes), antiseptic and cotton balls or antiseptic wipes, tourniquet, sterile gauze squares, sterile adhesive bandages

Method

1. Review the laboratory request form, and make sure you have the necessary supplies.

2. Greet the patient, confirm the patient's identity, and introduce yourself.

3. Explain the purpose of the procedure, and confirm that the patient has followed the physician's special instructions.

4. Make sure the patient is sitting in a venipuncture chair or is lying down.

5. Wash your hands. Put on examination gloves.

6. Prepare the needle holder/adapter assembly by inserting the threaded side of the needle into the adapter and twisting the adapter in a clockwise direction. Push the first collection tube into the other end of the needle holder/adapter until the outer edge of the collection tube stopper meets the guideline.

7. Ask the patient whether one arm is better than the other for the venipuncture. The chosen arm should be positioned slightly downward (Figure 48-6).

8. Apply the tourniquet to the patient's upper arm midway between the elbow and the shoulder. Wrap the tourniquet around the patient's arm and cross the ends. Holding one end of the tourniquet against the patient's arm, stretch the other end to apply pressure against the patient's skin. Pull a loop of the stretched end under the end held tightly against the patient's skin, as shown in Figure 48-7. The tourniquet should be

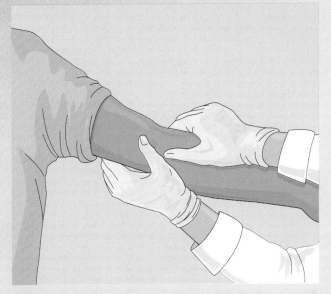

Figure 48-6. The patient's arm should be positioned slightly downward for a venipuncture.

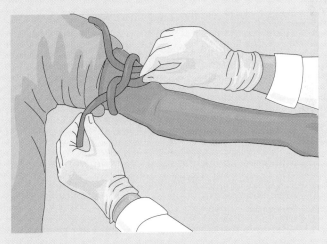

Figure 48-7. Applying a tourniquet makes it easier to find a patient's vein when you are drawing blood.

tight enough to cause the veins to stand out but should not stop the flow of blood. You should still be able to feel the patient's radial pulse. Ask the patient to make a fist and release it several times to make the veins in the forearm stand out more prominently.

9. Palpate the proposed site, and use your index finger to locate the vein, as shown in Figure 48-8. The vein will feel like a small tube with some

continued ⟶

Performing Venipuncture Using an Evacuation System *(continued)*

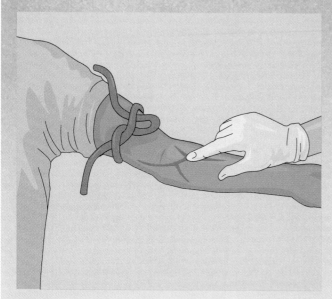

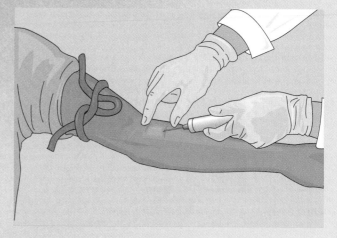

Figure 48-9. When performing venipuncture, hold the needle at a 15° angle.

Figure 48-8. Use your index finger to locate the vein.

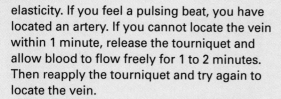

elasticity. If you feel a pulsing beat, you have located an artery. If you cannot locate the vein within 1 minute, release the tourniquet and allow blood to flow freely for 1 to 2 minutes. Then reapply the tourniquet and try again to locate the vein.

10. After locating the vein, clean the area with a cotton ball moistened with antiseptic or an antiseptic wipe. Use a circular motion to clean the area, starting at the center and working outward. Allow the site to air-dry, or use the same circular motion to wipe the area dry with a sterile gauze square.

11. Remove the plastic cap from the outer point of the needle cover, and ask the patient to tighten the fist. Hold the patient's skin taut above and below the insertion site. With a steady and quick motion, insert the needle—held at a 15° angle, bevel side up, and aligned parallel to the vein—into the vein (Figure 48-9). You will feel a slight resistance as the needle tip penetrates the vein wall. Penetrate to a depth of ¼ to ½ inch. Grasp the holder/adapter between your index and great (middle) fingers. Using your thumb, seat the collection tube firmly into place over the needle point, puncturing the rubber stopper. Blood will begin to flow into the collection tube.

12. Fill each tube until the blood stops running to ensure the correct proportion of blood to additives. Switch tubes as needed by pulling one tube out of the adapter and inserting the next in a smooth and steady motion. (The soft plastic cover on the inner point of the needle retracts as each tube is inserted and recovers the needle point as each tube is removed.)

13. Once blood is flowing steadily, ask the patient to release the fist, and untie the tourniquet by pulling the end of the tucked-in loop. The tourniquet should, in general, be left on no longer than 1 minute. (Longer periods may cause hemoconcentration, an increase in the blood-cell-to-plasma ratio, and invalidate test results.) You must remove the tourniquet before you withdraw the needle from the vein. (Removing the tourniquet releases pressure on the vein.)

14. As you withdraw the needle in a smooth and steady motion, place a sterile gauze square over the insertion site (Figure 48-10). Dispose of the needle immediately. Instruct the patient to hold the gauze pad in place with slight pressure. The patient should keep the arm straight and slightly elevated for several minutes.

15. If the collection tubes contain additives, you will need to invert them slowly several times to mix the chemical agent and the blood sample.

16. Label specimens and complete the paperwork.

continued ⟶

Performing Venipuncture Using an Evacuation System *(continued)*

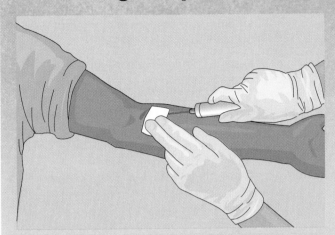

17. Check the patient's condition and the puncture site for bleeding. Replace the sterile gauze square with a sterile adhesive bandage.
18. Properly dispose of used supplies and disposable instruments, and disinfect the work area.
19. Remove the gloves and wash your hands.
20. Instruct the patient about care of the puncture site.
21. Document the procedure in the patient's chart.

Figure 48-10. Place a sterile gauze square over the insertion site as you withdraw the needle.

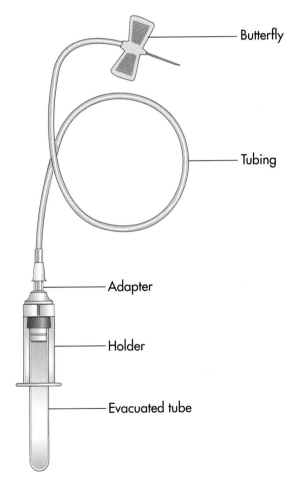

- Butterfly
- Tubing
- Adapter
- Holder
- Evacuated tube

Figure 48-11. Once inserted, the needle of a butterfly system remains undisturbed during specimen collection.

techniques do. A butterfly system can be used with an evacuated collection tube or a syringe (Figure 48-11).

Collection Tubes. No matter which method is used to collect blood, the samples must immediately be mixed with the appropriate additives in the correct collection tubes before they are transported to the laboratory for testing. The stoppers of the tubes are different colors, each color identifying the type of additives (if any) they contain (Figure 48-12).

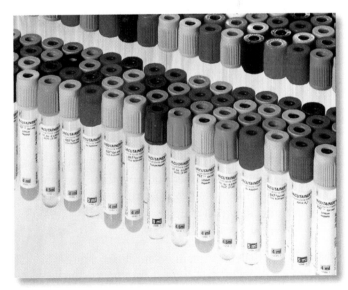

Figure 48-12. Special color-coded stoppers on collection tubes indicate which additives are present and, therefore, which types of laboratory tests may be performed on each blood specimen.

Collecting, Processing, and Testing Blood Specimens

TABLE 48-1　Blood-Collection Tubes

Stopper Color	Additive	Test Types
Yellow	Sodium polyanetholesulfonate	Blood cultures
Red	None	Blood chemistries, AIDS antibody, viral studies, serologic tests, blood grouping and typing
Red/black (tiger stripes)	Silicone serum separator	Tests requiring blood serum
Blue	Sodium citrate (anticoagulant)	Coagulation studies
Green	Sodium heparin (anticoagulant)	Electrolyte studies, arterial blood gases
Lavender	Ethylenediaminetetraacetic acid (EDTA) (anticoagulant)	Hematology studies
Gray	Potassium oxalate or sodium fluoride (anticoagulant)	Blood glucose

These additives must be compatible with the laboratory process that the sample will undergo. Each laboratory may choose which tubes to use for a particular test.

Additives include anticoagulants and other materials that help preserve or process a sample for particular types of testing. When you collect a blood sample, double-check that you are using the appropriate collection tubes for the tests ordered. You must also fill the tubes in a specific order to preserve the integrity of the blood sample. Each laboratory requires a specific order of draw for collection tubes. The National Committee for Clinical Laboratory Standards also publishes its recommended order of draw. Table 48-1, identifies collection tube stopper colors, additives present in the tubes, and types of tests, in a typical order of draw.

Engineered Safety Devices.　In response to the Needlestick Safety and Prevention Act, a number of engineered safety devices have been developed. These devices are intended to reduce the possibility of needlestick injuries (Figure 48-13). According to the National Institute for Occupational Safety and Health (NIOSH), the desired characteristics of engineered safety devices include the following:

- The performance of the device is reliable
- The device is easy to use, safe, and effective
- The device should be needleless when possible
- The device should either not have to be activated by the user or may be activated using only one hand
- Once the safety feature is activated, it cannot be deactivated

Procedure 48-1 details quality control procedures for collecting blood specimens.

In certain circumstances, some of these characteristics are not feasible. Drawing blood from an artery or a vein is not possible without the use of a needle. Several types of safety devices for collecting blood specimens have been

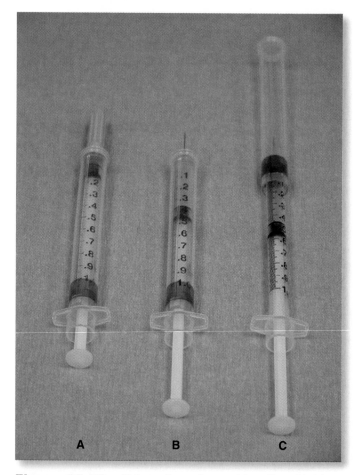

Figure 48-13.　Tuberculin syringe with safety shield: (a) syringe before use, (b) syringe during injection, and (c) safety shield engaged after injection.
Photo courtesy of Total Care Programming.

developed. These include:

- Retracting needles
- Hinged or sliding shields that cover phlebotomy and winged-steel (butterfly) needles

- Self-blunting phlebotomy and winged-steel needles
- Retractable lancets

Studies show that these devices, when used properly, have reduced needlestick injuries. NIOSH reports a 76% reduction of injuries with self-blunting needles, a 66% reduction with hinged needle shields, and a 23% reduction with sliding shields.

In addition to advocating the use of appropriate engineered safety devices, NIOSH also recommends that healthcare workers follow these precautions:

- Recap needles only when absolutely necessary
- Ensure the safe handling and disposal of sharps prior to beginning a procedure
- Dispose of used sharps promptly using approved sharps containers
- Report all needlestick injuries
- Inform their employer of workplace hazards
- Attend yearly blood-borne pathogen training
- Follow recommended infection control practices

Capillary Puncture. **Capillary puncture** requires a superficial puncture of the skin with a sharp point. Compared with venipuncture, capillary puncture releases a smaller amount of blood. The blood may be collected in small, calibrated glass tubes. It may also be collected on glass microscope slides or applied to reagent strips (or dipsticks), which are specially treated paper or plastic strips used in specific diagnostic tests.

Capillary puncture in adults and children is usually performed on the great (middle) finger or the ring finger. (Use the patient's nondominant hand for this procedure if possible.) The puncture should be made slightly off center on the pad of the fingertip. Capillary puncture in infants is usually performed on one of the outer edges of the underside of the heel. An alternate site for both children and adults is the lower part of the earlobe, unless the patient's ear is pierced.

Lancets. Lancets are used in the capillary puncture technique. This technique is employed when the amount of blood required for a specific procedure is not very large or when technical difficulties prevent use of the venipuncture technique. A **lancet** is a small, disposable instrument with a sharp point used to puncture the skin and make a shallow incision (between 2.0 and 3.0 mm deep for an adult and no deeper than 2.4 mm for an infant). The blood welling up from the incision is then collected.

Automatic Puncturing Devices. Automatic puncturing devices are loaded with a lancet. Because the depth to which they puncture the skin is mechanically controlled, they are more accurate than the traditional lancet method. These spring-loaded devices have disposable platforms that rest on the finger. Different platforms are used, depending on the desired depth of the puncture. Both the lancet and the platform should be discarded after use. Some companies also manufacture completely disposable devices, which come individually wrapped and are used only once.

Micropipettes. A pipette is a calibrated glass tube for measuring fluids. A **micropipette** is a small pipette that holds a small, precise volume of fluid. You will use micropipettes to collect capillary blood for some tests. Capillary tubes, with a single calibration mark, are also used to collect capillary blood for certain tests. Procedure 48-3 explains how to perform a capillary puncture and collect a sample of capillary blood.

PROCEDURE 48.3

Performing Capillary Puncture

Objective: To collect a capillary blood sample using the finger puncture method

OSHA Guidelines

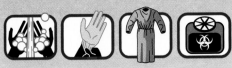

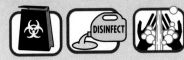

Materials: Capillary puncture device (lancet or automatic puncture device such as Autolet or Glucolet), antiseptic and cotton balls or antiseptic wipes, sterile gauze squares, sterile adhesive bandages, reagent strips, micropipettes, smear slides

Method

1. Review the laboratory request form, and make sure you have the necessary supplies.
2. Greet the patient, confirm the patient's identity, and introduce yourself.
3. Explain the purpose of the procedure, and confirm that the patient has followed the doctor's special instructions.
4. Make sure the patient is sitting in the venipuncture chair or is lying down.
5. Wash your hands. Put on examination gloves.

continued ⟶

Performing Capillary Puncture *(continued)*

6. Examine the patient's hands to determine which finger to use for the procedure. Avoid fingers that are swollen, bruised, scarred, or calloused. Generally, the ring and great (middle) fingers are the best choices. If you notice that the patient's hands are cold, you may want to warm them between your own, have the patient put them in a warm basin of water or under warm running water, or wrap them in a warm cloth. Warming the patient's hands improves circulation.

7. Prepare the patient's finger with a gentle "milking" or rubbing motion toward the fingertip. Keep the patient's hand below heart level so that gravity helps the blood flow.

8. Clean the area with a cotton ball moistened with antiseptic or an antiseptic wipe. Allow the site to air-dry, or wipe the area dry with a sterile gauze square.

9. Hold the patient's finger between your thumb and forefinger. Hold the lancet or automatic puncture device at a right angle to the patient's fingerprint, as shown in Figure 48-14. Puncture the skin on the pad of the fingertip with a quick, sharp motion. The depth to which you puncture the skin is generally determined by the length of the lancet point. Most automatic puncturing devices are designed to penetrate to the correct depth.

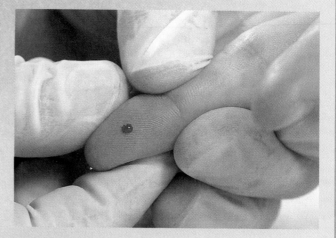

Figure 48-15. Apply steady pressure to the patient's finger, but do not milk it.

10. Allow a drop of blood to form at the end of the patient's finger. If the blood droplet is slow in forming, apply steady pressure (Figure 48-15). Avoid milking the patient's finger, because it dilutes the blood sample with tissue fluid and causes hemolysis.

11. Wipe away the first droplet of blood. (This droplet is usually contaminated with tissue fluids released when the skin is punctured.) Then fill the collection devices, as described.

    Micropipettes: Hold the tip of the tube just to the edge of the blood droplet. The tube will fill through capillary action. If you are preparing microhematocrit tubes, you need to seal one end of each tube with clay sealant. (See Procedure 48-5 for this process.)

    Reagent strips: With some reagent strips (dipsticks), you must touch the strip to the blood drop but not smear it; with other strips, you must smear it. Follow the manufacturer's guidelines.

    Smear slides: Gently touch the blood droplet to the smear slide and process the slide as described in Procedure 48-4.

12. After you have collected the required samples, dispose of the lancet immediately. Then wipe the patient's finger with a sterile gauze square (Figure 48-16). Instruct the patient to apply pressure to stop the bleeding.

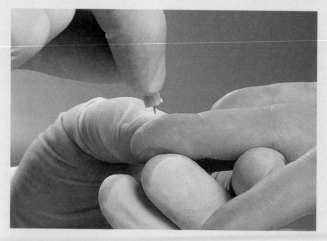

Figure 48-14. Hold the lancet or automatic puncture device at a right angle to the patient's fingerprint.

continued ⟶

Performing Capillary Puncture *(continued)*

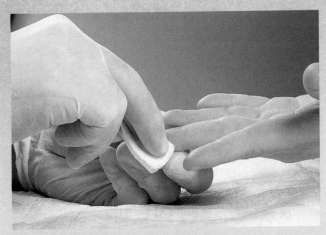

Figure 48-16. Use a sterile gauze square to wipe remaining blood from the patient's finger.

13. Label specimens and complete the paperwork. Some tests, such as glucose monitoring, must be completed immediately.

14. Check the puncture site for bleeding. If necessary, replace the sterile gauze square with a sterile adhesive bandage.

15. Properly dispose of used supplies and disposable instruments, and disinfect the work area.

16. Remove the gloves and wash your hands.

17. Instruct the patient about care of the puncture site.

18. Document the procedure in the patient's chart. (If the test has been completed, include the results.)

MICROTAINER Tubes. MICROTAINER tubes (manufactured by Becton Dickinson VACUTAINER Systems) are small plastic tubes that have a widemouthed collector, similar to a funnel, which allows blood to flow quickly and freely into the tube. Like collection tubes in an evacuation system, MICROTAINER tubes have different colored tops indicating which, if any, additives they contain.

Reagent Products. Several common tests do not require processing of fluid blood samples. For these tests, you may apply droplets of freshly collected blood to chemically treated paper or plastic reagent strips (dipsticks) or add freshly collected blood droplets to small containers holding chemicals that react in the presence of specific substances or microorganisms. Some of the blood tests performed in this way are those for determining blood glucose levels, sickle cell anemia, infectious mononucleosis, and rheumatoid arthritis.

Smear Slides. You may need to apply a drop of freshly collected blood to a prepared microscope slide for some tests. More commonly, a smear slide is prepared in the laboratory from a blood sample containing an anticoagulant, for examination under a microscope.

Responding to Patient Needs

Many patients are anxious when they have a blood test, and some patients have special needs or present special problems that make drawing blood challenging. Anxiety about blood tests may stem from a variety of concerns. Special needs may be related to a patient's age group or a medical condition. Some problems involve difficulty obtaining a blood sample or the patient's physiological or emotional response to a procedure. Being aware of possible sources of patient anxiety and understanding a wide range of special concerns can help you respond to patient needs with sensitivity and competence.

Patient Fears and Concerns

Some patients express their fears or concerns directly. Other patients ask questions that highlight their fears. Providing more information or a complete understanding is reassuring to many patients. For others, the information serves only to confuse, overwhelm, or create more fear. You must decide how much information to give each patient and be prepared to answer questions.

Patients sometimes ask questions that are not appropriate for you to answer. A patient may ask you about his prognosis, medical condition, blood type, or other medical information. It is not appropriate for you to discuss these topics with the patient. Tell the patient that only the physician can answer such questions. There are some commonly expressed fears and concerns to which you should respond, however.

Pain. The question that medical assistants performing phlebotomy probably hear most often is, Will this hurt? Never lie to a patient who asks this question. Inform the patient that he will feel a stick just as the lancet or point of the needle is inserted but that this pain goes away almost immediately. Tell a patient who seems particularly nervous to take a deep breath and let it out slowly. Also suggest that the patient focus on something else in the room or close his eyes and relax during the procedure.

A patient may express concern and report a previous unpleasant experience with blood testing. Listen to the patient's concerns. Describe what you will do to reduce discomfort and what the patient can do to be more at ease. Let the patient know that you will help him sit comfortably or lie down while the blood sample is being obtained. Tell the patient to let you know if he begins to feel lightheaded. You might also ask the patient whether one arm is better to use than the other. Many patients have had blood drawn before and can tell you which sites were successful. Consulting the patient helps the patient feel more in control and provides you with important information.

Bruises or Scars. Some patients may express fear of getting a bruise or scar from a blood test. Explain that some bruising is possible but that it will fade within a few days. Most bruising is caused by a hematoma, which occurs when blood leaks out of the vein and collects under the skin. Hematomas can be prevented by releasing the tourniquet before withdrawing the needle and applying proper pressure over the puncture site after the needle has been withdrawn. Bruising is common with fair-skinned patients. Scars, on the other hand, are unlikely.

Serious Diagnosis. Patient fears are not always rational. One fear that patients express is that the more tubes of blood you require, the more serious their condition must be. Patients may also fear that a blood test is being done to help the doctor diagnose an extremely serious disease.

You can help relieve a patient's fears by explaining that a blood test is one of the best ways to obtain an overall picture of health (emphasize health, not disease). Note that blood tests show what is normal about the blood as well as any abnormalities. You might also explain that several samples are being taken because the blood used in blood tests is processed in different ways; the blood collected for one test cannot be used in another.

Blood testing may also be done to determine how well and at what levels medications are acting in the blood. Explain that the doctor may want to see how much medication is in the blood to better manage the prescribed dosage. When a patient needs repeated tests for drug levels, explain that the tests show how the body is using the medication.

Contracting a Disease From the Procedure. Probably the greatest fear of patients undergoing blood tests is contracting HIV, AIDS, or hepatitis B virus (HBV). Although many people are now well informed about how AIDS and other serious diseases are contracted, it is understandable for a patient to worry about blood-borne pathogens. Do not dismiss the patient's concerns, and do not downplay the importance of following Universal Precautions.

Explain the precautions you will take to prevent the spread of infection. Allow the patient to see you wash your hands and put on new gloves before you begin to take the blood sample. Stress that the needle is sterile. Explain that you have not touched the needle and that it will be discarded when you finish. Let the patient see you put the needle in the sharps container.

Use this opportunity to educate the patient about the transmission of AIDS. Emphasize that AIDS, and other infections transmitted by blood, can be transmitted only when there is direct contact with contaminated blood or other body fluids. Explain that your gloves protect both you and the patient by providing a barrier to infection transmission from one person to another. Explain that your other protective equipment, such as goggles or a mask, also helps prevent the spread of infection.

Special Considerations

As you collect blood specimens, you will encounter a variety of patients, some of whom have special needs. You will find yourself in many different situations, some of them problematic. Some special needs and problematic situations are fairly common, and you must be prepared to deal with them.

Children. It is a challenge to explain blood-drawing procedures to children. Many children become visibly upset by the situation. If possible, it is best to talk with the parents or caregivers before working with the child. The adults can provide the best insight into how their child handles stressful situations.

Your primary concern when working with infants is to complete tests correctly. Because an infant's veins are often too small for adequate blood collection, the best site for drawing blood is usually the heel.

When working with children, address them directly. Speak clearly in a calm, soothing voice, and explain the procedure briefly in terms they can understand. If they ask whether the process will hurt, be honest. Very young children should be held by their parent or guardian or a coworker during a venipuncture or capillary puncture to prevent them from moving. If a child is extremely distressed, it may be best to go on to another patient while the child calms down.

After you have begun the procedure, give the child status reports such as, "We're almost finished!" and "You've been very brave." This information helps calm nervous parents or caregivers as well.

When the procedure is complete, offer a compliment on some aspect of the child's behavior. Gather your supplies and samples as quickly as possible to avoid alarming the child with the sight of blood-collection tubes. If parents or caregivers have questions, encourage them to discuss the tests with the child's physician.

Elderly Patients. The challenges presented by elderly patients may test your technical skills as well as your interpersonal skills. Physically, some older adults are frail and may not withstand blood-drawing procedures as easily as younger patients. Changes in skin condition often make elderly patients more prone to bruising and other injuries. Decreased circulation may make it difficult to collect enough blood for an adequate sampling. Elderly patients with impaired hearing may have trouble understanding instructions and answering questions. Patients with dementia may also be unable to understand what you are saying.

When you communicate with an elderly patient, speak in clear, low-pitched tones. High-pitched voices are more difficult for people with hearing impairments to understand. When asking questions, give the patient time to answer, and confirm the response to prevent misunderstandings. Avoid both overly simple yes or no questions that the patient might answer without thinking and overly complex questions that might confuse the patient. Take your time with the procedure, and explain it in language the patient can understand.

Patients at Risk for Uncontrolled Bleeding. Patients who have hemophilia or are taking blood-thinning medications are at risk for uncontrolled bleeding at the collection site. (Hemophilia is a disorder in which the blood does not coagulate at a wound or puncture site.) Be especially careful and alert as you follow the standard procedures for collecting a blood specimen. In addition, hold several gauze squares over the puncture site for at least 5 minutes to make sure bleeding has stopped completely. If uncontrolled bleeding does occur, call the physician immediately.

Difficult Patients. You may encounter a particular challenge in working with a patient either because of technical problems or because of personality issues. Being prepared for these situations is the best method for coping with them.

The Difficult Venipuncture. There will be times when you simply cannot get a good blood sample. If your first attempt at drawing blood fails, try again at another site. Give the patient (and yourself) a short break, and make an attempt on the other arm, for instance. Sometimes the veins in one arm are easier to work with than the veins in the other arm. If you cannot get a good sample on the second try, stop. Ask for assistance from your supervisor or the doctor.

Fainting Patients. It is impossible to predict which patients will have a reaction to a blood-drawing procedure. Generally, however, an ill patient is more likely to experience a reaction than a well patient. The best way to deal with this potential problem is to position every patient so that, if fainting does occur, no injury will result.

Have patients sit in a special venipuncture chair (Figure 48-17). These chairs are designed to help prevent patients from sliding to the floor in the event of fainting. If your office is not equipped with a venipuncture chair, have patients lie down on an examination table. A patient who has a history of fainting or feels ill should lie down with feet elevated or knees drawn up while you complete the procedure.

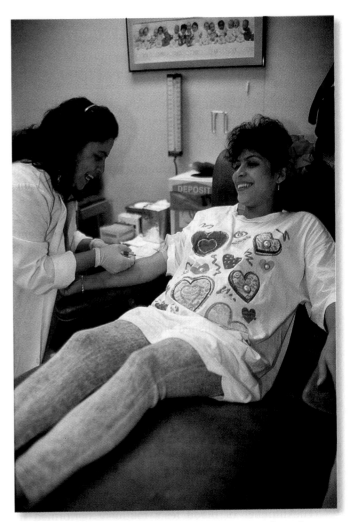

Figure 48-17. Venipuncture chairs are designed to make blood drawing easier and to prevent patients from falling if they should faint.

If a patient does faint and the needle is still in the vein, release the tourniquet and withdraw the needle quickly and steadily. Apply pressure to the site. Most people revive promptly, and no other action is required. Do not leave the patient alone. Notify the doctor that the patient fainted, and ask the doctor whether you should continue with the procedure.

If there is a more severe reaction, notify the appropriate staff member and remain with the patient. If the patient is in a chair and begins to slide out, raise the safety arm and gently lower the patient to the floor. Protect the patient's head at all times, and make sure the patient is breathing. The doctor should examine the patient before the patient is moved. Follow the doctor's instructions.

When the patient begins to recover, assist the person into a sitting position and then to a chair or couch. The patient should rest until feeling strong enough to walk—usually about 15 minutes. When the patient feels steady, take the patient to another area of the office, such as the patient reception area. At this point another staff member usually becomes responsible for the patient's care and determines when it is safe for the patient to leave.

Measuring Hematocrit Percentage After Centrifuge *(continued)*

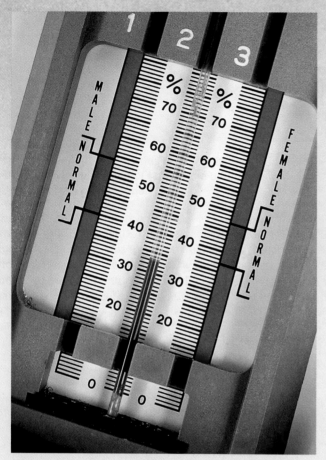

Figure 48-27. Compare the column of packed red blood cells in the microhematocrit tube with the hematocrit gauge to determine the hematocrit percentage.

9. Run the centrifuge for the required time, usually between 3 and 5 minutes. Allow the centrifuge to come to a complete stop before unsealing it.

10. Determine the hematocrit percentage by comparing the column of packed red blood cells in the microhematocrit tubes with the hematocrit gauge, as shown in Figure 48-27. Position each tube so that the boundary between sealing clay and red blood cells is at zero on the gauge. Some centrifuges are equipped with gauges, but others require separate handheld gauges.

11. Record the percentage value on the gauge that corresponds to the top of the column of red blood cells for each tube. Compare the two results. They should not vary by more than 3%. If you record a greater variance, at least one of the tubes was filled incorrectly, and you must repeat the test.

12. Calculate the average result by adding the two tube figures and dividing that number by 2.

13. Properly dispose of used supplies, and clean and disinfect the equipment and the area.

14. Remove the gloves and wash your hands.

15. Record the test result in the patient's chart. Be sure to identify abnormal results.

---

total blood volume represented by the RBCs. Average the readings of the two patient samples. (The samples should be within 3% of each other.)

Hemoglobin. Hemoglobin resides within the red blood cells. You will determine the concentration of hemoglobin in the blood by lysing (rupturing) the red blood cells (hemolysis) and evaluating the color of the sample. This procedure may be done with a hemoglobinometer—a handheld device that makes color evaluation less subjective than older methods of visual matching with color samples. Blood specimens mixed with a reagent, such as Drabkin's reagent, undergo a color reaction that can be quantified by reading color intensity in a photoelectric colorimeter.

Morphologic Studies. **Morphology** is the study of the shape or form of objects. A morphologic study of a blood sample can provide important information about a patient's condition. During a morphologic study on blood, a blood smear is examined, and the appearance and shape of cells in the sample are recorded. Special note is made of abnormal cell size, shape, or content and abnormal organization of cells. A morphologic study is often performed just after the differential count and platelet estimate on the same blood smear slide. Morphologic studies require special training and are not routinely done by medical assistants.

Coagulation Tests. A physician may order coagulation tests to identify potential bleeding problems before surgical procedures. A regular schedule of coagulation tests may be ordered to monitor therapeutic drug levels when a patient is receiving medications such as heparin or warfarin (Coumadin). Coagulation studies include the prothrombin time (PT) and partial thromboplastin time (PTT) tests. These tests are usually performed using automated

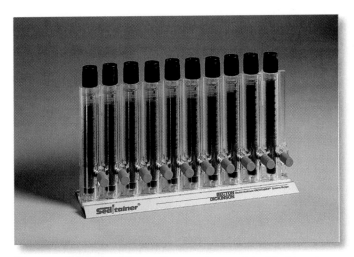

Figure 48-28. The sedimentation rack holds blood specimens steady and level for the ESR test.

devices such as the Coaguchek Plus, manufactured by Boehringer Mannheim Diagnostics, Indianapolis, Indiana. These systems monitor the changing pattern of light transmission through the sample as coagulation occurs. Medical assistants sometimes perform such coagulation studies.

Erythrocyte Sedimentation Rate. The nonautomated **erythrocyte sedimentation rate (ESR)** test measures the rate at which red blood cells, the heaviest blood component, settle to the bottom of a blood sample. You will transfer freshly collected, anticoagulated blood to a calibrated tube and place the tube in a sedimentation rack to run this test (Figure 48-28). You examine the tube an hour later to determine how far the red blood cells have fallen. Test results are recorded as millimeters per hour (mm/hr). Several standard testing systems are used, including the Westergren and Wintrobe systems. You must adhere closely to each manufacturer's instructions when using these systems, because ESR test results are sensitive to factors such as the temperature and freshness of the samples, precise position of the sample tube, and vibrations affecting the tube or the rack.

Chemical Tests

Blood chemistry analysis examines several dozen chemicals found in human blood. Tables 48-2 and 48-3 include many chemical tests on blood. Highly detailed studies are rarely performed in the POL because they require expensive, sophisticated equipment and techniques. Complex testing is also subject to strict CLIA '88 regulations that increase the administrative work and the need for more highly trained personnel. These types of tests, therefore, are commonly performed at an independent test laboratory. Automated equipment for analyzing blood chemistry, however, is becoming more available, less expensive, and simpler to operate than it was in the past. This trend makes it more likely that you may use automated equipment to perform some types of blood chemistry tests. Keeping abreast of new developments will help prepare you for possible changes in your laboratory duties.

Blood Glucose Monitoring. Some tests of blood chemistry are routinely performed in the POL. Blood glucose monitoring, for example, is often performed by a medical assistant or by a patient. Glucose monitoring systems require the use of sterile lancets to perform a capillary puncture. You will collect the blood on reagent strips that change color in accordance with glucose levels present in the blood. The level is determined either by comparing the color on the strip with color standards provided with the reagent strips or by feeding the strip into a handheld reading device. You will teach patients to perform this kind of test at home. Be sure to stress the importance of following the manufacturer's guidelines for correct operation of a testing device.

You will also teach patients and their families how to manage diabetes. This will include performing the blood glucose test, managing diet and exercise, self-monitoring for complications associated with diabetes, and additional resources for further education. See the Educating the Patient section.

Hemoglobin A1c. Another test used to monitor the health of patients with diabetes is the hemoglobin A1c test. This test measures the amount of glycosylated hemoglobin in the blood. When blood glucose levels are elevated, the glucose molecules bind with hemoglobin to form hemoglobin A1c (HgBA1c). Once HgBA1c is formed, it remains for the life of the red blood cell (90 to 120 days). This makes it a useful tool for monitoring the overall stability of the patient's blood glucose.

It is important for a patient to maintain a normal blood glucose level. Large fluctuations in blood sugar are problematic in patients with diabetes. These fluctuations can cause complications such as eye disease, stroke, renal failure, and cardiovascular disease. The HgBA1c test gives the physician a good overall picture of the patient's compliance to and the effectiveness of diabetes treatment.

There are several options for performing this test. The test may be sent to an outside reference laboratory with results available in 1 to 7 days. Some physicians' offices have the equipment necessary to perform this test in the office laboratory. These results are usually available in less than 10 minutes. Several home tests have recently become available. The patient can monitor his own HgBA1c levels, thus keeping a close watch on the efficiency of his diabetes treatment. FDA-approved home tests include:

- Bio-rad Micromat II Hemoglobin A1c Prescription Home Use Test
- Metrika A1c Now for Home Use
- Cholestech GDX A1c Test
- Provalis Diagnostics Glycosal II HBA1c
- Flex Site Diagnostics A1c at Home

Managing Diabetes

Diabetes affects an estimated 6 percent of the population, with more than 1 million newly diagnosed cases each year. In order to reduce the complications associated with diabetes, it is important for patients to maintain stable blood sugar. Proper patient education and medical care will help patients achieve this goal. As a medical assistant, you can assist patients and their families by providing them with information about diabetes that includes:

1. The risks and consequences associated with uncontrolled blood sugar. Patients whose blood sugar is unstable are at greater risk of developing the following conditions:
   - Loss of vision
   - Kidney failure
   - Heart disease
   - Nerve damage
   - Stroke

2. The patient's type of diabetes. Patients need to know the type of diabetes they have so that they can understand the type of treatment prescribed. The types of diabetes are:
   - Type I diabetes—An autoimmune disorder characterized by the body's inability to make enough insulin. Insulin is required for glucose utilization. Patients with Type I diabetes will need to take insulin daily.
   - Type II diabetes—The most common type of diabetes. Insulin is still being produced at normal levels but can no longer be utilized by the cells of the body. This causes a buildup of unused glucose in the blood. This type of diabetes is often controlled with careful diet management and increased exercise. There are also a number of oral medications used in the treatment of Type II diabetes.
   - Gestational diabetes—Develops only during pregnancy. This type of diabetes is generally managed through proper diet and exercise. Careful monitoring is important to reduce the risk of fetal complications. Women who have had gestational diabetes have an increased risk of developing Type II diabetes.

3. Maintaining proper diet and exercise. This should include:
   - Making proper food choices
   - Keeping a food diary
   - Reading food labels

- Choosing proper food exchanges
- Creating and implementing a routine exercise program

4. Routine self-monitoring of blood sugar and Hemoglobin A1c levels. Information should include:
   - The types of blood glucose monitors available. Figure 48-29 illustrates one type of blood glucose monitor, a glucometer.
   - Instructions on obtaining monitoring supplies
   - The number of times and the specific intervals at which blood sugar should be checked, based on individual needs and the physician's recommendations
   - Instructions on performing blood glucose testing
   - Guidelines on how to maintain a chart of blood glucose levels, including the time of day, associated meals and activities, and actual blood sugar values
   - Hemoglobin A1c monitoring. The patient should understand what Hemoglobin A1c

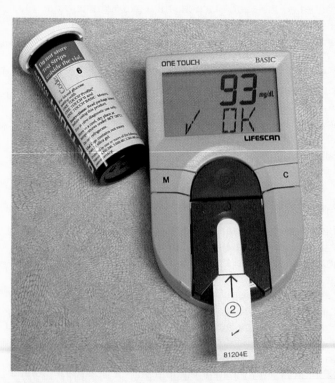

Figure 48-29. A hand-held glucometer is an important tool in helping patients manage diabetes.

continued ⟶

Educating the Patient

Managing Diabetes *(continued)*

is and why it is important to monitor these values.

- Normal (target) values for blood glucose and Hemoglobin A1c:
  - Blood glucose levels should remain between 90 and 130 mg/dl before meals and remain less than 180 mg/dl for 1 to 2 hours after a meal. Target ranges may be different for each patient. Consult with the physician about individual blood glucose levels.
  - Hemoglobin A1c is a test that shows the average amount of glucose in the blood over a three-month period. Ideally, this value should be less than 7%.

5. Symptoms of uncontrolled blood sugar. Patients need to be aware of the symptoms of both high and low blood sugar, both of which require immediate attention. Patients should test their blood sugar if any of the following occur:
   - Nausea, vomiting, or abdominal pain
   - Feeling tired all the time
   - Excessive thirst or dry mouth
   - Flushed skin
   - Confusion or difficulty thinking

6. Self-screening for complications of diabetes. Patients should be aware of the complications associated with diabetes and how to recognize them. Patients should be instructed to do the following:
   - Perform a daily foot inspection for sores
   - Recognize changes in vision
   - Recognize the symptoms of kidney failure, which include nausea, vomiting, yellow skin, and swelling of the hands and feet

- Recognizing early signs of nerve damage, which include numbness and tingling of the arms, hands, feet, or legs; dizziness; double vision; and drooping of the eyelid or lip

7. Additional sources of information. Patients should be encouraged to continue their education about diabetes. Providing patients with additional sources of information encourages them to take an active role in controlling their diabetes. Additional sources of information include:
   - American Association of Diabetes Educators
     1-800-338-DMED
     www.aadenet.org
   - American Diabetes Association
     1-800-DIABETES
     www.diabetes.org
   - American Dietetic Association
     1-800-877-1600
     1-800-366-1655 (consumer nutrition hotline in English and Spanish)
     www.eatright.org
   - Centers for Disease Control and Prevention Division of Diabetes Translation
     1-877-232-3422
     www.cdc.gov/diabetes
   - Juvenile Diabetes Foundation International
     1-800-JDF-CURE
     www.jdfcure.org
   - National Institute of Diabetes and Digestive and Kidney Diseases
     National Diabetes Information Clearinghouse
     301-654-3327
     www.niddk.hih.gov

Testing of HgBA1c should always be done in conjunction with routine blood glucose monitoring. Daily monitoring of blood glucose helps the patient with insulin therapy and diet maintenance. HgBA1c monitoring is important in assessing the patient's overall glucose levels. The advantages of this testing include:

- No pretesting preparation. The test may be done without regard to meals.
- Better overall assessment of long-term blood glucose control. Blood glucose testing gives information about glucose levels at one point in time. HgBA1c gives information over a period of 2 to 3 months.

Patients should have their HgBA1c levels checked two to four times per year. The target range for HgBA1c levels is less than 7%. Patients whose HgBA1c levels exceed 8% are at a greater risk for the complications associated with diabetes.

Serologic Tests

Serologic tests detect the presence of specific substances in a blood sample. The terms *serologic test* and *immunoassay* refer to the introduction of an antigen or antibody into the specimen and the detection of a specific reaction to the antigen or antibody. Serologic testing methods can be used to detect disease antibodies, drugs, hormones, and vitamins in the blood and to determine blood types. They are also used to test urine and other body fluids.

Immunoassays. Although medical assistants usually do not perform immunoassays, you should be familiar with several immunoassay methods that have common applications. These methods include:

- Western blot, in which antigens are blotted onto special filter paper for examination. Western blot tests are generally used to confirm HIV infection diagnosis.
- Radioimmunoassay (RIA), in which radioisotopes are used to "tag" antibodies. RIA tests are extremely sensitive and generally performed in a reference laboratory.
- Enzyme-linked immunosorbent assay (ELISA), in which enzyme-labeled antigens and substances that can absorb antigens generate reactions to specific antibodies. These reactions are identified through visual or photoelectric color detection. HIV infection is diagnosed using an ELISA test.
- Immunofluorescent antibody (IFA) test, in which dye, visible when the sample is examined under a fluorescent microscope, colors specific antibodies.

Rapid Screening Tests. Several serologic tests have been developed for quick processing. Some, such as early pregnancy tests performed on urine, are available for home use. When you use tests of this type or explain their use to a patient, keep in mind that the manufacturer's guidelines must be carefully followed to ensure accurate results.

Summary

Successful phlebotomy procedures require not only superior technical skills but also excellent interpersonal communication skills. When you are confident in your ability to perform venipuncture and capillary puncture techniques and in your understanding of common blood tests, you impart confidence to the patient. You should know what pretest instructions the patient should follow and what the patient can expect during the test.

As a medical assistant, you may be called on to complete certain testing procedures or to explain the purpose of tests to the patient. Therefore, it is important to understand the basics of blood composition and the common blood tests a patient might undergo. You can make the difference between a successfully drawn, accurately evaluated blood specimen and one that must be drawn again from a confused, unhappy patient.

CASE STUDY *QUESTIONS*

Now that you have completed this chapter, review the case study at the beginning of the chapter and answer the following questions:

1. What and where is the antecubital fossa?
2. What is the principle of the evacuated collection system?
3. How should you attempt to collect the blood on the second try?
4. What type of a blood test is a PT?
5. What could have caused the extensive bleeding this patient experienced after the venipuncture?

Discussion Questions

1. Describe the various functions of blood.
2. Identify the different methods of obtaining blood from a patient.
3. A complete blood count (CBC) consists of what components?
4. Identify the major components of whole blood.

Critical Thinking Questions

1. How would you adequately prepare a patient for drawing a blood test?
2. Identify the different blood collection tubes by their stopper color, additive, and the testing usually performed with those tubes.
3. What fears or concerns may you commonly encounter when you deal with patients who are having blood drawn?

Application Activities

1. With a partner, practice each step of the capillary puncture process on each other until you can smoothly execute each step. Critique each other's work.
2. Practice creating a smoothly drawn smear slide. Have a classmate critique your work.
3. With a classmate, role-play a situation in which a medical assistant must calm a child who is fearful about having a blood test. Then switch roles and offer suggestions for improving each other's communication skills.

Introduction

Nutrition is the process of how the body takes in and utilizes food and other sources of nutrients. It is a five-part process that includes intake, digestion, absorption, metabolism, and elimination. This chapter gives you an understanding of how a well-planned diet can lead to optimal health and well-being for your patients. You will also gain the knowledge needed to recognize the signs of illness related to diet.

CASE STUDY

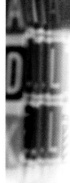

A 17-year-old female cheerleader is brought to her family doctor by her parents. As the medical assistant, you take her history and physical, noting that she has no medical problems. The patient mentions that she has a lack of interest in food because she is being "careful not to eat too many calories" so she can keep her weight down and have a chance to be head cheerleader next year. She tells you she plans to try out for a cheerleading scholarship next fall and is preparing for the competition.

You note her vital signs:

Blood pressure: 100/60
Height: 5'1"
Weight: 78 lbs.
Pulse rate: 40

She appears dehydrated and exhibits signs of muscle weakness.

As you read this chapter, consider the following questions:

1. What is the patient's probable diagnosis?
2. Do you think that the patient's attention to calorie intake is simply, as she says, preparation for the cheerleading competition?
3. Why is this patient experiencing muscle weakness?

The Role of Diet in Health

You need to know what effect food has on health so that you can help patients meet their dietary requirements. Food is the body's source of nutrients, or substances the body needs to function properly. As you study nutrition, you learn how the body uses nutrients as well as how and why people eat. People need specific types of foods to stay healthy or to regain their health after illness or surgery. People with specific conditions may also need to follow special diets.

You will work closely with the rest of the medical team to ensure that patients understand the role of diet in health and that they adhere to any diet prescribed by their physician or dietitian. A registered dietitian (RD) is a professional who uses the science of nutrition to design ways for people to obtain their optimal nourishment. Dietetics plays an important role in the health field. Dietitians work with physicians and the rest of the medical team to plan diets that are both therapeutic and realistic for patients.

Daily Energy Requirements

The human body requires the nutrients in food for three major purposes:

1. To provide energy

2. To build, repair, and maintain body tissues
3. To regulate body processes

A person's daily energy requirements depend on many factors. To understand the relationship of food to good health, you need to understand how the body uses food.

Metabolism

Food must be broken down before the body can use it. This process is an integral part of metabolism. Metabolism is the sum of all the cellular processes that build, maintain, and supply energy to living tissue. During metabolism body tissue is built up and broken down, and heat and energy are produced.

Metabolism takes place in two phases. In **anabolism,** substances such as nutrients are changed into more complex substances and used to build body tissues. In **catabolism,** complex substances, including nutrients and body tissues, are broken down into simpler substances and converted into energy. The body uses this energy to maintain and repair itself. Of the energy people get from the food they eat, about 25% is directly used for bodily functions, and the rest becomes heat.

Each person's body requires a minimal amount of nutrients to carry on a basic level of metabolism to live. Each

TABLE 49-1 Calories Burned per Hour in Selected Activities

Activity	120-lb Person	190-lb Person
Bicycling	360	570
Football (touch)	288	456
Calisthenics	324	516
Handball	456	720
Hiking	300	480
Running (10 mph)	720	1140
Skiing		
(downhill)	426	672
(cross-country)	564	888
Soccer	456	720
Swimming	228	366
Tennis	330	522
Volleyball	258	408
Walking (2 mph)	156	252

Adapted from Marvin R. Levy et al., *Life & Health: Targeting Wellness* (New York: McGraw-Hill, 1992).

person's daily nutritional requirements vary with age, weight, percentage of body fat, activity level, state of health, and other variables. The body's metabolic rate, or speed of metabolism, can also be affected by many factors, such as pregnancy, malnutrition, and disease.

Calories

The amount of energy a food produces in the body is measured in kilocalories. A kilocalorie, commonly called a **calorie,** is the amount of energy needed to raise the temperature of 1 kilogram of water by 1°C. Foods differ in the number of calories they contain. The more calories in a food, the more available energy it has. Calories are also used to measure the energy the body uses during all activities and metabolic processes.

As mentioned, people's daily nutritional needs differ, depending on variables of age, weight, percentage of body fat, activity level, and state of health. If people eat an excess of calories—more than the body can use—the excess is stored as fat in the body. Conversely, lowering caloric intake causes the body to burn off stored fat for energy.

Depending on the food's weight (in grams) or volume, each food has a value in calories. Therefore, you can count the number of calories a person consumes by monitoring food intake and adding up the calories in each food serving. You can use a food calorie counter, such as those often found in cookbooks and in nutrition books, to look up caloric values. A calorie counter tells you, for instance, that 1 cup of cooked carrots contains 50 calories or that 1 cup of cooked corn kernels contains 130 calories. Calories are also listed on the labels of food packages.

You can estimate the number of calories a person burns during certain activities by consulting a chart similar to Table 49-1. You can see how many more calories a 190-pound person burns than a 120-pound person does during the same activity.

Nutrients

The body needs a variety of nutrients for energy, growth, repair, and basic processes. Seven basic food components provide these nutrients and work together to help keep the body healthy:

1. Proteins
2. Carbohydrates
3. Fiber
4. Lipids
5. Vitamins
6. Minerals
7. Water

As the body digests foods that contain these components, it breaks them down so that it can use them. Of the seven components, only proteins, carbohydrates, and fats contain calories and provide the body with energy. The rest perform a variety of other essential functions.

Nutrition and Special Diets 973

functions. Depending on the relative amounts the body requires, minerals fall into two categories:

1. Major minerals that the body needs in fairly large quantities, including calcium, magnesium, and phosphorus
2. Trace minerals that the body needs in tiny amounts, including iron, iodine, zinc, selenium, copper, fluoride, chromium, manganese, and molybdenum

Minerals essential to good health include calcium, iron, iodine, zinc, copper, magnesium, phosphorus, fluoride, manganese, chromium, molybdenum, and selenium. Calcium, iron, and iodine are the minerals in which people are most often deficient. Most minerals are absorbed in the intestines, and any excess is eliminated.

Minerals With Recommended Dietary Allowances. There are several minerals for which RDAs have been established. These minerals are calcium, iron, iodine, zinc, magnesium, phosphorus, and selenium.

Calcium. Calcium builds healthy bones and teeth, aids in blood clotting, and helps nerves and muscles function properly. It is found in dairy products, green leafy vegetables, broccoli, legumes, and the soft bones of sardines and salmon (Figure 49-7).

Calcium deficiency can cause poor bone growth and tooth development in children, osteoporosis in adults, and poor blood clotting. The normal requirement is 800 to 1200 milligrams per day.

Iron. Iron, one of the most important nutrients, is essential for the production of red blood cells, which transport oxygen throughout the body. It is also a component of enzymes needed for energy production. Although iron is found in a wide variety of foods, it is the most frequently deficient nutrient in people's diets. Liver, meat, poultry, fish, egg yolks, fortified breads and cereals, dark green vegetables, and dried fruits are good dietary sources of iron (Figure 49-8), although less than 20% of it is usually absorbed.

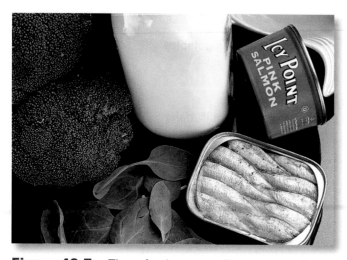

Figure 49-7. These foods are excellent sources of calcium, a mineral that is necessary for strong bones and teeth.

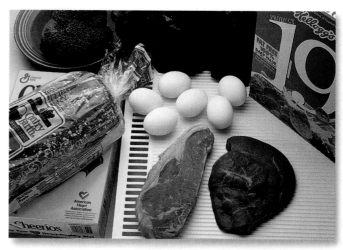

Figure 49-8. Iron, a mineral that is needed in small amounts, is found in a wide variety of foods.

Iron deficiency can cause anemia, a blood disorder that results in fatigue, weakness, and impaired mental abilities. At toxic levels iron may increase the risk of coronary heart disease. The daily requirement is 10 to 15 milligrams.

Iodine. Iodine plays a vital role in the activities of the thyroid hormones, which are involved in reproduction, growth, nerve and muscle function, and the production of new blood cells. Deficiency can cause an enlarged thyroid gland, known as goiter. Iodine can be obtained in seafood, iodized salt, and seaweed products. The daily requirement is 150 micrograms.

Zinc. Zinc promotes normal growth and wound healing and participates in many cell activities that involve proteins, enzymes, and hormones. It is found in liver, lamb, beef, eggs, oysters, and whole grain breads and cereals, although it is not always easily absorbed. Deficiency can result in growth retardation, impaired taste and smell, and reduced immune function. The daily requirement is 12 to 15 milligrams.

Magnesium. Magnesium activates cell enzymes, helps metabolize proteins and carbohydrates, maintains the structural integrity of the heart and other muscles, and aids in muscle contraction. Good sources include green leafy vegetables, nuts, legumes, bananas, and whole grain products. A deficiency may result from persistent vomiting or diarrhea, kidney disease, general malnutrition, alcoholism, and the use of certain medications. The daily requirement is 280 milligrams for women and 350 milligrams for men.

Phosphorus. Phosphorus is involved in bone and tooth formation, chemical reactions in the body, and energy production. It is found in dairy foods, animal foods, fish, cereals, nuts, and legumes. A deficiency of phosphorus can cause gastrointestinal, blood cell, and other disorders. Toxicity is harmful as well. The daily requirement is 800 milligrams for adults 25 and over.

Selenium. Selenium works with vitamin E to aid metabolism, growth, and fertility. It is found in seafood, kidney, liver, meats, grain products, and seeds. A daily dietary intake of 55 micrograms for women and 70 micrograms for men is recommended.

Minerals With Estimated Safe and Adequate Dietary Intakes. When data were sufficient to estimate a range of requirements—but insufficient for developing an RDA—the Food and Nutrition Board established a category of safe and adequate intakes for essential nutrients. The minerals in this category are copper, fluoride, chromium, manganese, and molybdenum.

Copper. Copper interacts with iron to form hemoglobin and red blood cells. It can be obtained through a wide variety of foods, such as liver, seafood, nuts and seeds, and whole grain products. Copper deficiency can cause anemia and central nervous system problems. The safe and adequate range of dietary copper for adults is 1.5 to 3.0 milligrams per day.

Fluoride. Fluoride is another contributor to bone and tooth formation, and it protects against tooth decay. Many municipal water supplies are fluoridated, and the mineral is also contained in saltwater fish, tea, and fluoridated toothpaste. Fluoride deficiency may predispose people to cavities and osteoporosis. Excess fluoride can cause discoloration and pitting of the teeth as well as other conditions. The range of safe and adequate intakes for adults is 1.5 to 4.0 milligrams per day.

Chromium. Chromium is essential for the body to use glucose, the primary food of cells. Foods containing chromium include calf's liver, American cheese, and wheat germ. A range of intakes between 50 and 200 micrograms per day is considered safe and adequate for adults.

Manganese. Manganese is part of several cell enzymes. It is also essential for bone formation and maintenance, insulin production, and nutrient metabolism. It is found in whole grain products, fruits, vegetables, and tea. A daily dietary intake of 2 to 5 milligrams for adults is recommended.

Molybdenum. Molybdenum helps in the metabolism of the mineral sulfur and the production of uric acid. The best sources are legumes, whole grains, milk, and organ meats such as liver and kidneys. The recommended range for dietary intake is 75 to 250 micrograms per day for adults.

Water

Water has no caloric value, but it contributes about 65% of body weight and is essential to the body's normal functioning. In general, water helps provide the body with other nutrients it needs and helps rid the body of what it does not need. Water has many functions, including these:

- Helping to maintain the balance of all the fluids in the body

- Lubricating the body's moving parts
- Dissolving chemicals and nutrients
- Aiding in digestion
- Helping to transport nutrients and secretions throughout the body
- Flushing out wastes
- Regulating body temperature through perspiration

The amount of water in the body directly affects the concentration and distribution of body fluids and all the functions related to them. The body maintains a careful balance between water consumed (in foods and beverages) and water lost (through urination, perspiration, and respiration). In a healthy fluid balance, water input equals water output. Measuring an ill person's level of water intake and output can help determine the best fluid replacement regimen to use.

People obtain most of their water from beverages such as tap water, milk, and fruit juices as well as coffee, tea, and soft drinks. On average, a person needs to drink six to eight glasses of water a day to maintain a healthy water balance. The daily need for water varies with size and age, the temperatures to which someone is exposed, the degree of physical exertion, and the water content of the foods one eats. Someone who is eating mostly foods with a high water content, such as fruits and vegetables, can drink a little less water than someone who is eating mostly foods with a low water content.

If people get too little water or lose too much water through vomiting, diarrhea, burns, or perspiration, they become dehydrated. Signs and symptoms of dehydration include dry lips and mucous membranes, weakness, lethargy, decreased urine output, and increased thirst. Severe dehydration can lead to hypovolemia, a reduction in the volume of blood in the body. Severe hypovolemia can result in inadequate blood pressure that affects the functioning of the heart, central nervous system, and various organs—a condition known as hypovolemic shock. If dehydration progresses so that water is lost from body cells, death usually occurs within a few days.

Procedure 49-1 explains how to educate patients to drink the right amount of water each day to prevent dehydration. Make sure patients know whether they are to drink extra fluids to replace fluids lost in an illness or to help rid the body of waste.

Principal Electrolytes and Other Nutrients of Special Interest

The principal electrolytes are essential to normal body functioning. Other nutrients, such as antioxidants, also merit special mention.

Principal Electrolytes. Although the principal electrolytes in the body—sodium, potassium, and chloride—are often excluded from lists of nutrients, they are essential dietary components. Electrolytes play an important role in maintaining body functions, such as normal heart rhythm.

PROCEDURE 49.2

Alerting Patients With Food Allergies to the Dangers of Common Foods

Objective: To explain how patients can eliminate allergy-causing foods from their diets

OSHA Guidelines: This procedure does not involve exposure to blood, body fluids, or tissues.

Materials: Results of the patient's allergy tests, patient's chart, pen, patient education materials

Method

1. Identify the patient and introduce yourself.
2. Discuss the results of the patient's allergy tests (if available), reinforcing the physician's instructions. List the foods the patient has been found to be allergic to. Provide the patient with a checklist of those foods.
3. Discuss with the patient the possible allergic reactions those foods can cause.
4. Talk about how the patient can avoid or eliminate those foods from the diet. Point out that the patient needs to be alert to avoid the allergy-causing foods not only in their basic forms but also as ingredients in prepared dishes and packaged foods. (Patients allergic to peanuts, for example, should avoid products containing peanut oil as well as peanuts.) Tell the patient to read labels carefully and to inquire

at restaurants about the use of those ingredients in dishes listed on the menu.

5. With the physician's or dietitian's consent, talk with the patient about the possibility of finding adequate substitutes for the foods if they are among the patient's favorites. Also discuss, if necessary, how the patient can obtain the nutrients in those foods from other sources (for example, the need for extra calcium sources if the patient is allergic to dairy products). Provide these explanations to the patient in writing, if appropriate, along with supplementary materials such as recipe pamphlets, a list of resources for obtaining food substitutes, and so on.
6. Discuss with the patient the procedures to follow if the allergy-causing foods are accidentally ingested.
7. Answer the patient's questions and remind the patient that you and the rest of the medical team are available if any questions or problems arise later on.
8. Document the patient education session or interchange in the patient's chart, indicate the patient's understanding, and initial the entry.

Patients With Diabetes. A special diet is one of the foundations of treatment for diabetes. Dietary guidelines for patients with diabetes must not only provide them with adequate nutrition but also keep their blood sugar level under control and interact appropriately with medication. Patient education is especially important, because patients with diabetes must comfortably maintain the dietary modifications over a lifetime.

The diet a physician or dietitian prescribes for someone with diabetes includes a specific number of calories, meals per day, amount of carbohydrates, and amounts of other nutrients. As a way to simplify the diet, a system of **food exchanges** is used. All food exchanges in a particular food category provide the same amounts of protein, fat, and carbohydrates. Food exchange lists can be obtained from a registered dietitian or the American Diabetes Association.

The list of exchanges is divided into six categories—vegetables, fruits, breads, meats, fats, and milk—and indicates how large a portion of each food in a category is equal to one "exchange" of food in that category. This information tells patients what portions of specific foods are

interchangeable and whether they are eating the correct amounts of those foods. The list includes a variety of foods from which patients make their selections. It is important that patients with diabetes not skip a meal, because skipping meals disturbs the balance of blood sugar and metabolism.

Patients with diabetes who are dependent on insulin should eat regular meals at consistent times. Skipping or delaying meals can result in hypoglycemia or an insulin reaction. Patients should work with a registered dietitian and their physician to create a meal plan that keeps blood glucose levels as close to normal as possible. The medical team specifies the proportion of carbohydrates and calories in meals, depending on the type of insulin patients use and the timing of injections.

Fiber is also important for patients who have diabetes. Fiber can sometimes prevent a sharp rise in blood glucose after a meal and may reduce the amount of insulin needed. It is therefore recommended that people with diabetes gradually increase their fiber intake until it is at about 45 grams per day.

Patients Who Are Elderly. Universal nutritional guidelines for aging patients have not been developed. It is known, however, that energy and metabolic requirements usually decline with age, which calls for some dietary modification. The Food and Nutrition Board of the National Academy of Science recommends a 10% decrease in caloric intake for people over age 50 compared with that of young adults. Men and women above age 75 should decrease their intake another 10% to 15%. The exact adjustment, however, depends on the individual patient's condition and needs.

Because protein requirements do not change, elderly patients should select foods that provide ample protein in a smaller quantity of food. To achieve daily nutritional goals, patients may require supplements for iron, calcium, and other minerals, such as phosphorus and magnesium.

Because aging is often accompanied by decreased gastrointestinal muscle tone, elderly patients should increase their intake of high-fiber foods and drink plenty of water. Although all people need a certain amount of fat in their diet to help the body absorb vitamins, too much may lead to atherosclerosis. Elderly individuals should therefore keep fat intake to 20% of their total calories.

Certain factors can impair or impede eating in this age group and may even lead to malnutrition. If you recognize any of these factors, discuss them with the patient's doctor:

- Physical factors, such as chewing difficulty caused by tooth loss or poorly fitting dentures, swallowing difficulty, and lack of appetite caused by altered taste, smell, or sight
- Medications, which may adversely affect food intake or nutrient use
- Social factors, including apathy toward food caused by depression, grief, or loneliness
- Economic factors, including homelessness or lack of money for food or transportation

Patients With Heart Disease. Coronary heart disease is caused by atherosclerosis, which usually results from hyperlipidemia, or an excess of lipids in the bloodstream. Left untreated, this condition can lead to angina, heart attack, or stroke.

Patients can significantly lower their risk by reducing their blood cholesterol levels and losing weight if they are overweight. Patients who have coronary heart disease usually must reduce their consumption of fats to a level that provides less than 30% of their total caloric intake. Saturated fats should provide less than 10% of caloric intake. Patients who have had a heart attack or are at increased risk for a heart attack are also encouraged to increase their consumption of soluble fiber.

As a medical assistant, your role with these patients is to encourage them to follow the nutritional regimen prescribed by the doctor. Do not recommend other dietary changes. Instead, educate patients about ways to reduce the amount of fat in their diets, such as by substituting skim milk for whole milk.

Patients With Hypertension. Hypertension (high blood pressure) is a condition that affects more than 20% of American adults. Nutritional therapy for patients with hypertension involves the following:

- Restricting sodium intake to 2 to 3 grams per day, especially in salt-sensitive individuals
- Increasing potassium intake through consumption of fresh fruits and vegetables
- Ensuring adequate calcium intake to meet an RDA of 800 milligrams
- Eliminating or reducing alcohol use
- Decreasing total fat intake and obtaining no more than 10% of calories from saturated fats

Patients With Lactose Sensitivity. Lactose is the sugar contained in human and animal milk. It must be broken down in the body by the enzyme lactase to enable the body to digest dairy products. In people from some parts of the world, lactase is present in the body until age 3 or 4, after which it all but disappears. As a result, after early childhood many people have trouble digesting foods that contain lactose and eliminate these foods from their diets. People who are especially sensitive to dietary lactose are often referred to as being lactose intolerant.

Chemical preparations can help a person digest lactose. Those preparations may be added to certain foods, such as ice cream, for lactose-sensitive people. If people with a lactose sensitivity choose to avoid dairy products, they need to be sure to obtain protein and calcium from other sources.

Patients Who Are Overweight. Overweight is a common problem: more than one-third of American adults are overweight. Overweight patients weigh 10% to 20% more than is recommended for their height and gender. Patients who are more than 20% overweight are considered obese. Obesity can lead to medical complications such as elevated blood cholesterol levels, hypertension, diabetes, joint problems, respiratory problems, and heart disease.

Approaches to Weight Loss. Overweight may be approached with dietary modification alone, but an exercise program is usually included. Behavior modification is also a common element of weight-loss programs. In a weight-loss program, foods should be proportioned in accordance with the Food Guide Pyramid, and the diet should be appealing and enjoyable. The goal is to have the patient decrease daily caloric intake and increase physical activity at an appropriate rate while remaining comfortable and healthy.

Weight loss will not occur unless patients expend more energy than they consume. A physician or dietitian can calculate each person's daily caloric needs and determine how many calories must be cut from the diet and how much activity must be increased to result in weight loss. Foods that are high in nutrients but low in calories are desirable.

The **behavior modification** facet of weight loss includes such methods as keeping a food diary to pinpoint overeating patterns, controlling the stimuli associated with overeating, and providing rewards for successful behavior.

TABLE 50-2 Selected Drug Categories *(continued)*

Drug Category	Examples Generic Name (Trade Name)	Action of Drug
Antipyretic	Acetaminophen (Tylenol) Acetylsalicylic acid, or aspirin	Reduces fever
Antiseptic	Isopropyl alcohol, 70% Povidone-iodine (Betadine)	Inhibits growth of microorganisms
Antitussive	Codeine Dextromethorphan hydrobromide (component of Robitussin DM)	Inhibits cough reflex
Bronchodilator	Albuterol (Proventil) Epinephrine (Epinephrine Mist) Salmeterol (Severent)	Dilates bronchi (airways in the lungs)
Cathartic (laxative)	Bisacodyl (Dulcolax) Casanthranol (Peri-Colace) Magnesium hydroxide (Milk of Magnesia)	Induces defecation, alleviates constipation
Contraceptive	Ethinyl estradiol and norgestimate (Ortho Cyclen) Norethindrone and ethinyl estradiol (Ortho-Novum) Norgestrel (Ovrette)	Reduces risk of pregnancy
Decongestant	Oxymetazoline HCl (Afrin) Phenylephrine HCl (Neo-Synephrine) Pseudoephedrine HCl (Sudafed)	Relieves nasal swelling and congestion
Diuretic	Bumetanide (Bumex) Furosemide (Lasix) Hydrochlorothiazide (Hydrodiuril) Mannitol	Increases urine output, reduces blood pressure and cardiac output
Expectorant	Guaifenesin (component of Robitussin)	Liquefies mucus in bronchi; allows expectoration of sputum, mucus, and phlegm
Hemostatic	Aminocaprocic acid (Amicar) Phytonadione or vitamin K_1 (Mephyton) Thrombin (Thrombogen)	Controls or stops bleeding by promoting coagulation
Hormone replacement	Hydrocortisone (Hydrocortone Acetate) for adrenocortical deficiency Insulin (Humulin) for pancreatic deficiency Levothyroxine sodium (Synthroid) for thyroid deficiency	Replaces or resolves hormone deficiency
Hypnotic (sleep-inducing) or sedative	Chloral hydrate (Noctec) Ethchlorvynol (Placidyl) Secobarbital sodium (Seconal Sodium)	Induces sleep or relaxation (depending on drug potency and dosage)

continued ⟶

TABLE 50-2 Selected Drug Categories (continued)

Drug Category	Examples Generic Name (Trade Name)	Action of Drug
Muscle relaxant	Carisoprodol (Rela or Soma) Cyclobenzaprine HCl (Flexeril)	Relaxes skeletal muscles
Mydriatic	Atropine sulfate (Allergan) for ophthalmic use Phenylephrine HCl (Alcon Efrin) for ophthalmic use or (Neo-Synephrine HCl) for nasal use	Constricts vessels of eye or nasal passage, raises blood pressure, dilates pupil of eye in ophthalmic preparations
Stimulant	Amphetamine sulfate (Benzadrine) for central nervous system Caffeine (No-Doz) for central nervous system; also component of many analgesic formulations and coffee	Increases activity of brain and other organs, decreases appetite
Vasoconstrictor	Dopamine HCl (Intropin) Norepinephrine bitartrate (Levophed)	Constricts blood vessels, increases blood pressure
Vasodilator	Enalopril (Vasotec) Lisinopril (Prinivil) Nitroglycerin (Nitrostat)	Dilates blood vessels, decreases blood pressure

Sources: *Physicians' Desk Reference; U.S. Pharmacopeia Dictionary.*
Note: Some drugs have a secondary category. When in doubt, check the *Physicians' Desk Reference* or *U.S. Pharmacopeia Dictionary.*

Indications and Labeling

An **indication** is the purpose or reason for using a drug. FDA-approved indications are part of a drug's **labeling.** Labeling also includes the form of the drug, such as tablet or liquid.

Regardless of category, some drugs may be used to treat several different conditions. Multiple uses are possible if the drug affects several body systems at once or if the drug's primary effect produces significant secondary effects in other body systems.

When a drug is used for multiple indications, one or more indications may not be in its labeling. Out-of-label prescribing is legal. Doctors who do it usually know from continuing education (seminars or journal articles) that such uses are generally accepted. For example, Benadryl (diphenhydramine) is an antihistamine used to treat allergic symptoms in both children and adults. Because it tends to make a patient sleepy but is safe for children, a pediatrician may use a low dose of Benadryl as a temporary sedative for a young child. Its use as a sedative, however, is not part of the labeling for Benadryl.

Another example of a drug with multiple uses is minoxidil. As a trade-name tablet, it is known as the antihypertensive Loniten; as a trade-name topical solution, it is known as the hair-growth stimulant Rogaine. In the case of minoxidil, both indications are approved, but the tablet labeling is for hypertension and the topical solution labeling is for hair growth.

It is important to be aware of these labeling considerations when dealing with questions from patients. Never assume that a drug is appropriate for only one use or that it is administered in only one form. Always consult the doctor or other sources of drug information before answering a patient's question.

Safety

The safety of a drug is determined by how many and what kinds of adverse effects are associated with it. An adverse effect may require immediate attention. It is not uncommon for a patient to call the physician's office with complaints of new symptoms soon after beginning therapy with a drug. Be alert for such complaints, because they could be signs of an adverse reaction to the drug or an interaction with another medication. These calls should be brought to the physician's attention. Some adverse effects are common whereas others are rare.

Efficacy

A patient may complain that a newly prescribed drug is not doing what the doctor said it would. There are a variety of explanations for such a complaint, including the following:

- The drug is working adequately, but the patient does not understand how it works
- The **dosage** (size, frequency, and number of doses) needs to be adjusted

- The drug has not yet reached a therapeutic level in the bloodstream
- The wrong drug was prescribed, or the wrong drug was dispensed by the pharmacy (this is rare, but possible)
- Some drugs work better in some patients than in others; not every drug is for everyone (this is particularly true of antihistamines)
- Some forms of a drug work better than others, such as tablets versus injection
- The generic drug does not work, but the trade-name drug does

Kinds of Therapy

There are several descriptive terms for drug therapy. Depending on a patient's condition, the physician may use drugs for any of the following kinds of therapy:

- Acute: Drug is prescribed to improve a life-threatening or serious condition, such as epinephrine for severe allergic reaction
- Empiric: Drug is prescribed according to experience or observation until blood or other tests prove another therapy to be appropriate, such as penicillin for suspected strep throat
- Maintenance: Drug is prescribed to maintain a condition of health, especially in chronic disease, such as insulin for diabetes mellitus
- Palliative: Drug is prescribed to reduce the severity of a condition or its accompanying pain, such as morphine for cancer
- Prophylactic: Drug is prescribed to prevent a disease or condition, such as immunizations or birth control drugs
- Replacement: Drug is prescribed to provide chemicals otherwise missing in a patient, such as hormone replacement therapy for a woman in menopause
- Supportive: Drug is prescribed for a condition other than the primary disease until that disease resolves, such as a corticosteroid for severe allergic reactions.
- Supplemental: Drug or nutrients are prescribed to avoid deficiency, such as iron for a woman who is pregnant

Toxicology

Toxicology is the study of the poisonous effects, or toxicity, of drugs, including adverse effects and drug interactions. Because you are likely to see evidence of immediate toxic effects only when administering a drug, this topic will be discussed in more detail in Chapter 51. You must be aware, however, of some possible toxic effects that may not be apparent right away:

- An adverse effect on a fetus when the drug crosses the placenta
- An adverse effect on infants when the drug passes easily into breast milk

- Adverse reactions reported in clinical trials, such as headache, drowsiness, gastric upset, or other effects
- An adverse effect in immunocompromised patients who are unable to metabolize a drug normally
- An adverse effect in pediatric or elderly patients or in patients with hypertension, diabetes mellitus, or other serious chronic conditions
- An adverse drug interaction when the drug is taken with another drug that is incompatible
- A carcinogenic (cancer-causing) effect in some patients

Nearly always, an adverse effect has been encountered in the clinical trials of a drug, and there will be mention of the adverse effect under that heading in the package insert or in accepted drug reference works. In the reports of clinical trials, however, the drug company must report *all* adverse effects noted during testing. As a result, effects that, at least theoretically, could not be caused by the drug are included. In dealing with patients who are about to begin drug therapy, it is best to avoid mentioning specific adverse effects associated with drugs. To do so could cause undue alarm, prompt patients to imagine they have the effects, or discourage patients from taking the needed medication. Always ask patients if they have any questions, and have the doctor answer patients' questions if they are drug related. Because patients will receive lists of adverse effects from the pharmacist, encourage them to discuss concerns with the pharmacist or to call the doctor's office. Also encourage patients to inform the doctor of adverse effects they experience after beginning drug therapy.

Sources of Drug Information

It is important to keep several up-to-date sources of drug information in the office for when you or the doctor need detailed information about a specific drug. Sources to refer to include the *Physicians' Desk Reference* (Figure 50-5),

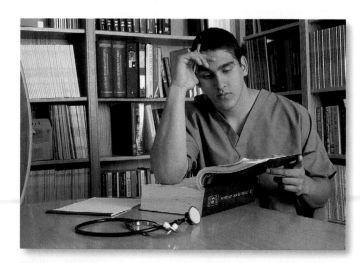

Figure 50-5. The *Physicians' Desk Reference* is one of several publications in which you can find current information on specific drugs.

Drug Evaluations, United States Pharmacopeia/National Formulary, and *American Hospital Formulary Service.*

Physicians' Desk Reference (PDR)

Medical Economics of Oradell, New Jersey, publishes the *Physicians' Desk Reference,* or *PDR,* annually, along with supplements twice a year. It sends the book free to doctors' offices and sells it through bookstores. The company also publishes separate editions for generic, nonprescription, and ophthalmologic drugs as well as a guide to drug interactions, adverse effects, and indications.

The *PDR* presents information provided by pharmaceutical companies about more than 2500 prescription drugs. The *PDR* has color-coded directories of drug categories, generic names, and trade names. It also lists each pharmaceutical company's name, address, emergency telephone number, and available products.

The drug information section is divided according to manufacturer, and the drugs are then grouped alphabetically within each manufacturer's subsection. The information closely resembles that on drug package inserts, which are illustrated in the Tips for the Office section. The package insert for each drug describes the drug, its purpose and effects (clinical pharmacology), indications, contraindications (conditions under which the drug should not be administered), warnings, precautions, adverse reactions, drug abuse and dependence, overdosage, dosage and administration, and how the drug is supplied (for example, tablets in different doses, liquid). Also included in this section are diagnostic compounds made by the drug companies.

A separate section of the *PDR* is devoted to color photographs of common drugs in various forms, also grouped by manufacturer. Other sections on poison control centers, controlled substances, and the system for reporting adverse reactions to vaccines could be important resources for you.

Drug Evaluations

Drug Evaluations is published once a year by the American Medical Association. It contains detailed information on more than 1000 drugs, including their names, efficacy, adverse reactions, and precautions.

United States Pharmacopeia/ National Formulary

The *United States Pharmacopeia/National Formulary,* or *USP/NF,* is the official source of drug standards in the United States and is published about every 5 years. By law, every drug sold under a name listed in the *USP/NF* must meet the strict standards of the *USP/NF.*

The *USP/NF* describes each drug approved by the federal government and lists its standards for purity, composition, and strength as well as its uses, dosages, and storage. The *NF* portion of the book provides the chemical formulas of the drugs.

American Hospital Formulary Service (AHFS)

The American Society of Hospital Pharmacists in Bethesda, Maryland, publishes the *American Hospital Formulary Service,* or *AHFS.* It sells the two-volume set by subscription and provides four to six supplements each year. The *AHFS* lists generic names and is divided into sections based on drug actions.

Regulatory Function of the FDA

After the FDA approves a drug, it continues its regulatory function to protect patients and consumers. The FDA reviews new-indication proposals (applications from companies for new indications for a drug), OTC proposals (applications for OTC status of a prescription drug), and further clinical trial results. If an adverse effect appears many times, for example, the FDA may withdraw the causative drug from the market.

Drug Manufacturing

The FDA also regulates drug manufacturing. It ensures that drugs shipped between states have the proper identity, strength, purity, and quality. Each manufacturer must consistently identify each drug by a particular color, form, shape, size, and label. It must produce every dose at the same tested strength, using the exact formula approved by the FDA. The manufacturer must also use high-quality, contaminant-free ingredients.

Nonprescription, or Over-the-Counter, Drugs

A nonprescription, or OTC, drug is one that the FDA has approved for use without the supervision of a licensed health-care practitioner. The consumer must follow the manufacturer's directions to use the drug safely. Some drugs, such as aspirin and vitamin supplements, have been OTC drugs for many years. The number of prescription drugs that have been granted OTC status is increasing. Although OTC drugs are safe when used as directed on the package, patient education contributes significantly to their safe use.

Prescription Drugs

A **prescription drug** is one that can be used only by order of a physician and must be dispensed by a licensed health-care professional, such as a pharmacist, physician, podiatrist, or licensed midwife. Some prescription drugs are dispensed as over-the-counter medications at much lower dosages.

Controlled Substances

A **controlled substance** is a drug or drug product that is categorized as potentially dangerous and addictive. The

Helping the Physician Comply With the Controlled Substances Act of 1970 *(continued)*

OMB Approval No. 1117-0007	DEPARTMENT OF JUSTICE/DRUG ENFORCEMENT ADMINISTRATION REGISTRANTS INVENTORY OF DRUGS SURRENDERED	PACKAGE No.

The following schedule is an inventory of controlled substances which is hereby surrendered to you for proper disposition.

FROM: *(Include Name, Street, City, State and ZIP Code in space provided below).*

Signature of applicant or authorized agent

Registrant's DEA Number

Registrant's Telephone Number

NOTE: CERTIFIED MAIL (Return Receipt Requested) IS REQUIRED FOR SHIPMENTS OF DRUGS VIA U.S. POSTAL SERVICE: See instructions on reverse of form.

NAME OF DRUG OF PREPARATION Registrants will fill in Columns 1, 2, 3, and 4 Only.	Number of Containers	CONTENTS *(Number of grams, tablets, ounces or other units per container)*	Controlled Substance Content *(Each Unit)*	FOR DEA USE ONLY		
				DISPOSITION	QUANTITY	
					GMS.	MGS.
1	*2*	*3*	*4*	*5*	*6*	*7*
1						
2						

The controlled substances surrendered in accordance with Title 21 of the Code of Federal Regulations, Section 1307.21, have been received in _____ packages purporting to contain the drugs listed on this inventory and have been: **(1) Forwarded tape-sealed without opening; (2) Destroyed as indicated and the remainder forwarded tape-sealed after verifying contents; (3) Forwarded tape-sealed after verifying

DATE: _____ 19 ____   DESTROYED BY: _____

**Strike out lines not applicable*   WITNESSED BY: _____

INSTRUCTIONS

1. List the name of the drug in column 1, the number of containers in column 2, the size of each container in column 3, and in column 4 the controlled substance content of each unit described in column 3; e.g., morphine sulfate tabs., 3 pkgs., 100 tabs., 1/4 gr. (16 mg.) or morphine sulfate tabs., 1 pkg., 83 tabs., 1/2 gr. (32 mg.), etc.

2. All packages included on a single line should be identical in name, content and controlled substance strength.

3. Prepare this form in quadruplicate. Mail two (2) copies of this form to the Special Agent in Charge, under separate cover. Enclose one additional copy in the shipment with the drugs. Retain one copy for your records. One copy will be returned to you as a receipt. No further receipt will be furnished to you unless specifically requested. Any further inquiries concerning these drugs should be addressed to the DEA District Office which serves your area.

4. There is no provision for payment for drugs surrendered. This is merely a service rendered to registrants enabling them to clear their stocks and records of unwanted items.

5. Drugs should be shipped tape-sealed via prepaid express or certified mail (return reciept requested) to Special Agent in Charge, Drug Enforcement Administration, of the DEA District Office which serves your area.

PRIVACY ACT INFORMATION

AUTHORITY: Section 307 of the Controlled Substances Act of 1970 (P.L. 91-513).
PURPOSE: To document the surrender of controlled substances which have been forwarded by registrants to DEA for disposal.
ROUTINE USES: This form is required by Federal Regulations for the surrender of unwanted Controlled Substances. Disclosures of information from this system are made to the following categories of users for the purposes stated.
    A. Other Federal law enforcement and regulatory agencies for law enforcement and regulatory purposes.
    B. State and local law enforcement and regulatory agencies for law enforcement and regulatory purposes.
EFFECT: Failure to document the surrender of unwanted Controlled Substances may result in prosecution for violation of the Controlled Substances Act.

Public reporting burden for this collection of information is estimated to average 30 minutes per response, including the time for reviewing instructions, searching existing data sources, gathering and maintaining the data needed, and completing and reviewing the collection of information. Send comments regarding this burden estimate or any other aspect of this collection of information, including suggestions for reducing this burden, to the Drug Enforcement Administration, Records Management Section, Washington, D.C. 20537; and to the Office of Management and Budget, Paperwork Reduction Project No. 1117-0007, Washington, D.C. 20503.

DEA Form – 41
(Jun. 1986)

Figure 50-9. Use DEA Form 41 to report disposal of controlled drugs.

PROCEDURE 50.2

Renewing the Physician's DEA Registration

Objective: To accurately complete DEA Form 224a to renew the physician's DEA registration on time

OSHA Guidelines: This procedure does not involve exposure to blood, body fluids, or tissues.

Materials: Calendar, tickler file (optional), DEA Form 224a, pen

Method

1. Calculate a period of 3 years from the date of the original registration or the most recent renewal. Note that date as the expiration date of the physician's DEA registration.

2. Subtract 45 days from the expiration date, and mark this date on the calendar as a reminder to submit renewal forms. You might also put a reminder to submit renewal forms in the physician's tickler file for that date.

3. If you receive registration renewal paperwork (DEA Form 224a) from the DEA well before the submission date, put it in a safe place until you can complete it and have the physician sign it.

4. If you do not receive renewal paperwork by the submission date, call your regional DEA office to request DEA Form 224a or send written notice that no form was received and a request for the renewal form to:

   Drug Enforcement Administration
   Registration Unit
   Central Station
   P.O. Box 28083
   Washington, DC 20038-8083

5. Before the expiration deadline, complete DEA Form 224a as instructed on the form, and have the physician sign it. Prepare or request a check for the fee.

6. Submit the original and one copy of the completed form with the appropriate fee to the DEA so that it will arrive before the deadline. Keep one copy for the office records.

---

do not apply to doctors who prescribe but neither administer nor dispense controlled drugs.

Dispensing Records. The dispensing record for Schedule II drugs must be kept separate from the patient's regular medical record. Each time a drug is administered or dispensed, the doctor must note the date, the patient's name and address, the drug, and the quantity dispensed.

The dispensing record for Schedules III through V drugs must include the same information. The record for these drugs may be kept in the patient's medical record unless the doctor charges for the drugs dispensed. All dispensing records must be kept for 2 years and are subject to inspection by the DEA.

Inventory Records. A doctor who regularly dispenses controlled drugs must also keep inventory records of all stock on hand. This regulation applies to all scheduled drugs. To take an inventory, count the amount of each drug on hand. Compare this amount with the amount of the drug ordered and the amount dispensed to patients.

The controlled drug inventory must be repeated every 2 years. You must include copies of invoices from drug suppliers in the inventory record. All inventories and records of Schedule II drugs must be kept separate from other records. Inventories and records of other controlled drugs must be separate or easily retrievable from ordinary business and professional records. All records on controlled drugs must be retained for 2 years and made available for inspection and copying by DEA officials if requested.

Disposing of Drugs. If the doctor asks you to dispose of any outdated, noncontrolled drugs, you may flush them down the toilet or put them in the trash, depending on state law. Incineration may be required for large amounts of injectable and topical drugs. In some instances the doctor may hire an outside company to incinerate the drugs. If not, you may ask the local hospital to incinerate them for you if this is permitted by state law.

If the doctor needs to dispose of controlled drugs, such as expired samples, obtain DEA Form 41 (Figure 50-9), called Registrants Inventory of Drugs Surrendered, which is available from the nearest DEA office. Complete the form, have the doctor sign it, and call the DEA to obtain instructions for disposal of the drugs. If you must ship them, use registered mail. After the drugs have been destroyed, the DEA will issue the doctor a receipt, which you should keep in a safe place.

If doctors terminate their medical practice, they must return their DEA registration certificate and any unused copies of DEA Form 222 to the nearest DEA office. To prevent unauthorized use, write the word *VOID* across the front of these forms. Regional DEA offices will tell doctors how to dispose of any remaining controlled drugs.

Common Abbreviations Used in Prescriptions

Abbreviation	Meaning	Abbreviation	Meaning
†	one	o.d.	once a day
††	two	O.D., OD	right eye
†††	three	oint	ointment
a̅	before	O.S., OS	left eye
A̅A̅, a̅a̅	of each	O.U., OU	both eyes
a.c., ac	before meals	oz	ounce
ad lib	as desired	p̅	after, past
amt	amount	p.c., pc	after meals
aq.	aqueous	per	by or with
b.i.d., BID, bid	twice a day	po, per os	by mouth
c̅	with	PRN, p.r.n., prn	whenever necessary
cap, caps	capsules	pt	pint
cc	cubic centimeter	Pt	patient
d	day	pulv	powder
D/C, d/c	discontinue	q.	every
Dil, dil	dilute	q.a.m., qam	every morning
dr	dram	q.d., qd	every day
Dr	doctor	q.h., qh	every hour
D/W	dextrose in water	q2h, q2	every 2 hours
Dx, dx	diagnosis	qhs	every night
Fl, fl, fld	fluid	q.i.d., qid	four times a day
gal	gallon	qns, QNS	quantity not sufficient
gm, Gm, g	gram	qod	every other day
gr	grain	qs	quantity sufficient
gt, gtt	drop(s)	℞, Rx	prescription, take
H, hr, h	hour	s̅	without
HS, h.s., hs	hour of sleep or at bedtime	SC, s.c., SQ, subq, SubQ	subcutaneous
IM	intramuscular	Sig	directions
IU	international unit	sol	solution
IV	intravenous	ss	one-half
kg	kilogram	stat, STAT	immediately
L, l	liter	subling, SL	sublingual
liq	liquid	S/W	saline in water
m, min	minim	tab	tablet
mcg, µg	microgram	Tbsp, tbsp	tablespoon
mEq	milliequivalent	t.i.d., tid	three times a day
mEq/L	milliequivalents per liter	tinc, tr, tinct	tincture
mg	milligram	top	topically
mL, ml	milliliter	tsp	teaspoon
mm	millimeter	ung, ungt	ointment
noc, noct	night	U	unit
npo, NPO	nothing by mouth	wt	weight
NS	normal saline		

Figure 50-10. Physicians use many abbreviations when they write prescriptions.

Writing Prescriptions

Any drug that is not available over the counter requires a prescription. According to the Controlled Substances Act, doctors may issue prescriptions for controlled drugs only in the schedules for which they are registered with the DEA.

You must be familiar with the terms and abbreviations used in prescriptions (Figure 50-10), and you must become familiar with the doctor's style of writing. With this knowledge, you will be able to administer the prescribed drugs accurately (if allowed in your state) and to discuss the prescription accurately with a patient or pharmacist.

Every prescription has four basic parts: the superscription, inscription, subscription, and signature.

1. The superscription includes the date, the patient's full name and address, and the symbol R̸, which means "take thou" in Latin.

2. The inscription is the name of the drug (either generic or trade name) and the amount. It usually specifies the amount of drug in each dose of capsules, tablets, or suppositories in milligrams, such as "Banthine 50 mg." The inscription for oral liquid drugs typically uses milligrams per milliliter, such as "codeine sulfate 15 mg/5 mL." The inscription usually gives the amount for creams, ointments, and topical liquids as a percentage, such as "Spectazole 1% cream."

3. The subscription contains the directions to the pharmacist. It includes the size of each dose, the total number or amount of the drug to be dispensed for this prescription, and the form of the drug, such as tablets.

4. The signature, or transcription, refers to patient instructions. These are nearly always written using the abbreviations shown in Figure 50-10. Instructions generally follow the abbreviation Sig, which means "mark" in Latin. Many of these instructions appear in Latin, which the pharmacist must translate. The pharmacist includes the translated patient instructions on the prescription drug label.

A prescription also includes these items:

- Doctor's name, office address and telephone number, and DEA registration number
- Doctor's signature
- Number of times the prescription can be refilled
- Indication of whether the pharmacist may substitute a generic version of a trade-name drug at the patient's request

Prescriptions may be typed or handwritten in ink or indelible pencil on a prescription blank. Prescriptions for multiple medications may be written on a different form than that used for a single medication (Figure 50-11). In some states a prescription for Schedule II drugs must be prepared in triplicate on an official Department of Justice prescription form. When this form is required, the doctor keeps one copy, and the pharmacist keeps the original and sends the endorsed second copy to the Department of Justice.

The doctor may have you prepare prescriptions for signing. Because the doctor is responsible for the accuracy of prescriptions, you must be sure to write them clearly and correctly.

Prescription Blanks. Prescription blanks make prescription writing convenient and efficient. They are usually preprinted with the doctor's name, address, telephone number, state license number, and DEA registration number. Most blanks also provide space for writing the patient's name and address, the date, and other information. Some blanks are printed on colored paper or have a background design to minimize the risk of alteration,

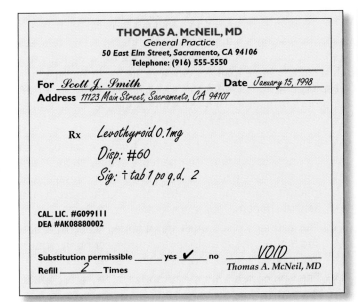

Figure 50-11. The physician may order drugs on a prescription blank (left) for a single medication or (right) for multiple medications.

CAUTION *Handle With Care*

Secure Handling of Prescription Pads

Because prescription pads are small, substance abusers can easily steal a single prescription sheet or an entire pad and use it to obtain controlled substances. To keep prescription pads secure, handle them with caution and follow these tips.

Storage and Use

- Keep all prescription pads, except the pad the physician is currently using, in a locked cabinet or a locked drawer in the physician's desk.
- Remind the physician to carry the current pad at all times or to keep it out of sight but easily accessible for writing prescriptions.
- Never ask the physician to sign prescription blanks in advance.
- Never use prescription blanks as notepaper.
- Suggest that the physician write prescribed amounts of medication in numerals and words—for example, "25 (twenty-five) capsules."

Printing and Preparation

- Order printing in colored ink that is not reproducible.

- Order prescription blanks with attached no-carbon-required duplicates to provide a permanent record of all prescriptions written. Keep the duplicate in the patient's record.
- Order tinted prescription blanks to allow easy detection of erasures or correction fluid.
- See to it that the phrase "℞ not valid for narcotics, barbiturates, or amphetamines" or "Not valid for Schedule II or III drugs" is preprinted in the center of each prescription blank. Use higher security and separate prescription blanks for these drugs.
- Do *not* allow the physician's DEA registration number to be preprinted on separate prescription blanks for Schedule II or III drugs.
- Have a sequencing number preprinted on all prescription blanks so that a missing blank will be noticed quickly.

---

counterfeiting, or loss. To prevent unauthorized use of prescription blanks, never leave them unattended. For tips on secure handling of prescription blanks, read the Caution: Handle With Care section.

If something about a prescription arouses suspicion, the pharmacist who receives it may call the doctor's office to verify it. You should be able to check the patient's records and tell the pharmacist whether the doctor wrote a prescription for that patient. If the prescription is a forgery, notify the doctor and, if she gives you authorization, notify the DEA.

The doctor should not use a prescription to obtain drugs for office stock. When the office needs drugs (other than Schedule II drugs), they should be obtained from a pharmacy with an order form. When the drugs are delivered, you should receive an invoice from the pharmacist.

Telephone Prescriptions. If requested by the doctor, you may telephone a new or renewal prescription to the patient's pharmacy. To do this, provide the pharmacist with the same information that would appear in a written prescription. You may not, however, telephone a prescription for a Schedule II drug. In an emergency situation, when a patient needs a drug immediately and no alternative is available, the doctor may telephone a prescription

for a Schedule II drug. The amount must be limited to the period of emergency, and a written prescription must be sent to the pharmacist within 72 hours. The pharmacist must notify the DEA if a written prescription does not arrive within the specified time.

Telephone prescription renewals are called in on a daily basis from patients and pharmacies. The renewal requests may be called into the receptionist or left on a designated phone mail system. It is the medical assistant's responsibility to handle the prescription renewals in an appropriate manner. Here are some guidelines for handling office prescription renewal requests:

- Proper messages must be taken from the call or from the message system. The patient's name, phone number, pharmacy phone number, medication, dosage, and amount must be recorded and verified from the patient's medical chart.
- The patient's chart must be obtained for verification and for the physician. Do not give a prescription request to the physician without the chart.
- The physician must authorize the prescription renewal.
- The prescription renewal must be documented in the chart after the medication is called into the pharmacy.

An example of charting is as follows:

11/24/03 RX: Zyrtec 10mg, one tablet QD HS, # 30, 6 refills._____st

Note: Every conversation you have with patients regarding medications must be written into the medical chart.

- Prescriptions must be called in to the pharmacy the day they are requested. It is good customer service to call the patient after you have called the prescription into the pharmacy.

Vaccines

A **vaccine** is a special preparation made from microorganisms and administered to a person to produce reduced sensitivity to, or increased immunity to, an infectious disease. Vaccines are stored with the office supply of drugs and require similar handling. If you work in a pediatrician's office, you will handle the vaccines for childhood diseases. In an adult practice you can expect to see influenza vaccines and vaccines for diseases to which patients might be exposed in foreign travel.

It is important to know how vaccines work in the immune system. Immunity is discussed in detail in Chapter 19. Immunizations, particularly those for children, are discussed in Chapter 20. Adverse reactions to medications and vaccines are discussed in Chapter 51.

Through the action of the immune system, a patient can be protected from—or made not susceptible to—a disease. This immunity results from the formation of antibodies that destroy or alter disease-causing agents.

Antibody Formation

The human body creates antibodies in response to an invasion by an antigen (foreign substance). When an antigen enters the body, specialized white blood cells (lymphocytes) produce antibodies, which in turn combine with the antigens to neutralize them. This action arrests or prevents the reaction or disease that the antigen otherwise would cause. Specific antibodies always fight specific antigens.

Antigens can be bacteria, viruses, or other organisms that enter the body in spite of its natural defenses. Toxins, pollens, and drugs can also be antigens if the body reacts to them by forming antibodies. (Allergens are antigens that induce an allergic reaction.)

Vaccines contain organisms that have been killed or attenuated (weakened) in a laboratory. Because the organisms have been weakened, they stimulate antibody formation but do not overpower the body and cause disease. They may, however, still be strong enough to cause slight inflammation at the injection site and a fever. Some vaccines, such as those for the influenza viruses, may even produce some of the lesser effects of the disease against which they provide protection.

Immunizations made from organisms are called vaccines. Those made from the toxins of organisms are called toxoids. Some immunizations, such as polio vaccine, last a lifetime. Others, such as tetanus toxoid, do not. In the latter case booster immunizations must be used to stimulate the lymphocytes to produce antibodies again.

Timing of Immunizations

The Advisory Committee on Immunization Practices, the American Academy of Pediatrics, and the American Academy of Family Physicians jointly publish a schedule for immunizations (discussed in Chapter 20). This schedule covers children from infancy through 16 years of age. Just as children receive immunizations before exposure to disease, adults may receive immunizations for influenza or other diseases, including those to which an adult could be exposed during travel.

Patients are sometimes immunized after exposure. For example, if patients have been exposed to a serious disease and there is too little time for them to produce antibodies, they may receive an antiserum that contains antibodies to the disease-carrying organism. These immunizations are made from human or animal serum. If bacterial toxins (rather than bacteria) cause the disease, the patient may receive an antitoxin.

Antiserums and antitoxins must be used cautiously. They are usually reserved for life-threatening infectious diseases. Because patients can be allergic to substances in animal antiserums and antitoxins, human serums are usually preferred.

An example of a postexposure immunization is one given to a patient who has been exposed to hepatitis B virus (HBV). This patient should be given the antiserum hepatitis B immune globulin (HBV-Ig) within 7 days after exposure and again 28 to 30 days later. Because HBV-Ig is made from human serum, it causes relatively few adverse reactions. Another example involves a patient who may have been exposed to tetanus (lockjaw) organisms as the result of an injury such as a puncture wound. This patient may receive tetanus immune globulin (T-Ig, a human product) or tetanus antitoxin. Because tetanus antitoxin is made from horse serum, it may cause serious reactions in patients who are allergic to horses or horsehair.

For every vaccine in your medical office, you must be familiar with the indications, contraindications, dosages, administration routes, potential adverse effects, and methods of storage and handling. You must carefully read the package insert provided with each vaccine and, when necessary, consult drug reference books for further information.

Patient Education About Drugs

Your role as teacher cannot be underestimated with regard to drugs. In addition to providing specific instructions about different categories of drugs, you need to give your attention to all the drugs a patient is taking, whether prescription or over-the-counter.

Over-the-Counter Drugs

Even though patients can obtain OTC drugs without a prescription, they need to know several important facts to use them safely. That is why you should plan an education session with any patient whose medical history reveals use of OTC drugs or for whom a doctor has suggested an OTC drug.

In your patient education sessions, caution patients not to treat themselves with OTC drugs as a way to avoid medical care. For example, OTC drugs are available to treat recurrent yeast infections. Nonetheless, a patient should consult a doctor the first time she develops an infection.

Also inform patients that OTC drugs, which provide safe dosages for self-care only when used as directed, may not produce enough therapeutic benefit in some cases. In other cases they may mask symptoms or aggravate the problem.

Inform patients that many OTC drugs contain more than one active ingredient. These extra ingredients, such as aspirin or caffeine, can cause allergic or other undesirable effects.

It is important to advise patients that interactions can occur when a person takes more than one OTC drug at a time or takes an OTC and a prescription drug together. These interactions can lead to adverse reactions. For example, a patient who takes the prescription blood thinner warfarin (Coumadin) to prevent blood clots must avoid taking aspirin for pain relief. Taking these drugs together increases the risk of uncontrolled bleeding.

Prescription Drugs

Before patients begin drug therapy, you must inform them of certain considerations (such as when to take the drug) and drug safety precautions. As part of your patient education, provide instructions orally and, if possible, in writing. For commonly prescribed drugs, you may use preprinted information sheets published by the American Medical Association. Some pharmacies now routinely provide an information sheet with each dispensed drug. Figure 50-12 shows a sample of a drug information sheet.

Encouraging the Complete Medication List. Advise patients to inform the doctor of all drugs—prescription and OTC—they use regularly or periodically. Also advise patients to include past and present use of alcohol and recreational drugs as well as herbal remedies. When patients have more than one doctor, tell them to inform each doctor about all medications they are taking. Encourage them to keep up-to-date medication lists with dosages (some patients keep this information on their home computers). This information can help patients and health-care professionals prevent and monitor for drug interactions.

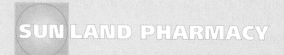

SUN LAND PHARMACY

Patient Name: Jean Cranston
RX#: 711428172
Drug: Albuterol Inhalation Aerosol

COMMON USES:
To treat asthma, bronchitis, and other lung diseases.

HOW SHOULD I USE IT?
Follow your doctor's and/or the package instructions. Shake well before each use. Rinse mouth after each inhalation to avoid dryness. If breathing has not improved in 20 minutes, call doctor.

ARE THERE ANY SIDE EFFECTS?
Very unlikely, but report: Flushing, trembling, headache, nausea, vomiting, rapid heartbeat, chest pain, weakness, dizziness.

HOW DO I STORE THIS?
Store at room temperature away from moisture and sunlight. Do not puncture. Do not store in the bathroom. Rinse and clean inhaler regularly as described in package instructions.

Figure 50-12. Many pharmacies provide consumers with drug information sheets that accompany their prescriptions.

Encouraging the Complete Adverse Reaction List. Tell patients to inform each of their doctors of any adverse reactions (including allergic reactions) they have had to drugs. Previous adverse reactions may prompt a doctor to adjust a dosage or select a different drug. A history of drug allergies may contraindicate the use of a particular drug.

Educating for Patient Compliance. To help ensure that patients comply with instructions, confirm that they completely understand the name, dosage, and purpose of each drug prescribed for them. If patients must take more than one drug at a time, be sure they know the correct and relevant information for each one. Also teach patients to inform other health-care providers whenever there is a change in their medication regimen. In addition, cover each of the following points when educating patients about drugs.

- Explain how and when to take each drug to ensure its safety and effectiveness. Some drugs should be taken with food to minimize gastrointestinal irritation. Others should be taken on an empty stomach for proper absorption and metabolism. Some drugs must be taken once a day in the morning; others should be taken three or four times a day. If patients' medication schedules are complex, suggest that they create a chart, calendar, or diary to remind them of what drug to take and when, or create a schedule for them.

- Tell patients how long to take each drug. In the case of antibiotics, advise them to take all of the drug as scheduled, even if they feel better before finishing it. In the case of medicines prescribed for chronic disease, advise patients that they will need to continue taking the medication unless the doctor tells them to stop. Be aware that some drugs, such as prednisone, must be tapered off slowly to prevent adverse reactions.

- Explain how to identify possible adverse effects of each drug and safety measures related to adverse effects. For example, instruct patients to avoid certain activities, such as driving or operating machinery, while taking a drug that causes drowsiness. Also tell them to call the doctor if they experience adverse effects or any unusual reactions. If appropriate, inform patients that misuse of the drug may lead to dependence, and mention the dangers of drug dependence.

- Tell patients not to save old medications or share them with anyone else. Old medications and those taken by people other than the patient for whom they were prescribed can cause severe, unexpected adverse effects. Advise patients to check the expiration date on all drugs and to flush expired ones down the toilet.

- Suggest that patients avoid alcohol when taking a drug unless the doctor or pharmacist indicates otherwise. Alcohol interacts with some drugs, causing adverse effects such as lethargy, confusion, or coma.

- Tell patients to ask their pharmacists where to store each medication. Some drugs must be refrigerated. Others should be kept in a dry, cool area. Drugs should not usually be kept in a hot, damp place, such as a bathroom. They must always be kept out of the reach of children.

- Tell patients to take their drugs in a well-lit area so they can read each drug label carefully before taking each dose. They should never assume that they are taking the right medication without reading the label on the container. If patients have poor vision, print the name of the drug and the dosage schedule clearly on a separate piece of paper or card to attach to the medication container.

- Instruct patients to call the doctor if they have any questions about their drug therapy.

Summary

Pharmacology is the study of drugs, or pharmaceuticals. The pharmacologist studies pharmacognosy, pharmacokinetics, pharmacodynamics, pharmacotherapeutics, and toxicology. Pharmacognosy is the study of the characteristics of natural drugs and their sources. Pharmacokinetics pertains to how the body absorbs, metabolizes, distributes, and excretes a drug. Pharmacodynamics relates to a drug's mechanism of action, or how it affects the body. Pharmacotherapeutics addresses the use of drugs to prevent or treat disease. Toxicology is the study of poisons and the toxic effects of drugs, including adverse effects or drug interactions.

Every drug has several names, including chemical, generic, and trade names. Based on its action, a drug can belong to one of many classifications. These data can be found in the *Physicians' Desk Reference* and other sources of drug information.

Patients can obtain nonprescription (over-the-counter) drugs without a physician's order. For prescription drugs, patients must have a physician's written (or oral) order. For drugs that have been classified as controlled substances because they are potentially dangerous and addictive, extensive regulations apply. The physician must be registered with the Drug Enforcement Administration and follow the legal requirements of the Controlled Substances Act of 1970 to administer, dispense, and prescribe these drugs.

Immunizations usually contain killed or weakened organisms. They are used to provide immunity against specific diseases. Childhood immunizations should follow a recommended schedule. Other immunizations should be given as the need arises.

No matter what type of drug a patient must take, your role as an educator is an important one. You need to teach patients about specific drugs and required safety precautions. When you educate a patient carefully and thoroughly about a drug, you enhance the likelihood of patient compliance and safety.

TABLE 51-3 Common Apothecaries' Equivalents

Measures of Volume	Measures of Weight
60 minims (min, ♏) = 1 fluidram (fl dr, f℥)	20 grains (gr) = 1 scruple (scr, ℈)
8 fl dr = 1 fluidounce (fl oz, f℥)	60 gr or 3 scr = 1 dram (dr, ℨ)
16 fl oz = 1 pint (pt)	8 dr = 1 ounce (oz, ℥)
2 pt = 1 quart (qt)	12 oz = 1 pound (℔)
4 qt = 1 gallon (gal)	

TABLE 51-4 Common Household Measurements

Measures of Volume
60 drops (gtt) = 1 teaspoon (tsp)
3 tsp = 1 tablespoon (tbsp)
6 tsp = 1 ounce (oz) or 2 tbsp
8 oz = 1 cup (c)
2 c = 1 pint (pt)
4 c = 1 quart (qt) or 2 pt

amount of the drug. For example, ASA gr X means "10 grains of acetylsalicylic acid (aspirin)." Note that in the metric system, the amount precedes the unit, whereas in the apothecaries' system, the amount follows the unit. Although this system is less popular than it once was, some doctors still use it.

Household System. The only household units of measurement that are used to measure drugs are units of volume. These include drops, teaspoons, tablespoons, ounces, cups, pints, quarts, and gallons. Common household equivalents are shown in Table 51-4.

Conversions Between Measurement Systems

At times you may need to convert from one measurement system to another. Because of the difference in basic units of measure, you must remember that conversions between systems are only approximate equivalents. If you use a conversion chart, read it carefully before administering a drug. Check it several times, and place a ruler under the line you are reading to be absolutely sure you are reading the chart properly. When you must calculate conversions instead of using a conversion chart, use either the ratio or the fraction method.

Basic Calculations. In some instances, you can use a basic formula to calculate drugs that have the same labels—such as milligrams and milligrams—and therefore do not require a conversion. The basic calculation that you would use looks like this:

$$\frac{\text{desired dose}}{\text{dose on hand}} \times \text{quantity of dose on hand}$$

Suppose that the physician orders aspirin, 10 grains. However, all that the office has on hand are 5-grain aspirins. Follow these steps to perform the basic calculation:

1. Verify that no conversion is necessary. In this example, because both measures are in grains, you do not need to convert the measurement.

2. Use the following formula and label all the parts:

$$\frac{\text{desired dose}}{\text{dose on hand}} \times \text{quantity of dose on hand}$$

$$\frac{10 \, \cancel{\text{gr}}}{5 \, \cancel{\text{gr}}} \times 1 \, \text{Tablet} = \frac{10}{5} = 2 \, \text{tablets}$$

Ratio Method. Suppose the doctor orders ASA gr X. Although this translates to 10 grains of aspirin in the apothecaries' system, the available tablets come in milligrams, a metric measurement. To convert from apothecaries' to metric measure, you must set up a ratio to solve for x, the unknown dose in milligrams. Follow these steps to convert the measurement.

1. Set up the first ratio:

$$x : 10 \, \text{gr}$$

2. Next set up the second ratio with the standard equivalent between the available and ordered measurements:

$$60 \, \text{mg} : 1 \, \text{gr}$$

3. Then use both ratios in a proportional equation that reads, x is to 10 gr as 60 mg is to 1 gr. Mathematically, this is written:

$$x : 10 \, \text{gr} :: 60 \, \text{mg} : 1 \, \text{gr}$$

4. Multiply the outer and then the inner parts of the proportion:

$$x \times 1 \, \text{gr} = 10 \, \text{gr} \times 60 \, \text{mg}$$

5. To solve for x, divide both sides of the equation by 1 gr, then do the arithmetic, canceling out like terms in

each numerator (top of the fraction) and denominator (bottom of the fraction):

$$\frac{x \times \cancel{1\,gr}}{\cancel{1\,gr}} = \frac{10\,\cancel{gr} \times 60\,mg}{1\,\cancel{gr}}$$

$$x = \frac{10 \times 60\,mg}{1}$$

$$x = \frac{600\,mg}{1}$$

$$x = 600\,mg$$

Fraction Method. Suppose the physician orders 300 mg of aspirin in the metric system. The tablets, however, are labeled in grains, an apothecaries' measure. To make this conversion, follow these steps.

1. Set up a fraction with the ordered dose on the top and the unknown amount on the bottom:

$$\frac{300\,mg}{x}$$

2. Next set up a fraction with the standard equivalent. Make sure that for this fraction you use units of measure on the top and the bottom that match the units of measure on the top and the bottom of the first fraction:

$$\frac{60\,mg}{1\,gr}$$

3. Then set up a proportion with both fractions:

$$\frac{300\,mg}{x} = \frac{60\,mg}{1\,gr}$$

4. Now cross multiply. Multiply the bottom left number by the top right number, and multiply the top left number by the bottom right number:

$$x \times 60\,mg = 300\,mg \times 1\,gr$$

5. To solve for x, divide both sides of the equation by 60, then do the arithmetic, canceling out like terms in the top and bottom of each fraction:

$$\frac{x \times \cancel{60\,mg}}{\cancel{60\,mg}} = \frac{300\,\cancel{mg} = 1\,gr}{60\,\cancel{mg}}$$

$$x = \frac{300 \times 1\,gr}{60}$$

$$x = \frac{300\,gr}{60}$$

$$x = 5\,gr$$

Calculations and Drug Doses

You may occasionally need to do some calculations to provide a prescribed drug dose. You can use the ratio method or the fraction method to calculate the dose. Because a patient's health or life can depend on your calculations, take the time to check and recheck your arithmetic. If you need extra practice in calculations, consider buying and using a dosage calculation workbook.

Ratio Method. Suppose the doctor orders 500 mg of ampicillin, but each tablet contains only 250 mg. To calculate how to provide this dose, follow these steps.

1. Set up a ratio with the unknown number of tablets and the amount of the drug ordered:

$$x : 500\,mg$$

2. Next set up a ratio with a single tablet and the amount of drug in a single tablet:

$$1\,tab : 250\,mg$$

3. Now put both of these ratios in a proportion:

$$x : 500\,mg :: 1\,tab : 250\,mg$$

4. Multiply the outer and then the inner parts of the proportion:

$$x \times 250\,mg = 500\,mg \times 1\,tab$$

5. To solve for x, divide both sides of the equation by 250 mg, then do the arithmetic, canceling out like terms in the top and bottom of each fraction:

$$\frac{x \times \cancel{250\,mg}}{\cancel{250\,mg}} = \frac{500\,\cancel{mg} \times 1\,tab}{250\,\cancel{mg}}$$

$$x = \frac{500\,tabs}{250}$$

$$x = 2\,tabs$$

As another example, the doctor orders 30 mg of Adalat, but each capsule contains only 10 mg. To calculate the prescribed drug dose using the ratio method, you would set up these equations:

$$x : 30\,mg$$

$$1\,cap : 10\,mg$$

$$x : 30\,mg :: 1\,cap : 10\,mg$$

$$x \times 10\,mg = 30\,mg \times 1\,cap$$

$$\frac{x \times \cancel{10\,mg}}{\cancel{10\,mg}} = \frac{30\,\cancel{mg} \times 1\,cap}{10\,\cancel{mg}}$$

$$x = \frac{30\,caps}{10}$$

$$x = 3\,caps$$

Fraction Method. For the same problem, you could use the fraction method to calculate how to provide the prescribed dose. Follow these steps for the fraction method.

1. Set up the first fraction with the dose ordered and the unknown number of capsules:

$$\frac{30\,mg}{x}$$

2. Set up the second fraction with the amount of drug in a capsule and a single capsule:

$$\frac{10\,\text{mg}}{1\,\text{cap}}$$

3. Then use both fractions in a proportion:

$$\frac{30\,\text{mg}}{x} = \frac{10\,\text{mg}}{1\,\text{cap}}$$

4. Cross multiply. Remember to multiply the bottom left number by the top right number and multiply the top left number by the bottom right number:

$$x \times 10\,\text{mg} = 30\,\text{mg} \times 1\,\text{cap}$$

5. To solve for x, divide both sides of the equation by 10 mg, then do the arithmetic, canceling out like terms in the top and bottom of each fraction:

$$\frac{x \times \cancel{10\,\text{mg}}}{\cancel{10\,\text{mg}}} = \frac{30\,\cancel{\text{mg}} \times 1\,\text{cap}}{10\,\cancel{\text{mg}}}$$

$$x = \frac{30\,\text{caps}}{10}$$

$$x = 3\,\text{caps}$$

As another example, the doctor orders 120 mg of Armour thyroid but each tablet contains only 30 mg. To calculate the prescribed drug dose using the fraction method, you would set up these equations:

$$\frac{120\,\text{mg}}{x}$$

$$\frac{30\,\text{mg}}{1\,\text{tab}}$$

$$\frac{120\,\text{mg}}{x} = \frac{30\,\text{mg}}{1\,\text{tab}}$$

$$x \times 30\,\text{mg} = 120\,\text{mg} \times 1\,\text{tab}$$

$$\frac{x \times \cancel{30\,\text{mg}}}{\cancel{30\,\text{mg}}} = \frac{120\,\cancel{\text{mg}} \times 1\,\text{tab}}{30\,\cancel{\text{mg}}}$$

$$x = \frac{120\,\text{tabs}}{30}$$

$$x = 4\,\text{tabs}$$

Pediatric Dosage Calculations

Most pediatric dosage calculations are based on the child's age or body weight. The common formulas used for pediatric dosage calculations are Clark's rule and Fried's rule.

Clark's Rule

$$\frac{\text{weight of child}}{150\,\text{lbs}} \times \text{adult dose} = \text{child's dose}$$

Fried's Rule

$$\frac{\text{age of child in months}}{150\,\text{lbs}} \times \text{average adult dose}$$

$$= \text{child's dose}$$

Example. Katie has just turned 3 years old and weighs 30 pounds. Her mother wants to know how much cough syrup to give Katie. The directions have worn off the bottle and she can only make out the dosage for adults: 2 teaspoons every 4 hours. How much cough syrup should Katie receive?

The calculation based on Clark's rule would look like this:

$$\frac{30}{150} \times 10\,\text{ml} = \text{Katie's dose}$$

$$\frac{1}{5} \times 10\,\text{ml} = 2\,\text{ml}$$

The calculation based on Fried's rule would look like this:

$$\frac{36}{150} \times 10\,\text{ml} = \text{Katie's dose}$$

$$0.24 \times 10\,\text{ml} = 2.4\,\text{ml}$$

Preparing to Administer a Drug

Drugs may be administered for either local or systemic effects. Generally, drugs that have local effects are applied directly to the skin, tissues, or mucous membranes. Drugs that produce systemic effects are administered by routes that allow the drug to be absorbed and distributed in the bloodstream throughout the body. The importance of extreme care with drug dose and route is described in the Caution: Handle With Care section.

Before prescribing the route of administration for a drug, the doctor considers the drug's mechanism of action (described in the section on pharmacodynamics in Chapter 50); the drug's characteristics, cost, and availability; and the patient's physical and emotional state. The different routes of administration are described in Table 51-5 and discussed later in this chapter.

Assessment

Although the doctor gives the order to administer a drug, much of the responsibility is yours. Because you will often interview the patient, you must be alert to—and inform the doctor of—any change in the patient's condition that could affect drug therapy.

Injection Site. Part of your assessment is to locate and inspect the injection site. Find the injection site by using anatomical landmarks. Inspect the skin by checking for the following conditions:

- Moles
- Birthmarks
- Traumatic injury
- Redness
- Rash
- Edema
- Cyanosis

Dose and Route in Drug Administration

In the 2003 AAMA Role Delineation Chart, drug preparation and administration are included among the basic clinical skills for patient care. They require close attention to detail, strong patient assessment skills, and expert technique.

You must give close attention to both dose and route of administration, especially when one depends on the other. Not only must you give extreme care to dose and route, but frequently you must also check and recheck the ordered form of the drug (for example, tablet or extended release capsule). In the following examples, this crucial relationship is illustrated.

1. Prochlorperazine (Compazine) is an antiemetic drug for acute nausea and vomiting. It is given to both children and adults. When the vomiting is so severe that a tablet or capsule cannot be swallowed, the drug is administered in injectable or suppository form. This drug is available in the following forms:

   - 10 mL multidose vials with 5 mg of drug per mL, written as 5 mg/mL
   - 2 mL single-dose vials 5 mg/mL
   - 4 fl oz bottles of syrup 5 mg/5 mL (5 mg/1 tsp)
   - 5 mg tablets
   - 10 mg tablets
   - 2 mL prefilled disposable syringes 5 mg/mL
   - 2½ mg suppositories
   - 5 mg suppositories
   - 25 mg suppositories
   - 10 mg extended release capsules
   - 15 mg extended release capsules

   Because so many forms of this drug are available, there is a high risk of error in choosing the correct form. In addition, the route of administration can determine how much drug is delivered in one dose. For example, note that suppositories are available in 2½-mg, 5-mg, and 25-mg forms. If the 2½-mg dose were written as

2.5 mg, there might be confusion with the 25-mg dose suppository. Thus the 2½-mg suppository is always written this way, even in the PDR. This clarification helps prevent a child's receiving the adult dose of 25 mg, which could result in serious complications to the central nervous system. This possible confusion is a good example of how much difference a decimal point can make.

Note also that in the syrup there is a 5-mg dose of drug per 5 mL (1 tsp), whereas in the other liquid forms (vials and prefilled syringes), there is a 5-mg dose of drug per 1 mL. The injectable form is five times more concentrated than the syrup. Therefore, if you were to administer the same amount of injectable liquid as syrup to a patient, you would give the patient five times more drug than in the syrup. Just as a child could be endangered with the 25-mg suppository, an adult could be endangered with the wrong form of liquid. Because elderly patients often receive syrup forms of medication, this instruction could be particularly confusing.

2. Allergy shots must be administered subcutaneously rather than intramuscularly to allow slower absorption of the serum. Within 30 minutes, a wheal and redness will appear if the patient has an allergic reaction. In such a case the patient requires further close monitoring. If the serum were injected intramuscularly, this reaction would not only be hidden (because of the deeper administration), it would also occur more rapidly (because of the faster rate of absorption). In fact, the patient could go into anaphylaxis, or anaphylactic shock, without any warning.

Check and recheck every order and drug label to prevent confusion and incorrect administration. This procedure is always worth the time it takes.

- Burns
- Tattoos
- Side of a mastectomy
- Paralyzed areas
- Warts

If you are unsure about any of these conditions, inform the physician.

Drug Allergies. During the assessment, it is important to ask the patient about any drug allergies. Even though you may see a patient on a regular basis, be in the habit of asking about drug allergies at every patient visit. Patients often see other physicians or specialists, who may have prescribed different medications. A patient could have had a drug reaction by a medication that has been prescribed by another physician. If applicable,

TABLE 51-5 Routes and Methods of Drug Administration

Route and Drug Forms	Method
Buccal route Tablets	Place drug between patient's gum and cheek. To ensure absorption, tell patient to leave tablet there until it dissolves and not to chew or swallow it. Tell the patient not to eat, drink, or smoke until tablet is completely dissolved.

Intradermal route
   Solutions
   Powders for reconstitution
	Administer drug by injection into upper layers of patient's skin.

Intramuscular route
   Solutions
   Powders for reconstitution
	Administer drug by injection into muscle.

Intravenous route
   Solutions (often in bags of 250, 500, or 1000 mL)
   Powders for reconstitution
   Blood and blood products
	Administer drug by injection or infusion into vein.

Inhalation therapy (nasal or oral)
   Aerosols
   Sprays
   Mists or steam
	Administer drug by inhalation to reach respiratory tract.

Oral route
   Tablets
   Capsules
   Liquids
   Lozenges
	Give drug to patient to swallow.

Ophthalmic (eye) or otic (ear) route
   Solutions
   Ointments
	Apply drug, usually as drops, in patient's eye or ear.

Rectal route
   Suppositories
   Solutions
	Insert suppository into rectum. Administer solution as enema, using tube and nozzle.

Subcutaneous route
   Solutions
   Powders for reconstitution
	Administer drug by injection into subcutaneous layer of skin.

Sublingual route
   Tablets
   Sprays
	Place drug under patient's tongue. To ensure absorption, tell patient to leave tablet there until it dissolves and not to chew or swallow it. Tell the patient not to eat, drink, or smoke until tablet is completely dissolved.

Topical route
   Ointments
   Lotions
   Creams
   Tinctures
   Powders
   Sprays
   Solutions
	Apply drug to patient's skin or rub into skin.

continued ⟶

TABLE 51-5 Routes and Methods of Drug Administration *(continued)*

Route and Drug Forms	Method
Transdermal route 　Patches	Apply drug to clean, dry, nonhairy area of skin.
Urethral route 　Solutions	Administer drug by instilling in bladder, using catheter.
Vaginal route 　Solutions 　Suppositories 　Ointments 　Foams 　Creams	Administer solution as douche, using tube and nozzle. Administer any other form by inserting into vagina with applicator.

document in the patient chart "NKDA" or "no known drug allergies."

Patient Condition. Before administering a drug, assess the patient's overall condition. For example, does the patient have a viral infection? Vaccines are not recommended if the patient has a viral infection such as a common cold. In addition, review the patient's drug list to ensure that any medications already being taken will not interfere with the ordered drug or route of administration. Also verify again that the ordered dose is appropriate for the patient's age and weight.

Patient Consent Form. Many physicians require that a patient sign a consent form before receiving an injection. This form provides general information regarding the medication or vaccine and lists the possible side effects or adverse reactions. If your physician requires a consent form, make sure that the patient signs the form and that you have answered any questions prior to giving the injection.

General Rules for Drug Administration

No matter what drug or administration route is ordered, follow these general rules when administering drugs.

- Give only the drugs the physician has ordered. Written orders are preferable, but oral orders are appropriate for emergencies. If you are unfamiliar with any aspect of a drug the physician orders, consult a drug reference work.
- Wash your hands before handling the drug. Prepare the drug in a well-lit area, away from distractions. Focus only on the task at hand.
- Calculate the dose if necessary. If you are unsure of your computation, ask another medical assistant, a nurse, or the physician to check it.
- Avoid leaving a prepared drug unattended, and never administer a drug that someone else has prepared.

- Ask the patient to state his name to ensure correct identification. Also ask the patient to tell you about any possible drug allergies. Do not rely on documentation in his chart; he may have developed a new allergy that has not yet been added to the record. Then verify any drug allergies in the chart.
- Be sure the physician is in the office when you administer a drug or vaccine. If the patient develops an anaphylactic reaction (sudden, severe allergic reaction) to the drug or vaccine, the physician must administer epinephrine. Some patients need to know how to administer this drug themselves. For information about epinephrine, see the Educating the Patient section.
- After administering the drug, ask the patient to remain in the facility for 10 to 20 minutes so that you can observe the patient for any unexpected effects. Give the patient specific instructions about the effects of the drug as well as general information about drug use.
- If the patient refuses to take the drug, flush it down the toilet. Do *not* return it to the original container. Be sure to document the refusal in the patient's record and tell the physician.
- If you make an error in drug administration, tell the physician immediately.
- Document immediately the drug and dose administered; never document administration before giving medicine.

To master your administration techniques, practice with classmates. When on the job, ask a coworker, perhaps a nurse or a more experienced medical assistant, to critique your technique.

Seven Rights of Drug Administration

When administering any drug, whether medication or vaccine, observe the seven "rights" of drug administration.

Using an Epinephrine Autoinjector

If you are working in a medical office that treats people with allergies, you must be familiar with epinephrine so that you can teach patients how to self-administer the drug. Epinephrine is a drug used to treat allergies so severe that exposure to the allergen may be life-threatening. The following reactions indicate the possibility of anaphylaxis, or anaphylactic shock, a severe allergic reaction:

- Flushing
- Sharp drop in blood pressure
- Hives
- Difficulty breathing
- Difficulty swallowing
- Convulsions
- Vomiting
- Diarrhea and abdominal cramps

If a patient with a severe allergy experiences any or all of these symptoms, the reaction can be fatal unless emergency treatment is given immediately. Therefore, patients who cannot always control their exposure to an allergen—for example, bee or wasp venom—must have access to an epinephrine autoinjector for emergency intramuscular use.

These injectors, which are prepackaged (Figure 51-1), deliver either 0.3 mg of epinephrine—a single dose for an adult—or 0.15 mg of epinephrine—a single dose for a child. A patient who is exposed to the allergen should use the injector if the allergy is confirmed or if the allergy is suspected and signs of anaphylaxis appear.

Teach the patient to follow these steps when using an autoinjector.

1. Remove the autoinjector from the packaging (box and/or plastic tube).
2. Pull back the gray cap.
3. Place the black tip of the injector on the outside of the upper thigh. (The injector can go through clothing.)

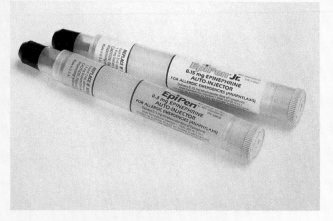

Figure 51-1. Epinephrine autoinjectors come prepackaged, containing the correct amount of the drug for an adult or a child (the junior unit).

4. Press firmly into the thigh and hold for 10 seconds.
5. Remove the autoinjector and massage the injection site for a few minutes.
6. Call your physician or go to the emergency room of a nearby hospital. An autoinjector is designed as emergency supportive therapy only. It is not a replacement or substitute for immediate medical or hospital care.

Make sure the patient is thoroughly familiar with the parts of the autoinjector, how to activate it, how to use it, and what to do next. Ask the patient to explain the use of the autoinjector to you, as if you had never seen one. This approach not only reinforces the patient's understanding of the process but also improves the patient's self-confidence and points out any possible misconceptions. If the patient is very young or otherwise unable to use the autoinjector reliably, teach a family member or companion how to perform the process.

Never deviate from these seven steps. Adhering to these rights helps ensure that you administer the drug correctly. The seven rights refer to the following:

1. Right patient
2. Right drug
3. Right dose
4. Right time
5. Right route
6. Right technique
7. Right documentation

Right Patient. Always check the name on the order for a drug or vaccine in the patient's chart; then ask the patient to tell you her name. Be especially careful with a forgetful or confused patient, because she might answer to any name. Have a confused patient state her name, or check her name with an attending family member.

Right Drug. Carefully compare the name of the prescribed drug or vaccine in the patient's chart with the label on the drug container. As you check the drug name on the label, look at the expiration date. Never use a drug that has passed this date.

If you are unfamiliar with the drug, look it up in the *PDR* or other drug reference. Also, never prepare a drug from a container with a damaged or handwritten label. To ensure accuracy, read the label three times:

1. When you obtain the drug container from the cabinet
2. When you pour or prepare the drug from the container
3. When you put the container back in the cabinet (before leaving the medication room)

Right Dose. Compare the dose on the order in the patient's chart with the dose you prepare. To obtain the right dose, read the label closely. Do not confuse the dose contained in one tablet with the number of tablets in the container.

Right Time. Be sure to give the drug at the right time. If it must be given after meals, make sure the patient has eaten recently. For certain drugs, you must ensure that it is the correct time of day and the correct time in a series of doses. Timing is crucial with allergy shots because of possible reactions.

Right Route. Double-check to make sure the administration route you are preparing to use matches the route the doctor ordered. Check that the patient can receive the drug by this route and that the route seems appropriate. For example, if the patient has an injury at the specified injection site, consult the doctor for a possible alternative site or a different route.

Right Technique. Always use the proper administration technique. If you have not given a drug or vaccine by the ordered route recently, review the technique before administering the drug.

Right Documentation. Document the procedure immediately after administering the drug or vaccine to the patient. Do not wait until later, and do not document before administration. Be sure to include the date, time, drug or vaccine name, dose, administration route, patient reaction, patient education about the drug, and your initials. If the drug is a controlled substance, also document it on the controlled substance inventory record. Remember that correct documentation demands neat handwriting that others who care for the patient can read easily.

Techniques of Administering Drugs

The doctor may ask you to administer drugs by one of the routes outlined in Table 51-5. Because most patients take a prescription to a pharmacy to be filled and then take oral drugs at home, you rarely need to administer these drugs in the office. You are likely, however, to be asked to do the following.

- Place drugs in the patient's mouth between the cheek and gum or under the tongue
- Administer a drug by any means other than by mouth (if permitted in your state)
- Demonstrate how to use an inhaler
- Apply topical drugs (those applied to the skin)
- Administer or assist in administering drugs into the urethra, vagina, or rectum
- Administer medications to the eye or ear

These duties require you to master a variety of techniques to give drugs safely by any route.

Oral Administration

Drugs for oral administration include tablets, capsules, lozenges, and liquids. These drugs are absorbed relatively slowly as they travel along the gastrointestinal (GI) tract.

Oral administration is contraindicated in patients who have severe nausea, are comatose, or cannot swallow. Certain drugs are ineffective when administered orally, because the digestive process changes them chemically to an ineffective form or does not deliver them to the bloodstream quickly enough.

Many drugs, however, are most effective when given orally. These include antibiotics, vitamins, throat lozenges, and cough syrups. Although these drugs are familiar to most people, as a medical assistant, you must follow certain steps to ensure that the patient understands the drug and that the drug is administered safely and effectively. The steps for oral administration are outlined in Procedure 51-1.

Buccal and Sublingual Administration

Although buccal and sublingual drugs are placed in the mouth, they do not continue along the GI tract. Instead, they dissolve and are absorbed in the **buccal** area (between the cheek and gum) or the **sublingual** area (under the tongue), where they are placed. The medication is absorbed through tissue that is rich in capillaries, and the drug enters the bloodstream directly. Because the drug does not pass into the stomach or intestines before absorption, it produces a therapeutic effect more quickly than do oral drugs.

Specially formulated tablets may be given by the buccal or sublingual routes. Except for the point at which you give the tablet to the patient, the steps for administering buccal and sublingual drugs are the same as those for drugs administered orally (as outlined in Procedure 51-1). When you administer buccal or sublingual medications, your role usually involves teaching the patient how to administer these medications at home.

For both buccal and sublingual administration, tell the patient not to chew or swallow the tablet. Tell the patient

Administering Oral Drugs

Objective: To safely administer an oral drug to a patient

OSHA Guidelines: This procedure does not involve exposure to blood, body fluids, or tissues.

Materials: Drug order (in patient chart), container of oral drug, small paper cup (for tablets, capsules, or caplets) or plastic calibrated medicine cup (for liquids), glass of water or juice, straw (optional), package insert or drug information sheet

Method

1. Identify the patient and wash your hands.
2. Select the ordered drug (tablet, capsule, or liquid).
3. Check the seven rights, comparing information against the drug order.
4. If you are unfamiliar with the drug, check the PDR or other drug reference, read the package insert, or speak with the physician. Determine whether the drug may be taken with or followed by water or juice.
5. Ask the patient about any drug or food allergies. If the patient is not allergic to the ordered drug or other ingredients used to prepare it, proceed.
6. Perform any calculations needed to provide the prescribed dose. If you are unsure of your calculations, check them with a coworker or the physician.

If You Are Giving Tablets or Capsules

7. Open the container and tap the correct number into the cap (Figure 51-2). Do not touch the inside of the cap because it is sterile. If you pour out too many tablets or capsules and you have not touched them, tap the excess back into the container.
8. Tap the tablets or capsules from the cap into the paper cup.
9. Recap the container.
10. Give the patient the cup along with a glass of water or juice. If the patient finds it easier to drink with a straw, unwrap the straw and place it in the fluid. If patients have difficulty swallowing pills, have them drink some water or juice before putting the pills in the mouth. This additional fluid makes the pills float and allows patients to swallow quickly.

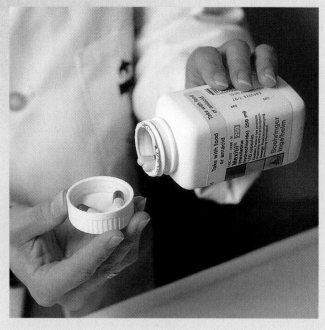

Figure 51-2. Tap tablets gently into the cap.

If You Are Giving a Liquid Drug

7. If the liquid is a suspension, shake it well.
8. Locate the mark on the medicine cup for the prescribed dose. Keeping your thumbnail on the mark, hold the cup at eye level and pour the correct amount of the drug. To prevent liquid drips from obscuring the label, keep the label side of the bottle on top as you pour (Figure 51-3), or put your palm over it.
9. After pouring the drug, place the cup on a flat surface, and check the drug level again. At eye level the base of the meniscus (the crescent-shaped form at the top of the liquid) should align with the mark that indicates the prescribed dose (Figure 51-4). If you poured out too much, discard it. Do not return it to the container because medicine cups are not sterile.
10. Give the medicine cup to the patient with instructions to drink the liquid. If appropriate, offer a glass of water or juice to wash down the drug.

continued ⟶

Administering Oral Drugs *(continued)*

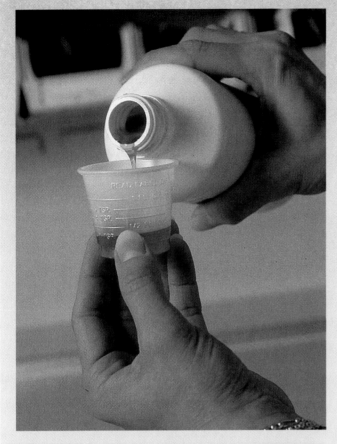

Figure 51-3. Pour a liquid drug into a calibrated medication cup.

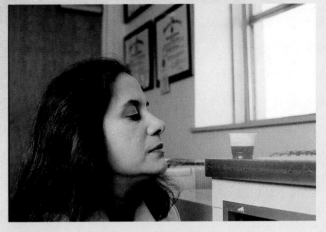

Figure 51-4. Read the measurement at eye level.

After You Have Given an Oral Drug

11. Wash your hands.
12. Give the patient an information sheet about the drug. Discuss the information with the patient and answer any questions she may have. If the patient has questions you cannot answer, refer her to the physician.
13. Document the drug administration with the date, time, drug name, dosage, expiration date, lot number, manufacturer, route, site, and significant patient reactions in the patient's chart. Also document patient education about the drug.

---

to place a buccal drug, such as hyoscyamine sulfate, between the cheek and gum until it dissolves, as shown in Figure 51-5. Explain that this area has a rich blood supply that promotes rapid drug absorption.

Tell the patient to place a sublingual drug, such as nitroglycerin, under the tongue until it dissolves, as shown in Figure 51-6. Explain that the capillaries in this area promote rapid drug absorption.

Instruct patients not to eat, drink, or smoke until after the tablet completely dissolves. Food and fluids wash the drug into the GI tract, slowing absorption or allowing gastric juices to destroy it. Smoking increases salivation, causing impaired absorption of the drug.

Remain with patients until their tablet dissolves to monitor for possible adverse reaction and to ensure that patients have allowed the tablet to dissolve in the mouth instead of chewing or swallowing it. Give patients an information sheet about the drug. Discuss it with them, and answer their questions. If they have questions you cannot answer, refer them to the doctor.

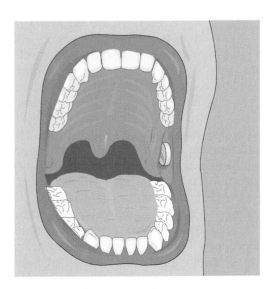

Figure 51-5. Place a buccal drug between the cheek and gum.

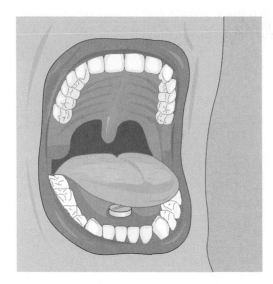

Figure 51-6. Place a sublingual drug under the tongue.

As always, immediately document the drug administration with the date, time, drug name, dose, route, site, and any significant patient reactions. Also document patient education about the drug.

Parenteral Administration

Parenteral administration is the administration of a substance such as a drug by muscle, vein, or any means other than through the GI tract (substances administered through the GI tract are usually given by mouth). It generally applies to giving drugs by injection. Although the parenteral route offers the advantage of rapid drug action, it has several potential drawbacks.

Parenteral administration poses more safety risks for the patient than administration by other routes. The reason is that after the drug has been injected, it cannot be retrieved. To reduce the risks, you must administer the drug expertly and observe the seven rights meticulously.

Parenteral administration increases your risk of potential exposure to blood-borne pathogens when performing injections and disposing of used needles. To minimize risks, follow Universal Precautions during injections. Also adhere to Occupational Safety and Health Administration (OSHA) and Environmental Protection Agency (EPA) regulations for disposing of contaminated needles and sharp items, as discussed in Chapter 19. Most offices provide a rigid, puncture-proof container for collecting disposable sharp instruments. This container should be self-sealing and have a lock-tight cap and a safety neck.

After using a needle, lancet, or syringe, immediately place it in the sharps container. To avoid puncturing yourself, do not force the needle, lancet, or syringe into the container. If you do accidentally stick yourself, notify the physician at once so you can be treated. OSHA requires medical follow-up for all workers who have been accidentally punctured.

Never let a sharps container become full. When the container is two-thirds full, seal it and follow your office procedure for container disposal.

Needles. When you administer a parenteral drug, you must select the appropriate needle, syringe, and drug form to use on the basis of the type of injection. The following are methods of injection:

- **Intradermal (ID),** or within the upper layers of the skin
- **Subcutaneous (SC),** or beneath the skin
- **Intramuscular (IM),** or within a muscle
- **Intravenous (IV),** or directly into a vein

Needles consist of a hub, hilt, shaft, lumen, point, and bevel (Figure 51-7). The hub of the needle fits onto the syringe. The needle tip is beveled (sloped at the opening). The bevel helps the needle cut through the skin with minimum trauma.

Needles are available in various gauges (inside diameters) and lengths (Figure 51-8). A needle's gauge is expressed with numbers. The smaller the number, the larger

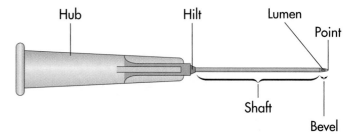

Figure 51-7. Understanding the parts of a needle will help you use it correctly.

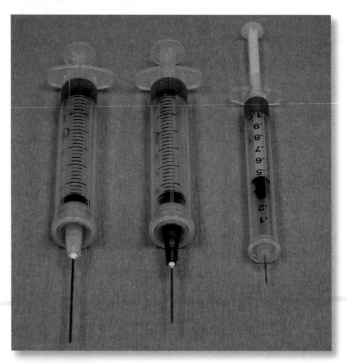

Figure 51-8. Choose a needle with a length, gauge, and bevel appropriate to the type of injection, the drug being injected, and the patient receiving the injection.

TABLE 51-6 Choosing a Needle

Type of Injection	Gauge of Needle	Length of Needle
Intradermal	25–26 gauge	⅜–½ inch
Subcutaneous	23–27 gauge	½–¾ inch
Intramuscular	18–23 gauge	1–3 inches

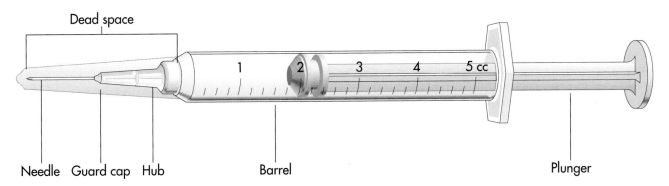

Figure 51-9. Know the parts of a standard syringe.

the gauge. For example, a 25-gauge needle is smaller than an 18-gauge needle. Use the right gauge for the type of injection and the viscosity (thickness) of the drug to be administered. For example, use a large-gauge needle for a highly viscous drug.

When selecting a needle, also consider its length. It must be long enough to penetrate the appropriate layers of tissue but not so long as to go too deep. Choose the correct needle length on the basis of the type of injection as well as the patient's size, amount of fatty tissue, and injection site. Table 51-6 lists the ranges of needle gauge and length typically used for intradermal, subcutaneous, and intramuscular injections.

Syringes. Syringes have two basic parts: a barrel and a plunger. The barrel is the calibrated cylinder that holds the drug. The plunger forces the drug through the barrel and out the needle, as shown in Figure 51-9. The syringe may be packaged with the needle attached and a guard cap over the needle, or the syringe and needle may be packaged separately.

Syringes come in many sizes and are calibrated according to how the syringe will be used. For example, the common 3-mL syringe is divided into tenths of a milliliter on one side and minims on the other. It is used to measure most drugs. A tuberculin (TB) syringe holds 1 mL and is calibrated in hundredths of a milliliter on one side and minims on the other for small doses of drugs (Figure 51-10). Insulin syringes are calibrated in units (U), commonly either 50 U or 100 U (Figure 51-10). Unlike other syringes, insulin syringes have permanently attached needles and no dead space (fluid remaining in the needle or syringe after the plunger is depressed fully). These differences help the patient self-administer the correct amount of insulin.

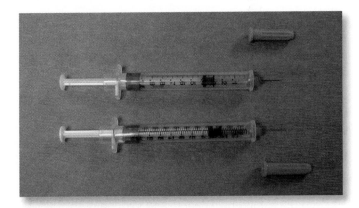

Figure 51-10. You may use the tuberculin syringe (top) to deliver small doses (up to 1.0 mL) of drugs. This insulin syringe (bottom) delivers precisely 100 U of insulin when filled with insulin of the proper concentration (100 U per mL).

Forms of Packaging for Parenteral Drugs. Parenteral drugs are supplied in the forms shown in Figure 51-11. They are ampules, cartridges, and vials.

- An ampule is a small glass or plastic container that is sealed to keep its contents sterile. It must be opened and used with care, as described in Procedure 51-2.
- A cartridge is a small barrel prefilled with a sterile drug. It slips into a special, reusable syringe assembly.
- A vial is a small bottle with a rubber diaphragm that can be punctured by needle. A vial contains a liquid or powder, which must first be reconstituted with a **diluent** (liquid used to dissolve and dilute a drug), as described in Procedure 51-3. It may contain a single or multiple dose. This procedure requires two needle and

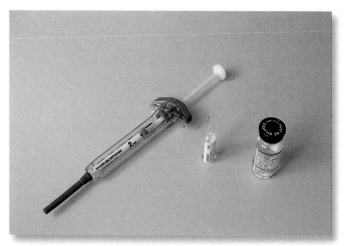

Figure 51-11. Injectable drugs may come in a cartridge (left), an ampule (center), or a vial (right).

syringe sets—one for inserting the diluent into the vial and another to draw and administer the reconstituted drug—to avoid using a contaminated needle. The first needle is considered contaminated when you set it down to mix the diluent and the drug.

Methods of Injection. Injections are the most common method of drug administration in a medical office. You need to be knowledgeable about all injection methods: intradermal, subcutaneous, intramuscular, and intravenous. You must also become proficient in administering intradermal, subcutaneous, and intramuscular injections, as permitted in your state.

Intradermal. An intradermal injection is administered into the upper layer of skin at an angle almost parallel to the skin, as described in Procedure 51-4. Common sites for intradermal injections are the forearm and back. Intradermal

PROCEDURE 51.2

Drawing a Drug From an Ampule

Objective: To safely open an ampule and draw a drug, using sterile technique

OSHA Guidelines

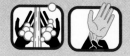

Materials: Ampule of drug, alcohol swab, 2-by-2-inch gauze square, small file (provided by the drug manufacturer), needle and syringe of the appropriate size

Method

1. Identify the patient. Wash your hands and put on examination gloves.
2. Gently tap the top of the ampule with your forefinger to settle the liquid to the bottom of the ampule.
3. Wipe the ampule's neck with an alcohol swab.
4. Wrap the 2-by-2-inch gauze square around the ampule's neck. Then snap the neck away from you (Figure 51-12). If it does not snap easily, score the neck with the small file and snap it again.
5. Insert the needle into the ampule without touching the side of the ampule.
6. Pull back on the plunger to aspirate (remove by vacuum or suction) the liquid. The drug is now ready for injection.

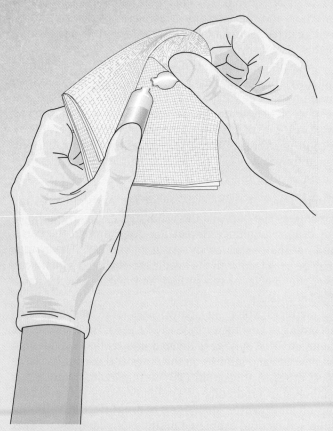

Figure 51-12. You must snap the neck of the ampule before inserting the needle.

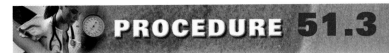
Reconstituting and Drawing a Drug for Injection

Objective: To reconstitute and draw a drug for injection, using sterile technique

OSHA Guidelines

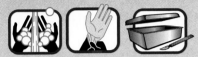

Materials: Vial of drug, vial of diluent, alcohol swabs, two disposable sterile needle and syringe sets of appropriate size, sharps container

Method

1. Identify the patient. Wash your hands and put on examination gloves.

2. Place the drug vial and diluent vial on the countertop. Wipe the rubber diaphragm of each with an alcohol swab.

3. Remove the cap from the needle and the guard from the syringe. Pull the plunger back to the mark that equals the amount of diluent needed to reconstitute the drug ordered. (This action aspirates air into the syringe.)

4. Puncture the diaphragm of the vial of diluent with the needle, and inject the air into the diluent. This action creates positive pressure that lets you draw the diluent easily (Figure 51-13). (If you do not add air, a vacuum forms, making it difficult to draw the diluent.)

5. Invert the vial and aspirate the diluent.

6. Remove the needle from the diluent vial, inject the diluent into the drug vial, and withdraw the needle. Properly dispose of this needle and syringe.

7. Roll the vial between your hands to mix the drug and diluent thoroughly. Do not shake the vial unless so directed on the drug label. When completely mixed, the solution in the vial should have no flakes. The solution will be clear or cloudy when completely mixed (depending on the drug).

8. Remove the cap and guard from the second needle and syringe.

9. Pull back the plunger to the mark that reflects the amount of drug ordered. Inject the air into the drug vial.

10. Invert the vial and aspirate the proper amount of the drug into the syringe (Figure 51-14). The drug is now ready for injection.

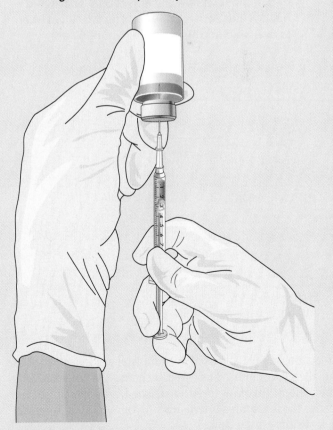

Figure 51-13. Injecting air into the diluent makes it easier to draw.

Figure 51-14. Invert the vial and draw the reconstituted drug.

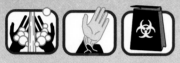

PROCEDURE 51.4

Giving an Intradermal Injection

Objective: To administer an intradermal injection safely and effectively, using sterile technique

OSHA Guidelines

Materials: Drug order (in patient's chart), alcohol swab, disposable needle and syringe of the appropriate size filled with the ordered dose of drug, sharps container

Method

1. Identify the patient. Wash your hands and put on examination gloves.
2. Check the seven rights, comparing information against the drug order.
3. Identify the injection site on the patient's forearm. To do so, rest the patient's arm on a table with the palm up. Measure 2 to 3 finger-widths below the antecubital space and a hand-width above the wrist. The space between is available for the injection (Figure 51-15).
4. Prepare the skin with the alcohol swab, moving in a circle from the center out.
5. Let the skin dry before giving the injection. Otherwise, you could introduce antiseptic under the skin, which could cause irritation and falsify intradermal test results.
6. Hold the patient's forearm, and stretch the skin taut with one hand.
7. With the other hand, place the needle—bevel up—almost flat against the patient's skin. Press the needle against the skin and insert it.
8. Inject the drug slowly and gently. You should see the needle through the skin and feel resistance. As the drug enters the upper layer of skin, a wheal (raised area of the skin) will form (Figure 51-16).
9. After the full dose of the drug has been injected, withdraw the needle. Properly dispose of used materials and the needle and syringe immediately.
10. Remove the gloves and wash your hands.
11. Stay with the patient to monitor for unexpected reactions.
12. Document the injection with the date, time, drug name, dosage, expiration date, lot number, manufacturer, route, site, and significant patient reactions in the patient's chart. Also document patient education about the drug.

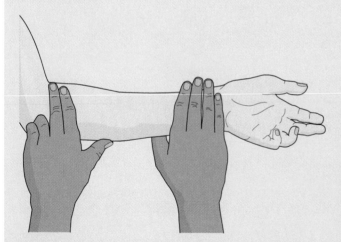

Figure 51-15. This space is available for intradermal injection sites.

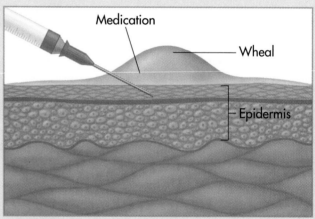

Figure 51-16. Medication collects under the skin, forming a wheal during an intradermal injection.

injections are usually used to administer a skin test, such as an allergy test or a TB test. When choosing an injection site on patients, avoid scarred, blemished, or hairy areas, because those features interfere with your ability to interpret test results on the skin.

The drug is injected under the top skin layer, and a little bubble or wheal is raised. If the body reacts to the drug, erythema (redness) and induration (hardening) occur. This reaction generally takes place 15 to 20 minutes after an allergy test and from 48 to 72 hours after a TB test.

Subcutaneous. Orally referred to as sub Q by most health-care professionals, a subcutaneous injection provides a slow, sustained release of a drug and a relatively long duration of action. Generally, 1 mL or less of a drug can be delivered by SC injection (Procedure 51-5). Various drugs, such as insulin and heparin, are commonly administered by SC injection.

Common subcutaneous injection sites include an area on the back between the shoulder blades, the outer sides of the upper arms and thighs, and the abdomen (except for a 2-inch area around the umbilicus). To prepare for an SC injection, select a site away from bones and blood vessels. Do not use an area that is edematous (swollen), scarred, or hardened or one that has a large amount of fat, because

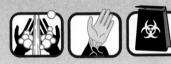

PROCEDURE 51.5

Giving a Subcutaneous Injection

Objective: To administer a subcutaneous injection safely and effectively, using sterile technique

OSHA Guidelines

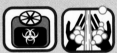

Materials: Drug order (in patient's chart), alcohol swabs, container of the ordered drug, disposable needle and syringe of the appropriate size, sharps container

Method

1. Identify the patient. Wash your hands and put on examination gloves.

2. Check the seven rights, comparing information against the drug order.

3. Prepare the drug and draw it up to the mark on the syringe that matches the ordered dose. Then pull the plunger back an additional 0.2 to 0.3 mL to create an air bubble. When you inject the drug, the air bubble helps seal the subcutaneous tissue (Figure 51-17).

4. Choose a site (Figure 51-18) and clean it with an alcohol swab, moving in a circle from the center out. Let the area dry.

5. Pinch the skin firmly to lift the subcutaneous tissue.

6. Position the needle—bevel up—at a 45° angle to the skin.

7. Insert the needle in one quick motion. Then release the skin, and aspirate by pulling back slightly on the plunger to check the needle placement (do not pull back if you are administering insulin or heparin). If pulling back

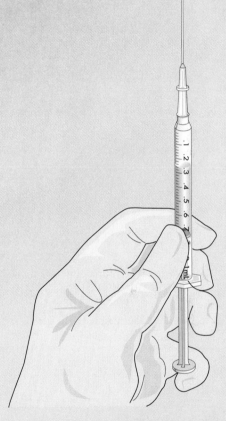

Figure 51-17. Pull back the plunger to create an air bubble in the syringe used in subcutaneous injection.

on the plunger produces blood, placement is incorrect and you must begin again with a fresh needle and syringe. If pulling back on the plunger produces no blood, placement is correct. Inject the drug slowly (Figure 51-19).

8. After the full dose of the drug has been injected, place an alcohol swab over the site, and withdraw the needle at the same angle you inserted it.

9. Apply pressure at the puncture site with the alcohol swab.

continued ⟶

Giving a Subcutaneous Injection *(continued)*

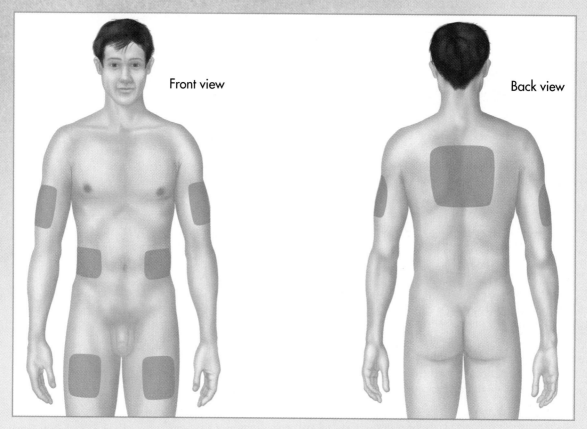

Figure 51-18. Many sites are available for subcutaneous injection.

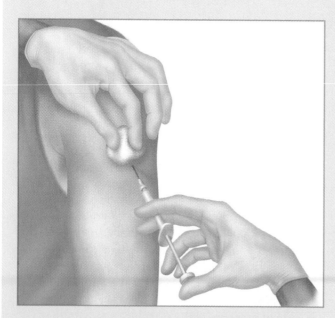

Figure 51-19. Perform a subcutaneous injection.

10. Massage the site gently to help distribute the drug, if indicated.
11. Properly dispose of the used materials and the needle and syringe.
12. Remove the gloves and wash your hands.
13. Stay with the patient to monitor for unexpected reactions.
14. Document the injection with the date, time, drug name, dosage, expiration date, lot number, manufacturer, route, site, and significant patient reactions in the patient's chart. Also document patient education about the drug.

these areas may not have the capillary network needed for absorption. When patients need regular SC injections, remember to rotate injection sites systematically. Begin the rotation pattern by giving injections in rows in the same area of the body (such as the abdomen). After all those sites have been used once, proceed to the next area on the body (such as the right leg), and follow a similar pattern there. Rotating sites promotes drug absorption and prevents hard subcutaneous lumps from forming.

At the injection site, ensure that you can pinch at least a 1-inch skin fold for the injection. If a patient is frail, dehydrated, or thin, you may need to use a site other than the back or abdomen to provide the necessary fold of skin.

Intramuscular. When a patient requires rapid drug absorption, you may be asked to administer an intramuscular injection, as described in Procedure 51-6. An IM injection usually irritates a patient's tissues less than an SC injection

and allows administration of a larger amount of drug, usually 3 to 5 mL in an adult.

Common IM injection sites include the dorsogluteal, ventrogluteal, vastus lateralis, and deltoid muscles, illustrated in Figure 51-20. Before giving an IM injection, identify the site carefully to prevent injury to blood vessels and nerves in the area. As with SC injections, rotate sites if the patient must receive regular or multiple IM injections.

Take into consideration the patient's layer of fat when choosing an IM injection site. You want the injection to penetrate beyond the fat layer to muscle. If, for example, a patient is heavy in the buttocks and thighs, the deltoid may be the best site for administering an IM injection.

When giving an IM injection to a pediatric patient, use the smallest gauge needle, usually 22 to 25 gauge. Also use the shortest length needle that will allow you to reach muscle, usually 1 inch.

PROCEDURE 51.6

Giving an Intramuscular Injection

Objective: To administer an intramuscular injection safely and effectively, using sterile technique

OSHA Guidelines

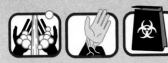
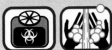

Materials: Drug order (in patient's chart), alcohol swabs, container of the ordered drug, disposable needle and syringe of the appropriate size, sharps container

Method

1. Identify the patient. Wash your hands and put on examination gloves.

2. Check the seven rights, comparing information against the drug order.

3. Prepare the drug and draw it up to the mark on the syringe that matches the ordered dose. Then pull the plunger back another 0.2 to 0.3 mL to add air. This air clears the drug from the needle and prevents drug seepage.

4. Choose a site (Figure 51-20) and gently tap it. Tapping stimulates the nerve endings and reduces pain caused by the needle insertion.

5. Clean the site with an alcohol swab, moving in a circle from the center out. Let the site dry.

6. Stretch the skin taut over the injection site.

7. Hold the needle and syringe at a 90° angle to the skin. Then insert the needle with a quick, dartlike thrust.

8. Release the skin and aspirate by pulling back slightly on the plunger to check the needle placement. If pulling back on the plunger produces blood, placement is incorrect and you must begin again with a fresh needle and syringe. If pulling back on the plunger produces no blood, placement is correct. Inject the drug slowly.

9. After the full dose of the drug has been injected, place an alcohol swab over the site. Then quickly remove the needle at a 90° angle.

10. Use the alcohol swab to apply pressure to the site and massage it, if indicated.

11. Properly dispose of used materials and the needle and syringe.

12. Remove the gloves and wash your hands.

13. Stay with the patient to monitor for unexpected reactions.

14. Document the injection with the date, time, drug name, dosage, expiration date, lot number, manufacturer, route, site, and significant patient reactions in the patient's chart. Also document patient education about the drug.

continued ———→

PROCEDURE 51.6

Giving an Intramuscular Injection *(continued)*

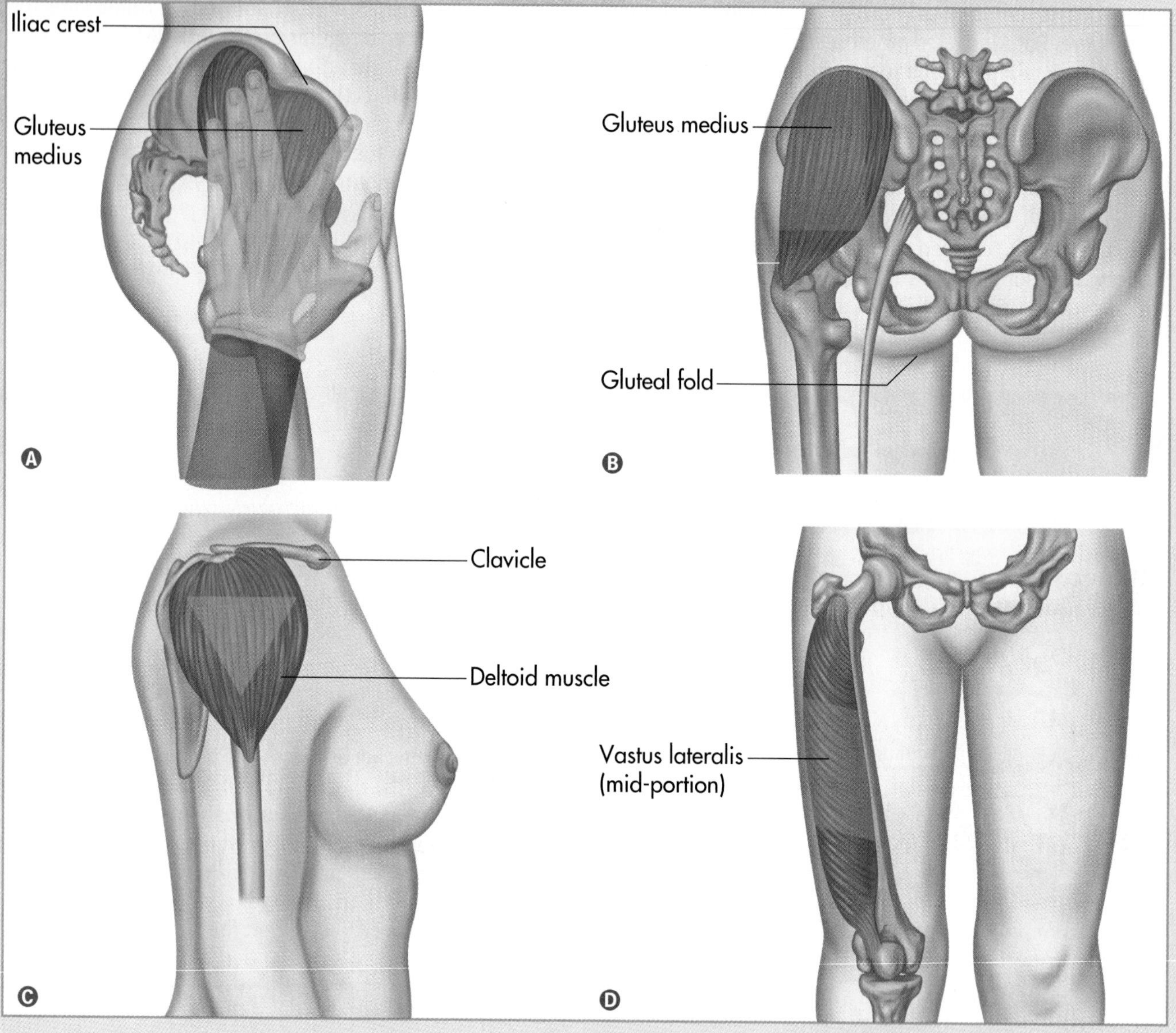

Figure 51-20. For intramuscular injection in an adult, use (a) the ventrogluteal site, (b) the dorsogluteal site, (c) the deltoid site, or (d) the vastus lateralis site.

Injection sites vary with age. For an infant or toddler, use the vastus lateralis muscle. For a child who has been walking for about a year, use the ventrogluteal or dorsogluteal site. For an older, well-developed child, use any adult site.

When injecting an IM drug that can irritate subcutaneous tissues, such as iron dextran (Imferon), use the **Z-track method,** illustrated in Figure 51-21. To do this, pull the skin and subcutaneous tissue to the side before inserting the needle at the site. After the drug is injected, release the tissue. This technique creates a zigzag path in the tissue layers, which prevents the drug from leaking into the subcutaneous tissue and causing irritation.

Intravenous. Although intravenous injections are not commonly performed in a medical office or by medical assistants, certain drugs may be administered this way. Drugs may also be mixed and dissolved into a **solution** (a homogeneous mixture of a solid, liquid, or gaseous substance in a liquid) and given by IV **infusion** (slow drip)

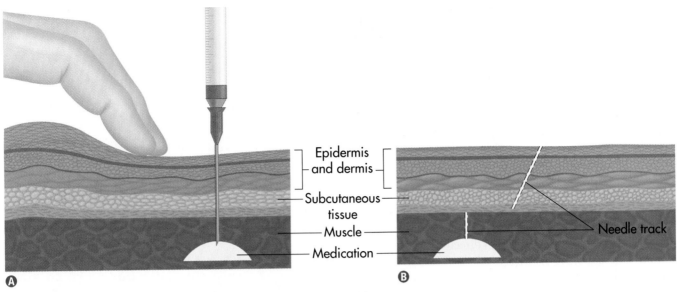

Figure 51-21. Use the Z-track method for IM injection of irritating solutions. (a) Pull the skin to one side before inserting the needle. (b) After injecting the drug, release the skin to seal off the needle track.

into a vein. Examples of IV drugs include powerful antibiotics, chemotherapeutic drugs, emergency drugs, and electrolytes. Because these drugs are introduced directly into the bloodstream, they produce an almost immediate effect. They also can cause sudden adverse reactions.

Although a doctor or nurse must administer an IV drug, you may assist by laying out supplies and equipment. When assisting with a venipuncture, gather the ordered drug and a tourniquet, bedsaver pad, gloves, iodine and alcohol swabs, venipuncture device, tape, and gauze pad, as ordered. Obtain other supplies and equipment, depending on the specific type of infusion or injection being administered.

Inhalation Therapy

Inhalation therapy can be administered through the mouth or nose. There are a number of disorders for which the physician may order an inhaler or aerosol form of medication. For example, an oral inhaler is frequently used by patients with asthma, whereas a nasal inhaler is frequently used for local treatment of nasal congestion. Nasal inhalers are also used to administer medicines for systemic effect, such as a vasopressin derivative for nocturnal bed-wetting.

Package inserts for inhaled drugs provide detailed descriptions of the correct procedure. If directed by the physician, however, you must teach the patient how to use an inhaler safely and correctly.

As with all drug administrations, check the seven rights, comparing information against the drug order. Ensure that you have the correct patient, the correct drug, and the correct form (oral or nasal) of inhaler. As you teach the patient, refer to the package insert, and show the patient where to find each step on the instruction sheet, so

that he will be familiar with the steps when administering the inhaler at home.

Check the label of the inhaler to determine whether the inhaler must be shaken thoroughly before administration. If shaking the inhaler is indicated, stress this point with the patient. Otherwise, the drug will not be evenly distributed in the inhaler, and its effectiveness will be jeopardized. If indicated, a nasal inhaler must be shaken before administration to each nostril.

Tell patients to follow these steps when administering a nasal inhaler.

1. Wash hands and blow the nose to clear the nostrils as much as possible before using the inhaler.
2. Tilt the head back, and with one hand, place the inhaler tip about ½ inch into the nostril.
3. Point the tip straight up toward the inner corner of the eye. Angling the inhaler downward makes the drug run down the back of the throat, causing a burning sensation.
4. Use the opposite hand to block the other nostril.
5. Inhale gently while quickly and firmly squeezing the inhaler.
6. Remove the inhaler tip and exhale through the mouth.
7. Shake the inhaler and repeat the process in the other nostril.

If indicated in the package insert, instruct patients to keep the head tilted back and not to blow their nose for several minutes. They can then wash their hands while you immediately document the inhaler administration with date, time, drug, dose, route, and any significant patient reactions. Also record your patient education about inhaler use.

Topical Application

Topical application is the direct application of a drug on the skin. Topical drugs can take the form of creams, lotions, **ointments** (salves), tinctures, powders, sprays, and solutions, which are used for their local effects. They include antibacterial and antifungal drugs as well as corticosteroids.

To apply a cream, lotion, or ointment, use long, even strokes with a cotton-tipped applicator when rubbing it into the skin. Follow the direction of the hair growth to avoid irritating the hair follicles and skin. To apply a powder, shake it on but do not rub it in.

A specialized type of topical administration that produces a systemic effect is the **transdermal** system (or patch). A drug administered through the transdermal patch is absorbed through the skin directly into the bloodstream. The patch slowly and evenly releases a systemic drug, such as scopolamine, nitroglycerin, estrogen, or fentanyl, through the skin. The patient receives a timed-release dose, usually over a day or several days.

Because the release of a drug from a transdermal patch is often crucial to a patient's health, the package inserts with transdermal medications are extremely detailed. You must instruct the patient to follow the instructions precisely and to be sure to change the patch on the prescribed schedule.

If the doctor directs you to provide some education, your goal is to teach the patient how to apply and remove a transdermal drug unit safely and effectively. Refer to the package insert as you teach, and show the patient where each step is located on the instruction sheet. This identification gives the patient the reference needed for changing the patch at home.

Before showing and administering the patch, check the seven rights, comparing information against the drug order. Wash your hands and instruct the patient to do the same when preparing for transdermal system application.

Some patches come sealed in a protective pouch. The plastic backing is easily peeled off once the patch is removed from the pouch. The plastic backing on patches without a protective pouch must be manipulated carefully to allow its removal. Show the patient how to bend the sides of the latter type of transdermal unit back and forth until the clear plastic backing snaps down the middle.

For either type of patch, demonstrate how to peel off the clear plastic backing to expose the sticky side of the patch. Then show the patient how to apply the patch to a reasonably hair-free site, such as the abdomen. Figure 51-22 shows how to apply both types of patches. Advise the patient to avoid using the extremities below the knee or elbow, skin folds, scar tissue, or burned or irritated areas. Estrogen patches are usually placed on the hip. Wash your hands and instruct the patient to do the same after applying a transdermal system at home.

To remove the patch, instruct the patient to gently lift and slowly peel it back from the skin. Then wash the skin with soap and water, dry the area with a towel, and wash the hands. Explain that the skin may appear red and warm, which is normal. Reassure the patient that the redness

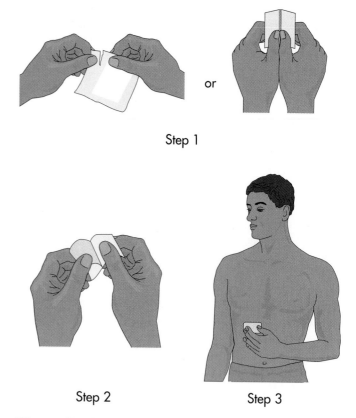

or

Step 1

Step 2   Step 3

Figure 51-22. To apply a transdermal patch, first either (1) remove it from the pouch, or bend the sides back and forth until the backing snaps; then (2) peel the backing off the patch; and (3) apply the patch, sticky side down, to a clean, relatively hairless site.

will disappear. Instruct the patient to notify the doctor if the redness does not disappear in several days or if a rash develops.

Tell the patient never to apply a new patch to the site just used. It is best to allow each site to rest between applications. Some transdermal systems call for waiting 7 days before using a site again. Be sure to check the package directions regarding site rotation.

Patients frequently ask whether they can apply lotion or talc to the area after removing the patch. Tell them they may do so if the skin is dry. After answering any other questions, immediately document the drug application with date, time, drug, dose, route, and any significant patient reactions. Also record your patient education about transdermal system application and removal.

If the physician order calls for you to apply a transdermal patch, it is important that you wear gloves during this procedure. Even though the procedure is not invasive, the medication can absorb into your skin. Wash your hands thoroughly after you apply the transdermal patch.

Urethral Administration

The urethral route is used when antibiotic and antifungal drugs are needed locally—that is, at the site of infection—for some urinary tract infections. Depending on the nature of the infection and the duration of drug action, the physician or a nurse may instill liquid drugs only one time or several times a day for a week. Urethral administration is used in both men and women.

Urethral drug administration requires passing a small-diameter urinary catheter into the bladder, instilling a drug through it, and clamping the catheter to let the drug bathe the urinary bladder walls. The materials needed for catheterization are included in a urinary catheter kit.

When the physician or nurse administers a urethral drug, you may assist with the following steps as directed.

1. Use sterile technique. Wash your hands and gather the necessary supplies. Depending on the amount of drug to be administered, you will need either a syringe without a needle or tubing and a bag. You will also need a urinary catheter kit, sterile gloves, the prescribed drug, a drape, and a bedsaver pad.
2. Check the seven rights, comparing information against the drug order, and explain the procedure and the drug order to the patient.
3. Assist the patient into the lithotomy position, and drape her to preserve her modesty while exposing the vulva.
4. Place a bedsaver pad under the buttocks.
5. Open the catheter kit.
6. Put on sterile gloves.
7. Cleanse the vulva as you would to perform catheterization, using the materials in the kit. As you sweep down with the antiseptic swab, watch for the urethral opening to "wink," which helps you locate it accurately.
8. The physician or nurse will insert the lubricated catheter. Tell the patient that she should feel pressure, not pain, and that the physician or nurse is going to attach the syringe to the catheter and insert the drug (or attach the tubing and bag to the catheter and let the drug run in by gravity).
9. After instilling the drug, the physician or nurse will clamp the catheter and leave the drug in place for the ordered amount of time.
10. Stay with the patient not only to ensure that she remains still but also to reassure her that the full feeling in the bladder is normal. She may also say she feels the need to urinate. Advise her that this feeling, too, is normal and is caused by the catheter.
11. When the time is up, unclamp the catheter, gently remove it, and allow the patient to urinate. Assist the patient as needed.
12. While the patient is dressing, immediately document the drug instillation with date, time, drug, dose, route, and any significant patient reactions.

Vaginal Administration

Physicians usually prescribe vaginal drugs to treat local fungal infections. The drugs may also be used for local bacterial infections. They are usually packaged as suppositories (the most common form), solutions, creams, ointments, and foams. Patients frequently ask about administering vaginal medications, and they usually administer such medications at home. Therefore, you must be prepared to provide detailed patient education for this route of administration. The physician may ask you to administer the first dose as a means of teaching a patient the method to use at home, or you may be asked to administer a one-time-only dose.

To administer a vaginal suppository, follow these steps.

1. Wash your hands and gather the following materials: the prescription or drug order in the patient's chart, a cloth or paper drape, a bedsaver pad, gloves, cotton balls, water-soluble lubricant, and the prescribed drug.
2. Check the seven rights, comparing information against the drug order, and explain the procedure and the drug order to the patient.
3. Give the patient the opportunity to empty her bladder before beginning.
4. Assist the patient into the lithotomy position, and drape her to preserve her modesty while exposing the vulva.
5. Place a bedsaver pad under the buttocks.
6. Put on sterile gloves.
7. Cleanse the perineum with soap and water, using one cotton ball per stroke, and cleanse the center last, while spreading the labia.
8. Lubricate the vaginal suppository applicator in lubricant spread on a paper towel.
9. While spreading the labia with one hand, insert the applicator with the other (the applicator should be about 2 inches into the vagina and angled toward the sacrum).
10. Release the labia and push the applicator's plunger to release the suppository into the vagina.
11. Remove the applicator, and wipe any excess lubricant off the patient.
12. Help her to a sitting position, and assist with dressing if needed.
13. Document the administration with date, time, drug, dose, route, and any significant patient reactions.

Follow the same steps, using an appropriate applicator, for vaginal drugs in the forms of creams, ointments, gels, and tablets. The liquid form of vaginal medication is administered by performing a **douche** (vaginal irrigation). This process is similar to giving a urethral drug, but it requires a special irrigating nozzle.

Rectal Administration

Certain medications, such as drugs used to treat constipation, nausea, and vomiting, may be administered by the rectal route. These medications may be given in the form of suppositories or enemas and may produce local or systemic effects.

Rectal Suppository. Administering rectal suppositories is rarely done in a doctor's office except on a pediatric patient. The doctor may, however, ask you to give a first suppository to an adult as a means of patient education. To do so, follow these steps.

1. Check the seven rights, comparing information against the drug order.
2. Explain the procedure and the drug order to the patient.
3. Give the patient the opportunity to empty the bladder before beginning.
4. Help the patient into Sims' position (shown in Chapter 38, Figure 38-1).
5. Lift the patient's gown to expose the anus.
6. Put on gloves and remove the wrapper from the suppository.
7. Lubricate the tapered end of the suppository with about 1 tsp of lubricant.
8. While spreading the patient's buttocks with one hand, insert the suppository—tapered end first—into the anus with the other hand.
9. Gently advance the suppository past the sphincter with your index finger. Before it passes the sphincter, the suppository may feel as if it is being pushed back out the anus. When it passes the sphincter, it seems to disappear.
10. Use tissues to remove excess lubricant from the area.
11. Remove your gloves and ask the patient to lie quietly and retain the suppository for at least 20 minutes.
12. When the treatment is completed, help the patient to a sitting, then standing, position.
13. Wash your hands and immediately document the drug administration with date, time, drug, dose, route, and any significant patient reactions.

Retention Enema. Retention enemas are usually not administered in a physician's office. You may, however, be asked to perform this procedure in an unusual circumstance, such as for a frail, elderly patient with fecal impaction. The steps for administering a retention enema are as follows.

1. Check the seven rights, comparing information against the drug order.
2. Help the patient lie on the left side and bend the right knee.
3. Put a bedsaver pad under the patient's left hip.
4. Place the tip of a syringe into a rectal tube. Let a little rectal solution flow through the syringe and tube. While holding the tip up, clamp the tubing.
5. Lubricate the end of the tube.
6. Spread the patient's buttocks, and slide the tube into the rectum about 4 inches.
7. After the tube is in place, slowly pour the rectal solution into the syringe, release the clamp, and let gravity move the solution into the patient.

8. When you have administered the ordered amount of solution, clamp the tube, then remove it.
9. Using tissues, apply pressure over the anus for 20 seconds to stifle the patient's urge to defecate.
10. Wipe any excess lubricant or solution from the area, and encourage the patient to retain the enema for the time ordered.
11. When the time has passed, help the patient use a bedpan or direct the patient to a toilet to expel the solution.
12. Wash your hands and immediately document the drug administration with date, time, drug, dose, route, and any significant patient reactions.

Administering Medications to the Eye or Ear

Doctors commonly administer eye medications to assist patients in eye tests, reduce pressure in the eyes, relieve eye pain, and treat eye infections and inflammation. Refer to Procedure 39-2 in Chapter 39 for instructions on how to administer eye medications. Although most eye medications are administered for local effect, some contain drugs that are absorbed systemically. To prevent systemic absorption, the doctor may request that you apply pressure with one finger just below the inner corner of each eye after instilling medications. Continue applying pressure for 2 to 3 minutes, as directed.

Doctors often administer eardrops to treat patients' ear infections or inflammation, relieve ear pain, or loosen earwax. Like eye medications, eardrops are ordered primarily for their local effects. They are not usually absorbed systemically, nor do they cause systemic effects. Procedure 39-5 in Chapter 39 describes how to administer eardrops.

Educating the Patient About Drug Administration

Educating patients about what drugs do to the body and what the body does to drugs is discussed in detail in Chapter 50. You need to provide additional patient education, however, with regard to routes of administration. This education is extremely important; a patient who does not administer a drug correctly or safely may put health or life at risk.

Reading the Drug Package Label

You must check the *PDR* for information about any drug with which you are not familiar. Likewise, before you teach a patient how to administer a drug, you must review the specific administration instructions for the drug in the *PDR*. An important aspect of this kind of information is teaching the patient how to read a prescription drug label. Instruct the patient to be particularly alert for special instructions and warning labels, such as those shown in Figure 51-23.

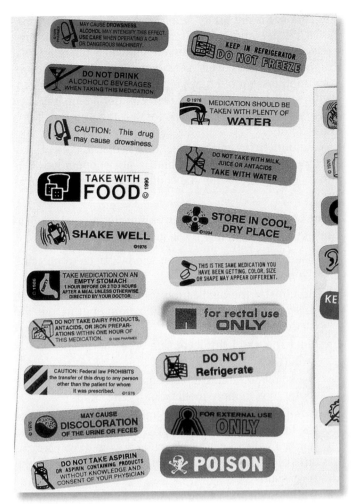

Figure 51-23. Teach the patient to heed warning labels and instructions on drug bottles.

Interactions

Drug interactions should not be confused with adverse effects of drugs, discussed in Chapter 50. Patient education with regard to interactions is important. Interactions may occur between two prescription or nonprescription drugs or between a drug and food and may cause serious effects. Explain that the greater the number of drugs the patient takes, the greater the chance of a drug interaction.

Drug-Drug Interactions. Most drug interactions affect the absorption, distribution, metabolism, or excretion of the drugs. In some cases drug-drug interactions can affect the results of laboratory tests. When two drugs are taken at the same time, there are several possible interactions.

- The effects of both drugs are increased, causing either a toxic or beneficial effect. For example, when alcohol is combined with diazepam (Valium), there is the potential toxic effect of severe central nervous system depression, because one drug intensifies the effect of the other. An example of a beneficial effect is the combination of acetaminophen and codeine, which increases the activity of both drugs, allowing the physician to

prescribe a lower dose of each. In fact, this combination of drugs is available in one tablet (Tylenol with codeine).

- The effects of both drugs are decreased, or one drug cancels out the effect of the other. For example, combining propanolol (Inderal) with albuterol (Proventil) causes each drug to lose its effectiveness.
- The effect of one of the drugs is increased by the other. For example, the effect of digoxin (Lanoxin) is increased by the presence of furosemide (Lasix), but the furosemide still works at the same degree of effectiveness as when administered alone.

To help prevent unintentional drug interactions, thoroughly assess the patient's medication use. Be sure to ask about medications prescribed by specialists as well as over-the-counter (OTC) drugs. Question the patient about past and present use of alcohol and recreational drugs as well as herbal remedies. Update the chart as needed. If you detect a potential for drug interactions, notify the physician.

Also teach patients about possible drug interactions and how to avoid or minimize them. For example, patients may need to take certain drugs at least 2 hours apart. Instruct patients to call the office if they think their drugs are interacting adversely.

Drug-Food Interactions. Interactions between a drug and food can alter a drug's therapeutic effect. For example, taking tetracycline with milk can reduce the drug's effectiveness because of decreased absorption from the GI tract. The drug-food interaction between a monoamine oxidase (MAO) inhibitor (such as Parnate, an antidepressant drug) and aged cheese or meat or other foods containing high levels of tyramine can produce a toxic effect. This interaction can cause a dangerous hypertensive crisis in which the patient's blood pressure rises quickly to dangerous levels, possibly leading to stroke and death.

Some drug-food interactions can affect the body's use of nutrients. For example, the cholesterol-lowering drugs cholestyramine resin and colestipol HCl may reduce the body's absorption of fat-soluble vitamins (A, D, E, and K) from food.

When teaching a patient about drug-food interactions, specify exactly which foods to avoid and when. For example, a patient may drink milk or eat food several hours before or after taking tetracycline, whereas a patient taking an MAO inhibitor must avoid foods that contain high levels of tyramine at all times. Explain what to expect if an interaction occurs, and describe how to deal with it.

Adverse Effects

Adverse effects or reactions associated with a drug and reported in the *PDR* are discussed briefly in the section on toxicology in Chapter 50. These responses are somewhat predictable and range from mild adverse reactions, such as stomach upset, to severe or life-threatening allergic responses. Unpredictable adverse effects can also occur; they are unique to each patient. Always advise the patient to report any change in overall health, because that change could be drug-related.

Elderly patients and patients with liver or kidney disease are more susceptible than others to adverse effects because these conditions affect drug metabolism and excretion. When drugs are not metabolized properly or excreted from the body quickly enough, drugs can reach toxic levels, even with normal doses.

To help prevent adverse effects, teach the patient to take the drug at the right time, in the right amount, and under the right circumstances. For example, the patient may need to take a cephalosporin with food to avoid nausea and diarrhea. Also teach the patient to recognize significant adverse effects and to call the office if any of them occur.

Special Considerations

Pediatric, pregnant, breast-feeding, or elderly patients or patients from different cultures require special considerations. When giving a drug to these patients, you must adjust patient care as needed.

Pediatric Patients

Children pose special challenges in drug administration and use. Their physiology and immature body systems may make drug effects less predictable because drugs are absorbed, distributed, metabolized, and excreted differently in children than in adults. Therefore, plan to observe a pediatric patient closely for adverse effects and interactions.

A child's small size may also increase the risk of overdose and toxicity. These factors may require dosage adjustments and careful measurement of small doses. To help administer drugs safely to pediatric patients, always check your calculations for providing a prescribed dose, and then ask a nurse or the doctor to double-check them.

Remember that administration sites and techniques for a child may differ from those for an adult. For example, fewer IM injection sites can be used for a young child. Also, the technique for eardrop administration varies slightly.

When dealing with an infant or young child, teach the parents—not the patient—about the drug. With an older child, include parents and patient in the teaching session. Be sure to use age-appropriate language when speaking to children.

It is important to use your therapeutic communication skills when working with pediatric patients. Pediatric patients are not like adults—they often have difficulty adjusting to medical procedures or illnesses. Children who do not understand what is happening to them can become problematic; some may see a physician visit as a punishment. It is important for you to be sensitive to the needs and reactions of pediatric patients. The first memorable exposure to an office visit will often determine how the child will react to physician visits for years to come.

Patience is important when working with pediatric patients. Infants and children can sense when you are irritated or annoyed. Pay close attention to your nonverbal communication as well as your verbal communication. New mothers are often apprehensive about invasive procedures when it concerns their children. Empathy and compassion are needed to ensure that the office visit is a pleasant one.

Administering medications to a pediatric patient may become a challenge if the child is not cooperative. It is important to ensure that the child receives the full dose as ordered.

Oral Medications. When administering oral medications to children, follow these guidelines:

- Use a calibrated dropper or spoon device to measure the ordered dose.
- Administer the medication to the side of the tongue; this method prevents the child from spitting out the medication.
- Hold the child until you are sure the medication is swallowed.
- If a small amount dribbles from the mouth, do not attempt to give more medication to the child.
- If the child vomits within 5 minutes and you can see the medication in the vomitus, you should readminister the medication after the child is calm. If you are unsure of readministering medication, consult with the physician.
- If the medication only comes in tablet form and the child is unable to swallow a tablet or capsule, verify in a drug reference to see if the medication can be crushed and given with food, such as applesauce.

Injections. Stress and anxiety will differ from child to child. When giving injections to pediatric patients, the following steps will help to ensure a smooth procedure:

- Distract the patient. Talk to the child while giving the injection. Often the injection is performed and over before the child realizes it.
- Praise the child. Say things that promote maturity and self-esteem.
- Use an anesthetic topical agent prior to the injection. This can be applied in the office or at home before the patient arrives in the office.
- Be swift. Do not allow a lot of time to pass before giving the injection. The faster the better.
- Try not to allow the child to see the syringe before giving the injection.

Pediatric Injection Sites. Pediatric patients have less muscle development than adults do, which limits the sites for intramuscular injections. The deltoid muscle is not developed enough for an injection and can be painful for the child. The sciatic nerve is larger in children; dorsogluteal injections are therefore not recommended because of the danger of hitting the sciatic nerve.

TABLE 51-7 Pregnancy Drug Risk Categories

Category	Meaning
A	Controlled studies in pregnant women have failed to demonstrate risk to the fetus.
B	There is no evidence of risk in humans, either because human findings show no risk or because there are no human findings but animal findings are negative.
C	Human studies are lacking, and animal findings are either positive for fetal risk or lacking as well. However, potential benefits may justify the potential risk.
D	There is positive evidence of risk. Nevertheless, potential benefits may outweigh the potential risk.
X	Fetal risk clearly outweighs any possible benefit to the patient.
NR	No rating is available.

Source: *2004* Physicians' Desk Reference, Thompson Healthcare.

The vastus lateralis and ventrogluteal sites are recommended for infants and children. The vastus lateralis site is good because it is a large and thick muscle that is developed before the child begins to walk. It is also the most desirable site for infants and children because it is not near major nerves and blood vessels. The vastus lateralis site is an easier site if you need to incorporate restraining methods.

The most common injections given to pediatric patients are vaccines. Most vaccines are given intramuscularly with a 25-gauge, ⅝-inch needle. Use your critical thinking and best judgment when selecting a needle.

Restraining Methods. Sometimes a pediatric patient will need to be restrained in order for you to administer an injection. Two medical assistants may be needed to safely restrain a child while giving an injection. Common restraining methods include the following:

- Have the child "hug the mother." The mother holds the child in front of her, with the child's thighs extended on either side of her torso. As the mother is talking to her child, make the injection in the vastus lateralis.
- Weight-bearing restraining is better than muscular control. Have the child sit on the edge of the exam table and use your weight to immobilize the child's legs against the table.

Pregnant Patients

When dealing with pregnant patients, remember that you are caring for two patients at once: the mother and her fetus. When you give the mother a drug, you may also be giving it to the fetus.

In addition, pregnancy-related changes in the mother's body can affect drug absorption, distribution, metabolism, and excretion. It is extremely important to double-check the drug in the *PDR* for toxicology or pregnancy warnings and to assess the patient carefully for therapeutic and adverse effects of the drug.

Some drugs can cause physical defects in the fetus if the mother takes them during pregnancy (especially in the first trimester). For this reason, you must be aware of the pregnancy drug risk categories (Table 51-7). These categories, established by the Food and Drug Administration (FDA), are based on the degree to which available information has ruled out risk to the fetus balanced against the drug's potential benefits to the patient. If the physician orders a high-risk drug for a pregnant patient, double-check the order with the physician before administering the drug.

Patients Who Are Breast-Feeding

Some drugs are excreted in breast milk and can thus be ingested by a breast-feeding infant. This ingestion can be dangerous because infants have immature body systems and cannot metabolize and excrete drugs that are safe for the mother. Some drugs, such as sedatives, diuretics, and hormones, can reduce the mother's flow of breast milk.

Whenever a drug is ordered for a patient who is breast-feeding, check a drug reference to see whether the drug is contraindicated during lactation. If so, consult the doctor. If not, teach the mother to recognize signs of adverse drug effects in her infant. If a mother must take a drug that affects lactation, advise her to supplement breast-feedings with infant formula.

Elderly Patients

Age-related changes in the body can affect drug absorption, metabolism, distribution, and excretion. These normal changes can be exaggerated by various diseases or disorders. Therefore, as people age, they have an increased risk of drug toxicity, adverse effects, or lack of therapeutic effects. Because of this risk, be especially alert when assessing an elderly patient who is on drug therapy.

Many elderly patients have complex, chronic diseases with unusual symptoms. This situation can make it difficult to tell whether a problem is caused by a drug. Listen closely to elderly patients and their family members; they are more likely to notice subtle changes than you are.

Patient *and family* education is important with elderly patients, particularly if they engage in polypharmacy (take several medications concurrently). Polypharmacy is common in elderly patients, and possible drug-drug interactions can be severe, as described in the Caution: Handle With Care section.

If an elderly patient is forgetful or confused, talk to the doctor about simplifying the medication schedule to reduce the risk of drug administration errors or omissions. Suggest the use of pill-organizing devices to help prevent forgotten doses or overdoses. If the patient has vision problems, provide drug instruction sheets in large type. To do this, either type instructions on a word processor in a large type size, enlarge the instructions on a photocopier, or clearly handwrite the instructions in large block letters. You might also contact a local association for the blind or visually impaired for devices and tips.

Patients From Different Cultures

Although cultural background is not likely to affect a drug's action in the body, it can affect a patient's understanding of drug therapy and compliance with it. For example, a patient who speaks little or no English cannot benefit from instructions given in English. To remedy this problem, obtain drug information sheets in the languages that are commonly spoken by patients of the practice. Use simple gestures and drawings to clarify difficult words or concepts. Also try to find a family member of the patient who speaks English.

To improve compliance, ask about the patient's feelings regarding medications and home remedies. Depending on cultural background, the patient may be more likely to use teas, poultices, and other home remedies than prescription or nonprescription drugs. If it appears that home remedies are not likely to affect the prescribed medication, tell the patient that it is all right to continue using the home remedies. Suggest adding the drug to the patient's usual routine to help it work better. Your cultural sensitivity may greatly increase the patient's compliance.

Charting Medications

Whenever a patient receives some form of treatment, such as medication, a record is kept of that treatment. Special problems or circumstances are also recorded, such as new symptoms, the patient's own statements, and how the patient tolerated the medications or treatment.

Most charting in the physician's office is documented on a progress note. As you learned in Chapter 9, a progress note is a document that is organized in a chronological sequence by date. The progress note is important because it serves as a communication tool that is utilized by all allied health-care members who are connected to that patient. The medical record is considered a legal document and is taken as proof that care was administered to the patient. All chart entries must be factual, accurate, complete, current,

CAUTION *Handle With Care*

Avoiding Unsafe Polypharmacy

Before administering any drug by any route, you must know every drug, both prescription and nonprescription, that the patient is taking. Many patients, especially elderly ones, visit several doctors. It is entirely possible that each doctor may prescribe one or more drugs without being aware of other drugs the patient is taking. This practice can result in polypharmacy, which means taking several drugs at once. Polypharmacy can be safe, but if the doctor is unaware of the total drug profile, serious drug interactions can result.

When asking patients to identify *all* other drugs they are taking, including OTC drugs, keep in mind that patients may forget to mention all their medicines or OTC drugs to the doctor. Drugs that patients often forget to mention include antacids (such as Tums or Rolaids), birth control pills (some women do not think of these as medication), and medicines that are used only as needed, such as medicine for migraine headaches.

To help prompt patients about drugs they may have forgotten, ask patients who have seen an orthopedist or cardiologist whether pain medication has been prescribed. Ask women who have seen a gynecologist if they are using a patch or other form of hormone replacement therapy. Ask women of an appropriate age whether there is any chance they are pregnant. Ask a pregnant woman whether she is taking prenatal vitamin and mineral supplements. If a patient has been referred to any other doctor for any reason, ask whether that doctor prescribed medication.

After determining the total drug profile, you should:

- Update the patient's record.
- Consider possible drug interactions, consulting the *PDR* or other drug reference if needed.
- Inform the doctor of your findings.

organized, and confidential. Avoid using words or statements that can be interpreted as your opinion. For example, if a patient gags and spits up cough syrup that you just administered, you would not write that the patient did not like the taste of the medication; you would simply state, "patient experienced difficulty in swallowing medication and expelled medication." Avoid terms like "appear" or "seems," which can lead you to draw assumptions without objective data to support them. Use abbreviations when appropriate because they allow you to say a great deal in a small space. Learn them well and use them carefully so that others can understand your notes. It is also useful and professional to learn the proper medical terms for symptoms and body functions.

Charting is not difficult, but it requires some practice. Review your office's charts to keep consistent with the charting methods used in them. Your own charting will be appropriate if you follow a few simple rules:

- Before you begin, make sure you have the right chart.
- Chart medications directly from the physician order.
- Be specific. Do not write "Gave Demerol for pain in the evening." Instead, write "(Date), Demerol 100 mg given IM in right upper outer quadrant of gluteus maximus for c/o sharp pain in left arm, lot number, expiration date, initials."
- Do not leave gaps or skip lines. If an entry does not fill a complete line, draw a straight line to fill the gap. Put your signature or initials at the right side directly after the note.
- If you make an error, do not erase it. Draw a line through the mistake. It should still be visible, so do not black it out. Initial it and write the word "error" on the line, then rechart the information correctly.
- Never use ditto marks.
- Write only in blue ink, never in pencil or another color ink.
- Write neatly in longhand.
- Spelling must be accurate.
- Use abbreviations and correct symbols.
- When you are unsure about charting, ask the physician.

Here is an example of a charted medication on a progress note:

When documenting an injection, you must include the following information:

- Date
- Name of patient
- Medication given
- Dose
- Route
- Location
- Lot number and expiration date
- Manufacturer
- Patient instructions and any other circumstances
- Initials

Nonpharmacologic Pain Management

Because of drug interactions, adverse effects, or the risk of dependence, many patients prefer not to take drugs to relieve chronic pain. To meet their needs, some practices now offer nonpharmacologic methods for managing pain, such as biofeedback, guided imagery, and relaxation exercises, in addition to traditional drug therapy. (For other alternative treatments, see Chapter 43.)

Biofeedback requires equipment that measures physical indicators of stress and relaxation, such as the galvanic skin response or pulse rate. This equipment provides feedback to help the patient recognize stress and relaxation responses and, ultimately, to control them. Biofeedback can help a patient learn to evoke relaxation, which helps block pain perception.

Guided imagery helps patients relax by teaching them to envision themselves in a calm, nurturing, wonderful place. Some cancer patients are taught to envision the cancer cells being eaten by healthy cells. Audiotapes and videotapes are available to help lead patients through these mental exercises.

Relaxation exercises involve learning special breathing techniques. Patients also learn how to relax different muscle groups.

Date	Patient Name: Jane Doe	DOB 12/12/63	Progress Note
11/29/03	PPD, .1cc given ID, Rt. Forearm, Lot # 222-01, Exp. Date 12/05, ABC Pharmaceutical Co. Pt to return to office in 48–72 hours for screening results Patient tolerated well---ST/RMA		

Summary

As a medical assistant, you must be prepared to administer drugs safely and effectively. Before you can do so, however, you must be familiar with the metric, apothecaries', and household systems of measurement. You must also be able to convert measures from one system to another and perform calculations to provide a prescribed dose. For both of these skills, you can use the ratio or fraction method.

When preparing to administer a drug, assess the patient for contraindications, and observe the general rules and seven rights of drug administration. Depending on the prescription, the drug may be administered by the oral, buccal, sublingual, intradermal, subcutaneous, intramuscular, nasal, topical, transdermal, vaginal, or rectal routes or as eyedrops or eardrops. If directed, assist the physician or nurse with urethral administration and IV drug injection or infusion.

Patient education is an important responsibility related to drug administration. You may need to instruct patients in the proper use of a prescribed drug. In addition, you may have to teach them to prevent or to recognize and report drug interactions and adverse effects.

Some patients require special consideration when receiving drugs. These include pediatric, pregnant, breast-feeding, and elderly patients as well as patients from different cultures.

Nonpharmacologic methods for managing chronic pain are gaining acceptance. Patients who are interested in learning about such methods should ask the physician for further information.

CASE STUDY *QUESTIONS*

Now that you have completed this chapter, review the case study at the beginning of the chapter. Detail what you think the medical assistant should do next and why.

Discussion Questions

1. What effects may drug interactions produce?
2. Why should you observe the seven rights every time you prepare and administer a drug?
3. Compare subcutaneous and intramuscular drug administration in terms of technique and possible dosage levels.
4. Why is proper needle selection important when administering an injection?

Critical Thinking Questions

1. A foreign patient is in the office, and the physician has ordered a PPD. You ask the patient if he has had a reaction to a TB screen before, and the patient responds by telling you he has had the BCG vaccination as a child. What is BCG? What should you do? What can happen if you administer the PPD?
2. A patient in her first trimester of pregnancy calls the office saying she has acid indigestion. She says that before her pregnancy, she used to take Tagamet for acid indigestion and wants to know if it is safe to take it now. How can you find this information, and what should you do once you find it?
3. Mr. Lance, age 29, visits the office for his regular IM injection. As you are making a routine assessment, he tells you that the last time the drug was administered, he had a bad reaction to it. What should you do?

Application Activities

1. Perform the necessary calculations for the following conversions. Use a table of equivalents, if needed.
   a. 350 mL = _____ L
   b. 0.17 g = _____ mg
   c. 3 tbsp = _____ tsp
   d. ½ tsp = _____ gtt
   e. 2 fl dr = _____ mL
2. Using the ratio or fraction method, calculate the following to provide a prescribed drug dose.
   a. The doctor orders 60 mg of acetaminophen with codeine, but each tablet contains only 15 mg. How many tablets should the patient take?
   b. The doctor orders 300 mg of theophylline anhydrous, but each tablet contains only 100 mg. How many tablets should the patient take?
   c. The doctor orders 5 mg of glyburide, but each tablet contains only 1.25 mg. How many tablets should the patient take?
3. Using the basic formula of dose desired/dose on hand × quantity = dose, calculate the following to provide a prescribed drug dose.
   a. The doctor orders 250 mg of a drug. You have 100-mg scored tablets on hand. How many tablets will you give the patient?
   b. An injectable antibiotic is packaged as 100,000 units per cc. The doctor orders 400,000 units. How many packages will you administer parenterally to the patient?

CHAPTER 52

Electrocardiography and Pulmonary Function Testing

KEY TERMS

calibration syringe
cardiac cycle
deflection
depolarization
electrocardiogram (ECG)
electrocardiograph
electrocardiography
electrode
forced vital capacity (FVC)
Holter monitor
lead
polarity
pulmonary function test
spirometer
spirometry
stylus

AREAS OF COMPETENCE

2003 Role Delineation Study

CLINICAL

Fundamental Principles

- Apply principles of aseptic technique and infection control

Diagnostic Orders

- Perform diagnostic tests

Patient Care

- Prepare patient for examinations, procedures, and treatments

CHAPTER OUTLINE

- The Medical Assistant's Role in Electrocardiography and Pulmonary Function Testing
- Anatomy and Physiology of the Heart
- The Conduction System of the Heart
- The Electrocardiograph
- Preparing to Administer an ECG
- Applying the Electrodes and the Connecting Wires
- Operating the Electrocardiograph
- Troubleshooting: Artifacts and Other Problems
- Completing the Procedure
- Interpreting the ECG
- Exercise Electrocardiography (Stress Testing)
- Ambulatory Electrocardiography (Holter Monitoring)
- Anatomy and Physiology of the Respiratory System
- Pulmonary Function Testing
- Spirometry
- Performing Spirometry

OBJECTIVES

After completing Chapter 52, you will be able to:

52.1 Describe the anatomy and physiology of the heart.
52.2 Explain the conduction system of the heart.
52.3 Describe the basic patterns of an electrocardiogram (ECG).
52.4 Identify the components of an electrocardiograph and what each does.
52.5 Explain how to position the limb and precordial electrodes correctly.
52.6 Describe in detail how to obtain an ECG.

52.7 Identify the various types of artifacts and potential equipment problems and how to correct them.

52.8 Discuss how the ECG is interpreted.

52.9 Define exercise electrocardiography.

52.10 Explain the procedure of Holter monitoring.

52.11 Describe the anatomy and physiology of the lungs.

52.12 Describe various types of spirometers.

52.13 Describe the procedure of performing spirometry.

Introduction

It is not uncommon for patients to have cardiovascular or respiratory problems when they consult physicians. As a medical assistant, you may be responsible for performing screening and/or diagnostic testing in the physician's office. To correctly perform testing on the cardiac or respiratory system, you need to review the anatomy and physiology of the heart and the respiratory system. This chapter introduces you to the electrocardiograph instrument and how to administer an electrocardiogram. You will also learn how to apply electrocardiograph electrodes and wires, operate the instrument, and troubleshoot problems that can occur while recording the heart's electrical activity. Because many physicians perform more complex cardiac diagnostic testing, you will also learn about Holter monitors and stress testing. Pulmonary function testing is more commonplace now in physician's offices, and this chapter introduces you to the basics of performing a spirometry.

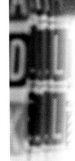

CASE STUDY

A 57-year-old woman has been having chest pain, discomfort in the chest, and a slight shortness of breath since the previous morning. She chose to come to the office where you are employed rather than the emergency room because she didn't think her symptoms were too severe. The physician orders an ECG and spirometry after reviewing the patient's history. The ECG reveals nonspecific wave changes, and the spirometry shows that the FVC is slightly decreased. The physician then orders a Holter monitor to be placed on the patient and requests that she be scheduled for an exercise electrocardiography.

As you read this chapter, consider the following questions:

1. What does the abbreviation ECG stand for? What is the diagnostic value of the ECG?
2. What is another name for a spirometry? What does FVC designate?
3. Why were the Holter monitor and stress tests ordered for this patient?

The Medical Assistant's Role in Electrocardiography and Pulmonary Function Testing

Electrocardiography and pulmonary function testing are two procedures you may be required to perform in a medical office. **Electrocardiography** is the process by which a graphic pattern is created from the electrical impulses generated within the heart as it pumps. It is often performed to evaluate symptoms of heart disease, to detect abnormal heart rhythms, to evaluate a patient's progress after a heart attack, or to check the effectiveness or side effects of certain medications. Electrocardiography is sometimes performed as part of a general examination.

Pulmonary function tests (PFTs) measure and evaluate a patient's lung capacity and volume. Such tests are commonly performed when a person suffers from shortness of breath, but they may also be performed as part of a general examination. Pulmonary function tests can help detect and diagnose pulmonary problems. They are also used to monitor certain respiratory disorders and to evaluate the effectiveness of treatment.

Anatomy and Physiology of the Heart

A description of the anatomy and physiology of the heart will help you better understand electrocardiography. It will also help you make sense of the electrical activity that electrocardiography records.

Anatomy of the Heart

The heart is a muscular pump that circulates blood throughout the body, carrying oxygen and nutrients to the tissues and removing waste products. The pumping action begins in the muscle tissue of the heart, called the myocardium.

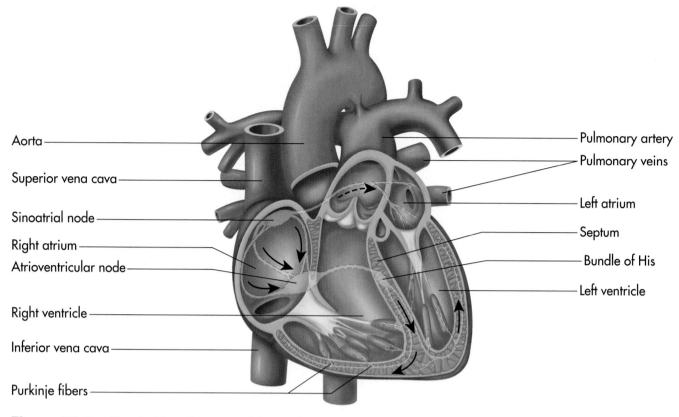

Aorta

Superior vena cava

Sinoatrial node

Right atrium

Atrioventricular node

Right ventricle

Inferior vena cava

Purkinje fibers

Pulmonary artery

Pulmonary veins

Left atrium

Septum

Bundle of His

Left ventricle

Figure 52-1. Electrical impulses control the cardiac conduction system. Each impulse begins in the sinoatrial node, progresses to the atrioventricular node, and then travels through the bundle of His, the right and left bundle branches, and the Purkinje fibers.

The heart is actually a double pump. The right side of the heart receives blood from the body by way of the superior vena cava and the inferior vena cava. From there, the pulmonary arteries deliver blood to the lungs, where the blood exchanges carbon dioxide for oxygen. Oxygenated blood flows into the left side of the heart through the pulmonary veins. Once in the heart, blood is pumped into the aorta, which pumps oxygenated blood to all parts of the body.

The heart has four sections, or chambers: two upper receiving chambers, the atria (singular, atrium), and two lower pumping chambers, the ventricles (Figure 52-1). Valves between each atrium and ventricle prevent blood from regurgitating (backing up) into the atrium while the ventricle contracts. Similar valves between the ventricles and the arteries into which they pump (the aorta and the pulmonary arteries) prevent blood from regurgitating into the ventricles when they relax. A partition, the septum, divides the heart into right and left sides.

Physiology of the Heart

The heart is divided into separate chambers that work as a single unit. Contraction of the atria, followed by contraction of the ventricles, moves the blood. This contraction phase is called systole. Systole is followed by a relaxation phase, called diastole. When you take someone's blood pressure, you are measuring the pressure during the contraction

(systolic) and relaxation (diastolic) phases. This sequence of contraction and relaxation makes up a complete heartbeat, known as the **cardiac cycle.** Each cycle lasts an average of 0.8 second.

All the fibers in the cardiac muscle are interconnected and act as one muscle. Consequently, when one fiber is stimulated to contract, the entire group of fibers contracts. This property plays an important role in the conduction system of the heart.

The Conduction System of the Heart

The cardiac cycle is regulated by specialized tissues in the heart wall, shown in Figure 52-1, that transmit electrical impulses. These electrical impulses cause the heart muscle to contract and relax.

Transmission of electrical impulses in the heart begins in the sinoatrial (SA) node, also called the sinus node or the pacemaker of the heart. The sinoatrial node is a small bundle of heart muscle tissue in the superior wall of the right atrium that specializes in producing electrical impulses. The sinoatrial node sets the rhythm (or pattern) of the heart's contractions.

When the electrical impulse for muscle contraction is generated, it travels throughout the muscle of each atrium, causing atrial contraction. The impulse then travels to the atrioventricular (AV) node, another mass of specialized conducting cells, similar to those of the SA node. The AV node is located at the bottom of the right atrium, near the junction of the ventricles (the septum), where transmission of the impulse is slightly delayed. This delay gives the atria time to completely contract and fill the ventricles with blood.

The atrioventricular node then passes the impulse to the bundle of His (named after the Swiss physician Wilhelm His Jr. [1863–1934]), located in the septum between the ventricles. The bundle of His acts as a relay station, sending the impulse through a series of bundle branches to a network of cardiac conducting muscle fibers. These specialized muscle fibers, called Purkinje fibers (named after the Czech physiologist Jan Evangelista Purkinje [1787–1869]), are located in the ventricle walls. When the impulse reaches the Purkinje fibers, the ventricles contract.

Conduction and Electrocardiography

Electrocardiography records the transmission, magnitude, and duration of the various electrical impulses of the heart. Before you can understand how electrocardiography works, you must understand **polarity,** the condition of having two separate poles, one of which is positive and the other negative. A resting cardiac cell is polarized; that is, there is a negative charge inside and a positive charge outside. When the cardiac cell loses its polarity (a natural occurrence), depolarization occurs. **Depolarization** is the electrical impulse that initiates a chain reaction resulting in contraction. This wave of depolarization flows from the SA node to the ventricles and can be detected by **electrodes,** or electrical impulse sensors, that are placed on specific areas on the surface of the body. During electrocardiography, electrodes detect and record the electrical activity of the heart, including disturbances or disruptions in its rhythm.

Depolarization is always followed by a period of electrical recovery called **repolarization,** when polarity is restored. Following repolarization, the heart returns to a resting, polarized state. The electrical cycle is then repeated, leading to another cardiac cycle.

The Basic Pattern of the Electrocardiogram

The waves of electrical impulses responsible for the cardiac cycle produce a series of waves and lines on an **electrocardiogram** (abbreviated **ECG** or **EKG**), which is the tracing made by an **electrocardiograph,** an instrument that measures and displays these impulses (Figure 52-2). These peaks and valleys, called waves or **deflections,** are labeled with the letters P, Q, R, S, T, and U. Each letter represents a specific part of the pattern, as explained in Table 52-1. The recognition of abnormalities in the size of the waves or the various time intervals can aid in the diagnosis of certain types of heart problems.

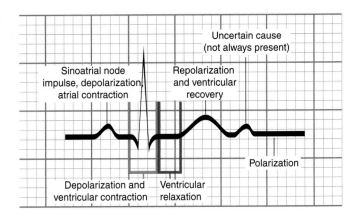

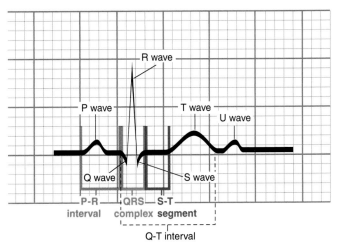

Figure 52-2. This ECG tracing shows the pattern of one cardiac cycle in a normal heart. These specific electrical impulses (top) represent the cycle of cardiac contraction and relaxation. The waves and lines (bottom) represent specific parts of the pattern.

The Electrocardiograph

Each type of electrocardiograph works in the same way. The electrical impulses produced by the heart can be detected through the skin; these impulses are measured, amplified, and recorded on the ECG. Detection begins with electrodes that conduct and transmit the electrical impulses to the electrocardiograph through insulated wires. An amplifier increases the signal, making the heartbeat visible. The **stylus,** a penlike instrument, records this movement on the ECG paper. The impulses received through various combinations of electrodes constitute different **leads,** or views of the electrical activity of the heart, that are recorded on the ECG.

Types of Electrocardiographs

Several different types of electrocardiographs are in use today. Two types are shown in Figure 52-3. The standard machine is a 12-lead electrocardiograph, which records the electrical activity of the heart simultaneously from 12 different views. A single-channel electrocardiograph records the electrical activity of one lead, and consequently, one

TABLE 52-1 Parts of the ECG

Name	Appearance	Represents
P wave	Small upward curve	Sinoatrial node impulse, wave of depolarization through atria, and resultant contraction
QRS complex	Includes Q, R, and S waves	Contraction (following depolarization) of ventricles; QRS complex is larger than P wave because ventricles are larger than atria
Q wave	Downward deflection	Impulse traveling down septum toward Purkinje fibers
R wave	Large upward spike	Impulse going through left ventricle
S wave	Downward deflection	Impulse going through both ventricles
T wave	Upward curve	Recovery (repolarization) of ventricles; repolarization of atria is not obvious because it occurs while ventricles are contracting and producing QRS complex
U wave	Small upward curve sometimes found after T wave	May be seen in normal individuals, in patients who experience slow recovery of Purkinje fibers, or in patients who have low potassium levels or other metabolic disturbances
P–R interval	Includes P wave and straight line connecting it to QRS complex	Time it takes for electrical impulse to travel from SA node to AV node
Q–T interval	Includes QRS complex, S–T segment, and T wave	Time it takes for ventricles to contract and recover, or repolarize
S–T segment	Connects end of QRS complex with beginning of T wave	Time between contraction of ventricles and recovery

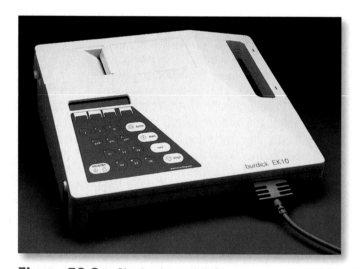 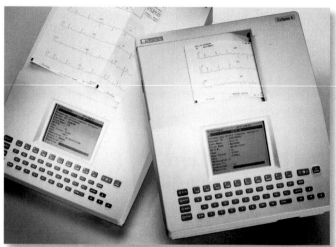

Figure 52-3.   Single-channel (left) and multichannel (right) electrocardiographs are used to obtain an ECG.

view of the heart's electrical activity at a time. The record is printed on a long, thin strip of ECG paper. The most common single-channel units allow you to attach all electrodes at the same time and obtain a manual or automatic printout of individual leads. Some older units use fewer electrodes,

requiring you to systematically attach, remove, and reposition the electrodes to obtain recordings from different leads.

The newer multichannel units record more than one lead at a time. These machines use wider paper and more than one stylus to record the leads.

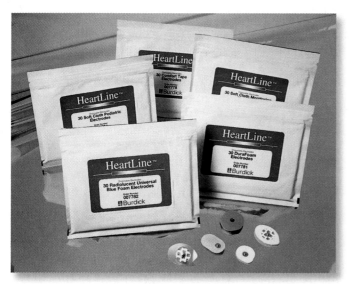

Figure 52-4. Disposable electrodes are available in several varieties.

Electrodes and Electrolyte Products

Electrodes are attached to the patient's skin during electrocardiography. There are several types of electrodes, including metal plate, suction bulb, and disposable electrodes. Disposable electrodes (Figure 52-4) are the most widely used.

The skin does not conduct electricity well. Consequently, an electrolyte (a substance that enhances transmission of electric current) is needed with each electrode. Disposable electrodes come with an electrolyte preparation in place, but you must apply an electrolyte to reusable electrodes. Electrolytes are available in the form of gels, lotions, and solutions and disposable pads impregnated with electrolyte (Figure 52-5).

When performing routine electrocardiography, you place electrodes on ten areas of the body: one each on the right arm (RA), left arm (LA), right leg (RL), and left

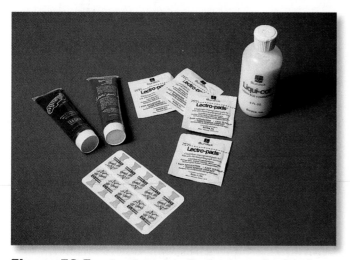

Figure 52-5. An electrolyte (in the form of gel, lotion, solution, or impregnated pad) must be applied to each electrode.

leg (LL) and six on specific locations on the chest wall. The right leg is designated as the ground. You will move the fifth electrode to six different positions on the chest for successive readings. Evaluating different leads, that is, the electrical activity measured through various combinations of electrodes, enables the physician to pinpoint the origin of certain problems.

Leads

Each lead provides an image of the electrical activity of the heart from a different angle. Together, the images give the doctor a full picture of electrical activity moving up and down, left and right, and forward and backward through the heart. Monitoring the electrodes on the arms and legs in two different ways produces six leads that record electrical impulses that move up and down and left and right. The electrodes that are placed on the chest provide six more leads, showing electrical activity moving forward and backward (from the front of the body toward the back and vice versa).

Each lead is given a specific designation and code. The 12 leads are usually marked automatically on the ECG.

Limb Leads. Of the six leads that directly monitor electrodes on the arms and legs, three are standard leads and three are augmented leads. The standard leads each monitor two limb electrodes, recording electrical activity between them. These leads are also called bipolar leads, because they monitor two electrodes. The augmented leads monitor one limb electrode and a point midway between two other limb electrodes, recording electrical activity between the monitored electrode and the midway point. Because they directly monitor only one electrode, augmented leads are also called unipolar leads. The electrical activity recorded by these leads is very slight, requiring the machine to augment (amplify) the tracings to produce readable waves and lines on the ECG paper.

Precordial Leads. The six precordial, or chest, leads are unipolar leads. The electrodes are placed across the chest in a specific pattern (Figure 52-6). Each precordial lead monitors one electrode and a point within the heart. The precordial leads are each designated by a letter and a number. The designations for the 12 leads of a routine ECG are shown in Table 52-2. The table also indicates which electrodes and points are monitored by each lead. A common system of marking codes completes the information in the table. Other coding systems are in use; be sure to follow office policy or the doctor's preference when you code an ECG.

ECG Paper

ECG paper is provided in a long, continuous roll. If the paper is designed for use with a single-channel electrocardiograph, it is just wide enough for a single trace. Other ECG papers can accommodate several traces at once; these papers are used with multichannel electrocardiography. ECG paper consists of two layers and is both heat- and pressure-sensitive. The

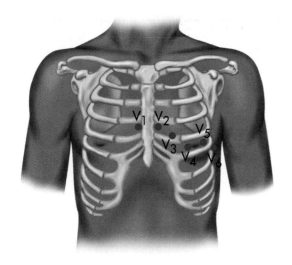

V₁ Fourth intercostal space (between the ribs), to the right of the sternum (breastbone)

V₂ Fourth intercostal space, to the left of the sternum

V₄ Fifth intercostal space, on the left midclavicular line

V₃ Fifth intercostal space, midway between V₂ and V₄

V₆ Fifth intercostal space, on the left midaxillary line

V₅ Fifth intercostal space, midway between V₄ and V₆

Figure 52-6. Six precordial electrodes are arranged in specific positions on the chest. Notice that electrode V_4 must be positioned before V_3 and V_6 before V_5.

heated stylus on the electrocardiograph serves as a "pen" that records the ECG pattern on the paper.

ECG paper (Figure 52-7) is marked with light and dark lines or with dots and lines. The pattern is standardized to permit uniform interpretation by any physician. Each small square, or square area delineated by dots, measures 1 mm by 1 mm. Each large square measures 5 mm by 5 mm.

The vertical, or short, axis of the paper records the voltage, or strength of the impulse; the horizontal axis measures time. Normally the paper moves through the machine at a speed of 25 mm per second. This means that the distance across 1 small square represents 0.04 second. The distance across 1 large square represents 0.2 second. The distance across 5 large squares represents 1.0 second. In 1 minute (60 seconds), the paper advances 300 large squares, or 1500 mm (150 cm).

Each electrocardiograph is standardized before use so that one small square represents 0.1 millivolt (mV). One large square represents 0.5 mV, and two large squares represent 1.0 mV.

Electrocardiograph Controls

The location of certain knobs and buttons on an electrocardiograph may vary from model to model. Certain features, however, are common to most machines. These include the standardization control, speed selector, sensitivity control, lead selector, centering control, stylus temperature control, marker control, and on/off switch.

Standardization Control. Before you obtain an ECG, you must correctly standardize the machine. The standardization control uses a 1-mV impulse to produce a standardization mark on the ECG paper. When you press the standardization control, the stylus should move up ten small squares, or 10 mm (1 cm) and remain there for

TABLE 52-2 ECG Lead Designations and Marking Codes

Lead	Electrodes and Points Monitored	Marking Codes
Standard limb		
I	RA and LA	•
II	RA and LL	••
III	LA and LL	•••
Augmented limb		
aVR	RA and (LA-LL)	-
aVL	LA and (RA-LL)	--
aVF	LL and (RA-LA)	---
Precordial		
V_1	V_1 and (LA-RA-LL)*	-•
V_2	V_2 and (LA-RA-LL)*	-••
V_3	V_3 and (LA-RA-LL)*	-•••
V_4	V_4 and (LA-RA-LL)*	-••••
V_5	V_5 and (LA-RA-LL)*	-•••••
V_6	V_6 and (LA-RA-LL)*	-••••••

*The point within the heart is identified by averaging the readings from the electrodes.

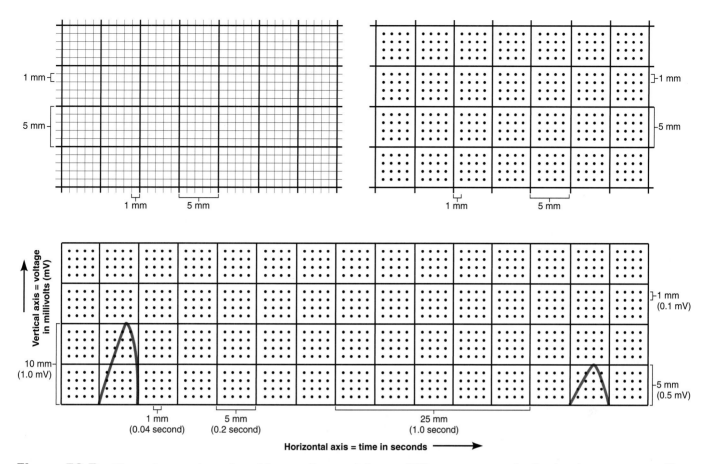

Figure 52-7. The pattern and spacing of lines or lines and dots on ECG paper are standardized and represent specific units of voltage and time.

0.08 second (two small squares, or 2 mm). If it does not, the instrument must be adjusted before you use it.

Speed Selector. The paper is normally set to run at 25 mm per second for adults. When you run an ECG on infants and children or on adults with a rapid heartbeat, the deflections may appear too close together. In these cases you may need to adjust the speed to 50 mm per second to separate the peaks and create a tracing that is easier to read. If you must set the speed at 50 mm per second, note it on the strip. Otherwise, a speed of 25 mm per second is assumed. In any case do not change the speed selection unless the doctor directs you to do so.

Sensitivity Control. The sensitivity control adjusts the height of the standardization mark and the tracing. It is normally set on 1. When the height of an ECG tracing is too high to fit completely on the paper, however, adjust this control to ½ to reduce the size of both the standardization mark and the tracing by one-half. For tracings that have very low peaks, set this control on 2 to double the standardization mark and the height of the tracing. Note this change on the strip.

Lead Selector. Most newer electrocardiographs have a setting that enables a standard 12-lead tracing to run

automatically. All machines, however, have a lead selector that allows you to run each lead individually, in case you need to repeat a strip containing artifacts (erroneous marks or defects) during a run.

Centering Control. The centering control allows you to adjust the position of the stylus, which must be centered on the paper. (Centering the stylus simplifies the process of measuring wave heights for the person who interprets the ECG.)

Stylus Temperature Control. Another control allows you to adjust the temperature of the stylus. A higher temperature results in a heavier line, whereas a lower temperature results in a lighter, thinner line. The line should be clear without being so dark that it bleeds or smears on the ECG paper.

Marker Control. Most older machines have a marker control that allows you to place marking codes (Table 52-2) on the ECG paper to identify the lead during each run. Many newer machines do this automatically.

On/Off Switch. The on/off switch turns the machine on and off. Most machines have an indicator light that signals when the power is on.

Preparing to Administer an ECG

You must obtain a good-quality tracing when performing electrocardiography. To do so, you must be able to recognize an artifact or a generally defective ECG tracing when you see one. Proper technique is also essential to help you obtain the best-quality tracing. The following sections guide you through the process. The steps in obtaining a standard 12-lead ECG using a single-channel electrocardiograph are listed in Procedure 52-1.

Preparing the Room and Equipment

Be sure the room and equipment are properly set up before you begin to administer electrocardiography. The accuracy of an ECG can sometimes be affected by electric currents emitted from nearby machines. Although some electrocardiographs have filters to minimize outside electrical interference, it is always a good idea to perform electrocardiography in a room where all other electrical equipment is turned off. This equipment includes air conditioners, refrigerators, and fans as well as laboratory and diagnostic equipment.

The room should be in a quiet location, protected from interruptions. Because the patient must partially disrobe, adjust the room temperature to a comfortable level.

The examining table should be sturdy and comfortable. If the table is made of metal, it must be padded so the patient does not come in contact with any metal parts during the procedure.

Before using the electrocardiograph, check the date of its last inspection. Each machine should be periodically inspected and certified safe to use for a specific period of time. Using a machine only within this time period helps ensure your safety and that of the patient. Be sure to turn the machine on ahead of time to allow the stylus to warm up.

Preparing the Patient

Introduce yourself to the patient, explain the procedure, and answer any questions the patient has. Follow the steps described in Procedure 52-1 as you prepare the patient for

---

PROCEDURE 52.1

Obtaining an ECG

Objective: To obtain a graphic representation of the electrical activity of a patient's heart

OSHA Guidelines

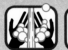

Materials: Electrocardiograph, ECG paper, electrodes, electrolyte preparation, wires, patient gown, drape, blanket, pillows, gauze pads, alcohol, moist towel, disposable shaving supplies (if needed)

Method

1. Turn on the electrocardiograph and, if necessary, allow the stylus to heat up.
2. Identify the patient, introduce yourself, and explain the procedure.
3. Wash your hands.
4. Ask the patient to disrobe from the waist up and remove jewelry, socks or stockings, and shoes.

If the electrodes will be placed on the patient's legs, have the patient roll up his or her pant legs. Sometimes the electrodes are placed on the sides of the lower abdomen—check the manufacturer's instructions. Provide a gown if the patient is female, and instruct her to wear the gown with the opening in front.

5. Assist the patient onto the table and into a supine position. Cover the patient with a drape (and a blanket if the room is cool). If the patient experiences difficulty breathing or cannot tolerate lying flat, use a Fowler's or semi-Fowler's position, adjusting with pillows under the head and knees for comfort if needed.
6. Tell the patient to rest quietly and breathe normally. Explain the importance of lying still to prevent false readings.
7. Wash the patient's skin, using gauze pads moistened with alcohol. Then rub it vigorously with dry gauze pads to promote better contact of the electrodes.
8. If the patient's leg or chest hair is dense, put on examination gloves, and shave the areas where

continued ⟶

Obtaining an ECG *(continued)*

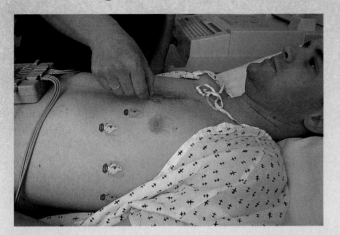

Figure 52-8. Place electrodes at the specified locations on the chest, arms, and legs.

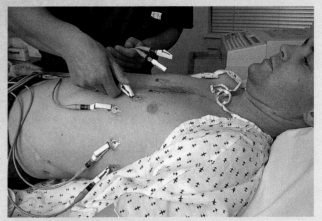

Figure 52-9. Attach wires and cables, draping wires over the patient to avoid tension that can result in artifacts.

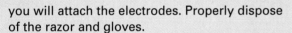

you will attach the electrodes. Properly dispose of the razor and gloves.

9. Apply electrodes to fleshy portions of the limbs, making sure that the electrodes on one arm and leg are placed similarly to those on the other arm and leg (Figure 52-8). The direction that the tabs (where the wires are fastened) are facing will vary. For disposable electrodes, peel off the backings, and press them into place. Reusable electrodes are rarely used.

10. Apply the precordial electrodes at specified locations on the chest.

11. Attach wires and cables, making sure all wire tips follow the patient's body contours.

12. Check all electrodes and wires for proper placement and connection; drape wires over the patient to avoid creating tension on the electrodes that could result in artifacts (Figure 52-9).

13. Enter the patient data into the electrocardiograph. Press the on, run, or record button. Older machines may require the following steps:

    a. Set the paper speed to 25 mm per second or as instructed.

    b. Set the sensitivity setting to 1 or as instructed.

    c. Turn the lead selector to standardization mode.

    d. Adjust the stylus so the baseline is centered.

    e. Press the standardization button. The stylus should move upward above the baseline 10 mm (two large squares).

14. Run the strip.

    a. If the machine has an automatic feature, set the lead selector to automatic.

    b. For manual tracings, turn the lead selector to standby mode. Select the first lead (I), and record the tracing. Switch the machine to standby, and then repeat the procedure for all 12 leads.

15. Check tracings for artifacts.

16. Correct problems and repeat any tracings that are not clear.

17. Disconnect the patient from the machine.

18. Remove the tracing from the machine, and label it with the patient's name, the date, and your initials.

19. Disconnect the wires from the electrodes, and remove the electrodes from the patient.

20. Clean the patient's skin with a moist towel.

21. Assist the patient into a sitting position.

22. Allow a moment for rest, and then assist the patient from the table.

23. Assist the patient in dressing if necessary, or allow the patient privacy to dress.

24. Wash your hands.

25. Record the procedure in the patient's chart.

26. Properly dispose of used materials and disposable electrodes. Clean reusable electrodes, if used.

27. Clean and disinfect the equipment and the room according to OSHA guidelines.

Allaying Patient Anxiety About Having Electrocardiography

The most common reason for a patient's anxiety is not knowing what to expect from electrocardiography. The patient may be fearful of being hooked up to an electrical device and worried about receiving an electric shock.

Calmly and simply explain the procedure in detail, both before you begin and while you prepare the patient for the test. Assure her that it is a safe procedure that will last about 10 to 15 minutes. Explain that the machine measures the electrical activity of the heart and that no outside electricity will pass through the body. It is also helpful to explain why the doctor has ordered the procedure, without giving any diagnosis or prognosis.

Above all, talk to and listen to the patient. Encourage her to express her concerns and ask questions. Respond to the patient's concerns and questions calmly, fully, and respectfully.

Ensuring Patient Comfort

Ensuring that the patient is comfortable will help her feel more at ease. It will also result in less body movement and a more accurate ECG.

Each patient is an individual. You will need to find out from the patient what is and is not comfortable for her. First make sure the room temperature is right for the patient. If she says the room feels too cool, provide an extra blanket to prevent chills. Being chilly can make a patient shiver and increase her anxiety. If the patient says she feels too warm, do not provide a blanket.

Next ensure that the patient is comfortable on the examining table. Placing a small pillow under the head can help. Make sure, however, that the pillow does not touch the shoulders or raise them off the table. For most patients, placing a pillow under the knees helps relax the abdomen and lower extremities and prevents lower-back pain. Try this arrangement and let the patient decide whether it contributes to or detracts from her comfort. If the patient has trouble breathing, shift her into a Fowler's or semi-Fowler's position. Ask the patient which position is more comfortable, and use the position she chooses. If the patient chooses a position other than supine, be sure to note the position in her chart.

---

electrocardiography. Keep in mind that some patients are apprehensive about undergoing electrocardiography. Anxiety often stems from the fear of receiving an electric shock from the machine. See the Caution: Handle With Care section for ways to allay a patient's anxiety about having an ECG.

Applying the Electrodes and the Connecting Wires

You must prepare the patient's skin before applying the electrodes. Proper contact between an electrode and the skin allows for proper conduction of the impulses. Follow the steps described in Procedure 52-1 as you prepare the patient's skin. Depending on your office policy, you may be required to shave chest or leg hair if it is dense to ensure proper contact. Because you may be exposed to blood or broken skin when shaving a patient, observe Universal Precautions and wear gloves to prevent contact with potentially contaminated body fluids.

Electrodes

Disposable electrodes are the most commonly used type of electrode. Disposable electrodes come with the electrolyte product already applied. Simply remove the adhesive backing and press the electrode firmly into place on the skin. This type of electrode has largely replaced the metal plate and suction bulb electrodes from previous models. Because the electrolyte gel is prepackaged and measured, artifacts occurring from the placement of unequal amounts of electrolyte have been minimized.

Positioning the Electrodes

You must position electrodes at ten locations on the body (Figure 52-10). Remember, if the electrocardiograph has only five electrodes, you will need to move the fifth electrode to six different positions on the patient's chest to obtain the necessary tracings.

Limb Electrodes. Placement of limb electrodes need not be exact. Limb electrodes are most commonly placed on the inside of the fleshy part of the calf muscle and on the outside of the upper arm, but they are sometimes placed on the thigh and above the wrist. It is generally better to place arm electrodes on the upper arm because this reduces the amount of artifact caused by arm movement. Attach the electrodes to a smooth and fleshy part of each limb to ensure optimal conduction of impulses. Limb electrodes must always be placed at the same level on both arms and on both legs. If a patient has had a leg amputated, both leg electrodes should be placed on the thighs.

Precordial Electrodes. Unlike the limb electrodes, the precordial electrodes must be placed at specific locations

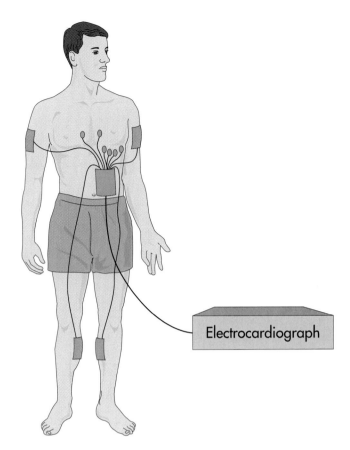

Figure 52-10. There are ten electrode positions for electrocardiography.

on the chest to obtain accurate readings. These locations specify intercostal spaces, the spaces between the ribs. Intercostal spaces are numbered from top to bottom. Refer to Figure 52-6 for the exact description of each location.

Determine the position for the first precordial electrode (V_1) by counting to the fourth intercostal space to the right of the sternum (breastbone). The V_1 electrode should be placed over this space, directly adjacent to the sternum. After you have this electrode in place, use it as a guide to position the other electrodes.

Place the V_2 electrode in the fourth intercostal space to the left of the sternum in the same manner. Note that the V_1 and V_2 positions may not line up exactly; one may be higher than the other. Perfect symmetry is rare in the human body.

Next place the V_4 electrode in the fifth intercostal space, where it intersects an imaginary line drawn straight down from the middle of the clavicle (midclavicular line). When the V_4 electrode is in place, place the V_3 electrode midway between V_2 and V_4 in the fifth intercostal space.

Place the V_6 electrode in the fifth intercostal space, directly below the middle of the armpit (midaxillary line). Place the last electrode (V_5) in the fifth intercostal space, midway between V_4 and V_6.

Attaching the Wires

After placing the electrodes, attach the wires that connect the electrodes to the electrocardiograph. Numbers and letters on the wires correspond to numbers and letters for the electrodes. For example, RA stands for right arm, LL stands for left leg, and so on. The precordial electrode wires are labeled V_1 through V_6. Connect the limb wires first, then the precordial wires, in the sequence already described. Some wires are also color-coded.

Depending on the type of electrodes you use, connect the wires to the electrodes by snapping, clipping, or screwing the wire tips tightly in place. Wires should follow the patient's body contours and lie flat against the body. Drape the wires over the patient to avoid putting tension on the electrodes, which could cause interference. You may also bundle the wires together to form a single cable.

Operating the Electrocardiograph

Before running the ECG, remind the patient to remain as still as possible and not to talk. Be sure the patient is comfortable. A comfortable patient is less likely to move around and cause artifacts on the ECG tracing.

Standardizing the Electrocardiograph

Follow the steps described in Procedure 52-1 as you standardize the electrocardiograph. The stylus should move upward above the baseline 10 mm (two large squares) when you press the standardization button. If it does not, you must see to it that the instrument is adjusted before continuing.

Running the ECG

You can now run the ECG. On most newer machines, turning the lead selector to the automatic mode produces a standard 12-lead strip. Because each lead provides a specific view of the heart's electrical activity, each of the 12 leads has a characteristic tracing (Figure 52-11).

Manual ECGs. If your office has a machine without an automatic setting, you must manually run the ECG for each of the 12 leads. You may also be required to repeat certain leads manually if artifacts are detected.

To run a manual ECG, standardize the machine as already outlined. Then turn the lead selector to standby mode. Some older machines may require you to stop the paper before selecting the first lead (I) using the lead selector. Push the marking button on the machine to indicate the lead if the machine does not do this automatically. Allow the strip to run for four to five cardiac cycles, taking about 3 to 5 seconds. Turn the machine back to the standby mode; stop the paper if necessary, and repeat the procedure for leads II and III, the augmented leads, and the precordial leads. Remember to standardize the machine for consistency before running each lead.

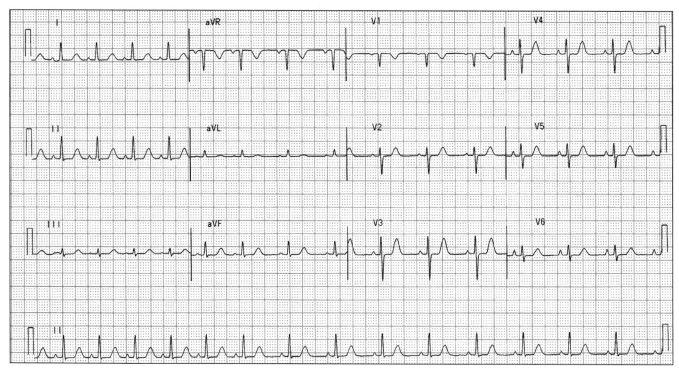

Figure 52-11. The tracing from each lead will differ. The long tracing of a single lead along the bottom is the rhythm strip. (Courtesy of Burdick, Inc., Milton, Wisconsin)

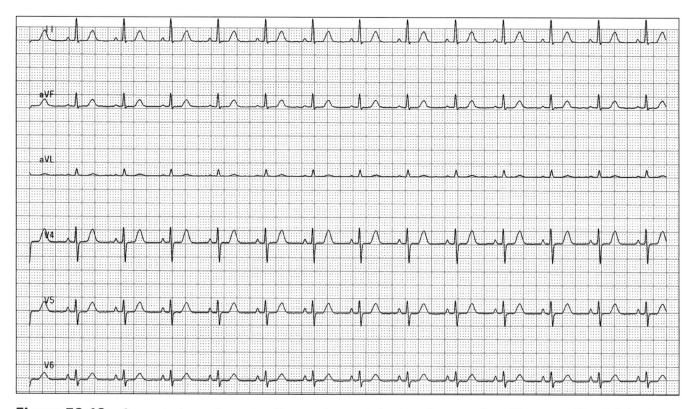

Figure 52-12. Some electrocardiographs allow you to run six leads at the same time. (Courtesy of Burdick, Inc.)

Many physicians request another strip on lead II to assess for rhythm. Some physicians choose a different lead for the rhythm strip. Run the rhythm strip on the requested lead to produce a strip that is at least 2 feet long so rhythmic abnormalities can be easily recognized.

Multiple-Channel Electrocardiographs. Some electrocardiographs have multiple channels that can record three, four, or six leads simultaneously (Figure 52-12). Electrode placement is the same for these types of electrocardiographs.

Checking the ECG Tracing

After running the 12 leads and before disconnecting the patient from the machine, check all tracings to make sure they are clear and free of artifacts. If any of the leads do not appear on a tracing, it may mean that a wire has come loose. In this case reconnect the wire, and repeat the tracing. Repeat any tracings that are not clear.

Also check that all tracings are contained within the boundaries of the paper and that no waves peak above the edges of the paper. If this happens, recenter the stylus if it is positioned too high, or set the sensitivity selector to ½ before repeating the tracing. In the reverse situation—where very low peaks appear—set the sensitivity selector to 2 to increase the height of the peaks.

If the peaks in a tracing are too close together, increase the paper speed to 50 mm per second. Increasing the speed separates the peaks and makes the tracing easier to read.

Make a note on the ECG tracing whenever it is necessary to adjust sensitivity or speed settings. This information is vital to the interpretation of the test.

Troubleshooting: Artifacts and Other Problems

To ensure high-quality tracings, it is essential to recognize artifacts and identify sources of interference. You must also know how to correct them.

Artifacts

Artifacts are caused by improper technique, poor conduction, outside interference, or improper handling of a tracing. If artifacts are present on an ECG tracing, the doctor may not be able to make an accurate diagnosis of the patient's condition. Recognizing the presence of an artifact in the baseline during setup allows you to correct the problem before the tracing is recorded.

There are several types of artifacts. Among the common ones you may see are a wandering baseline or a flat line. You may also see marks that are not characteristic of a tracing; large, erratic spikes; or uniform, small spikes. Table 52-3 outlines these artifacts and summarizes possible causes and solutions.

TABLE 52-3 Correcting ECG Artifacts

Problem	Possible Causes	Solutions
Wandering baseline	Inadequately warmed stylus	Allow electrocardiograph to warm up
	Poor skin preparation	Repeat skin preparation and electrode placement
	Loose electrode	Reapply electrode
	Improper electrode placement	Reapply electrode
	Dirty or corroded electrode	Clean and reapply electrode/replace electrode
	Somatic interference	Help patient relax and be comfortable
	Pickup of breathing movement	Reposition electrode
	Tension on electrode	Drape wires over patient
Flat line	Detached/loose wire or cable	Reattach wires/cable
	Wrong selector switch setting	Check/change selector switch setting
	Crossed wires	Check/switch wires
	Short circuit in wires	Check/replace broken equipment
	Cardiac arrest	Check pulse/respiration; begin CPR
Marks not part of tracing	Careless handling	Handle carefully
	Use of paper clips	Use a rubber band
	Wet hands	Ensure hands are dry
	Improper mounting	Mount properly
Uniform, small spikes	AC interference	Turn off/unplug other electrical equipment; remove patient's watch
	Improper electrode placement	Reapply electrode
	Inadequate grounding	Check grounding
	Dirty electrode	Clean and reapply electrode
Large, erratic spikes	Somatic interference	Help patient relax and be comfortable
	Loose/dry electrode	Reapply electrode
	Electrode placed over bone	Reposition electrode

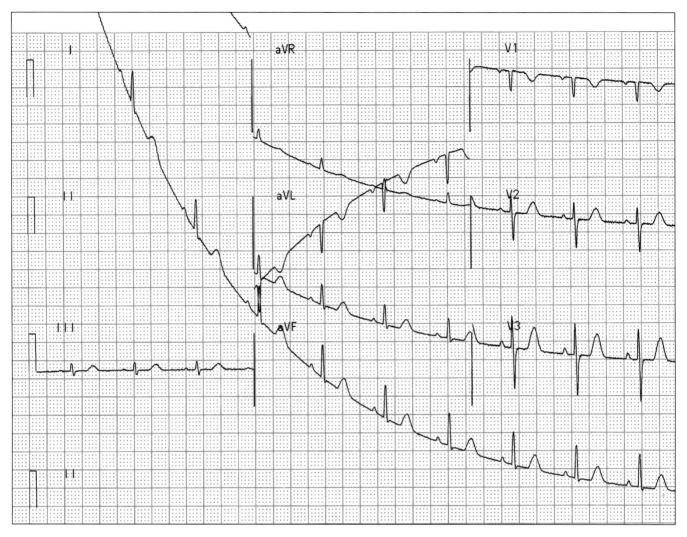

Figure 52-13. A wandering baseline may be caused by somatic interference or a mechanical problem. (Courtesy of Burdick, Inc.)

Wandering Baseline. A wandering baseline, shown in Figure 52-13, is identified by a shift in the baseline from the center position for that lead. Causes include somatic interference and a variety of mechanical problems. Mechanical problems may be an inadequately warmed stylus, improper application of electrodes (too loose or incorrectly placed), dirty or corroded electrodes, tension on electrodes caused by a dangling wire, inadequate or unevenly applied electrolyte products, inadequate skin preparation, or the presence of creams or lotions on the skin.

Having the patient lie still can reduce somatic interference. Proper skin preparation and electrode placement are also essential. When the appointment for electrocardiography is made, instruct the patient to use no creams or lotions, deodorant, perfume, or powder. Be sure to include specific instructions in patient education materials, and ask the patient whether any of these substances were used before the procedure. If so, clean each area of electrode placement thoroughly with alcohol to avoid conduction disturbances.

Flat Line. A flat line on the tracing of one of the leads (Figure 52-14) is typically caused by a loose or disconnected wire. If flat lines occur on more than one lead, two of the wires may have been switched. If flat lines occur on all leads, the patient cable may be loose or disconnected, or there may be a break (short) somewhere in the unit. On the other hand, a flat line on all leads can be an indication of cardiac arrest. Always assess the patient's pulse and respiration first when flat lines occur on all leads.

Extraneous Marks. Because ECG graph paper is sensitive to heat and pressure, it can easily be damaged. Any marks on the paper that are not part of the tracing are referred to as extraneous marks. These marks can be caused by careless handling, such as using paper clips to hold the tracing together or handling the tracing with wet hands.

Causes of Artifacts

You can use the line of the tracing to identify the cause of artifacts. Then you can take steps to eliminate the particular type of interference involved.

Alternating Current (AC) Interference. AC interference occurs when the electrocardiograph picks up a

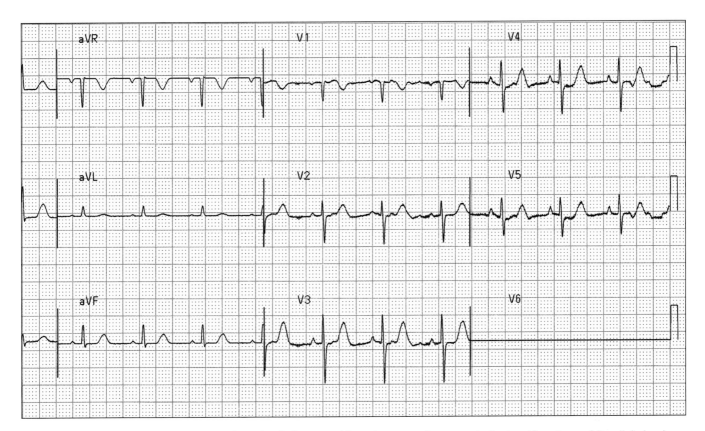

Figure 52-14. A flat line on one of the leads is caused by a loose or disconnected wire. (Courtesy of Burdick, Inc.)

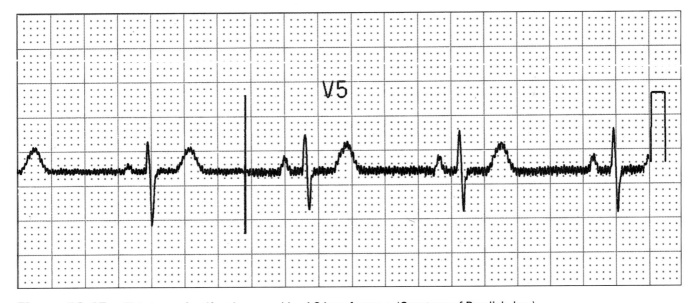

Figure 52-15. This type of artifact is caused by AC interference. (Courtesy of Burdick, Inc.)

small amount of electric current given off by another piece of electrical equipment. The line of the tracing will be jagged, consisting of a series of uniform, small spikes (Figure 52-15). Many of the newer electrocardiographs have filters to reduce or eliminate most of this interference.

AC interference can often be eliminated by turning off or unplugging other appliances in the room. It is also helpful to keep the examining table away from the wall, because wiring in the wall can contribute to AC interference.

If these remedies do not work, check to see whether the electrodes are dirty or attached improperly or whether the machine is incorrectly grounded.

Somatic Interference. Somatic interference is caused by muscle movement. Tensing of voluntary muscles, shifting of body position, tremors, or even talking requires muscular contractions that generate electrical impulses.

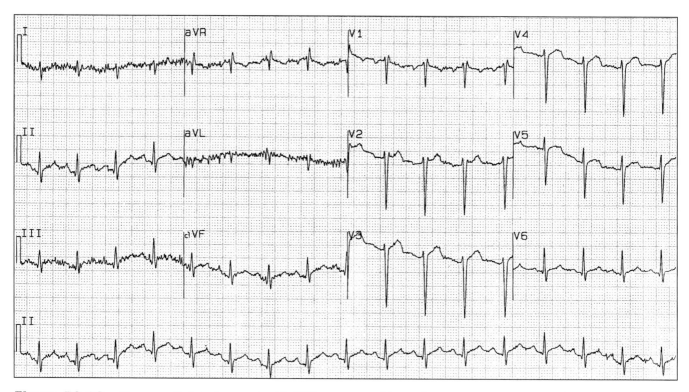

Figure 52-16. The somatic interference in this ECG was caused by patient tremors. (Courtesy of Burdick, Inc.)

A sensitive electrocardiograph detects these impulses. The result is erratic movement of the stylus during the tracing, leading to large, erratic spikes and a shifting baseline (Figure 52-16).

Eliminate this type of interference by reminding the patient to remain still and to refrain from talking. To reduce the chance of shivering, be sure the room temperature is comfortable. Make the patient comfortable to reduce shifting and moving.

Placing the limb electrodes closer to the trunk of the body—on the upper arms, close to the shoulder, and on the upper thighs—can reduce interference. Reducing patient anxiety by explaining the procedure can also help reduce somatic interference.

Certain nervous system disorders, such as Parkinson's disease, cause patients to experience involuntary movements that can cause interference. Placing the limb electrodes closer to the trunk of the body is often helpful; however, it may be necessary to interrupt the tracing until the tremors subside.

Identifying the Source of Interference

The source of interference on an ECG can often be identified by checking the tracings obtained on leads I, II, and III. If there is a problem with a particular limb electrode, the interference will be prominent in two leads. For prominent interference in the following pairs of leads, check the limb electrode indicated:

- Leads I and II, right arm electrode
- Leads I and III, left arm electrode
- Leads II and III, left leg electrode

If the cause of the artifact or the source of interference cannot be determined, stop the machine and notify your supervisor or the physician of the problem. Do not disconnect the patient from the electrocardiograph.

Completing the Procedure

When you are sure the quality of all ECG tracings is acceptable, disconnect the patient from the machine. First remove the tracing from the machine, and label it with the patient's name, the date, and your initials. Loosely roll long tapes from single-channel machines with the printed side facing in, and secure them with a rubber band. Do not use paper clips because they can cause extraneous marks on the tracing.

Next, disconnect the wires from the electrodes, and remove the electrodes from the patient. Wipe excess electrolyte from the patient's skin with a moist towel. Assist the patient to a sitting position, allowing a moment's rest before assisting the patient from the table. Help the patient dress if necessary, or allow the patient privacy to dress. Remove disposable paper covers from the table and pillows, clean surfaces according to OSHA guidelines, and discard all disposable materials in a biohazardous waste container.

Equipment Maintenance

If your machine has reusable electrodes, wipe off the electrolyte product, and wash the electrodes and rubber straps with a mild detergent. Metal plate electrodes must be polished with a fine grade of scouring powder. Do not use steel wool or metal-base polish because they will cause artifacts. Rinse the electrodes well, and dry them thoroughly before storing.

Mounting the Tracing

There are many types of ECG mounts or holders for single-channel ECG tracings. These mounts form a permanent record of the ECG and allow the doctor to read tracings from all 12 leads at once. Mounts are not typically necessary for multiple-channel ECG tracings because these are compact records of several leads. Several types of mounts are available, including slotted folders and folders with self-adhesive surfaces.

Interpreting the ECG

As a medical assistant, you are not responsible for interpreting an ECG. Knowing something about how ECGs are interpreted, however, may allow you to recognize a problem that requires immediate attention. Some of the features that are assessed by means of an ECG include heart rhythm, heart rate, the length and position of intervals and segments, and wave changes. A series of ECGs are often taken before a physician makes a diagnosis. The tracings are compared for changes in a patient's condition, progress, or response to a specific medication.

Heart Rhythm

The ECG is the best way to assess heart rhythm—the regularity of the heartbeat. A normal heart rhythm is indicated on the ECG by regularly spaced complexes. In a regularly spaced complex, the distance between one P wave and the next P wave—or one R wave and the next R wave—is consistent. The physician assesses the patient's rhythm by viewing the rhythm strip you obtain from lead II.

Irregularities in heart rhythm are called **arrhythmias.** Some arrhythmias do not cause problems, but many of them can be dangerous. It is important, therefore, to detect these irregularities with an ECG.

Heart Rate

The heart rate can easily be determined by counting the number of QRS complexes in a 6-second strip of the tracing (30 large squares at 25 mm per second) and multiplying by 10. Irregularities in heart rate may result from conduction abnormalities or reactions to certain drugs.

Intervals and Segments

Variations in the length and position of the intervals and segments can indicate many heart conditions, including conduction disturbances and **myocardial infarction,** or

heart attack. For example, following a heart attack, the S–T segment will be elevated in the tracing for a period of time. Thus, the ECG can be used to determine not only the occurrence of a heart attack but also the approximate time it occurred. Electrolyte disturbances in the blood and drug reactions can also affect intervals and segments.

Wave Changes

The direction of certain waves may vary, depending on which lead is being viewed. Normally each wave should have a similar appearance in each of the leads. Changes in the height, width, or direction of a wave may indicate a problem. During the early stages of a heart attack, for example, the T wave forms a large peak. Not long afterward the T wave inverts and appears below the baseline.

Exercise Electrocardiography (Stress Testing)

The resting ECG does not always provide a doctor with enough information to diagnose a problem. Exercise electrocardiography, more commonly known as a stress test, assesses the heart's conduction system during exercise, when the demand for oxygen increases. This test measures a patient's response to a constant or increasing workload.

A stress test may be performed on a patient who has had surgery or a heart attack to determine how the heart is functioning. It is sometimes used to screen a patient for heart disease and to determine a patient's ability to undertake an exercise program.

During the procedure the patient is required to walk on a treadmill, pedal a stationary bicycle, or walk on a stair-stepping ergonometer while ECG readings are taken (Figure 52-17). An ergonometer measures work performed. You are responsible for preparing the patient for electrocardiography and monitoring blood pressure throughout the procedure. The test continues until the patient reaches a target heart rate, experiences chest pain or fatigue, or develops complications, such as tachycardia or dysrhythmia.

A patient who undergoes stress testing is often suspected of having a heart problem or is recovering from a heart attack or surgery. Consequently, there may be a risk of cardiac distress, heart attack, or cardiac arrest during testing. Because of the risks, the patient must be monitored by a physician throughout the test. Emergency medication and equipment, such as a defibrillator, must always be present in the room. The patient must sign an informed consent form before the procedure.

Because of the potential risk, patients may be apprehensive about the test. As a medical assistant, you can be instrumental in helping them feel comfortable about undergoing the procedure and in making the procedure as

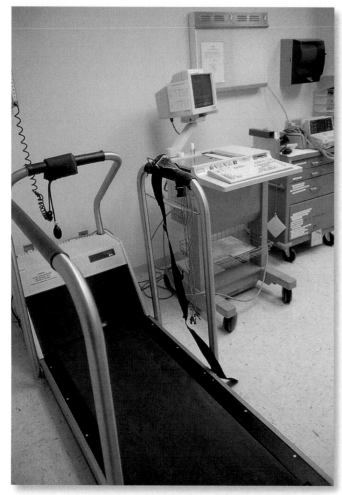

Figure 52-17. During a stress test, the patient exercises on special equipment to see how well the heart handles increased physical demands.

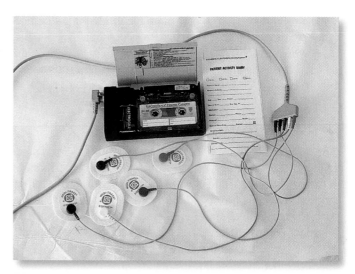

Figure 52-18. The Holter monitor is used to determine electrical activity of a patient's heart over a 24-hour period.

safe as possible for them. See the Caution: Handle With Care section for ways to help a patient safely undergo stress testing.

Ambulatory Electrocardiography (Holter Monitoring)

Patients who experience intermittent chest pain or discomfort may have a normal resting ECG and a normal stress test. When this is the case, the electrical activity of the patient's heart can be monitored over a 24-hour period of normal activity to help diagnose the problem. A special monitor, the Holter monitor, is used for this purpose.

Function of the Holter Monitor

The **Holter monitor** is an electrocardiography device that includes a small cassette recorder worn around a patient's waist or on a shoulder strap to record the heart's electrical activity. The monitor is connected to electrodes on the patient's chest (Figure 52-18). During the testing period, the patient is asked to perform usual daily activities and to keep a written log of activities undertaken and of stress or symptoms experienced. To aid in the diagnosis, some monitors allow patients to press an event button to mark the area on the recording whenever symptoms appear.

The patient returns to the office at the end of the 24-hour test period to have the monitor and electrodes removed. The tape is analyzed by a microcomputer in the office or at a reference laboratory, and a printout of the results is prepared. When the tracing has been evaluated, the doctor can correlate cardiac irregularities, such as arrhythmias or S–T segment changes, with the activities and symptoms listed in the patient's diary.

In addition to its role as a diagnostic tool, Holter monitoring can be used to evaluate the status of a patient who is recovering from a heart attack. It can indicate progress or the need to change therapy or modify the rehabilitation plan.

Patient Education

It is absolutely essential that the patient continue normal activities during Holter monitoring. Give the patient the following additional instructions.

- Record all activities, emotional upsets, physical symptoms, and medications taken.
- Wear loose-fitting clothing that opens in the front while wearing the monitor.
- Avoid going near magnets, metal detectors, and high-voltage areas, and avoid using electric blankets during the monitoring period. These devices and areas can interfere with the recording.
- Avoid getting the monitor wet. Do not take a bath or shower. A sponge bath is permissible.

Show the patient how to check the monitor to make sure it is working properly. This step is particularly important if

Ensuring Patient Safety During Stress Testing

Some risk is involved in exercise electrocardiography, because patients who most commonly undergo the test may either already have cardiac problems or be suspected of having them. The risk of having a heart attack during a stress test, however, is less than 1 in 500, and the risk of death is less than 1 in 10,000. Still, some patients may be apprehensive about the procedure because of the risks.

You can help educate and prepare patients for stress tests and assist them during the procedure. One way to help is to ask patients to wear comfortable shoes and clothes. In addition, there are several ways to help these patients be less fearful of the procedure while helping to ensure their safety.

A patient who has recently suffered a heart attack may be particularly afraid to undergo stress testing. A stress test may, however, be the only way the physician can accurately determine the functional ability of the patient's heart and assess his physical limitations. This information is vital to preventing future heart attacks.

By informing the patient of what symptoms he may expect during the test—including fatigue, slight breathlessness, an increased heart rate, and increased perspiration—the patient will be better able to cope with the test. Make it clear that an advance warning of adjustments in the procedure, such as an increased workload, will be given.

Assure the patient that there are few risks associated with the test and that the test may be stopped if he experiences chest pain or extreme fatigue. Patients will relax and follow instructions better when they know that the procedure can be controlled. Tell the patient that both you and the physician will be monitoring his vital signs during and after the procedure and that all safety precautions will be taken. Explain the presence of the safety equipment—for example, the crash cart with medication, equipment, and supplies.

During the test, remember to talk to and listen to the patient. Even symptoms not related to cardiac symptoms should be reported, and the patient should be encouraged to report any symptoms. Observe the patient for signs of distress and inform the physician immediately if such symptoms appear.

---

any of the electrodes seem loose. Instruct the patient to inform the office if there are any problems.

Connecting the Patient

Holter monitors have either three or five electrodes, depending on the unit. As with a resting ECG, correct placement of the electrodes is necessary for accurate readings.

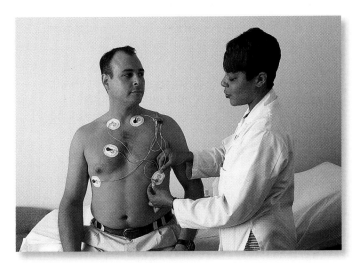

Figure 52-19. Taping the wires to the patient's chest reduces the chance that tension on a wire or electrode will produce artifacts on the ECG.

Because the electrodes must stay in place for 24 hours, you may need to shave the areas where the electrodes are attached to permit optimum adherence. The wires may be connected to the electrodes before they are attached to minimize patient discomfort.

After the electrodes and wires are attached and the monitor is in place, tape the wires to the patient's chest to eliminate tension on the wires or electrodes (Figure 52-19). Be sure that the unit has a fresh battery, that a cassette tape has been inserted, and that the unit is turned on. The steps in performing Holter monitoring are outlined in Procedure 52-2.

Anatomy and Physiology of the Respiratory System

Pulmonary function tests are used to evaluate a patient's lung volume and capacity. A description of the anatomy and physiology of the respiratory system will help clarify pulmonary function testing and the problems it is used to diagnose.

Anatomy of the Respiratory System

The respiratory system is composed of the nose, pharynx, larynx, trachea, two bronchi, and the lungs. The bronchi branch into bronchioles and eventually into alveoli. In the

PROCEDURE 52.2

Holter Monitoring

Objective: To monitor the electrical activity of a patient's heart over a 24-hour period to detect cardiac abnormalities that may go undetected during routine electrocardiography or stress testing

OSHA Guidelines

Materials: Holter monitor, battery, cassette tape, patient diary or log, alcohol, gauze pads, disposable shaving supplies, disposable electrodes, hypoallergenic tape, drape, electrocardiograph

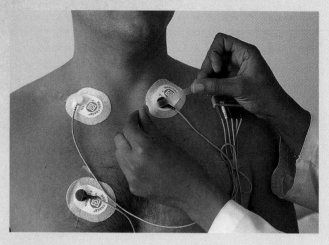

Figure 52-20. Correctly connecting the patient to the Holter monitor is essential.

Method

1. Identify the patient, introduce yourself, and explain the procedure.
2. Ask the patient to remove clothing from the waist up; provide a drape if necessary.
3. Wash your hands and assemble the equipment.
4. Assist the patient into a comfortable position (sitting or supine).
5. If the patient's body hair is particularly dense, put on examination gloves and shave the areas where the electrodes will be attached. Properly dispose of the razor and the gloves.
6. Clean the electrode sites with alcohol and gauze.
7. Rub each electrode site vigorously with a dry gauze square to help electrodes adhere to the skin.
8. Attach wires to the electrodes, and peel off the paper backing on the electrodes. Apply as indicated (Figure 52-20), pressing firmly to ensure that each electrode is securely attached and is making good contact with the skin.
9. Attach the patient cable.
10. Insert a fresh battery, and position the unit (Figure 52-21).
11. Tape wires, cable, and electrodes as necessary to avoid tension on the wires as the patient moves.

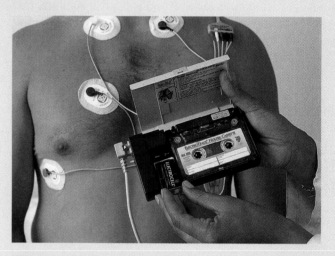

Figure 52-21. Make sure the monitor has a fresh battery and cassette tape.

12. Insert the cassette tape, and turn on the unit.
13. Confirm that the cassette tape is actually running (Figure 52-22). Indicate the start time in the patient's chart.
14. Instruct the patient on proper use of the monitor and how to enter information in the diary. Caution the patient not to alter any diary entries; it is crucial to know what the patient is doing at all times.

continued →

Holter Monitoring *(continued)*

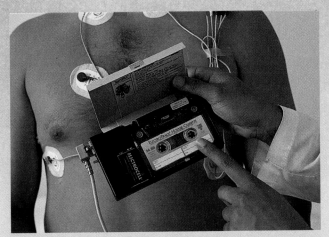

Figure 52-22. Observe the cassette to make sure the tape is moving through the recording unit.

15. Schedule the patient's return visit for the same time on the following day.
16. On the following day remove the electrodes, discard them, and clean the electrode sites.
17. Wash your hands.
18. Remove the cassette and obtain a printout of the tracing according to office procedure.

alveoli, external respiration—the exchange of gases between the air and the blood—occurs. Figure 52-23 shows the lungs, bronchi, and alveoli in detail.

Physiology of the Respiratory System

There are two levels of respiration: external and internal. External respiration involves two processes: ventilation and diffusion. Ventilation is the movement of air in and out of the lungs. It results from the contraction and relaxation of the respiratory muscles. The major respiratory muscle is the diaphragm. Other respiratory muscles, including the intercostal muscles (between the ribs), are found in the walls of the chest and back.

Inspiration, or breathing in, results when the respiratory muscles contract. The diaphragm pushes down toward the abdomen when it contracts, while the other respiratory muscles help expand the chest outward and upward. Both actions serve to decrease the pressure within the alveoli so that it is less than the atmospheric pressure. The result is the flow of air into the lungs.

Expiration, or breathing out, results from relaxation of the respiratory muscles and a consequent increase in pressure within the alveoli. As a result, air flows out of the lungs. Expiration is normally a passive process. During fast, hard breathing, however, the abdominal muscles push the diaphragm upward, and certain chest and back muscles pull the ribs downward and inward to decrease the size of the chest cavity and help force the air out.

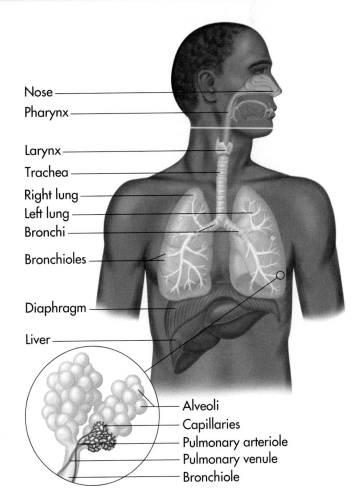

Figure 52-23. Knowing how the respiratory system works will help you understand the application of spirometry.

Diffusion is a passive process wherein oxygen and carbon dioxide cross the capillary and alveolar membranes to enter the capillaries or alveoli. Oxygen diffuses from the alveolar air into the blood, because there is a higher concentration in the alveoli than in the blood. Carbon dioxide, at a higher concentration in the blood, diffuses across the membranes into the alveoli.

Perfusion, or internal respiration, is the exchange of oxygen in the blood for carbon dioxide in the cells of body tissues and organs. Perfusion, diffusion, and ventilation occur simultaneously, as the circulatory system moves the blood from the lungs to the body cells and back.

Pulmonary Function Testing

Pulmonary function tests (PFTs) evaluate lung volume and capacity. These tests are commonly used to evaluate shortness of breath and can help detect and classify pulmonary disorders. They may also be performed as part of a general examination. PFTs are used to monitor conditions such as asthma, certain allergies, cystic fibrosis, and chronic obstructive pulmonary disease (COPD), a chronic lung disorder. The tests are also used to evaluate the effectiveness of particular treatments on a patient's lung function.

Career Opportunities

Respiratory Therapist

To gain medical assistant credentials, you must fulfill the requirements of either the American Association of Medical Assistants (for a Certified Medical Assistant) or the American Medical Technologists (for a Registered Medical Assistant). After obtaining your medical assistant certification or registration, you may wish to acquire additional skills in specialty areas through course work or on-the-job training. Although this course work or training may not lead to an additional certification or degree, it will enable you to expand your role in the medical office and advance your career as the demand for skilled health professionals increases.

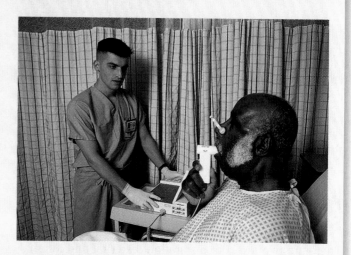

Skills and Duties

A respiratory therapist diagnoses, treats, and cares for people who have difficulty breathing. Some of his patients are people with chronic lung problems, such as asthma, bronchitis, emphysema, and chronic obstructive pulmonary disease. Others may have difficulty breathing as the result of complications caused by a heart attack, an accident, cystic fibrosis, lung cancer, or acquired immunodeficiency syndrome (AIDS). Some infants who are born prematurely have difficulty breathing and may need respiratory therapy, which may include the use of apnea monitors and oxygen tents.

A respiratory therapist works under the supervision of a physician. Duties include both diagnostic and therapeutic tasks. For example, to diagnose a breathing problem, the therapist analyzes samples of a patient's breath or blood for levels of oxygen, carbon dioxide, and other gases. He also measures the capacity of a patient's lungs to determine whether they are working properly and performs stress tests and other studies of the cardiopulmonary system.

Once a problem is diagnosed, the respiratory therapist may use a variety of treatment options. He may use equipment such as oxygen respirators and oxygen tents to administer oxygen to help the patient breathe. He may administer medication in aerosol form to treat breathing disorders. The respiratory therapist may also set up and maintain mechanical ventilation, such as artificial airways, for patients who cannot breathe on their own.

In addition to diagnosis and treatment of breathing disorders, the respiratory therapist may be responsible for patient education to promote healthy breathing. Education duties may include:

- Teaching smoking cessation programs to help prevent breathing problems associated with smoking.
- Conducting rehabilitation activities, such as low-impact aerobics, to help patients increase their lung capacity.

continued ⟶

Spirometry

Spirometry is a test used to measure breathing capacity. An instrument called a **spirometer** measures the air taken in by and expelled from the lungs. Several different measurements related to lung volume and capacity can be made with a spirometer (Table 52-4). Some of these measurements are made directly by the spirometer; others are calculated.

Forced Vital Capacity

Many measurements can be obtained during one particular maneuver—obtaining the **forced vital capacity (FVC),** the greatest volume of air that can be expelled when a person performs rapid, forced expiration. To obtain the FVC, ask the patient to take as deep a breath as possible and to exhale into the spirometer as quickly and completely as possible. You can determine the lung's ability to function by taking into account the volume of air expelled and the time it takes to perform this maneuver.

Types of Spirometers

Many types of spirometers are used in physicians' offices. Each consists of a mouthpiece or a mouthpiece and a tube to carry air to the machine, a mechanism to measure the volume or flow of air, and a means of calculating and printing the results.

Computerized spirometers are available that can measure air volume and airflow, perform various calculations, and print a graphic representation of the information. Figure 52-24 shows a computerized spirometer.

Mechanical spirometers directly measure either the air volume displaced or airflow. Spirometers that directly measure airflow calculate air volume using flow rate and time values. The flow-sensing spirometer illustrated in Figure 52-25 calculates airflow by counting the rotations of a turbine.

Performing Spirometry

The technique for performing pulmonary function testing is similar for all types of spirometers. Successful spirometry depends on proper patient preparation and consistent technique in performing the procedure and analyzing the results. The steps involved in measuring forced vital capacity using a spirometer are described in detail here and outlined in Procedure 52-3.

Patient Preparation

When patients are scheduled for pulmonary function tests, inform them that the following conditions and activities may affect the test's accuracy:

- Viral infection or acute illness within the previous 2 to 3 weeks
- Serious medical condition, such as a recent heart attack
- Recent use of a prescribed medication if test order calls for spirometry before and after prescribed medication

TABLE 52-4 Pulmonary Function Tests

Lung Capacity Tests	Definition
Vital capacity (VC)	Total volume of air that can be exhaled after maximum inspiration
Inspiratory capacity (IC)	Amount of air that can be inhaled after normal expiration
Functional residual capacity (FRC)	Amount of air remaining in lungs after normal expiration
Total lung capacity (TLC)	Total volume of lungs when maximally inflated
Forced vital capacity (FVC)	Greatest volume of air that can be expelled when person performs rapid, forced expiratory maneuver
Forced expiratory volume (FEV)	Volume of air expelled in first, second, or third second of FVC maneuver
Peak expiratory flow rate (PEFR)	Greatest rate of flow during forced expiration
Forced expiratory flow (FEF)	Average rate of flow during middle half of FVC
Maximal voluntary ventilation (MVV)	Greatest volume of air breathed per unit of time
Tidal volume (T_V)	Amount of air inhaled or exhaled during normal breathing
Minute volume (MV)	Total amount of air expired per minute
Inspiratory reserve volume (IRV)	Amount of air inspired over above-normal inspiration
Expiratory reserve volume (ERV)	Amount of air exhaled after normal expiration
Residual volume (RV)	Amount of air remaining in lungs after forced expiration

Adapted from *Illustrated Guide to Diagnostic Tests* (Springhouse, PA: Springhouse, 1998).

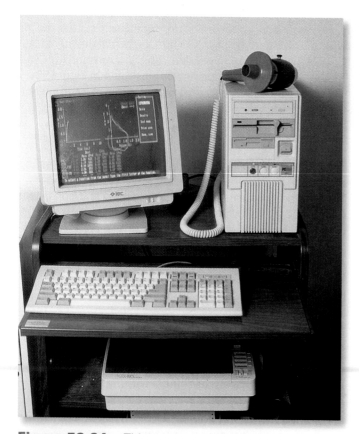

Figure 52-24. This computerized spirometer measures air volume and airflow.

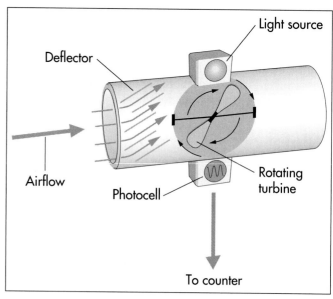

Figure 52-25. One type of flow-sensing spirometer uses a turbine to measure airflow directly from the lungs.

- Use of a sedative or opioid substance before the test
- Smoking or eating a heavy meal within 1 hour of taking the test

Review the conditions and activities with patients again on the day of the test to ensure that none apply. If

PROCEDURE 52.3

Measuring Forced Vital Capacity Using Spirometry

Objective: To determine a patient's forced vital capacity using a volume-displacing spirometer

OSHA Guidelines

Materials: Adult scale with height bar, spirometer, patient tubing (tubing that runs from the mouthpiece to the machine), mouthpiece, nose clip, disinfectant

Method

1. Prepare the equipment. Ensure that the paper supply in the machine is adequate.
2. Calibrate the machine as necessary.
3. Identify the patient and introduce yourself.
4. Check the patient's chart to see whether there are special instructions to follow.
5. Ask whether the patient has followed instructions.
6. Wash your hands and put on examination gloves.
7. Measure and record the patient's height and weight.
8. Explain the proper positioning.
9. Explain the procedure.
10. Demonstrate the procedure.
11. Turn on the spirometer, and enter applicable patient data and the number of tests to be performed.
12. Ensure that the patient has loosened any tight clothing, is comfortable, and is in the proper position. Apply the nose clip.
13. Have the patient perform the first maneuver, coaching when necessary.
14. Determine whether the maneuver is acceptable.
15. Offer feedback to the patient and recommendations for improvement if necessary.
16. Have the patient perform additional maneuvers until three acceptable maneuvers are obtained.
17. Record the procedure in the patient's chart, and place the chart and the test results on the physician's desk for interpretation.
18. Ask the patient to remain until the physician reviews the results.
19. Properly dispose of used materials and disposable instruments.
20. Sanitize and disinfect patient tubing and reusable mouthpiece and nose clip.
21. Clean and disinfect the equipment and room according to OSHA guidelines.

there are no contraindications, weigh and measure patients. Use simple terms to explain the procedure and its purpose. Have them loosen tight clothing so they will be comfortable and their breathing will not be restricted in any way. The procedure is performed with patients sitting down. Make sure their legs are not crossed and that both feet are flat on the floor.

Explain that they need to wear a nose clip or hold the nose tightly closed to be sure that they will inhale and exhale through the mouth. The mouthpiece of the unit may be a disposable cardboard tube or a reusable rubber one that can be disinfected after use. If disposable mouthpieces are used, instruct patients to avoid biting down on them, because that will obstruct the flow of air. Be sure patients form a tight seal around the mouthpiece with their lips. Dentures normally help maintain a tight seal; however, they should be removed if they hinder the process.

Proper Positioning. Instruct patients to keep their chin and neck in the correct position during the procedure. The chin should be slightly elevated and the neck slightly

extended. Bending the chin to the chest tends to restrict the flow of air and should be avoided (Figure 52-26). Some bending at the waist is acceptable.

Explaining and Demonstrating the Procedure. Tell patients to take the deepest breath possible, insert the mouthpiece into the mouth, form a tight seal, and then blow into the mouthpiece as hard and as fast as possible to completely exhale. Tell them to exhale as long as they can to force air from the lungs. Remind them that the initial force of their exhalation must be strong to get a valid reading. Demonstrate the procedure to show how the test is done correctly.

Performing the Maneuver

You can improve patients' performance during the maneuver by actively and forcefully coaching them. Urge patients to blow hard and to continue blowing. After a maneuver, give them feedback on their performance, and indicate corrective actions they can take to improve the next maneuver.

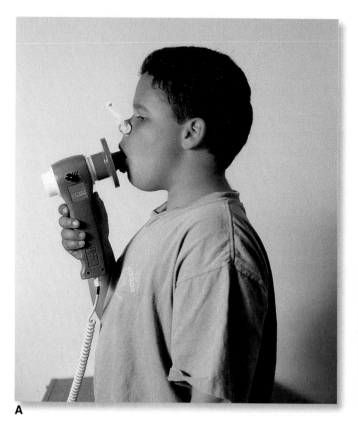
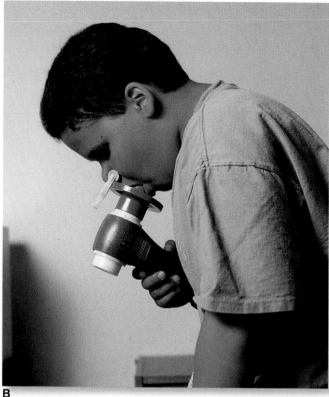

A   **B**

Figure 52-26. The patient must maintain the proper position during a pulmonary function test. (a) The chin should be slightly elevated and the neck slightly extended. (b) The neck should not approach the chest.

Some spirometers indicate whether a particular maneuver was of adequate force and duration to be measured. Adequate force does not, however, indicate that the maneuver was acceptable. An acceptable maneuver must have the following five features:

1. No coughing, particularly during the first second
2. A quick and forceful start
3. An adequate length of time (a minimum of 6 seconds)
4. A consistent and fast flow with no variability
5. Consistency with other maneuvers

Spirometry tracings plot volume and time. You will need to obtain three acceptable maneuvers, which may require more than three attempts. Observe the patient for signs of breathing difficulty, dizziness, light-headedness, or changes in pulse and blood pressure. If necessary, allow the patient to rest briefly before continuing. Notify the physician immediately if symptoms are severe.

Determining the Effectiveness of Medication.
Spirometry is often used to determine the effectiveness of certain medications that a patient is taking. You will perform two sets of maneuvers if this determination is required. Instruct the patient to refrain from taking the prescribed medication on the day of the test. Before performing the test, confirm that the patient has followed this instruction. Conduct the first set of maneuvers, ensuring that they are acceptable. After obtaining the results, instruct the patient to take the prescribed medication. Allow the medication to take effect, and then perform a second set of maneuvers. Comparing the two sets of readings shows whether the medication has effectively improved the patient's lung function. Some computerized spirometers can graph both sets of readings together to simplify the comparison (Figure 52-27).

Special Considerations. On occasion you may have to deal with an uncooperative patient, one who cannot understand or follow directions, or one who cannot perform the procedure. In these situations patience and skill are essential to obtaining an acceptable spirometry tracing.

The doctor may be able to convince an uncooperative patient to perform the maneuver. You can help by taking a no-nonsense approach, perhaps stating that the doctor needs these test results to help the patient. Patients who cannot understand or follow directions—the very young, the very old, those who have limited proficiency in English, or those with a hearing impairment—may need extra attention and patience to obtain acceptable results. Explain the procedure in simple terms, and repeat instructions as necessary. If, after eight attempts, the patient is unable to perform the procedure, stop and report the situation to the doctor.

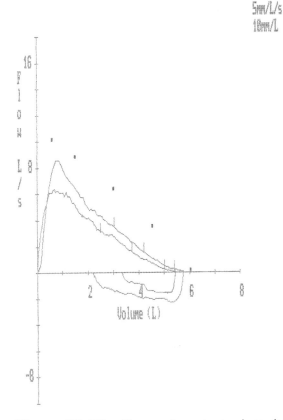

5mm/L/s
10mm/L   Pred ...
         Pre- —
         Post —

Figure 52-27. These spirometry tracings show air volume per second before and after use of a medication.

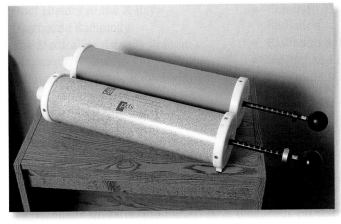

Figure 52-28. A calibration syringe delivers a fixed volume of air.

The Importance of Calibration

Spirometers should be calibrated each day they are used to ensure accurate readings. You may be required to perform this procedure. Calibration of a spirometer requires the use of a standardized measuring instrument called a **calibration syringe** (Figure 52-28). When the plunger is pulled back, this syringe contains a fixed volume of air. Connect the syringe to the patient tubing (the tubing that runs from the mouthpiece to the machine), and depress the plunger to inject the entire volume of air. The reading on the spirometer should be within ±3% of the stated volume. It is important to keep a calibration logbook for each spirometer.

While calibrating the spirometer, you can detect leaks by checking the volume/time graph. The volume should remain at a steady reading. If the volume declines with time, there is a leak somewhere in the system.

Infection Control

After a patient completes the pulmonary function test, you must clean the spirometer thoroughly to prevent transmission of microorganisms. If disposable mouthpieces and nose clips are used, discard them in a biohazardous waste container. If reusable mouthpieces and nose clips are used, clean and disinfect them between patients. Also change patient tubing between patients. Thoroughly clean and disinfect patient tubing before reusing it. Most important, wash your hands thoroughly before and after performing a pulmonary function test.

What the Results Reveal

Pulmonary function tests help the doctor evaluate ventilatory function of the lungs and chest wall. They are good screening tools for pulmonary disorders, such as pulmonary edema, chronic obstructive pulmonary disease, and asthma. These tests also help the doctor determine the nature of a patient's disorder, such as narrowing or obstruction of the airways. Pulmonary function tests can determine the severity of a patient's problem and response to therapy or medication.

Summary

Electrocardiography and pulmonary function testing play a vital role in the diagnosis and treatment of cardiac and pulmonary disease. As a medical assistant, you may be required to perform these procedures in the medical office.

To understand electrocardiography, you need to know the basics of the conduction system of the heart and the components of an electrocardiograph. To obtain accurate electrocardiogram readings, you must properly place the electrodes and be able to recognize artifacts and correct them.

Likewise, to provide accurate assessments of pulmonary function, you must use proper technique and recognize the acceptability of a spirometric maneuver. Because patient compliance is crucial for accurate results, effective patient education is vital to the process.

well as your role as a medical assistant in this testing. Safety issues for the administration of radiologic testing are discussed, as is the proper handling and storage of the actual films. In addition, you learn about preparing and instructing patients for the more common radiology procedures.

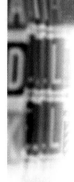

CASE STUDY

A 42-year-old woman has arrived at the office for her annual physical, part of which involves scheduling her to have a mammogram performed. The patient completes the procedure, which comes back revealing a small, abnormal density. The physician asks you to schedule the patient for a CT scan of the breast, which also reveals an abnormal mass. The patient decides that she wants to be more aggressive in determining if the small mass is cancerous, so you now schedule a mammotest, which is used to determine that the mass is benign with no evidence of cancer.

As you read this chapter, consider the following questions:

1. What special instructions should be given to the patient before her mammogram?
2. How is a CT scan performed?
3. When preparing a patient for a CT scan, what allergies should be disclosed during the patient interview?
4. Why was a mammotest requested by the physician?
5. What education requirements must you fulfill in order to work as a radiographer/sonographer?

Brief History of the X-Ray

In 1895 Wilhelm Konrad Roentgen (1845–1923) discovered the x-ray, or roentgen ray, a type of electromagnetic wave. It has a high energy level, traveling at the speed of light (186,000 miles per second), and an extremely short wavelength (one-billionth of an inch) that can penetrate solid objects. X-rays react with photographic film to produce a permanent record (x-ray, or radiograph). The x-ray image is lightest where the film is struck by the most x-ray energy. Differences in tissue densities produce the x-ray image, with the least dense being lightest and the most dense being darkest on the film.

Today there are both diagnostic and therapeutic uses for x-rays and radioactive substances. Radiologic technologists are trained medical personnel who are certified to perform certain radiologic procedures upon completion of a radiology curriculum lasting 2 to 4 years. Some radiologic technologists receive further training in radiology subspecialties, such as ultrasound, mammography, magnetic resonance imaging, and nuclear medicine. Radiographers, sonographers, radiation therapists, and nuclear medicine technologists are all radiologic technologists. Invasive radiologic procedures or procedures requiring a high degree of expertise are nearly always performed by a radiologist, a physician who specializes in radiology. A radiologist is also the physician who interprets the films for other physicians. Other specialists who perform radiologic procedures, either alone or with the assistance of a radiologist, include cardiologists, orthopedists, obstetricians, and oncologists.

Diagnostic Radiology

Diagnostic radiology is the use of x-ray technology for diagnostic purposes. Radiologic tests sometimes use contrast media as well as special techniques or instruments for viewing internal body structures and functions. A **contrast medium** is a substance that makes internal organs denser and blocks the passage of x-rays to the photographic film. Introducing contrast media into certain structures or areas of the body can provide a clearer image of organs and tissues and indications of how well they are functioning. Contrast media include gases (air, oxygen, or carbon dioxide), heavy metal salts (barium sulfate or bismuth carbonate), and iodine compounds. They can be administered orally, parenterally (for example, intravenously), or by routes that introduce them into an organ or body cavity (for example, by insertion). Types of diagnostic imaging include x-rays, computed tomography (CT), nuclear medicine, magnetic resonance imaging (MRI), and ultrasound.

Invasive Procedures

Diagnostic tests can be invasive or noninvasive. An **invasive** procedure (such as angiography) requires a radiologist to insert a catheter, wire, or other testing device into a patient's blood vessel or organ through the skin or a body orifice. All invasive tests require surgical aseptic technique. Some procedures, including angiography, are performed in a hospital or same-day surgical facility. The patient may need general anesthesia for some procedures. The anesthetist must closely monitor the patient who is under

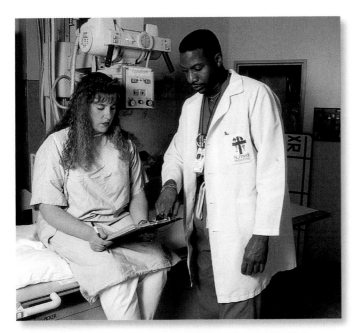

Figure 53-1. A standard x-ray is one of the most frequently performed radiologic tests.

anesthesia during and after the test for life-threatening complications, such as anaphylaxis.

Noninvasive Procedures

Noninvasive procedures, such as standard x-rays or ultrasound, use other technologies to view internal structures. They do not require inserting devices, breaking the skin, or the degree of monitoring needed with invasive procedures.

The most familiar equipment used for diagnostic imaging is the conventional x-ray machine, as shown in Figure 53-1. This machine consists of a table, an x-ray tube, a control panel, and a high-voltage generator. Other equipment used for diagnostic radiology includes instruments specifically designed for the test. Examples are a mammography unit, a scanner for CT, and a transducer for ultrasound.

The Medical Assistant's Role in Diagnostic Radiology

You may deal with diagnostic radiology in a radiology facility or in a medical office. Your duties in a radiology facility will include assisting a radiologic technologist or a radiologist in performing diagnostic radiologic procedures. Depending on the scope of practice in your state, you may be allowed to learn how to operate certain x-ray equipment. Even if you are not allowed to assist with an x-ray procedure or to operate x-ray equipment, you will probably provide preprocedure and postprocedure care of the patient.

Your duties in a medical facility, such as an orthopedic office, may include assisting a radiologic technologist in

performing x-ray procedures. In an obstetric practice, you might assist a physician in performing an ultrasound examination of a pregnant woman. Even if you work in a medical office that does no radiologic testing, you must still provide a certain amount of preprocedure care. To properly explain a test to a patient and to assist a radiologic technologist or radiologist in performing a test, you must have a basic understanding of x-ray technology. You may also need in-service training to ensure accuracy and patient safety for some procedures.

Preprocedure Care

Preprocedure care varies somewhat, depending on the test. In general, however, you may do the following:

- Schedule the patient's appointment, if necessary. Inform the patient of the location, date, and time of the procedure.
- Provide preparation instructions. Advise the patient about diet restrictions or requirements (such as fasting or drinking liquids) as well as medication requirements (such as taking a laxative). Always check with the radiology facility for specific requirements, and be sure the patient receives this information.
- Explain the procedure to the patient briefly and clearly. Use proper terminology and nontechnical language, but do not talk down to the patient. Reinforce the doctor's reason for requesting the procedure, and provide any available written information about the test. Inform the patient about the length of the examination, about possible side effects or safety precautions and warnings, and about injections or uncomfortable steps.
- Ask pertinent questions. Obtain a medication history from the patient (current medications could interfere with some procedures). If the patient is a woman of childbearing age, ask whether she is pregnant or whether there is any chance she could be pregnant. Report the answers to the physician in a medical office or to the radiologic technologist in a radiology facility.

Care During and After the Procedure

If you work in a radiology facility, your responsibilities include preparing and guiding the patient through the procedure. You may also assist the radiologic technologist or the radiologist in performing the procedure by placing, removing, and developing film in the x-ray machine. Procedure 53-1 describes the general process of assisting with a radiologic procedure.

You may care for a patient and assist the radiologic technologist or radiologist during a wide variety of x-ray and other diagnostic imaging tests. Although requirements vary depending on the procedure, you will probably be

PROCEDURE 53.1

Assisting With an X-Ray Examination

Objective: To assist with a radiologic procedure under the supervision of a radiologic technologist

OSHA Guidelines: This procedure does not involve exposure to blood, body fluids, or tissue. You must wear a radiation exposure badge (dosimeter), however, and will be required to wear a garment containing a lead shield if you remain in the room during the operation of x-ray equipment

Materials: X-ray examination order, x-ray machine, x-ray film and holder, x-ray film developer, drape, patient shield

Method

1. Check the x-ray examination order and equipment needed.
2. Identify the patient and introduce yourself.
3. Determine whether the patient has complied with the preprocedure instructions.
4. Explain the procedure and the purpose of the examination to the patient.
5. Instruct the patient to remove clothing and all metals (including jewelry) as needed, according to body area to be examined, and to put on a gown. Explain that metals may interfere with the image. Ask whether the patient has any surgical metal or a pacemaker, and report this

information to the radiologic technologist. Leave the room to ensure patient privacy.

Note: Steps 6 through 11 are nearly always performed by a radiologic technologist.

6. Position the patient according to the x-ray view ordered.
7. Drape the patient and place the patient shield appropriately.
8. Instruct the patient about the need to remain still and to hold the breath when requested.
9. Leave the room or stand behind a lead shield during the exposure.
10. Ask the patient to assume a comfortable position while the films are developed. Explain that x-rays sometimes must be repeated.
11. Develop the films.
12. If the x-ray films are satisfactory, instruct the patient to dress and tell the patient when to contact the physician's office for the results.
13. Label the dry, finished x-ray films, place them in a properly labeled envelope, and file them according to the policies of your office.
14. Record the x-ray examination, along with the final written findings, in the patient's chart.

---

asked to perform many of the duties described in Procedure 53-1. Although you are unlikely to position the patient, you should know that the position relative to the x-ray source determines the path of the x-rays and the sorts of images that result. Figure 53-2 illustrates common x-ray pathways and the images produced.

Common Diagnostic Radiologic Tests

A variety of radiologic imaging tests are available. Table 53-1 identifies some of the most frequently ordered tests and the disorders they are used to diagnose.

Contrast Media in Diagnostic Tests

Various procedures involve the use of contrast media to visualize body structures and observe their function. These procedures include angiography, arthrography, barium enema, barium swallow, cholangiography, cholecystography, fluoroscopy, intravenous pyelography, magnetic resonance imaging (sometimes), myelography, nuclear medicine studies, and retrograde pyelography.

As mentioned, contrast media can be administered by mouth, by needle or catheter into a blood vessel, or by a route that introduces the medium into an organ or body cavity (for example, into the colon). A contrast medium can cause adverse effects in some patients. Common adverse effects with oral agents include mild and transient abdominal cramping, constipation, nausea, vomiting, diarrhea, skin rashes, itching, heartburn, dizziness, and headache. Intravenous agents cause some of the same adverse effects as well as localized injection-site reactions and more serious reactions such as anaphylaxis. Because many contrast media contain iodine, a common allergen, patients should be questioned about known allergies to iodine or shellfish, which contain iodine, before procedures involving the use of contrast media. All patients should be observed during such procedures for signs of allergic reaction.

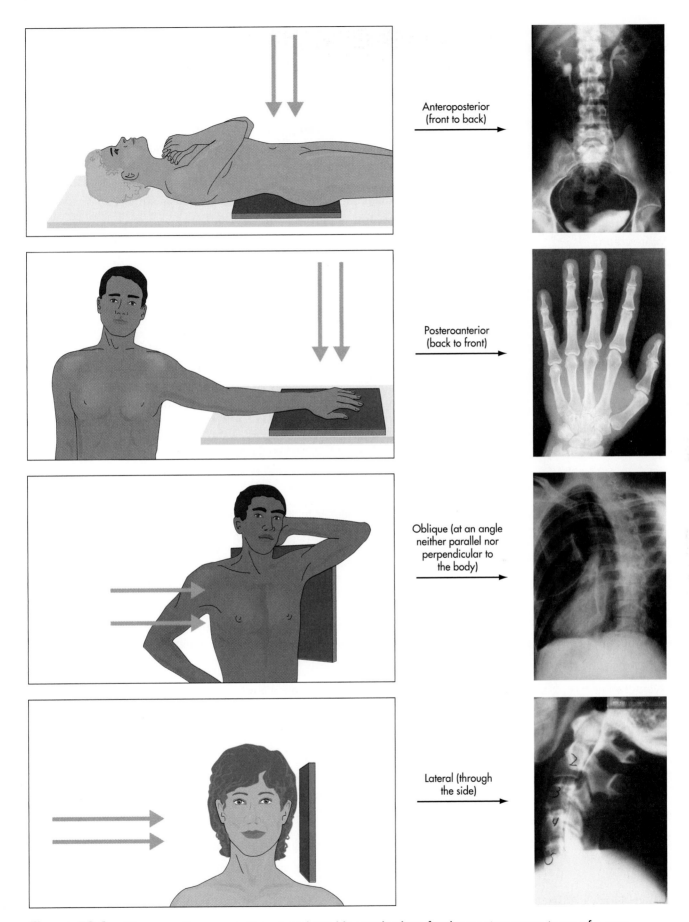

Figure 53-2. These are the x-ray pathways and resulting projections for the most common types of x-rays.

Anteroposterior
(front to back)

Posteroanterior
(back to front)

Oblique (at an angle
neither parallel nor
perpendicular to
the body)

Lateral (through
the side)

TABLE 53-1 Common Radiologic Tests and Disorders Diagnosed

Test	Disorders Diagnosed/Treated
Angiography	
Cardiovascular	Status of blood flow, collateral circulation, malformed vessels, aneurysm, narrowing or blockages of vessels, presence of hemorrhage
Cerebral	Aneurysm, hemorrhage, evidence of cerebrovascular accident, arteriosclerosis
Gastrointestinal (GI)	Upper gastrointestinal bleeding
Pulmonary	Pulmonary emboli (especially when lung scan is inconclusive), evaluation of pulmonary circulation in some heart conditions before surgery
Renal	Abnormalities of blood vessels in urinary system
Arthrography	Joint conditions
Barium enema (lower GI series)	Obstructions, ulcers, polyps, diverticulosis, tumor, and motility problems of colon or rectum
Barium swallow (upper GI series)	Obstructions, ulcers, polyps, diverticulosis, tumor, and motility problems of esophagus, stomach, duodenum, and small intestine
Cholangiography, cholecystography	Gallstones, gallbladder or common bile duct stones or obstructions; ability of gallbladder to concentrate and store dye
Computed tomography (CT)	Aortic and heart aneurysms, disorders of liver and biliary systems, renal and pulmonary tumors, brain abnormalities (tumors, blood clots, evidence of cerebrovascular accident, outlines of brain ventricles), GI tract lesions, GI disorders (acute pseudocyst of pancreas, abdominal abscesses, biliary obstruction), breast diseases and disorders, spinal disorders; to guide biopsy procedures
Fluoroscopy	Structure, process, and function of organs in motion to detect abnormalities
Intravenous pyelography (IVP) (excretory urography)	Urinary system abnormalities, including renal pelvis, ureters, and bladder (for example, kidney stones); abnormal size, shape, or structure of kidneys, ureters, or bladder; space-occupying lesions; pyelonephrosis; hydronephrosis; trauma to the urinary system
KUB (kidneys, ureters, bladder) radiography	Size, shape, and position of urinary organs; urinary system diseases or disorders; kidney stones
Magnetic resonance imaging (MRI)	Cancerous tissue, atherosclerotic tissue, blood clots, tumors, and deformities, particularly of the heart valves, brain, spine, and joints
Mammography	Breast tumors and lesions
Myelography	Irregularities or compression of spinal cord
Nuclear medicine (radionuclide imaging)	Abnormal function (defects), lesions, or disorders of bone, brain, lungs, kidneys, liver, pancreas, thyroid, and spleen
Radiation therapy	Treatment of cancer
Retrograde pyelogram	Obstruction of ureters, bladder, or urethra (including tumors, stones, strictures, or blood clots); perinephritic abscess
Stereoscopy	Fractures, dense areas that indicate a tumor or increased pressure within the skull
Thermography	Breast tumors, breast abscesses, fibrocystic breast disease
Ultrasound	Abnormalities of gallbladder, liver, spleen, heart, kidneys, gonads, blood vessels, and lymph system; fetal conditions (including number of fetuses; age and sex of fetus; fetal development, position, and deformities)
Xeroradiography	Breast cancer, abscesses, lesions, calcifications

Fluoroscopy

X-rays can cause certain chemicals to fluoresce, or emit visible light. When x-rays penetrate a body structure and are directed onto a fluorescent screen, they produce an image the radiologist can view either directly or through special glasses. Usually, fluoroscopic procedures are performed by a radiologist rather than by a radiology technician or a medical assistant.

Many diagnostic procedures involve fluoroscopy, which allows viewing of internal organ movement or the movement of a contrast medium, such as barium sulfate, while the contrast medium travels through the alimentary canal. Fluoroscopy also guides the radiologist in locating a precise internal area that needs to be recorded on film.

Fluoroscopic images are sometimes photographed for further study. Photofluorography is a series of these photographs that records the body's internal movements over time. Cinefluorography is a motion picture of the images.

Angiography

Angiography requires a physician (usually a radiologist) to insert a catheter into the patient's vein (venography) or artery (arteriography). The test may be performed jointly by a radiologist and a vascular surgeon or other specialist. Typically, the femoral, brachial, or carotid artery is evaluated. The physician guides the catheter tip to the vessel being examined. Then the physician injects a contrast medium through the catheter and takes a series of x-rays to assess the vessel's blood flow and condition.

Because this procedure requires insertion of a catheter into a blood vessel and the use of local anesthesia, the patient is admitted to a hospital or same-day surgical facility. The physician who performs the examination provides the patient with instructions immediately before the procedure. You will, however, schedule the procedure, and you can encourage the patient to ask questions. Radiology facilities usually have information sheets for each procedure. If the patient has questions you cannot answer or if you have any doubt about preprocedure instructions, check with your supervisor.

Arthrography

Arthrography is performed by a radiologist, who uses a contrast medium and fluoroscopy to help diagnose abnormalities or injuries in the cartilage, tendons, or ligaments of the joints—usually the knee or shoulder. When preparing patients for arthrography or assisting with the procedure, follow these guidelines:

- Describe the procedure to patients, and inform them that the examination will take about 1 hour. Ask patients about possible allergies to contrast media, iodine, or shellfish. If they have any of these allergies, inform the radiologist immediately.

- Explain to patients that no special preprocedure preparations are necessary.

- Tell patients the doctor will first inject a local anesthetic to numb the area being examined. Then the doctor will inject the contrast medium (dye, air, or both) into the joint and will use a fluoroscope to evaluate the joint's function. Inform patients who are having a knee examined that the doctor may ask them to walk a few steps to spread the contrast medium.

- After the test is completed, advise patients that for 1 or 2 days they may experience some pain or swelling, particularly if the joint is exercised. Tell them to rest and avoid putting strain on the joint.

Barium Enema (Lower GI Series)

A **barium enema** is performed by a radiologist, who instills barium sulfate through the anus into the rectum and then into the colon, to help diagnose and evaluate obstructions, ulcers, polyps, diverticulosis, tumors, or motility problems of the colon or rectum. This procedure is called a lower GI (gastrointestinal) series, a series of x-rays of the colon and rectum. The two types of barium enema techniques are single-contrast, in which only barium is instilled into the colon, and double-contrast, in which air is forced into the colon to distend the tissue. The air may be added while the barium is present, after it has been expelled, or both. The double-contrast technique makes structures more visible by fluoroscopy and allows identification of small lesions. The digestive tract must be totally empty, requiring the patient to thoroughly cleanse the tract with a series of preparatory steps and to have nothing by mouth for 8 hours before the test, except for one cup of clear liquid on the morning of the test. In most facilities a nurse assists with a barium enema, but you may assist the patient before and after the procedure. If you do assist with a barium enema, you will have various responsibilities before, during, and after the procedure.

Before the Procedure. Include the following steps when you instruct a patient about the preparation for a barium enema:

- Schedule the patient's appointment in the morning so he can sleep through most of the period during which his digestive tract must be empty and thus avoid experiencing hunger unnecessarily.

- Describe the procedure to the patient, and tell him the examination will take 1 to 2 hours. Ask about possible allergies to contrast media, iodine, or shellfish, and report such allergies to the radiologist.

- Explain to the patient the importance of following the preparation instructions so the colon and rectum are free of residual material. (Residual material in the colon or rectum could cause blockages or shadows, resulting in an inaccurate test.) Preprocedure preparation on the day before the examination includes following an all-liquid diet beginning in the morning (coffee, tea, carbonated beverages, sherbet, clear gelatin, strained fruit juice, bouillon, clear broths, or tomato juice; milk is not permitted) and taking pre-scribed amounts of electrolyte solution or other laxa-tive preparations and fluids on a specified schedule. Tell the patient he may have one cup of coffee, tea, or water on the morning of the examination.

During the Procedure.   Follow these steps when as-sisting during a barium enema:

- Have the patient undress and put on a gown.
- Tell the patient to expect some discomfort during the examination, as well as frequent side-to-side turning.
- Have the patient lie on his side. The radiologist inserts the enema tip, which is designed to help the patient hold the liquid, into the rectum and instills the barium sulfate into the colon. If the patient experiences cramp-ing or the urge to defecate during instillation of the barium, instruct him to relax the abdominal muscles by breathing slowly and deeply through the mouth.
- Instruct the patient to remain still and hold his breath when x-rays are taken. Using a fluoroscope, the doctor observes the barium as it flows through the lower bowel and periodically takes x-rays while the patient is placed in various positions. You may be asked to as-sist with placing the patient in these positions.
- Tell the patient if a double-contrast study is being per-formed. Explain that air will be introduced into the colon to expand the colon tissue. Also tell the patient that the combination of air and barium provides a clearer view of structures than only one contrast medium would provide and allows possible identifica-tion of small lesions if they are present.
- Tell the patient that when the doctor has completed the barium portion of the examination, including x-rays with both barium and air, the patient should use the toilet and expel as much barium as possible. Ex-plain that if enough barium is expelled, the doctor may take a final x-ray of the empty colon.
- Have the patient wait to dress until the doctor tells you that no additional x-rays are needed.

After the Procedure.   After the radiologist has com-pleted the barium enema, instruct the patient in postpro-cedure care. Tell the patient the following:

- He may now have a regular meal.
- The residual barium may make his stools appear whitish or lighter than usual, but this is normal.
- The barium may cause constipation, so he should drink extra water to help relieve constipation and to eliminate remaining barium sulfate. The physician may order a laxative to be taken if constipation is not relieved within 1 or 2 days.

Barium Swallow (Upper GI Series)

A **barium swallow** involves oral administration of a barium sulfate drink to help diagnose and evaluate

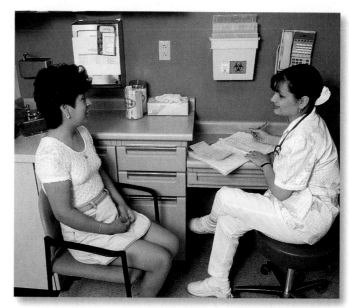

Figure 53-3.   Preprocedure instruction is essential to a successful barium swallow procedure.

obstructions, ulcers, polyps, diverticulosis, tumors, or motility problems of the esophagus, stomach, duodenum, and small intestine. This test is called an upper GI series. In preparation for this test, the patient can have nothing by mouth for at least 8 hours before the test. You will have various responsibilities before, during, and after the procedure.

Before the Procedure.   When instructing a patient about the preparation for an upper GI series (Figure 53-3), include the following steps:

- Schedule the patient's appointment in the morning so she can sleep through most of the period during which her digestive tract is empty and thus avoid experienc-ing hunger unnecessarily.
- Describe the procedure to the patient, and tell her the examination will take about 1 hour. If x-rays of the small bowel are needed, the test may take several hours. Ask about possible allergies to contrast media, iodine, or shellfish, and report such allergies to the radiologist.
- Explain to the patient the importance of following the preparation instructions so that the stomach is empty. Preprocedure requirements include having nothing by mouth (food or liquids) after midnight the night before the examination and no breakfast the morning of the examination. If the patient's small bowel is to be eval-uated, also tell her to take the prescribed laxative preparation between 2:00 and 4:00 P.M. the day before the examination.
- Instruct the patient not to swallow water when brush-ing her teeth or rinsing her mouth and, if applicable, to stop smoking, because nicotine stimulates gastric secretions and can affect the test results.

Radiographer/Sonographer

To gain medical assistant credentials, you must fulfill the requirements of either the American Association of Medical Assistants (for a Certified Medical Assistant) or the American Medical Technologists (for a Registered Medical Assistant). After obtaining your medical assistant certification or registration, you may wish to acquire additional skills in specialty areas through course work or on-the-job training. Although this course work or training may not lead to an additional certification or degree, it will enable you to expand your role in the medical office and advance your career as the demand for skilled health professionals increases.

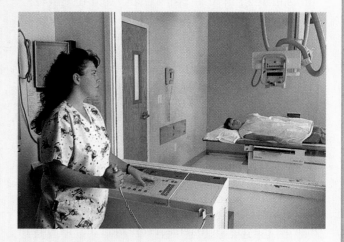

Skills and Duties

Radiographers and sonographers obtain images of internal organs, tissues, bones, and blood vessels. Physicians use these images to diagnose disease or to monitor health status.

A radiographer uses x-rays to produce the images. The radiographer positions the patient for imaging, covering parts of the body that are not to be x-rayed with a lead drape to protect them from the radiation. She then positions the x-ray machine, sets the controls, and makes the requested number of exposures.

The resulting black-and-white images can reveal whether a patient has a broken bone, tumor, ulcer, or other condition. Sometimes the radiographer or a physician administers a special material before the imaging process to make organs and blood vessels more visible on the x-ray film. The physician, usually a radiologist, examines the film and makes a diagnosis.

Sonographers use ultrasound machines that rely on sound waves rather than electromagnetic radiation to produce the images. The images are displayed on a television screen and can be videotaped or printed on film for further review by the physician.

The sonographer prepares the patient by applying a sound-enhancing gel. She then strokes the machine's handheld pad across the gel to create the image. She must be well-versed in anatomy to determine which parts of the image are important as she records measurements and data from the examination. Again, the physician uses the image to make a diagnosis and prescribe treatment if needed.

Sonographers can specialize in a variety of fields. Because sound waves are considered safe, sonography is frequently used in obstetrics and gynecology to take pictures of a fetus in the womb. Sonographers may also specialize in echocardiography, where they focus on heart problems.

Workplace Settings

Radiographers and sonographers most often work in hospitals. Some are employed in clinics, physicians' offices, and imaging centers. Radiographers may also work in dentists' offices, in mobile units, or in private industry. People in this field generally work 40-hour weeks, including some nights, weekends, and holidays.

Education

To become a radiographer or sonographer, you must complete an accredited 2- to 4-year program in radiography/sonography from an accredited vocational school, college, or university. (For those who are already employed in health care, a 1-year certificate program may be available.) Typically, such a program provides instruction in physics, biology, anatomy, medical terminology, radiation safety, and imaging techniques. The program may also include brief courses in nuclear medicine, computed tomography, magnetic resonance imaging, and radiation therapy—each of which can be further studied as a specialty.

After completing the program, you may take a national registry examination from the American Registry of Radiologic Technologists. The disciplines of sonography, nuclear medicine, and radiation therapy require a national registration examination for entry-level work. Radiographers must also have a license from the state to practice.

Where to Go for More Information

American Society of Radiologic Technologists
15000 Central Avenue SE
Albuquerque, NM 87123
(505) 298-4500

Society of Diagnostic Medical Sonographers
12770 Coit Road, Suite 508
Dallas, TX 75251
(214) 239-7367

During the Procedure. When assisting during an upper GI series, take the following steps:

- Have the patient undress and put on a gown.
- Explain to the patient that she will be drinking a barium sulfate drink that tastes chalky and resembles a milk shake.
- Have the patient stand and drink part of the barium. The radiologist will use a fluoroscope to observe the flow of the barium and to assess the functioning of the esophagus, stomach, duodenum, and small intestine as the barium passes through the structures. (The doctor will then direct the patient to drink additional barium and continue to observe the function of the various structures.)
- Place the patient on the x-ray table, and move her to different positions (if medical assistants are permitted to do so in your state) as instructed by the doctor, to allow x-rays to be taken of the upper digestive tract. Instruct the patient to remain still and hold her breath when x-rays are taken.

After the Procedure. After the physician completes the upper GI series, instruct the patient in postprocedure care. Give the patient the following information:

- She may now have a regular meal.
- Her stools may appear whitish or lighter than usual as the barium is eliminated, but this is normal.
- Sometimes another examination may be required after 24 hours to determine whether the barium has moved into the large intestine. If this test is indicated, tell the patient to follow a liquid diet (coffee, tea, carbonated beverages, sherbet, clear gelatin, strained fruit juices, bouillon, clear broths, or tomato juice; milk is not permitted) and to return in 24 hours.

Cholecystography and Cholangiography

Two similar tests performed by a radiologist are cholecystography and cholangiography. Both tests involve use of a contrast medium to view parts of the gallbladder.

Cholecystography. A radiologist uses cholecystography to detect gallstones and other abnormalities of the gallbladder. The doctor x-rays the patient's gallbladder after the patient has ingested an oral contrast medium. Cholecystography is usually used when ultrasound does not provide enough information for a diagnosis. You will be responsible for preparing the patient for the procedure and assisting during the procedure.

Before the Procedure. When instructing a patient about preparing for a cholecystography, follow these guidelines:

- Schedule the patient's appointment in the morning so he can sleep through most of the period during which

his digestive tract is empty and thus avoid experiencing hunger unnecessarily.

- Describe the procedure to the patient, and explain that the examination will take about 1 to 2 hours. Ask the patient about possible allergies to contrast media, iodine, or shellfish, and report them to the radiologist.
- Explain to the patient the diet restrictions necessary to prepare for the test. Tell the patient to have a fat-free dinner (dry toast, tea, fruit, gelatin dessert) the evening before the examination. He should not smoke or have any food or liquids after midnight, and he should have no breakfast the morning of the examination.
- Instruct the patient to take the oral contrast medium (usually in tablet form) beginning about 2 hours after dinner or as prescribed by the doctor. The tablets should be taken one at a time, 5 minutes apart, with a small amount of water, until six tablets have been taken. Explain to the patient that the contrast agent may cause nausea or diarrhea but that nothing should be taken for these conditions. In the case of severe nausea, the doctor may prescribe an antiemetic; diarrhea is an expected result of the contrast medium used for this test.
- Some doctors also order a laxative for the patient to take the day before the examination.

During and After the Procedure. When assisting during a cholecystography, take the following steps:

- Have the patient undress and put on a gown.
- Have the patient lie on the x-ray table in the supine position (face up).
- Explain that the radiologist will take x-rays of the gallbladder, which will be filled with the contrast medium the patient took the night before. Then the radiologist will use a fluoroscope to study the gallbladder's function. A functioning gallbladder absorbs the contrast agent properly.
- Next give the patient a specially prepared fatty meal, which should stimulate the gallbladder to empty bile into the duodenum. After about 1 hour, the doctor takes more x-rays to study the gallbladder's function. A functioning gallbladder empties the contrast medium properly. A nonfunctioning gallbladder may indicate, for example, the presence of gallstones or obstruction of the bile ducts.
- After the examination advise the patient to return to a normal diet and to drink plenty of fluids to replace those lost with diarrhea.

Cholangiography. Cholangiography is similar to cholecystography and is performed by a radiologist to evaluate the function of the bile ducts. It involves injection of the contrast medium directly into the common bile duct (during gallbladder surgery) or through a T tube (after gallbladder surgery or during radiologic testing). X-rays are taken immediately after injection. Use the guidelines for cholecystography. In addition, follow these steps:

- Describe the procedure to the patient, and tell him the examination will take about 2 to 3 hours. Ask the patient about possible allergies to contrast media, iodine, or shellfish, and report them to the radiologist.
- Explain the preparation instructions to the patient. Tell the patient to eat a light evening meal the night before the examination, to take a laxative (as prescribed by the doctor), and to have no food or liquids after midnight. He should also have no solid food the morning of the examination.

Conventional Tomography and Computed Tomography

Conventional tomography produces tomograms, and computed tomography produces CT scans. These two techniques are frequently confused. Computers are involved in producing both kinds of images, but the computers are different and have different functions.

Conventional tomography uses a computerized x-ray camera that moves back and forth in an arc over the patient to produce a series of views of a body part. The computer sets the angle and layer for each arc; the camera produces one view per arc.

In CT scans produced by computed tomography, the x-ray camera rotates completely around the patient, and the computer compiles one cross-sectional view from each rotation of the camera. The patient is lying on a special table that gradually moves through the doughnut-shaped machine containing the rotating camera. Figure 53-4 compares the two kinds of images (tomogram and CT scan) with those produced by x-ray, magnetic resonance imaging (MRI), and myelography.

The preparation is essentially the same for the two procedures. Reassure the patient that he will not be inserted into an enclosed space, as is the case in magnetic resonance imaging. The patient will be able to see around the room during the test.

Tomograms and CT scans are used to diagnose abnormalities in almost all body structures, including the head, kidneys, heart, chest, liver, biliary tract, pancreas, GI tract, spine, pelvis, bones, and breast. When preparing the patient for a tomogram or a CT scan, use the following guidelines:

- Ask the patient about possible allergies to contrast media, iodine, or shellfish, and report them to the radiologist.
- Tell the patient that he will be placed on a table that moves through the scanner for CT scans or on an x-ray table for tomograms.
- Inform the patient that the procedure will last about 45 to 90 minutes and that he must lie still while the scans are taken. The patient may breathe normally while the CT scans are taken but must hold his breath for each of the tomograms.

- If a contrast medium will be used, advise the patient that it will be injected into a vein in the arm or on the back of the hand (except with a CT scan of the spine) to enhance detail of the structure being evaluated.
- If the patient is having a CT scan of the head or chest, instruct him not to eat anything for 4 hours or drink any liquids for 2 hours before the examination. Explain that he may experience mild nausea after injection of the contrast medium if the stomach is too full.
- If the patient is having tomograms or a CT scan of the abdomen or pelvis, tell him to obtain a preparation kit from the office or hospital the day before the examination. This kit includes a special drink the patient must take the night before the examination that helps outline the intestines. Inform the patient that the drink should not produce a laxative effect or any discomfort.
- Tell the patient to remove metallic objects that could interfere with the path of the x-rays. Also, ask if the patient has skin staples or metallic prostheses that could interfere.
- Inform the patient that a written report of the results should be available within 24 hours of the test and that a report will be sent to his primary care physician (or the referring physician).

Heart X-Ray

An x-ray of the heart, using a contrast medium, may be necessary to show the configuration of the heart and to reveal cardiac enlargement and aortic dilation. Angiography of the heart is called angiocardiography, in which a contrast medium is injected into a major blood vessel. X-rays are taken while the medium flows through the heart, lungs, and major vessels. Coronary arteriography uses a dye inserted through a catheter that has been passed through an artery to the heart. Both procedures require hospital admission, usually in a day surgery or ambulatory surgery unit.

Intravenous Pyelography

Also known as excretory urography, **intravenous pyelography (IVP)** is performed by a radiologist who injects a contrast medium into a vein. The doctor then takes a series of x-rays as the contrast medium travels through the kidneys, ureters, and bladder. IVP is used to evaluate urinary system abnormalities or trauma to the urinary system. In most facilities a nurse assists with IVP, but you may assist the patient before the procedure. If you assist with IVP, you will have several responsibilities both before and during the procedure.

Before the Procedure. When instructing a patient about the preparation for an IVP, include the following steps:

- Schedule the patient's appointment in the morning so she can sleep through most of the period during which her digestive tract is empty and thus avoid experiencing hunger unnecessarily.

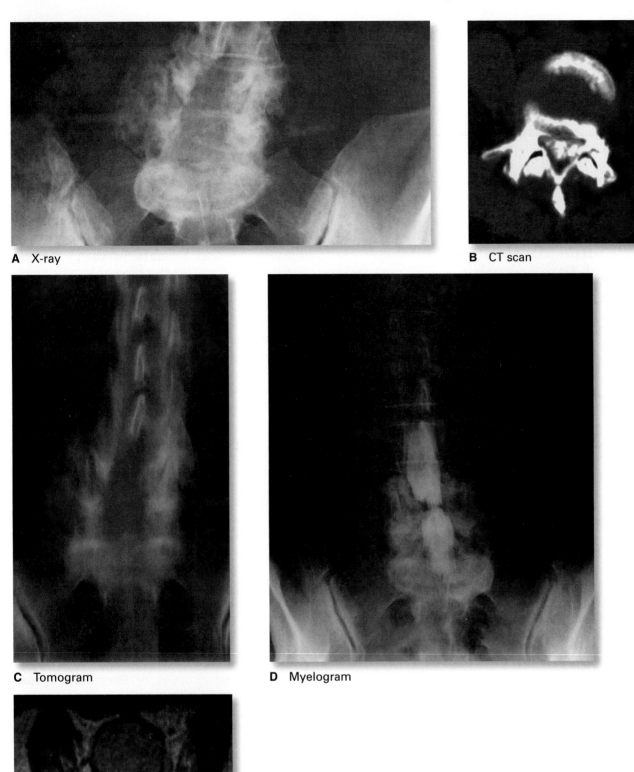

A X-ray

B CT scan

C Tomogram

D Myelogram

E MRI

Figure 53-4. These images of part of one patient's spine indicate scoliosis, degenerative disk disease, and osteoarthritis. Various techniques and x-ray pathways were involved: (a) x-ray, anteroposterior; (b) CT scan, full rotation; (c) tomogram, anteroposterior arc; (d) myelogram, posteroanterior; and (e) MRI, full rotation.

- Describe the procedure to the patient, and tell her that the examination will take about 1½ hours. Ask about possible allergies to contrast media, iodine, or shellfish, and report such allergies to the radiologist.
- Explain the importance of adhering to the preparation instructions, so that the bowel is free of any material that could obstruct the view of the urinary organs. Tell the patient to follow a liquid diet (coffee, tea, carbonated beverages, sherbet, clear gelatin, strained fruit juice, bouillon, clear broths, or tomato juice, but no milk) the day before the examination. The patient should take the prescribed amount of electrolyte solution or other laxative preparation as specified the night before the examination and have no food or liquids after midnight and no breakfast the morning of the examination. Some physicians also order an enema to be taken about 2 hours before the examination.

During and After the Procedure. When assisting during an IVP, you will generally proceed in this manner:

- Have the patient undress and put on a gown.
- Explain that a contrast medium will be injected into her vein (usually in the arm). Instruct her to inform the physician if she notices shortness of breath or itching after injection of the dye. This type of symptom can indicate an allergic reaction.
- Have the patient lie on the x-ray table, and move her to different positions as instructed by the physician, to allow x-rays to be taken of the urinary tract as the contrast medium is excreted. Instruct the patient to remain still and hold her breath when x-rays are taken.
- Note that some physicians place a compression device on the abdomen, which helps hold the contrast medium in the kidneys and ureters by exerting moderate pressure.
- After the physician takes the series of x-rays to evaluate urinary system function, ask the patient to urinate, and explain that a final x-ray will be taken.
- Inform the patient that she may resume a normal diet after the test and that the contrast medium will be eliminated in the urine.

Retrograde Pyelography

Retrograde pyelography is similar to the IVP, except that the doctor injects the contrast medium through a urethral catheter. This procedure, which evaluates function of the ureters, bladder, and urethra, is often used for patients with poor kidney function. Follow the same preparation and assistance instructions as for the IVP.

KUB (Kidneys, Ureters, and Bladder) Radiography

Also called a flat plate of the abdomen, **KUB radiography** is an x-ray of the abdomen used to assess the size, shape,

and position of the urinary organs; to evaluate urinary system diseases or disorders; and to determine the presence of kidney stones. It can also be helpful in determining the position of an intrauterine device (IUD) or in locating foreign bodies in the digestive tract. No patient preparation is required. A KUB x-ray is taken by a radiologic technologist; thus, you follow the guidelines you would use for a patient having any type of standard, noninvasive x-ray.

Magnetic Resonance Imaging (MRI)

Nonionizing radiation and a strong magnetic field are combined in magnetic resonance imaging to allow the physician to examine internal structures and soft tissues of any area of the body. The combination of nonionizing radiation and magnetic field, which allows the MRI scanner to produce images based primarily on the water content of tissues, appears to have no harmful effects on the patient. The test may be performed with or without contrast. You will be responsible for preparing the patient for an MRI and assisting with the procedure.

Before the Procedure. When instructing a patient about preparing for an MRI, include the following steps:

- If a contrast medium is going to be used, ask the patient and inform the radiologist about possible allergies to contrast media, iodine, or shellfish.
- Screen the patient to determine whether any internal metallic materials are present. (This is especially important because a magnetic field is involved in creating the image.) Ask about a pacemaker, brain or aneurysm clips, brain or heart surgery, shunts and heart valves, other surgeries, and shrapnel or metal fragments (particularly in an eye).
- Ask the patient whether he is or has been a metalworker. If so, he may carry metal slivers, chips, or filings under his nails or skin.
- Describe the procedure to the patient, and explain that the examination will take between 45 minutes and 2 hours.
- Tell the patient he does not need to fast before the examination or follow any preprocedure diet, unless he is having an MRI of the pelvis. In that case instruct him to have no solid food for 6 hours and no liquids for 4 hours before the examination. Inform the patient that he may take prescription medications.
- Explain that he will not be required to drink an oral contrast preparation but that he should avoid caffeine for 4 hours before the examination. (Instruct women not to wear eye makeup the day of the examination, because eye makeup often contains metallic ingredients.)
- Tell the patient that he will probably have no side effects from the examination but that some nausea may occur as a result of the contrast medium.

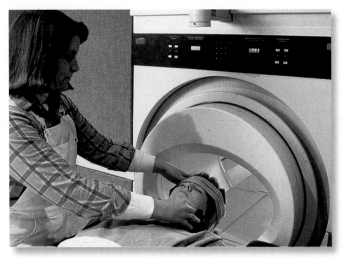

Figure 53-5. A patient who is claustrophobic or unable to lie still may require sedation during an MRI.

During and After the Procedure. When assisting during an MRI, you will need to follow these specific steps:

- Inform the patient that he may wear street clothing, unless it has metallic thread, metal stays or grippers, or thick elastic. Tell the patient that he will probably be asked to undress, however, and put on a gown.

- Have the patient lie on the padded table.

- Explain that the table will be placed inside a long, narrow tube about 22 inches in diameter and that he will hear a loud knocking noise as the machine scans. Warn the patient to remain still to avoid blurring the image and the consequent need for a retake. Note that physicians commonly order sedation for patients who are claustrophobic or cannot lie still for a long period (Figure 53-5).

- Advise the patient that although the technician will not be in the scanning room during the examination, she will maintain contact with a camera and a microphone. The patient may speak to the technician at any time in case of a problem, but he is encouraged to be still for each series.

- Inform the patient that his primary care physician or referring doctor should have a preliminary report of test results within about 24 hours.

Mammography

Mammography, the x-ray examination of the internal breast tissues, helps in diagnosing breast abnormalities (Figure 53-6). A specially trained radiologic technologist takes mammograms. Types of mammography include film-screen, thermography, diaphanography, and ultrasonography (ultrasound). Diaphanography is produced by directing a high-intensity light through the breast or soft tissue; images are then produced on a screen (a process called transillumination). Unlike other forms of mammography, diaphanography does not require ionizing radiation.

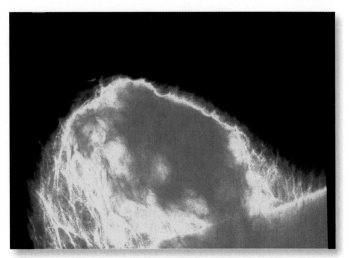

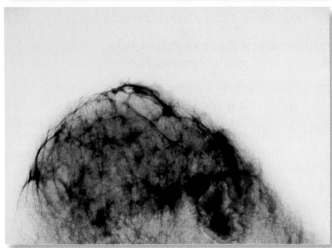

Figure 53-6. Mammograms can reveal the presence of tumors that are not detected by other means. The upper mammogram indicates normal breast tissue, whereas the lower suggests a malignancy.

You will have several responsibilities during both setup and patient care before and after mammography. A medical assistant does not assist during mammography in most states. Instead, you will prepare the patient for the procedure and ease her fears. The Educating the Patient section provides information on this topic.

Mammotest Biopsy Procedure

When a mammogram reveals an abnormality in the breast tissue, it is often treated in one of two ways—either the abnormality is followed for a period of time to see if there are any significant changes or a surgical excision biopsy is performed. Because so many abnormalities revealed by mammography are benign and present no health risk, physicians now perform stereotactic breast biopsies, which are less painful and less invasive than conventional excisional biopsies. The procedure is performed by a physician and a radiologic technologist and is similar to mammography except that the patient is lying face down rather than standing. The breast is compressed with a

Educating the Patient

Preprocedure Care for Mammography

A patient who is scheduled for mammography must know the guidelines to follow before the examination. You can help educate the patient by instructing her in the following preprocedure care:

- The mammography should be scheduled for the first week after the patient's menstrual cycle. This timing helps minimize discomfort from compression of the breasts and ensures that the breasts are in their most normal state.

- No special preprocedure diet or medication requirements are necessary, but the patient should consider avoiding caffeine for 7 to 10 days before the examination (in some patients caffeine may cause swelling and soreness that would heighten discomfort during the procedure). Have the patient decrease caffeine intake gradually, however, to avoid getting headaches.

- The patient should shower or bathe as close as possible to the time of the mammography and wear loose clothing that is easy to remove. A blouse and pants or skirt work best to allow undressing only to the waist.

- The patient should not use deodorants, powders, or perfumes on the breasts or underarm areas

before the examination, because these products could produce a false result on the x-ray.

In addition to providing these instructions, you may need to reassure a patient who is fearful about mammography. Explain that although mammography is uncomfortable, it is usually not painful. Describing how the procedure is performed may alleviate the patient's fears. Provide the patient with the following information:

- The procedure usually takes 15 to 20 minutes.
- A lead apron will be placed on the patient's abdominal area to protect her from unnecessary radiation exposure.
- The patient will be positioned in front of the machine. The technician will compress the left breast between the machine plates and take two x-rays—one horizontal view and one vertical view—of the left breast.
- The technician will then position and compress the right breast between the machine plates. Two x-rays will be taken of the right breast.
- If needed, the physician may order a mild pain reliever after the procedure to alleviate discomfort or aching.

compression paddle to confirm that the area of the breast with the lesion is correctly centered in the paddle window. A computer is used to help determine the exact positioning of the biopsy needle, and the physician takes a small sample of tissue to be examined by a pathologist for the presence of malignant cells. The attending physician later contacts the patient with the test results.

Myelography

Myelography is a kind of fluoroscopy of the spinal cord. The physician performs a lumbar puncture, removes some cerebrospinal fluid (CSF), and instills a contrast medium to evaluate spinal abnormalities, such as compression of the spinal cord. Sometimes the physician performs pneumoencephalography, which involves instilling air after removal of the CSF to allow visualization of the cerebral cavities.

The physician who performs myelography or pneumoencephalography must be skilled in performing lumbar puncture—most likely a radiologist, neurologist, neurosurgeon, or anesthetist. A radiologic technologist is typically the only other person present for the test. Although

myelography is not used as frequently as it was before the invention of CT and MRI, it is still performed when these newer techniques do not provide enough information about the spinal canal. Myelography may be reserved for cases in which the clinical findings are unusual or the scanning results uncertain.

Nuclear Medicine

Also known as radionuclide imaging, **nuclear medicine** involves use of radionuclides, or radioisotopes (radioactive elements or their compounds). The radionuclides are administered orally, intravenously, or through routes that introduce them into organs or body cavities. The purpose is to evaluate the bone, brain, lungs, kidneys, liver, pancreas, thyroid, or spleen. Sometimes the entire body is scanned for "hot spots," or places where the radioisotope is concentrated.

For common nuclear medicine scans, the technician uses a scanner called a gamma camera. This scanner detects radiation from the radioisotope and converts it into an image (called a scintiscan or scintigram) to be photographed or displayed on a screen (see Figure 53-7). Some

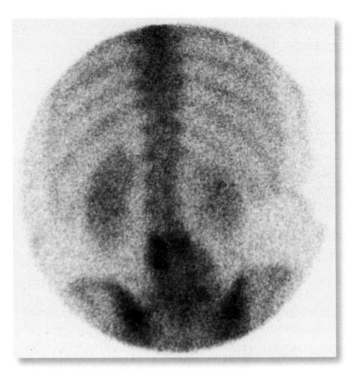

Figure 53-7. This bone scan of the spine (same patient as in Figure 53-4) shows the uptake of the radioactive contrast medium, which is darkest in the areas of inflammation.

images are produced immediately, whereas others may take up to several days. Radionuclide imaging exposes patients to lower doses of radiation than some radiologic techniques, because the amount of ionizing radiation in the isotope is less than that emitted from x-ray cameras.

Other nuclear medicine procedures include single photon emission computed tomography (SPECT), positron emission tomography (PET), and MUGA (multiple gated acquisition) scan.

- **SPECT** is often used to locate and determine the extent of brain damage from a stroke. The gamma camera detects signals induced by gamma radiation, and a computer converts these signals into either two- or three-dimensional images that are displayed on a screen.
- **PET** entails injecting isotopes combined with other substances involved in metabolic activity, such as glucose. These special isotopes emit positrons, which a computer processes and displays on a screen. PET is especially useful for diagnosing brain-related conditions, such as epilepsy, mental illnesses, and Parkinson's disease.
- The **MUGA scan** evaluates the condition of the heart's myocardium. It can be done while the patient is at rest or in stress (exercise) and involves the injection of radioisotopes that concentrate in the myocardium. The gamma camera allows the physician to measure ventricular contractions to evaluate the patient's heart wall.

When preparing a patient for a nuclear medicine procedure, describe the procedure and tell her how long the examination will take. Explain any preparation requirements and other special instructions, and tell the patient she will need to wait the required length of time for the uptake of the radioisotope. Length of examination and requirements for common scans are as follows:

- A bone scan lasts about 1 hour; it is done 2 to 3 hours after a 15-minute injection; the patient drinks 1 quart of liquid between the injection and the scan; a normal diet is permitted
- A liver/spleen or lung scan lasts approximately 1 hour; there are no diet restrictions
- A kidney scan lasts about 2 hours; there are no diet restrictions
- A thyroid uptake and scan test usually requires 2 days; the patient takes a capsule of contrast medium in the morning and has the scan on the first day; the patient returns 24 hours later for the second scan; there are no diet restrictions, except that the patient must have no fish because of its natural iodine content

Stereoscopy

Used primarily to study the skull, **stereoscopy** is an x-ray procedure that uses a specially designed microscope (stereoscopic, or Greenough, microscope) with double eyepieces and objectives to take films at different angles. Stereoscopy identifies fractures and dense areas to produce three-dimensional images. The images, which have depth as well as height and width, can indicate a tumor or increased pressure within the skull. No special preparation is required. Follow the guidelines you would use with any other noninvasive x-ray.

Thermography

Thermography is performed to diagnose breast tumors, breast abscesses, and fibrocystic breast disease. The procedure uses an infrared camera to take photographs that record variations in skin temperature as dark (cool areas), light (warm areas), or shades of gray (areas with temperatures between cool and warm). Tumors or inflammations produce more heat than healthy tissues and therefore show up lighter on these photographs; areas with lack of circulation are cooler than tissues with adequate circulation and show up as dark. Because no preparation requirements are necessary for this test, you need only to schedule the procedure and to assist as needed with reassurance during the examination.

Ultrasound

Ultrasound directs high-frequency sound waves through the skin over the area of the body being examined and produces an image based on the echoes. A radiologist or

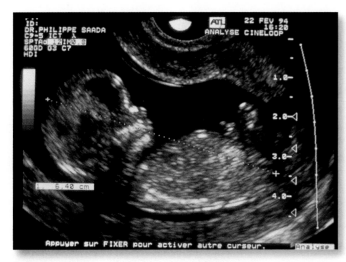

Figure 53-8. Ultrasound is commonly used to evaluate the health of a developing fetus.

an ultrasound radiologic technologist coats the body area with a special gel and passes a transducer (instrument similar to a microphone) over the area. As the transducer passes back and forth over the area, it picks up echoes from the sound waves, which a computer converts into an image on a screen. Ultrasound is used to detect abnormalities in the gallbladder, liver, spleen, heart, and kidneys. It is also safe to use in obstetrics to evaluate the developing fetus or to detect multiple fetuses, because it does not expose the patient (or the fetus) to radiation (Figure 53-8). In this case the obstetrician may perform the test in the office.

One form of ultrasound, called Doppler echocardiography, involves sound waves that echo against the flow of blood through vessels. Doppler echocardiography is usually performed by a cardiologist to determine whether blood flow is laminar (normal) or turbulent (disturbed).

When preparing the patient for an ultrasound or assisting with the examination, follow these guidelines:

- Describe the procedure to the patient and inform her that the examination will take about ½ to 2 hours, depending on the type of ultrasound. For example, a cardiac ultrasound takes about 1½ hours; pelvic, 1 to 2 hours; and abdominal, ½ to 1 hour.
- Explain the preparation requirements, which vary according to the type of ultrasound. Tell a patient who is having a gallbladder or liver ultrasound not to eat for several hours before the test. Tell a pregnant patient to drink the prescribed amount of water 1 hour before the examination and not to void. Advise a patient having a pelvic ultrasound to take the prescribed laxative (if indicated), drink three to four glasses of water within 1 hour, and not to void within 1 hour of the test. If the patient is having an abdominal ultrasound, instruct her to take a laxative the night before the examination and not to have any food or fluids for 8 hours before the test.

- Advise the patient to wear loose clothing that is easy to remove.

Xeroradiography

Xeroradiography is used to diagnose breast cancer, abscesses, lesions, and calcifications. The xeroradiographic x-rays are developed with a powder toner, similar to the toner in photocopiers, and the image is processed on specially treated xerographic paper. Xeroradiography uses lower exposure times and less radiation than standard x-rays.

Common Therapeutic Uses of Radiation

Used therapeutically, radiology is called **radiation therapy.** Radiation therapy is used to treat cancer by preventing cellular reproduction. The two types of radiation therapy are teletherapy and brachytherapy. **Teletherapy** allows deep penetration and is used primarily for deep tumors; it is done on an outpatient basis. The patient experiences minimal side effects, and superficial tissues are not damaged.

Localized cancers are treated with **brachytherapy.** In this technique the radiologist places temporary radioactive implants close to or directly into cancerous tissue. Both the staff and patient are subject to radiation exposure. Therefore, radiation safety precautions must be closely followed. When preparing the patient for radiation therapy, follow these guidelines:

- Describe the procedure to the patient, and explain how long the procedure will take, as determined by the radiologist and oncologist according to the diagnosis and the condition of the patient.
- Inform the patient that the radiologist or oncologist will explain the possible side effects of the treatment. Common side effects include nausea, vomiting, hair loss, ulceration of mucous membranes, weakness, and malaise. Other possible effects include localized burns on tissue and damage to organs in the path of treatment. Encourage the patient to discuss with the doctor (or the oncology nurse specialist) measures to relieve or minimize stress and discomfort.
- Advise the patient to immediately report any other symptoms to the doctor.

Radiation Safety and Dose

For many years after the discovery of the x-ray, the seriousness of radiation hazards was not addressed. In the 1920s the government of Great Britain took the first steps to limit x-ray exposure. Since World War II, studies have been performed, mostly on the effects of high-dose radiation.

Other studies on the effects of background radiation and nonradiologic versus radiologic (x-ray–related) risks have enabled scientists to assess the risks of diagnostic x-rays. Results from these studies show the risk of excess radiation from routine x-rays to be minimal.

Reducing Patient Exposure

Advances in diagnostic imaging technology, as well as limits to radiation exposure, have helped reduce the dose of radiation to which a patient is exposed during a diagnostic procedure. Another way to reduce the risk of excessive radiation exposure lies with the physician, who must assess the benefit-to-risk ratio when recommending a diagnostic radiology procedure. Because radiation has a cumulative effect, the physician must have valid medical reasons for ordering the test, particularly if the patient has recently had other x-rays. Some types of x-rays, such as mammograms, should be repeated regularly, however, because of their potential to prevent or promote treatment of life-threatening disorders.

According to a 1993 report by the National Council on Radiation Protection and Measurements (NCRP) titled *Limitation of Exposure to Ionizing Radiation,* one of the earliest pieces of legislation in the United States to limit occupational radiation exposure was enacted in the 1930s. The first legislation to limit public exposure, however, was not enacted until the 1950s. The NCRP report of 1993 set guidelines for protection from radiation in and out of the workplace. The two primary objectives outlined in the report are to prevent serious general tissue damage from radiation by limiting radiation dose to levels below known thresholds for such damage and to reduce the risk of cancer and genetic effects to a level that is balanced by potential benefits to the individual and society.

Because exposure to radiation always poses some degree of risk, the NCRP recommends that any activity involving radiation exposure be justified, or balanced against the expected benefits to society. Furthermore, the NCRP recommends that the cost, or detriment, to society from such activities be kept *as low as reasonably achievable* (ALARA) and that individual dose limits be applied to ensure that justification and ALARA principles do not result in unacceptable levels of risk for individuals or groups.

The NCRP has developed detailed lists on radiation doses to achieve the primary objectives stated in the report. There are separate specific limits for occupational exposure and public exposure.

Safety Precautions

Understanding and following standard safety precautions are crucial for protection from radiation exposure. These precautions are essential to the health and safety of both medical personnel and patients.

Personnel Safety. If you work in a medical facility that performs radiologic tests, you are at risk for excessive

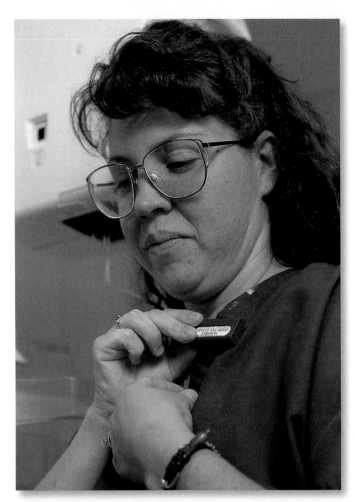

Figure 53-9. A radiation exposure badge contains a film that registers the levels of radiation to which a medical staff member is exposed at work.

radiation exposure. To protect yourself from radiation exposure, you must adhere to the following specific guidelines:

- You (and other members of the medical staff) must always wear a radiation exposure badge, or dosimeter, which is a sensitized piece of film in a holder (Figure 53-9). You must have the badge checked regularly by specially qualified personnel, who measure the degree of radiation uptake on the film to determine the amount of radiation to which you have been exposed.

- Make sure that all equipment is in good working order and is checked routinely for radiation leakage and any other problems.

- Be aware that the technician and any other staff members present when equipment is operating should always wear a garment that contains a lead shield.

Patient Safety. You must follow all rules governing patient safety from radiation exposure. The Educating the Patient section explains safety measures and information that help protect a patient from exposure to unnecessary radiation.

Educating the Patient

Safety With X-Rays

You are responsible for teaching the patient about x-ray safety. You will need to obtain pertinent patient history data, answer questions, and provide basic information on x-rays, possible side effects, and other important guidelines. Consider the following points when teaching the patient about x-ray safety.

Patient History

- Ask the patient about x-rays received in the past, including how many and what type, and about the possibility of exposure to radiation in the home, school, or workplace. Explain that the effects of radiation exposure are cumulative; that is, the effects are related to total exposure over the lifetime as well as to exposure from each procedure.

- Ask a female patient about the possibility of pregnancy. Use the 10-day rule—take an x-ray only within 10 days of the last menstrual period to avoid taking an x-ray of a patient who is unknowingly pregnant. If the patient knows that she is pregnant, do not schedule an x-ray unless approved by the radiologist.

- Inform the patient about possible side effects of radiation exposure. These effects include fetal abnormality or genetic mutation in a fetus (when a patient is pregnant) and the depression of bone marrow activity, which decreases the production of red blood cells and white blood cells.

Patient Questions

- Always answer questions in simple, easy-to-understand language; make explanations brief and clear. Do not use complex medical terms; however, do include proper terminology. Offer written information about the test, if available.

- Answer fully any questions about examinations, including descriptions of procedures; the doctor's reason for ordering them; their length, side effects, injections or other uncomfortable aspects; preprocedure requirements; cost and insurance issues; and availability of test results.

- Help the patient reduce fear or anxiety surrounding the scheduled test and feel comfortable and informed about the procedure.

General X-Ray Information

- Be aware of the most current guidelines established by the American College of Radiology. Always keep up with new studies on the risks of radiation exposure.

- Encourage the patient to ask questions about the need for x-rays ordered by the doctor and risks associated with those x-rays.

- If the patient's employer requires annual x-rays or a potential employer asks for preemployment x-rays, advise the patient to question the necessity of these tests. Suggest that the patient find out whether the doctor has x-rays on file that could be submitted.

- Advise the patient to discuss testing options with the doctor. For instance, if the doctor orders fluoroscopy, the patient might ask whether standard x-rays can be taken instead, because fluoroscopy often represents a higher risk for exposure to radiation than do standard x-rays. (Mobile x-ray examinations often pose a higher exposure risk as well.)

- Advise the patient to ask questions about x-ray safety standards in the office or hospital in which the tests are to take place.

- Tell the patient to avoid dental x-rays that are performed with wide-beamed plastic cones; narrow-beamed cones are more exact and less dangerous. In addition, educate the patient about the opinions of the American Dental Association and the National Conference of Dental Radiology, both of which believe that x-rays should not be performed solely for insurance claim purposes.

- Advise the patient to always ask for a lead apron over organs not being studied.

- Tell the patient to avoid retakes of x-rays because of blurriness or shadows (which are caused by movements or breathing) by remaining still when instructed to do so during x-ray examinations.

- Explain to the patient the importance of x-rays in proper diagnosis of disorders. Inform the patient about the constant improvements in equipment and x-ray procedures and the much lower doses of radiation now used in these procedures.

- Advise the patient to keep a family record of x-ray examinations.

- Educate a female patient without breast disease on the correct schedule for mammography examinations. The patient should have a baseline mammogram between ages 35 and 40; a mammogram every 1 to 2 years between ages 40 and 49; and an annual mammogram after age 50.

- Also tell the patient to see a doctor immediately if she notices a breast mass, lump, or nipple discharge.

deliver a drug. Researchers hope to expand this technology to other parts of the body, such as the liver or blood vessels.

Summary

Diagnostic tests are an important part of medical care because they help doctors diagnose a variety of diseases and disorders. As a medical assistant, you will be asked to assist with patient care before, and sometimes during and after, diagnostic radiology procedures. Your responsibilities include providing instructions and explanations to patients, preparing patients for various tests, and assisting the doctor or technician with the procedures. Your duties may also include storing and filing x-rays.

Safety is a vital concern with radiologic tests. Understanding and following safety precautions will help you ensure your patients' health and well-being as well as your own.

CHAPTER 53

CASE STUDY QUESTIONS

Now that you have completed this chapter, review the case study at the beginning of the chapter and answer the following questions:

1. What special instructions should be given to the patient before her mammogram?
2. How is a CT scan performed?
3. When preparing a patient for a CT scan, what allergies should be disclosed during the patient interview?
4. Why was a mammotest requested by the physician?
5. What education requirements must you fulfill in order to work as a radiographer/sonographer?

Discussion Questions

1. Which common diagnostic radiologic tests may be ordered for gastrointestinal complaints and symptoms?
2. What special preprocedure instructions should be provided to a patient scheduled for a mammogram?
3. What guidelines must be followed for the proper storage of x-rays?

Critical Thinking Questions

1. What are the differences between invasive and noninvasive diagnostic radiology tests?
2. In general, what preprocedure care should be given to patients for whom radiology procedures have been ordered?

3. When scheduling a patient for an MRI, you must note whether the patient has any internal metallic elements (such as a pacemaker, clips, pins, shrapnel, etc.). Explain why this information is important.
4. A patient who is scheduled for a series of x-rays tells you he is concerned about the amount of radiation he will be receiving. What would you say to ease this patient's fears?

Application Activities

1. Write a list of instructions to give to a patient who is going to have an upper GI series. Exchange lists with a classmate, and evaluate each other's work.
2. With another student, role-play a situation in which a medical assistant is preparing a patient for an MRI of the pelvis. Then switch roles and critique each other's technique.
3. With another student, role-play a situation in which a medical assistant is training a new coworker in how to document and file x-rays. Have your classmate evaluate the thoroughness of your instructions.

MEDICAL ASSISTANT PROGRAM

EXTERNSHIP TRAINING PLAN

NAME:	INTERNSHIP PERIOD: / / TO / /
SITE NAME:	ADDRESS:
ON-SITE EMPLOYER REPRESENTATIVE:	PHONE #:

DIRECTIONS: THIS TRAINING PLAN WILL SERVICE TO SPECIFY THE APPLICATIONS AND EXPERIENCES THAT ARE TO BE SECURED DURING THEIR TRAINING. UPON COMPLETION OF THEIR TRAINING, PLEASE INDICATE YOUR APPRAISAL OF THE STUDENTS' PERFORMANCE BY DRAWING A CIRCLE AROUND THE NUMBER CORRESPONDING WITH THE ACHIEVEMENT LEVEL AS FOLLOWS:

1 = UNSATISFACTORY, 2 = FAIR, 3 = VERY GOOD, 4 = OUTSTANDING.

CIRCLE THE UA IF THE STUDENT WILL BE UNAVAILABLE TO DO THIS PROCEDURE, AND THE NA IF THIS IS NOT APPLICABLE TO THE STUDENTS' STUDIES.

EXTERNSHIP GOALS & OBJECTIVES/PERFORMANCE RATING SCALE

DURING THE EXTERNSHIP PERIOD, THE STUDENT WILL:

A.	DEVELOP EFFECTIVE "FRONT OFFICE" SKILLS INCLUSIVE OF SUCH ACTIVITIES AS; PATIENT COMMUNICATION, MEDICAL RECORDS, BILLING & COLLECTIONS, INSURANCE PROCESSING, AND COMPUTERIZED BUSINESS FUNCTIONS	1	2	3	4	UA	NA
B.	ACCURATELY MEASURE AND RECORD VITAL SIGNS, UTILIZING PROPER TECHNIQUE	1	2	3	4	UA	NA
C.	PERFORM STANDARD EKG RECORDING/ MOUNTING PER SITE PROTOCOL	1	2	3	4	UA	NA
D.	DEVELOP PROFICIENCY IN PARENTERAL MEDICATION ADMINISTRATION (INTRADERMAL, SUBQ, INTRAMUSCULAR)	1	2	3	4	UA	NA
E.	DEVELOP PROFICIENCY AND TECHNIQUE IN PERFORMING VENIPUNCTURE USING THE EVACUATED TUBE SYSTEM	1	2	3	4	UA	NA
F.	DEMONSTRATE EFFECTIVE SPECIMEN COLLECTION TECHNIQUE AND DIAGNOSTIC PROCEDURES (i.e., URINALYSIS, BLOOD SUGAR, CHOLESTEROL, ETC.)	1	2	3	4	UA	NA

SIDE 1 OF 2

Figure 54-4. A form such as this one may be used by the clinical preceptor to evaluate a student's externship performance. (continued)

PROFESSIONAL ATTRIBUTES	PERFORMANCE RATING SCALE					
A. ORAL COMMUNICATIONS	1	2	3	4	UA	NA
B. ORGANIZATION & SAFETY	1	2	3	4	UA	NA
C. DEPENDABILITY & SELF-DIRECTION	1	2	3	4	UA	NA
D. COOPERATIVENESS	1	2	3	4	UA	NA
E. RECORDKEEPING	1	2	3	4	UA	NA
F. COLLABORATIVENESS/TEAMWORK	1	2	3	4	UA	NA
G. PATIENT RAPPORT/CONSIDERATION	1	2	3	4	UA	NA
H. ATTENDANCE/PUNCTUALITY	1	2	3	4	UA	NA

WHAT IS YOUR OVERALL OPINION OF THIS STUDENT'S PERFORMANCE?

( ) UNSATISFACTORY ( ) POOR ( ) FAIR ( ) GOOD ( ) VERY GOOD ( ) OUTSTANDING

THIS WILL CERTIFY THAT THE INTERN HAS COMPLETED ( ) HOURS AT THE SITE.

COMMENTS:

ON-SITE EVALUATOR'S SIGNATURE: _____

DATE: _____

SIDE 2 OF 2

THIS PAGE IS STRICTLY FOR THE USE OF EDUCATION

TOTAL GOALS AND OBJECTIVE POINTS		_____/_____
# OBJECTIVES EVALUATED	=	_____ AVG POINTS
TOTAL ATTRIBUTE POINTS		_____/_____
# ATTRIBUTES EVALUATED	=	_____ AVG POINTS

AVERAGE OF TOTAL POINTS = _____

GRADE POINT SCALE

A = 3.5–4.0

B = 2.5–3.4

C = 2.0–2.4

F = 1.9 OR LESS   FINAL GRADE = _____

PROGRAM DIRECTOR SIGNATURE: _____

DATE: _____

Figure 54-4. (continued)

improve that performance. You are not expected to know everything on your externship, but you are expected to be open to suggestions and ideas. It is not considered professional to question clinical preceptors during the learning experience. You may be exposed to some procedures that are not performed exactly as you were taught. Do not argue with preceptors about their skills. There is usually more than one way to get the desired result in patient care.

Your behavior is expected to be as professional as if you were an employee there. Foul language and inappropriate conversation is not tolerated in any workplace. You are expected to be professional with the patients under all circumstances. Medical facilities expect you to demonstrate empathy and compassion to every patient. Proper verbal skills and grammar are expected at all times. Do not use slang when communicating with office staff and patients. Personal phone calls should not be made during working hours; do not use the facility phone. Cell phones and pagers should be turned off during working hours.

Attendance.

You are expected to report to your externship *every day* that you are assigned to a schedule. It is your responsibility to have several alternates to baby-sitting and transportation. Employers are seeking dependable and punctual medical staff and would not tolerate attendance problems with their own staff. In the event of an emergency, you are expected to report a call-off to the medical facility and the school two hours before the beginning of your shift, as would any other employee. Many medical facilities will not tolerate absenteeism or tardiness from an externship student, and they may ask the school to remove the student from the site.

Adhere to the facility's policy regarding breaks. Take breaks only when it is appropriate to do so. If you smoke, refrain from smoking during working hours and do not smoke in patient entrances. Lunch breaks are permitted under facility policies.

Professional Appearance.

Medical facilities expect you to appear as a medical professional. Most require a uniform that consists of a scrub top and bottom and a lab jacket. Your scrubs should be clean, pressed, and well fitting. Shoes should be clean, white, and in good repair. Your name tag or badge should always be worn and visible to patients. Nails should be trimmed and polished in good taste in pale and neutral colors. Many medical facilities will not accept students with artificial nails, such as acrylics. Facial and tongue piercings are not acceptable when working with patients, and visible tattoos must be covered. Your hair should be a natural color and pulled back from your face and off your collar. Makeup should be conservative and in good taste. Perfumes and colognes should be avoided because patients with respiratory conditions or allergies may not be able to tolerate them.

Remember that you as a medical assisting student on an externship represent several things:

- The school you attend. It is important to maintain a good reputation in the medical community. You will depend on the reputation of the school to obtain a job.
- The profession of medical assisting. Participating in a medical assisting externship gives you an opportunity to represent the profession of medical assisting to patients and the community.
- Yourself. First impressions are lasting impressions. Make your first impression to the medical community an outstanding one.

Initiative and Willingness to Learn.

During your externship, accept all assignments with enthusiasm and grace, no matter how mundane. These tasks are often a test on how well you accept orders and work within a medical team. Ask for additional work if you are idle, and look for tasks that need to be done. Keep a notebook and record the office policies and procedures. Be prepared to observe and participate in office procedures.

Preparing to Find a Position

The next phase of beginning your new career is seeking a position as a medical assistant. Most accredited schools have a career services department. Its primary focus is job placement after graduation. The department's counselors will assist you in writing your résumé, improving your interviewing skills, and learning about positions in your field. Many employers will contact a school's career services department to recruit medical personnel. It is important to work closely with the career services department in the beginning of your career to assist you in obtaining your first position.

Seeking Employment

In addition to working with a career services department, you can take advantage of a number of other resources in seeking employment within the field of medical assisting. These resources include classified ads, Internet sites, employment services, and networking with classmates and others.

Classified Ads and Internet Sites.

Many prospective employers use classified advertisements in area newspapers to alert potential applicants to a career opportunity within their organization. The advertisement usually describes the duties and responsibilities of the position as well as the type of education and experience preferred.

When you are first beginning to seek a medical assisting position, don't become discouraged if you see advertisements asking for a specified amount of experience, such as 2 years. You must realize that employers place ads seeking an experienced candidate, but many will consider a new graduate because experienced candidates are not always available. Becoming credentialed will help you bridge the gap of experience. A local newspaper's classified advertisements are often a good place to start your search. There is usually a separate section listing health-related jobs.

It is important to explore all the possibilities when seeking employment opportunities. A medical assistant is qualified for a number of positions. New graduates can apply for the following positions:

- Unit secretary in hospitals
- Phlebotomist in labs
- Patient care associate or patient care technician in hospitals

- Entry-level medical coding and billing
- Customer service representative in medical-related companies
- Clinical or administrative position in physician offices

The Internet is another useful tool when seeking employment. Web sites often allow job seekers to post résumés online and to respond to advertisements that are posted by employers locally or statewide.

Employment Services.

Employment and temporary agencies provide assistance in locating a specific job. Both types of agencies have a variety of job openings on file. Agencies also place classified ads. You should call to make an appointment with an employment counselor. Agencies usually require you to fill out an application, take a basic health-care test, and provide a résumé. If the agency has positions that match your skills, it contacts the employer. If the service has no appropriate listings, it will place your résumé on file.

Employment services are an excellent way to gain experience and select a position. You are given an opportunity to try out the office or facility at little commitment on your part. Many permanent opportunities can result from a temporary job assignment.

Networking.

Networking involves making contacts with relatives, friends, and acquaintances who may have information about how to find a job in your field. People in your network may be able to give you job leads or tell you about openings. Word-of-mouth referrals—finding job information by talking with other people—can be very helpful. Other people may be able to introduce you to others who work in, or know people who work in, your field. Networking is a valuable tool. It can advance your career even while you are employed.

Joining a medical assisting organization and attending conferences are the easiest ways to network. Attend an organization's local chapter meetings and talk with as many people as possible. Remember to bring a pen and a notebook. Be prepared to exchange information with other attendees. Remember, networking is an exchange of information—it is not one-sided. What you learn through networking may enable you to provide others with information to help their job search or further their career.

Your classmates are often a good source of networking. It is important to build lasting friendships with your classmates and keep in touch after graduation. Oftentimes they will know of positions as they gain employment. Networking begins in the classroom.

Creating a Résumé

Your résumé is a vital part of the employment process. It provides potential employers with information about your educational and work history and other aspects of your background.

Components of a Résumé.

In order to create a well-rounded, informative résumé, you need to include a wide variety of information about your background.

Personal Information. Include your name, address, telephone number, cell phone number, and e-mail address. Do not include your marital status or the number of children you have. You should not include your height, weight, interests, or hobbies unless you think they are relevant to the position.

Professional Objective. A professional objective is a brief, general statement that demonstrates a career goal. An example of an effective, professional objective is the following: "To work as a medical assistant, applying skills in patient relations and laboratory work while gaining increasing responsibility." If you want to list a specific career objective, such as applying your medical assisting skills in a pediatric medical facility, it would be best to mention it in the cover letter and not on your résumé.

Employment Experience. List the title of your most recent or last job first, the dates you were employed there, and a brief description of your duties. Choose jobs that have been the most beneficial to your working career. Do not clutter your résumé with needless details or irrelevant jobs. You can elaborate on specific duties in your cover letter and in the interview. Only include jobs you have held for a longer period of time, such as six months to a year.

Educational Background. In providing your educational history, list your highest degree first, the school attended, the dates, and the major field of study. Include educational experience that may be relevant to the job, such as certification, licensing, advanced training, and intensive seminars. Do not list individual classes on your résumé. If you have taken special classes that relate directly to the job you are seeking, list them in your cover letter.

Awards and Honors. List the awards and honors that are related to your career or that indicate excellence. Perfect attendance, academic honors, and student of the month are excellent traits that employers are seeking. Highlight this information prominently rather than writing it as an afterthought. You can make the most impact by displaying your best qualities at the beginning of this section.

Campus and Community Activities. List activities that show leadership abilities and a willingness to contribute. Include any volunteer work that you may have performed.

Professional Memberships and Activities. List any professional memberships that are related to your career. Student memberships are available through the American Medical Technologists (AMT) and the American Association of Medical Assistants (AAMA). You can contact the AMT and request a copy of the student by-laws and directions on how to form a student membership in your school. The AAMA provides continuing education through their local chapters. They sponsor local meetings periodically throughout the year. Employers like medical professionals who are involved in their disciplines. It demonstrates a commitment and dedication to their chosen field.

Summary of Skills. As you learn clinical and administrative skills, you will want to list them on your résumé. Under headings such as "Clinical Skills" or "Administrative Skills," list the skills you have acquired in school and on your externship. Some examples of clinical skills are the following:

- EKG
- Venipuncture
- Urinalysis
- Parenteral injections
- Aseptic technique
- Bandaging and first aid
- CPR
- Triage and vital statistics

Some examples of administrative skills are the following:

- ICD-9 and CPT coding
- Insurance claim form processing, HCFA
- Practice management software, Medisoft
- Pegboard accounting
- Typing, 45 wpm
- Microsoft Office software

References. Prior to the end of your externship, meet with your preceptor and ask for a **reference**. A reference is a recommendation for employment from the facility and the preceptor. A reference can be in the form of a letter from the facility, preceptor, or physician, or it can be a request to include these people on your reference list. It is professional to always ask before you list someone as a reference. References are important to career building because employers often like to inquire about a person prior to offering them employment. Your first references in medical assisting are your instructors and then the externship facility.

You will want three to five references, including employment, academic, and character references. Ask instructors for a general letter before you finish your program. Fellow members of professional associations or your classmates can provide character references, and your externship can provide an employment reference. Make certain that you ask your references for permission to use their names and phone numbers. Do not print your references on the bottom of your résumé. List them on a separate sheet of paper so that you can update the list as needed. On the bottom of your résumé, you should type "References available on request."

Choosing a Résumé Style. Three different résumé styles have been developed, each of which has specific advantages and disadvantages. You will want to choose a style or combination of styles that best describes your strengths and skills.

Functional Résumé. A **functional résumé** highlights specialty areas of your accomplishments and strengths. You can organize these in an order that supports your objective. Functional résumés are useful when you change careers, reenter the job market after an absence, or have had a variety of different, unconnected work experiences. Functional résumés are often not appropriate in highly traditional fields such as teaching, law, or health care, where the specific employers are the main interest. A sample of a functional résumé is shown in Figure 54-5.

Chronological Résumé. A **chronological résumé** is used by individuals who have job experience. List your most recent job first, and end with your first job. Chronological résumés are best when you stay in the same field as your prior jobs and when your employment history shows growth and development. Do not use a chronological résumé if you have gaps in your work history, if you have changed careers, if you have been in the same job for many years, or if you are looking for your first job. Figure 54-6 illustrates a chronological résumé.

Targeted Résumé. A **targeted résumé** is best if you are focused on a specific job target. The résumé should contain a clear, concise objective about what you are looking for. This résumé should list your skills, academic achievements, student honors, and other pertinent information that correlates with your objective. This type of information adds substance to your résumé when you have just graduated and do not have relevant job experience. Because the targeted résumé is an academic-type résumé, your skills, achievements, and community and volunteer work—your most significant assets—should be listed first. A sample of a targeted résumé is shown in Figure 54-7.

Résumé Writing Tips. Pay close attention to detail as you create your résumé. Here are some suggestions to help you:

- Organize your information by using a worksheet. List all the addresses, dates, phone numbers, and supervisors of previous positions that you have held. Write down brief descriptions of all the responsibilities and duties of your positions.

- List your educational institutions and their addresses, your dates of attendance, and the type of diploma or degree, including your major.

- Choose a résumé format that best describes your experience, education, and achievements.

- Use a computer and save your résumé on a disk.

- Proofread all spelling and grammar. Your completed résumé should be perfect. Do not rely on the spell-checking feature of your computer. Proofread your résumé line by line, and request that someone else also proofread your résumé.

- Select a high-quality résumé paper that is the standard size of 8½ by 11, with a weight between 16 and 25 pounds. Use an ivory or white paper with matching envelopes.

Donna Turner-Smith
18 Kingsley Road
Olmsted Falls, OH 44138
(440) 555-4279

PUBLIC HEALTH EDUCATION:
Instructed community groups on HIV awareness.
Instructed volunteers on how to set up community programs on domestic violence
Facilitated workshops for parents of teenagers
Provided in-services for public school teachers on signs and symptoms of
substance abuse

COUNSELING:
Consulted with social workers on individual cases for suspected child abuse
Worked with parents from abused homes
Counseled individual abused children

ORGANIZATIONAL:
Grant writing for federal funds for HIV awareness programs
Served as a liaison for transitional shelters for victims of domestic violence
Served as a liaison between community health agencies and public schools

PROFESSIONAL WORK HISTORY:
1990–1997   Project SAFE, Plymouth, Michigan
             HIV Public Health Instructor

1997–2004   Department of Child Health and Safety, Cleveland, Ohio
             Public Health Educator

EDUCATION:
1990 B.S. Sociology, Eastern Michigan University, Ypsilanti, Michigan

References available upon request

Figure 54-5. A functional résumé is often used by people who are reentering the job market.

- Use clear and concise statements and sentences. Your writing should reflect a positive and confident tone. For example, if you are describing your duties as a server, use sentences that focus on customer service, cash management, and the training and development of new servers. Avoid using the word "I" because the reader already knows that the résumé is referring to you.

- Be truthful and honest about your strengths and abilities. Do not mislead or exaggerate any skills, talents, or experience.

Procedure 54-1 provides information on how to write a résumé.

Writing a Cover Letter

A cover letter is an introduction to your résumé. It is a tool that markets your résumé as well as your skills and abilities. Cover letters are just as important as your résumé in your job search. An effective cover letter motivates the employer to review the résumé and interview the candidate.

Your cover letter should be direct and to the point. It should be no longer than one page and is typed on paper that matches your résumé. If possible, your cover letter should be addressed to a specific person in the organization. You can call the hospital or facility and ask to whom you should address the letter. If a name is not available,

Anthony Dalton
1234 West 25th Street
Park Ridge, NJ 07656
(201) 555-8311

WORK EXPERIENCE:

September, 2000–Present   NORTH BERGEN CLINIC FOUNDATION

Lead Medical Assistant for Cardiology practice
Patient preparation
EKG and Holter Monitor
Assist with Stress Testing
Patient follow-up

June, 1997–September, 2000   ST. JOSEPH HOSPITAL

Phlebotomist–inpatient and outpatient

March, 1997–June, 1997   ST. JOSEPH HOSPITAL

Medical Assisting Externship
Administrative and clinical responsibilities utilizing all
medical assisting skills in the Emergency department.

- Patient Triage
- Foley catheters
- EKG
- Specimen collection
- Patient intake
- Insurance verification

EDUCATION AND CERTIFICATIONS:

Associate of Applied Science Degree, June 1997, Bergen Community College,
Paramus, New Jersey, 07645

Certified Medical Assistant, August, 1997

References available upon request

Figure 54-6.   A chronological résumé lists a person's job history in chronological order.

it is acceptable to address the letter to "Human Resource Manager" or "Recruitment Manager." Research the facility or hospital prior to writing the letter. This information can help you tailor your letter to show how your qualifications and interests directly relate to the needs of the company or medical facility. Make sure the description of your qualifications and interests reflects the words used by the company in the advertisement. Always be truthful about the information in the cover letter; employers often verify all facts presented in your résumé and cover letter. Check each cover letter for errors in spelling, grammar, and punctuation. An example of a cover letter is shown in Figure 54-8.

Sending a Résumé

When sending a résumé, make sure you have the correct name, address, and zip code of the facility. This information should be typed on a matching envelope. Many word-processing programs have an envelope template feature that allows you to print an envelope using the address in your cover letter. Do not hand-write envelopes; professionally

Kelly Adamson
220 Terrace Avenue
Mooresburg, TN 37811
(423) 555-2657

CAREER OBJECTIVE:

To obtain a challenging position as a medical assistant in a growth oriented ambulatory care facility

ACHIEVEMENTS:

Registered Medical Assistant
Certified Phlebotomy Technician
Registered Medical Office Specialist
Graduate of an Accredited Medical Assistant Program
OSHA Compliance Officer
American Heart BLS Instructor

SKILLS AND CAPABILITIES:

Front office and Clinical Medical Assistant Patient Triage
Specimen Collection Venipuncture
EKG and Holter Monitor Parenteral Injections
ICD-9 and CPT Coding Medical Billing

PROFESSIONAL EXPERIENCE:

September, 2000–Present   Affiliated Physician Network, Mooresburg, Tennessee
     Medical Assistant/Office Coordinator
June, 1996–September, 2000   Partners in Internal Medicine, Mooresburg, Tennessee
     Medical Assistant

EDUCATION:

Sanford Brown Institute, Diploma, Medical Assisting 1996

AFFILIATIONS:

American Medical Technologists

References available upon request

Figure 54-7.   A targeted résumé is often used by a person who is focusing on a specific job target.

appearing mail is often opened first. Make sure that you attach sufficient postage.

When you fax a résumé, verify the fax number and person or department you are faxing to. Make sure your name is on all the faxed pages. If your fax machine provides a fax completion printout, save it to verify that the fax was delivered.

Some classified ads request that you send your résumé via e-mail. In order to send your résumé in electronic form, you must first have an account with an Internet service provider (ISP). You will be asked by the ISP to select a log-in, or screen, name. Do not use a casual name for your log-in prospective employers will see your log-in name in their in-box. Instead, choose a name that is conservative and professional. Most e-mail programs have an attachment feature that will allow you to send a word-processing document via e-mail. Verify that your e-mail was sent by checking your sent items or your out-box.

members who answer the phone (especially children) know proper phone etiquette and how to take a written message. When a prospective employer calls with an interview invitation, write down the interviewer's name, company or practice name, day, time, and location of the interview.

Interview Planning and Strategies

Just as the résumé is important for opening the door to opportunity, the job interview itself is critical for allowing you to present yourself professionally and to clearly articulate why you are the best person for the job. As you learned in Chapter 4, being successful in a medical assisting career is centered on communication—both verbal and nonverbal. These communication skills will be assets during your job interviews. The following list provides some strategies that will help you improve your interviewing skills:

- Practice interviewing. Rehearse possible questions and be prepared to answer them directly. Have a friend or family member interview you as you sit in front of a mirror and observe your body language.

- Anticipate question types. Expect open-ended questions such as, What are your strengths? What are your weaknesses? Tell me about your best work experience. Can you give me an example how you have worked with others to solve a problem? Decide in advance what information and skills are pertinent to the position and reveal your strengths. For example, you could say, "While I was at school, I learned to get along with a diverse group of people."

- Learn about the company. Be prepared; research the company or medical facility. What is the type of specialty? How many physicians are there?

- Dress appropriately. Because much communication is nonverbal, dressing appropriately for the interview is important. In most situations, you will be safe if you wear clean, pressed, conservative business clothes in neutral colors. Do not wear current fashions or fad clothing to an interview. Pay special attention to grooming. Keep makeup light, and wear little jewelry. Make sure that your hair and nails are clean and styled conservatively. Do not carry a large purse, backpack, books, coat, or hat. Leave extra clothing in an outside office, and simply carry a pen, your portfolio with extra copies of your résumé, and a small pad for taking notes.

- Be punctual. A good first impression is important and can be lasting. If you arrive late for the interview, a prospective employer may conclude that you will be late in arriving to work. Make certain you know the location and the time of the interview. Allow time for traffic, parking, and other preliminaries.

- Be professional. Being too familiar in your manner can be a barrier to a professional interview. Never call anyone by his or her first name unless you are asked to.

Know the interviewer's title and the pronunciation of his or her name. Do not sit down until the interviewer does.

- Exhibit appropriate interview behavior. Always greet the interviewer with a smile. The interview is an opportunity to sell yourself to the employer. Offer your hand for a firm, confident handshake, and be alert to the interviewer's body language. The flow of conversation during an interview should be natural. Maintain eye contact, pay attention to the interviewer, and show interest. Ask intelligent questions that you have prepared before the interview. Remember, the interview is an opportunity for both the prospective employer and the prospective employee to gather information and make a good impression. In addition to reviewing the experience listed on your résumé, the interviewer will evaluate your personality and behavior. At the same time, you will be observing the office and learning more about the position. Try to be aware of the office's atmosphere, its equipment and supplies, and the attitudes of the staff. Does it seem like a pleasant, professional place to work? Request a tour of the facility, and ask yourself if you would be happy in that work environment.

- Be poised and relaxed. Avoid nervous habits such as tapping your pencil, playing with your hair, or covering your mouth with your hand. Watch language such as "you know," "ah," "stuff like that." Use proper grammar and pronunciation as you talk with the interviewer—do not use slang. Do not smoke, chew gum, fidget, or bite your nails.

- Maintain comfortable eye contact. Look the interviewer in the eye and speak with confidence. Your eyes reveal much about you; use them to show interest, confidence, poise, and sincerity. Use other nonverbal techniques such as a firm handshake to reinforce your confidence.

- Relate your experience to the job. Use every question as an opportunity to show how your skills relate to the job. Use examples taken from school, previous jobs, your externship, volunteer work, leadership in student organizations, and personal experience to indicate that you have the personal qualities, aptitude, and skills needed for this job.

- Be honest. While it is important to be confident and stress your strengths, it is equally important to your sense of integrity to be honest. Dishonesty always catches up to you sooner or later. Someone will verify your background, so do not exaggerate your accomplishments, grade point average, or experience.

- Focus on how you can benefit the company. Don't ask about benefits, salary, or vacations until you are offered the job. During a first interview, try to show how you can contribute to the organization. Do not appear to be too eager to move up through the company or suggest that you are more interested in gaining experience than in contributing to the company.

PROCEDURE 54.2

Writing Thank-You Notes

Objective: To write an appropriate, professional thank-you note after an interview or externship

Materials: Paper; pen; dictionary; thesaurus; computer or word processor; #10 business envelope

Method

1. Write the letter within 2 days of the interview or completion of the externship. Begin by writing the date at the top of the letter.

2. Write the name of the person who interviewed you (or who was your mentor in the externship). Include credentials and title, such as Dr. or Director of Client Services. Write the complete address of the office or organization.

3. Start the letter with "Dear Dr., Mr., Mrs., Miss, or Ms. _____:"

4. In the first paragraph, thank the interviewer for his time and for granting the interview. Discuss some specific impressions, for example, "I found the interview and tour of the facilities an enjoyable experience. I would welcome the opportunity to work in such a state-of-the-art medical setting." If you are writing to thank your mentor for her time during your externship and

for allowing you to perform your externship at her office, practice, or clinic, discuss the knowledge and experience you gained during the externship.

5. In the second paragraph, mention the aspects of the job or externship that you found most interesting or challenging. For a job interview thank-you note, state how your skills and qualifications will make you an asset to the staff. When preparing an externship thank-you letter, mention interest in any future positions.

6. In the last paragraph, thank the interviewer for considering you for the position. Ask to be contacted at his earliest convenience regarding his employment decision.

7. Close the letter with "Sincerely," and type your name. Leave enough space above your typewritten name to sign your name.

8. Type your return address in the upper left corner of the #10 business envelope. Then type the interviewer's name and address in the envelope's center, apply the proper postage, and mail the letter.

- Close the interview on a positive note. Thank the interviewer for his or her time, shake hands, and say that you are looking forward to hearing from him or her. On the way out of the office, thank the staff members involved in the interview. Ask for a business card from anyone whom you think you might want to send a thank-you note. After leaving the interview, write down any additional information you want to remember. Every interview provides you with information about the medical assisting profession. Even if an interview does not result in a job, you will have met new people, developed a larger network of professional contacts, and gained valuable interviewing experience.

- Follow up with a letter. After an interview, it is professional to send a thank-you letter to the person or persons from the company who conducted your interview. You should send this letter within two days of the interview. It may be brief, but it should express your appreciation for the opportunity to have met with the interviewer, reaffirm your interest in the organization, and state your desire to remain a part of the selection process. By sending a thank-you letter, you display common business courtesy, which can make a

difference in the employer's hiring decision. Even if you are not interested in continuing the interview and selection process, you should thank the employer for holding the interview. Procedure 54-2 explains how to write and send a thank-you letter.

- Complete an application. Some employers ask you to complete an employment application at an interview even when you provide a résumé. You can use your résumé to help you complete the application. Fill out the application neatly. Spell all words correctly, and read and follow the instructions on the form carefully. Your application represents you; it must make a good first impression. Fill in all sections of the application—do not write "see résumé." An example of an application is shown in Figure 54-9.

- Comply with other aspects of the application process. As part of the application process, employers are required by federal law to request documents that prove your identity and eligibility to work in the United States. To maintain the safety and confidentiality of the medical office, hospital, or laboratory, employers may also check your police record, credit rating, and history of chemical or alcohol abuse. A drug screen

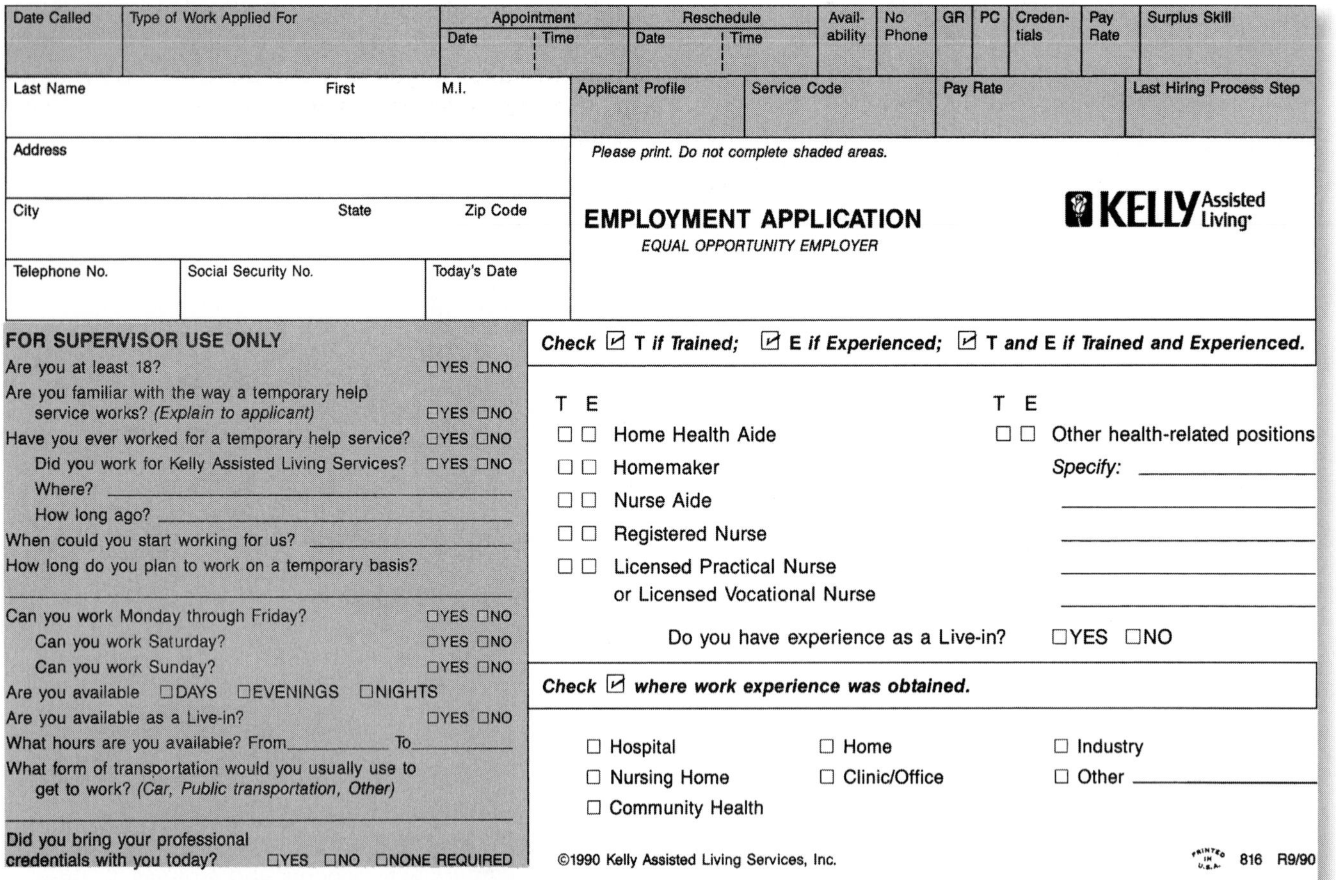
Date Called | Type of Work Applied For | Appointment Date Time | Reschedule Date Time | Availability | No Phone | GR | PC | Credentials | Pay Rate | Surplus Skill

Last Name | First | M.I. | Applicant Profile | Service Code | Pay Rate | Last Hiring Process Step

Address

Please print. Do not complete shaded areas.

City | State | Zip Code

EMPLOYMENT APPLICATION

EQUAL OPPORTUNITY EMPLOYER

KELLY Assisted Living®

Telephone No. | Social Security No. | Today's Date

FOR SUPERVISOR USE ONLY

Are you at least 18? ☐YES ☐NO

Are you familiar with the way a temporary help service works? *(Explain to applicant)* ☐YES ☐NO

Have you ever worked for a temporary help service? ☐YES ☐NO

Did you work for Kelly Assisted Living Services? ☐YES ☐NO

Where? ____

How long ago? ____

When could you start working for us? ____

How long do you plan to work on a temporary basis?

____

Can you work Monday through Friday? ☐YES ☐NO

Can you work Saturday? ☐YES ☐NO

Can you work Sunday? ☐YES ☐NO

Are you available ☐DAYS ☐EVENINGS ☐NIGHTS

Are you available as a Live-in? ☐YES ☐NO

What hours are you available? From____ To____

What form of transportation would you usually use to get to work? *(Car, Public transportation, Other)*

____

Did you bring your professional credentials with you today? ☐YES ☐NO ☐NONE REQUIRED

Check ☑ T if Trained; ☑ E if Experienced; ☑ T and E if Trained and Experienced.

T E

☐ ☐ Home Health Aide

☐ ☐ Homemaker

☐ ☐ Nurse Aide

☐ ☐ Registered Nurse

☐ ☐ Licensed Practical Nurse or Licensed Vocational Nurse

T E

☐ ☐ Other health-related positions

Specify: ____

Do you have experience as a Live-in? ☐YES ☐NO

Check ☑ where work experience was obtained.

☐ Hospital ☐ Home ☐ Industry

☐ Nursing Home ☐ Clinic/Office ☐ Other ____

☐ Community Health

©1990 Kelly Assisted Living Services, Inc. PRINTED IN U.S.A. 816 R9/90

Figure 54-9. Job applicants are often asked to fill out an application form like the one shown here. (Reprinted with permission from Kelly Assisted Living Services, Inc.)

may be requested. You may be asked to provide the needed documents or to give the employer authorization to obtain them.

Interview Questions

In order to prepare for your interview, you can anticipate that you may be asked any of the following questions:

- I see from your résumé that you graduated from ABC School. What did that school have to offer you that others did not?
- What is your five-year goal?
- Tell me about yourself.
- What do you consider to be your greatest strengths and weaknesses?
- How would your instructors describe you?
- What qualifications do you have that make you a good candidate for this position?
- How could you make a contribution to this facility?
- How well do you work with others?
- What is your concept of a team environment?
- How well do you work under pressure?
- Will you be able to work overtime?
- Do you have the flexibility to work various shifts?
- What has been your major accomplishment to date?
- Why did you choose medical assisting as your career?
- Do you have any questions that you would like to ask?

It is helpful to be prepared with any questions that you may have for the interviewer about the position or the facility. Questions about salary and benefits are not appropriate in a first interview.

An interviewer may ask you questions that you are not obligated to answer. These questions refer to age, race, sexual orientation, marital status, or number of children. Even if the questions sound harmless or the interviewer seems nonjudgmental, these questions have nothing to do with your skills or abilities. If the interviewer asks even one of these questions, you should reconsider whether you want to work for the organization.

If you are asked an inappropriate question during an interview, be polite and remain professional in declining to answer. You may simply state that you do not believe the requested information is necessary for the employer to evaluate your qualifications for the job. Try to move the discussion onto a more relevant topic.

Reasons for Not Being Hired

Employers in business were asked to list reasons for not hiring a job candidate. The 15 biggest complaints are the following:

1. Poor appearance, not being dressed properly, and being poorly groomed
2. Acting like a know-it-all
3. Not communicating clearly as well as poor voice, diction, and grammar
4. Lack of planning for the interview, with no purpose or goals communicated
5. Lack of confidence or poise
6. No interest in or enthusiasm for the job
7. Not being active in extracurricular school programs
8. Being interested only in the best salary offer
9. Poor school record, either in academics, attendance, or both
10. Unwillingness to begin in an entry-level position
11. Making excuses about an unfavorable record
12. No tact
13. No maturity
14. No curiosity about the job
15. Being critical of past employers

Salary Negotiations

Medical assisting salaries are varied and differ by geographic area. When you are a new graduate, you will begin your career as an entry-level medical assistant. As you gain experience, your compensation will reflect that. Salary ranges are determined by geographic location, medical specialty, years of experience, credentialing, and the job description.

The first step in determining your compensation needs is to know how much income is required to meet your living expenses. You will need to prepare a budget. Keep track of your overall expenditures and living expenses. Itemizing your basic living expenses can help you to prepare a budget. These living expenses can include:

- Rent
- Car payments or anticipated car payments
- Car insurance
- Food
- Utilities
- Student loans
- Credit cards
- Clothing
- Child care
- Other

Establishing a budget will give you an idea of the amount of income you may need. Once your budget is established,

you have a negotiating benchmark. Employers will often ask you what you are looking for with regard to salary. If you answer directly, you may risk either quoting yourself out of a job or leaving money on the table. The best response to this question is to ask the employer the range of the position. Most positions have a low-to-high range. For example, the range for a specific position could be between $23,000 and $32,000 annually. Once you know the range, quote a little higher than what your budgetary amount is, which will give the employer room to negotiate down if necessary. Allow the employer to bring up salary first.

On the Job

Once you have a job, you must learn how to be an effective employee. There are many ways that your initiative enables the medical team in the office, hospital, clinic, or laboratory to function effectively. You must identify the important skills in your daily duties, stay competitive and marketable through continuing education, and integrate constructive criticism from your employee evaluations into your daily work and annual goals.

Employee Evaluations

Employee evaluations are usually held annually. An initial employment review generally occurs after a probationary period of 90 days. Evaluations describe an employee's performance. A completed evaluation is placed in an official record of employment. In most situations, the employee and the employer meet to discuss the employee's performance. The purpose of an annual evaluation should be to check the goals and values of both the employer and the employee to make sure they support each other.

An employee evaluation form typically outlines the most important qualities and abilities needed for the job. It evaluates the employee's strengths and weaknesses. This form may help determine whether an employee is worthy of a merit raise, which is a raise based on performance (as opposed to a cost-of-living raise). The quantity and quality of work are assessed on this form, as are initiative, judgment, and cooperation.

Continuing Education

After completing a medical assisting program, you should continue your education, setting specific educational advancement goals on a yearly basis. For example, you may decide to obtain further education to learn more about the medical specialty in which you work.

As medical research expands its discoveries and as new technologies emerge, the necessity for self-education increases. You must read to stay abreast of updates in medicine. The need for more highly specialized training presents you with an opportunity for growth in your education and career. Medical publications are the best source for the latest medical information (Figure 54-10). Local and state

APPENDIX III

Latin and Greek Equivalents Commonly Used in Medical Terms

abdomen venter
adhesion adhaesio
and et
arm brachium; brachion (Gr*)
artery arteria
back dorsum
backbone spina
backward retro; opistho (Gr)
bend flexus
bile bilis; chole (Gr)
bladder vesica, cystus
blister vesicula
blood sanguis; haima (Gr)
body corpus; soma (Gr)
bone os, ossis; osteon (Gr)
brain encephalon
break ruptura
breast mamma; mastos (Gr)
buttock gloutos (Gr)
cartilage cartilago; chondros (Gr)
cavity cavum
chest pectoris, pectus; thorax (Gr)
child puer, puerilis
choke strangulo
corn clavus
cornea kerat (Gr)
cough tussis
deadly lethalis
death mors
dental dentalis
digestive pepticos
disease morbus
dislocation luxatio
doctor medicus
dose dosis (Gr)
ear auris; ous (Gr)
egg ovum
erotic erotikos (Gr)
exhalation exhalatio, expiro
external externus
extract extractum
eye oculus; ophthalmos (Gr)
eyelid palpebra
face facies
fat adeps; lipos (Gr)
female femella
fever febris
finger (or toe) digitus
flesh carnis, caro
foot pes
forehead frons
gum gingiva
hair capillus, pilus; thrix (Gr)

hand manus; cheir (Gr)
harelip labrum fissum; cheiloschisis (Gr)
head caput; kephale (Gr)
health sanitas
hear audire
heart cor; kardia (Gr)
heat calor; therme (Gr)
heel calx, talus
hysterics hysteria
infant infans
infectious contagiosus
injection injectio
intellect intellectus
internal internus
intestine intestinum; enteron (Gr)
itching pruritis
jawbone maxilla
joint vertebra; arthron (Gr)
kidney ren, renis; nephros (Gr)
knee genu
kneecap patella
lacerate lacerare
larynx guttur
lateral lateralis
limb membrum
lip labium, labrum; cheilos (Gr)
listen auscultare
liver jecur; hepar (Gr)
loin lapara
looseness laxativus
lung pulmo; pneumon (Gr)
male masculinus
malignant malignons
milk lac
moisture humiditas
month mensis
monthly menstruus
mouth oris, os; stoma, stomato (Gr)
nail unguis; onyx (Gr)
navel umbilicus; omphalos (Gr)
neck cervix; trachelos (Gr)
nerve nervus; neuron (Gr)
nipple papilla; thele (Gr)
no, none nullus
nose nasus; rhis (Gr)
nostril naris
nourishment alimentum
ointment unguentum
pain dolor; algia (Gr)
patient patiens
pectoral pectoralis
pimple pustula

poison venenum
powder pulvis
pregnant praegnans, gravida
pubic bone os pubis
pupil pupilla
rash exanthema (Gr)
recover convalescere
redness rubor
rib costa
ringing tinnitus
scaly squamosus
sciatica sciaticus; ischiadikos (Gr)
seed semen
senile senilis
sheath vagina; theke (Gr)
short brevis; brachys (Gr)
shoulder omos (Gr)
shoulder blade scapula
side latus
skin cutis; derma (Gr)
skull cranium; kranion (Gr)
sleep somnus
solution solutio
spinal spinalis
stomach stomachus; gaster (Gr)
stone calculus
sugar saccharum
swallow glutio
tail cauda
taste gustatio
tear lacrima
testicle testis; orchis (Gr)
thigh femur
throat fauces; pharynx (Gr)
tongue lingua; glossa (Gr)
tooth dens; odontos (Gr)
touch tactus
tremor tremere
twin gemellus
ulcer ulcus
urine urina; ouran (Gr)
uterus hystera (Gr)
vagina vagina; kolpos (Gr)
vein vena; phlebos, phleps (Gr)
vertebra spondylos (Gr)
vessel vas
wash diluere
water aqua
wax cera
weak debilis
windpipe arteria aspera
wrist carpus; karpos (Gr)

* Parenthetical "Gr" means the preceding term is Greek. Other terms in the column are Latin.

1138

APPENDIX IV
Abbreviations Commonly Used in Medical Notations

a before
a.c. before meals
AD right ear
ADD attention deficit disorder
ADL activities of daily living
ad lib as desired
ADT admission, discharge, transfer
AIDS acquired immunodeficiency syndrome
a.m.a. against medical advice
AMA American Medical Association
amp. ampule
amt amount
aq., AQ water; aqueous
AS left ear
ausc. auscultation
AU both ears
ax axis
Bib, bib drink
b.i.d., bid, BID twice a day
BM bowel movement
BP, B/P blood pressure
BPC blood pressure check
BPH benign prostatic hypertrophy
BSA body surface area
c., c̄ with
Ca calcium; cancer
cap, caps capsules
CBC complete blood (cell) count
cc cubic centimeter
C.C., CC chief complaint
CDC Centers for Disease Control and Prevention
CHF congestive heart failure
chr chronic
CNS central nervous system
Comp, comp compound
COPD chronic obstructive pulmonary disease
CP chest pain
CPE complete physical examination
CPR cardiopulmonary resuscitation
CSF cerebrospinal fluid
CT computed tomography
CV cardiovascular
d day
d/c, D/C discontinue, discharge
D & C dilation and curettage
DEA Drug Enforcement Administration
Dil, dil dilute
DM diabetes mellitus
DOB date of birth

DTP diptheria-tetanus-pertussis vaccine
Dr. doctor
DTs delirium tremens
D/W dextrose in water
Dx, dx diagnosis
ECG, EKG electrocardiogram
ED emergency department
EEG electroencephalogram
EENT eyes, ears, nose, and throat
EP established patient
ER emergency room
ESR erythrocyte sedimentation rate
FBS fasting blood sugar
FDA Food and Drug Administration
FH family history
Fl, fl, fld fluid
F/u follow-up
Fx fracture
GBS gallbladder series
GI gastrointestinal
Gm gram
gr grain
gt, gtt drops
GTT glucose tolerance test
GU genitourinary
GYN gynecology
HB, Hgb hemoglobin
HEENT head, ears, eyes, nose, throat
HIV human immunodeficiency virus
HO history of
h.s., hs, HS hour of sleep/at bedtime
Hx history
ICU intensive care unit
I & D incision and drainage
I & O intake and output
IM intramuscular
inf. infusion; inferior
inj injection
IT inhalation therapy
IUD intrauterine device
IV intravenous
KUB kidneys, ureters, bladder
L1, L2, etc. lumbar vertebrae
lab laboratory
liq liquid
LLL left lower lobe
LLQ left lower quadrant
LMP last menstrual period
LUQ left upper quadrant
MI myocardial infarction
MM mucous membrane
MRI magnetic resonance imaging

MS multiple sclerosis
NB newborn
NED no evidence of disease
no. number
noc, noct night
npo, NPO nothing by mouth
NPT new patient
NS normal saline
NSAID nonsteroidal anti-inflammatory drug
NTP normal temperature and pressure
N & V nausea and vomiting
NYD not yet diagnosed
OB obstetrics
OC oral contraceptive
o.d. once a day
OD overdose
O.D., OD right eye
oint ointment
OOB out of bed
OPD outpatient department
OPS outpatient services
OR operating room
O.S., OS left eye
OTC over-the-counter
O.U., OU both eyes
P & P Pap smear (Papanicolaou smear) and pelvic examination
PA posteroanterior
Pap Pap smear
Path pathology
p.c., pc after meals
PE physical examination
per by, with
PH past history
PID pelvic inflammatory disease
p/o postoperative
POMR problem-oriented medical record
PMFSH past medical, family, social history
PMS premenstrual syndrome
p.r.n., prn, PRN whenever necessary
Pt patient
PT physical therapy
PTA prior to admission
PVC premature ventricular contraction
pulv powder
q. every
q2, q2h every 2 hours
q.a.m., qam every morning

1139

q.d., qd every day

q.h., qh every hour

qhs every night, at bedtime

q.i.d., QID four times a day

qns, QNS quantity not sufficient

qod every other day

qs, QS quantity sufficient

RA rheumatoid arthritis; right atrium

RBC red blood cells; red blood (cell) count

RDA recommended dietary allowance, recommended daily allowance

REM rapid eye movement

RF rheumatoid factor

RLL right lower lobe

RLQ right lower quadrant

R/O rule out

ROM range of motion

ROS/SR review of systems/systems review

RUQ right upper quadrant

RV right ventricle

Rx prescription, take

SAD seasonal affective disorder

s.c., SC, SQ, subq, SubQ subcutaneously

SIDS sudden infant death syndrome

Sig directions

sig sigmoidoscopy

SOAP subjective, objective, assessment, plan

SOB shortness of breath

sol solution

S/R suture removal

ss, $\overline{ss}$ one-half

Staph staphylococcus

stat, STAT immediately

STD sexually transmitted disease

Strep streptococcus

subling, SL sublingual

surg surgery

S/W saline in water

SX symptoms

T1, T2, etc. thoracic vertebrae

T & A tonsillectomy and adenoidectomy

tab tablet

TB tuberculosis

TBS, tbs. tablespoon

TIA transient ischemic attack

t.i.d., tid, TID three times a day

tinc, tinct, tr tincture

TMJ temporomandibular joint

top topically

TPR temperature, pulse, and respiration

tsp teaspoon

TSH thyroid stimulating hormone

Tx treatment

U unit

UA urinalysis

UCHD usual childhood diseases

UGI upper gastrointestinal

ung, ungt ointment

URI upper respiratory infection

US ultrasound

UTI urinary tract infection

VA visual acuity

VD venereal disease

Vf visual field

VS vital signs

WBC white blood cells; white blood (cell) count

WNL within normal limits

wt weight

y/o year old

APPENDIX V
Symbols Commonly Used in Medical Notations

Apothecaries' Weights and Measures

℥ minim
℈ scruple
ʒ dram
fʒ fluidram
℥ ounce
f℥ fluidounce
O pint
℔ pound

Other Weights and Measures

\# pounds
° degrees
′ foot; minute
″ inch; second
μm micrometer
μ micron (former term for micrometer)
mμ millimicron; nanometer
μg microgram
mEq milliequivalent
mL milliliter
dL deciliter
mg% milligrams percent; milligrams per 100 mL

Abbreviations

a̅a̅, A̅A̅ of each
c̅ with

M mix (Latin *misce*)
m- meta-
o- ortho-
p- para-
p̅ after
s̅ without
ss, s̅s̅ one-half (Latin *semis*)

Mathematical Functions and Terms

\# number
+ plus; positive; acid reaction
− minus; negative; alkaline reaction
± plus or minus; either positive or negative; indefinite
× multiply; magnification; crossed with, hybrid
÷, / divided by
= equal to
≈ approximately equal to
> greater than; from which is derived
< less than; derived from
≮ not less than
≯ not greater than
≤ equal to or less than
≥ equal to or greater than
≠ not equal to
√ square root
$^3\sqrt{}$ cube root
∞ infinity

: ratio; "is to"
∴ therefore
% percent
π pi (3.14159)—the ratio of circumference of a circle to its diameter

Chemical Notations

Δ change; heat
⇌ reversible reaction
↑ increase
↓ decrease

Warnings

Ⓒ Schedule I controlled substance
Ⓒ Schedule II controlled substance
Ⓒ Schedule III controlled substance
Ⓒ Schedule IV controlled substance
Ⓒ Schedule V controlled substance
☤ poison
☢ radiation
☣ biohazard

Others

℞ prescription; take
□, ♂ male
○, ♀ female
ī one
īī two
īīī three

APPENDIX VI
Professional Organizations and Agencies

American Academy of Dental Practice Administrators
1063 Whippoorwill Lane
Palatine, IL 60067
(312) 934-4404

American Academy of Medical Administrators
30555 Southfield Road, Suite 150
Southfield, MI 48076
(313) 540-4310

American Academy of Ophthalmology
655 Beach Street
San Francisco, CA 94109
(415) 561-8500

American Academy of Pediatrics
PO Box 927
Elk Grove, IL 60009-0927
(708) 228-5005

American Association for Medical Transcription
PO Box 576187
Modesto, CA 95355
(209) 527-9620

American Association for Respiratory Care
11030 Ables Lane
Dallas, TX 75229
(214) 243-2272

American Association of Medical Assistants
20 N. Wacker Drive, Suite 1575
Chicago, IL 60606
(312) 899-1500

American Cancer Society
777 Third Avenue
New York, NY 10017
(212) 586-8700

American College of Cardiology
9111 Old Georgetown Road
Bethesda, MD 20814
(301) 897-5400

American College of Physicians
2011 Pennsylvania Avenue, NW
Washington, DC 20006
(202) 261-4500

American Diabetes Association
Two Park Avenue
New York, NY 10016
(212) 683-7444

American Dietetic Association
216 West Jackson Boulevard, Suite 800
Chicago, IL 60606-6995
(800) 366-1655

American Health Information Management Association
(formerly the American Medical Record Association)
233 N. Michigan Avenue, Suite 2150
Chicago, IL 60601-5800
(312) 233-1100

American Heart Association
National Center
7272 Greenville Avenue
Dallas, TX 75231-4596
(800) 242-8721, or call your local center

American Hospital Association
One North Franklin, Suite 2706
Chicago, IL 60606
(312) 422-3000

American Lung Association
1740 Broadway
New York, NY 10019
(212) 315-8700

American Medical Association
Division of Allied Health Education and Accreditation
515 North State Street
Chicago, IL 60610
(312) 464-5000

American Medical Technologists
710 Higgins Road
Park Ridge, IL 60068
(847) 823-5169

American Occupational Therapy Association
4720 Montgomery Lane
PO Box 31220
Bethesda, MD 20824-1220
(301) 948-9626

American Pharmacists Association
2215 Constitution Avenue, NW
Washington, DC 20037-2985
(202) 628-4410

American Physical Therapy Association
1111 North Fairfax Street
Alexandria, VA 22314
(703) 684-2782

American Red Cross
17th and D Streets, NW
Washington, DC 20006
(202) 728-6400, or call your local chapter

American Red Cross
HIV/AIDS Education, Health and Safety Services
8111 Gatehouse Road, 6th Floor
Falls Church, VA 22042
(703) 206-7180

American Society for Cardiovascular Professionals
120 Falcon Drive, Unit 3
Fredericksburg, VA 22408
(540) 891-0079

American Society for Clinical Laboratory Science
7910 Woodmont Avenue, Suite 1301
Bethesda, MD 20814
(301) 657-2768

American Society of Clinical Pathologists
2100 West Harrison Street
Chicago, IL 60612
(312) 738-1336

American Society of Hand Therapists
401 North Michigan Avenue
Chicago, IL 60611
(312) 321-6866

American Society of Phlebotomy Technicians
PO Box 1831
Hickory, NC 28603
(704) 322-1334

American Society of Radiologic Technologists
15000 Central Avenue SE
Albuquerque, NM 87123
(505) 298-4500

The Arthritis Foundation
1314 Spring Street, NW
Atlanta, GA 30309
(404) 872-7100

Association of Surgical Technologists
7108-C South Alton Way
Englewood, CO 80112
(303) 694-9130

Association of Technical Personnel in Ophthalmology
50 Lee Road
Chestnut Hill, MA 02167
(617) 232-4433

Asthma and Allergy Foundation of America
1717 Massachusetts Avenue, Suite 305
Washington, DC 20036
(202) 265-0265

International Society for Clinical Laboratory Technology
818 Olive Street, Suite 918
St. Louis, MO 63101
(314) 241-1445

Joint Commission on Allied Health Personnel in Ophthalmology
2025 Woodlane Drive
St. Paul, MN 55125-2995
(800) 284-3937

Medical Group Management Association
104 Inverness Terrace East
Englewood Cliffs, CA 80112
(313) 799-1111

National Accrediting Agency for Clinical Laboratory Services
8410 West Bryn Mawr Avenue, Suite 670
Chicago, IL 60631
(312) 714-8880

National AIDS Hotline
215 Park Avenue South, Suite 714
New York, NY 10003
(800) 342-AIDS
(800) 344-SIDA (Spanish)

National Association of Medical Staff Services
PO Box 23590
Knoxville, TN 37933-1590
(615) 531-3571

National Cancer Institute
9000 Rockville Pike
Building 31, Room 10A18
Bethesda, MD 20205
(800) 4-CANCER

National Clearinghouse for Alcohol and Drug Information
PO Box 2345
Rockville, MD 20852
(301) 468-2600

National Health Council
1730 Street NW, Suite 500
Washington, DC 20036
(202) 785-3910

National Health Information Center
PO Box 1133
Washington, DC 20013-1133
(800) 336-4797

National Institute of Mental Health
Office of Communications
6001 Executive Boulevard, Room 8184, MSC 9663
Bethesda, MD 20892-9663
(301) 443-4513

National Institute on Aging
Building 31, Room 5C27
31 Center Drive, MSC 2292
Bethesda, MD 20892
(301) 496-1752

National Kidney Foundation
30 East 33rd Street
New York, NY 10016
(212) 889-2210

National Mental Health Association
2001 N. Beauregard Street, 12th Floor
Alexandria, VA 22311
(703) 684-7722

National Organization for Rare Disorders
100 Route 37, PO Box 8923
New Fairfield, CT 06812
(800) 999-NORD

National Phlebotomy Association
5615 Landover Road
Hyattsville, MD 20784
(301) 386-4200

National Rehabilitation Association
633 South Washington Street
Alexandria, VA 22314
(703) 836-0850

National Society for Histotechnology
4201 Northview Drive, Suite 502
Bowie, MD 20716-1073
(301) 262-6221

President's Council on Physical Fitness and Sports
Department of Health and Human Services
Washington, DC 20001
(202) 272-3421

Society of Diagnostic Medical Sonographers
12770 Coit Road, Suite 508
Dallas, TX 75251
(214) 239-7367

Glossary

Note: (†) Pronunciation from Stedman's Medical Dictionary 26th edition, all others from American Heritage 4th edition, in case you need to consult.

10× lens (tĕn) A magnifying lens in the ocular of a microscope that magnifies an image ten times. (45*)

24-hour urine specimen (twĕn´tē fôr our yŏŏr´ĭn spĕs´ə-mən) A urine specimen collected over a 24-hour period and used to complete a quantitative and qualitative analysis of one or more substances, such as sodium, chloride, and calcium. (47)

abandonment (ə-băn´dən-mənt) A situation in which a health-care professional stops caring for a patient without arranging for care by an equally qualified substitute. (3)

ABA number (nŭm´bər) A fraction appearing in the upper right corner of all printed checks that identifies the geographic area and specific bank on which the check is drawn. (18)

abduction (ab-dŭk´shŭn)(†) Movement away from the body. (26)

abscess (ăb´sĕs´) A collection of pus (white blood cells, bacteria, and dead skin cells) that forms as a result of infection. (42)

absorption (əb-sôrp´shən) The process by which one substance is absorbed, or taken in and incorporated, into another, as when the body converts food or drugs into a form it can use. (50)

access (ăk´sĕs) The way patients enter and exit a medical office (13)

accessibility (ăk-sĕs´ə-bĭl´ĭ-tē) The ease with which people can move into and out of a space. (22)

accounts payable (ə-kounts´ pā´-ə-bəl) Money owed by a business; the practice's expenses. (17)

accounts receivable (ə-kounts´ rĭ-sē´və-bəl) Income or money owed to a business. (17)

accreditation (ə-krĕd´ĭ-tā´shən) The documentation of official authorization or approval of a program. (1)

acetylcholine (as-e-til-kō´lēn)(†) A neurotransmitter released by the parasympathetic nerves onto organs and glands for resting and digesting. (26)

acetylcholinesterase (as´e-til-kō-lin-es´ter-ās) An enzyme within the nervous system that hydrolyzes acetylcholine to acetate and choline. (26)

acid-fast stain (ăs´ĭd făst stān) A staining procedure for identifying bacteria that have a waxy cell wall. (46)

acids (ăs´ĭds) Electrolytes that release hydrogen ions in water. (23)

acinar cells (as´i-nar sĕlz)(†) Cells in the pancreas that produce pancreatic juice. (31)

acquired immunodeficiency syndrome (AIDS) (ə-kwīrd im´yū-nō-dē-fish´en-sē sĭn´drōm´)(†) The most advanced stage of HIV infection; it severely weakens the body's immune system. (29)

acromegaly (ak-rō-meg´ă-lē)(†) A disorder in which too much growth hormone is produced in adults. (32)

acrosome (ak´rō-sōm)(†) An enzyme-filled sac covering the head of a sperm that aids in the penetration of the egg during fertilization. (35)

action potential (ăk´shən pə-tĕn´shəl) The flow of electrical current along the axon membrane. (27)

active file (ăk´tĭv fīl) A file used on a consistent basis. (10)

active listening (ăk´tĭv lĭs´ənĭng) Part of two-way communication, such as offering feedback or asking questions; contrast with **passive listening**. (4)

active transport (ak-tiv trans-pórt) The movement of a substance across a cell membrane from an area of low concentration to an area of high concentration. (23)

acupuncturist (ăk´yŏŏ-pŭngk´chər-ĭst) A practitioner of acupuncture. The acupuncturist uses hollow needles inserted into the patient's skin to treat pain, discomfort, or systemic imbalances. (2)

acute (ə-kyŏŏt´) Having a rapid onset and progress, as acute appendicitis. (40)

addiction (ă-dĭk´shun)(†) A physical or psychological dependence on a substance, usually involving a pattern of behavior that includes obsessive or compulsive preoccupation with the substance and the security of its supply, as well as a high rate of relapse after withdrawal. (36)

add-on code (ăd´on´ kōd) A code indicating procedures that are usually carried out in addition to another procedure. Add-on codes are used together with the primary code. (16)

adduction (ă-dŭk´shŭn)(†) Movement toward the body. (26)

adenoids (ăd´n-oidz´) See **pharyngeal tonsils**. (31)

administer (ăd-mĭn´ĭ-stər) To give a drug directly by injection, by mouth, or by any other route that introduces the drug into the body. (50)

adrenocorticotropic hormone (ă-drē´nō-kōr´ti-kō-trōpik hōr´mōn) Hormone that stimulates the adrenal cortex to release its hormones. (32)

advance scheduling (ăd-văns skĕj´ŏŏl-ĭng) Booking an appointment several weeks or even months in advance. (12)

aerobes (âr´ōbs´) Bacteria that grow best in the presence of oxygen. (46)

aerobic respiration (â-rō´bĭk rĕs´pə-rā´shən) A process that requires large amounts of oxygen and uses glucose to make ATP. (26)

afebrile (ā-feb´ril)(†) Having a body temperature within one's normal range. (37)

afferent arterioles (ăf´ər-ənt ar-tēr´ē-ōlz)(†) Structures that deliver blood to the glomeruli of the kidneys. (34)

affiliation agreement (ə-fĭl´ē-ā´shən ə-grē´mənt) An agreement that externship participants must sign that states the expectations of the facility and the expectations of the student. (54)

agar (ä´gär´) A gelatinlike substance derived from seaweed that gives a culture medium its semisolid consistency. (46)

age analysis (āj ə-năl´ĭ-sĭs) The process of clarifying and reviewing past due accounts by age from the first date of billing. (17)

agenda (ə-jĕn´də) The list of topics discussed or presented at a meeting, in order of presentation. (12)

agent (ā´-jənt) (legal) A person who acts on a physician's behalf while performing professional tasks; (clinical) an active principle or entity that produces a certain effect, for example, an infectious agent. (3)

---

* Parenthetical numbers indicate the chapter in which the entry is a key term or is first defined in context. Entries not followed by a chapter number are important terms related to material covered but not specifically defined in the text.

agglutination (ă-glū-ti-nā´shŭn) (†) The clumping of red blood cells following a blood transfusion. (28)

aggressive (ə-grĕs´ĭv) Imposing one's position on others or trying to manipulate them. (4)

agranular leukocyte (ă-grăn´-yu-lər lū´kŏ-sīt) (†) A type of leukocyte (white blood cell) with a solid nucleus and clear cytoplasm; includes lymphocytes and monocytes. (48)

agranulocyte (ă-grăn´yū-lō-sīt) (†) See **agranular leukocyte.** (28)

albumins (ăl-byōō´mĭns) The smallest of the plasma proteins. Albumins are important for pulling water into the bloodstream to help maintain blood pressure. (28)

aldosterone (al-dos´ter-ōn) (†) A hormone produced in the adrenal glands that acts on the kidney. It causes the body to retain sodium and excrete potassium. Its role is to maintain blood volume and pressure. (32)

alimentary canal (ăl´ə-mĕn´tə-rē kə-năl´) The organs of the digestive system that extend from the mouth to the anus. (31)

allele (ə-lēl´) Any one of a pair or series of **genes** that occupy a specific position on a specific **chromosome.** (23)

allergen (ăl´ər-jən) An antigen that induces an allergic reaction. (29)

allergist (ăl´ər-jĭst) A specialist who diagnoses and treats physical reactions to substances including mold, dust, fur, pollen, foods, drugs, and chemicals. (2)

allowed charge (ə-loud´ chärj) The amount that is the most the payer will pay any provider for each procedure or service. (15)

alopecia (ăl´ə-pē´shə) The clinical term for baldness. (24)

alphabetic filing system (ăl´fə-bĕt´ĭkəl fī´lĭng sĭs´təm) A filing system in which the files are arranged in alphabetic order, with the patient's last name first, followed by the first name and middle initial. (10)

Alphabetic Index (ăl´fə-bĕt´ĭk ĭn´dĕks´) One of two ways diagnoses are listed in the ICD-9-CM. They appear in alphabetic order with their corresponding diagnosis codes. (16)

alveolar glands (al-vē´ō-lär glăndz) (†) Glands that make milk under the influence of the hormone **prolactin.** (35)

alveoli (ăl-vē´ə-lī´) Clusters of air sacs in which the exchange of gases between air and blood takes place; located in the lungs. (30)

American Association of Medical Assistants (AAMA) (ə-mĕr´ĭkən ə-sō´sē-ā´shən mĕd´ĭ-kəl ə-sĭs´tənts) The professional organization that certifies medical assistants and works to maintain professional standards in the medical assisting profession. (1)

Americans With Disabilities Act (ADA) (ə-mĕr´ĭ-kəns dĭs´ə-bĭl´ĭ-tēs ăkt) A U.S. civil rights act forbidding discrimination against people because of a physical or mental handicap. (13)

amblyopia (am-blē-ō´pē-ă) (†) Poor vision in one eye without a detectable cause. (33)

amino acids (ə-mē´nō ăs´ĭds) Natural organic compounds found in plant and animal foods and used by the body to create protein. (49)

amnion (ăm´nē-ən) The innermost membrane enveloping the embryo and containing amniotic fluid. (35)

anabolism (ə-năb´ə-lĭz´əm) The stage of metabolism in which substances such as nutrients are changed into more complex substances and used to build body tissues. (49)

anaerobe (ăn´ə-rōb´) A bacterium that grows best in the absence of oxygen. (46)

anal canal (ā´nəl kə-năl´) The last few centimeters of the rectum. (31)

anaphylaxis (an´ă-fī-lak´sis) A severe allergic reaction with symptoms that include respiratory distress, difficulty in swallowing, pallor, and a drastic drop in blood pressure that can lead to circulatory collapse. (29)

anatomical position (ăn´ə-tŏm´ĭ-kəl pə-zĭsh´ən) When the body is standing upright and facing forward with the arms at the side and the palms of the hands facing forward. (23)

anatomy (ə-năt´ə-mē) The scientific term for the study of body structure. (23)

anemia (ə-nē´mē-ə) A condition characterized by low red blood cell count. This condition decreases the ability to transport oxygen throughout the body. (28)

anergic reaction (an-er´jik rē-ăk´shən) A lack of response to skin testing that indicates the body's inability to mount a normal response to invasion by a pathogen. (21)

anesthesia (ăn´ĭs-thē´zhə) A loss of sensation, particularly the feeling of pain. (42)

anesthetic (ăn´ĭs-thĕt´ĭk) A medication that causes anesthesia. (42)

anesthetist (ă-nes´thĕ-tist) (†) A specialist who uses medications to cause patients to lose sensation or feeling during surgery. (2)

aneurysm (ăn´yə-rĭz´əm) A serious and potentially life-threatening bulge in the wall of a blood vessel. (28)

angiography (an-jē-og´ră-fē) (†) An x-ray examination of a blood vessel, performed after the injection of a contrast medium, that evaluates the function and structure of one or more arteries or veins. (41)

angiotensin II (an-jē-ō-ten´sin tōō) (†) A hormone that raises blood pressure and causes the secretion of another hormone called **aldosterone.** (34)

annotate (ăn´ō-tāt´) To underline or highlight key points of a document or to write reminders, make comments, and suggest actions in the margins. (7)

anorexia nervosa (ăn´ə-rĕk´sē-ə nûr-vō´sə) An eating disorder in which people starve themselves because they fear that if they lose control of eating they will become grossly overweight. (49)

antagonist (ăn-tăg´ə-nĭst) A muscle that produces the opposite movement of the **prime mover.** (26)

antecubital space (an-te-kyū´bi-tăl spās) The inner side or bend of the elbow; the site at which the brachial artery is felt or heard when a pulse or blood pressure is taken. (37)

anterior (ăn-tîr´ē-ər) Anatomical term meaning toward the front of the body; also called ventral. (23)

antibodies (ăn´tĭ-bod´ēs) Highly specific proteins that attach themselves to foreign substances in an initial step in destroying such substances, as part of the body's defenses. (19)

antidiuretic hormone (an´tē-dī-yū-ret´ik hôr´mōn´) (†) A hormone that increases water reabsorption, which decreases urine production and helps to maintain blood pressure. (32)

antigen (an´tĭ-jən) A foreign substance that stimulates white blood cells to create antibodies when it enters the body. (19)

antihistamines (ăn´tē-hĭs´tə-mēnz) Medications used to treat allergies. (29)

antimicrobial (an´tē-mī-krō´bē-ăl) (†) An agent that kills microorganisms or suppresses their growth. (46)

antioxidants (ăn´tē-ŏk´sī-dənt) Chemical agents that fight cell-destroying chemical substances called free radicals. (49)

antiseptic (ăn′tĭ-sĕp′tĭk) A cleaning product used on human tissue as an anti-infection agent. (20)

anuria (an-yū′rē-ă)(†) The absence of urine production. (47)

aortic valve (ā-ôr′tĭk vălv) Heart valve that is a semilunar valve and that is situated between the left ventricle and the aorta. (28)

apex (ā′pĕks) The left lower corner of the heart, where the strongest heart sounds can be heard. (37)

apical (ap′i-kăl)(†) Located at the **apex** of the heart. (37)

apocrine gland (ap′ō-krin glănd)(†) A type of sweat gland. It produces a thicker type of sweat than other sweat glands and contains more proteins. (24)

aponeurosis (ap′ō-nū-rō′sis)(†) A tough, sheet-like structure that is made of fibrous connective tissue. It typically attaches muscles to other muscles. (26)

appendicitis (ə-pĕn′dĭ-sī′tĭs) Inflammation of the appendix. (31)

appendicular (ap′en-dik′yū-lăr) The division of the skeletal system that consists of the bones of the arms, legs, pectoral girdle, and pelvic girdle. (25)

approximation (ə-prŏk′sə-mā′shən) The process of bringing the edges of a wound together, so the tissue surfaces are close, to protect the area from further contamination and to minimize scar and scab formation. (42)

aqueous humor (ā′kwē-əs hyōō′mər) A liquid produced by the eye's ciliary body that fills the space between the cornea and the lens. (33)

arbitration (är′bĭ-trā′shən) A process in which opposing sides choose a person or persons outside the court system, often someone with special knowledge in the field, to hear and decide a dispute. (3)

areflexia (ā-rē-flek′sē-ă)(†) The absence of **reflexes.** (27)

areola (ă-rē′ō-lă)(†) The pigmented area that surrounds the nipple. (35)

arrector pili (ă-rek′tŏr pī′lī)(†) Muscles attached to most hair follicles and found in the dermis. (24)

arrhythmia (ə-rĭth′mē-ə) Irregularity in heart rhythm. (28)

arterial blood gases (är-tîr′ē-əl blŭd găs′ses) A test that measures the amount of gases, such as oxygen and carbon dioxide, dissolved in arterial blood. (40)

arthrography (ar-throg′ră-fē)(†) A radiologic procedure performed by a radiologist, who uses a contrast medium and fluoroscopy to help diagnose abnormalities or injuries in the cartilage, tendons, or ligaments of the joints—usually the knee or shoulder. (53)

arthroscopy (är-thŏs′kə-pē) A procedure in which an orthopedist examines a joint, usually the knee or shoulder, with a tubular instrument called an arthroscope; also used to guide surgical procedures. (41)

articular cartilage (ar-tik′yu-lăr kär′tl-ij)(†) The cartilage that covers the **epiphysis** of long bones. (25)

artifact (är′tə-făkt′) Any irrelevant object or mark observed when examining specimens or graphic records that is not related to the object being examined; for example, a foreign object visible through a microscope or an erroneous mark on an ECG strip. (45)

ascending colon (ə-sĕnd′ĭng kō′lən) The segment of the large intestine that runs up the right side of the abdominal cavity. (31)

ascending tracts (ə-sĕnd′ĭng trăkts) The tracts of the spinal cord that carry sensory information to the brain. (27)

asepsis (ă-sep′sis)(†) The condition in which pathogens are absent or controlled. (19)

assault (ə-sôlt′) The open threat of bodily harm to another. (3)

assertive (ə-sûrt′tĭv) Being firm and standing up for oneself while showing respect for others. (4)

asset (ăs′ĕt′) An item owned by the practice that has a dollar value, such as the medical practice building, office equipment, or accounts receivable. (18)

assignment of benefits (ə-sĭn′mənt bĕn′ə-fĭts) An authorization for an insurance carrier to pay a physician or practice directly. (15)

astigmatism (ə-stĭg′mə-tĭz′əm) A condition in which the cornea has an abnormal shape, which causes blurred images during near or distant vision. (33)

atherosclerosis (ăth′ə-rō-sklə-rō′sĭs) The accumulation of fatty deposits along the inner walls of arteries. (28)

atlas (ăt′ləs) The first cervical vertebra. (25)

atoms (ăt′əmz) The simplest units of all matter. (23)

atria (ā′trē-ă)(†) [*Singular:* atrium] Chambers of the heart that receive blood from the veins and circulate it to the ventricles. (28)

atrial natriuretic peptide (ā′trē-əl nā′trē-yū-ret′ik pep′tĭd)(†) A hormone secreted by the heart that regulates blood pressure. (32)

atrioventricular bundle (ā′trē-ō-ven-trik′yū-lar bŭn′dl)(†) A structure that is located between the ventricles of the heart and that sends the electrical impulse to the Purkinje fibers. (28)

atrioventricular node (ā′trē-ō-ven-trik′yū-lar nōd) A node that is located between the atria of the heart. After the electrical impulse reaches the atrioventricular node, the atria contract and the impulse is sent to the ventricles. (28)

audiologist (aw-dē-ol′ōjist)(†) A health-care specialist who focuses on evaluating and correcting hearing problems. (39)

audiometer (aw-dē-om′ē-ter) An electronic device that measures hearing acuity by producing sounds in specific frequencies and intensities. (39)

auditory tube (ô′dĭ-tôr′ē tōōb) A structure that connects the middle ear to the throat. Also called the **eustachian tube.** (33)

auricle (ôr′ĭ-kəl) The outside part of the ear, made of cartilage and covered with skin. (33)

auscultated blood pressure (ô′skəl-tāt-ĕd blŭd prĕsh′ər) Blood pressure as measured by listening with a stethoscope. (37)

auscultation (ô′skəl-t ā′shən) The process of listening to body sounds. (38)

authorization (ô′thər-ĭ-zā′shən) A form that explains in detail the standards for the use and disclosure of patient information for purposes other than treatment, payment, or health-care operations. (3)

autoclave (aw′tō-klāv)(†) A device that uses pressurized steam to sterilize instruments and equipment. (20)

automated external defibrillator (AED) (ô′tə-mā′tĭd ĭk-stûr′nəl dē-fĭb′ri-lā-ter) A computerized defibrillator programmed to recognize lethal heart rhythms and deliver an electrical shock to restore a normal rhythm. (44)

autonomic (ô′tə-nŏm′ĭk) A division of the peripheral nervous system that connects the central nervous system to viscera such as the heart, stomach, intestines, glands, blood vessels, and bladder. (27)

autosome (ô′tə-sōm′) A chromosome that is not a sex chromosome. (23)

axial (ăk′sē-əl) The division of the skeletal system that consists of the skull, vertebral column, and rib cage. (25)

axilla (ăk-sĭl′ə) Armpit; one of the four locations for temperature readings. (37)

axis (ak′-səs) The second vertebra of the neck on which the head turns. (25)

axon (ăk′sŏn′) A type of nerve fiber that is typically long and branches far from the cell body. Its function is to send information away from the cell body. (27)

bacillus (ba-sĭl′ŭs)(†) A rod-shaped bacterium. (46)

bacterial spore (băk-tîr′ē̆l spôr) A primitive, thick-walled reproductive body capable of developing into a new individual; resistant to killing through disinfection. (19)

balance billing (băl′əns bĭl′ĭng) Billing a patient for the difference between a higher usual fee and a lower allowed charge. (15)

barium enema (bâr′ē-əm ĕn′ə-mə) A radiologic procedure performed by a radiologist who administers barium sulfate through the anus, into the rectum, and then into the colon to help diagnose and evaluate obstructions, ulcers, polyps, diverticulosis, tumors, or motility problems of the colon or rectum; also called a lower GI (gastrointestinal) series. (53)

barium swallow (bâr′ē-əm swŏl′ō) A radiologic procedure that involves oral administration of a barium sulfate drink to help diagnose and evaluate obstructions, ulcers, polyps, diverticulosis, tumors, or motility problems of the esophagus, stomach, duodenum, and small intestine; also called an upper GI (gastrointestinal) series. (53)

baroreceptors (bar′ō-rē-sep′ters)(†) Structures, located in the aorta and carotid arteries, that help regulate blood pressure. (28)

bases (bā′sēz′) Electrolytes that release hydroxyl ions in water. (23)

basophil (bā-sō-fil)(†) A type of granular leukocyte that produces the chemical histamine, which aids the body in controlling allergic reactions and other exaggerated immunologic responses. (28)

battery (băt′ə-rē) An action that causes bodily harm to another. (3)

behavior modification (bĭ-hāv′yər mŏd′ə-fĭ-kă-shən) The altering of personal habits to promote a healthier lifestyle. (49)

benefits (bĕn′ə-fĭts) Payments for medical services. (15)

bicarbonate ions (bī-kar′bon-āt ī′onz) Elements formed when carbon dioxide gets into the bloodstream

and reacts with water. In the alimentary canal, these ions neutralize acidic chyme arriving from the stomach. (30)

bicuspids (bī-kŭs′pĭds) Teeth with two cusps. There are two in front of each set of molars. (31)

bicuspid valve (bī-kŭs′pĭd vălv) Heart valve that has two cusps and that is located between the left atrium and the left ventricle. Also known as the mitral valve. (28)

bile (bīl) A substance created in the liver and stored in the gallbladder. Bile is a bitter yellow-green fluid that is used in the digestion of fats. (31)

bilirubin (bili-rū′bin)(†) A bile pigment formed by the breakdown of hemoglobin in the liver. (28)

bilirubinuria (bil′i-rū-bi-nū′rē-ă)(†) The presence of bilirubin in the urine; one of the first signs of liver disease or conditions that involve the liver. (47)

birthday rule (bûrth′dā′rōōl) A rule that states that the insurance policy of a policyholder whose birthday comes first in the year is the primary payer for all dependents. (15)

biliverdin (bil-i-ver′din)(†) A pigment released when a red blood cell is destroyed. (28)

biochemistry (bī′ō-kĕm′ĭ-strē) The study of matter and chemical reactions in the body. (23)

bioethics (bī-ō-ĕth′ĭks) Principles of right and wrong in issues that arise from medical advances. (3)

biohazard symbol (bī-ō-hăz′ərd sĭm′bəl) A symbol that must appear on all containers used to store waste products, blood, blood products, or other specimens that may be infectious. (45)

biohazardous materials (bī-ō-hăz′ərd-əs mə-tîr′ə-əls) Biological agents that can spread disease to living things. (19)

biohazardous waste container (bī-ō-hăz′ərd-əs wāst kən-tā′nər) A leakproof, puncture-resistant container, color-coded red or labeled with a special biohazard symbol, that is used to store and dispose of contaminated supplies and equipment. (19)

biopsy (bī′ŏp′sē) The process of removing and examining tissues and cells from the body. (29)

biopsy specimen (bī′ŏp′sē spĕs′ə-mən) A small amount of tissue removed from the body for examination under a microscope to diagnose an illness. (42)

bioterrorism (bī-ō′tĕr′ə-rĭz′əm) The intentional release of a biologic agent

with the intent to harm individuals. (44)

blastocyst (blas′tō-sist) A **morula** that travels down the uterine tube to the uterus and is invaded with fluid. It then implants into the wall of the uterus. (35)

blood-borne pathogen (blŭd-bôrn păth′ə-jən) A disease-causing microorganism carried in a host's blood and transmitted through contact with infected blood, tissue, or body fluids. (21)

blood-brain barrier (blŭd brān băr′ē-ər) A structure that is formed from tight capillaries to protect the tissues of the central nervous system from certain substances. (27)

B lymphocyte (bē lĭm′fə-sīt) A type of nongranular leukocyte that produces antibodies to combat specific pathogens. (48)

body language (bŏd′ē lăng′gwĭj) Non-verbal communication, including facial expressions, eye contact, posture, touch, and attention to personal space. (4)

bookkeeping (bōōk′kē′pĭng) The systematic recording of business transactions. (18)

bone conduction (bōnkən-dŭk′shən) The process by which sound waves pass through the bones of the skull directly to the inner ear, bypassing the outer and middle ears. (39)

botulism (bŏch′ə-lĭz′əm) A life-threatening type of food poisoning that results from eating improperly canned or preserved foods that have been contaminated with the bacterium *Clostridium botulinum*. (26)

brachial artery (brāk′ē-ăl är′tə-rē) An artery that provides a palpable pulse and audible vascular sounds in the antecubital space (the bend of the elbow). (37)

brachytherapy (brak-ē-thăr′ă-pē′)(†) A radiation therapy technique in which a radiologist places temporary radioactive implants close to or directly into cancerous tissue; used for treating localized cancers. (53)

brain stem (brān stĕm) A structure that connects the cerebrum to the spinal cord. (27)

breach of contract (brēch kŏn′trăkt′) The violation of or failure to live up to a contract's terms. (3)

bronchi (brŏn′kī) The two branches of the trachea that enter the lungs. (30)

bronchial tree (brŏng′kē-al trē) A series of tubes that begins where the distal end of the trachea branches. (30)

bronchioles (brŏng′kē-ōlz) A part of the respiratory tract that branches from the tertiary bronchi. (30)

buccal (bŭk′ăl)(†) Between the cheek and gum. (51)

bulbourethral glands (bŭl′bō-yū-rē′thrăl glăndz)(†) Glands that lie beneath the prostate and empty their fluid into the urethra. Their fluid aids in sperm movement. (35)

buffy coat (buf′ē kōt) The layer between the packed red blood cells and plasma in a centrifuged blood sample; this layer contains the white blood cells and platelets. (48)

bulimia (boo-lē′mē-ə) An eating disorder in which people eat a large quantity of food in a short period of time (bingeing) and then attempt to counter the effects of bingeing by self-induced vomiting, use of laxatives or diuretics, and/or excessive exercise. (49)

burnout (′bər-naůt) The end result of prolonged periods of stress without relief. Burnout is an energy-depleting condition that can affect one's health and career. It can be common for those who work in health care. (4)

bursitis (bər-sī′tĭs) Inflammation of a bursa. (25)

calcaneus (kal-kā′nē-ŭs)(†) The largest tarsal bone; also called the heel bone. (25)

calcitonin (kal-si-tō′nin) A hormone produced by the thyroid gland that lowers blood calcium levels by activating osteoblasts. (32)

calibrate (kăl′ə-brāt) to determine the caliber of (37)

calibration syringe (kăl′ə-brā′shən sə-rĭnj′) A standardized measuring instrument used to check and adjust the volume indicator on a spirometer. (52)

calorie (kăl′ə-rē) A unit used to measure the amount of energy food produces; the amount of energy needed to raise the temperature of 1 kg of water by 1°C. (49)

calyces (kā′lĭ-sēz′) Small cavities of the renal pelvis of the kidney. (34)

canaliculi (kan-ă-lik′yū-lī) Tiny canals that connect lacunae to each other. (25)

capillary (kăp′ə-lĕr′ē) Branches of arterioles and the smallest type of blood vessel. (28)

capillary puncture (kăp′ə-lĕr′ē pŭngk′chər) A blood-drawing technique that requires a superficial

puncture of the skin with a sharp point. (48)

capitation (kăp′ĭ-tā′shən) A payment structure in which a health maintenance organization prepays an annual set fee per patient to a physician. (15)

carboxypeptidase (kar-bok-sē-pep′ti-dās) (†) A pancreatic enzyme that digests proteins. (31)

carcinogen (kär-sĭn′ə-jən) A factor that is known to cause the formation of cancer. (29)

cardiac catheterization (kär′dē-ăk′ kath′ě-ter-ĭ-zā′shun)(†) A diagnostic method in which a catheter is inserted into a vein or artery in the arm or leg and passed through blood vessels into the heart. (41)

cardiac cycle (kär′dē-ăk′ sī′kəl) The sequence of contraction and relaxation that makes up a complete heartbeat. (52)

cardiologist (kär′dē-ŏl′ə-jĭst) A specialist who diagnoses and treats diseases of the heart and blood vessels (cardiovascular diseases). (2)

carditis (kar-dī′tis)(†) Inflammation of the heart. (28)

carpal (kär′pəl) Bones of the wrist. (25)

carpal tunnel syndrome (kär′pəl tŭn′əl sĭn′drōm′) A painful disorder caused by compression of the median nerve in the carpal tunnel of the wrist. (25)

carrier (kăr′ē-ər) A reservoir host who is unaware of the presence of a pathogen and so spreads the disease while exhibiting no symptoms of infection. (19)

cast (kăst) A rigid, external dressing, usually made of plaster or fiberglass, that is molded to the contours of the body part to which it is applied; used to immobilize a fractured or dislocated bone. (44) Cylinder-shaped elements with flat or rounded ends, differing in composition and size, that form when protein from the breakdown of cells accumulates and precipitates in the kidney tubules and is washed into the urine. (47)

catabolism (kə-tăb′ə-lĭz′əm) The stage of metabolism in which complex substances, including nutrients and body tissues, are broken down into simpler substances and converted into energy. (49)

cataracts (kăt′ə-răkts′) Cloudy areas that form in the lens of the eye that prevent light from reaching visual receptors. (33)

cash flow statement (kăsh flō stā′mənt) A statement that shows the cash on

hand at the beginning of a period, the income and disbursements made during the period, and the new amount of cash on hand at the end of the period. (18)

cashier's check (kă-shîrz′ che′k) A bank check issued by a bank on bank paper and signed by a bank representative; usually purchased by individuals who do not have checking accounts. (18)

catheterization (kath′ě-ter-ĭ-zǎ′shun)(†) The procedure during which a catheter is inserted into a vessel, an organ, or a body cavity. (47)

caudal (kôd′l) See **inferior**. (23)

CD-ROM (sē′dē′rŏm′) A compact disc that contains software programs; an abbreviation for "compact disc—read-only memory." (6)

cecum (sē′kəm) The first section of the large intestine. (31)

cell body (sĕl bŏd′ē) The portion of the neuron that contains the nucleus and organelles. (27)

cell membrane (sĕl mĕm′brăn′) The outer limit of a cell that is thin and selectively permeable. It controls the movement of substances into and out of the cell. (23)

cells (sĕlz) The smallest living units of structure and function. (23)

cellulitis (sel-yū-lī′tis) Inflammation of cellular or connective tissue. (24)

cellulose (sĕl′yə-lōs′) A type of carbohydrate that is found in vegetables and cannot be digested by humans; commonly called fiber. (31)

Celsius (centigrade) (sĕl′sē-əs) One of two common scales for measuring temperature; measured in degrees Celsius, or °C. (37)

Centers for Medicare and Medicaid Services (CMS) (sĕn′tərs mĕd′ĭ-kâr′ mĕd′ĭ-kād′ sûr′vĭs-əz) A congressional agency designed to handle Medicare and Medicaid insurance claims. It was formerly known as the Health Care Financing Administration. (15)

central nervous system (CNS) (sĕn′trəl nûr′vəs sĭs′təm) A system that consists of the brain and the spinal cord. (27)

central processing unit (CPU) (sĕn′trəl prŏs′es′ĭng yoo′nĭt) A microprocessor, the primary computer chip responsible for interpreting and executing programs. (6)

centrifuge (sĕn′trə-fyooj′) A device used to spin a specimen at high speed until it separates into its component parts. (45)

cerebellum (sĕr´ə-bĕl´əm) An area of the brain inferior to the cerebrum that coordinates complex skeletal muscle coordination. (27)

cerebrospinal fluid (CSF) (ser´ē-brō-spī´năl floo´ĭd) The fluid in the sub-arachnoid space of the meninges and the central canal of the spinal cord. (27)

cerebrum (sĕr´ə-brəm) The largest part of the brain; it mainly includes the cerebral hemispheres. (27)

Certificate of Waiver tests (sər-tĭf´ĭ-kĭt wā´vər tĕsts) Laboratory tests that pose an insignificant risk to the patient if they are performed or interpreted incorrectly, are simple and accurate to such a degree that the risk of obtaining incorrect results is minimal, and have been approved by the Food and Drug Administration for use by patients at home; laboratories performing only Certificate of Waiver tests must meet less stringent standards than laboratories that perform tests in other categories. (45)

certified check (sûr´tə-fīd´ chĕk) A payer's check written and signed by the payer, which is stamped "certified" by the bank. The bank has already drawn money from the payer's account to guarantee that the check will be paid. (18)

Certified Medical Assistant (CMA) (sûr´tə-fīd´ mĕd´ĭ-kəl ə-sĭs´tənt) A medical assistant whose knowledge about the skills of medical assistants, as summarized by the 2003 AAMA Role Delineation Study areas of competence, has been certified by the Certifying Board of the American Association of Medical Assistants (AAMA). (1)

cerumen (sə-roo´mən) A waxlike substance produced by glands in the ear canal; also called earwax. (38)

cervical enlargement (sûr´vĭ-kəl in-lär´j-mənt) The thickening of the spinal cord in the neck region. (27)

cervical orifice (sûr´vĭ-kəl ôr´ə-fĭs) The opening of the uterus through the cervix into the vagina. (35)

cervicitis (ser-vi-sī´tis) Inflammation of the cervix. (35)

cervix (sûr´vĭks) The lowest portion of the uterus that extends into the vagina. (35)

chain of custody (chān kŭs´tə-dē) A procedure for ensuring that a specimen is obtained from a specified individual, is correctly identified, is under the uninterrupted control of authorized personnel, and has not been altered or replaced. (44)

CHAMPVA (Civilian Health and Medical Program of the Veterans Administration) (sĭ-vĭl´yən hĕlth mĕd´ĭ-kəl prō´grăm vĕt´ər-enz ăd-mĭn´ĭ-strā´shən) A type of health insurance that covers the expenses of families (dependent spouses and children) of veterans with total, permanent, and service-connected disabilities. It also covers the surviving families of veterans who die in the line of duty or as a result of service-connected disabilities. (15)

chancre (shang´ker)(†) A painless ulcer that may appear on the tongue, the lips, the genitalia, the rectum, or elsewhere. (21)

charge slip (chärj slĭp) The original record of services performed for a patient and the charges for those services. (18)

check (chĕk) A bank draft or order written by a payer that directs the bank to pay a sum of money on demand to the payee. (18)

chemistry (kĕm´ĭ-strē) The study of the composition of matter and how matter changes. (23)

chemoreceptor (kē´mō-rĭ-sĕp´tôr) Any cell that is activated by a change in chemical concentration and results in a nerve impulse. The olfactory or smell receptors in the nose are an example of a chemoreceptor. (33)

chief cells (chēf sĕlz) Cells in the lining of the stomach that secrete **pepsinogen**. (31)

chief complaint (chēf kəm-plān´t) The patient's main issue of pain or ailment. (36)

chiropractor (kī´rə-prăk´tôr) A physician who uses a system of therapy, including manipulation of the spine, to treat illness or pain. This treatment is done without drugs or surgery. (2)

cholangiography (kō-lan-jē-og´rä-fē)(†) A test that evaluates the function of the bile ducts by injection of a contrast medium directly into the common bile duct (during gallbladder surgery) or through a T-tube (after gallbladder surgery or during radiologic testing) and taking an x-ray. (53)

cholecystography (kō-lē-sis-tog´rä-fē)(†) A gallbladder function test performed by x-ray after the patient ingests an oral contrast agent; used to detect gallstones and bile duct obstruction. (41)

cholesterol (kə-lĕs´tə-rôl) A fat-related substance that the body produces in the liver and obtains from dietary sources; needed in small amounts to carry out several vital functions. High levels of cholesterol in the blood increase the risk of heart and artery disease. (49)

chordae tendineae (kôr´dē ten-din´ā)(†) Cord-like structures that attach the cusps of the heart valves to the papillary muscles in the ventricles. (28)

choroid (kôr´oid´) The middle layer of the eye, which contains the iris, the ciliary body, and most of the eye's blood vessels. (33)

chromosome (krō´mə-sōm´) Thread-like structures comprised of DNA. (23)

chronic (krŏn´ĭk) Lasting a long time or recurring frequently, as in chronic osteoarthritis. (40)

chronic obstructive pulmonary disease (COPD) (krŏn´ĭk ob-strŭk´tĭv pŏol´mə-nĕr´ē dĭ-zēz´) A disease characterized by the presence of airflow obstruction due to chronic bronchitis or emphysema. It is typically progressive. Cigarette smoking is the leading cause. (30)

chronological résumé (krŏn´ə-lŏj´ĭ-kəl rĕz´ōo-mā´) The type of résumé used by individuals who have job experience. Jobs are listed according to date, with the most recent being listed first. (54)

chylomicron (kī-lō-mī´kron) The least dense of the lipoproteins; it functions in lipid transportation. (28)

chyme (kīm)(†) The mixture of food and gastric juice. (31)

chymotrypsin (kī-mō-trip´sin)(†) A pancreatic enzyme that digests proteins. (31)

ciliary body (sĭl´ē-ĕr´ē bŏd´ē) A wedge-shaped thickening in the middle layer of the eyeball that contains the muscles that control the shape of the lens. (33)

circumduction (ser-kŭm-dŭk´shŭn) Moving a body part in a circle; for example, tracing a circle with your arm. (26)

cirrhosis (sĭ-rō´sĭs) A long-lasting liver disease in which normal liver tissue is replaced with nonfunctioning scar tissue. (31)

civil law (sĭv´əl lô) Involves crimes against persons. A person can sue another person, business, or the government. Judgments often require a payment of money. (3)

clarity (klăr´ĭ-tē) Clearness in writing or stating a message. (7)

class action lawsuit (klăs-ăk´shən lô´sōot´) A lawsuit in which one or more people sue a company or other legal entity that allegedly wronged all of them in the same way. (17)

clavicle (klăv´ĭ-kəl) A slender, curved long bone that connects the sternum and the scapula; also called the collar bone. (25)

clean-catch midstream urine specimen (klēn-kăch mĭd´strēm yōor´ĭn spĕs´ə-mən) A type of urine specimen that requires special cleansing of the external genitalia to avoid contamination by organisms residing near the external opening of the urethra and is used to identify the number and types of pathogens present in urine; sometimes referred to as midvoid. (47)

clearinghouse (klĭr´ĭng-hous´) A group that takes nonstandard medical billing software formats and translates them into the standard EDI formats. (15)

cleavage (klē´vĭj) The rapid rate of mitosis of a zygote immediately following fertilization. (35)

clinical coordinator (klĭn´ĭ-kəl kō-ôr´dn-ā´tor) The person associated with the medical assisting school that procures externship sites and qualifies them to ensure that they provide a thorough educational experience. (54)

clinical diagnosis (klĭn´ĭ-kəl dī´əg-nō´sĭs) A diagnosis based on the signs and symptoms of a disease or condition. (38)

clinical drug trial (klĭn´ĭ-kəl drŭg trī´əl) An internationally recognized research protocol designed to evaluate the efficacy or safety of drugs and to produce scientifically valid results. (21)

Clinical Laboratory Improvement Amendments (CLIA '88) (klē´ə) A law enacted by Congress in 1988 that placed all laboratory facilities that conduct tests for diagnosing, preventing, or treating human disease or for assessing human health under federal regulations administered by the Health Care Financing Administration (HCFA) and the Centers for Disease Control and Prevention (CDC). (1)

clitoris (klĭt´ər-ĭs) Located anterior to the urethral opening in females. It contains erectile tissue and is rich in sensory nerves. (35)

closed file (klōzd fīl) A file for a patient who has died, moved away, or for some other reason no longer consults the office for medical expertise. (10)

closed posture (klōzd pŏs´chər) A position that conveys the feeling of not being totally receptive to what is being said; arms are often rigid or folded across the chest. (4)

cluster scheduling (klŭs´tər skĕj´ōol-ĭng) The scheduling of similar appointments together at a certain time of the day or week. (12)

coagulation (kō-ăg´yə-lā´shən) The process by which a clot forms in blood. (28)

coccus (kŏk´əs) A spherical, round, or ovoid bacterium. (46)

coccyx (kŏk´sĭks) A small, triangular-shaped bone consisting of three to five fused vertebrae. (25)

cochlea (kŏk´lē-ăr) A spiral-shaped canal in the inner ear that contains the hearing receptors. (33)

code linkage (kōd lĭng´kĭj) Analysis of the connection between diagnostic and procedural information in order to evaluate the medical necessity of the reported charges. This analysis is performed by insurance company representatives. (16)

coinsurance (kō-ĭn-shōor´əns) A fixed percentage of covered charges paid by the insured person after a deductible has been met. (15)

colitis (kə-lī´tĭs) Inflammation of the colon. (31)

colonoscopy (kō-lon-os´ kŏ-pē)(†) A procedure used to determine the cause of diarrhea, constipation, bleeding, or lower abdominal pain by inserting a scope through the anus to provide direct visualization of the large intestine. (41)

colony (kōl´ə-nē) A distinct group of microorganisms, visible with the naked eye, on the surface of a culture medium. (46)

color family (kūl´ər făm´ə-lē) A group of colors that share certain characteristics, such as warmth or coolness, allowing them to blend well together. (13)

colposcopy (kol-pos´kŏ-pē)(†) The examination of the vagina and cervix with an instrument called a colposcope to identify abnormal tissue, such as cancerous or precancerous cells. (40)

common bile duct (kŏm´ən bīl dŭkt) Duct that carries bile to the duodenum. It is formed from the merger of the cystic and hepatic ducts. (31)

compactible file (kəm-păkt´-əbəl fīl) Files kept on rolling shelves that slide along permanent tracks in the floor and are stored close together or stacked when not in use. (10)

complement (kŏm´plə-mənt) A protein present in serum that is involved in specific defenses. (29)

complete proteins (kəm-plēt´ prō´tēn´) Proteins that contain all nine essential amino acids. (49)

complex carbohydrates (kəm-plĕks´ kär´bō-hī´drāt´s) Long chains of sugar units; also known as polysaccharides. (49)

complex inheritance (kəm-plĕks´ ĭn-hĕr´ĭ-təns) The inheritance of traits determined by multiple genes. (23)

compliance plan (kəm-plī´əns plăn) A process for finding, correcting, and preventing illegal medical office practices. (16)

compound (kŏm´pound´) A substance that is formed when two or more atoms of more than one element are chemically combined. (23)

compound microscope (kŏm´pound´ mī´krə-skōp´) A microscope that uses two lenses to magnify the image created by condensed light focused through the object being examined. (45)

computed tomography (kəm-pyōōt´ĕd tō-mogra-fē)(†) A radiographic examination that produces a three-dimensional, cross-sectional view of an area of the body; may be performed with or without a contrast medium. (41)

conciseness (kən-sīs´nəs) Brevity; the use of no unnecessary words. (7)

concussion (kən-kŭsh´ən) A jarring injury to the brain; the most common type of head injury. (44)

conductive hearing loss (kon-dŭk-tiv´ hēr´ing lôs)(†) A type of hearing loss that occurs when sound waves cannot be conducted through the ear. Most types are temporary. (33)

condyle (kon´dīl)(†) Rounded articular surface on a bone. (25)

cones (kōnz) Light-sensing nerve cells in the eye, at the posterior of the retina, that are sensitive to color, provide sharp images, and function only in bright light. (33)

conflict (kŏn´flĭkt´) An opposition of opinions or ideas. (4)

conjunctiva (kŏn´jŭngk-tī´və) The protective membrane that lines the eyelid and covers the anterior of the sclera, or the white of the eye. (33)

conjunctivitis (kən-jŭngk´tə-vī´tĭs) A contagious infection of the conjunctiva caused by bacteria, viruses, and allergies. The symptoms may include discharge, red eyes, itching, and swollen eyelids; also commonly called pinkeye. (33)

connective (kə-nĕk´tĭv) A tissue type that is the framework of the body. (23)

consumable (kən-soo′mə-bəl) Able to be emptied or used up, as with supplies. (22)

consumer education (kən-soo′mər ĕj′ə-ka-shən) The process by which the average person learns to make informed decisions about goods and services, including health care. (14)

constructive criticism (kən-stre′k-tiv kr′i-tə-si-zəm) A type of critique that is aimed at giving an individual feedback about his or her performance in order to improve that performance. (54)

contagious (kən-tā′jəs) Having a disease that can easily be transmitted to others. (13)

contaminated (kən-tăm′ə-nāt′ĕd) Soiled or stained, particularly through contact with potentially infectious substances; no longer clean or sterile. (1)

contract (kŏn′trăct′) A voluntary agreement between two parties in which specific promises are made. (3)

contraindication (kŏn′trə-ĭn′dĭ-kā′-shən) A symptom that renders use of a remedy or procedure inadvisable, usually because of risk. (20)

contrast medium (kŏn′trast′ mē′dē-əm) A substance that makes internal organs denser and blocks the passage of x-rays to photographic film. Introducing a contrast medium into certain structures or areas of the body can provide a clear image of organs and tissues and highlight indications of how well they are functioning. (53)

controlled substance (kən-trōld′ sŭb′stəns) A drug or drug product that is categorized as potentially dangerous and addictive and is strictly regulated by federal laws. (50)

control sample (kən-trōl′ săm′pəl) A specimen that has a known value; used as a comparison for test results on a patient sample. (45)

contusion (kon-tū′shŭn)(†) A closed wound, or bruise. (44)

conventions (kən-vĕn′shənz) A list of abbreviations, punctuation, symbols, typefaces, and instructional notes appearing in the beginning of the ICD-9. The items provide guidelines for using the code set. (16)

convolutions (kŏn′və-loo′shənz) The ridges of brain matter between the sulci; also called **gyri**. (27)

coordination of benefits (kō-ôr′dn-ā′shən bĕn′ə-fĭts) A legal principle that limits payment by insurance companies to 100% of the cost of covered expenses. (15)

co-payment (kō-pā′mənt) A small fee paid by the insured at the time of a medical service rather than by the insurance company. (15)

cornea (kôr′nē-ə) A transparent area on the front of the outer layer of the eye that acts as a window to let light into the eye. (33)

coronary sinus (kôr′ə-nĕr′ē sī′nəs) The large vein that receives oxygen-poor blood from the cardiac veins and empties it into the right atrium of the heart. (28)

corpus callosum (kôr′pəs ka-l′ō-səm) A thick bundle of nerve fibers that connects the cerebral hemispheres. (27)

corpus luteum (kôr′pŭs lū-tē′um)(†) A ruptured follicle cell in the ovary following ovulation. (35)

cortex (kôr′tĕks′) The outermost layer of the cerebrum. (27)

cortisol (kôr′ti-sol)(†) A steroid hormone that is released when a person is stressed. It decreases protein synthesis. (32)

costal (kos′tăl)(†) Cartilage that attaches true ribs to the sternum. (25)

counter check (koun′tər chĕk) A special bank check that allows a depositor to draw funds from his own account only, as when he has forgotten his checkbook. (18)

courtesy title (kûr′tĭ-sē tĭt′l) A title used before a person's name, such as Dr., Mr., or Ms. (7)

cover sheet (kŭr′ər shēt) A form sent with a fax that provides details about the transmission. (5)

coxal (koks-al′)(†) Pertaining to the bones of the pelvic girdle. The coxa is composed of the ilium, ischium, and pubis. (25)

CPT See *Current Procedural Terminology.* (16)

cranial (krā′-nē-ăl)(†) See **superior.** (23)

cranial nerves (krā′nē-ăl nûrvs)(†) Peripheral nerves that originate from the brain. (27)

crash cart (krăsh kärt) A rolling cart of emergency supplies and equipment. (44)

creatine phosphate (krē′ă-tēn fos′fāt)(†) A protein that stores extra phosphate groups. (26)

credit (krĕd′ĭt) An extension of time to pay for services, which are provided on trust. (17)

credit bureau (krē′-dit byür′-o) A company that provides information about the credit worthiness of a person seeking credit. (17)

cricoid cartilage (krī′koyd kär′tl-ĭj)(†) A cartilage of the larynx that forms most of the posterior wall and a small part of the anterior wall. (30)

crime (krīm) An offense against the state committed or omitted in violation of public law. (3)

criminal law (krĭm′ə-nəl lô) Involves crimes against the state. When a state or federal law is violated, the government brings criminal charges against the alleged offender. (3)

cross-reference (krôs′rĕf′ər-əns) The notation within the ICD-9 of the word *see* after a main term in the index. The *see* reference means that the main term first checked is not correct. Another category must then be used. (16)

cross-referenced (krôs′rĕf′ər-ənsd) Filed in two or more places, with each place noted in each file; the exact contents of the file may be duplicated, or a cross-reference form can be created, listing all the places to find the file. (10)

cross-training (krós-trā′-ning) The acquisition of training in a variety of tasks and skills. (1)

cryotherapy (krī′ō-thĕr′ə-pē) The application of cold to a patient's body for therapeutic reasons. (43)

cryosurgery (krī′ō-sûr′jə-rē) The use of extreme cold to destroy unwanted tissue, such as skin lesions. (42)

crystals (krĭs′təls) Naturally produced solids of definite form; commonly seen in urine specimens, especially those permitted to cool. (47)

culture (kŭl′chər) In the sociological sense, a pattern of assumptions, beliefs, and practices that shape the way people think and act. (38) To place a sample of a specimen in or on a substance that allows microorganisms to grow in order to identify the microorganisms present. (46)

culture and sensitivity (C and S) (kŭl′chər sĕn′sĭ-tĭv′ə-tē) A procedure that involves culturing a specimen and then testing the isolated bacteria's susceptibility (sensitivity) to certain antibiotics to determine which antibiotics would be most effective in treating an infection. (46)

culture medium (kŭlchər mē′de-əm) A substance containing all the nutrients a particular type of microorganism needs to grow. (46)

***Current Procedural Terminology* (CPT) (kûr′ənt prə-sē′jər-əl tûr′mə-nŏl′ə-jē)** A book with the most commonly used system of procedure codes. It is the HIPAA-required code set for physicians' procedures. (16)

cursor (kûr'sər) A blinking line or cube on a computer screen that shows where the next character that is keyed will appear. (6)

Cushing's disease (kush'ingz dĭ-zēz') A condition in which a person produces too much **cortisol** or has used too many steroid hormones. Some of the signs and symptoms include buffalo hump obesity, a moon face, and abdominal stretch marks; also called hypercortisolism. (32)

cuspids (kŭs'pĭdz) The sharpest teeth; they act to tear food. (31)

cyanosis (sī'ə-no'sĭs) A bluish color of skin that results when the supply of oxygen is low in the blood. (24)

cycle billing (sī'kəl bĭl'ĭng) A system that sends invoices to groups of patients every few days, spreading the work of billing all patients over the month while billing each patient only once. (17)

cystic duct (sĭs'tĭk dŭkt) The duct from the gallbladder that merges with the hepatic duct to form the common bile duct. (31)

cystitis (sis-tī'tis)(†) Inflammation of the urinary bladder caused by infection. (34)

cytokines (sī'tō-kīnz) A chemical secreted by T lymphocytes in response to an antigen. Cytokines increase T and B cell production, kill cells that have antigens, and stimulate red bone marrow to produce more white blood cells. (29)

cytokinesis (sī'tō-ki-nē'sis)(†) Splitting of the cytoplasm during cell division. (23)

cytoplasm (sī'tə-plăz'əm) The watery intracellular substance that consists mostly of water, proteins, ions, and nutrients. (23)

damages (dăm'ijz) Money paid as compensation for violating legal rights. (17)

database (dā'tə-bās) A collection of records created and stored on a computer. (6)

dateline (dāt'līn') The line at the top of a letter that contains the month, day, and year. (7)

debridement (dā-brēd-mont')(†) The removal of debris or dead tissue from a wound to expose healthy tissue. (42)

decibel (dĕs'ə-bəl) A unit for measuring the relative intensity of sounds on a scale from 0 to 130. (39)

deductible (dĭ-dŭk'tə-bəl) A fixed dollar amount that must be paid by the insured before additional expenses are covered by an insurer. (15)

deep (dēp) Anatomical term meaning closer to the inside of the body. (23)

defamation (dĕf'ə-mā'shən) Damaging a person's reputation by making public statements that are both false and malicious. (3)

defecation reflex (def-ē-kā'shun rē'flĕks') The relaxation of the anal sphincters so that feces can move through the anus in the process of elimination. (31)

deflection (dĭ-flĕk'shən) A peak or valley on an electrocardiogram. (52)

dehydration (dē-hī'drā'shən) The condition that results from a lack of adequate water in the body. (44)

dementia (dĭ-mĕn'shə) The deterioration of mental faculties from organic disease of the brain. (14)

dendrite (dĕn'drīt') A type of nerve fiber that is short and branches near the cell body. Its function is to receive information from the neuron. (27)

deoxyhemoblobin (dē-oks-ē-hē-mō-glō'bin)(†) A type of hemoglobin that is not carrying oxygen. It is darker red in color than hemoglobin. (28)

dependent (dĭ-pĕn'dənt) A person who depends on another person for financial support. (18)

depolarization (dē-pō'lăr-i-za-shun)(†) The loss of polarity, or opposite charges inside and outside; the electrical impulse that initiates a chain reaction resulting in contraction. (52)

depolarized (dē-pō'lăr-īzd)(†) A state in which sodium ions flow to the inside of the cell membrane, making the outside less positive. Depolarization occurs when a neuron responds to stimuli such as heat, pressure, or chemicals. (27)

depression (dĭ'-pre-shan) The lowering of a body part. (26)

dermatitis (dûr'mə-tī'tis) Inflammation of the skin. (24)

dermatologist (der-mă-tol'ō-jist)(†) A specialist who diagnoses and treats diseases of the skin, hair, and nails. (2)

dermis (dûr'mis) The middle layer of the skin, which contains connective tissue, nerve endings, hair follicles, sweat glands, and oil glands. (24)

descending colon (dĭ-sĕnd'ĭng kō'lən) The segment of the large intestine after the transverse colon that descends the left side of the abdominal cavity. (31)

descending tracts (dĭ-sĕnd'ĭng trăkts) Tracts of the spinal cord that carry motor information from the brain to muscles and glands. (27)

detrusor muscle (dē-trŭs'or mŭs'əl) A smooth muscle that contracts to push urine from the bladder into the urethra. (34)

diabetes mellitus (dī'ə-bē'tĭs mə-lī'təs) Any of several related endocrine disorders characterized by an elevated level of glucose in the blood, caused by a deficiency of insulin or insulin resistance at the cellular level. (32)

diagnosis (Dx) (dī'əg-no'sĭs) The primary condition for which a patient is receiving care. (16)

diagnosis code (dī'əg-nō'sĭs kōd) The way a diagnosis is communicated to the third-party payer on the healthcare claim. (16)

diagnostic radiology (dī'əg-nos'tik rā'dē-ŏl'ə-jē) The use of x-ray technology to determine the cause of a patient's symptoms. (53)

diapedesis (dī'ă-pē-dē'sis)(†) The squeezing of a cell through a blood vessel wall. (28)

diaphragm (dī'ə-frăm') A muscle that separates the thoracic and abdominopelvic cavities. (23)

diaphysis (dī'-af'i-sis) The shaft of a long bone. (25)

diastolic pressure (dī'ə-stŏl'ĭk prĕsh'ər) The blood pressure measured when the heart relaxes. (28)

diathermy (dī'ə-thŭr'mē) A type of heat therapy in which a machine produces high-frequency waves that achieve deep heat penetration in muscle tissue. (43)

diencephalon (dī-en-sef'ă-lon)(†) A structure that includes the thalamus and the hypothalamus. It is located between the cerebral hemispheres and is superior to the brain stem. (27)

differential diagnosis (dĭf'ə-rĕn'shəl dī'əg-nō'sĭs) The process of determining the correct diagnosis when two or more diagnoses are possible. (38)

differently abled (dĭf'ər-ənt-lē ā'bəld) Having a condition that limits or changes a person's abilities and may require special accommodations. (13)

diffusion (di-fyū'zhŭn)(†) The movement of a substance from an area of high concentration to an area of low concentration. (23)

digital examination (dĭj'ĭ-tl ĭg-zam'ə-nā'shən) Part of a physical examination in which the physician inserts one or two fingers of one hand into the opening of a body canal such as the vagina or the rectum; used to palpate canal and related structures. (38)

diluent (dĭl′yoo-ənt) A liquid used to dissolve and dilute another substance, such as a drug. (51)

disaccharide (dī-sak′ă-rīd)(†) A type of carbohydrate that is a simple sugar. (31)

disability insurance (dĭs′ə-bĭlĭ-tē ĭn-shoor′əns) Insurance that provides a monthly, prearranged payment to an individual who cannot work as the result of an injury or disability. (15)

disbursement (dĭs-bûrs′mənt) Any payment of funds made by the physician's office for goods and services. (8)

disclaimer (dĭs-klā′mər) A statement of denial of legal liability. (5)

disclosure (dĭ-sklō′zhər) The release of, the transfer of, the provision of access to, or the divulgence in any manner of patient information. (3)

disclosure statement (dĭ-sklō′zhər stāt′mənt) A written description of agreed terms of payment; also called a federal Truth in Lending statement. (17)

disinfectant (dĭs′ĭn-fĕk′tănt) A cleaning product applied to instruments and equipment to reduce or eliminate infectious organisms; not used on human tissue. (20)

disinfection (dĭs′ĭn-fĕk′shən) The destruction of infectious agents on an object or surface by direct application of chemical or physical means. (19)

dislocation (dĭs′lō-kā′shən) The displacement of a bone end from a joint. (44)

dispense (dĭ-spĕns′) To distribute a drug, in a properly labeled container, to a patient who is to use it. (50)

distal (dĭs′təl) Anatomical term meaning farther away from a point of attachment or farther away from the trunk of the body. (23)

distal convoluted tubule (dĭs′təl kon′vō-lū-ted tū′byūl) The last twisted section of the renal tubule; it is located after the loop of Henle. Several of these tubules merge together to form collecting ducts. (34)

distribution (dĭs′trĭ-byoo′shən) The biochemical process of transporting a drug from its administration site in the body to its site of action. (50)

diverticulitis (dī′ver-tik-yū-lī′tis)(†) Inflammation of the diverticuli, which are abnormal dilations in the intestine. (31)

DNA (dē′ĕn-ā′) A nucleic acid that contains the genetic information of cells. (23)

doctor of osteopathy (dok′tər ŏs′tē-ŏp′ə-thē) A doctor who focuses special attention on the musculoskeletal system and uses hands and eyes to identify and adjust structural problems, supporting the body's natural tendency toward health and self-healing. (2)

documentation (dŏk′yə-mən-tā′shən) The recording of information in a patient's medical record; includes detailed notes about each contact with the patient and about the treatment plan, patient progress, and treatment outcomes. (9)

dorsal (dôr′səl) See **posterior.** (23)

dorsal root (dôr′səl root) A portion of a spinal nerve that contains axons of sensory neurons only. (27)

dorsiflexion (dôr-si-flek′shŭn)(†) Pointing the toes upward. (26)

dosage (dōs′āj) The size, frequency, and number of doses. (50)

dose (dōs) The amount of a drug given or taken at one time. (50)

dot matrix printer (dŏt mā′trĭks prĭn′tər) An impact printer that creates characters by placing a series of tiny dots next to one another. (6)

double-booking system (dŭb′əl book′ĭng sĭs′təm) A system of scheduling in which two or more patients are booked for the same appointment slot, with the assumption that both patients will be seen by the doctor within the scheduled period. (12)

douche (doosh) Vaginal irrigation, which can be used to administer vaginal medication in liquid form. (51)

drainage catheter (drā′nĭj kăth′ĭ-tər) A type of catheter used to withdraw fluids. (47)

dressings (drĕs′ĭngs) Sterile materials used to cover a surgical or other wound. (42)

ductus arteriosus (dŭk′tŭs ar-tēr-ē-ō′sus)(†) The connection in the fetus between the pulmonary trunk and the aorta. (35)

ductus venosus (duk′tŭs ven-ō′sus)(†) A blood vessel that allows most of the blood to bypass the liver in the fetus. (35)

duodenum (doo′ə-dē′nəm) The first section of the small intestine. (31)

durable item (door′ə-bəl ī′təm) A piece of equipment that is used repeatedly, such as a telephone, computer, or examination table; contrast with **expendable item.** (8)

durable power of attorney (door′ə-bəl pouər ə-tûr′nē)(†) A document naming the person who will make decisions regarding medical care on behalf of another person if that person becomes unable to do so. (3)

dwarfism (dwôrf′ĭzm) A condition in which too little growth hormone is produced, resulting in an abnormally small stature. (32)

dysmenorrhea (dis-men-ōr-ē′ă)(†) Severe menstrual cramps that limit daily activity. (35)

dyspnea (disp-nē′ă)(†) Difficult or painful breathing. (37)

ear ossicles (îr os′i-kl)(†) Three tiny bones called the malleus, the incus, and the stapes located in the middle ear cavity. They are the smallest bones of the body. (33)

eccrine gland (ek′rin glănd)(†) The most numerous type of sweat gland. Eccrine sweat glands produce a watery type of sweat and are activated primarily by heat. (24)

echocardiography (ek′ō-kar-dē-og′ră-fē)(†) A procedure that tests the structure and function of the heart through the use of reflected sound waves, or echoes. (41)

E code (ē kŏd) A type of code in the ICD-9. E-codes identify the external causes of injuries and poisoning. (16)

ectoderm (ek′tō-derm)(†) The primary germ layer that gives rise to nervous tissue and some epithelial tissue. (35)

eczema (ĕk′sə-mə) Inflammatory condition of the skin. (24)

edema (ĭ-dē′mə) An excessive buildup of fluid in body tissue. (28)

editing (ĕd′ĭt-ĭng) The process of ensuring that a document is accurate, clear, and complete; free of grammatical errors; organized logically; and written in the appropriate style. (7)

effectors (ĭ-fĕk′tərs) Muscles and glands that are stimulated by motor neurons in the peripheral nervous system. (27)

efferent arterioles (ĕf′ər-ənt ar-tēr′ē-ōlz)(†) Structures that deliver blood to peritubular capillaries that are wrapped around the renal tubules of the nephron in the kidneys. (34)

efficacy (ĕf′ĭ-kə-sē) The therapeutic value of a procedure or therapy, such as a drug. (50)

efficiency (ĭ-fĭsh′ən-sē) The ability to produce a desired result with the least effort, expense, and waste. (8)

electrocardiogram (ECG or EKG) (ĭ-lĕk′trō-kär′dē-ə-grăm′) The tracing made by an **electrocardiograph.** (52)

electrocardiograph (ĭ-lĕk′trō-kär′dē-ə-grăf′) An instrument that measures and displays the waves of electrical impulses responsible for the cardiac cycle. (52)

electrocardiography (ĭ-lĕk′trō-kär′dē-ŏg′rə-fē) The process by which a graphic pattern is created to reflect the electrical impulses generated by the heart as it pumps. (52)

electrocauterization (ĭ-lĕk′trō-kô′tər-ĭ-zā′shən) The use of a needle, probe, or loop heated by electric current to remove growths such as warts, to stop bleeding, and to control nosebleeds that either will not subside or continually recur. (42)

electrodes (ĭ-lĕk′trōds′) Sensors that detect electrical activity. (52)

electroencephalography (ĭ-lĕk′trō-ĕn-sĕf′ə-lŏg′rə-fē) A procedure that records the electrical activity of the brain as a tracing called an electroencephalogram, or EEG, on a strip of graph paper. (41)

electrolytes (ĭ-lĕk′trə-līts) Substances that carry electrical current through the movement of ions. (23)

electromyography (ĭ-lĕk′trō-mī-ŏg′rə-fē) A procedure in which needle electrodes are inserted into some of the skeletal muscles and a monitor records the nerve impulses and measures conduction time; used to detect neuromuscular disorders or nerve damage. (41)

electron microscope (ĭ-lĕk′trŏn mī′krə-skōp′) A microscope that uses a beam of electrons instead of a beam of light; can magnify an image several million times. (45)

electronic data interchange (EDI) (ĭ-lĕk-trŏn′ĭk dā′tə ĭn′tər-chānj′) Transmitting electronic medical insurance claims from providers to payers using the necessary information systems. (15)

electronic mail (ĭ-lĕk′trŏn′ĭks) A method of sending and receiving messages through a computer network; commonly known as e-mail. (6)

electronic transaction record (ĭ-lĕk′trŏn′ĭk trăn-săk′shən rĭ-kôrd) The standardized codes and formats used for the exchange of medical data. (3)

elevation (e-lə-vā′shən) The raising of a body part. (26)

embolism (ĕm′bə-lĭz′əm) An obstruction in a blood vessel. (40)

embolus (ĕm′bə-ləs) A portion of a thrombus that breaks off and moves through the bloodstream. (28)

embryonic period (em-brē-on′ik pîr′ē-əd) (†) The second through eighth weeks of pregnancy. (35)

E/M code (ē/ĕm kōd) Evaluation and management codes that are often considered the most important of all CPT codes. The E/M section guidelines explain how to code different levels of services. (16)

empathy (ĕm′pə-thē) Identification with or sensitivity to another person's feelings and problems. (4)

employment contract (ĕm-ploi′mənt kŏn′trăkt′) A written agreement of employment terms between employer and employee that describes the employee's duties and the considerations (money, benefits, and so on) to be given by the employer in exchange. (18)

enclosure (ĕn-klō′zhərz) Materials that are included in the same envelope as the primary letter. (7)

endocardium (en-dō-kar′dē-ŭm) (†) The innermost layer of the heart. (28)

endochondral (en-dō-kon′drăl) (†) A type of ossification in which bones start out as cartilage models. (25)

endocrine gland (ĕn′də-kra-n glănd) A gland that secretes its products directly into tissue, fluid, or blood. (23)

endocrinologist (ĕn′də-kra-nŏl′ə-jĭst) A specialist who diagnoses and treats disorders of the endocrine system, which regulates many body functions by circulating hormones that are secreted by glands throughout the body. (2)

endoderm (ĕn′dō-derm) (†) The primary germ layer that gives rise to epithelial tissues only. (35)

endogenous infection (ĕn′-dŏj′ə-nəs ĭn-fĕk′shən) An infection in which an abnormality or malfunction in routine body processes causes normally beneficial or harmless microorganisms to become pathogenic. (19)

endolymph (ĕn′dō-limf) (†) A fluid in the inner ear. When this fluid moves, it activates hearing and equilibrium receptors. (33)

endometriosis (ĕn′dō-mē-trē-ō′sis) (†) A condition in which tissues that make up the lining of the uterus grow outside the uterus. (35)

endometrium (ĕn′dō-mē′trē-ŭm) (†) The innermost layer of the uterus. It

undergoes significant changes during the menstrual cycle. (35)

endomysium (ĕn′dō-mĭz′ē-ŭm) (†) A connective tissue covering that surrounds individual muscle cells. (26)

endorse (ĕn-dôrs′) To sign or stamp the back of a check with the proper identification of the person or organization to whom the check is made out, to prevent the check from being cashed if it is stolen or lost. (18)

endoscopy (ĕn-dôs′kə-pē) Any procedure in which a scope is used to visually inspect a canal or cavity within the body. (41)

endosteum (en-dos′tē-ŭm) (†) A membrane that lines the medullary cavity and the holes of spongy bone. (25)

enunciation (ĭ-nŭn′sē-ā′shən) Clear and distinct speaking. (11)

enzyme immunoassay (EIA) (ĕn′zīm im′yū-nō-as′ā) (†) The detection of substances by immunological methods. This method involves an antigen, an antibody specific for the antigen, and a second antibody conjugated to an enzyme. (47)

enzyme-linked immunosorbent assay (ELISA) test (ĕn′zīm-lĭngkt im′yū-nō-sōr′bent ăs′ā tĕst) (†) A blood test that confirms the presence of antibodies developed by the body's immune system in response to an initial HIV infection. (21)

eosinophil (ē-ō-sin′ō-fil) (†) A type of granular leukocyte that captures invading bacteria and antigen-antibody complexes through phagocytosis. (48)

epicardium (ep-i-kar′dē-ŭm) (†) The outermost layer of the wall of the heart. Also known as the **visceral pericardium.** (28)

epidermis (ĕp′ĭ-dûr′mĭs) The most superficial layer of the skin. (24)

epididymis (ep-i-did′i-mis) (†) An elongated structure attached to the back of the testes and in which sperm cells mature. (35)

epididymitis (ep-i-did-i-mī′tis) (†) Inflammation of an **epididymis.** Most cases result from infection. (35)

epiglottic cartilage (ep-i-glot′ik kär′tl-ĭj) (†) A cartilage of the larynx that forms the framework of the epiglottis. (30)

epiglottis (ep-i-glot-ī′tis) (†) The flap-like structure that closes off the larynx during swallowing. (30)

epilepsy (ĕp′ə-lĕp′sē) A condition that occurs when parts of the brain receive a burst of electrical signals that disrupt normal brain function; also called **seizures.** (27)

epimysium (ep-i-mis´ē-ŭm)(†) A thin covering that is just deep to the fascia of a muscle. It surrounds the entire muscle. (26)

epinephrine (ĕp´ə-nĕf´rĭn) An injectable medication used to treat anaphylaxis by causing vasoconstriction to increase blood pressure. (29) A hormone secreted from the adrenal glands. It increases heart rate, breathing rate, and blood pressure. (32)

epiphyseal disk (ep-i-fiz´ē-ăl dĭsk)(†) A plate of cartilage between the **epiphysis** and the **diaphysis.** (25)

epiphysis (e-pif´i-sis)(†) The expanded end of a long bone. (25)

epistaxis (ĕp´i-stak´sis) Nosebleed. (44)

epithelial tissue (ep-i-thē´lē-ĕl tĭsh´ōō)(†) A tissue type that lines the tubes, hollow organs, and cavities of the body. (23)

erectile tissue (ĭ-rĕk´təl tĭsh´ōō) A highly specialized tissue located in the shaft of the penis. It fills with blood to achieve an erection. (35)

erythema (er-i-thē´mă) Redness of the skin. (43)

erythroblastosis fetalis (ĕ-rith´rō-blas-tō´sis fe´tăl-is)(†) A serious anemia that develops in a fetus with Rh-positive blood as a result of antibodies in an Rh-negative mother's body. (28)

erythrocytes (i-rĭth´rə-sīt´s) Red blood cells. (28)

erythrocyte sedimentation rate (ESR) (i-rĭth´rə-sīt´ sĕd´ə-mən-tā´shən rāt) The rate at which red blood cells, the heaviest blood component, settle to the bottom of a blood sample. (48)

erythropoietin (ĕ-rith-rō-poy´ē-tin)(†) A hormone secreted by the kidney and is responsible for regulating the production of red blood cells. (28)

esophageal hiatus (i-sŏf´ə-jē´əl) Hole in the diaphragm through which the esophagus passes. (31)

established patient (i-stăb´lisht pā´shənt) A patient who has seen the physician within the past three years. This determination is important when using E/M codes. (16)

estrogen (ĕs´trə-jən) A female sex hormone; when produced during ovulation, estrogen causes a buildup of the lining of the uterus (womb) to prepare it for a possible pregnancy. (32)

ethics (ĕth´ĭks) General principles of right and wrong, as opposed to requirements of law. (3)

ethmoid (ĕth´moyd)(†) Bones located between the sphenoid and nasal bone that form part of the floor of the cranium. (25)

etiologic agent (ē´tē-ə-lŏj´ĭk ā´jənt) A living microorganism or its toxin that may cause human disease. (46)

etiquette (ĕt´ĭ-ket´) Good manners. (11)

eustachian tube (yōō-stā´shən tōōb) An opening in the middle ear, leading to the back of the throat, that helps equalize air pressure on both sides of the eardrum. (39)

eversion (ē-ver´zhŭn)(†) Turning the sole of the foot laterally. (26)

exclusion (ĭk-sklōozh´ən) An expense that is not covered by a particular insurance policy, such as an eye examination or dental care. (15)

excretion (ĭk-skrē´shən) The elimination of waste by a discharge; in drug metabolism, the manner in which a drug is eliminated from the body. (50)

exocrine gland (ĕk´sə-krĭn glănd) A gland that secretes its product into a duct. (23)

exogenous infection (ĕk-sŏj´ə-nəs ĭn-fĕk´shən) An infection that is caused by the introduction of a pathogen from outside the body. (19)

expendable item (ĭk-spĕn´dəbəl ī´təm) An item that is used and must then be restocked; also known collectively as supplies. Contrast with **durable item.** (8)

expiration (ĕk´spə-rā´shən) The process of breathing out; also called exhalation. (30)

expressed contract (ĭk-sprĕst´ kŏn´trăct) A contract clearly stated in written or spoken words. (3)

extension (ĭk-stĕn´shən) An unbending or straightening movement of the two elements of a jointed body part. (26)

external auditory canal (ĭk-stûr´nəl ô´dĭ-tôr´ē kə-năl´) Canal that carries sound waves to the tympanic membrane; commonly called the ear canal. (33)

externship (ĭk-stûrn´shĭp) A period of practical work experience performed by a medical assisting student in a physician's office, hospital, or other health-care facility. (1)

extrinsic eye muscles (ĭk-strĭn´sĭk ĭ mŭs´əlz) The skeletal muscles that move the eyeball. (33)

facsimile machine (făk-sĭm´ə-lē mə-shēn´) A piece of office equipment used to send a facsimile, or fax, over telephone lines from one modem to another; more commonly called a fax machine. (11)

facultative (fak-ŭl-tā´tiv)(†) Able to adapt to different conditions; in microbiology, able to grow in environments either with or without oxygen. (46)

Fahrenheit (făr´ən-hīt) One of two common scales used for measuring temperature; measured in degrees Fahrenheit, or °F. (37)

fallopian tubes (fə-lō´pē-ən tūbz) Tubes that extend from the uterus on each side and that open near an ovary. (35)

family practitioner (făm´ə-lē prăk-tĭsh´ə-nər)(†) A physician who does not specialize in a branch of medicine but treats all types and ages of patients; also called a general practitioner. (2)

fascia (fash´ē-ă)(†) A structure that covers entire skeletal muscles and separates them from each other. (26)

fascicle (făs´ĭ-kəl) Sections of a muscle divided by connective tissue called perimysium. (26)

febrile (fĕb´rəl) Having a body temperature above one's normal range. (37)

feces (fē´sēz) Material found in the large intestine and made from leftover chyme. Faces are eventually eliminated through the anus. (31)

feedback (fēd´băk´) Verbal and nonverbal evidence that a message was received and understood. (4)

fee-for-service (fē fôr sûr´vĭs) A major type of health plan. It repays policyholders for the costs of health care that are due to illness and accidents. (15)

fee schedule (fē skĕj´ōol) A list of the costs of common services and procedures performed by a physician. (15)

felony (fĕl´ə-nē) A serious crime, such as murder or rape, that is punishable by imprisonment. In certain crimes, a felony is punishable by death. (3)

femoral (fem´ŏ-răl)(†) Relating to the femur or thigh. (23)

femur (fē´mər) The bone in the upper leg; commonly called the thigh bone. (25)

fenestrated drape (fĕn´ĭ-strāt´ĕd drāp) A drape that has a round or slitlike opening that provides access to the surgical site. (38)

fertilization (fer´til-i-zā´shŭn) The process in which an egg unites with a sperm. (35)

fetal period (fēt´l pîr´ē-əd) A period that begins at week nine of pregnancy and continues through delivery of the offspring. (35)

fiber (fī´bər) The tough, stringy part of vegetables and grains, which is not absorbed by the body but aids in a variety of bodily functions. (49)

fibrinogen (fī-brin′ō-jen) (†) A protein found in plasma that is important for blood clotting. (28)

fibroid (fī′broid′) A benign tumor in the uterus composed of fibrous tissue. (35)

fibromyalgia (fī-brō-mī-al′jē-ă) (†) A condition that exhibits chronic pain primarily in joints, muscles, and tendons. (26)

fibula (fĭb′yə-lə) The lateral bone of the lower leg. (25)

file guide (fīlgīd) A heavy cardboard or plastic insert used to identify a group of file folders in a file drawer. (10)

filtration (fĭl-trā′shən) A process that separates substances into solutions by forcing them across a membrane. (23)

fimbriae (fĭ′m-brē-ə) Fringe-like structures that border the entrances of the **fallopian tubes.** (35)

first morning urine specimen (fûrst môr′nĭng yŏŏr′ĭn spĕs′ə-mən) A urine specimen that is collected after a night's sleep; contains greater concentrations of substances that collect over time than specimens taken during the day. (47)

fixative (fĭk′sə-tĭv) A solution sprayed on a slide immediately after the specimen is applied. It is used to preserve and hold the cells in place until a microscopic examination is performed. (22)

flexion (flek′shŭn) (†) A bending movement of the two elements of a jointed body part. (26)

floater (flō′tər) A nonsterile assistant who is free to move about the room during surgery and attend to unsterile needs. (42)

fluidotherapy (flŏŏ′ĭd-ōthĕr′ə-pē) A technique for stimulating healing, particularly in the hands and feet, by placing the affected body part in a container of glass beads that are heated and agitated with hot air. (43)

follicle (fŏl′ĭ-kəl) An accessory organ of the skin that is found in the dermis and the sites at which hairs emerge. (24)

follicle-stimulating hormone (FSH) (fŏl′ĭ-kəl stim′yū-lā-ting hôr′mōn′) A hormone that in females stimulates the production of estrogen by the ovaries; in males, it stimulates sperm production. (32)

follicular cells (fə-lĭ′-kyə-lər selz) Small cells contained in the primordial follicle along with a large cell called a primary **oocyte.** (35)

folliculitis (fŏ-lik-yū-lī′tis) (†) Inflammation of the hair follicle. (24)

fomite (fō′mĭt) (†) An inanimate object, such as clothing, body fluids, water, or food, that may be contaminated with infectious organisms and thus serve to transmit disease. (19)

fontanel (făn-tə-n′el) The soft spot in an infant's skull that consists of tough membranes that connect to incompletely developed bone. (25)

food exchange (fŏŏd ĭks-chānj′) A unit of food in a particular food category that provides the same amounts of protein, fat, and carbohydrates as all other units of food in that category. (49)

foramen magnum (fə-rā′-mən mag-nəm) The large hole in the occipital bone that allows the brain to connect to the spinal cord. (25)

foramen ovale (fō-rā′men ō-va′lē) (†) A hole in the fetal heart between the right atrium and the left atrium. (35)

forced vital capacity (FVC) (fôrst vīt′l kə-păs′ĭ-tē) The greatest volume of air that a person is able to expel when performing rapid, forced expiration. (52)

formalin (fōr-mă-lin) (†) A dilute solution of formaldehyde used to preserve biological specimens. (42)

formed elements (fôrmd ĕl′ə-mənts) Red blood cells, white blood cells, and platelets; comprise 45% of blood volume. (48)

formulary (fōr′myū-lā-rē) (†) An insurance plan's list of approved prescription medications. (15)

fraud (frôd) An act of deception that is used to take advantage of another person or entity. (3)

fracture (frăk′chər) Any break in a bone. (41)

frequency (frē′kwən-sē) The number of complete fluctuations of energy per second in the form of waves. (39)

frontal (frŭn′tl) Anatomical term that refers to the plane that divides the body into anterior and posterior portions. Also called coronal. (23)

full-block letter style (fŏŏl blŏk lĕt′ər stīl) A letter format in which all lines begin flush left; also called block style. (7)

functional résumé (fŭngk′shə-nəl rĕz′ōō-mā′) A résumé that highlights specialty areas of a person's accomplishments and strengths. (54)

fungus (fŭng′gəs) A eukaryotic organism that has a rigid cell wall at some stage in the life cycle. (46)

gait (gāt) The way a person walks, consisting of two phases: stance and swing. (43)

ganglia (găng′glē-ə) Collections of neuron cell bodies outside the central nervous system. (27)

gastic juice (găs′trĭk jüs) Secretions from the stomach lining that begin the process of digesting protein. (31)

gastritis (gă-strī′tĭs) Inflammation of the stomach lining. (31)

gastroenterologist (găs′trō-ĕn-ter-ol′ō-jist) (†) A specialist who diagnoses and treats disorders of the entire gastrointestinal tract, including the stomach, intestines, and associated digestive organs. (2)

gastroesophageal reflux disease (GERD) (gas′trō-ē-sof′ă-jē′ălrē′flĕks dĭ-zēz′) A condition that occurs when stomach acids are pushed into the esophagus and cause heartburn. (31)

gene (jĕn) A segment of DNA that determines a body trait. (23)

general physical examination (jĕn′ər-əl fĭz′ĭ-kəl ĭg-zăm′ə-nā′shən) An examination performed by a physician to confirm a patient's health or to diagnose a medical problem. (22)

generic name (jə-nĕr′ĭk nām) A drug's official name. (50)

gerontologist (jĕr′ən-tŏl′ə-jist) A specialist who studies the aging process. (2)

giantism (jī′an-tizm) (†) A condition in which too much growth hormone is produced in childhood, resulting in an abnormally increased stature. (32)

glans penis (glanz pē′nĭs) A cone-shaped structure at the end of the penis. (35)

glaucoma (glou-kō′mə) A condition in which too much pressure is created in the eye by excessive aqueous humor. This excess pressure can lead to permanent damage of the optic nerves, resulting in blindness. (33)

global period (glō′bəl pîr′ē-əd) The period of time that is covered for follow-up care of a procedure or surgical service. (16)

globulins (glob′yū-lin) (†) Plasma proteins that transport lipids and some vitamins. (28)

glomerular capsule (glō-măr′yū-lăr kăp′səl) (†) A capsule that surrounds the **glomerulus** of the kidney. (34)

glomerular filtrate (glō-măr′yū-lăr fĭl′trāt′) (†) The fluid remaining in the **glomerular capsule** after **glomerular filtration.** (34)

glomerular filtration (glō-măr′yū-lăr fĭl-trā′shən) (†) The process by which urine forms in the kidneys as blood moves through a tight ball of capillaries called the glomerulus. (34)

glomerulonephritis (glō-mār′yŭ-lō-nef-rī′tis) (†) An inflammation of the glomeruli of the kidney. (34)

glomerulus (glō-mār′yŭ-lŭs) (†) A group of capillaries in the renal corpuscle. (34)

glottis (glot′is) (†) The opening between the vocal cords. (30)

glucagon (gloō′kǝ-gŏn′) A hormone that increases glucose concentrations in the bloodstream and slows down protein synthesis. (32)

glycogen (glī′kǝ-jǝn) An excess of glucose that is stored in the liver and in skeletal muscle. (31)

glycosuria (glī-kō-sū′rē-ă) (†) The presence of significant levels of glucose in the urine. (47)

gonads (gō′nǎdz) The reproductive organs; namely, in women, the ovaries, and in men, the testes. (32)

gonadotropin-releasing hormone (GnRH) (gō′nad-ō-trō′pinrī-lēs′ĭng hôr′mōn′) Hormone that stimulates the anterior pituitary gland to release **follicle stimulating hormone (FSH)**. (35)

goniometer (gō-nē-ă′-me-tǝr) A protractor device that measures range of motion. (43)

gout (gowt) (†) A medical condition characterized by an elevated uric acid level and recurrent acute arthritis. (25)

G-protein (jē-prō′tēn) (†) A substance that causes enzymes in the cell to activate following the activation of the hormone-receptor complex in the cell membrane. (32)

gram-negative (grăm′nĕg′ǝ-tĭv) Referring to bacteria that lose their purple color when a decolorizer has been added during a Gram's stain. (46)

gram-positive (grăm′pŏz′ĭ-tĭv) Referring to bacteria that retain their purple color after a decolorizer has been added during a Gram's stain. (46)

Gram's stain (grămz stān) A method of staining that differentiates bacteria according to the chemical composition of their cell walls. (46)

granular leukocyte (grăn′yǝ-lǝr loō′kǝ-sīt′) A type of leukocyte (white blood cell) with a segmented nucleus and granulated cytoplasm; also known as a polymorphonuclear leukocyte. (48)

granulocyte (gran′yŭ-lō-sīt) (†) See **granular leukocyte.** (28)

Grave's disease (grāvz dĭ-zēz′) A disorder in which a person develops antibodies that attack the thyroid gland. (32)

gray matter (grā mǎt′ǝr) The inner tissue of the brain and the spinal cord that is darker in color than **white matter.** It contains all the bodies and dendrites of nerve cells. (27)

gross earnings (grōs ûr′nĭngz) The total amount an employee earns before deductions. (18)

growth hormone (GH) (grōth hôr′mōn′) A hormone that stimulates an increase in the size of the muscles and bones of the body. (32)

gustatory receptors (gǝ′s-tǝ-tör-ē ri-se′p-tǝr) Taste receptors that are found on taste buds. (33)

gynecologist (gī′nĭ-kŏl′ǝ-jĭst) A specialist who performs routine physical care and examinations of the female reproductive system. (2)

gyri (jī′rī) (†) The ridges of brain matter between the sulci; also called **convolutions.** (27)

hapten (hap′tĕn) (†) Foreign substances in the body too small to start an immune response by themselves. (29)

HCPCS Level II codes (ăch sē pē sē ĕs lĕv′ǝl toō kōdz) Codes that cover many supplies such as sterile trays, drugs, and durable medical equipment; also referred to as national codes. They also cover services and procedures not included in the CPT. (16)

hairy leukoplakia (hâr′ē lū-kō-plā′kē-ă) (†) A white lesion on the tongue associated with AIDS. (21)

hard copy (härd kŏp′ē) A readable paper copy or printout of information. (6)

hardware (härd′wâr′) The physical components of a computer system, including the monitor, keyboard, and printer. (6)

hazard label (hăz′ǝrd lā′bǝl) A shortened version of the Material Safety Data Sheet; permanently affixed to a hazardous substance container. (45)

Health Care Common Procedure Coding System (HCPCS) (hĕlth kâr kŏm′ǝn prǝ-sē′jǝr kōd′ĭng sĭs′tǝm) A coding system developed by the Centers for Medicare and Medicaid Services that is used in coding services for Medicare patients. (16)

health maintenance organization (HMO) (hĕlth mān′tǝ-nǝns ôr′gǝ-nĭ-zā′shǝn) A health-care organization that provides specific services to individuals and their dependents who are enrolled in the plan. Doctors who enroll in an HMO agree to provide certain services in exchange for a prepaid fee. (15)

helper T-cells (hĕl′pǝr tē′sĕlz) White blood cells that are a key component of the body's immune system and that work in coordination with other white blood cells to combat infection. (21)

hematemesis (hē′-mǎ-tem′ē-sis) The vomiting of blood. (44)

hematocrit (hē′mǎ-tō-krit) (†) The percentage of the volume of a sample made up of red blood cells after the sample has been spun in a centrifuge. (48)

hematology (hēmǝ-tŏl′ǝ-jē) The study of blood. (48)

hematoma (hē′mǝ-tō′mǝ) A swelling caused by blood under the skin. (44)

hematuria (hē-mǎ-tu′rē-ă) (†) The presence of blood in the urine. (47)

hemocytoblast (hē′mǎ-tō-sī′tō-blast) (†) Cells of the red bone marrow that produce most red blood cells. (28)

hemoglobin (hē′mǝ-glō′bĭn) A protein that contains iron and bonds with and carries oxygen to cells; the main component of erythrocytes. (24)

hemoglobinuria (hē′mō-glō-bi-nū′rē-ă) (†) The presence of free **hemoglobin** in the urine; a rare condition caused by transfusion reactions, malaria, drug reactions, snake bites, or severe burns. (47)

hemolysis (hē-mol′ĭ-sis) (†) The rupturing of red blood cells, which releases hemoglobin. (48)

hemorrhoids (hĕm′ǝ-roidz′) Varicose veins of the rectum or anus. (31)

hemostasis (hē′mō-stā-sis) (†) The stoppage of bleeding. (28)

hepatic duct (hĭ-pǎt′ĭk dŭkt) A duct that leaves the liver carrying bile and merges with the cystic duct to form the common bile duct. (31)

hepatic lobule (he-pǎt′ĭk lob′yŭl) (†) Smaller divisions within the lobes of the liver. (31)

hepatic portal system (he-pat′ik pôr′tl sĭs′tǝm) (†) The collection of veins carrying blood to the liver. (28)

hepatic portal vein (hĭ-pǎt′ĭk pôr′tl vān) A blood vessel that carries blood from the other digestive organs to the **hepatic lobules.** (31)

hepatitis (hĕp′ǝ-tī′tĭss) Inflammation of the liver usually caused by viruses or toxins. (31)

hepatocytes (hep′ǎ-tō-sītz) (†) The cells within the lobules of the liver. Hepatocytes process nutrients in the blood and make bile. (31)

hernia (hûr′nē-ǝ) The protrusion of an organ through the wall that usually contains it, such as a hiatal or inguinal hernia. (31)

herpes simplex (her´pēz sĭm´plĕks) (†) A medical condition characterized by an eruption of one or more groups of vesicles on the lips or genitalia. (24)

herpes zoster (her´pēz zos´ter) (†) A medical condition characterized by an eruption of a group of vesicles on one side of the body following a nerve root. (24)

hierarchy (hī´ə-rär´kē) A term that pertains to Abraham Maslow's hierarchy of needs. This hierarchy states that human beings are motivated by unsatisfied needs and that certain lower needs must be satisfied before higher needs can be met. (4)

hilum (hī´lŭm) (†) The indented side of a lymph node. (28) The entrance of the renal sinus that contains the renal artery, renal vein, and ureter. (34)

HIPAA (Health Insurance Portability and Accountability Act) (hĭp´ə) A set of regulations whose goals include the following: (1) improving the portability and continuity of health-care coverage in group and individual markets; (2) combating waste, fraud, and abuse in health-care insurance and health-care delivery; (3) promoting the use of a medical savings account; (4) improving access to long-term care services and coverage; and (5) simplifying the administration of health insurance. (1)

Holter monitor (hol´tər mŏn´ĭ-tər) An electrocardiography device that includes a small portable cassette recorder worn around a patient's waist or on a shoulder strap to record the heart's electrical activity. (52)

homeostasis (hō´mē-ō-stā´sĭs) A balanced, stable state within the body. (4)

homologous chromosome (hŏ-mŏl´ō-gŭs krō´mə-sōm´) (†) Members in each pair of chromosomes. (23)

hormone (hôr´mōn´) A chemical secreted by a cell that affects the functions of other cells. (32)

hospice (hŏs´pĭs) Volunteers who work with terminally ill patients and their families. (4)

human chorionic gonadotropin (HCG) (hyōō´mən kō-rē-on´ik gō´nad-ō-trō´pin) A hormone secreted by cells of the embryo after implantation. It maintains the corpus luteum in the ovary so it will continue to secrete estrogen and progesterone. (35)

human immunodeficiency virus (HIV) (hyōō´mən im´yū-nō-dē-fish´en-sē vī´rəs) A retrovirus that gradually destroys the body's immune system and causes AIDS. (29)

humerus (hyü´-mə-rəs) The bone of the upper arm. (25)

humors (hyōō´mərz) Fluids of the body. (29)

hydrotherapy (hī´drə-thĕr´ə-pē) The therapeutic use of water to treat physical problems. (43)

hyoid (hī´-óid) The bone that anchors the tongue. (25)

hyperextension (hī´per-eks-ten´shŭn) (†) Extension of a body part past the normal anatomical position. (26)

hyperglycemia (hī´pər-glī-sē´mē-ə) High blood sugar. (44)

hyperopia (hī-per-ō´pē-ă) A condition that occurs when light entering the eye is focused behind the retina; commonly called farsightedness. (33)

hyperpnea (hī-per-nē´ă) (†) Abnormally deep, rapid breathing. (37)

hyperreflexia (hī´per-rē-flek´sē-ă) Reflexes that are stronger than normal reflexes. (27)

hypertension (hī´pər-tĕn´shan) High blood pressure. (28)

hyperventilation (hī´pər-vĕn´tl-ā´shən) The condition of breathing rapidly and deeply. Hyperventilating decreases the amount of carbon dioxide in the blood. (30)

hypodermis (hī´pə-dûr´mĭs) The subcutaneous layer of the skin that is largely made of adipose tissue. (24)

hypoglycemia (hī´pō-glī-sē´mē-ə) Low blood sugar. (44)

hyporeflexia (hī´pō-rē-flek´sē-ă) (†) A condition of decreased reflexes. (27)

hypotension (hī´pō-tĕn´shan) Low blood pressure. (37)

hypothalamus (hī´pō-thăl´ə-məs) A region of the **diencephalon**. It maintains homeostasis by regulating many vital activities such as heart rate, blood pressure, and breathing rate. (27)

hypovolemic shock (hī´per-vō-lē´mē-ă shŏk) (†) A state of shock resulting from insufficient blood volume in the circulatory system. (44)

hysterectomy (hĭs´tə-rĕk´tə-mē) Surgical removal of the uterus. (35)

ICD-9 See *International Classification of Diseases, Ninth Revision, Clinical Modification.* (16)

icon (ī´kŏn´) A pictorial image; on a computer screen, a graphic symbol that identifies a menu choice. (6)

identification line (ī-dĕn´tə-fĭ-kā´shən līn) A line at the bottom of a letter containing the letter writer's initials and the typist's initials. (7)

ileocecal sphincter A structure that controls the movement of **chime** from the **ileum** to the **cecum.** (31)

ileum (ĭl´ē-əm) The last portion of the small intestine. It is directly attached to the large intestine. (31)

ilium (ĭ´-lē-əm) The most superior part of the hip bone. It is broad and flaring. (25)

immunity (ĭ-myōōn´ĭ-tē) The condition of being resistant or not susceptible to pathogens and the diseases they cause. (19)

immunization (ĭm´yū-nĭ-zā-shən) The administration of a vaccine or toxoid to protect susceptible individuals from communicable diseases. (20)

immunocompromised (ĭm´yū-nō-kom´pro-mīzd) (†) Having an impaired or weakened immune system. (21)

immunofluorescent antibody (IFA) test (ĭm´yū-nō-flūr-es´ent ăn´tĭ-bŏd-ē tĕst) (†) A blood test used to confirm enzyme-linked immunosorbent assay (ELISA) test results for HIV infection. (21)

immunoglobulins (ĭm´yū-nō-glob´yū-linz) (†) A class of structurally related proteins that include IgG, IgA, IgM, and IgE; also called **antibodies.** (29)

impetigo (ĭm´pĭ-tī´gō) A contagious skin infection usually caused by germs commonly called staph and strep. (24)

implied contract (ĭm-plīd kŏn´trăct´) A contract that is created by the acceptance or conduct of the parties rather than the written word. (3)

impotence (ĭm´pŏ-tens) (†) A disorder in which a male cannot maintain an erect penis to complete sexual intercourse; also called erectile dysfunction. (35)

inactive file (ĭn-ăk´tĭv fīl) A file used infrequently. (10)

incision (ĭn-sĭzh´ən) A surgical wound made by cutting into body tissue. (42)

incisors (ĭn-sī´zərz) The most medial teeth. They act as chisels to bite off food. (31)

incomplete proteins (ĭn´kəm-plēt´ prō´tēnz´) Proteins that lack one or more of the essential amino acids. (49)

incontinence (in-kon´ti-nens) (†) The involuntary leakage of urine. (34)

incus (ĭng´kəs) A small bone in the middle ear, located between the malleus and the stapes; also called the anvil. (39)

indication (ĭn´dĭ-kā´shən) The purpose or reason for using a drug, as approved by the FDA. (50)

induration The process of hardening or of becomming hard. (20)

infection (ĭn-fĕk´shən) The presence of a pathogen in or on the body. (29)

infectious waste (ĭn-fĕk´shəs wāst) Waste that can be dangerous to those who handle it or to the environment; includes human waste, human tissue, and body fluids as well as potentially hazardous waste, such as used needles, scalpels, and dressings, and cultures of human cells. (13)

inferior (ĭn-fîr´ē-ər) Anatomical term meaning below or closer to the feet; also called caudal. (23)

inflammation (ĭn´flə-mā´shən) The body's reaction when tissue becomes injured or infected. The four cardinal signs are redness, heat, pain, and swelling. (29)

informed consent form (ĭn-fôrmd´ kən-sĕnt fôrm) A form that verifies that a patient understands the offered treatment and its possible outcomes or side effects. (9)

infundibulum (ĭn-fŭn-dĭb´yū-lŭm)(†) The funnel-like end of the uterine tube near an ovary. It catches the secondary oocyte as it leaves the ovary. (35)

infusion (ĭn-fyū´zhŭn)(†) A slow drip, as of an intravenous solution into a vein. (51)

ink-jet printer (ĭngk´jĕt´ prĭn´tər) A nonimpact printer that forms characters by using a series of dots created by tiny drops of ink. (6)

inner cell mass (ĭn´ər sĕl măs) A group of cells in a blastocyte that gives rise to an embryo. (35)

inorganic (ĭn´ôr-găn´ĭk) Matter that generally does not contain carbon and hydrogen. (23)

insertion (ĭn-sûr´shən) An attachment site of a skeletal muscle that moves when a muscle contracts. (26)

inspection (ĭn-spĕk´shən) The visual examination of the patient's entire body and overall appearance. (38)

inspiration (in(†)-spə-rā´-shən) The act of breathing in; also called inhalation. (30)

insulin (ĭn´sə-lĭn) A hormone that regulates the amount of sugar in the blood by facilitating its entry into the cells. (32)

interactive pager (ĭn´tər-ăk´tĭv pāj´ər) A pager designed for two-way communication. The pager screen displays a printed message and allows the physician to respond by way of a mini keyboard. (5)

intercalated disc (in-ter´kă-lā-ted disk)(†) A disk that connects groups of cardiac muscles. This disc allows the fibers in that group to contract and relax together. (26)

interferon (in-ter-fēr´on)(†) A protein that blocks viruses from infecting cells. (29)

interim room (ĭn´tər-ĭm rōōm) A room off the patient reception area and away from the examination rooms for occasions when patients require privacy. (13)

***International Classification of Diseases, Ninth Revision, Clinical Modification* (ICD-9)** (ĭn´tər-năsh´ə-nəl klăs´ə-fĭ-kā´shən dĭ-zēz´əz nīnth rĭ-vĭzh´ən klĭn´ĭ-kəl mŏd´ə-fĭ-kā´shən) Code set that is based on a system maintained by the World Health Organization of the United Nations. The use of the ICD-9 codes in the health-care industry is mandated by **HIPAA** for reporting patients' diseases, conditions, and signs and symptoms. (16)

Internet (ĭn´tər-nĕt´) A global network of computers. (6)

interneuron (in´ter-nū´ron)(†) A structure found only in the central nervous system that functions to link sensory and motor neurons together. (27)

internist (ĭn-tûr´nĭst) A doctor who specializes in diagnosing and treating problems related to the internal organs. (2)

interpersonal skills (ĭn´tər-pûr´sə-nəl skĭlz) Attitudes, qualities, and abilities that influence the level of success and satisfaction achieved in interacting with other people. (4)

interphase (ĭn´ter-fāz)(†) The state of a cell carrying out its normal daily functions and not dividing. (23)

interstitial cell (in-ter-stish´əl sĕl) A cell located between the seminiferous tubules that is responsible for making testosterone. (35)

intestinal lipase (ĭn-tĕs´tĭ-n lĭp´ās) An enzyme that digests fat. (31)

intradermal (ID) (ĭn´tră-der´măl) Within the upper layers of the skin. (51)

intradermal test (ĭn´tră-der´măl tĕst) An allergy test in which dilute solutions of allergens are introduced into the skin of the inner forearm or upper back with a fine-gauge needle. (41)

intramembranous (in-tra-me´m-bra-nəs) A type of ossification in which bones begin as tough fibrous membranes. (25)

intramuscular (IM) (in´tră-mŭs´kyū-lăr) Within muscle; an IM injection allows administration of a larger amount of a drug than a subcutaneous injection allows. (51)

intraoperative (ĭn´tră-ŏp´ər-ə-tĭv) Taking place during surgery. (42)

intravenous IV (ĭn´tra-vē´nəs) Injected directly into a vein. (51)

intravenous pyelography (IVP) (ĭn´tra-vē´nəs pī´ē-log´ră-fē)(†) A radiologic procedure in which the doctor injects a contrast medium into a vein and takes a series of x-rays of the kidneys, ureters, and bladder to evaluate urinary system abnormalities or trauma to the urinary system; also known as excretory urography. (53)

intrinsic factor (in-trĭn´zĭk făk´tər) A substance secreted by **parietal cells** in the lining of the stomach. It is necessary for vitamin B$_{12}$ absorption. (31)

invasive (ĭn-vā´sĭv) Referring to a procedure in which a catheter, wire, or other foreign object is introduced into a blood vessel or organ through the skin or a body orifice. Surgical asepsis is required during all invasive tests. (53)

inventory (ĭn´vən-tôrē) A list of supplies used regularly and the quantities in stock. (8)

inversion (ĭn-vûr´zhən) Turning the sole of the foot medially. (26)

invoice (ĭn´vois´) A bill for materials or services received by or services performed by the practice. (8)

ions (ī´ənz) Positively or negatively charged particles. (23)

iris (ī´rĭs) The colored part of the eye, made of muscular tissue that contracts and relaxes, altering the size of the pupil. (33)

ischium (is´-kē-əm) A structure that forms the lower part of the hip bone. (25)

islets of Langerhans (ī´lĭt lan´ger-hans) Structures in the pancreas that secrete insulin and glucagon into the bloodstream. (32)

itinerary (ī-tĭn´ə-rĕr´ē) A detailed travel plan listing dates and times for specific transportation arrangements and events, the location of meetings and lodgings, and phone numbers. (12)

jaundice (jôn´dĭs) A condition characterized by yellowness of the skin, eyes, mucous membranes, and excretions; occurs during the second stage of hepatitis infection. (21)

jejunum (jə-jōō´nəm) The mid-portion and the majority of the small intestine. (31)

journalizing (jûr′nə-līz′ĭng) The process of logging charges and receipts in a chronological list each day; used in the single-entry system of bookkeeping. (18)

juxtaglomerular apparatus (jŭks′tă-glō-mer′yū-lăr ăp′ə-răt′əs)(†) A structure contained in the nephron and made up of the macula densa and **juxtaglomerular cells.** (34)

juxtaglomerular cells (jŭks′tă-glō-mer′yū-lăr sělz) Enlarged smooth muscle cells in the walls of either the afferent or efferent arterioles. (34)

Kaposi's sarcoma (kap′ō-sēz sar-kō′mă) Abnormal tissue occurring in the skin, and sometimes in the lymph nodes and organs, manifested by reddish-purple to dark blue patches or spots on the skin. (21)

keratin (kĕr′ə-tĭn) A tough, hard protein contained in skin, hair, and nails. (24)

keratinocyte (kĕ-rat′i-nō-sīt)(†) The most common cell type in the epidermis of the skin. (24)

key (kē) The act of inputting or entering information into a computer. (7)

KOH mount (kā′ō-āch mount) A type of mount used when a physician suspects a patient has a fungal infection of the skin, nails, or hair and to which potassium hydroxide is added to dissolve the keratin in cell walls. (46)

Krebs cycle (krěbz sī′kəl) Also called the citric acid cycle. This cycle generates ATP for muscle cells. (26)

KUB radiography (kā′yōō-bē rā′dē-og′rə-fē)(†) The process of x-raying the abdomen to help assess the size, shape, and position of the urinary organs; evaluate urinary system diseases or disorders; or determine the presence of kidney stones. It can also be helpful in determining the position of an intrauterine device (IUD) or in locating foreign bodies in the digestive tract; also called a flat plate of the abdomen. (53)

kyphosis (kī-fō′sis) A deformity of the spine characterized by a bent-over position; more commonly called humpback. (38)

labeling (lā′bəl-ĭng) Information provided with a drug, including FDA-approved indications and the form of the drug. (50)

labia majora (lā′bē-ă mă′jôr-ă) The rounded folds of adipose tissue and skin that serve to protect the other female reproductive organs. (35)

labia minora (lā′bē-ă mĭ′nôr-ă) The folds of skin between the labia majora. (35)

labyrinth (lăb′ə-rĭnth′) The inner ear. (39)

laceration (lăs′ə-rā′shən) A jagged, open wound in the skin that can extend down into the underlying tissue. (42)

lacrimal apparatus (lăk′rə-məl ăp′ə-răt′əs) A structure that consists of the lacrimal glands and nasolacrimal ducts. (33)

lacrimal gland (lăk′rə-məl glănd) A gland in the eye that produces tears. (33)

lactase (lăk′tās)(†) An enzyme that digests sugars. (31)

lactic acid (lăk′tĭk ăs′ĭd) A waste product that must be released from the cell. It is produced when a cell is low on oxygen and converts pyruvic acid. (26)

lactogen (lak′tō-jen) Substance secreted by the placenta that stimulates the enlargement of the mammary glands. (35)

lacunae (lə-kü-na) Holes in the matrix of bone that hold osteocytes. (25)

lag phase (lăg fāz) The initial phase of wound healing, in which bleeding is reduced as blood vessels in the affected area constrict. (42)

lamella (lə-me′-lə) Layers of bone surrounding the canals of osteons. (25)

lancet (lăn′sĭt) A small, disposable instrument with a sharp point used to puncture the skin and make a shallow incision; used for capillary puncture. (48)

laryngopharynx (lă-ring′gō-far-ingks)(†) The portion of the pharynx behind the **larynx.** (31)

larynx (lăr′ĭngks) The part of the respiratory tract between the pharynx and the trachea that is responsible for voice production; also called the voice box. (30)

laser printer (lā′zər prĭn′tər) A high-resolution printer that uses a technology similar to that of a photocopier. It is the fastest type of computer printer and produces the highest-quality output. (6)

lateral (lăt′ər-əl) A directional term that means farther away from the midline of the body. (23)

lateral file (lăt′ər-əl fīl) A horizontal filing cabinet that features doors that flip up and a pull-out drawer, where files are arranged with sides facing out. (10)

law (lô) A rule of conduct established and enforced by an authority or governing body, such as the federal government. (3)

law of agency (lô ā′jən-sē) A law stating that an employee is considered to be acting on the physician's behalf while performing professional duties. (3)

lead (lēd) A view of a specific area of the heart on an electrocardiogram. (52)

lease (lēs) To rent an item or piece of equipment. (5)

legal custody (lēgəl kŭs′tə-dē) The court-decreed right to have control over a child's upbringing and to take responsibility for the child's care, including health care. (17)

lens (lěnz) A clear, circular disc located in the eye, just posterior to the iris, that can change shape to help the eye focus images of objects that are near or far away. (39)

letterhead (lět′ər-hěd′) Formal business stationery, with the doctor's (or office's) name and address printed at the top, used for correspondence with patients, colleagues, and vendors. (7)

leukemia (lōō-kē′mē-ə) A medical condition in which bone marrow produces a large number of white blood cells that are not normal. (28)

leukocytes (lōō-kə-sīt′s) White blood cells. (28)

leukocytosis (lŭ′kō-sī-tō′sis)(†) A white blood cell count that is above normal. (28)

leukopenia (lŭ′kō-pē′nē-ă)(†) A white blood cell count that is below normal. (28)

liable (lī′ə-bəl) Legally responsible. (3)

liability insurance (lī′ə-bĭl′ĭ-tē ĭn-shōōr′əns) A type of insurance that covers injuries caused by the insured or injuries that occurred on the insured's property. (15)

lifetime maximum benefit (līf′tīm′ măk′sə-məm běn′ə-fĭt) The total sum that a health plan will pay out over the patient's life. (15)

ligament (lĭg′ə-mənt) A tough, fibrous band of tissue that connects bone to bone. (25)

ligature (lĭg′ə-chōōr′) Suture material. (42)

limited check (lĭm′ĭ-tĭd chěk) A check that is void after a certain time limit; commonly used for payroll. (18)

lingual frenulum (ling′gwăl fren′yū-lŭm)(†) A flap of mucosa that holds the body of the tongue to the floor of the oral cavity. (31)

lingual tonsils (ling′gwăl ton′silz)(†) Two lumps of lymphatic tissue on the back of the tongue that act to destroy bacteria and viruses. (31)

linoleic acid (lin-ō-lē´ik as´id)(†) An essential fatty acid found in corn and sunflower oils. (31)

lipoproteins (lip-ō-prō´tēnz) Large molecules that are fat-soluble on the inside and water-soluble on the outside and carry lipids such as cholesterol and triglycerides through the bloodstream. (49)

living will (liv´ing wil) A legal document addressed to a patient's family and health-care providers stating what type of treatment the patient wishes or does not wish to receive if he becomes terminally ill, unconscious, or permanently comatose; sometimes called an advance directive. (3)

lobe (lōb) The frontal, parietal, temporal, or occipital regions of the cerebral hemisphere. (27)

locum tenens (lō´kum těn´ens)(†) A substitute physician hired to see patients while the regular physician is away from the office. (12)

loop of Henle (lōōp hen´lē) The portion of the renal tubule that curves back toward the renal corpuscle and twists again to become the distal convoluted tubule. (34)

lumbar enlargement (lŭm´bər ěn-lärj´mənt) The thickening of the spinal cord in the low back region. (27)

lunula (lŭ´nū-lă) The white half-moon–shaped area at the base of a nail. (24)

lupus erythematosis (lōō´pəs er-ə-the´-tō-səs) An autoimmune disorder in which a person produces antibodies that target the person's own cells and tissues. (29)

luteinizing hormone (LH) (lŭ´tē-in-iz-ing hôr´mōn´)(†) Hormone that in females stimulates ovulation and the production of estrogen; in males, it stimulates the production of testosterone. (32)

lymph (limf) A pale fluid found between cells that is collected by the lymphatic system and returned to the bloodstream. (28)

lymphedema (limf´e-dē´mă) The blockage of lymphatic vessels that results in the swelling of tissue from the accumulation of lymphatic fluid. (29)

lymphocyte (lim´fō-sīt)(†) An agranular leukocyte formed in lymphatic tissue. Lymphocytes are generally small. See **T lymphocyte** and **B lymphocyte**. (28)

lysozyme (lī´sō-zīm)(†) An enzyme in tears that destroys pathogens on the surface of the eye. (29)

macrophage (măk´rə-fāj´) A type of phagocytic cell found in the liver, spleen, lungs, bone marrow, and connective tissue. Macrophages play several roles in humoral and cell-mediated immunity, including presenting the antigens to the lymphocytes involved in these defenses; also known as monocytes while in the bloodstream. (19)

macula densa (mak´yū-lă den´sa)(†) An area of the distal convoluted tubule that touches afferent and efferent arterioles. (34)

macular degeneration (mak´yū-lăr dē-jen-er-ā´shŭn)(†) A progressive disease that usually affects people over the age of 50. It occurs when the retina no longer receives an adequate blood supply. (33)

magnetic resonance imaging (măg-nět´ik rěz´ə-nəns ĭ-māj´ing) A viewing technique that uses a powerful magnetic field to produce an image of internal body structures. (41)

maintenance contract (mān´tə-nəns kŏn´trăkt´) A contract that specifies when a piece of equipment will be cleaned, checked for worn parts, and repaired. (5)

major histocompatibility complex (MHC) (mā´jər his´tō-kom-pat-i-bil´i-tē kəm-plěks) A large protein complex that plays a role in T cell activation. (29)

malignant (mə-lĭg´nənt) A type of tumor or neoplasm that is invasive and destructive and that tends to metastasize; it is commonly known as cancerous. (29)

malleus (măl´ē-əs) A small bone in the middle ear that is attached to the eardrum; also called the hammer. (39)

malpractice claim (măl-prăk´tĭs klām) A lawsuit brought by a patient against a physician for errors in diagnosis or treatment. (3)

maltase (mawl-tās) An enzyme that digests sugars. (31)

mammary glands (mam´ă-rē glăndz) Accessory organs of the female reproductive system that secrete milk after pregnancy. (35)

mammography (mă-mŏg´rə-fē) X-ray examination of the breasts. (53)

managed care organization (MCO) (măn´ijd kâr ôr´gə-nĭ-zā´shən) A health-care business that, through mergers and buyouts, can deliver health care more cost-effectively. (1)

mandible (man´-də-bəl) A bone that forms the lower portion of the jaw. (25)

manipulation (mə-nĭp´yə-la´shən) The systematic movement of a patient's body parts. (38)

marrow (mer´-ō) A substance that is contained in the medullary cavity. In adults, it consists primarily of fat. (25)

massage therapist (mə-säzh´thěr´ə-pĭst) An individual who is trained to use pressure, kneading, and stroking to promote muscle and full-body relaxation. (2)

mastoid process (mas´-tó´id pr´ä-ses) A large bump on each temporal bone just behind each ear. It resembles a nipple, hence the name mastoid. (25)

Material Safety Data Sheet (MSDS) (mə-tîr´ē-əl sāf´tē dā´tə shět) A form that is required for all hazardous chemicals or other substances used in the laboratory and that contains information about the product's name, ingredients, chemical characteristics, physical and health hazards, guidelines for safe handling, and procedures to be followed in the event of exposure. (8)

matrix (mā´trĭks) The basic format of an appointment book, established by blocking off times on the schedule during which the doctor is able to see patients. (12) The material between the cells of connective tissue. (23)

matter (măt´er) Anything that takes up space and has weight. Liquids, solids, and gases are matter. (23)

maturation phase (măch´ə-rā´shən fāz) The third phase of wound healing, in which scar tissue forms. (42)

maxillae (mak-si´-lə) A bone that forms the upper portion of the jaw. (25)

Mayo stand (mā´ō stănd) A movable stainless steel instrument tray on a stand. (42)

medial (mē´dē-əl) A directional term that describes areas closer to the midline of the body. (23)

Medicaid (měd´ĭ-kād´) A federally funded health cost assistance program for low-income, blind, and disabled patients; families receiving aid to dependent children; foster children; and children with birth defects. (15)

medical asepsis (měd´ĭ-kəl ə-sěp´sĭs) Measures taken to reduce the number of microorganisms, such as hand washing and wearing examination gloves, that do not necessarily eliminate microorganisms; also called clean technique. (42)

medical practice act (mĕd´ĭ-kəl prăk´tĭs ăkt) A law that defines the exact duties that physicians and other healthcare personnel may perform. (40)

Medicare (mĕd´ĭ-kâr´) A national health insurance program for Americans aged 65 and older. (15)

Medicare + Choice Plan (mĕd´ĭ-kâr´ chois plăn) Medicare benefit in which beneficiaries can choose to enroll in one of three major types of plans instead of the **Original Medicare Plan.** (15)

Medigap (mĕd´ĭ-găp´) Private insurance that Medicare recipients can purchase to reduce the gap in coverage—the amount they would have to pay from their own pockets after receiving Medicare benefits. (15)

medullary cavity (me´-de-ler-ē ka´-və-tē) The canal that runs through the center of the **diaphysis.** (25)

megakaryocytes (meg-ă-kar´ē-ō-sĭts)(†) Cells within red blood marrow that give rise to platelets. (28)

meiosis (mī-ō´sis)(†) A type of cell division in which each new cell contains only one member of each chromosome pair. (23)

melanin (mĕl´ə-nĭn) A pigment that is deposited throughout the layers of the epidermis. (24)

melanocyte (mĕl´ă-nō-sīt)(†) A cell type within the epidermis that makes the pigment **melanin.** (24)

melatonin (mĕl´ə-tō´nĭn) A hormone that helps to regulate circadian rhythms. (32)

membrane potential (mĕm´brăn´ pə-tĕn´shəl) The potential inside a cell relative to the fluid outside the cell. (27)

meninges (mĕ-nĭn´jēz)(†) Membranes that protect the brain and spinal cord. (27)

meningitis (mĕn´ĭn-jī´tĭs) An inflammation of the **meninges.** (27)

meniscus (mə-nĭs´kəs) The curve in the air-to-liquid surface of a liquid specimen in a container. (37)

menopause (mĕn´ə-pôz´) The termination of the menstrual cycle due to the normal aging of the ovaries. (35)

menses (mĕn´sēz) The clinical term for menstrual flow. (35)

menstral cycle (mĕn´strōō-əl sī´kəl) The female reproductive cycle. It consists of regular changes in the uterine lining that lead to monthly bleeding. (35)

mensuration (mĕn´sə-rā´-shən) The process of measuring. (38)

mesoderm (mez´ō-derm)(†) The primary germ layer that gives rise to connective tissue and some epithelial tissue. (35)

metabolism (mĭ-tăb´ə-lĭz´əm) The overall chemical functioning of the body, including all body processes that build small molecules into large ones (anabolism) and break down large molecules into small ones (catabolism). (23)

metacarpals (me-tə-k̆ar-pəl) The bones that form the palms of the hand. (25)

metastasis (mə-tăs´tə-sĭs) The transfer of abnormal cells to body sites far removed from the original tumor. (41)

metatarsals (mĕt´ə-tär´salz) The bones that form the front of the foot. (25)

microbiology (mī´krō-bī-ŏl´ə-jē) The study of microorganisms. (46)

microfiche (mī´krō-fēsh´) Microfilm in rectangular sheets. (5)

microfilm (mī´krə-fĭlm´) A roll of film stored on a reel and imprinted with information on a reduced scale to minimize storage space requirements. (5)

microorganism (mī´krō-ôr´gə-nĭz´əm) A simple form of life, commonly made up of a single cell and so small that it can be seen only with a microscope. (19)

micropipette (mī´krō-pī-pet´) A small pipette that holds a small, precise volume of fluid; used to collect capillary blood. (48)

microvilli (mī´krō-vil´-ī)(†) Structures found in the lining of the small intestine. They greatly increase the surface area of the small intestine so it can absorb many nutrients. (31)

micturition (mik-chū-rish´ŭn)(†) The process of urination. (34)

midsagittal (mid´saj´i-tăl)(†) Anatomical term that refers to the plane that runs lengthwise down the midline of the body, dividing it into equal left and right halves. (23)

minerals (mĭn´ər-əlz) Natural, inorganic substances the body needs to help build and maintain body tissues and carry on life functions. (49)

minutes (mi-nōōtz´) A report of what happened and what was discussed and decided at a meeting. (12)

mirroring (mĭr´ər-ĭng) Restating in your own words what a person is saying. (36)

misdemeanor (mĭs´dĭ-mē´nər) A less serious crime such as theft under a certain dollar amount or disturbing the peace. A misdemeanor is punishable by fines or imprisonment. (3)

mitosis (mī-tō´sĭs) A type of cell division that produces ordinary body, or somatic, cells; each new cell receives a complete set of paired chromosomes. (23)

mitral valve (mī´trăl vălv)(†) See **bicuspid valve.** (28)

mobility aids (mō´bəl-ə-tē ādz) Devices that improve one's ability to move from one place to another; also called mobility assistive devices. (43)

modeling (mŏd´l-ĭng) The process of teaching the patient a new skill by having the patient observe and imitate it. (14)

modem (mō´dəm) A device used to transfer information from one computer to another through telephone lines. (6)

modified-block letter style (mŏd´ə-fīd blŏk lĕt´ər stīl) A letter format similar to full-block style, except that the dateline, complimentary closing, signature block, and notations are aligned and begin at the center of the page or slightly to the right of center. (7)

modified-wave schedule (mŏd´ə-fīd wāv skĕj´ōol) A scheduling system similar to the wave system, with patients arriving at planned intervals during the hour, allowing time to catch up before the next hour begins. (12)

modifier (mŏd´ə-fī´ər) One or more two-digit codes assigned to the five-digit main code to show that some special circumstance applied to the service or procedure that the physician performed. (16)

molars (mō´lərz) Back teeth that are flat and are designed to grind food. (31)

mold (mōld) Fungi that grow into large, fuzzy, multicelled organisms that produce spores. (46)

molecule (mŏl´ĭ-kyōōl´) The smallest unit into which an element can be divided and still retain its properties; it is formed when atoms bond together. (23)

money order (mŭn´ē ôr´dər) A certificate of guaranteed payment, which may be purchased from a bank, a post office, or some convenience stores. (18)

monocytes (mŏn´ō-sīts)(†) A large white blood cell with an oval or horseshoe-shaped nucleus that defends the body by phagocytosis; develops into a macrophage when it moves from blood into other tissues. (28)

monosaccharide (mon-ō-sak′ă-rīd)(†) A type of carbohydrate that is a simple sugar. (31)

mons pubis (m′änz py′ü-bəs) A fatty area that overlies the public bone. (35)

moral values (môr′əl văl′yōoz) Values or types of behavior that serve as a basis for ethical conduct and are formed through the influence of the family, culture, or society. (3)

mordant (môr′dnt) A substance, such as iodine, that can intensify or deepen the response a specimen has to a stain. (46)

morphology (môr-fŏl′ə-jē) The study of the shape or form of objects. (48)

morula (môr′u-lă)(†) A zygote that has undergone cleavage and results in a ball of cells. (35)

motherboard (mŭth′ər-bôrd′) The main circuit board of a computer that controls the other components in the system. (6)

motor (mō′tər) Efferent neurons that carry information from the central nervous system to the effectors. (27)

mucocutaneous exposure (myü-kō-kyü′-tā-nē-əs ik-spō′-zhər) Exposure to a pathogen through mucous membranes. (21)

mucosa (myōo-kō′sə) The innermost layer of the wall of the alimentary canal. (31)

mucous cells (myōo′kəs sĕlz) Cells that are found in the salivary glands and the lining of the stomach and that secrete mucous. (31)

MUGA scan (mŭg′ə skăn) A radiologic procedure that evaluates the condition of the heart's myocardium; it involves injection of radioisotopes that concentrate in the myocardium, followed by the use of a gamma camera to measure ventricular contractions to evaluate the patient's heart wall. (53)

multimedia (mŭl′tē-mē′dē-ə) More than one medium, such as in graphics, sound, and text used to convey information. (6)

multitasking (mŭl′tē-tăs′kĭng) Running two or more computer software programs simultaneously. (6)

multi-unit smooth muscle (mŭl′ta-yōo′nĭt smōoth mŭs′əl) A type of smooth muscle that is found in the iris of the eye and in the walls of blood vessels. (26)

murmur (mûr′mər) An abnormal heart sound heard when the ventricles contract and blood leaks back into the atria. (28)

muscle tissue (mŭs′əl tĭsh′ōo) A tissue type that is specialized to shorten and elongate. (23)

muscle fatigue (mŭs′əl fa-tēg′) A condition caused by a buildup of lactic acid. (26)

muscle fiber (mŭs′əl fī′bər) Muscle cells that are called fibers because of their long lengths. (26)

muscular dystrophy (mŭs′kyə-lər dis′trŏ-fē)(†) A group of inherited disorders characterized by a loss of muscle tissue and by muscle weakness. (26)

mutation (myōo-ta′shən) An error that sometimes occurs when DNA is duplicated. When it occurs, it is passed to descendent cells and may or may not affect them in harmful ways. (23)

myasthenia gravis (mī-as-thē′nē-ă grav′is) An autoimmune disorder that is characterized by muscle weakness. (26)

myelin (mī′ə-lĭn) A fatty substance that insulates the axon and allows it to send nerve impulses quickly. (27)

myelography (mī′ĕ-log′ră-fē) An x-ray visualization of the spinal cord after the injection of a radioactive contrast medium or air into the spinal subarachnoid space (between the second and innermost of three membranes that cover the spinal cord). This test can reveal tumors, cysts, spinal stenosis, or herniated disks. (41)

myocardial infarction (mī-ō-kär′dē-ăl ĭn-fark′shən) A heart attack that occurs when the blood flow to the heart is reduced as a result of blockage in the coronary arteries or their branches. (28)

myocardium (mī-ō-kär′dē-əm) The middle and thickest layer of the heart. It is made primarily of cardiac muscle. (28)

myofibrils (mī-ō-fī′brils)(†) Long structures that fill the sarcoplasm of a muscle fiber. (26)

myoglobin (mī-ō-glō′bin)(†) A pigment contained in muscle cells that stores extra oxygen. (26)

myoglobinuria (mī′ō-glō-bi-nūrē-ă) The presence of myoglobin in the urine; can be caused by injured or damaged muscle tissue. (47)

myometrium (mī′ō-mē′trē-ŭm)(†) The middle, thick muscular layer of the uterus. (35)

myopia (mī-ō′pē-ə) A condition that occurs when light entering the eye is focused in front of the retina; commonly called nearsightedness. (33)

myxedema (mik-se-dē′mă)(†) A severe type of hypothyroidism that is most common in women over the age of 50. (32)

nail bed (nāl bĕd) The layer beneath each nail. (24)

narcotic (när-kŏt′ĭk) A popular term for an opioid and term of choice in government agencies; see **opioid**. (50)

nasal (nā′zəl) Relating to the nose. The nasal bones fuse to form the bridge of the nose. (25)

nasal conchae (nā′zəl kon′kē)(†) Structures that extend from the lateral walls of the nasal cavity. (30)

nasal mucosa (nā′zəl myōo-kō′sə) The lining of the nose. (38)

nasal septum (nā′zəl sĕp′təm) A structure that divides the nasal cavity into a left and right portion. (30)

nasolacrimal duct (nā-zō-lăk′rə-məl dŭkt) A structure located on the medial aspect of each eyeball. These ducts drain tears into the nose. (33)

nasopharynx (nā′zō-far′ingks)(†) The portion of the pharynx behind the nasal cavity. (31)

natural killer (NK) cells (năch′ər-el kĭl′ər selz) Non-B and non-T lymphocytes. NK cells kill cancer cells and virus-infected cells without previous exposure to the antigen. (29)

needle biopsy (nĕd′l bī′ŏp′sē) A procedure in which a needle and syringe are used to aspirate (withdraw by suction) fluid or tissue cells. (42)

negligence (nĕg′lĭ-jəns) A medical professional's failure to perform an essential action or performance of an improper action that directly results in the harm of a patient. (3)

negotiable (nĭ-gō′shē-ə-bəl) Legally transferable from one person to another. (18)

neonatal period (nē-ō-nā′tăl pîr′ē-əd)(†) The first four weeks of the postnatal period of an offspring. (35)

neonate (nē′ə-nāt′) An infant during the first four weeks of life. (35)

nephrologist (ne-frol′ō-jĭst)(†) A specialist who studies, diagnoses, and manages diseases of the kidney. (2)

nephrons (nef′ronz)(†) Microscopic structures in the kidneys that filter blood and form urine. (34)

nerve fiber (nûrv fī′bər) A structure that extends from the cell body. It consists of two types: axons and dendrites. (27)

nerve impulse (nûrv ĭm′pŭls′) Electrochemical messages transmitted from neurons to other neurons and effectors. (27)

nervous tissue (nûr′vəs tĭsh′oo) A tissue type located in the brain, spinal cord, and peripheral nerves. (23)

net earnings (nĕt ûr′nĭngz) Take-home pay, calculated by subtracting total deductions from gross earnings. (18)

network (nĕt′wûrk′) A system that links several computers together. (6)

networking (nĕt′wûrk′ĭng) Making contacts with relatives, friends, and acquaintances that may have information about how to find a job in your field. (54)

neuralgia (noo-răl′jə) A medical condition characterized by severe pain along the distribution of a nerve. (27)

neuroglial cell (nū-rog′lē-əl sĕl) (†) Non-neuronal type of nervous tissue that is smaller and more abundant than neurons. Neuroglial cells support neurons. (27)

neurologist (noo-rəl′ə-jē) A specialist who diagnoses and treats disorders and diseases of the nervous system, including the brain, spinal cord, and nerves. (2)

neuron (noor′ŏn′) A nerve cell; it carries nerve impulses between the brain or spinal cord and other parts of the body. (23)

neurotransmitter (noor′ō-trăns′mĭt-ər) A chemical within the vesicles of the synaptic knob that is released into the postsynaptic structures when a nerve impulse reaches the synaptic knob. (27)

neutrophil (nū′trō-fil) (†) A type of granular leukocyte that aids in phagocytosis by attacking bacterial invaders; also responsible for the release of pyrogens. (28)

new patient (noo pā′shənt) Patient that, for CPT reporting purposes, has not received professional services from the physician within the past three years. (16)

nocturia (nok-tū′rē-ă) (†) Excessive nighttime urination. (47)

noncompliant (nŏn′kəm-plī′ent) The term used to describe a patient who does not follow the medical advice given. (9)

noninvasive (non-in-vā′siv) (†) Referring to procedures that do not require inserting devices, breaking the skin, or monitoring to the degree needed with invasive procedures. (53)

nonsteroidal hormone (non-stĕr′oyd-al hôr′mōn′) (†) A type of hormone made of amino acids and proteins. (32)

norepinephrine (nôr′ep-i-nef′rin) (†) A neurotransmitter released by sympathetic neurons onto organs and glands for fight-or-flight (stressful) situations. (26)

normal flora (nôr′məl flô′ră) Beneficial bacteria found in the body that create a barrier against pathogens by producing substances that may harm invaders and using up the resources pathogens need to live. (19)

no-show (nō shō) A patient who does not call to cancel and does not come to an appointment. (12)

nosocomial infection (nos-ō-kō′mē-ăl ĭn-fĕk-shən) An infection contracted in a hospital. (20)

Notice of Privacy Practices (NPP) (nō′tĭs prī′və-sē prăk′tis-əs) A document that informs patients of their rights as outlined under HIPAA. (3)

nuclear medicine (noo′klē-ər mĕd′i-sĭn) The use of radionuclides, or radioisotopes (radioactive elements or their compounds), to evaluate the bone, brain, lungs, kidneys, liver, pancreas, thyroid, and spleen; also known as radionuclide imaging. (53)

nucleases (nū′klē-ās-ez) Pancreatic enzymes that digest nucleic acids. (31)

nucleus (noo′klē-əs) (†) The control center of a cell; contains the chromosomes that direct cellular processes. (23)

numeric filing system (noo-mĕr′ĭk fī′lĭng sĭs′təm) A filing system that organizes files by numbers instead of names. Each patient is assigned a number in the order in which she joins the practice. (10)

O and P specimen (ō ənd pē spĕs′ə-mən) An ova and parasites specimen, or a stool sample, that is examined for the presence of certain forms of protozoans or parasites, including their eggs (ova). (46)

objective (əb-jĕk′tĭv) Pertaining to data that is readily apparent and measurable, such as vital signs, test results, or physical examination findings. (9)

objectives (ob-jek′tĭvs) The set of magnifying lenses contained in the nosepiece of a compound microscope. (45)

occipital (ŏk-sĭp′ĭ-tl) Relating to the back of the head. The occipital bone forms the back of the skull. (25)

occult blood (ə-kŭlt blŭd) Blood contained in some other substance, not visible to the naked eye. (22)

ocular (ŏk′yə-lər) An eyepiece of a microscope. (45)

oil-immersion objective (oili-mûr′zhən əb-jĕk′tĭv) A microscope objective that is designed to be lowered into a drop of immersion oil placed directly above the prepared specimen under examination, eliminating the air space between the microscope slide and the objective and producing a much sharper, brighter image. (45)

ointment (oint′mənt) A form of topical drug; also known as a salve. (51)

Older Americans Act of 1965 (ōl′dər ə-mĕr′ĭ-kəns ăkt) A U.S. law that guarantees certain benefits to elderly citizens, including health care, retirement income, and protection against abuse. (13)

olfactory (ŏl-făk′tə-rē) Relating to the sense of smell. (33)

oliguria Insufficient production (or volume) of urine. (47)

oncologist (ŏn-kŏl′ə-jĭst) A specialist who identifies tumors and treats patients who have cancer. (2)

onychectomy (ŏn-i-kek′tō-mē) The removal of a fingernail or toenail. (42)

oocyte (ōō-sīt) (†) The immature egg. (35)

oogenesis (ō-ō-jen′ĕ-sis) (†) The process of egg cell formation. (35)

open-book account (ō′pən book ə-kount′) An account that is open to charges made occasionally as needed. (17)

open hours scheduling (ō′pən ourz skĕj ōol-ĭng) A system of scheduling in which patients arrive at the doctor's office at their convenience and are seen on a first-come, first-served basis. (12)

open posture (ōpən pŏs′chər) A position that conveys a feeling of receptiveness and friendliness; facing another person with arms comfortably at the sides or in the lap. (4)

ophthalmologist (ŏf-thəl-mŏl′ə-jĭst) A medical doctor who is an eye specialist. (39)

ophthalmoscope (of-thal′mōskōp) (†) A hand-held instrument with a light; used to view inner eye structures. (41)

opioid (ō′-pē-òid) A natural or synthetic drug that produces opium-like effects. (50)

optic chiasm (ŏp′tĭk kī′azm) (†) A structure located at the base of the brain where parts of the optic nerves cross. It carries visual information to the brain. (32)

optical microscope (ŏp′ti-kəl mī′krə-skōp′) A microscope that uses light, concentrated through a condenser and focused through the object being examined, to project an image. (45)

opportunistic infection (ŏp′ər-tōōnĭs′tĭk ĭn-fĕk-shən) Infection by microorganisms that can cause disease only when a host's resistance is low. (19)

optometrist (ŏp-tŏm′ĭ-trĭst) A trained and licensed vision specialist who is not a physician. (39)

orbicularis oculi (ōr-bik′yū-lā′ris ok′yū-lī) The muscle in the eyelid responsible for blinking. (33)

orbit (ôr′bĭt) The eye socket, which forms a protective shell around the eye. (39)

organ (ôr′gan) Structure formed by the organization of two or more different tissue types that carries out specific functions. (23)

organelle (ôr′gə-nəl′) A structure within a cell that performs a specific function. (23)

organic (ôr-găn′ĭk) Pertaining to matter that contains carbon and hydrogen. (23)

organism (ôr′gə-nĭz′əm) A whole living being that is formed from organ systems. (23)

organ system (ôr′gan sĭs′təm) A system that consists of organs that join together to carry out vital functions. (23)

origin (ôr′ə-jĭn) An attachment site of a skeletal muscle that does not move when a muscle contracts. (26)

Original Medicare Plan (ə-rĭj′ə-nəl mĕd′ĭ-kâr′ plăn) The Medicare fee-for-service plan that allows the beneficiary to choose any licensed physician certified by Medicare. (15)

oropharynx (ōr′ō-far′ingks)(†) The portion of the pharynx behind the oral cavity. (31)

orthopedist (ôr′thə-pēdĭst) A specialist who diagnoses and treats diseases and disorders of the muscles and bones. (2)

OSHA (Occupational Safety and Health Act) (ō′shə) A set of regulations designed to save lives, prevent injuries, and protect the health of workers in the United States. (1)

osmosis (ŏz-mō′sĭs) The diffusion of water across a semipermeable membrane such as a cell membrane. (23)

ossification (ä-sə-fə-kā′-shən) The process of bone growth. (25)

osteoblast (os′tē-ō-blast)(†) Bone-forming cells that turn membrane into bone. They use excess blood calcium to build new bone. (25)

osteoclast (os′tē-ō-klast)(†) Bone-dissolving cells. When bone is dissolved, calcium is released into the bloodstream. (25)

osteocyte (äs′-tē-ə-sīt) A cell of osseous tissue; also called a bone cell. (25)

osteon (äs′-tē-ən) Elongated cylinders that run up and down the long axis of bone. (25)

osteopathic manipulative medicine (OMM) (ŏs′tē-ō-păth′ĭk mə-nĭp′ū-lā′tĭv mĕd′ĭ-sĭn) A system of hands-on techniques that help relieve pain, restore motion, support the body's natural functions, and influence the body's structure. Osteopathic physicians study OMM in addition to medical courses. (2)

osteoporosis (ŏs′tē-ō-pə-rō′sĭs) An endocrine and metabolic disorder of the musculoskeletal system, more common in women than in men, characterized by hunched-over posture. (40)

osteosarcoma (os′tē-ō-sar-kō′mă) A type of bone cancer that originates from osteoblasts, the cells that make bony tissue. (25)

otologist (ō-tol′ŏ-jist)(†) A medical doctor who specializes in the health of the ear. (39)

otorhinolaryngologist (ō-tō-rī′nōlar-ing-gol′ŏ-jist) A specialist who diagnoses and treats diseases of the ear, nose, and throat. (2)

out guide (out gīd) A marker made of stiff material and used as a placeholder when a file is taken out of a filing system. (10)

oval window (ō′val wĭn′dō) The beginning of the inner ear. (33)

overbooking (ō′vər-bōōk′ĭng) Scheduling appointments for more patients than can reasonably be seen in the time allowed. (12)

ovulation (ō′vyə-lā′shən) The process by which the ovaries release one ovum (egg) approximately every 28 days. (35)

oxygen debt (ŏk′sĭ-jən) A condition that develops when skeletal muscles are used strenuously for a minute or two. (26)

oxyhemoglobin (oks-ē-hē-mō-glō′bin)(†) Hemoglobin that is bound to oxygen. It is bright red in color. (28)

oxytocin OT (ok-sē-tō′sin)(†) A hormone that causes contraction of the uterus during childbirth and the ejection of milk from mammary glands during breast-feeding. (32)

packed red blood cells (păkt rĕd blud sĕlz) Red blood cells that collect at the bottom of a centrifuged blood sample. (48)

palate (pal′ăt)(†) The roof of the mouth. (31)

palatine (pa′-lə-tĭn) Bones that form the anterior potion of the roof of the mouth and the **palate.** (25)

palatine tonsils (pal′ă-tĭn tŏn′sils)(†) Two masses of lymphatic tissue located at the back of the throat. (31)

palpation (păl-pā′shən) A type of touch used by health-care providers to determine characteristics such as texture, temperature, shape, and the presence of movement. (38)

palpatory method (pal-pā′tôr′ē mĕth′əd) Systolic blood pressure measured by using the sense of touch. This measurement provides a necessary preliminary approximation of the systolic blood pressure to ensure an adequate level of inflation when the actual auscultatory measurement is made. (37)

palpitations (păl′pĭ-tā′shənz) Unusually rapid, strong, or irregular pulsations of the heart. (44)

pancreatic amylase (pan-krē-at′ik am′il-ās)(†) An enzyme that digests carbohydrates. (31)

pancreatic lipase (pan-krē-at′ik lip′ās)(†) An enzyme that digests lipids. (31)

panel (păn′əl) Tests frequently ordered together that are organ or disease oriented. (16)

papillae (pə-pĭl′ē) The "bumps" of the tongue in which the taste buds are found. (33)

paranasal sinuses (par-ă-nā′zəl sĭ′nŭs-ĕz) Air-filled spaces within skull bones that open into the nasal cavity. (30)

parasite (păr′ə-sīt′) An organism that lives on or in another organism and relies on it for nourishment or some other advantage to the detriment of the host organism. (46)

parasympathetic (păr′ə-sĭm′pə-thĕt′ĭk)(†) A division of the autonomic nervous system that prepares the body for rest and digestion. (27)

parathyroid hormone (par-ă-thī′royd hôr′mōn′)(†) A hormone that helps regulate calcium levels in the bloodstream. (35)

parenteral nutrition (pă-ren′ter-əl nōō-trĭsh′ən) Nutrition obtained when specially prepared nutrients are injected directly into patients' veins rather than taken by mouth. (49)

paresthesias (par-es-thē′zē-əs)(†) Abnormal sensations ranging from burning to tingling. (27)

parietal Bones that form most of the top and sides of the skull. (25)

parietal cells (pă-rī′ĕ-tăl sĕlz) Stomach cells that secrete hydrochloric acid, which is necessary to convert **pepsinogen** to **pepsin.** Parietal cells also secrete **intrinsic factor,** which is necessary for vitamin B$_{12}$ absorption. (31)

parietal pericardium (pă-rī′ĕ-tăl per-i-kar′dē-ŭm)(†) The layer on top of the visceral pericardium. (28)

parotid glands (pă-rot′id glăndz)(†) The largest of the salivary glands. The parotid glands are located beneath the skin just in front of the ears. (31)

participating physicians (pär-tĭs′ə-pāt′ĭng fĭ-zĭsh′ənz) Physicians who enroll in managed care plans. They have contracts with MCOs that stipulate their fees. (15)

passive listening (păs′ĭv lĭs′ən-ĭng) Hearing what a person has to say without responding in any way; contrast with **active listening.** (4)

patch test (păch tĕst) An allergy test in which a gauze patch soaked with a suspected allergen is taped onto the skin with nonallergenic tape; used to discover the cause of contact dermatitis. (41)

patella (pə-tĕ′lə) The bone commonly referred to as the kneecap. (25)

pathogen (păth′ə-jən) A microorganism capable of causing disease. (19)

pathologist (pă-thŏl′ə-jĭst) A medical doctor who studies the changes a disease produces in the cells, fluids, and processes of the entire body. (2)

patient compliance (pā′shənt kəm-plī′əns) Obedience in terms of following a physician's orders. (38)

patient ledger card (pā′shənt lĕj′ər kärd) A card containing information needed for insurance purposes, including the patient's name, address, telephone number, Social Security number, insurance information, employer's name, and any special billing instructions. It also includes the name of the person who is responsible for charges if this is anyone other than the patient. (18)

patient record/chart (pā′shənt rĕk′ərd/chärt) A compilation of important information about a patient's medical history and present condition. (9)

payee (pā-ē′) A person who receives a payment. (18)

payer (pā′ər) A person who pays a bill or writes a check. (18)

pay schedule (pā skĕj′ōōl) A list showing how often an employee is paid, such as weekly, biweekly, or monthly. (18)

pectoral girdle The structure that attaches the arms to the axial skeleton. (25)

pediatrician (pē′dē-ə-trĭshən) A specialist who diagnoses and treats childhood diseases and teaches parents skills for keeping their children healthy. (2)

pegboard system (pĕg′bôrd sĭs′təm) A bookkeeping system that uses a lightweight board with pegs on which forms can be stacked, allowing each transaction to be entered and recorded on four different bookkeeping forms at once; also called the one-write system. (18)

pelvic girdle The structure that attaches the legs to the axial skeleton. (25)

pepsin (pep′sin)(†) An enzyme that allows the body to digest proteins. (31)

pepsinogen (pep-sin′ō-jen)(†) Substance that is secreted by the chief cells in the lining of the stomach and becomes **pepsin** in the presence of acid. (31)

peptidases (pep′ti-dās-ez)(†) Enzymes that digest proteins. (31)

percussion (pər-kŭsh′ən) Tapping or striking the body to hear sounds or feel vibration. (38)

percutaneous exposure (per-kyū-tā′nē-ŭs ĭk-spō′zhər)(†) Exposure to a pathogen through a puncture wound or needlestick. (21)

pericardium (per-i-kar′dē-ŭm)(†) A membrane that covers the heart and large blood vessels attached to it. (28)

perilymph (per′i-limf)(†) A fluid in the inner ear. When this fluid moves, it activates hearing and equilibrium receptors. (33)

perimetrium The thin layer that covers the myometrium of the uterus. (35)

perimysium (per-i-mis′ē-ŭm)(†) The connective tissue that divides a muscle into sections called fascicles. (26)

periosteum The membrane that surrounds the **diaphysis** of a bone. (25)

peripheral nervous system (pə-rĭf′ər-əl nûr′vəs sĭs′təm) A system that consists of nerves that branch off the central nervous system. (27)

peristalsis (pĕr′ĭ-stôl′sĭs) The rhythmic muscular contractions that move food through the digestive tract. (26)

personal space (pûr′sə-nəl spās) A certain area that surrounds an individual and within which another person's physical presence is felt as an intrusion. (4)

petty cash fund (pĕt′ē kăsh fŭnd) Cash kept on hand in the office for small purchases. (18)

phagocyte (făg′ə-sīt′) A specialized white blood cell that engulfs and digests pathogens. (19)

phagocytosis (fag′ō-sī-tō′sis)(†) The process by which white blood cells defend the body against infection by engulfing invading pathogens. (29)

phalanges The bones of the fingers. (25)

pharmaceutical (fär′mə-sōō′tĭ-kəl) Pertaining to medicinal drugs. (50)

pharmacodynamics (far′mă-kō-dī-nam′iks)(†) The study of what drugs do to the body: the mechanism of action, or how they work to produce a therapeutic effect. (50)

pharmacognosy (far-mă-kog′nō-sē)(†) The study of characteristics of natural drugs and their sources. (50)

pharmacokinetics (far′mă-kō-kinet′iks)(†) The study of what the body does to drugs: how the body absorbs, metabolizes, distributes, and excretes the drugs. (50)

pharmacology (fär′ma-kŏl′ə-jē)(†) The study of drugs. (50)

pharmacotherapeutics (far′mă-kō-thĕr′ə-pyōō′tĭks) The study of how drugs are used to treat disease; also called clinical **pharmacology.** (50)

pharyngeal tonsils (fă-rĭn′jē-ăl tŏn′səls)(†) Two masses of lymphatic tissue located above the palatine tonsils; also called adenoids. (31)

pharynx (făr′ĭngks) Structure below the mouth and nasal cavities that is an organ of the respiratory system as well as the digestive system. (30)

phenylketonuria (PKU) (fen′il-kē′tō-nū′rē-ă)(†) A genetically inherited disorder in which the body cannot properly metabolize the nutrient phenylalanine, resulting in the buildup of phenylketones in the blood and their presence in the urine. The accumulation of phenylketones results in mental retardation. (23)

philosophy (fĭ-lŏs′ə-fē) The system of values and principles an office has adopted in its everyday practice. (14)

phlebotomy (flĭ-bŏt′ə-mē) The insertion of a needle or cannula (small tube) into a vein for the purpose of withdrawing blood. (48)

photometer (fō-tŏm′ĭ-trē) An instrument that measures light intensity. (45)

physiatrist (fiz-ī′ă-trist)(†) A physical medicine specialist, who diagnoses and treats diseases and disorders with physical therapy. (2)

physical therapy (fĭz´ĭ-kəl thĕr´ə-pē) A medical specialty that uses cold, heat, water, exercise, massage, traction, and other physical means to treat musculoskeletal, nervous, and cardiopulmonary disorders. (43)

physician assistant (PA) (fĭ-zĭsh´ən ə-sĭs´tənt) A health-care provider who practices medicine under the supervision of a physician. (2)

physician's office laboratory (POL) (fĭ-zĭsh´ənz ŏ´fĭs lăb´rə-tôr´ē) A laboratory contained in a physician's office; processing tests in the POL produces quick turnaround and eliminates the need for patients to travel to other test locations. (45)

physiology (fĭz´ē-ŏl´ə-jē) The science of the study of the body's functions. (23)

pineal body (pĭn´ē-ăl bŏd´ē) A small gland located between the cerebral hemispheres that secretes melatonin. (32)

pitch (pĭch) The high or low quality in the sound of a person's speaking voice. (11)

placenta (plə-sĕn´tə) An organ located between the mother and the fetus. It permits the absorption of nutrients and oxygen. In some cases, harmful substances such as viruses are absorbed through the placenta. (35)

plantar flexion (plăn´tăr flĕk´shŭn)(†) Pointing the toes downward. (26)

plasma (plăz´mə) The fluid component of blood, in which formed elements are suspended; makes up 55% of blood volume. (48)

plastic surgeon (plăs´tĭk sûr´jən) A specialist who reconstructs, corrects, or improves body structures. (2)

platelets (plāt´lĭts) Fragments of cytoplasm in the blood that are crucial to clot formation; also called thrombocytes. (48)

pleura (plŭr´ă)(†) The membranes that surround the lungs. (30)

pleuritis A condition in which the **pleura** become inflamed, which causes them to stick together. It can also cause an excess amount of fluid to form between the membranes. (30)

plexus (plĕk´səs) A structure that is formed when spinal nerves fuse together. It includes the cervical, brachial, and lumbosacral nerves. (27)

pneumothorax (nū-mō-thôr´aks)(†) The presence of air or gas in the pleural cavity. The lung typically collapses with pneumothorax. (30)

polar body (pō´lər bŏd´ē) A nonfunctional cell that is one of two small cells formed during the division of an oocyte. (35)

polarity (pō-lăr´ĭ-tē) The condition of having two separate poles, one of which is positive and the other, negative. (52)

polarized (pō´lə-rīzd´) The state in which the outside of a cell membrane is positively charged and the inside is negatively charged. Polarization occurs when a neuron is at rest. (27)

polysaccharide (pol-ē-sak´ă-rīd)(†) A type of carbohydrate that is a starch. (31)

POMR (pē´ō-ĕm-är) The problem-oriented medical record system for keeping patients' charts. Information in a POMR includes the database of information about the patient and the patient's condition, the problem list, the diagnostic and treatment plan, and progress notes. (9)

portfolio (pôrt-fō´lē-ō) A collection of an applicant's résumé, reference letters, and other documents of interest to a potential employer. (1)

positron emission tomography A radiologic procedure that entails injecting isotopes combined with other substances involved in metabolic activity, such as glucose. These special isotopes emit positrons, which a computer processes and displays on a screen. (53)

posterior (pŏ-stîr´ē-ar) Anatomical term meaning toward the back of the body. Also called dorsal. (23)

postnatal period (pōst-nā´tăl pîr´ē-əd)(†) The period following childbirth. (35)

postoperative (pōst-ŏp´ər-ə-tĭv) Taking place after a surgical procedure. (42)

posture (pŏs´chər) Body position and alignment. (43)

power of attorney (pou´ər ə-tûr´nē) The legal right to act as the attorney or agent of another person, including handling that person's financial matters. (18)

practitioner (prăk-tĭsh´ə-nər) One who practices a profession. (1)

preferred provider organization (PPO) (prĭ-fûrd´ prə-vī´dər or´gə-nĭ-zā´shən) A managed care plan that establishes a network of providers to perform services for plan members. (15)

premenstrual syndrome (PMS) (prē-mĕn´(†)-strə-wal sĭn´-drōm) A syndrome that is a collection of symptoms that occur just before the menstrual period. (35)

premium (prĕ´mē-əm) The basic annual cost of health-care insurance. (15)

prenatal period (prē-nā´tăl pîr´ē-əd)(†) The period that includes the embryonic and fetal periods until the delivery of the offspring. (35)

preoperative (prē-ŏp´ər-ə-tĭv) Taking place prior to surgery. (42)

prepuce (prē´pŭs)(†) A piece of skin in the uncircumcized male that covers the glans penis. (35)

presbyopia (prez-bē-ōpe´-ă) A common eye disorder that results in the loss of lens elasticity. Presbyopia develops with age and causes a person to have difficulty seeing objects close up. (33)

prescribe (prĭ-skrīb´) To give a patient a prescription to be filled by a pharmacy. (50)

prescription (prĭ-skrĭp´shən) A physician's written order for medication. (50)

prescription drug (prĭ-skrĭp´shən drŭg) A drug that can be legally used only by order of a physician and must be administered or dispensed by a licensed health-care professional. (50)

primary care physician (prī´mĕr´ē kâr fĭ-zĭsh´ən) A physician who provides routine medical care and referrals to specialists. (2)

primary germ layer (prī´mĕr´ē jûrm lā´ər) An inner cell mass that organizes into layers: the ectoderm, mesoderm, and endoderm. (35)

prime mover (prīm mōō´vər) The muscle responsible for most of the movement when a body movement is produced by a group of muscles. (26)

primordial follicle (prī-môr´dĕl-ăl fŏl´ĭ-kəl)(†) A structure that develops in the ovarian cortex of a female infant before she is born. (35)

Privacy Rule (prī´və-sē rōōl) Common name for the **HIPAA** Standard for Privacy of Individually Identifiable Health Information, which provides the first comprehensive federal protection for the privacy of health information. The Privacy Rule creates national standards to protect individuals' medical records and other personal health information. (3)

procedure code (prə-sē´jər kōd) Codes that represent medical procedures, such as surgery and diagnostic tests, and medical services, such as an examination to evaluate a patient's condition. (16)

proctoscopy (prok-tŏs´kō-pē) An examination of the lower rectum and anal canal with a 3-inch instrument called a proctoscope to detect hemorrhoids, polyps, fissures, fistulas, and abscesses. (41)

proficiency testing program (prə-fĭsh'ən-cē tĕst'ĭng prō'grăm') A required set of tests for clinical laboratories; the tests measure the accuracy of the laboratory's test results and adherence to standard operating procedures. (45)

progesterone (prō-jĕs'tə-rōn') A female steroid hormone primarily produced by the ovary. (32)

prognosis (prŏg-nō'sĭs) A prediction of the probable course of a disease in an individual and the chances of recovery. (38)

prolactin (PRL) (prō-lak'tin)(†) A hormone that stimulates milk production in the mammary glands. (32)

proliferation phase (prə-lĭf'ər-ā'shən fāz) The second phase of wound healing, in which new tissue forms, closing off the wound. (42)

pronation (prō-nā'shŭn)(†) Turning the palms of the hand downward. (26)

pronunciation (prə-nun'cē-ā'shən) The sounding out of words. (11)

proofreading (prōōf'rēd'ing) Checking a document for formatting, data, and mechanical errors. (7)

prostaglandin (pros-tă-glan'din)(†) A local hormone derived from lipid molecules. Prostaglandins typically do not travel in the bloodstream to find their target cells because their targets are close by. This hormone has numerous effects, including uterine stimulation during childbirth. (32)

prostate gland (prŏs'tāt' glănd) A chestnut-shaped gland that surrounds the beginning of the urethra in the male. (35)

prostatitis (pros-tă-tī'tis) Inflammation of the prostate gland, which can be acute or chronic. (35)

protected health information (PHI) (prə-tĕkt-əd hĕlth ĭn'fər-mă'shən) Individually identifiable health information that is transmitted or maintained by electronic or other media, such as computer storage devices. The core of the **HIPAA Privacy Rule** is the protection, use, and disclosure of protected health information. (3)

proteinuria (prō-tē-nū'rē-ă) An excess of protein in the urine. (47)

protozoan (prō'-tə-zō'ən) A single-celled eukaryotic organism much larger than a bacterium; some protozoans can cause disease in humans. (46)

protraction (prō-trăk'shən) Moving a body part anteriorly. (26)

proximal (prok'si-măl)(†) Anatomical term meaning closer to a point of attachment or closer to the trunk of the body. (23)

proximal convoluted tubule (prok'si-măl kon'vō-lū-ted tū'byūl)(†) The portion of the renal tubule that is directly attached to the glomerular capsule and becomes the loop of Henle. (34)

psoriasis (sə-rī'ə-sĭs) A common skin condition characterized by reddish-silver scaly lesions most often found on the elbows, knees, scalp, and trunk. (24)

puberty (pyōō'bər-tē) The period of adolescence when a person begins to develop secondary sexual traits and reproductive functions. (40)

pulmonary circuit (pool'mə-nĕr'ē sûr'kĭt) The route that blood takes from the heart to the lungs and back to the heart again. (28)

pulmonary trunk (pool'mə-nĕr'ē trŭngk) A large artery that branches into the pulmonary arteries and carries blood to the lungs. (28)

pulmonary valve (pool'mə-nĕr'ē vălv) A heart valve that is a semilunar valve. It is situated between the right ventricle and the pulmonary trunk. (28)

pubis (pyü'-bəs) The area that forms the front of a hip bone. (25)

pulmonary function test (pool'mə-nĕr'ē fŭngk'shən tĕst) A test that evaluates a patient's lung volume and capacity; used to detect and diagnose pulmonary problems or to monitor certain respiratory disorders and evaluate the effectiveness of treatment. (52)

puncture wound (pŭngk'chər wound) A deep wound caused by a sharp, pointed object. (42)

punitive damages (pyōō'nĭ-tĭv dăm'ĭjz) Money paid as punishment for intentionally breaking the law. (17)

pupil (pyōō'pəl) The opening at the center of the iris, which grows smaller or larger as the iris contracts or relaxes, respectively; it regulates the amount of light that enters the eye. (33)

purchase order (pûr'chĭs ôr'dər) A form that authorizes a purchase for the practice. (8)

purchasing groups (pur'chĭs-ĭng grōōps) Groups of medical offices associated with a nearby hospital that order supplies through the hospital to obtain a quantity discount. (8)

Purkinje Fibers (per'kin-jē fĭ'bərz) Cardiac fibers that are located in the lateral walls of the ventricles. (28)

pyelonephritis (pī'ĕ-lō-ne-frī-tis)(†) A urinary tract infection that involves one or both of the kidneys. (34)

pyrogens (pī'ō-jenz)(†) Fever-producing substances released by neutrophils. (48)

quadrants (kwŏd'rəntz) Four equal sections, such as those into which the abdomen is figuratively divided during an examination. (38)

qualitative analysis (kwŏl'ĭ-tā'tĭv ə-năl'ĭ-sĭs) In microbiology, identification of bacteria present in a specimen by the appearance of colonies grown on a culture plate. (46)

qualitative test response (kwŏl'ĭ-tā'tĭv tĕst rĭ-spŏns') A test result that indicates the substance tested for is either present or absent. (45)

quality assurance program (kwŏl'ĭ-tē ə-shōōr'əns prō'gram') A required program for clinical laboratories designed to monitor the quality of patient care, including quality control, instrument and equipment maintenance, proficiency testing, training and continuing education, and standard operating procedures documentation. (45)

quality control (QC) (kwŏl'ĭ-tē kən-trōl') An ongoing system, required in every physician's office, to evaluate the quality of medical care provided. (46)

quality control program (kwŏl'ĭ-tē kən-trōl' prō'grăm') A component of a quality assurance program that focuses on ensuring accuracy in laboratory test results through careful monitoring of test procedures. (45)

quantitative analysis (kwŏn'tĭ-tā'tĭv ə-năl'ĭ-sĭs) In microbiology, a determination of the number of bacteria present in a specimen by direct count of colonies grown on a culture plate. (46)

quantitative test results (kwŏn'tĭ-tā'tĭv tĕst rĭ-zŭltz') The concentration of a test substance in a specimen. (45)

quarterly return (kwŏr'tar-lē rĭ-tûrn') The Employer's Quarterly Federal Tax Return, a form submitted to the IRS every 3 months that summarizes the federal income and employment taxes withheld from employees' paychecks. (18)

radial artery (rā'dē-əl är'tə-rē) An artery located in the groove on the thumb side of the inner wrist, where the pulse is taken on adults. (37)

radiation therapy (rā′dē-ā′shən thĕr′ə-pē) The use of x-rays and radioactive substances to treat cancer. (53)

radiologist (rā′dē-ŏl′ə-jĭst) A physician who specializes in taking and reading x-rays. (2)

radius (rā-dā-əs) The lateral bone of the forearm. (25)

random access memory (RAM) (răn′dəm ăk′sĕs mĕm′ə-rē) The temporary, or programmable, memory in a computer. (6)

random urine specimen (răn′dəm yŏŏr′ĭn spĕs′ ə-mən) A single urine specimen taken at any time of the day; the most common type of sample collected. (47)

range of motion (ROM) (rānj mō′shən) The degree to which a joint is able to move. (43)

rapport (ră-pôr′) A harmonious, positive relationship. (4)

read only memory (ROM) (rēd ōn′lē mĕm′ə-rē) A computer's permanent memory, which can be read by the computer but not changed. It provides the computer with the basic operating instructions it needs to function. (6)

reagent (rē-ā′jənt) A chemical or chemically treated substance used in test procedures and formulated to react in specific ways when exposed under specific conditions. (45)

reconciliation (rĕk′ən-sĭl′ē-ā′shən) A comparison of the office's financial records with bank records to ensure that they are consistent and accurate; usually done when the monthly checking account statement is received from the bank. (18)

records management system (rĭ-kôrdz măn′ĭj-mənt sĭs′təm) How patient records are created, filed, and maintained. (10)

recovery position (rĭ-kŭv′ər-ē pə-zĭsh′ən) The position a person is placed in after receiving first aid for choking or cardiopulmonary resuscitation. (44)

rectum (rĕk′təm) The last section of the sigmoid colon that straightens out and becomes the anal canal. (31)

reference (rĕf′ər-əns) A recommendation for employment from a facility or a preceptor. (54)

reference laboratory (rĕf′ər-əns lăb′rə-tôr′ē) A laboratory owned and operated by an organization outside the physician's practice. (45)

referral (rĭ-fûr′əl) An authorization from a medical practice for a patient to have specialized services performed by another practice;

often required for insurance purposes. (15)

reflex (rē′flĕks′) A predictable automatic response to stimuli. (27)

refraction examination (rĭ-frăk′shən ĭg-zăm′ə-nā′shən) An eye examination in which the patient looks through a succession of different lenses to find out which ones create the clearest image. (41)

refractometer (rĕ-frak-tom′ĕ-ter)(†) An optical instrument that measures the refraction, or bending, of light as it passes through a liquid. (47)

Registered Medical Assistant (RMA) (rĕj′ĭ-stərd mĕd′ĭ-kəl ə-sĭs′tənt) A medical assistant who has met the educational requirements and taken and passed the certification examination for medical assisting given by the American Medical Technologists (AMT). (1)

relaxin (rē-lak′sin)(†) A hormone that comes from the corpus luteum. It inhibits uterine contractions and relaxes the ligaments of the pelvis in preparation for childbirth. (35)

remittance advice (RA) (rĭ-mĭt′ns ăd-vīz′) A form that the patient and the practice receive for each encounter that outlines the amount billed by the practice, the amount allowed, the amount of subscriber liability, the amount paid, and notations of any service not covered, including an explanation of why that service is not covered; also called an explanation of benefits. (15)

renal calculi (rē′nəl kăl′kyə-lī′) Kidney stones. (34)

renal column (rē′nəl kŏl′əm) The portion of the **renal cortex** between the **renal pyramids.** (34)

renal corpuscle (rē′nəl kôr′pə-səl) Corpuscle that is composed of the glomerulus and the glomerular capsule. The filtration of blood occurs here. (34)

renal cortex (rē′nəl kôr′tĕks′) The outermost layer of the kidney. (34)

renal medulla (rē′nəl mĭ-dŭl′ə) The middle portion of the kidney. (34)

renal pelvis (rē′nəl pĕl′vĭs) The internal structure of the kidney. Urine flows from the renal pelvis down the ureter. (34)

renal pyramids (rē′nəl pĭr′ə-mĭdz) Triangular-shaped areas in the medulla of the kidney. (34)

renal sinus (rē′nəl sī′nəs) The medial depression of a kidney. (34)

renal tubule (rē′nəl tū′byūl) Structure that extends from the glomerular

capsule of a nephron and is comprised of the proximal convoluted tubule, the loop of Henle, and the distal convoluted tubule. (34)

renin (ren′in)(†) A hormone secreted by the kidney that helps to regulate blood pressure. (34)

repolarization (rē′pō-lăr-i-zā′shŭn)(†) The process of returning to the original polar (resting) state. (27)

reputable (rĕpyə-tə-bəl) Having a good reputation. (8)

requisition (rĕk′wĭ-zĭsh′ən) A formal request from a staff member or doctor for the purchase of equipment or supplies. (8)

reservoir host (rĕz′ər-vwär′ hōst) An animal, insect, or human whose body is susceptible to growth of a pathogen. (19)

respiratory volume (rĕs′pər-ə-tôr′ē vŏl′yŏŏm) The different volumes of air that move in and out of the lungs during different intensities of breathing. These volumes can be measured to assess the healthiness of the respiratory system. (30)

resource-based relative value scale (RBRVS) (rē′sôrs′ bāst rĕl′ə-tĭv văl′yŏŏ skāl) The payment system used by Medicare. It establishes the relative value units for services, replacing the providers' consensus on usual fees. (15)

résumé (rĕz′ŏŏ-mā′) A typewritten document summarizing one's employment and educational history. (1)

retention schedule (rĭ-tĕn′shən skĕj′ŏŏl) A schedule that details how long to keep different types of patient records in the office after they have become inactive or closed and how long the records should be stored. (10)

retina (rĕt′n-ə) The inner layer of the eye; contains light-sensing nerve cells. (33)

retraction (rĭ-trăk′shən) Moving a body part posteriorly. (26)

retrograde pyelography (rĕt′rə-grād′ pī′ē-lŏg′ră-fē)(†) A radiologic procedure in which the doctor injects a contrast medium through a urethral catheter and takes a series of x-rays to evaluate function of the ureters, bladder, and urethra. (53)

retroperitoneal (re-trō-per-ə-ə-nē′-əl) An anatomical term that means behind the peritoneal cavity. It is where the kidneys lie. (34)

return demonstation (rĭ-tûrn′ dĕm′ən-strā′shən) Participatory teaching method in which the technique is first described to the patient and then demonstrated to the patient; the patient is then asked to repeat the demonstration. (14)

rhabdomyolysis (rab′dō-mĭ-ol′ĭ-sĭs) (†) A condition in which the kidneys have been damaged due to toxins released from muscle cells. (26)

Rh antigen (är′ăch an′tĭ-jən) A protein first discovered on the red blood cells of rhesus monkeys, hence the name Rh. (28)

RhoGAM (rō′găm) A medication that prevents an Rh-negative mother from making antibodies against the Rh antigen. (28)

RNA (är′ĕn-ā′) A nucleic acid used to make protein. (23)

rods (rŏdz) Light-sensing nerve cells in the eye, at the posterior of the retina, that function in dim light but do not provide sharp images or detect color. (33)

rosacea (rō-zā′shē-ă) (†) A condition characterized by chronic redness and acne over the nose and cheeks. (24)

rotation (rō-tā′shən) Twisting a body part. (26)

route (rōōt) The way a drug is introduced into the body. (51)

sacrum (sa′-krəm) A triangular-shaped bone that consists of five fused vertebra. (25)

sagittal (saj′i-tăl) (†) An anatomical term that refers to the plane that divides the body into left and right portions. (23)

salutation (săl′yə-tā′shən) A written greeting, such as "Dear," used at the beginning of a letter. (7)

sanitization (săn′ĭ-tĭ-zā′shən) (†) A reduction of the number of microorganisms on an object or a surface to a fairly safe level. (19)

sarcolemma (sar′kō-lem′ă) The cell membrane of a muscle fiber. (26)

sarcoplasm The cytoplasm of a muscle fiber. (26)

sarcoplasmic reticulum (sar-kō-plaz′mik re-tik′yū-lŭm) The endoplasmic reticulum of a muscle fiber. (26)

SARS (severe acute respiratory syndrome) (särz) A severe and acute respiratory illness characterized by fever and a nonproductive cough that progresses to the point at which insufficient oxygen is present in the blood. (38)

saturated fat (săch′ə-rā′tĭd făt) Fats, derived primarily from animal sources, that are usually solid at room temperature and that tend to raise blood cholesterol levels. (49)

scabies (skā′bēz) Skin lesions that are very itchy and caused by a burrowing mite. Scabies is most commonly found between the fingers and on the genitalia. (24)

scanner (skăn′ər) An optical device that converts printed matter into a format that can be read by the computer and inputs the converted information. (6)

scapula (sk′a-pyə-la) Thin, triangular-shaped, flat bones located on the dorsal surface of the rib cage; also called shoulder blades. (25)

Schwann cell (shwahn sĕl) (†) A neuroglial cell whose cell membrane coats the axons. (27)

sciatica (sī-ăt′ĭ-kə) Pain in the low back and hip radiating down the back of the leg along the sciatic nerve. (27)

sclera (sklîr′ə) The tough, outermost layer, or "white," of the eye, through which light cannot pass; covers all except the front of the eye. (33)

scoliosis (skŏ′lē-ō′sĭs) A lateral curvature of the spine, which is normally straight when viewed from behind. (25)

scratch test (skrăch tĕst) An allergy test in which extracts of suspected allergens are applied to the patient's skin and the skin is then scratched to allow the extracts to penetrate. (41)

screening (skrēn′ĭng) Performing a diagnostic test on a person who is typically free of symptoms. (14)

screen saver (skrēn sā′vər) A program that automatically changes the monitor display at short intervals or constantly shows moving images to prevent burn-in of images on the computer screen. (6)

scrotum (skrō′təm) In a male, the sac of skin below the pelvic cavity that contains the testes. (35)

sebaceous (sĭ-bā′shəs) A type of oil gland found in the dermis. (24)

sebum (sē′bŭm) (†) An oily substance produced by sebaceous glands. (24)

Security Rule (sĭ-kyŏŏr′ĭ-tē rōōl) The technical safeguards that protect the confidentiality, integrity, and availability of health information covered by **HIPAA**. The Security Rule specifies how patient information is protected on computer networks, the Internet, disks, and other storage media. (3)

seizure (sē′zhər) A series of violent and involuntary contractions of the muscles; also called a convulsion. (27)

sella turcica (sel′ă tŭr′sē-kă) (†) A deep depression in the sphenoid bone where the pituitary gland sits. (25)

semen (sē′mən) Sperm and the various substances that nourish and transport them. (35)

semicircular canals (sĕm′ē-sûr′kyə-lər kə-nălz′) Structures in the inner ear that help a person maintain balance; each of the three canals is positioned at right angles to the other two. (33)

seminal vesicles (sem′-năl ves′i-klz) (†) A pair of convoluted tubes that lie behind the bladder. These tubes secrete a fluid that provides nutrition for the sperm. (35)

seminiferous tubules (sem′i-nif′er-ŭs tū′byūlz) (†) These tubes contain spermatogenic cells and are located in the lobules of the testes. (35)

sensorineural hearing loss (sen′sōr-i-nūr′ăl hîr′ĭng lôs) This type of hearing loss occurs when neural structures associated with the ear are damaged. Neural structures include hearing receptors and the auditory nerve. (33)

sensory (sĕn′sə-rē) Afferent neurons that carry sensory information from the periphery to the central nervous system. (27)

sensory adaptation (sĕn′sə-rē ăd′ăp-tā′shən) A process in which the same chemical can stimulate receptors only for a limited amount of time until the receptors eventually no longer respond to the chemical. (33)

septic shock (sĕp′tĭk shŏk) A state of shock resulting from massive, widespread infection that affects the blood vessels' ability to circulate blood. (44)

sequential order (sĭ-kwĕn′shəl ôr′dər) One after another in a predictable pattern or sequence. (10)

serosa (se-rō′să) (†) The outermost layer of the alimentary canal; also known as the visceral peritoneum. (31)

serous cells (sēr′ŭs sĕlz) (†) One of two types of cells that make up the salivary glands. These cells secrete a watery fluid that contains amylase. (31)

serum (sēr′ŭm) (†) The clear, yellow liquid that remains after a blood clot forms; it is separated from the clotted elements by centrifugation. (48)

service contract (sûr′vĭs kŏn′trăkt) A contract that covers services for equipment that are not included in a standard maintenance contract. (5)

sex chromosome (sĕks krō′mə-sōm′) Chromosome of the 23rd pair. (23)

sex-linked trait (sĕks lĭngk trāt) Traits that are carried on the sex chromosomes, or X and Y chromosomes. (23)

sigmoid colon (sig-móid ko-lən) An S-shaped tube that lies between the **descending colon** and the **rectum**. (31)

sigmoidoscopy (sig´moy-dos´kŏ-pē) A procedure in which the interior of the sigmoid area of the large intestine, between the descending colon and the rectum, is examined with a sigmoidoscope, a lighted instrument with a magnifying lens. (41)

sign (sīn) An objective or external factor, such as blood pressure, rash, or swelling, that can be seen or felt by the physician or measured by an instrument. (9)

simplified letter style (sĭm´plə-fīd´ lĕt´ər stīl) A modification of the full-block style in which the salutation and complimentary closing are omitted and a subject line typed in all capital letters is placed between the address and the body of the letter. (7)

single-entry account (sĭng´gəl-ĕn´trē ə-kount´) An account that has only one charge, usually for a small amount, for a patient who does not come in regularly. (17)

sinoatrial node (sī´nō-ā´trē-əl nōd)(†) A small bundle of heart muscle tissue in the superior wall of the right atrium that sets the rhythm (or pattern) of the heart's contractions; also called sinus node or pacemaker. (28)

sinusitis (sī´nə-sī´tĭs) Inflammation of the lining of a sinus. (30)

skinfold test (skĭn´ tĕst) A method of measuring fat as a percentage of body weight by measuring the thickness of a fold of skin with a caliper. (49)

slit lamp (slĭt lămp) An instrument composed of a magnifying lens combined with a light source; used to provide a minute examination of the eye's anatomy. (41)

smear (smîr) A specimen spread thinly and unevenly across a slide. (46)

SOAP (sōp) An approach to medical records documentation that documents information in the following order: S (**subjective** data), O (**objective** data), A (assessment), P (plan of action). (9)

software (sôft´wâr´) A program, or set of instructions, that tells a computer what to do. (6)

solution (sə-lōō´shən) A homogeneous mixture of a solid, liquid, or gaseous substance in a liquid, such as a dissolved drug in liquid form. (51)

somatic (sō-măt´ĭk) A division of the peripheral nervous system that connects the central nervous system to skin and skeletal muscle. (27)

SPECT (spĕkt) Single photon emission computed tomography; a radiologic procedure in which a gamma camera detects signals induced by gamma radiation and a computer converts these signals into two- or three-dimensional images that are displayed on a screen. (53)

speculum (spĕk´yə-ləm) An instrument that expands the vaginal opening to permit viewing of the vagina and cervix. (40)

spermatids (sperm´mă-tidz)(†) Immature sperm before they develop their flagella (tails). (35)

spermatocytes (sperm´mă-tō-sīts)(†) The cells that result when **spermatogonia** undergo mitosis. (35)

spermatogenesis (sperm´mă-tō-jenĕ´-sis)(†) The process of sperm cell formation. (35)

spermatogenic cells (sperm´mă-tō-jenĭk sĕlz)(†) The cells that give rise to sperm cells. (35)

spermatogonia (sperm´mă-tō-gōnĕ´-ă)(†) The earliest cell in the process of **spermatogenesis**. (35)

sphenoid A bone that forms part of the floor of the cranium. (25)

sphincter (sfĭngk´tər) A valve-like structure formed from circular bands of muscle. Sphincters are located around various body openings and passages. (26)

sphygmomanometer (sfĭg´mō-mănom´ĕ-ter)(†) An instrument for measuring blood pressure; consists of an inflatable cuff, a pressure bulb used to inflate the cuff, and a device to read the pressure. (37)

spinal nerves (spī´nəl nûrvs)(†) Peripheral nerves that originate from the spinal cord. (27)

spirillum (spī-ril´ŭm)(†) A spiral-shaped bacterium. (46)

spirometer (spī-rom´ĕ-ter)(†) An instrument that measures the air taken in and expelled from the lungs. (52)

spirometry (spī-rom´ĕ-trē)(†) A test used to measure breathing capacity. (52)

splint A device used to immobilize and protect a body part. (44)

splinting catheter (splĭnt´ĭng kăth´ĭ-tər) A type of catheter inserted after plastic repair of the ureter; it must remain in place for at least a week after surgery. (47)

sprain (sprān) An injury characterized by partial tearing of a ligament that supports a joint, such as the ankle. A sprain may also involve injuries to tendons, muscles, and local blood vessels and contusions of the surrounding soft tissue. (44)

stain (stăn) In microbiology, a solution of a dye or group of dyes that impart a color to microorganisms. (46)

standard (stăn´dərd) A specimen for which test values are already known; used to calibrate test equipment. (45)

Standard Precautions (stăn´dərd prī-kô´shənz) A combination of Universal Precautions and Body Substance Isolation guidelines; used in hospitals for the care of all patients. (19)

stapes (stā´pēz) A small bone in the middle ear that is attached to the inner ear; also called the stirrup. (39)

statement (stāt´mənt) A form similar to an invoice; contains a courteous reminder to the patient that payment is due. (17)

statute of limitations (stăch´ōōt lĭmĭ-tā´shənz) A state law that sets a time limit on when a collection suit on a past-due account can legally be filed. (17)

stereoscopy (ster-ē-os´kŏ-pē)(†) An x-ray procedure that uses a specially designed microscope (stereoscopic, or Greenough, microscope) with double eyepieces and objectives to take films at different angles and produce three-dimensional images; used primarily to study the skull. (53)

sterile field (stĕr´əl fēld) An area free of microorganisms used as a work area during a surgical procedure. (42)

sterile scrub assistant (stĕr´əl skrŭb ə-sĭs´tənt) An assistant who handles sterile equipment during a surgical procedure. (42)

sterilization (stĕr´ə-lĭ-zā´shən) The destruction of all microorganisms, including bacterial spores, by specific means. (19)

sterilization indicator (stĕr´ə-lĭ-zā´shən ĭn´dĭ-kā´shən) A tag, insert, tape, tube, or strip that confirms that the items in an autoclave have been exposed to the correct volume of steam at the correct temperature for the correct amount of time. (20)

steroid hormone (stĭr´oid´ hôr´mōn´) A hormone derived from steroids that are soluble in lipids and can cross cell membranes very easily. (32)

sternum (st´ər-nəm) A bone that forms the front and middle portion of the rib cage; also called the breastbone or breast plate. (25)

stethoscope (stĕth´ə-skōp´) An instrument that amplifies body sounds. (37)

strabismus (strə-bĭz´məs) A condition that results in a lack of parallel visual axes of the eyes; commonly called crossed eyes. (33)

strain (strān) A muscle injury that results from overexertion or overstretching. (44)

stratum basale (straf´ŭm bā-sā´le)(†) The deepest layer of the epidermis of the skin. (24)

stratum corneum (straf´ŭm kōr´nē-ŭm) (†) The most superficial layer of the epidermis of the skin. (24)

stressor (stres´or)(†) Any stimulus that produces stress. (32)

stress test (strĕs tĕst) A procedure that involves recording an electrocardiogram while the patient is exercising on a stationary bicycle, treadmill, or stair-stepping ergometer, which measures work performed. (41)

striations (strī-ā´shŭns)(†) Bands produced from the arrangement of filaments in myofibrils in skeletal and cardiac muscle cells. (26)

stroke (strōk) A condition that occurs when the blood supply to the brain is impaired. It may cause temporary or permanent damage. (44)

stylus (stī´ləs) A penlike instrument that records electrical impulses on ECG paper. (52)

subarachnoid space (sŭb-ă-rak´noyd spās) (†) An area between the arachnoid mater and the pia mater. (27)

subclinical case (sŭb-klin´i-kăl kās)(†) An infection in which the host experiences only some of the symptoms of the infection or milder symptoms than in a full case. (19)

subcutaneous (SC) (sŭb´kyoo-tăne-əs) Under the skin. (24)

subjective (səb-jĕk´tĭv) Pertaining to data that is obtained from conversation with a person or patient. (9)

sublingual (sŭb-ling´gwăl)(†) Under the tongue. (51)

sublingual gland (sŭb-ling´gwăl glănd)(†) The smallest of the salivary glands. (31)

submandibular gland (sŭb-man-dib´yū-lăr glănd)(†) The gland that is located in the floor of the mouth. (31)

submucosa (sŭb-mū-kō´să)(†) The layer of the alimentary canal located between the mucosa and the muscular layer. (31)

subpoena (sə-pĕnə) A written court order that is addressed to a specific person and requires that person's presence in court on a specific date at a specific time. (3)

substance abuse (sŭb´stəns ə-byooz´) The use of a substance in a way that is not medically approved, such as using diet pills to stay awake or consuming large quantities of cough syrup that contains codeine. Substance abusers are not necessarily addicts. (36)

sucrose (sū´krōs)(†) An enzyme that digests sugars. (31)

sulci (sŭl´si)(†) The grooves on the surface of the cerebrum. (27)

superbill (soo´pər-bĭl´) A form that combines the charges for services rendered, an invoice for payment or insurance co-payment, and all the information for submitting an insurance claim. (17)

superficial (soo´pər-fĭsh´əl) Anatomical term meaning closer to the surface of the body. (23)

superior (soo´-pîr´-ē-ər) Anatomical term meaning above or closer to the head; also called cranial. (23)

supernatant (sū-per-nā´tănt)(†) The liquid portion of a substance from which solids have settled to the bottom, as with a urine specimen after centrifugation. (47)

supination (sū´pi-nā´shŭn)(†) Turning the palm of the hand upward. (26)

surgeon (sûr´jən) A physician who uses hands and medical instruments to diagnose and correct deformities and treat external and internal injuries or disease. (2)

surgical asepsis (sûr´jə-kəl ă-sep´sis)(†) The elimination of all microorganisms from objects or working areas; also called sterile technique. (42)

susceptible host (sə-sĕp´təbal hōst) An individual who has little or no immunity to infection by a particular organism. (19)

suture (soo´chər) Fibrous joints in the skull. (25) A surgical stitch made to close a wound. (42)

symmetry (sĭm´ĭ-trē) The degree to which one side of the body is the same as the other. (38)

sympathetic (sĭm´pə-thĕt´ĭk) A division of the autonomic nervous system that prepares organs for fight-or-flight (stressful) situations. (27)

symptom (sĭm´təm) A subjective, or internal, condition felt by a patient, such as pain, headache, or nausea, or another indication that generally cannot be seen or felt by the doctor or measured by instruments. (9)

synaptic knob (si-nap´tik nŏb)(†) The end of the axon branch. (27)

synergist (sĭn´ər-jist´) Muscles that help the **prime mover** by stabilizing joints. (26)

synovial (sin-ō-vā-əl) A type of joint, such as the elbow or knee, that is freely moveable. (25)

systemic circuit (sĭ-stĕm´ĭk sûr´kĭt) The route that blood takes from the heart through the body and back to the heart. (28)

systolic pressure (sĭ-stŏl´ĭk prĕsh´ər) The blood pressure measured when the left ventricle of the heart contracts. (28)

tab (tăb) A tapered rectangular or rounded extension at the top of a file folder. (10)

Tabular List (tăb´yə-lər lĭst) One of two ways that diagnoses are listed in the **ICD-9.** In the Tabular List, the diagnosis codes are listed in numerical order with additional instructions. (16)

tachycardia (taki-kar´dē-ă)(†) Rapid heart rate, generally in excess of 100 beats per minute. (44)

tachypnea Abnormally rapid breathing. (37)

targeted résumé (tär´gĭt-əd rĕz´oo-mā´) A résumé that is focused on a specific job target. (54)

tarsals (tär´-səlz) Bones of the ankle. (25)

taste bud (tāst bŭd) A structure that is made of taste cells (a type of chemoreceptor) and supporting cells. (33)

tax liability (tăk lī´ə-bĭl´ĭ-tē) Money withheld from employees' paychecks and held in a separate account that must be used to pay taxes to appropriate government agencies. (18)

telephone triage (tĕl´ə-fōn´ trē-äzh´) A process of determining the level of urgency of each incoming telephone call and how it should be handled. (11)

teletherapy (tel-ē-thăr´əpē)(†) A radiation therapy technique that allows deeper penetration than brachytherapy; used primarily for deep tumors. (53)

teletype (TTY) device (tĕl´ə-tīp) A specially designed telephone that looks very much like a laptop computer with a cradle for the receiver of a traditional telephone. It is used by the hearing impaired to type communications onto a keyboard. (13)

template (tĕm´plĭt) A guide that ensures consistency and accuracy. (7)

temporal (tem´-p(a)-rəl) Bones that form the lower sides of the skull. (25)

tendon (tĕn´dən) A cordlike fibrous tissue that connects muscle to bone. (26)

terminal (tûr´mə-nəl) Fatal. (21)

testes (tĕs´tēz) The primary organs of the male reproductive system. Testes produce the hormone **testosterone**. (35)

testosterone (tĕs-tŏs´tə-rōn´) A hormone produced by the testes that maintains the male reproductive structures and male characteristics such as deep voice, body hair, and muscle mass. (32)

tetanus (tĕt´n-əs) A disease caused by *clostridium tetani* living in the soil and water; more commonly called lockjaw. (26)

thalamus (thăl´ə-məs) Structure that acts as a relay station for sensory information heading to the cerebral cortex for interpretation; a subdivision of the **diencephalon**. (27)

therapeutic team (thĕr´ə-pyōō´tĭk tēm) A group of physicians, nurses, medical assistants, and other specialists who work with patients dealing with chronic illness or recovery from major injuries. (43)

thermography (ther-mog´ră-fē)(†) A radiologic procedure in which an infrared camera is used to take photographs that record variations in skin temperature as dark (cool areas), light (warm areas), or shades of gray (areas with temperatures between cool and warm); used to diagnose breast tumors, breast abscesses, and fibrocystic breast disease. (53)

thermotherapy (ther´mō-thăr´ă-pē)(†) The application of heat to the body to treat a disorder or injury. (43)

third-party check (thûrd pär´tē chĕk) A check made out to one recipient and given in payment to another, as with one made out to a patient rather than the medical practice. (18)

third-party payer (thûrd pär´tē pā´ər) A health plan that agrees to carry the risk of paying for patient services. (15)

thrombocytes (throm´bō-sīts) See **platelets**. (48)

thrombophlebitis (throm´bō-flĕ-bī´tis) (†) A medical condition that most commonly occurs in leg veins when a blood clot and inflammation develop. (28)

thrombus (throm´bəs) A blood clot that forms on the inside of an injured blood vessel wall. (28)

thymosin (thĭm´ō-sin)(†) A hormone that promotes the production of certain lymphocytes. (32)

thymus gland (thī´məs glănd) A gland that lies between the lungs. It secretes a hormone called **thymosin**. (32)

thyroid cartilage (thī´roid´ kär´tl-ĭj) The largest cartilage in the larynx. It forms the anterior wall of the larynx. (30)

thyroid hormone (thī´roid´ hôr´mōn´) A hormone produced by the thyroid gland that increases energy production, stimulates protein synthesis, and speeds up the repair of damaged tissue. (32)

thyroid stimulating hormone (thī´roid´ stim´yū-lā-ting hôr´mōn´) A hormone that stimulates the thyroid gland to release its hormone. (32)

tibia (ti-bē´ə) The medial bone of the lower leg; commonly called the shin bone. (25)

tickler file (tĭk´lər fīl) A reminder file for keeping track of time-sensitive obligations. (10)

timed urine specimen (tīmd yōōr´in spĕs´ə-mən) A specimen of a patient's urine collected over a specific time period. (47)

time-specified scheduling (tīm spĕs´ə-fīd skĕj´ōōl-ĭng) A system of scheduling where patients arrive at regular, specified intervals, assuring the practice a steady stream of patients throughout the day. (12)

tinnitus (ti-nī´tus)(†) An abnormal ringing in the ear. (33)

tissue (tĭsh´ōō) A structure that is formed when cells of the same type organize together. (23)

T lymphocyte (tē lĭm´fə-sīt) A type of nongranular leukocyte that regulates immunologic response; includes helper T cells and suppressor T cells. (48)

topical (tŏp´ĭ-kəl) Applied to the skin. (42)

tort (tôrt) In civil law, a breach of some obligation that causes harm or injury to someone. (3)

tower case (tou´ər kās) A vertical housing for the system unit of a personal computer. (6)

toxicology (tŏk´sĭ-kŏl´ə-jē) The study of poisons or poisonous effects of drugs. (50)

trachea (trā´kē-ə) The part of the respiratory tract between the larynx and the bronchial tree that is tubular and made of rings of cartilage and smooth muscle; also called the windpipe. (30)

tracking (trăk´ĭng) (financial) Watching for changes in spending so as to help control expenses. (18)

traction (trăk´shən) The pulling or stretching of the musculoskeletal system to treat dislocated joints, joints afflicted by arthritis or other diseases, and fractured bones. (43)

trade name (trād nām) A drug's brand or proprietary name. (50)

transcription (trăn-skrĭp´shən) The transforming of spoken notes into accurate written form. (9)

transcutaneous absorption (trans-kyū-tăn´ē-ŭs əb-sorp´shən)(†) Entry (as of a pathogen) through a cut or crack in the skin. (22)

transdermal (trans-der´mel) A type of topical drug administration that slowly and evenly releases a systemic drug through the skin directly into the bloodstream; a transdermal unit is also called a patch. (51)

transfer (trăns-fûr´) To give something, such as information, to another party outside the doctor's office. (9)

transverse (trăns-vûrs´) Anatomical term that refers to the plane that divides the body into superior and inferior portions. (23)

transverse colon (trăns-vûrs´ kō´lən) The segment of the large intestine that crosses the upper abdominal cavity between the ascending and descending colon. (31)

traveler's check (trăv´əlz chĕk) A check purchased and signed at a bank and later signed over to a payee. (18)

treatment, payments and operations (TPO) (trēt´mənt pā´mənts ŏp´ə-rā´shəns) The portion of **HIPAA** that allows the provider to use and share patient health-care information for treatment, payment, and operations (such as quality improvement). (3)

triage (trē-äzh´) To assess the urgency and types of conditions patients present as well as their immediate medical needs. (2)

TRICARE (trī´kâr) A program that provides health-care benefits for families of military personnel and military retirees. (15)

trichinosis (trik-i-nō´sis)(†) A disease caused by a worm that is usually ingested from undercooked meat. (26)

tricuspid valve (trī-kŭs´pid vălv)(†) A heart valve that has three cusps and is situated between the right atrium and the right ventricle. (28)

triglycerides (trī-glĭs´ə-rīd´z) Simple lipids consisting of glycerol (an alcohol) and three fatty acids. (49)

trigone (trī´gōn)(†) The triangle formed by the openings of the two ureters and the urethra in the internal floor of the bladder. (34)

troubleshooting (trŭb´əl-shōō´tĭng) Trying to determine and correct a problem without having to call a service supplier. (5)

trypsin (trĭp'sĭn)(†) A pancreatic enzyme that digests proteins. (31)

tubular reabsorption (tŭ'byŭ-lăr)(†) The second process of urine formation in which the glomerular filtrate flows into the proximal convoluted tubule. (34)

tubular secretion (tŭ'byŭ-lăr sĭ-krē'shən)(†) The third process of urine formation in which substances move out of the blood in the peritubular capillaries into renal tubules. (34)

tutorial (tōō-tôr'ē-əl) A small program included in a software package designed to give users an overall picture of the product and its functions. (6)

tympanic membrane (tĭm-păn'ĭk mĕm'brăn') A fibrous partition located at the inner end of the ear canal and separating the outer ear from the middle ear; also called the eardrum. (33)

tympanic thermometer (tim-pan'ik ther-mom'ĕ-ter) A type of electronic thermometer that measures infrared energy emitted from the tympanic membrane. (37)

ulna (əl'-nə) The medial bone of the lower arm. (25)

ultrasonic cleaning (ŭl'trə-sŏn'ĭk klēn'ĭng) A method of sanitization that involves placing instruments in a cleaning solution in a special receptacle that generates sound waves through the cleaning solution, loosening contaminants. Ultrasonic cleaning is safe for even very fragile instruments. (20)

ultrasound The noninvasive therapuetic or diagnostic use of ultrasound for examination of internal body structures. (53)

umbilical cord (ŭm-bĭl'ĭ-kəl kôrd) The rope-like connection between the fetus and the placenta. It contains the umbilical blood vessels. (35)

underbooking (ŭn'dər-bōōkĭng) Leaving large, unused gaps in the doctor's schedule; this approach does not make the best use of the doctor's time. (12)

uniform donor card (yōō'nə-fôrm' dŏnər kärd) A legal document that states a person's wish to make a gift upon death of one or more organs for medical research, organ transplants, or placement in a tissue bank. (3)

unit price (yōō'nĭt prīs) The total price of a package divided by the number of items that comprise the package. (8)

Universal Precautions (yōō'nə-vur'səl prĭ-kō'shənz) Specific precautions required by the Department of Health and Human Services' Centers for Disease Control and Prevention (CDC) to prevent health-care workers from exposing themselves and others to infection by blood-borne pathogens. (19)

unsaturated fats (ŭn-săch'ə-rā'tĭd făts) Fats, including most vegetable oils, that are usually liquid at room temperature and tend to lower blood cholesterol. (49)

urea (yōō-rē'ə) Waste product formed by the breakdown of proteins and nucleic acids. (34)

ureters (yōō-rē'tərz) Long, slender, muscular tubes that carry urine from the kidneys to the urinary bladder. (34)

urethra (yōō-rē'thrə) The tube that conveys urine from the bladder during urination. (34)

uric acid (yōō'ĭk as'id) Waste product formed by the breakdown of proteins and nucleic acids. (34)

urinalysis (yōōr'ə-năl'ĭ-sĭs) The physical, chemical, and microscopic evaluation of urine to obtain information about body health and disease. (47)

urinary catheter (yōōr'ə-nĕr'ē kăth'ĭ-tər) A sterile plastic tube inserted to provide urinary drainage. (47)

urinary pH (yōōr'ə-nĕr'ē pē'ăch) A measure of the degree of acidity or alkalinity of urine. (47)

urine specific gravity (yōōr'ĭn spĭ-sĭf'ĭk grăv'ĭ-tē) A measure of the concentration or amount (total weight) of substances dissolved in urine. (47)

urobilinogen (yŭr-ō-bī-lin'ō-jen)(†) A colorless compound formed by the breakdown of hemoglobin in the intestines. Elevated levels in urine may indicate increased red blood cell destruction or liver disease, whereas lack of urobilinogen in the urine may suggest total bile duct obstruction. (47)

urologist (yōō-rŏl'ə-jĭst) A specialist who diagnoses and treats diseases of the kidney, bladder, and urinary system. (2)

use (yōōz) The sharing, employing, applying, utilizing, examining, or analyzing of individually identifiable health information by employees or other members of an organization's workforce. (3)

uterus (yōō'tər-əs) A hollow, muscular organ that functions to receive an embryo and sustain its development; also called the womb. (35)

uvula (yōō'vyə-lə) The part of the soft palate that hangs down in the back of the throat. (31)

vaccine (văk-sēn') A special preparation made from microorganisms and administered to a person to produce reduced sensitivity to, or increased immunity to, an infectious disease. (50)

vagina (və-jī'nə) A tubular organ that extends from the uterus to the labia. (35)

vaginitis (vaj-i-nī'tis)(†) Inflammation of the vagina characterized by an abnormal vaginal discharge. (35)

varicose veins (văr'i-kōs vānz)(†) Distended veins that result when vein valves are destroyed and blood pools in the veins, causing these veins to dilate. (28)

vas deferens (văs' dĕf'ər-ənz) A tube that connects the epididymis with the urethra and that carries sperm. (35)

vasectomy (və-sĕk'tə-mē) A male sterilization procedure in which a section of each vas deferens is removed. (41)

vasoconstriction (vă'sō-kon-strik'shŭn) (†) The constriction of the muscular wall of an artery to increase blood pressure. (28)

vasodilation (vă-sō-dī-lā'shŭn)(†) The widening of the muscular wall of an artery to decrease blood pressure. (28)

V code (vē kōd) A code used to identify encounters for reasons other than illness or injury, such as annual checkups, immunizations, and normal childbirth. (16)

vector (vĕk'tər) A living organism, such as an insect, that carries microorganisms from an infected person to another person. (19)

venipuncture (ven'i-pŭnk-chŭr)(†) The puncture of a vein, usually with a needle, for the purpose of drawing blood. (48)

ventilation (vĕn'tə-lā'shən) Moving air in and out of the lungs; also called breathing. (30)

ventral (vĕn'trəl) See **anterior**. (23)

ventral root (vĕn'trəl rōōt) A portion of the spinal nerve that contains axons of motor neurons only. (27)

ventricle (vĕn'trĭ-kəl) Interconnected cavities in the brain filled with cerebrospinal fluid. (27)

ventricular fibrillation (ven-trik'yū-lăr fī-bri-lā'shŭn) An abnormal heart rhythm that is the most common cause of cardiac arrest. (44)

verbalizing (vûr´bə-līz´-ĭng) Stating what you believe the patient is suggesting or implying. (36)

vermiform appendix (uer´mi-fōrm ə-pĕn´dĭks)(†) A structure made mostly of lymphoid tissue and projecting off the cecum. It is commonly referred to as simply the appendix. (31)

vertical file (vûr´tĭ-kəl fil) A filing cabinet featuring pull-out drawers that usually contain a metal frame or bar equipped to handle letter- or legal-sized documents in hanging file folders. (10)

vesicles (vĕs´ĭ-kəlz) Small sacs within the synaptic knobs that contain chemicals called neurotransmitters. (27)

vestibular glands (ves-tĭb´yū-lăr glăndz)(†) Glands that secrete mucus into the vestibule of the female during sexual excitement. (35)

vestibule (vĕs´tə-byōōl´) The area in the inner ear between the semicircular canals and the cochlea. (33)

vial (vī´əl) A small glass bottle with a self-sealing rubber stopper. (42)

vibrio (†)(vĭb´rē-ō) A comma-shaped bacterium. (46)

virulence (vĭr´yə-ləns) A microorganism's disease-producing power. (19)

virus (vī´rəs) One of the smallest known infectious agents, consisting only of nucleic acid surrounded by a protein coat; can live and grow only within the living cells of other organisms. (46)

visceral pericardium (vĭs´er-ăl per-i-kar´dē-ŭm)(†) The innermost layer of the pericardium that lies directly on top of the heart; also known as the **epicardium**. (28)

visceral smooth muscle (vĭs´ar-əl smōōth mŭs´əl) A type of smooth muscle containing sheets of muscle that closely contact each other. It is found in the walls of hollow organs such as the stomach, intestines, bladder, and uterus. (26)

vitamins (vī´tə-mĭnz) Organic substances that are essential for normal body growth and maintenance and resistance to infection. (49)

vitreous humor (vĭt´rē-əs hyōō´mər) A jellylike substance that fills the part of the eye behind the lens and helps the eye keep its shape. (33)

voice mail (vois māl) An advanced form of answering machine that allows a caller to leave a message when the phone line is busy. (5)

void (void) (legal) A term used to describe something that is not legally enforceable. (3)

volume (vŏl´yōōm) The amount of space an object, such as a drug, occupies. (51)

vomer (vō´-mər) A thin bone that divides the nasal cavity. (25)

voucher check (vou´chər chĕk) A business check with an attached stub, which is kept as a receipt. (18)

walk-in (wôk´ĭn) A patient who arrives without an appointment. (12)

warranty (wôk´ən-tē) A contract that specifies free service and replacement of parts for a piece of equipment during a certain period, usually a year. (5)

warts (wôrts) Flesh-colored skin lesions with distinct round borders that are raised and often have small fingerlike projections; also called verruca. (24)

wave scheduling (wāv skĕj´ōōl-ĭng) A system of scheduling in which the number of patients seen each hour is determined by dividing the hour by the length of the average visit and then giving that number of patients appointments with the doctor at the beginning of each hour. (12)

Western blot test (wĕs´tərn blŏt tĕst) A blood test used to confirm enzyme-linked immunosorbent assay (ELISA) test results for HIV infection. (21)

wet mount (wĕt mount) A preparation of a specimen in a liquid that allows the organisms to remain alive and mobile while they are being identified. (46)

white matter (hwīt măt´ər) The outer tissue of the spinal cord that is lighter in color than **gray matter**. It contains myelinated axons. (27)

whole blood (hōl blŭd) The total volume of plasma and formed elements, or blood in which the elements have not been separated by coagulation or centrifugation. (48)

whole-body skin examination (hōl bŏd´ē skĭn ĭg-zăm´ə-nā´shən) An examination of the visible top layer of the entire surface of the skin, including the scalp, genital area, and areas between the toes, to look for lesions, especially suspicious moles or precancerous growths. (41)

Wood's light examination (wŏŏdz līt ĭg-zăm´ə-nā´shən) A type of dermatologic examination in which a physician inspects the patient's skin under an ultraviolet lamp in a darkened room. (41)

written-contract account (rĭt´n kŏn´trăkt´ ə-kount´) An agreement between the physician and patient stating that the patient will pay a bill in more than four installments. (17)

X12 837 Health Care Claim (hĕlth kâr klām) An electronic claim transaction that is the **HIPAA** Health Care Claim or Equivalent Encounter Information ("HIPAA claim"). (15)

xeroradiography (zē´rō-rā´dē-og´rä-fē)(†) A radiologic procedure in which x-rays are developed with a powder toner, similar to the toner in photocopiers, and the x-ray image is processed on specially treated xerographic paper; used to diagnose breast cancer, abscesses, lesions, or calcifications. (53)

xiphoid process (zif´oyd prŏs´ĕs)(†) The lower extension of the breastbone. (44)

yeast (yēst) A fungus that grows mainly as a single-celled organism and reproduces by budding. (46)

yolk sac (yōk săk) The sac that holds the materials for the nutrition of the embryo. (35)

zona pellucida (zō´nă pe-lū´sid-ă)(†) A layer that surrounds the cell membrane of an egg. (35)

zygomatic (zī-gə-m´a-tik) The bones that form the prominence of the cheeks. (25)

zygote (zī´gō) The cell that is formed from the union of the egg and sperm. (35)

Z-track method (zē´trăk mĕth´əd) A technique used when injecting an intramuscular (IM) drug that can irritate subcutaneous tissue; involves pulling the skin and subcutaneous tissue to the side before inserting the needle at the site, creating a zigzag path in the tissue layers that prevents the drug from leaking into the subcutaneous tissue and causing irritation. (51)

Photo Credits

Fig. 48.28: © Terry Wild Studio; Fig. 48.29, Fig. 48.30, Fig. 48.31, Fig. 48.32: Courtesy Becton Dickinson.

CHAPTER 49

Fig. 49.1: © Spangler Studio/Merrill Property; Fig. 49.2, Fig. 49.3: Ken Lax; Fig. 49.4: © Tom Dunham; Fig. 49.5, Fig. 49.6: © Elaine Shay/Merrill Property; Fig. 49.7, Fig. 49.8: Ken Lax; Fig. 49.9, Fig. 49.10: © David Kelly Crow; Fig. 49.11, Fig. 49.12: Ken Lax; Fig. 49.19: Robert Matthews.

CHAPTER 50

Fig. 50.2: © David Kelly Crow; Fig. 50.3a: © R.J. Erwin/Photo Researchers, Inc.; Fig. 50.3b: © Andrew McClenaghan/SPL/Photo Researchers, Inc.; Fig. 50.4: © Terry Wild Studio; Fig. 50.5: © David Kelly Crow.

CHAPTER 51

Fig. 51.1: Center Laboratories; Fig. 51.2, Fig. 51.3, Fig. 51.4: © Cliff Moore; Fig. 51.8, Fig. 51.10: Courtesy of Total Care Programming; Fig. 51.11, Fig. 51.23: © Cliff Moore.

CHAPTER 52

Fig. 52.3a–b, Fig. 52.4: Courtesy Burdick, Inc.; Fig. 52.5: © Cliff Moore; Fig. 52.8, Fig. 52.9: © David Kelly Crow Fig. 52.17: © Cliff Moore; Fig. 52.18, 52.19, Fig. 52.20, Fig. 52.21, Fig. 52.22: © David Kelly Crow; Page 1082: © Robert Crandall/Medical Images, Inc.; Fig. 52.24, Fig. 52.26a–b, Fig. 52.28: © Cliff Moore.

CHAPTER 53

Fig. 53.1: © Cliff Moore; Fig. 53.2a–d: © Martin M. Rotker; Fig. 53.3: © Cliff Moore; Page 1097: © David Kelly Crow; Fig. 53.4a: Courtesy of Radiology Affiliates of Central NJ, PA; Mercerville, NJ; Fig. 53.4b: Courtesy of Virtual Healthscan; Fig. 53.4c: Courtesy of Mercer Medical Center, Dept. of Radiology, Trenton, NJ; Fig. 53.4d: Courtesy of Virtual Healthscan; Fig. 53.4e: Courtesy of MRI Center at Lawrenceville, NJ; Fig. 53.5: © NIH/Science Source/Photo Researchers, Inc.; Fig. 53.6a: © Stephen Gerard/Science Source/Photo Researchers, Inc.; Fig. 53.6b: © Scott Camazine/Photo Researchers, Inc.; Fig. 53.7: Courtesy of Mercer Medical Center, Dept. of Radiology, Trenton, NJ; Fig. 53.8: © P. Sadda/Eurelios/SPL/Photo Researchers, Inc.; Fig. 53.9, Fig. 53.11: © Cliff Moore.

CHAPTER 54

Fig. 54.10: © David Kelly Crow.

Text and Line Art Credits

CHAPTER 1

Context (pg 18–19) The Medical Assistant Role Delineation Chart, courtesy of the American Association of Medical Assistants.

CHAPTER 3

Fig. 3.1: *Source:* Medicolegal Forms With Legal Analysis, American Medical Association, © 1991; Fig. 3.6: The AAMA's Code of Ethics, (Reprinted with permission of the American Association of Medical Assistants.). Context (pg 40) The Four Ds of Negligence, courtesy of the American Medical Association (AMA).

CHAPTER 4

Table 4.1: From *YOUR PERFECT RIGHT: Assertiveness and Equality in Your Life and Relationships, 8th Edition* © 2001 by Robert E. Alberti and Michael L. Emmons. Reproduced for Ramutkowski et al. by permission of Impact Publishers, Inc., PO Box 6016, Atascadero, CA 93423. Further reproduction prohibited. Context (pg 76) "Preventing Burnout." Section adapted from *The Stress Solution* by Lyle H. Miller, PhD and Alma Dell Smith, PhD, American Psychological Association, 1997.

CHAPTER 6

Fig. 6.5: Windows 2000-Screen shot reprinted by permission from Microsoft Corporation; Fig. 6.6: I. Hoffmann + Associates Inc. (H + a) Image from the Epilepsy CD-ROM of the H + a Medical Series. All rights reserved; Fig. 6.7: Screen capture Corel Corporations.

CHAPTER 10

Table 10.1: Adapted from William A. Sabin, *The Gregg Reference Manual,* 8th ed. (Columbus, OH: Glencoe/McGraw-Hill, 1996), 288–295.

CHAPTER 14

Context (pg 244) Data for in-home deaths of people of all ages, provided by National Safety Council.

CHAPTER 15

Fig. 15.1: *Source:* Mercer's National Survey of Employer Sponsored Health Plans, 2003. Copyright 2003, The Managed Care Information Center; Fig. 15.4: *Source:* Blue Cross and Blue Shield Association; Fig. 15.7: *Source:* Center for Medicare and Medicaid Services.

CHAPTER 16

Fig. 16.1: *Source:* International Classification of Diseases, Ninth Revision, Clinical Modification, 2004, Volumes 1 and 2. International Classification of Diseases, Ninth Revision, Clinical Modification http://www.cdc.gov/nchs/about/otheract/icd9/abticd9.htm; Fig. 16.2: *Source:* American Medical Association, *Current Procedural Terminology,* copyright 2003.

CHAPTER 20

Fig. 20.12: Adult immunization, (National Coalition for Adult Immunization. Reprinted with permission.).

CHAPTER 21

Table 21.1: Source: Centers for Disease Control and Prevention; Table 21.2: Source: US Department of Health and Human Services; Food and Drug Administration and AIDSInfo; Table 21.3: Source: *"State Health Facts Online,"* The Henry J. Kaiser Family Foundation, www.kff.org. This information was reprinted with permission from the Henry J. Kaiser Family Foundation. The Kaiser Family Foundation, based in Menlo Park, California, is a nonprofit, independent national health care philanthropy and is not associated with Kaiser Permanente or Kaiser Industries.

CHAPTER 23

Fig. 23.2: Seeley- *Essentials of Anatomy and Physiology* 5th ed. McGraw-Hill © 2005; Fig. 23.6: Shier- *Hole's Essentials of Human Anatomy and Physiology* 8th ed. McGraw-Hill © 2003; Fig. 23.7: Shier- *Hole's Essentials of Human Anatomy and Physiology* 8th ed. McGraw-Hill © 2003; Fig. 23.8: Shier- *Hole's Essentials of Human Anatomy and Physiology* 8th ed. McGraw-Hill © 2003; Fig. 23.9: Shier- *Hole's Essentials of Human Anatomy and Physiology* 8th ed. McGraw-Hill © 2003; Fig. 23.10: Shier- *Hole's Essentials of Human Anatomy and Physiology* 8th ed. McGraw-Hill © 2003; Fig. 23.11: Shier- *Hole's Essentials of Human Anatomy and Physiology* 8th ed. McGraw-Hill © 2003; Fig. 23.12: Shier- *Hole's Essentials of Human Anatomy and Physiology* 8th ed. McGraw-Hill © 2003; Fig. 23.13: Shier- *Hole's Essentials of Human Anatomy and Physiology* 8th ed. McGraw-Hill © 2003.

CHAPTER 24

Fig. 24.1: Shier- *Hole's Essentials of Human Anatomy and Physiology* 8th ed. McGraw-Hill © 2003; Fig. 24.4: Shier- *Hole's Essentials of Human Anatomy and Physiology* 8th ed. McGraw-Hill © 2003; Fig. 24.5: Mader-*Understanding Human Anatomy and Physiology* 4th ed. McGraw-Hill © 2001; Fig. 24.6: Shier- *Hole's Essentials of Human Anatomy and Physiology* 8th ed. McGraw-Hill © 2003.

CHAPTER 25

Fig. 25.1: Shier- *Hole's Essentials of Human Anatomy and Physiology* 8th ed. McGraw-Hill © 2003; Fig. 25.3: Shier- *Hole's Essentials of Human Anatomy and Physiology* 8th ed. McGraw-Hill © 2003; Fig. 25.4: Shier- *Hole's Essentials of Human Anatomy and Physiology* 8th ed. McGraw-Hill © 2003; Fig. 25.5: Mader-*Understanding Human Anatomy and Physiology* 4th ed. McGraw-Hill © 2001; Fig. 25.6: Shier- *Hole's Essentials of Human Anatomy and Physiology* 8th ed. McGraw-Hill © 2003; Fig. 25.7: Shier- *Hole's Essentials of Human Anatomy and Physiology* 8th ed. McGraw-Hill © 2003; Fig. 25.8: Shier- *Hole's Essentials of Human Anatomy and Physiology* 8th ed. McGraw-Hill © 2003; Fig. 25.9: Shier- *Hole's Essentials of Human Anatomy and Physiology* 8th ed. McGraw-Hill © 2003; Fig. 25.10: Saladin- *Anatomy and Physiology: The Unity of Form and Function* 3rd ed. McGraw-Hill © 2004; Fig. 25.11: Saladin- *Anatomy and Physiology: The Unity of Form and Function* 3rd ed. McGraw-Hill © 2004; Fig. 25.12: Shier- *Hole's Essentials of Human Anatomy and Physiology* 8th ed. McGraw-Hill © 2003.

CHAPTER 26

Fig. 26.1: Shier- *Hole's Essentials of Human Anatomy and Physiology* 8th ed. McGraw-Hill © 2003; Fig. 26.2: Shier- *Hole's Essentials of Human Anatomy and Physiology* 8th ed. McGraw-Hill © 2003; Fig. 26.3: Shier- *Hole's Essentials of Human Anatomy and Physiology* 8th ed. McGraw-Hill © 2003; Fig. 26.4: Shier- *Hole's Essentials of Human Anatomy and Physiology* 8th ed. McGraw-Hill © 2003; Fig. 26.5: Shier- *Hole's Essentials of Human Anatomy and Physiology* 8th ed. McGraw-Hill © 2003; Fig. 26.6: Shier- *Hole's Essentials of Human Anatomy and Physiology* 8th ed. McGraw-Hill © 2003; Fig. 26.7: Shier- *Hole's Essentials of Human Anatomy and Physiology* 8th ed. McGraw-Hill © 2003; Fig. 26.8: Shier- *Hole's Essentials of Human Anatomy and Physiology* 8th ed. McGraw-Hill © 2003; Fig. 26.9: Shier- *Hole's Essentials of Human Anatomy and Physiology* 8th ed. McGraw-Hill © 2003.

CHAPTER 27

Fig. 27.2: Shier- *Hole's Essentials of Human Anatomy and Physiology* 8th ed. McGraw-Hill © 2003; Fig. 27.3: Shier- *Hole's Essentials of Human Anatomy and Physiology* 8th ed. McGraw-Hill © 2003; Fig. 27.4: Shier- *Hole's Essentials of Human Anatomy and Physiology* 8th ed. McGraw-Hill © 2003; Fig. 27.5: Mader-*Understanding Human Anatomy and Physiology* 4th ed. McGraw-Hill © 2001; Fig. 27.6: Saladin- *Anatomy and Physiology: The Unity of Form and Function* 3rd ed. McGraw-Hill © 2004; Fig. 27.7: Shier- *Hole's Essentials of Human Anatomy and Physiology* 8th ed. McGraw-Hill © 2003; Fig. 27.8: Shier- *Hole's Essentials of Human Anatomy and Physiology* 8th ed. McGraw-Hill © 2003.

CHAPTER 28

Fig. 28.1: Shier- *Hole's Essentials of Human Anatomy and Physiology* 8th ed. McGraw-Hill © 2003; Fig. 28.2: Shier- *Hole's Essentials of Human Anatomy and Physiology* 8th ed. McGraw-Hill © 2003; Fig. 28.3: Shier- *Hole's Essentials of Human Anatomy and Physiology* 8th ed. McGraw-Hill © 2003; Fig. 28.4: Shier- *Hole's Essentials of Human Anatomy and Physiology* 8th ed. McGraw-Hill © 2003; Fig. 28.5: Shier- *Hole's Essentials of Human Anatomy and Physiology* 8th ed. McGraw-Hill © 2003;

Fig. 28.6: Shier- *Hole's Essentials of Human Anatomy and Physiology* 8th ed. McGraw-Hill © 2003;
Fig. 28.8: Shier- *Hole's Essentials of Human Anatomy and Physiology* 8th ed. McGraw-Hill © 2003;
Fig. 28.10: Shier- *Hole's Essentials of Human Anatomy and Physiology* 8th ed. McGraw-Hill © 2003;
Fig. 28.11: Shier- *Hole's Essentials of Human Anatomy and Physiology* 8th ed. McGraw-Hill © 2003;
Fig. 28.12: Shier- *Hole's Essentials of Human Anatomy and Physiology* 8th ed. McGraw-Hill © 2003;
Fig. 28.13: Shier- *Hole's Essentials of Human Anatomy and Physiology* 8th ed. McGraw-Hill © 2003;
Fig. 28.14: Shier- *Hole's Essentials of Human Anatomy and Physiology* 8th ed. McGraw-Hill © 2003;
Fig. 28.20: Shier- *Hole's Essentials of Human Anatomy and Physiology* 8th ed. McGraw-Hill © 2003;
Fig. 28.21: Shier- *Hole's Essentials of Human Anatomy and Physiology* 8th ed. McGraw-Hill © 2003;
Fig. 28.23: Shier- *Hole's Essentials of Human Anatomy and Physiology* 8th ed. McGraw-Hill © 2003;
Fig. 28.24: Shier- *Hole's Essentials of Human Anatomy and Physiology* 8th ed. McGraw-Hill © 2003;
Fig. 28.25: Shier- *Hole's Essentials of Human Anatomy and Physiology* 8th ed. McGraw-Hill © 2003;
Fig. 28.26: Shier- *Hole's Essentials of Human Anatomy and Physiology* 8th ed. McGraw-Hill © 2003;
Fig. 28.27: Shier- *Hole's Essentials of Human Anatomy and Physiology* 8th ed. McGraw-Hill © 2003;
Fig. 28.28: Shier- *Hole's Essentials of Human Anatomy and Physiology* 8th ed. McGraw-Hill © 2003;
Fig. 28.29: Shier- *Hole's Essentials of Human Anatomy and Physiology* 8th ed. McGraw-Hill © 2003.

CHAPTER 29
Fig. 29.1: Shier- *Hole's Essentials of Human Anatomy and Physiology* 8th ed. McGraw-Hill © 2003;
Fig. 29.2: Shier- *Hole's Essentials of Human Anatomy and Physiology* 8th ed. McGraw-Hill © 2003.

CHAPTER 30
Fig. 30.1: Mader-*Understanding Human Anatomy and Physiology* 4th ed. McGraw-Hill © 2001;
Fig. 30.2: Mader-*Understanding Human Anatomy and Physiology* 4th ed. McGraw-Hill © 2001;
Fig. 30.3: Mader-*Understanding Human Anatomy and Physiology* 4th ed. McGraw-Hill © 2001. Context (pg 546) Scale to determine the severity of snoring, adapted from The Mayo Clinic's Sleep Disorders Center.

CHAPTER 31
Fig. 31.1: Shier- *Hole's Essentials of Human Anatomy and Physiology* 8th ed. McGraw-Hill © 2003;
Fig. 31.2: Shier- *Hole's Essentials of Human Anatomy and Physiology* 8th ed. McGraw-Hill © 2003;
Fig. 31.3: Shier- *Hole's Essentials of Human Anatomy and Physiology* 8th ed. McGraw-Hill © 2003;
Fig. 31.4: Shier- *Hole's Essentials of Human Anatomy and Physiology* 8th ed. McGraw-Hill © 2003;
Fig. 31.5: Shier- *Hole's Essentials of Human Anatomy and Physiology* 8th ed. McGraw-Hill © 2003;
Fig. 31.6: Shier- *Hole's Essentials of Human Anatomy and Physiology* 8th ed. McGraw-Hill © 2003;
Fig. 31.7: Shier- *Hole's Essentials of Human Anatomy and Physiology* 8th ed. McGraw-Hill © 2003;
Fig. 31.8: Shier- *Hole's Essentials of Human Anatomy and Physiology* 8th ed. McGraw-Hill © 2003;
Fig. 31.9: Shier- *Hole's Essentials of Human Anatomy and Physiology* 8th ed. McGraw-Hill © 2003;
Fig. 31.10: Shier- *Hole's Essentials of Human Anatomy and Physiology* 8th ed. McGraw-Hill © 2003;
Fig. 31.11: Shier- *Hole's Essentials of Human Anatomy and Physiology* 8th ed. McGraw-Hill © 2003;
Fig. 31.12: Shier- *Hole's Essentials of Human Anatomy and Physiology* 8th ed. McGraw-Hill © 2003.

CHAPTER 32
Fig. 32.1: Shier- *Hole's Essentials of Human Anatomy and Physiology* 8th ed. McGraw-Hill © 2003;

Fig. 32.2: Shier- *Hole's Essentials of Human Anatomy and Physiology* 8th ed. McGraw-Hill © 2003.

CHAPTER 33
Fig. 33.1: Shier- *Hole's Essentials of Human Anatomy and Physiology* 8th ed. McGraw-Hill © 2003;
Fig. 33.2: Mader-*Understanding Human Anatomy and Physiology* 4th ed. McGraw-Hill © 2001;
Fig. 33.3: Mader-*Understanding Human Anatomy and Physiology* 4th ed. McGraw-Hill © 2001;
Fig. 33.4: Shier- *Hole's Essentials of Human Anatomy and Physiology* 8th ed. McGraw-Hill © 2003;
Fig. 33.5: Shier- *Hole's Essentials of Human Anatomy and Physiology* 8th ed. McGraw-Hill © 2003.

CHAPTER 34
Fig. 34.1: Shier- *Hole's Essentials of Human Anatomy and Physiology* 8th ed. McGraw-Hill © 2003;
Fig. 34.2: Shier- *Hole's Essentials of Human Anatomy and Physiology* 8th ed. McGraw-Hill © 2003;
Fig. 34.3: Shier- *Hole's Essentials of Human Anatomy and Physiology* 8th ed. McGraw-Hill © 2003;
Fig. 34.4: Shier- *Hole's Essentials of Human Anatomy and Physiology* 8th ed. McGraw-Hill © 2003;
Fig. 34.5: Shier- *Hole's Essentials of Human Anatomy and Physiology* 8th ed. McGraw-Hill © 2003;
Fig. 34.6: Shier- *Hole's Essentials of Human Anatomy and Physiology* 8th ed. McGraw-Hill © 2003.

CHAPTER 35
Fig. 35.1: Shier- *Hole's Essentials of Human Anatomy and Physiology* 8th ed. McGraw-Hill © 2003;
Fig. 35.2: Shier- *Hole's Essentials of Human Anatomy and Physiology* 8th ed. McGraw-Hill © 2003;
Fig. 35.3: Shier- *Hole's Essentials of Human Anatomy and Physiology* 8th ed. McGraw-Hill © 2003;
Fig. 35.4: Shier- *Hole's Essentials of Human Anatomy and Physiology* 8th ed. McGraw-Hill © 2003;
Fig. 35.5: Shier- *Hole's Essentials of Human Anatomy and Physiology* 8th ed. McGraw-Hill © 2003;
Fig. 35.6: Shier- *Hole's Essentials of Human Anatomy and Physiology* 8th ed. McGraw-Hill © 2003;
Fig. 35.7: Shier- *Hole's Essentials of Human Anatomy and Physiology* 8th ed. McGraw-Hill © 2003;
Fig. 35.8: Shier- *Hole's Essentials of Human Anatomy and Physiology* 8th ed. McGraw-Hill © 2003;
Fig. 35.9: Shier- *Hole's Essentials of Human Anatomy and Physiology* 8th ed. McGraw-Hill © 2003;
Fig. 35.10: Shier- *Hole's Essentials of Human Anatomy and Physiology* 8th ed. McGraw-Hill © 2003;
Fig. 35.11: Shier- *Hole's Essentials of Human Anatomy and Physiology* 8th ed. McGraw-Hill © 2003.

CHAPTER 37
Fig. 37.8: *Source:* Kathryn Booth, *Health Care Science Technology*, 1st ed. Peoria, IL: Glencoe/McGraw-Hill, 2004.

CHAPTER 38
Fig. 38.11: Adapted from The National Cancer Institute includes these instructions and illustrations in the brochure *Breast Exams: What You Should Know* (NIH Publications No. 90-2000).

CHAPTER 39
Fig. 39.3: (Richmond International, Inc. Boca Raton, Florida); Fig. 39.4: (Richmond International, Inc.); Fig. 39.5: (Richmond International, Inc.); Fig. 39.7: (Richmond International, Inc.).

CHAPTER 40
Fig. 40.2: From Corbin et. al., *Concepts of Physical Fitness* 11/e © 2003 The McGraw-Hill Companies. Reprinted by permission. All rights reserved; Fig. 40.14: From Seeley *Anatomy & Physiology* 6th ed. © 2003 The McGraw-Hill Companies. Reprinted by permission. All rights reserved.

CHAPTER 42
Fig. 42.20: *Source:* Keir, Wise, and Krebs, *Medical Assisting Administrative and Clinical Competencies*, 5th ed. 2003, p. 763.

CHAPTER 43
Fig. 43.6: *Source:* McGraw-Hill *Health Care Science Technology* by Booth, 2004; Fig. 43.8: teaching a patient to walk with crutches, borrowed from McGraw-Hill *Health Care Science Technology* by Booth, 2004.

CHAPTER 44
Fig. 44.20: *Source: Glencoe Health Care Science Technology,* Booth 2004, p. 98; Fig. 44.21: *Source: Glencoe Health Care Science Technology,* Booth 2004, p. 101, Fig. 4.8.

CHAPTER 45
Fig. 45.11: (Courtesy of Medical Chemical Corp.)

CHAPTER 46
Table 46.3: Source: Centers for Disease Control, Health Topics A to Z. Atlanta, Georgia, 2003 http://www.cdc.gov/health/default.htm.

CHAPTER 48
Fig. 48.3: Source: Adapted from Norbert W. Tietz, ed., *Clinical Guide to Laboratory Tests*, 3rd ed. (Philadelphia: W.B. Saunders, 1995.)

CHAPTER 49
Table 49.1: Adapted from Marvin R. Levy et. al., *Life & Health: Targeting Wellness* (New York: McGraw-Hill, 1992; Table 49.3: Reprinted with permission from (Recommended Dietary Allowances: 10th Edition) © (1989) by the National Academy of Sciences, courtesy of the National Academies Press, Washington, D.C.; Table 49.4: Source: Nutrition and Your Health: *Dietary Guidelines for Americans*, 5th ed. (Washington, DC: U.S. Department of Agriculture and U.S. Department of Health and Human Services, 2000.); Table 49.5: Source: *Nutrition and Your Health: Dietary Guidelines for Americans*, 5th ed. (Washington, DC: U.S. Department of Agriculture and U.S. Department of Health and Human Services, 2000.); Fig. 49.14: *Source:* 1998 American Dietetic Association. Reprinted with permission.

CHAPTER 50
Table 50.1: Adapted from "The Top 200 Prescriptions for 200 by Number of US Prescriptions Dispensed." RxList: The Internet Drug Index, www.rxlist.com.; Table 50.2: Sources: *Physicians' Desk Reference: U.S. Pharmacopeia Dictionary;* Table 50.3: Source: U.S. Department of Justice, *Physician's Manual*, March 1990.

CHAPTER 51
Table 51.7: Source: *2004 Physicians' Desk Reference*, Thompson Healthcare.

CHAPTER 52
Fig. 52.11: Courtesy of Burdick, Inc., Milton, Wisconsin; Fig. 52.12: Courtesy of Burdick, Inc; Fig. 52.13: Courtesy of Burdick, Inc; Fig. 52.14: Courtesy of Burdick, Inc; Fig. 52.15: Courtesy of Burdick, Inc; Fig. 52.16: Courtesy of Burdick, Inc. Table 52.4: Adapted from *Illustrated Guide to Diagnostic Tests* (Springhouse, PA: Springhouse, 1998).

CHAPTER 54
Fig. 54.9: (reprinted with permission from Kelly Assisted Living Services, Inc.) Context (pg. 1130) *Source: Peak Performance: Success in College and Beyond*, 4th ed., Sharon K. Ferret, McGraw-Hill, 2003. Text (pg. 1131) *Source:* Highline Community College, Counceling/Career Center, Des Moines, WA.

Index

Page numbers in **boldface** indicate figures. Page numbers followed by (b) indicate box features, (p) procedures, and (t) tables, respectively.

Appointment scheduling system
advance scheduling, 217
cluster scheduling, 217, 217(p)
combination scheduling, 217
computerized scheduling, **217**, 217–218
double-booking system, 214
modified-wave scheduling, 214, **216**
open-hours scheduling, 214
time-specified scheduling, 214, **215**
wave scheduling, 214
Approximated, wound healing, 760, 761(b)
Aquatic therapy, 787(b)
Aqueous humor, 575, **576**, 669, **670**
Arachnoid mater, 496
Arbitration, 41
Areas of competence (AOC), 18
administrative procedures, 83(b), 119(b), 156(b), 176(b), 210(b), 256(b), 785(b)
communication skills, 5(b), 59(b), 100(b), 119(b), 156(b), 196(b), 240(b), 256(b), 611(b), 628(b), 645(b), 668(b), 694(b), 785(b), 908(b), 936(b), 1027(b), 1113(b)
diagnostic orders, 668(b), 723(b), 850(b), 877(b), 908(b), 936(b), 1060(b)
fundamental principles, 37(b), 349(b), 371(b), 394(b), 420(b), 645(b), 694(b), 757(b), 785(b), 850(b), 877(b), 908(b), 936(b), 1027(b), 1060(b)
instruction, 240(b), 349(b), 371(b), 394(b), 645(b), 668(b), 694(b), 723(b), 785(b), 811(b), 971(b), 1000(b), 1027(b)
legal concepts, 21(b), 37(b), 59(b), 156(b), 226(b), 256(b), 371(b), 394(b), 420(b), 611(b), 694(b), 757(b), 850(b), 877(b), 1000(b), 1027(b), 1089(b)
operational functions, 83(b), 100(b), 140(b), 312(b), 757(b), 1000(b)
patient care, 156(b), 256(b), 349(b), 420(b), 611(b), 628(b), 645(b), 668(b), 694(b), 723(b), 757(b), 811(b), 877(b), 1000(b), 1027(b), 1060(b), 1089(b)
practice finances, 293(b), 312(b)
professionalism, 5(b), 21(b), 59(b), 196(b), 210(b), 394(b), 645(b), 785(b), 811(b), 1000(b), 1113(b)
Areflexia, 501
Areola, 599, **599**
Arm, microscope, **853**, 855
Arms
bones of, **466**, 471–472
muscles of, 485, 487, **487**
Aromatherapy, 808(b)
Arrector pili, 459
Arrhythmias, 527(b)
Arterial blood gases, 698
Arterial blood pressure, 634
Arteries, 512, **512**
disorders of, 730(t)
major, 514, 514(t), **515**
Arterioles, 512
Arteriosclerosis, 730(t)
Arthritis, 702(t), 751(t)
rheumatoid, 539(b)
Arthritis Foundation, **251**
Arthrography, 750, 1094(t), 1095
Arthroscopy, 750, **750**
Articular cartilage, 465
Artifacts, microscope, 855(b)
Artifacts on ECG, 1073–1076, 1073(t), **1074–1076**
Artificial active immunity, 354, **354**, 536
Artificial passive immunity, 354, **354**, 536
Art therapy, 787(b)
Ascending colon, 559, **560**

Ascending tracts, 496
Ascorbic acid, 979(t)
ASCP. *See* American Society of Clinical Pathologists (ASCP)
Asepsis, 349–370. *See also* Infection-control techniques; Universal precautions
aseptic handwashing, 358, 359(p)
Bloodborne Pathogens Standard, 366
body's defenses against pathogens, 352–355
breaking cycle of infection, 357
cycle of infection, **355**, 355–357
defined, 357
disinfecting work surfaces, 360–361, **361**
history of infectious disease prevention, 350–352
infectious laundry waste disposal, 362(b)–363(b)
medical, 357–358, 766–767
in minor surgery, 765–771
OSHA Blood-borne Pathogens Standard, 361, 363(t)
patient education about disease prevention, 367–368
sanitizing, disinfecting and sterilizing instruments, 360
surgical, 357, 358, 360, 767–771
Aseptic meningitis, 384
As low as reasonably achievable (ALARA) principle, 1106
Aspartate aminotransferase, 960(t)
Aspirin, children's use of, 706, 708
Assault, 39
Assertiveness skills, 67, 67(t)
Assessment
before drug administration, 1032–1035
of patient in medical emergency, 813, 815(p)
in SOAP, 167
Assets, in double-entry bookkeeping system, 319
Assignment of benefits statement, 268
Associate degrees in nursing (ADN), 30
Association of Surgical Technologists, 759(b)
Association of Technical Personnel, 673(p)
Associations, as patient education resource, **251**, 252
Asthma, 546(b), 831
Asthma and Allergy Foundation of America, **251**
Astigmatism, 578(b), 749–750
Atherosclerosis, 527(b), 528(b), 730(t)
hyperlipidemia, 699, **699**
Athlete, injured, 799(b)
Athletes foot, 883
Atlas, 471
Atoms, 437, **437**
ATP (adenosine triphosphate), 480–481
Atrial natriuretic peptide, 569
Atrioventricular bundle, 511, **511**
Atrioventricular node, 511, **511**, 1062, 1062–1063
Atrium, 508, **509**, 1062, **1062**
Attention
to details, as medical assistant skill, 15
in telephone techniques, 204
Attention deficit hyperactivity disorder (ADHD), 447(b), 708
Attention line, 124
Attitude, of medical assistant, 17
Attorneys, handling calls from, 202
Audiologist, 687
Audiometer, 684, **685**
Auditory tube, 579, **580**
Aura, 503(b)
Auricle, 681, **683**
Auscultation, in general physical examination, 657

Authorization of disclosure form, 53, 57
Autoclave, 45, **376**, 376–381, 377(p)–378(p), 380(p), 771, 852
cleaning autoclave and work area, 379
general procedures for, 376
general steps in running, 380(p)
overcrowding, 381
performing quality control, 379
preheating, 378
preventing incomplete sterilization, 379
settings for, 378–379
steam level guidelines, 381
storing sterilized supplies, 379
temperature guidelines, 381
timing guidelines for, 379, 381
wrapping and labeling items in, 376, 377(p)–378(p), 378
Automated external defibrillator (AED), 835, **835**
Automated menu telephone system, 86, 86(b)
Automatic puncturing devices, 951
Automation equipment, office
adding machines and calculators, 90
check writers, 93
dictation-transcription equipment, 92–93, 92(p)
microfilm and microfiche readers, **94**, 94–95
paper shredders, **93**, 93–94
photocopiers, 89–90
postage meters, **90**, 90–91, 91(p)
postage scales, 91–92
Autonomic nervous system, **500**, 500–501
Autosomes, 447
Autricle, 579, **580**
Awakening Phase of burnout, 76
Axial skeleton, 465, **466**
Axilla, 630
Axillary crutches, 803
Axillary temperature, 630, 632
Axis, 471
Axons, 493–494, **494**

Baccalaureate nurse, 30
Bachelor of science in nursing (BSN), 30
Bacillus, 880–881, **882**
Backup systems, for office equipment, 97
Bacteria. *See also* Infectious diseases
classification and identification of, 880–882, **881**, 881(t), **882**
drug-resistant, 387
gram-negative, 881(t)
gram-positive, 881(t)
as microorganisms, 352
normal flora, 352
sexually transmitted diseases (STDs), 602
shape of, 880–881
as source for drugs, 1004
special groups of, 881
staining procedures and, 881
testing urine for, 925(t)
in urine specimens, 932
Bacterial infections
stool samples for suspected, 893
transmitted by airborne droplets, 647(t)
Bacterial meningitis, 384–385, 833
Bacterial spores, 360
Balance, ear and, 683
Balance billing, 268
Balasa, Donald A., 8
Bandages
after surgery, 780
storage of, 143
wounds, **829**
Banking
accepting checks, 321
electronic, 323–324, 327–328

endorsing checks, 322, **322**
establishing procedures for, 313
making deposits, 322–323, **323**, 324(p)
reconciling bank statements, 323
telephone, 327(b)
writing checks, 321
Bank statements, reconciling, 323, 326(p)–327(p)
Barbiturates, abuse of, 619(t)
Bargaining, as stage of death, 72
Barium enema, 738, 1094(t), 1095–1096
Barium swallow, 738, **738**, 1094(t), 1096, 1098
Baroreceptors, 514
Basal cell carcinoma, 456(b)–457(b), **457**, 734, **734**
Bases, 442
Basic HIV/AIDS Program, 397(b)
Basophils, 520, **520**, 938, **938**, 959(t), 961, 963
Battered women, 619
Battery, defined, 39
Battery power backup, 97
B cells, 354, **534**, 534–535, **535**
Beepers, 87
Behavior modification, for weight loss, 989–990
Bell's palsy, 502(b), 742(t)
Benadryl, 1011
Benefits
explanation of, 266
health insurance, 257
review for allowed, 266
Benign tumor, 743
Benzalkonium chloride, 775
Benzodiazepine, 1014, 1014(t)
abuse of, 619(t)
Beta-carotene, 983, 996(b)
Betadine, 775
Bethesda system of classification, 715, 716(t)
Bicarbonate ions, 545
Bicuspids, 554, **555**
Bicuspid valve, 509, **509**
Bile, 517, 558
Bile ducts, cholangiography, 1098–1099
Bilirubin, 517, 960(t)
testing urine for, **48**, 925(t), 926–927
Bilirubinuria, 926
Biliverdin, 517
Billing. *See also* Collections
accepting payment, 296–297
basic accounting for, 294
coding, billing, and insurance specialist, 309(b)
credit arrangements, 306–310
determining appropriate fees, 294
ethical behavior and, 49
insurance fraud and, 288
managing billing cycles, 298, 301
preparing invoices, 298, **299**
processing charge slips, 294, **295**, 296
software for, 108
standard payment procedures and, 294–298
standard procedures for, 298–301
telephone inquiries, 201
using superbill, 298, **300**, 301(p)
Billing service, independent, 298
Binders, 180
Biochemistry, 443–444
Bioethics, 49–50
Biofeedback, 808(b), 1057
Biogenesis, 351
Biohazard labels, 860, **860**
Biohazardous materials, 360
refrigerator for, 425(b)
storage of, 425(b)
Biohazardous waste, 382
disposal of, 45, **46**, 767, 869(p)
infectious laundry waste, 362(b)–363(b)

processing devices, 105
safeguarding confidential
files, 114
security issues, 114–115
Security Rule of HIPAA, 53–54
selecting equipment, 112
software, 106–112, 113
storage devices, 105–106
storage of files on, 188
system care and maintenance, 115
types of, 102–103
upgrading office system, 112–113
viruses, 114–115
word processing program to create
form letter, 108(p)
Conciseness
in patient records, 165, 620
telephone techniques and, 198
of writing style, 125
Concussion, 824, 824(b)
Condom, 718
AIDS prevention and use of, 403
Conduction system of heart,
1062–1063
Conductive hearing loss, 581, 684
Condyles, 470
Cones, 575, 670
Conference calls, 207
Confidentiality. *See also* Privacy
for electronic claims
transmission, 276
fax machines and, 208
leaving messages on answering/fax
machines, 85, 88
legal obligation for, 44
mandatory disclosure, 56–57
notifying those at risk for
sexually transmitted disease,
55(b)–56(b)
patient confidentiality statement,
246–247
patient records, 165, 173–174, 620
securing confidential files on
computer, 114
taking messages and maintaining
patient, 206
telephone calls and, 198, 202
Conflict, with coworkers and dealing
with, 74
Confusion, elderly patients and, 71–72
Congenital heart disease, 708
Congestive heart failure, 528(b)
Conjunctivas, 576
Conjunctivitis, 578(b), 747
Connective tissue, 449–451, **450**
Consciousness, state of, and
neurological examination, 501
Consent form
drug administration, 1035
as preoperative procedure, 771
urine specimens, 917, **917**
Consideration, in communication, 65
Constipation, 562(b), 739(t)
constipation-diarrhea cycle, 699
Constipation-diarrhea cycle, 699
Constructive criticism, 1117, 1119
Consumable supplies, 429
Consumer education, 243
Contact dermatitis, 733
*Contagiousness of Puerperal Fever,
The*(Holmes), 351
Contagious patients
in reception area, 230
reception area and, 238
Contaminated supplies, 14
Continuing education, 1131–1132
laboratory testing, 872
Continuing education credits, 50
Contraception, 606–607, 718–719,
1007(t), 1010(t)
Contracts
breach of, 40, 41
defined, 39
employment, 339, 342
legal elements of, 39–40, 339, 342
medical assistant contract, 342
types of, 40

Contraindications, immunizations,
390–391
Contrast baths, 798
Contrast media, 1090, 1093
Contrast sensitivity, 674, **676,** 678(p)
Controlled substances, 1013–1019,
1015(p)–1019(p)
Comprehensive Drug Abuse
Prevention and Control Act,
1014
defined, 1013
disposing of drugs, **1018,** 1019
doctor registration and, 1015,
1015(p)–1016(p), 1019(p)
drug security, 1015
labeling, 1014, **1014**
legal issues, 43
ordering, 1015, **1017**
record keeping for, 1015, 1019
schedules of, 1014, 1014(t)
writing prescriptions, 1021–1023
Controlled Substances Act (CSA), 1014
Control samples, 870
Conventional records, 165
Conventional tomography, 1099
Conventions, of ICD-9-CM, 282–283
Conversion factor, 266
Conversions
between measurement systems,
1030–1031
metric conversion for height, **640**
metric conversions for weight, **640**
for temperature, **630**
Convolutions, 497
Coordination of benefits, 264, 264(t)
Co-payment, 257–258
Copier machines, 89–90
Copper, 981
Cords, in examination room,
safety of, 430
Cornea, 575, **576,** 669, **670**
Corneal abrasions, 747
Corneal ulcers, 747
Coronal, 441, **441**
Coronary artery disease, 528(b), 730(t)
Coronary catheterization, 519(b)
Coronary sinus, 512
Coronary spasms, 518(b)
Corpus callosum, 497
Corpus luteum, 600
Correcting patient records, 171, 172(p)
Correspondence, 119–130.
See also Letters; Mail
basic rules of writing, 131(t)
business letter, **122,** 122–124
editing, 128
effective writing for, 125
general formatting guidelines for
letters, 124–125
letter styles, 125, **126, 127**
in patient record, 162
professionalism and, 120
proofreading, 128–130
punctuation style, 124
reference books for, 125, 128
signing letters, 130
style and language usage for, 128
supplies, choosing, 120–122
templates for, 122
types of, 122
written, 122–130
Cortex, 498
Cortisol, 567, 569
Corynebacterium diphtheriae, 887(t)
Costochondritis, 519(b)
Cotton fiber bond paper, 121
Coumadin, 966
Counter check, 330
Courier services, 137
Courtesy, telephone techniques and,
198, 204
Courtesy title, 123
Cover letter, writing, 1123–1124, **1127**
Cover sheet, for faxes, 88, **88**
Coverslip, 855
Coworkers, communicating with,
73–74

Coxal bones, **466,** 473, **473**
CPR, performing, 836(p)–838(p)
CPR instructor, 834(b)
CPT, 283, **284,** 285
add-on codes, 285
Category II codes, Category III codes
and Unlisted procedures, 285
evaluation and management codes
(E/M codes), 285
laboratory procedures, 285–286
locating a code, 287(p)
modifiers, 285
surgical procedures, **284,** 285
Crabs, 602
Crafts therapy, 787(b)
Cranial, 439, **440,** 440(t), 441, **441**
Cranial bones, 470, **471**
Cranial cavity, 441, **443**
Cranial nerves, 499
assessment of, 740
tests of, 501
Craniosacral therapy, 808(b)
Crash cart, 813
stocking, 814(p)
Creatine kinase (CK), 960(t)
Creatine phosphate, 480
Creatinine, 961(t)
Credentials, 8–9
Credit
arrangements for, 306–310
following laws governing extension
of credit, 307–310
performing credit check, 306–307
unilateral decision, 310
Credit bureau report, 306–307, **307**
Credit cards, accepting payment in,
296–297, **297**
Credit check, performing, 306–307
Cretinism, 735
Crib death, 709
Cricoid cartilage, 542, **544**
Crime, 39
Criminal law, 39
Criminal penalties, of HIPAA
violations, 54
Critical thinking skills
of medical assistant, 15
during patient interview,
616(p)–617(p)
CRNA. *See* Certified registered nurse
anesthetist (CRNA)
Crohn's disease, 562(b)
Cross-references, 185, 281
Cross-trained, 14
Croup, 383, 383(t)
Crutches, 803–807
gaits for, 803–804, **806–807**
measuring patient for, 803
teaching patient to use, 805(p)
Cryosurgery, 762
Cryotherapy, 791–793, 794(p)
administering, 792–793, 794(p)
defined, 791
factors affecting use of,
791–792, 792(t)
principles of, 792
Crystals, in urine specimens,
931–932, **933**
CT scans. *See* Computed
tomography (CT)
Cultural differences and considerations
communicating for general physical
examination and, 652, 653(p)
communicating with patients and,
68–70, 70(b)
drug administration, 1056
eye contact, 64
nutrition and diet patient
education, 998
patient education, 248–249, 417
view of illness, symptoms and
treatment expectations, 70(b)
Culture, 652
Culture, microorganism, 886
Culture and sensitivity
(C and S), 891
Culture media, 886, 901

Culture plate
incubating, 903
inoculating, 901–903
Culture (specimen)
collecting, 891–896
culturing specimens in medical
office, 900–904
determining antimicrobial
sensitivity, 904–905
interpreting, 903–904
in steps to diagnosis infection,
885–886, 891
CULTURETTE Collection and
Transport system, 892, **892**
Curettes, 763, **763**
Current Procedural Terminology, 283,
284, 285
Cursor, 103
Cushing's syndrome, 570(b), 736
Cuspids, 554, **555**
Customary fees, 294
Customer service
defined, 60
importance of, 60–61
Cutting instruments, 762–763, **763**
Cyanosis, 456
Cyberspace Hospital, 111(t)
Cycle billing, 298, 301
Cystic duct, 558, **558**
Cystic fibrosis, 448(b)
Cystine crystals, **933**
Cystitis, 589(b), 755
Cystometry, 754
Cystoscopy, 754
Cysts, ovarian, 720(t)
Cytokines, 534
Cytokinesis, 445
Cytomegalovirus (CMV), 410,
699, 961(t)
Cytoplasm, 444, 963

Daily log, in single-entry bookkeeping
system, **314,** 314–315
Damages, negligence and, 40
Dance therapy, 787(b)
Data, in SOAP, 167
Database, 107
in POMR, 165
Database management software, 108
Data elements, 269, 271, 275(b)
Data errors, in correspondences, 128
Dateline, **122,** 122–123
Death, stages of dying, 72
Debridement, 760
Debt collection. *See* Collections
Decibels, 685
Decongestant, 1010(t)
Decontamination, OSHA regulations, 45
Decor, in reception area, 228–229
Deductible, 257
Deductions, payroll, 334
Deep, anatomical terms, 439,
440, 440(t)
Deep-vein thrombosis (DVT),
698–699
Deer ticks, **884**
Defamation, 39
Defecation reflex, 560
Defense Enrollment Eligibility
Reporting System (DEERS), 261
Defense mechanisms, 66–67
Deficiency needs, 62
Deflections, 1063
Dehydration, 831
Delayed treatment, 40
Dementia, 248
Dendrites, 493–494, **494**
Denial
as defense mechanism, 66
elderly patients and, 71–72
as stage of death, 72
Dental assistant, 31
Dental office administrator, 116(b)
Deoxyhemoglobin, 517
Dependents, 331–332
Depolarization, 1063
Depolarized, 495